OKU®

5

Orthopaedic Knowledge Update®

Shoulder and Elbow

OKU®

5

Orthopaedic Knowledge Update®

Shoulder and Elbow

EDITOR:
Gregory P. Nicholson, MD
Associate Professor of Orthopedic Surgery
Midwest Orthopedics at Rush
Rush University Medical Center
Chicago, Illinois

Wolters Kluwer

AAOS
American Academy of Orthopaedic Surgeons

AAOS

AMERICAN ACADEMY OF ORTHOPAEDIC SURGEONS

Staff

American Academy of Orthopaedic Surgeons

Anna Salt Troise, MBA: *Chief Education Strategist*

Hans Koelsch, PhD: *Director, Publishing*

Lisa Claxton Moore: *Senior Manager, Editorial*

Steven Kellert: *Senior Editor*

Wolters Kluwer Health

Brian Brown: *Director, Medical Practice*

Stacey Sebring: *Senior Development Editor*

Emily Buccieri: *Senior Editorial Coordinator*

Erin Cantino: *Portfolio Marketing Manager*

David Saltzberg: *Production Project Manager*

Stephen Druding: *Design Coordinator*

Beth Welsh: *Senior Manufacturing Coordinator*

TNQ Technologies: *Prepress Vendor*

The material presented in the *Orthopaedic Knowledge Update®: Shoulder and Elbow, Fifth Edition* has been made available by the American Academy of Orthopaedic Surgeons for educational purposes only. This material is not intended to present the only, or necessarily best, methods or procedures for the medical situations discussed, but rather is intended to represent an approach, view, statement, or opinion of the author(s) or producer(s), which may be helpful to others who face similar situations. Some drugs or medical devices demonstrated in Academy courses or described in Academy print or electronic publications have not been cleared by the Food and Drug Administration (FDA) or have been cleared for specific uses only. The FDA has stated that it is the responsibility of the physician to determine the FDA clearance status of each drug or device he or she wishes to use in clinical practice. Furthermore, any statements about commercial products are solely the opinion(s) of the author(s) and do not represent an Academy endorsement or evaluation of these products. These statements may not be used in advertising or for any commercial purpose.

ISBN 978-1-9751-4773-0

Library of Congress Control Number: Cataloging in Publication data available on request from publisher.

Printed in China

Published 2021 by the American Academy of Orthopaedic Surgeons
9400 West Higgins Road
Rosemont, Illinois 60018

Bone and Joint Initiative USA

CCS0620

Acknowledgments

Editorial Board, Orthopaedic Knowledge Update®: Shoulder and Elbow 5

Editor

Gregory P. Nicholson, MD
Associate Professor of Orthopedic Surgery
Midwest Orthopedics at Rush
Rush University Medical Center
Chicago, Illinois

Section Editors

Mark S. Cohen, MD *(Elbow Trauma, Fracture, and Reconstruction)*
Professor
Director, Hand and Elbow Section
Director, Orthopaedic Education
Rush University Medical Center
Department of Orthopaedic Surgery
Chicago, Illinois

T. Bradley Edwards, MD *(Principles of Clinical Information)*
Chief of Shoulder Surgery
Fondren Orthopedic Group
Texas Orthopedic Hospital
Houston, Texas

Ranjan Gupta, MD *(Arthroscopy)*
Professor and Chief of Shoulder Surgery
Department of Orthopaedic Surgery, Anatomy & Neurobiology, and Biomedical Engineering
University of California, Irvine
Irvine, California

Sumant "Butch" Krishnan, MD *(The Rotator Cuff)*
Director, The Shoulder Center
Baylor University Medical Center at Dallas
Associate Professor, Department of Surgery
Texas A&M Health Science Center College of Medicine
Dallas, Texas

Augustus D. Mazzocca, MS, MD *(Arthroscopy)*
Director and Professor of Orthopaedic Surgery
Department of Orthopaedic Surgery
UCONN Musculoskeletal Institute
University of Connecticut
Farmington, Connecticut

Edward G. McFarland, MD *(Miscellaneous Shoulder and Elbow Topics)*
Wayne H. Lewis Professor of Shoulder Surgery
Director Division of Shoulder and Elbow Surgery
Department of Orthopedic Surgery
The Johns Hopkins University
Baltimore, Maryland

Parick J. McMahon, MD *(Basic Science)*
Chief of Orthopedic Surgery
VA Pittsburgh Healthcare System
Clinical Professor, University of Pittsburgh
Pittsburgh, Pennsylvania

Brent J. Morris, MD *(Principles of Clinical Information)*
Shoulder and Elbow Surgeon
Baptist Health Lexington Orthopedics and Sports Medicine
Baptist Health Lexington
Lexington, Kentucky

Anand M. Murthi, MD *(Trauma and Fractures)*
Chief, Shoulder and Elbow Surgery
Director, Shoulder and Elbow Fellowship and Research
Professor of Orthopaedic Surgery, Georgetown University School of Medicine
Department of Orthopaedics and Sports Medicine
MedStar Union Memorial Hospital
Baltimore, Maryland

CAPT Matthew T. Provencher, MD, MC, USNR *(Instability and Athletic Injuries)*
Professor of Surgery and Orthopaedics
The Steadman Clinic, Shoulder Knee and Sports Surgery
The Steadman Philippon Research Institute
Vail, Colorado

Contributors

Daniel Aaron, MD
Department of Orthopedics & Physical Rehabilitation
University of Massachusetts
Amherst, Massachusetts

Joseph A. Abboud, MD
Professor of Shoulder and Elbow Surgery
Department of Orthopaedic Surgery
The Sidney Kimmel Medical College
Thomas Jefferson University
Philadelphia, Pennsylvania

Julie E. Adams, MD
Professor
Department of Orthopaedic Surgery
University of Tennessee College of Medicine - Chattanooga
Erlanger Orthopaedic Institute
Chattanooga, Tennessee

William R. Aibinder, MD
Assistant Professor
Director, Shoulder & Elbow Surgery
Department of Orthopaedic Surgery & Rehabilitation Medicine
SUNY Downstate Health Sciences University
Brooklyn, New York

Tjarco D. Alta, MD, PhD
Department of Orthopaedic Surgery
Spaarne Gasthuis
Haarlem/Hoofddorp
The Netherlands

James R. Andrews, MD
Orthopaedic Surgeon
Andrews Institute for Orthopaedics & Sports Medicine
Gulf Breeze, Florida

Michael E. Angeline, MD
Mercy Health
Janesville, Wisconsin

Robert A. Arciero, MD, FAAOS
Professor, Orthopaedic Surgery
Department of Orthopaedics
University of Connecticut Health
Farmington, Connecticut

George S. Athwal, MD, FRCSC
Professor
Department of Surgery
Western University
London, Ontario, Canada

Knut Beitzel, MD
Shoulder Surgery
ATOS Clinic
Cologne, Germany

John-Erik Bell, MD, MS
Associate Professor of Orthopaedic Surgery
Department of Orthopaedic Surgery
Dartmouth-Hitchcock Medical Center
Lebanon, New Hampshire

Pascal Boileau, MD
University Institute of Locomotion and Sports
Hôpital Pasteur 2
University Côte d'Azur
Nice, France

James P. Bradley, MD
Professor, Orthopaedic Surgery
University of Pittsburgh Medical Center
Head Team Physician, Pittsburgh Steelers
Pittsburgh, Pennsylvania

E. David Bravos, MD
Assistant Professor
Department of Anesthesiology and Critical Care Medicine
Johns Hopkins Hospital
Baltimore, Maryland

Stephen S. Burkhart, MD
Burkhart Research Institute for Orthopaedics and TSAOG Orthopaedics
San Antonio, Texas

Paul Cagle, MD
Leni and Peter May Department of Orthopedics
Icahn School of Medicine at Mount Sinai
New York, New York

John A. Carrino, MD, MPH
Professor of Radiology
Vice Chairman, Department of Radiology
Weill Cornell Medicine
New York, New York

Aaron M. Chamberlain, MD, MSc, MBA
Associate Professor
Department of Orthopedic Surgery
Washington University School of Medicine
St. Louis, Missouri

Emilie V. Cheung, MD
Associate Professor
Orthopedic Surgery
Stanford University
Redwood City, California

Paul J. Christo, MD, MBA
Associate Professor
Division of Pain Medicine
Department of Anaesthesiology & Critical Care Medicine
Johns Hopkins University School of Medicine
Baltimore, Maryland

Christopher R. Chuinard, MD, MPH, FAOA, FAAOS
Shoulder and Elbow Surgeon
Great Lakes Orthopaedic Center
Traverse City, Michigan

Brandon Cincere, MD
Clinical Assistant Professor
Department of Orthopaedics UT COM
Hip, Shoulder, Knee Arthroscopy and Sports Medicine
University of Tennessee at Chattanooga
Chattanooga, Tennessee

Terry Bradly Clay, MD
Department of Orthopaedic Surgery
University of South Alabama
Mobile, Alabama

Brian J. Cole, MD, MBA
Associate Chairman and Professor, Department of Orthopedics
Rush University Medical Center
Chicago, Illinois

John G. Costouros, MD
Private Practice
Mowry Avenue
Fremont, California

Richard E. Debski, PhD
Professor
Departments of Bioengineering and Orthopaedic Surgery
University of Pittsburgh
Pittsburgh, Pennsylvania

Maj. Travis J. Dekker, MD, MC, USAF
Orthopaedic Surgeon
Assistant Professor
Uniformed Services University of Health Sciences
Eglin Air Force Base, Florida

Joshua S. Dines, MD
Associate Professor
Orthopedic Surgery
Weill Cornell Medical College
Associate Attending
Sports Medicine/Shoulder Service
Hospital for Special Surgery
New York, New York

Jeffrey R. Dugas, MD
American Sports Medicine Institute
Birmingham, Alabama

T. Bradley Edwards, MD
Chief of Shoulder Surgery
Fondren Orthopedic Group
Texas Orthopedic Hospital
Houston, Texas

Kelly Fitzpatrick, DO
Assistant Professor
Orthopaedic Surgery
Uniformed Services University of Health Sciences
William Beaumont Army Medical Center
El Paso, Texas

Evan Flatow, MD
Professor
Department of Orthopaedics
Mount Sinai School of Medicine
New York, New York

Mark A. Frankle, MD
Chief, Shoulder and Elbow Service
Director, Shoulder and Elbow Fellowship
Florida Orthopaedic Institute
Clinical Professor
Department of Orthopaedic Surgery
University of South Florida Morsani College of Medicine
Tampa, Florida

Lisa G.M. Friedman, MD, MA
Midwest Orthopaedics at Rush
Rush University Medical Center
Chicago, Illinois

Jan Fritz, MD, PD, DABR
Associate Professor of Radiology
Division Chief, Musculoskeletal Radiology
Department of Radiology
NYU Grossman School of Medicine
New York, New York

Shawn M. Gargac, MSBE
R&D Director
US Upper Extremities
Wright Medical Group N.V.
Columbia City, Indiana

Raffaele Garofalo, MD
Director, Upper Limb Unit
F. Miulli Hospital
Acquaviva delle fonti- BA, Italy

Grant E. Garrigues, MD
Associate Professor of Orthopaedic Surgery
Midwest Orthopaedics at Rush
Rush University Medical Center
Co-team Physician, Chicago White Sox
Co-team Physician, Chicago Bulls
Chicago, Illinois

Reuben Gobezie, MD
Founding, Director
Shoulder and Elbow Surgery
Cleveland Shoulder Institute
Beachwood, Ohio

Andrew Green, MD
Professor of Orthopaedic Surgery
Chief of Division of Shoulder and Elbow Surgery
The Warren Alpert Medical School
Brown University
Providence, Rhode Island

Meares Green, DO
UNC Orthopedics at Goldsboro
Goldsboro, North Carolina

Michael J. Griesser, MD
Fellow
Department of Orthopaedic Surgery
The Cleveland Clinic Foundation
Cleveland, Ohio

James E. Hammond, DO, ATC
CDR MC USN
Chairman of Orthopedic Surgery
Naval Medical Center Portsmouth
Portsmouth, Virginia

Robert U. Hartzler, MD, MS
Shoulder and Elbow Surgeon, TSAOG Orthopaedics
Clinical Assistant Professor
Baylor College of Medicine Sports Medicine Fellowship Program
San Antonio, Texas

Hill Hastings II, MD
Emeritus Clinical Professor
Orthopedic Surgery
Telluride, Colorado

Armodios M. Hatzidakis, MD
Private Practice
Western Orthopaedics
Denver, Colorado

Eric D. Haunschild, BS
Rush University Medical Center
Chicago, Illinois

Jonah Hebert-Davies, MD
Harborview Medical Center
Department of Orthopedics
University of Washington
Seattle, Washington

Brian W. Hill, MD
Shoulder & Elbow Clinical Fellow
Department of Orthopaedic Surgery
Rothman Orthopaedic Institute
Thomas Jefferson University Hospitals
Philadelphia, Pennsylvania

Perry O. Hooper, DO
Orthopaedic Sports Medicine Surgeon
Southern Orthopaedic Surgeons
Montgomery, Alabama

C. Scott Humphrey, MD
Director, ISERF Shoulder and Elbow Fellowship
Humphrey Shoulder Clinic
Eagle, Idaho

James A. Hurt III, MD, FAAOS
Assistant Professor Orthopaedic Surgery and Sports Medicine
Department of Orthopaedic Surgery
University of Mississippi Medical Center
Jackson, Mississippi

Mohammad A. Issa, MD
Interventional Pain Physician (Position)
Department of PM&R
Riverside Hospital-Rush University Care Network
Greater Chicago, Illinois

Rolando Izquierdo, MD
Assistant Professor
OrthoIllinois
Rosalind Franklin Medical School
Algonquin, Illinois

Nicholas Jarmon, MD
Core Assistant Professor
Department of Orthopaedics
Hackensack Meridian School of Medicine
Spring Lake, New Jersey

James A. Johnson, PhD, PEng
Professor
Graham King Musculoskeletal Research Chair
Western University, Faculty of Engineering
Mechanical and Materials Engineering
Department of Surgery
London, Ontario, Canada

Cameron Kia, MD
Resident
Orthopaedic Surgery
University of Connecticut
Farmington, Connecticut

W. Ben Kibler, MD
Medical Director
Shoulder Center of Kentucky
Lexington Clinic
Lexington, Kentucky

Graham J.W. King, MD, MSc, FRCSC, FAAOS
Professor, Department of Surgery
University of Western Ontario
London, Ontario, Canada

Steven Klepps, MD
Orthopedic Surgeon
Department of Orthopedic Surgery
Ortho Montana, St. Vincent's Hospital
Billings, Montana

Sumant "Butch" Krishnan, MD
Director
The Shoulder Center
Baylor University Medical Center
Dallas, Texas

Rudy Kovachevich, MD
Orthopedic Surgeon
Orthopedic Centers of Colorado
Denver, Colorado

Ryan J. Leiphart, BS
Graduate Research Assistant
Department of Bioengineering
University of Pennsylvania
Philadelphia, Pennsylvania

Devin Lemmex, MD, FRCSC
Assistant Professor
Department of Surgery
University of Manitoba/Pan Am Clinic
Winnipeg, Manitoba

Ian K.Y. Lo, MD, FRCSC
Assistant Professor, Chief Shoulder and Elbow Surgery
Section of Orthopaedic Surgery
University of Calgary
Calgary, Alberta

Temilola Majekodunmi, MD
Project Coordinator
Baylor Scott and White Research Institute
Dallas, Texas

Keisuke Matsuki, MD
Sports Medicine & Joint Center
Funabashi Orthopaedic Hospital
Funabashi, Chiba

Luke T. Mattar, BS
Graduate Student Researcher
Department of Bioengineering
University of Pittsburgh
Pittsburgh, Pennsylvania

Augustus D. Mazzocca, MS, MD
Director of the UCONN Musculoskeletal Institute
Professor of Orthopaedic Surgery
Orthopaedic Surgery
University of Connecticut
Storrs, Connecticut

Brett McCoy, MD
Fellow
Orthopaedic Surgery
The Cleveland Clinic Foundation
Cleveland, Ohio

Peter J. Millett, MD, MSc
Orthopaedic Surgeon; Chief Medical Officer (CMO)
The Steadman Clinic
Steadman Philippon Research Institute
Vail, Colorado

Anthony Miniaci, MD
Department of Orthopaedic Surgery
Cleveland Clinic
Sports Health Center
Garfield Heights, Ohio

Lukas N. Muench, MD
Resident
Orthopaedic Sports Medicine
Technical University of Munich
Munich, Germany

Stephanie Muh, MD
Deputy Chief, Orthopaedic Surgery Service - Henry Ford West Bloomfield Hospital
Associate Program Director - Sports Medicine Fellowship
Department of Orthopaedic Surgery
Henry Ford Health System
Detroit, Michigan

Joseph B. Newton, BS
Graduate Research Assistant
Department of Bioengineering
University of Pennsylvania
Philadelphia, Pennsylvania

Phillip T. Nigro, MD
Shoulder and Elbow Surgeon
UChicago Medicine Medical Group
Chicago, Illinois

Robert P. Nirschl, MD, MS
Founding Chairman
Nirschl Orthopaedic Center
Arlington, Virginia

Carl Nunziato, MD
Resident Physician
Department of Surgery and Perioperative Care
Dell Medical School at the University of Texas at Austin
Austin, Texas

Daniel F. O'Brien, MD
Chief Resident Orthopaedics
Department of Orthopaedics
University of Connecticut Health
Farmington, Connecticut

Robert Stephen Otte, MD
Coastal Orthopedics
Bradenton, Florida

Randall J. Otto, MD
Shoulder and Elbow Surgeon
Signature Orthopedics
Adjunct Assistant Professor
Department of Orthopaedic Surgery
Saint Louis University School of Medicine
St. Louis, Missouri

Brett D. Owens, MD
Professor of Orthopaedic Surgery
Department of Orthopaedic Surgery
Brown University Alpert Medical School
Providence, Rhode Island

Bradford Parsons, MD
Leni and Peter May Department of Orthopedics
Icahn School of Medicine at Mount Sinai
New York, New York

Brendan Patterson, MD, MPH
Assistant Professor
Department of Orthopedic Surgery and Rehabilitation
Carver College of Medicine
University of Iowa
Iowa City, Iowa

Liam A. Peebles, BA
Research Coordinator
Orthopaedic Clinical Outcomes
Steadman Philippon Research Institute
Vail, Colorado

CAPT Matthew T. Provencher, MD, MC, USNR
Professor of Surgery and Orthopaedics
Orthopaedic Surgeon; Fellowship Director
The Steadman Clinic, Shoulder Knee and Sports Surgery
Steadman Philippon Research Institute
Vail, Colorado

Patric Raiss, MD
Professor
Head of Shoulder and Elbow Surgery
OCM
Munich, Germany

Mustafa S. Rashid, MB, ChB, MSc, PhD
Specialist Registrar
Nuffield Department of Orthopaedics, Rheumatology, and Musculoskeletal Sciences (NDORMS)
University of Oxford
Oxford, England

Ali Rashidi, MD
Postdoctoral Research Fellow in Radiology
Russell H. Morgan Department of Radiology and Radiological Science
Johns Hopkins University
Baltimore, Maryland

David Ring, MD, PhD
Professor
Department of Surgery and Perioperative Care
Dell Medical School at the University of Texas at Austin
Austin, Texas

Christopher P. Roche, MSBE, MBA
Vice President, Extremities BU
Exactech, Inc.
Gainesville, Florida

Anthony Romeo, MD
Chief of Orthopedics
Rothman Orthopaedic Institute
New York, New York

Marc Safran, MD
Professor
Orthopedic Surgery
Stanford University
Redwood City, California

Felix H. Savoie III, MD, FAAOS, FAOA
Ray Haddad Professor and Chair
Department of Orthopaedic Surgery
Tulane University
New Orleans, Louisiana

Aaron Sciascia, PhD, ATC, PES, SMTC
Associate Professor
Department of Exercise and Sport Science
Eastern Kentucky University
Richmond, Kentucky

Brett Shore, MD
Orthopaedic Surgeon
Southern California Permanente Medical Group
Kaiser – Panorama City
Panorama City, California

Daniel Grant Schwartz, MD
Shoulder and Elbow Surgeon
The Polyclinic
Seattle, Washington

Douglas Scott, MD
Beaufort Orthopedics Sports & Spine Center
Hilton Head, South Carolina

Benjamin W. Sears, MD
Private Practice
Western Orthopaedics
Denver, Colorado

Louis J. Soslowsky, PhD
Fairhill Professor
Department of Orthopaedic Surgery
University of Pennsylvania
Philadelphia, Pennsylvania

Trenton Sprenkle, DO
Orthopedic Resident
Department of Orthopedic Surgery
University of North Dakota
Fargo, North Dakota

Umasuthan Srikumaran, MD
Associate Professor
Department of Orthopeadic Surgery
Johns Hopkins School of Medicine
Baltimore, Maryland

Scott P. Steinmann, MD
Professor and Chair
Department of Orthopaedic Surgery
University of Tennessee College of Medicine - Chattanooga
Erlanger Orthopaedic Institute
Chattanooga, Tennessee
Emeritus Professor
Department of Orthopedic Surgery
Mayo Clinic
Rochester, Minnesota

Michael A. Stone, MD
Assistant Professor
Shoulder & Elbow Surgery
Department of Orthopaedics
Cedars-Sinai Medical Center
Los Angeles, California

Hiroyuki Sugaya, MD
Chairman
Sports Medicine & Joint Center
Funabashi Orthopaedic Hospital
Funabashi, Chiba

Satoshi Takeuchi, MD
Research Fellow
Department of Orthopaedic Surgery
University of Pittsburgh
Pittsburgh, Pennsylvania

Jennifer Tangtiphaiboontana, MD
University of California, San Francisco
Orthopaedic Trauma Institute
San Francisco, California

Robert Z. Tashjian, MD
Professor, Department of Orthopaedics
University of Utah
Salt Lake City, Utah

Geoffrey S. Van Thiel, MD, MBA
Associate Professor
OrthoIllinois
Rush University Medical Center
University of Illinois
Rockford, Illinois

Fotios Paul Tjoumakaris, MD
Professor, Orthopaedic Surgery
Sidney Kimmel College of Medicine
Thomas Jefferson University
Philadelphia, Pennsylvania

John M. Tokish, MD
Professor, Mayo Clinic
Department of Orthopedic Surgery
Director, Orthopedic Sports Medicine Fellowship
Team Orthopedic Surgeon, Arizona Coyotes Hockey Club
Phoenix, Arizona

Michael T. Torchia, MD, MS
Resident Physician
Department of Orthopaedic Surgery
Dartmouth-Hitchcock Medical Center
Lebanon, New Hampshire

Scott Trenhaile, MD
Associate Professor
OrthoIllinois
University of Illinois
Rockford, Illinois

Gilles Walch, MD
Department of Shoulder Surgery
Centre Orthopédique Santy
Hôpital Privé Jean Mermoz
Lyon, France

Taylor J. Wiley, MD
Peninsula Orthopaedic Associates
Salisbury, Maryland

Joshua Wright-Chisem, MD
Resident, Orthopaedic Surgery
Hospital for Special Surgery
New York, New York

Ken Yamaguchi, MD, MBA
Sam and Marilyn Fox Distinguished Professor of Orthopedic Surgery
Department of Orthopedic Surgery
Washington University School of Medicine
St. Louis, Missouri

Preface

The field of shoulder and elbow surgery continues to rapidly expand and evolve. This fifth edition of *Orthopaedic Knowledge Update® (OKU®): Shoulder and Elbow* is focused on the most recent advances in this area of orthopaedics. It is written for practicing orthopaedic surgeons and presents, in a concise yet thorough manner, the most recent literature on the shoulder and the elbow and the advances in all areas of shoulder and elbow surgery. Shoulder and elbow specialists will also find this edition useful, along with residents and fellows, who will benefit from the knowledge and expertise of a world-class group of section editors and authors.

New to this edition is an update on the design and biomechanics of reverse shoulder arthroplasty. The expanded indications and longer term results of reverse arthroplasty are addressed. New information on the biologics and indications and outcomes of these adjuncts to healing has been included. New chapters on the imaging of the shoulder specifically for the evaluation of the glenoid in instability and degenerative disease have been added. As all upper extremity surgeons know, pain syndromes, which are difficult to diagnose and manage, can occur. The chapter on complex regional pain syndrome and causalgia provides an update on current terminology, thought, diagnosis, and management. A chapter on both basic and advanced elbow arthroscopy is included. New information on management of elbow and shoulder injuries in throwing athletes is in this edition of OKU.

In the past 5 years, the advent of the superior capsular reconstruction for rotator cuff–deficient shoulders has become more common. This edition brings the early science and results to the reader. The section on rotator cuff includes chapters that discuss treatment and the most recent science on tendon healing and possible augmentations to improve rotator cuff healing.

The section editors are leaders in their fields and have selected a dedicated team of chapter authors, and they all have done a remarkable job in writing, editing, and preparing *OKU®: Shoulder and Elbow 5*. I am deeply grateful for their efforts and contributions to this project. The staff at the American Academy of Orthopaedic Surgeons (AAOS) has been invaluable in moving this project forward and helping me as the editor to bring this new fifth edition to publication. I am grateful for the opportunity to be the editor of this project and honored to have been chosen to lead this project. I would like to thank all the authors, section editors, contributors, and AAOS staff for their excellent effort. I hope that the information put forth is a valuable resource for all who manage shoulder and elbow conditions.

Gregory P. Nicholson, MD
Editor

Table of Contents

Section 3: The Rotator Cuff

Section Editor:
Sumant "Butch" Krishnan, MD

Section 4: Arthroscopy

Section Editors:
Augustus D. Mazzocca, MS, MD and Ranjan Gupta, MD

Section 5: Principles of Clinical Information

Section Editors:
T. Bradley Edwards, MD and Brent J. Morris, MD

Section 1

Basic Science

Section Editor:

Patrick J. McMahon, MD

Chapter 1

Anatomy and Function of the Shoulder Structures

Richard E. Debski, PhD • Satoshi Takeuchi, MD • Luke T. Mattar, BS

ABSTRACT

The shoulder is composed of osseous and soft-tissue structures that allow for joint mobility and stability throughout ranges of motion. Soft tissues such as the rotator cuff and glenohumeral capsule provide dynamic and static stabilization, respectively, whereas bones provide structural stability and points of attachment for soft tissues. Understanding the structure and function of the relevant anatomy, as well as the variability between patients, is important for diagnosing injuries and performing surgical procedures to help restore normal anatomy.

Keywords: bony morphology; glenohumeral capsule; kinematics; labrum; rotator cuff

Introduction

The shoulder has a larger range of motion than any other major joint in the musculoskeletal system. This range of motion primarily is attributed to the organization of the bony and soft-tissue structures that provide mobility and stability. Because the bony structures provide minimal stability, the muscles and the passive soft-tissue structures must maintain stability while the muscles move the arm. Shoulder motion involves the entire shoulder complex, including the scapulothoracic joint, which acts as a base for upper extremity motion.

Osseous Anatomy

Humeral Head

The proximal humerus has an ellipsoidal humeral head that forms part of the glenohumeral joint. The humeral head is covered with hyaline articular cartilage, and the anatomic neck of the humerus is marked by a bony transition from cartilage to the metaphyseal border. The retroversion angle of the humeral head is defined as the orientation of the articular surface with respect to the sagittal plane. The most widely used reference is between the transepicondylar axis of the elbow and the anterior-posterior axis at the cartilage or metaphyseal border[1-3] (**Figure 1**). The anatomic neck of the humerus is used as a reference for osteotomy during shoulder arthroplasty; the retroversion angle of the humeral head has been described as having great variability.[4,5]

A three-dimensional study using surface topographic data from 24 humeral heads found that the mean radius of curvature of the articular surface was 23.9 mm (range, 22.5 to 25.8 mm).[2] The deviation from sphericity was 0.2 mm (range, 0.15 to 0.26 mm), which is 0.9% of the radius of curvature. Retroversion of the humeral head at the midpoint between the superior and inferior margins was 18.6° (range, 2.5° to 40°), but the angle varied with the location of the measurement (**Figure 2**). The study concluded that a reference at a central point anteriorly along the cartilage may be a useful landmark for re-creating the version calculated using the centroid of the articular surface.[2]

In throwing athletes, the two shoulders appear to have different glenohumeral ranges of motion. Specifically, a greater external rotation and a loss of internal rotation were found in the dominant shoulder than in the nondominant shoulder.[6] Range of motion and laxity of the glenohumeral joint as well as humeral head and glenoid version in the dominant and nondominant shoulders were studied in 25 professional pitchers and 25 nonthrowing control athletes. Humeral and glenoid retroversion increased in the dominant shoulder of the throwing athletes compared with the nondominant shoulder. External rotation increased in the dominant shoulder at 90° and 45° of abduction and decreased in internal rotation at 90°. The nonthrowing athletes had no significant side-to-side difference in any parameter. Increased humeral retroversion was considered to be an adaptive change because of the rotational force and

None of the following authors or any immediate family member has received anything of value from or has stock or stock options held in a commercial company or institution related directly or indirectly to the subject of this chapter: Dr. Debski, Dr. Takeuchi, and Mr. Mattar.

This chapter is adapted from Fujimaki Y, Araki D, Debski RE: Anatomy and function of the shoulder structures, in Nicholson GP, ed: *Orthopaedic Knowledge Update: Shoulder and Elbow*, ed 4. Rosemont, IL, American Academy of Orthopaedic Surgeons, 2013, pp 3-11.

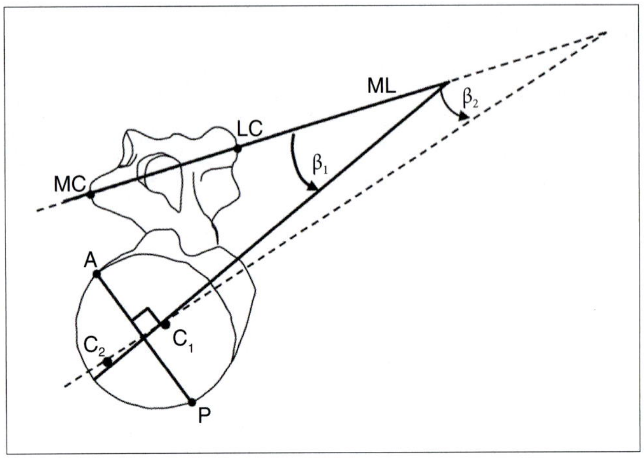

FIGURE 1 Schematic drawing showing retroversion definition based on the transepicondylar axis and the cartilage-calcar interface in the sagittal plane and the centroid of the articular surface. A to P = axial plane, β_1 = retroversion angle from the cartilage-calcar interface, β_2 = retroversion angle from the centroid of the articular surface, C_1 = centroid of the sphere representing the articular surface, C_2 = centroid of the articular surface, LC = lateral epicondyle, MC = medial epicondyle, ML = transepicondylar line. (Reprinted from J Shoulder Elbow Surg 21[5]. Harrold F, Wigderowitz C: A three-dimensional analysis of humeral head retroversion, 612-617. Copyright © 2012 Journal of Shoulder and Elbow Surgery Board of Trustees. doi:10.1016/j.jse.2011.04.005.)

became obvious between ages 9 and 10 years.[7] Interestingly, left-handed throwers showed significantly smaller side-to-side difference of humeral retroversion compared with right-handed throwers. This may be caused by the differences in throwing mechanics between right-handed and left-handed throwers.[8]

The implication of this altered arc of motion is that a physiologic adaptation of the dominant shoulder as a result of repetitive microtrauma leads to selective stretching of the anterior capsule and tightening of the posterior capsule. Adaptation can also occur in osseous structures because of the applied stresses. Surgeons should carefully examine high-level overhead athletes to determine their side-to-side difference in range of motion and bony characteristics.

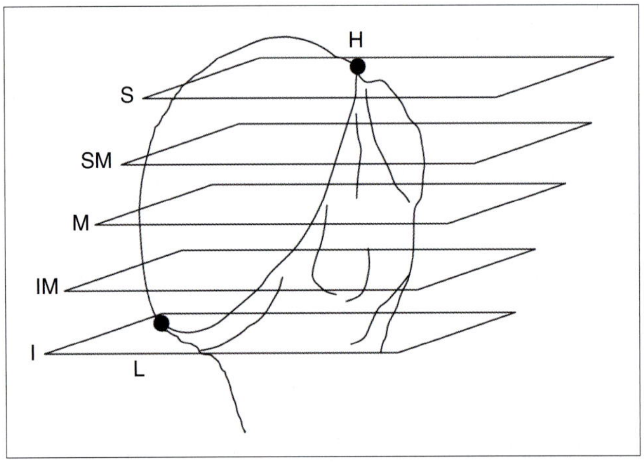

FIGURE 2 Schematic drawing showing the division of the humeral head into six sections by five parallel planes running orthogonal to the shaft axis. H = superiormost point on the cartilage-calcar interface, I = inferior plane, IM = inferior middle plane, L = inferiormost point on the cartilage-calcar interface, M = middle plane, S = superior plane, SM = superior middle plane. (Reprinted from J Shoulder Elbow Surg 21[5]. Harrold F, Wigderowitz C: A three-dimensional analysis of humeral head retroversion, 612-617. Copyright © 2012 Journal of Shoulder and Elbow Surgery Board of Trustees. doi:10.1016/j.jse.2011.04.005.)

Bicipital Groove

The bicipital groove has been used as a landmark during surgical fracture repair or prosthesis alignment during shoulder arthroplasty.[9,10] A morphometric study of 50 dry humeri found an average groove length of 8.1 cm (range, 6.7 to 10.4 cm), which corresponded to 25.4% (range, 16.3% to 32.5%) of the width of the humerus. The width at the midpoint of the groove was 10.1 mm (range, 7.3 to 15.5 mm), which corresponded to 49.7% to 54.5% of the width of the humerus. The 4.0-mm depth of the groove corresponded to 18.8% of the depth of the humerus. The angle formed by the walls of the bicipital groove was 106°. No correlation could be found among these parameters.[11]

Glenoid

The glenoid is a comma-shaped concave projection that extends laterally from the scapular body and acts as the socket of the glenohumeral joint. CT is commonly used to evaluate the effect on glenoid retroversion of scapular rotation in the coronal and sagittal planes. Measurements are made using a coordinate system for each scapula based on three anatomic landmarks: the center of the glenoid fossa, the point on the vertebral border at which the scapular spine intersects the medial border of the scapula, and the most distal point of the inferior scapular angle.[12] The anatomic glenoid version was found to be 2.0° (±3.8°) when it was evaluated independently from the resting position of the scapula. The difference between anatomic glenoid version and clinical glenoid version was found to depend on the position of the scapula in the original axial CT images, and it averaged 6.9° (range, 0.1° to 22.5°). These results suggest that malalignment of 1° of the scapula in the coronal or the sagittal plane creates inaccuracies in the measurement of glenoid version. The plane of axial reconstruction must be taken into account when CT is used to evaluate glenoid version.[12]

Biomechanically, glenoid version has implications on glenohumeral joint stability. Decreased glenoid retroversion was significantly related to the anterior instability compared with the healthy controls.[13] On the other hand,

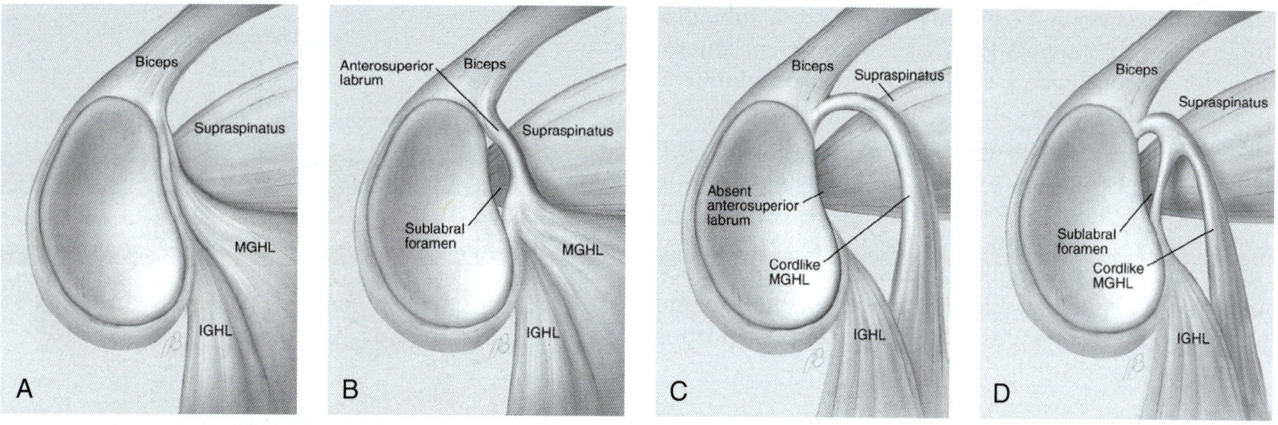

FIGURE 3 Schematic drawings showing the normal anatomy of the labrum (**A**), an isolated sublabral foramen (**B**), a sublabral foramen with a cordlike middle glenohumeral ligament (**C**), and a cordlike middle glenohumeral ligament without tissue at the anterosuperior labrum (**D**). IGHL = inferior glenohumeral ligament, MGHL = middle glenohumeral ligament.

compared with the healthy controls, the shoulders with posterior instability had more than 5° of the glenoid retroversion.[14] Thus, glenoid version should be evaluated in individuals considered at risk for shoulder dislocation, as well as in the planning of shoulder surgery.

Labral and Capsular Anatomy

Glenoid Labrum

The glenoid labrum is composed of a rim of fibrous tissue with a fibrocartilaginous transition zone that acts as a passive stabilizer by adding depth to the shallow glenoid fossa. It also serves as a primary attachment site for the glenohumeral capsule and the long head of the biceps tendon (LHBT).[15]

The labral outline is ovoid, conforming to the underlying glenoid rim, and is most firmly attached to the glenoid posteroinferiorly.[16] The contributions of the glenoid labrum to glenohumeral joint stability have been well described.[17,18] Superior labrum anterior to posterior (SLAP) lesions increasingly are recognized as a source of pain and instability in the shoulder. Labral lesions such as SLAP lesions are being more commonly diagnosed with MRI or shoulder arthroscopy, and, as a result, an accurate understanding of normal labral variations has become crucial[19] (**Figure 3**).

Several studies suggest that there is a wide variability in the anatomy of the anterosuperior portion of the labrum. A clinical study of 546 patients undergoing shoulder arthroscopy found that 73 patients (13.4%) had an anatomic variation in the anterosuperior labrum, including a sublabral foramen only in 18 patients (3.3%), a sublabral foramen with a cordlike middle glenohumeral ligament in 47 patients (8.6%), and an absence of labral tissue in the anterosuperior portion of the labrum with a cordlike middle glenohumeral ligament in 8 patients (1.5%).[20] The presence of one of these variations was positively associated with anterosuperior labral fraying, an abnormal superior glenohumeral ligament, and increased passive internal rotation with the arm in 90° of abduction (**Figure 4**).

A study of 691 patients found that 98 patients (14.2%) had one of three distinct anatomic variations in the anterosuperior portion of the labrum, classified as a

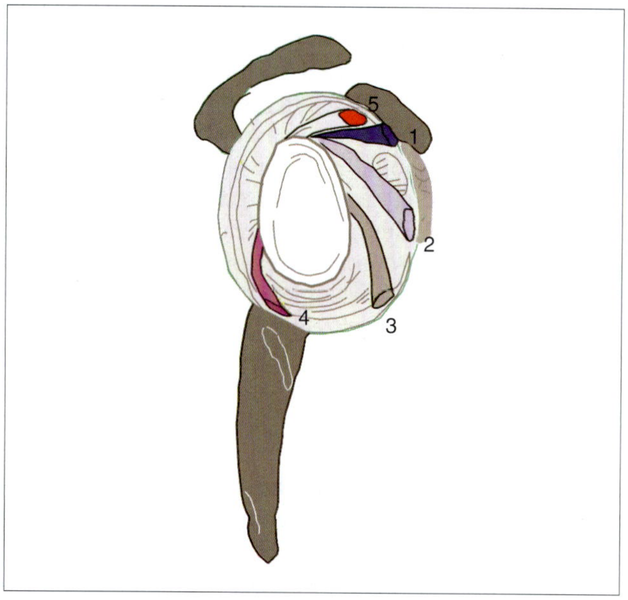

FIGURE 4 Schematic drawing showing the capsular ligaments of a right shoulder. 1 = superior glenohumeral ligament, 2 = middle glenohumeral ligament, 3 = anterior band of inferior glenohumeral ligament, 4 = posterior band of inferior glenohumeral ligament, 5 = long head of the biceps tendon

sublabral recess (in 17 patients [2.46%]), a sublabral foramen (in 53 patients [7.67%]), or an absent anterosuperior labrum with a cordlike middle glenohumeral ligament (in 28 patients [4.05%]).[21] Two of the variations, the sublabral foramen and the absent anterosuperior labrum with a cordlike middle glenohumeral ligament, had a significant relationship with a type II SLAP lesion. Even though labral variations do not appear to contribute to instability, they may allow increased internal rotation and predispose the shoulder to lesions of the superior glenohumeral ligament and the anterosuperior portion of the labrum.

Glenohumeral Capsule

The glenohumeral capsule surrounds the glenohumeral joint, maintains the synovial environment, and provides stability at the extremes of the range of motion.[22,23] Current references describe the superior, middle, and inferior glenohumeral ligaments as thickenings of the anterior joint capsule that reinforce the anterior-inferior part of the capsule and directly connect the humeral head to the glenoid fossa (**Figure 5**).

Experimental and computational investigations typically have isolated discrete ligamentous regions, but recent data suggest that the regions of the glenohumeral capsule have significant interactions and function multiaxially.[24-26] Finite element models were used to determine the distribution of maximum principal strain and deformed shape of the glenohumeral capsule at the apprehension position while a 25-N anterior load was applied to the humerus, with and without mechanical connection of the regions.[26] The results suggested that the regions of the capsule commonly described as glenohumeral ligaments have significant interactions when transferring forces between the scapula and humerus. Discrete capsular regions should not be isolated for experimental or computational analysis of glenohumeral capsule function. Instead, the glenohumeral capsule should be evaluated as a continuous sheet of fibrous tissue. The material properties of the glenohumeral capsule were found to be similar in directions parallel and perpendicular to the glenohumeral ligaments.[25] This finding further supported the concept of a continuous sheet of fibrous tissue.

An anatomic study with a histologic examination of 27 specimens concluded that the superior glenohumeral ligament is a constant macroscopic structure consisting of direct and oblique fibers.[27] The study suggested that the function of the superior glenohumeral ligament is not only to connect and stabilize the glenohumeral joint but also to place and stabilize the LHBT from its origin through the insertion into the biceps groove.

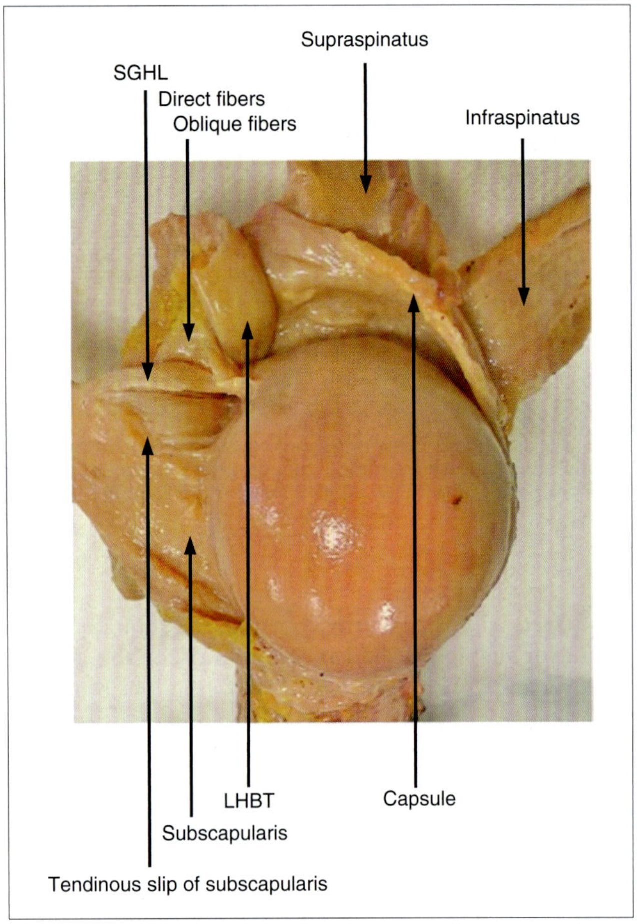

FIGURE 5 Photograph showing a right-shoulder humeral head and the surrounding structures of the capsule, ligaments, and rotator cuff tendons. LHBT = long head of biceps tendon, SGHL = superior glenohumeral ligament

Shoulder dislocations are a common injury in the young active population with most dislocations occurring in the anterior direction. Anterior dislocations may result in permanent deformation of the glenohumeral capsule, potentially leading to glenohumeral joint instability.[28] Reoccurring dislocations further damage the capsular tissue and may alter glenohumeral joint kinematics.

Muscle and Tendon Anatomy

Rotator Cuff

The rotator cuff consists of the tendons of the supraspinatus, infraspinatus, subscapularis, and teres minor muscles, which stabilize and move the glenohumeral joint (**Figure 6**). Shoulder stability is one of the primary functions of the rotator cuff muscles. During abduction of the arm, the rotator cuff pulls the humeral head into the glenoid to allow the large deltoid muscle to elevate the arm.[29]

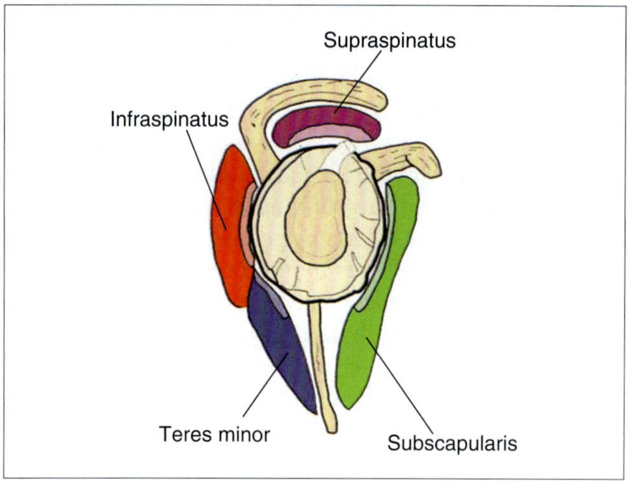

FIGURE 6 Schematic drawing showing the rotator cuff tendons: the supraspinatus, on the superior part of rotator cuff; the infraspinatus and the teres minor, on the posterior (rear) part; and the subscapularis on the anterior part.

This motion is called concavity compression. Without the action of the rotator cuff, the humeral head would translate superiorly out of the glenoid, and the deltoid would be less efficient. The glenoid fossa is most susceptible to shear force perturbation in the anterior-to-posterior direction because the glenoid fossa is less deep than it is in the superior-to-inferior direction.[30] In a normal shoulder, the combined antagonistic forces of the subscapularis anteriorly and the infraspinatus and teres minor posteriorly function to compress the humeral head onto the glenoid. A cadaver analysis found glenohumeral instability superiorly when rotator cuff paralysis of the infraspinatus, subscapularis, and teres minor tendons was simulated.[31]

Supraspinatus

The supraspinatus arises from the supraspinous fossa above the scapular spine. The accepted belief is that the supraspinatus and other tendons of the rotator cuff insert on the greater and lesser tuberosities lateral to the anatomic neck of the humerus. This pattern has been recently questioned, however. The supraspinatus was found to have a long tendinous portion in the anterior half of the muscle, which always inserted into the anteriormost area of the highest impression on the greater tuberosity; in 21% of the specimens, it also inserted into the superiormost area of the lesser tuberosity.[32] The footprint of the supraspinatus was found to be triangular, with an average maximum medial-to-lateral length of 6.9 mm and an average maximum anterior-to-posterior width of 12.6 mm. In contrast, the infraspinatus had a long tendinous portion in the superior half of the muscle, which was curved anteriorly and extended to the anterolateral area of the highest impression of the greater tuberosity. The footprint of the infraspinatus was trapezoidal, with an average maximum medial-to-lateral length of 10.2 mm and an average maximum anterior-to-posterior width of 32.7 mm. Thus, the footprint of the supraspinatus on the greater tuberosity was found to be much smaller than previously believed; this area of the greater tuberosity actually is occupied by a substantial amount of the infraspinatus. The researchers suggested that rotator cuff tears previously believed to involve only the supraspinatus tendon may have a substantial infraspinatus component.[32]

Contraction of the supraspinatus leads to shoulder abduction at the glenohumeral joint. The supraspinatus is the primary agonist muscle for shoulder abduction during the first 10° to 15° of the arc. Beyond 30° of abduction, the deltoid muscle becomes the main abductor. The supraspinatus muscle helps in resisting the inferior gravitational forces across the shoulder caused by the weight of the upper limb.[33]

Rotator cuff tears commonly occur in the supraspinatus tendon and are a serious clinical problem responsible for approximately 70% of clinical visits regarding shoulder pain.[34] Surgical repair of rotator cuff tears is generally prescribed following failure of nonsurgical treatment; however, postoperative retear is a common issue with incidence ranging between 20% and 70%.[35] The inability to reproduce the native tendon-to-bone interface may lead to stress concentrations because of commonly used suture-anchor repair techniques. Adhesive films are a promising new technique that may be used to restore load transfer mechanisms of the native enthesis in rotator cuff tear repairs.[36]

Infraspinatus

The infraspinatus is a thick triangular muscle that occupies the infraspinatus fossa on the scapula. The muscle arises by thick fibers from the medial two-thirds of the infraspinatus fossa and by tendinous fibers from the ridges on its surface; the muscle also arises from the infraspinatus fascia that covers it and separates it from the teres major and the teres minor.[37] The fibers converge to form a tendon that glides over the lateral border of the spine of the scapula, passes across the posterior region of the glenohumeral capsule, and inserts into the middle impression on the greater tubercle of the humerus.

The primary function of the infraspinatus is to horizontally extend and laterally rotate the humerus at the shoulder joint. When the arm is fixed, the infraspinatus abducts the inferior angle of the scapula. The infraspinatus and the teres minor externally rotate the shoulder and assist in extension of the glenohumeral joint.[37] A 2011 study examined the instantaneous moment arms of subregions in several muscles that cross the glenohumeral joint in axial rotation of the humerus during coronal plane abduction and sagittal plane flexion.[38] The study found that the inferior infraspinatus and the teres minor were the most important external rotators.

Subscapularis

The subscapularis originates from the anterior surface of the scapula, passing laterally beneath the coracoid and the scapular neck and becoming tendinous at the level of the glenoid. At its insertion, the tendinous portion of the subscapularis blends with the fibers of the glenohumeral capsule and inserts into the lesser tuberosity. The remaining insertion consists of muscle and is below the lesser tuberosity. The morphology of the subscapularis insertion was found to be broad proximally and tapered distally in a comma shape.[39] The insertion was found to consist of a proximal tendinous part and a distal muscular part. With the exception of the bare area at the proximal end, the measured values were significantly greater in specimens from men than from women.

The subscapularis muscle is the largest and strongest muscle of the rotator cuff. The subscapularis rotates the head of the humerus medially (in internal rotation). When the arm is raised, the subscapularis draws the humerus forward and downward.[40] The subscapularis also prevents anterior displacement of the humeral head. The inferior subscapularis was found to be the most important internal rotator.[38] The diagnosis of subscapularis injuries can be difficult, and the ability to assess some tears may be limited during arthroscopy or open surgery. An MRI study of subscapularis tendon tears compared with normal anatomy found diagnostic imaging to be important for diagnosing and evaluating the extent of subscapularis injury.[40] Clinicians must understand several unusual types of subscapularis tendon tears. A full-thickness tear may be difficult to appreciate because of overlying scar tissue attaching to the greater tuberosity and mimicking intact tendon fibers. Even an extensive subscapularis tendon tear may lack tendon retraction because of the stabilizing effect of the coracohumeral ligament or an intact inferior subscapularis attachment. The coracohumeral ligament also inserts on the anterior portion of the greater tuberosity, and its presence and support may be a reason for most supraspinatus tendon tears beginning on the undersurface and a bit posterior to the biceps tendon.[41,42] Scar tissue may prevent leakage of contrast material on magnetic resonance arthrography.

Teres Minor

The upper two-thirds of the teres minor arise from the dorsal surface of the axillary border of the scapula. The remaining one-third arises from two aponeurotic laminae, one of which separates the teres minor from the infraspinatus muscle, and the other separates it from the teres major muscle. The fibers of the teres minor run obliquely upward and downward into the lowest portion of the greater tuberosity. In a study of 31 cadaver shoulders, it was found that approximately half of the shoulders had a distinct fascial compartment surrounding the teres minor muscle, and the other half had a combined fascia surrounding both the infraspinatus and teres minor muscles.[43] All shoulders had a stout fascial sling at the inferior glenoid neck. The primary motor nerve branch to the teres minor always traveled between this sling and the teres minor muscle after making a sharp bend. These findings may have implications for understanding isolated teres minor muscle atrophy.

In addition to their function in adduction, extension, and transverse extension, the infraspinatus and the teres minor work in tandem with the posterior deltoid to externally rotate the humerus.

Biceps

The LHBT originates from the superior glenoid labrum and the supraglenoid tubercle and has an intra-articular portion that passes over the humeral head before leaving the glenohumeral joint through the bicipital groove.[44] The origin is continuous with and contributes to the glenoid labrum. The small head of the biceps originates at the coracoid, and the muscle belly from each origin converges to form the biceps muscle proper.[45]

The origin of the LHBT from the superior glenoid labrum and the supraglenoid tubercle was found to vary in a study of 101 cadaver shoulders.[46] Four origin types were described: entirely posterior, in 28 shoulders; posterior dominant, in 56 shoulders; equal, in 17 shoulders; and entirely anterior, in none of the shoulders. In all shoulders, the LHBT was found to originate from both the glenoid labrum and supraglenoid tubercle. Information from this study can aid clinicians in assessing the origin of the LHBT and treating pathologies such as SLAP lesions.

The size of the LHBT also varies. The intra-articular portion typically is wide and flat, and the extra-articular portion is smaller and rounder. The tendon is approximately 5 to 6 mm in diameter and 9 cm in length.[45] The anterior circumflex humeral artery provides the blood supply of the articular portion of the LHBT. The more distal portion of the tendon is avascular to accommodate its sliding motion within its sheath in the bicipital groove.[47]

From the neutral arm position, the LHBT slides up to 18 mm in and out of the glenohumeral joint during forward flexion and internal rotation.[48] The LHBT functions in shoulder flexion, extension, abduction, internal rotation, external rotation, and anterior stabilization.

Scapulothoracic Joint Function

The scapula serves as a base for glenohumeral joint motion, allowing the rotator cuff to function as a link in the kinematic chain between the thorax and the arm. Humerothoracic motion is generated by both the scapulothoracic and glenohumeral joints (**Figure 7**). Motion of the scapula on the thorax is essential for normal function of the upper extremity.[49] The scapulothoracic joint is not a diarthrodial joint. However, a significant amount of motion occurs between the scapula and the thorax during arm motion. In shoulder abduction, 2° of every 3° occur at the glenohumeral joint and 1° occurs at the scapulothoracic joint.[50] The coordinated motion during arm movement is called the scapulohumeral rhythm.

In a study using electromagnetic motion sensors and surface electrodes to detect muscle activity in 20 healthy subjects, the orientation and the position of the scapula on the thorax were found to be different when the arm was elevated actively rather than passively.[51] Decreased levels of muscle activity during passive elevation resulted in altered scapulothoracic kinematics, including upward rotation and external rotation of the scapula. The greatest effect was noted through the midrange of arm elevation. Significantly more upward rotation of the scapula occurred when the arm was raised actively rather than passively. This finding reinforces the important role of the trapezius and serratus anterior muscles in producing scapular upward rotation, especially throughout the midrange of arm elevation. These muscles and the upward rotation of the scapula, especially in the midrange of arm elevation, should be carefully assessed during physical examination.

An in vivo MRI study assessed the three-dimensional motion of the scapula from 90° of external rotation to 90° of internal rotation with the humerus in 90° of abduction.[52] The scapulothoracic joint was found to contribute approximately 12.5% of the motion during the

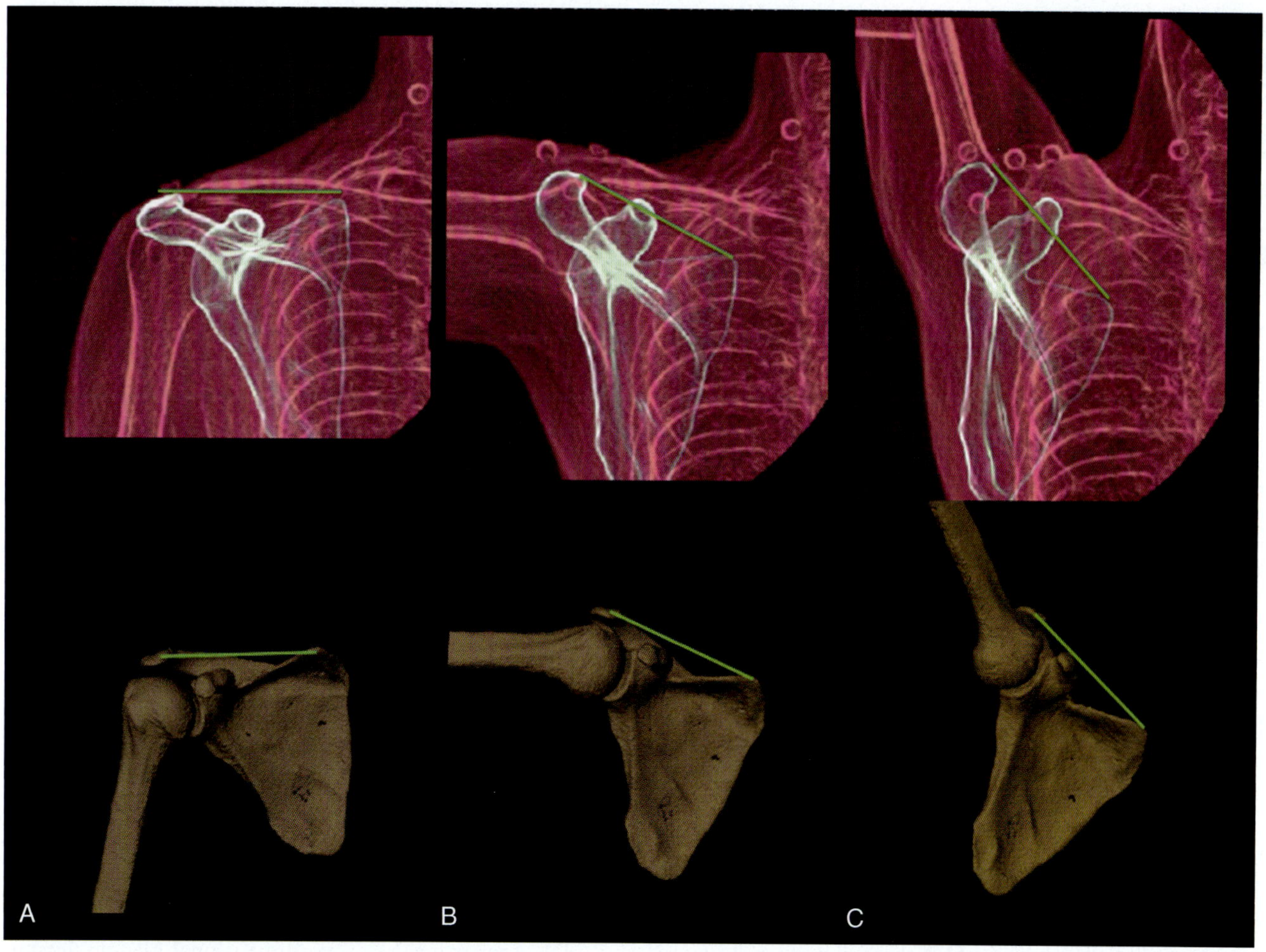

FIGURE 7 Fluoroscopic images (top row) and corresponding three-dimensional bone models (bottom row) showing scapulothoracic motion in three positions (green lines): neutral position (**A**), 90° of abduction (**B**), and maximum elevation (**C**).

entire motion. As the arm position changed from 90° of external rotation to 60° of internal rotation, most of the movement was from the glenohumeral joint. At more than 60° of internal rotation, the scapula began to markedly tilt in the anterior direction.[52] These findings reinforce the concept that scapulothoracic motion is important for normal function of the shoulder.

SUMMARY

The shoulder consists of a complex arrangement of osseous and soft-tissue structures that provide a large range of motion and maintain stability. The complex anatomy varies greatly among individuals and must be properly modeled to understand normal and pathologic function. To properly restore normal anatomy and joint function, surgeons must account for a patient's anatomic variability during diagnostic and surgical procedures.

KEY STUDY POINTS

- Bony morphology of the humerus is influenced by the repetitive loads experienced during development.
- The orientation of the glenoid in the coronal and sagittal planes has an effect on joint stability.
- The glenohumeral capsule should be evaluated as a continuous sheet of fibrous tissue and is permanently deformed during joint dislocation with increasing effects following multiple dislocations that affect joint stability.
- The rotator cuff is responsible for providing concavity compression that stabilizes the glenohumeral joint during elevation, and the ability to reproduce the native tendon-to-bone interface during surgical repair of rotator cuff tears is vital for restoring normal joint function.
- The motion of the scapula on the thorax is important for normal joint function, and this motion as well as the trapezius and serratus anterior should be carefully assessed during physical examination, especially in the midrange of arm elevation.

Annotated References

1. Crockett HC, Gross LB, Wilk KE, et al: Osseous adaptation and range of motion at the glenohumeral joint in professional baseball pitchers. *Am J Sports Med* 2002;30(1):20-26.

2. Harrold F, Wigderowitz C: A three-dimensional analysis of humeral head retroversion. *J Shoulder Elbow Surg* 2012;21(5):612-617.

3. Hill JA, Tkach L, Hendrix RW: A study of glenohumeral orientation in patients with anterior recurrent shoulder dislocations using computerized axial tomography. *Orthop Rev* 1989;18(1):84-91.

4. Robertson DD, Yuan J, Bigliani LU, Flatow EL, Yamaguchi K: Three-dimensional analysis of the proximal part of the humerus: Relevance to arthroplasty. *J Bone Joint Surg Am* 2000;82(11):1594-1602.

5. Pearl ML, Volk AG: Retroversion of the proximal humerus in relationship to prosthetic replacement arthroplasty. *J Shoulder Elbow Surg* 1995;4(4):286-289.

6. Kvitne RS, Jobe FW, Jobe CM: Shoulder instability in the overhand or throwing athlete. *Clin Sports Med* 1995;14(4):917-935.

7. Kurokawa D, Yamamoto N, Ishikawa H, et al: Differences in humeral retroversion in dominant and nondominant sides of young baseball players. *J Shoulder Elbow Surg* 2017;26:1083-1087.

   This study assessed when humeral retroversion in the dominant and nondominant sides of baseball players appeared. Humeral retroversion was found to decrease with age in the nonthrowing side but not in the throwing side. In addition, the side-to-side difference of humeral retroversion in the baseball players became obvious at the fourth grade timepoint.

8. Takeuchi S, Yoshida M, Sugimoto K, Tsuchiya A, Takenaga T, Goto H: The differences of humeral torsion angle and the glenohumeral rotation angles between young right-handed and left-handed pitchers. *J Shoulder Elbow Surg* 2019;28(4):678-684.

   The difference of humeral torsion angle between right- and left-handed throwers was investigated in 65 young baseball pitchers (age, 9 to 12 years) using ultrasonography. Humeral torsion angle of the throwing limb was significantly greater than that of the nonthrowing limb in the right-handed throwers, but no significant difference was observed in the left-handed throwers.

9. Angibaud L, Zuckerman JD, Flurin PH, Roche C, Wright T: Reconstructing proximal humeral fractures using the bicipital groove as a landmark. *Clin Orthop Relat Res* 2007;458:168-174.

10. Itamura J, Dietrick T, Roidis N, Shean C, Chen F, Tibone J: Analysis of the bicipital groove as a landmark for humeral head replacement. *J Shoulder Elbow Surg* 2002;11(4):322-326.

11. Wafae N, Atencio Santamaria LE, Vitor L, Pereira LA, Ruiz CR, Wafae GC: Morphometry of the human bicipital groove (sulcus intertubercularis). *J Shoulder Elbow Surg* 2010;19(1):65-68.

12. Bryce CD, Davison AC, Lewis GS, Wang L, Flemming DJ, Armstrong AD: Two-dimensional glenoid version measurements vary with coronal and sagittal scapular rotation. *J Bone Joint Surg Am* 2010;92(3):692-699.

13. Hohmann E, Tetsworth K: Glenoid version and inclination are risk factors for anterior shoulder dislocation. *J Shoulder Elbow Surg* 2015;24(8):1268-1273.

Glenoid version was investigated using MRI in patients with anterior glenohumeral joint instability and compared with a control group. Significantly smaller retroversion was observed in the study group than the control group. Level of evidence: II.

14. Privitera DM, Siegel EJ, Miller LR, Sinz NJ, Higgins LD: Glenoid version and its relationship to glenohumeral instability and labral tears. *J Shoulder Elbow Surg* 2016;25(7):1056-1063.

Glenoid version was measured with MRI in patients with unidirectional instability or labral tears. Patients with posterior pathology had 5° more retroversion than control subjects.

15. Dunham KS, Bencardino JT, Rokito AS: Anatomic variants and pitfalls of the labrum, glenoid cartilage, and glenohumeral ligaments. *Magn Reson Imaging Clin N Am* 2012;20(2):213-228, x.

16. Stoller D: *Magnetic Resonance Imaging in Orthopaedics and Sports Medicine*. Philadelphia, PA, Lippincott Williams & Wilkins, 2007.

17. Moseley H, Overgaard B: The anterior capsular mechanism in recurrent anterior dislocation of the shoulder. Morphological and clinical studies with special reference to the glenoid labrum and gleno-humeral ligaments. *J Bone Joint Surg Br* 1962;44:913-927.

18. Pagnani MJ, Deng XH, Warren RF, Torzilli PA, Altchek DW: Effect of lesions of the superior portion of the glenoid labrum on glenohumeral translation. *J Bone Joint Surg Am* 1995;77(7):1003-1010.

19. Powell SE, Nord KD, Ryu RKN: The diagnosis, classification, and treatment of SLAP lesions. *Oper Tech Sports Med* 2012;20:46-56.

20. Rao AG, Kim TK, Chronopoulos E, McFarland EG: Anatomical variants in the anterosuperior aspect of the glenoid labrum: A statistical analysis of seventy-three cases. *J Bone Joint Surg Am* 2003;85-A(4):653-659.

21. Kanatli U, Ozturk BY, Bolukbasi S: Anatomical variations of the anterosuperior labrum: Prevalence and association with type II superior labrum anterior-posterior (SLAP) lesions. *J Shoulder Elbow Surg* 2010;19(8):1199-1203.

22. Burkart AC, Debski RE: Anatomy and function of the glenohumeral ligaments in anterior shoulder instability. *Clin Orthop Relat Res* 2002;400:32-39.

23. Tischer T, Vogt S, Kreuz PC, Imhoff AB: Arthroscopic anatomy, variants, and pathologic findings in shoulder instability. *Arthroscopy* 2011;27(10):1434-1443.

24. Moore SM, Stehle JH, Rainis EJ, McMahon PJ, Debski RE: The current anatomical description of the inferior glenohumeral ligament does not correlate with its functional role in positions of external rotation. *J Orthop Res* 2008;26:1598-1604.

25. Rainis EJ, Maas SA, Henninger HB, McMahon PJ, Weiss JA, Debski RE: Material properties of the axillary pouch of the glenohumeral capsule: Is isotropic material symmetry appropriate? *J Biomech Eng* 2009;131(3):031007.

26. Moore SM, Ellis B, Weiss JA, McMahon PJ, Debski RE: The glenohumeral capsule should be evaluated as a sheet of fibrous tissue: A validated finite element model. *Ann Biomed Eng* 2010;38(1):66-76.

27. Kask K, Poldoja E, Lont T, et al: Anatomy of the superior glenohumeral ligament. *J Shoulder Elbow Surg* 2010;19(6):908-916.

28. Pickett A, Svoboda S: Anterior glenohumeral instability. *Sports Med Arthrosc Rev* 2017;25(3):156-162.

The normal anatomic variants and pathologic changes associated with anterior glenohumeral stability are discussed with respect to current treatment paradigms.

29. Harryman DT II, Sidles JA, Clark JM, McQuade KJ, Gibb TD, Matsen FA III: Translation of the humeral head on the glenoid with passive glenohumeral motion. *J Bone Joint Surg Am* 1990;72(9):1334-1343.

30. Wuelker N, Korell M, Thren K: Dynamic glenohumeral joint stability. *J Shoulder Elbow Surg* 1998;7(1):43-52.

31. Thompson WO, Debski RE, Boardman ND III, et al: A biomechanical analysis of rotator cuff deficiency in a cadaveric model. *Am J Sports Med* 1996;24(3):286-292.

32. Mochizuki T, Sugaya H, Uomizu M, et al: Humeral insertion of the supraspinatus and infraspinatus. New anatomical findings regarding the footprint of the rotator cuff. *J Bone Joint Surg Am* 2008;90(5):962-969.

33. Ackland DC, Pandy MG: Lines of action and stabilizing potential of the shoulder musculature. *J Anat* 2009;215(2):184-197.

34. Piper CC, Hughes AJ, Ma Y, Wang H, Neviaser AS: Operative versus nonoperative treatment for the management of full-thickness rotator cuff tears: A systematic review and meta-analysis. *J Shoulder Elbow Surg* 2018;27(3):572-576.

Level I and II research studies comparing surgical versus nonsurgical management of full-thickness rotator cuff tears were examined. Small improvements on PRO scores were found, suggesting larger studies with longer follow-up are required to determine whether clinical relevant differences occur between these treatments.

35. Honda H, Gotoh M, Kanazawa T, et al: Hyaluronic acid accelerates tendon-to-bone healing after rotator cuff repair. *Am J Sports Med* 2017;45(14):3322-3330.

Tendon-to-bone healing in the rotator cuff repair model was enhanced with HA, suggesting that HA-activated MSCs may have a crucial role in the healing process.

36. Linderman SW, Golman M, Gardner TR, et al: Enhanced tendon-to-bone repair through adhesive films. *Acta Biomater* 2018;70:165-176.

    A combined modeling and experimental validation protocol was used to determine the ability of adhesive films to improve current rotator cuff repair techniques. Increases in load tolerance of approximately 25% to 40% were observed over a 2.6 cm^2 supraspinatus repair footprint, which may lead to decreased risk of repair failure.

37. Clemente C: *Gray's Anatomy of the Human Body*. Philadelphia, PA, Lea & Febiger, 1985, vols 233-234.

38. Ackland DC, Pandy MG: Moment arms of the shoulder muscles during axial rotation. *J Orthop Res* 2011;29(5):658-667.

39. Ide J, Tokiyoshi A, Hirose J, Mizuta H: An anatomic study of the subscapularis insertion to the humerus: The subscapularis footprint. *Arthroscopy* 2008;24(7):749-753.

40. Morag Y, Jamadar DA, Miller B, Dong Q, Jacobson JA: The subscapularis: Anatomy, injury, and imaging. *Skeletal Radiol* 2011;40(3):255-269.

41. Clark JM, Harryman DT II: Tendons, ligaments, and capsule of the rotator cuff. Gross and microscopic anatomy. *J Bone Joint Surg Am* 1992;74(5):713-725.

42. Keener JD, Hsu JE, Steger-May K, Teefey SA, Chamberlain AM, Yamaguchi K: Patterns of tear progression for asymptomatic degenerative rotator cuff tears. *J Shoulder Elbow Surg* 2015;24(12):1845-1851.

    The patterns of rotator cuff tear size progression in degenerative rotator cuff tears were evaluated for tears with and without anterior supraspinatus tendon disruption. Most degenerative rotator cuff tears did not involve the anterior supraspinatus tendon. However, tear progression risks are similar for each tear type.

43. Chafik D, Galatz LM, Keener JD, Kim HM, Yamaguchi K: Teres minor muscle and related anatomy. *J Shoulder Elbow Surg* 2013;22(1):108-114.

    The complex anatomy surrounding the teres minor muscle was evaluated.

44. Ghalayini SR, Board TN, Srinivasan MS: Anatomic variations in the long head of biceps: Contribution to shoulder dysfunction. *Arthroscopy* 2007;23(9):1012-1018.

45. Elser F, Braun S, Dewing CB, Giphart JE, Millett PJ: Anatomy, function, injuries, and treatment of the long head of the biceps brachii tendon. *Arthroscopy* 2011;27(4):581-592.

46. Tuoheti Y, Itoi E, Minagawa H, et al: Attachment types of the long head of the biceps tendon to the glenoid labrum and their relationships with the glenohumeral ligaments. *Arthroscopy* 2005;21(10):1242-1249.

47. Ahrens PM, Boileau P: The long head of biceps and associated tendinopathy. *J Bone Joint Surg Br* 2007;89(8):1001-1009.

48. Braun S, Millett PJ, Yongpravat C, et al: Biomechanical evaluation of shear force vectors leading to injury of the biceps reflection pulley: A biplane fluoroscopy study on cadaveric shoulders. *Am J Sports Med* 2010;38(5):1015-1024.

49. Kibler WB, McMullen J: Scapular dyskinesis and its relation to shoulder pain. *J Am Acad Orthop Surg* 2003;11(2):142-151.

50. Karduna AR, McClure PW, Michener LA: Scapular kinematics: Effects of altering the Euler angle sequence of rotations. *J Biomech* 2000;33(9):1063-1068.

51. Ebaugh DD, McClure PW, Karduna AR: Three-dimensional scapulothoracic motion during active and passive arm elevation. *Clin Biomech (Bristol, Avon)* 2005;20(7):700-709.

52. Koishi H, Goto A, Tanaka M, et al: In vivo three-dimensional motion analysis of the shoulder joint during internal and external rotation. *Int Orthop* 2011;35(10):1503-1509.

Chapter 2

Preclinical Knowledge of Rotator Cuff Tendons and Healing

Ryan J. Leiphart, BS • Joseph B. Newton, BS • Louis J. Soslowsky, PhD

ABSTRACT

The four rotator cuff tendons—subscapularis, supraspinatus, infraspinatus, and teres minor—stabilize the glenohumeral joint. The supraspinatus is the most researched because of its susceptibility to injury. The increased injury risk of the supraspinatus tendon is likely due to its complex loading environment, compositional heterogeneity, and interactions with other rotator cuff tendons. Additionally, systemic alterations such as high cholesterol, diabetes, and smoking increase the risk of injury to this tendon. Animal models have been used to better understand the molecular mechanisms underlying rotator cuff degeneration and repair. Degeneration may be due to altered loading environments and catabolic imbalances. Progression of this degeneration can lead to fatty infiltration and damage to other tissues in the shoulder joint. Repair strategies are often most successful when performed early after injury, but rehabilitation protocols must be well-timed during the various stages of tendon healing to ensure the best functional outcomes.

Keywords: degeneration; rehabilitation; repair; tendinopathy; tendon rupture

Introduction

The shoulder is one of the most complex regions of the human musculoskeletal system. The ball-and-socket shape of the glenohumeral joint allows it to have a greater range of motion than any other joint. The intricacy and mobility of the glenohumeral joint likely cause the high risk of rotator cuff tendon injury, leading to pain, disability, and economic loss. The high incidence of shoulder injury and degeneration provides motivation for clinicians and scientists to investigate the biology, pathology, and management of these conditions. Recent studies of rotator cuff tendons have focused on molecular mechanisms, including factors that influence biomechanics, causes of deterioration, and interactions between biologic structures and mechanical function. Clinical studies, animal models, and new imaging techniques provide insight into rotator cuff tendon healing, which guide the selection of repair techniques, postoperative care, and rehabilitation.

Dr. Soslowsky or an immediate family member has received research or institutional support from Embody, Marine Polymer Technology, and Orthofix, Inc. Neither of the following authors nor any immediate family member has received anything of value from or has stock or stock options held in a commercial company or institution related directly or indirectly to the subject of this chapter: Mr. Leiphart and Mr. Newton.

Anatomy, Composition, and Structure of the Rotator Cuff

The four main muscles that make up the rotator cuff are the supraspinatus, infraspinatus, teres minor, and subscapularis. These muscles stabilize the glenohumeral joint and allow arm movement. Each tendon of these muscles inserts into the proximal end of the humerus. Of these tendons, the supraspinatus is most often injured. This increased injury rate is often attributed to the tendon's vulnerable location under the coracoacromial arch and poor vascularity. For this reason, most research on rotator cuff tendon injury and healing has focused on the supraspinatus.

Type I collagen accounts for 85% of the dry weight of the rotator cuff tendons; however, the supraspinatus contains a relatively high amount of type III collagen and glycosaminoglycans. The supraspinatus tendon undergoes significant compression and expresses extracellular matrix proteins often found in cartilage. Investigators have quantified the distributions and locations of specific proteoglycans in the supraspinatus tendon.[1] Decorin, associated with tension-bearing regions, was found in constant concentrations across the tendon. Aggrecan and biglycan, associated with regions of compression and active remodeling, respectively, were more abundant in the anterior and posterior regions than the medial region. Because the anterior region is the most susceptible

This chapter is adapted from Ilkhani-Pour S, Dunkman AA, Soslowsky LJ: Basic science of rotator cuff tendons and healing, in Nicholson GP, ed: *Orthopaedic Knowledge Update: Shoulder and Elbow*, ed 4. Rosemont, IL, American Academy of Orthopaedic Surgeons, 2013, pp 13-29.

to injury, understanding proteoglycan concentrations at this location is particularly valuable.

Most rotator cuff injuries occur at the tendon-to-bone transition zone, known as the enthesis, of the supraspinatus. This region endures significant stress concentrations because of the sharp gradient of material transitioning from tendon to bone. Understanding these properties from an engineering perspective is critical to improving treatments and surgical techniques. The insertion site has been characterized as having four distinct zones; however, the material transition is continuous. Tendon proper is the zone most like the midsubstance of the tendon and primarily contains well-aligned type I collagen fibers. The second zone, fibrocartilage, primarily contains type II and III collagen and increased proteoglycan content. As the enthesis continues, mineralization increases dramatically. The final two zones are described as mineralized fibrocartilage and bone. Quantification of transitional zone mineral composition revealed linear increases in the mineral-to-collagen ratio and crystalline organization across the insertion site[2] (**Figure 1**). The failure of repair and postoperative healing to re-create and restore this gradation contributes to the high retear rate.

Tendon Biomechanics

The mechanical function of the rotator cuff includes primary stabilization of the shoulder joint and secondary movement of the shoulder. Rotator cuff tendons have nonlinear, viscoelastic, and heterogeneous material properties. Understanding these biomechanical properties provides insight into rotator cuff tear prevention, repair, and rehabilitation. Recent advances include technologies to measure in vivo rotator cuff deformation, quantification of uninjured tendon material properties, interactions between rotator cuff tendons, and appreciation for the effects of systemic alterations on rotator cuff tendon mechanics.

In Vivo Measurements

In vivo imaging techniques are useful in evaluating rotator cuff tendon healing. In roentgen stereophotogrammetry, markers inserted into the materials of interest are analyzed using static radiographic image pairs. Stainless steel suture used as a marker in ovine rotator cuff tendon accurately measured migration to approximately 1 mm in distance.[3] This technique may be appropriate for tracking gap formation after surgical repair. Similarly, low-dosage CT was used to measure the position of markers implanted in patients.[4] This technique was accurate to within 0.7 mm. Intermarker distances were influenced by arm position and the location of the bead within the rotator cuff. These methods can only be used with static imaging and cannot be used to assess the functional properties of the tissue. To overcome this limitation, biplane radiographic analysis uses high-speed radiographic images to track implanted tantalum beads and measure dynamic deformation of rotator cuff tissue. In an in vivo canine model, this technique distinguished an intact repair, an unsuccessful repair, and a control infraspinatus.[5] The intact tendon repair contracted approximately 19% and became 70% stiffer over 28 weeks. The unsuccessful repair did not contract despite a stiffening of the scar tissue. This system is accurate to within 0.1 mm and is useful for functional analysis of in vivo tissue deformations. Two-dimensional speckle tracking echocardiography has been applied to intact, healthy supraspinatus tendons to determine the in vivo strains.[6] This technique detected differences in strain between the superficial (bursal) and deep (articular) sides of the supraspinatus tendon as well as different responses of the tendon to isotonic and isometric muscle contractions. Improvements in imaging in vivo rotator cuff tendon mechanics lead to new insights into treatment of tendon injuries.

Material Properties

Finite element models allow computational analysis of the rotator cuff mechanical environment. A three-dimensional finite element model of the supraspinatus tendon showed that maximum tensile stress occurs on the articular side of the anterior edge of the tendon. This result is corroborated by the frequency of tears at this site.[7] Although this analysis was the first to use a three-dimensional finite element model of the supraspinatus, it was limited by its assumptions of isotropy and homogeneity. In vitro mechanical testing of human cadaver supraspinatus tendons found that the tissue has highly inhomogeneous and nonlinear mechanical properties.[8,9] Tensile modulus is the ratio of stress to strain, with a higher modulus indicating the material is more difficult to deform. Tensile moduli values and fiber alignment were region dependent within the tendon during tensile loading, whether longitudinal (parallel to fibers) or transverse (orthogonal to fibers). In longitudinal loading, samples taken from the posterior portion of the supraspinatus tendon had lower tensile moduli than samples from the anterior or medial tendon. No moduli differences existed between bursal- and articular-side regions. Similarly, collagen fibers were most disorganized in posterior samples and most aligned in medial samples (**Figure 2**). Tendon material property measurements can distinguish between a normal and a torn rotator cuff tendon. Biopsies from patients with a massive rotator cuff tear revealed a significantly lower storage modulus than that of healthy tendons.[10] Storage modulus measures the stored elastic energy in viscoelastic materials. Torn tendons are mechanically weaker, and storage modulus may be a useful parameter for future studies. Decreased mechanical properties may predispose a massive tear to repair failure.

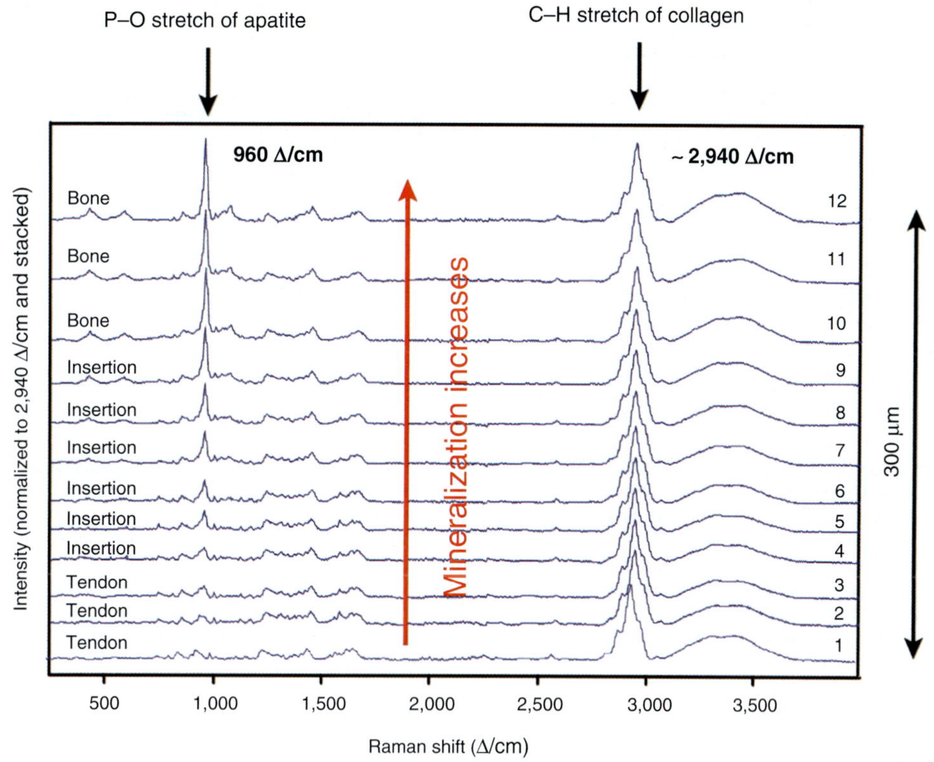

FIGURE 1 Diagram showing the use of Raman spectroscopy to quantify mineral composition across the rat shoulder tendon-bone insertion site. All spectra are normalized by the C–H stretch of collagen and then stacked along the *y*-axis for better comparison. The mineral content, represented by the P–O stretch of apatite at 960 Δ/cm, can be seen to gradually increase along the traverse from tendon to bone. (Reproduced with permission from Wopenka B, Kent A, Pasteris JD, Yoon Y, Thomopoulos S: The tendon-to-bone transition of the rotator cuff: A preliminary Raman spectroscopic study documenting the gradual mineralization across the insertion in rat tissue samples. *Appl Spectrosc* 2008;62[12]:1285-1294. doi:10.1366/000370208786822179.)

Mechanical Interactions Between Tendons

Rotator cuff tendons work together in vivo to provide stability and motion to the glenohumeral joint. For this reason, a set of studies investigated the mechanical interactions between the supraspinatus and infraspinatus tendons. Human cadaver shoulders were dissected, leaving the supraspinatus and infraspinatus tendons intact. Supraspinatus-applied loads and tear sizes, glenohumeral abduction angles, joint rotation angles, and the presence or absence of a supraspinatus repair were investigated to determine their effect on supraspinatus and infraspinatus tendon strains.[11-13] Multiple regression models using these variables found that the glenohumeral abduction angle and the supraspinatus tendon load were significant predictors of infraspinatus and supraspinatus tendon strains.[14] These findings suggest that tear propagation may be reduced by limiting loading and keeping the arm at 30° abduction in neutral rotation. This has implications for postrepair management.

Systemic Alterations

Researchers have sought to understand the risk factors associated with rotator cuff tendinopathy and tearing. Recently, the role of systemic alterations, including sex differences, high cholesterol, diabetes, age-related bone loss, and smoking, have been examined.

There is conflicting clinical evidence on whether sex is a risk factor for rotator cuff tendon tears. In uninjured rats, male supraspinatus tendons demonstrated increased stiffness under static loading relative to female tendons.[15] However, male tendons were less stiff under dynamic loading. This may contribute to the reasons for the increased prevalence of acute rotator cuff tendon tears in males.[16]

In a clinical study, patients with a rotator cuff tear had significantly higher levels of total cholesterol, triglycerides, and low-density lipoproteins than those who had shoulder pain without a tear[17] (**Figure 3**). Deposits of

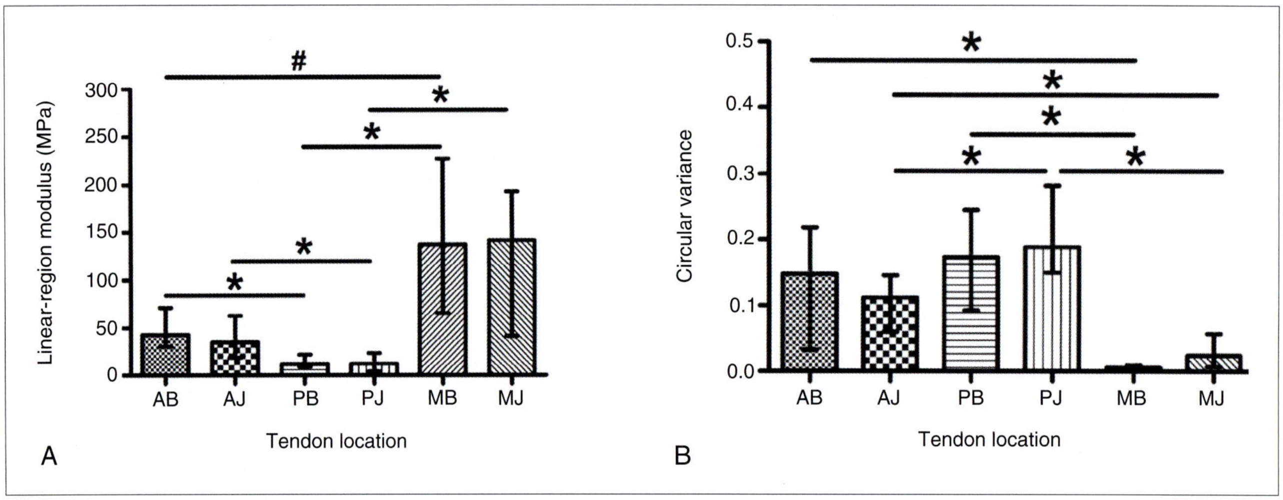

FIGURE 2 Diagrams depicting regional variations in tensile modulus and collagen organization. Both plots depict median and interquartile ranges. **A**, The elastic modulus of the supraspinatus tendon varies regionally. Posterior samples have consistently lower modulus values than medial and anterior samples. **B**, Circular variance, a measure of the disorganization of collagen fibers, is inhomogeneous across the supraspinatus tendon. The more aligned regions tend to have a higher modulus, whereas the more disorganized regions (with higher circular variance) tend to have lower modulus values. * = significant, # = trend, AB = anterior bursa, AJ = anterior joint, MB = medial bursa, MJ = medial joint, PB = posterior bursa, PJ = posterior joint. (Adapted with permission from Lake SP, Miller KS, Elliott DM, Soslowsky LJ: Effect of fiber distribution and realignment on the nonlinear and inhomogeneous mechanical properties of human supraspinatus tendon under longitudinal tensile loading. *J Orthop Res* 2009;27[12]:1596-1602. © Orthopaedic Research Society. Published by Wiley Periodicals, Inc. doi:10.1002/jor.20938.)

cholesterol (xanthomata) in the tendon or the extracellular matrix may alter the tendon's mechanics, increasing its susceptibility to injury or impairing its healing. In addition, the well-known restriction of blood flow in patients with hypercholesterolemia may further diminish the poor vascularity of the rotator cuff tendon. This study identified a correlation between high cholesterol and rotator cuff tears but did not establish causation. Research using animal models suggests that hypercholesterolemia reduces the elastic modulus of aged tendons.[18]

Earlier findings that patients with diabetes have decreased bone mass and diminished fracture healing led researchers to induce hyperglycemia in rats to model the effect of diabetes in tendon-to-bone healing after surgical repair. As anticipated, the repair sites of the hyperglycemic rats appeared qualitatively inferior, had significantly reduced collagen fiber organization and fibrocartilage formation, and failed under approximately half the load of repair sites in control animals. Special considerations are therefore needed for patients with poorly controlled glycemic levels.[19]

Estrogen deficiency causes greater bone resorption, resulting in decreased bone density. Rats that received a bilateral ovariectomy had decreased bone density at the supraspinatus enthesis.[20] Ovariectomized rats that received diphosphonate had increased density and a significantly higher failure stress. All estrogen-deficient rats (regardless of whether they received diphosphonate) had poorer fibrocartilage and insertion-site organization, increased stiffness, and an increased tensile modulus compared with control animals. Increasing a patient's bone density may help prevent repair failure.

Recent research has evaluated the effect of nicotine on the mechanical properties of healthy supraspinatus tendons in a rat model. The supraspinatus tendons of nicotine-dosed rats had a significantly higher elastic modulus than those of control animals, and the researchers speculated that this factor may relate to the increased risk of tearing among those who smoke tobacco.[21]

Tendon Degeneration and Tears

Animal Models

The rat shoulder is the most widely used animal model of the human rotator cuff. The bony anatomy of the rat shoulder closely mimics that of humans, with the supraspinatus passing underneath the acromion. Rat shoulder function also parallels that of the human shoulder. Because of the position of the rat scapula, forward flexion in the rat shoulder is comparable to abduction in humans. Supporting this notion, an acute rotator cuff tendon detachment was found to alter rat gait.[22] Decreased stride length at both early and late time points is consistent with reduced supraspinatus function. A second tendon detachment led to additional detrimental effects. This gait analysis technique was modified in a follow-up study to include force plates that measure ground reaction forces during rat locomotion.[23] After unilateral supraspinatus detachment and repair, gait

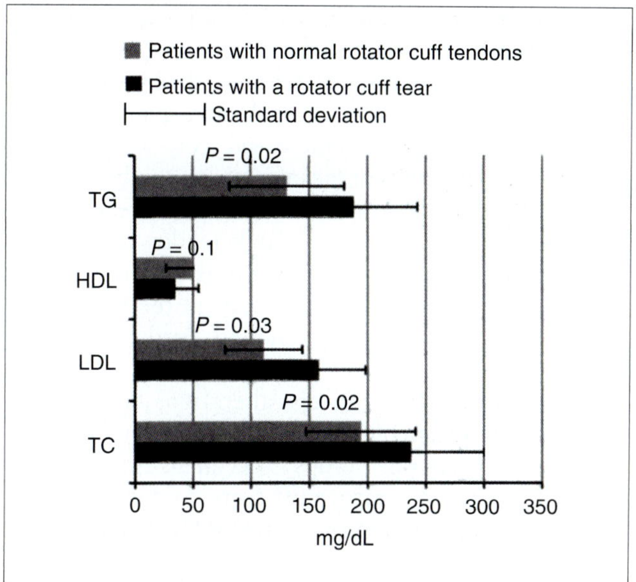

FIGURE 3 Diagram showing the findings of a clinical study comparing levels of triglyceride (TG), high-density lipoproteins (HDL), low-density lipoproteins (LDL), and total cholesterol (TC) in patients with normal rotator cuff tendons and patients with a rotator cuff tear. The patients with a rotator cuff tear had a higher incidence of hypercholesterolemia than those with normal rotator cuff tendons. (Adapted with permission from Abboud JA, Kim JS: The effect of hypercholesterolemia on rotator cuff disease. *Clin Orthop Relat Res* 2010;468[6]:1493-1497. doi:10.1007/s11999-009-1151-9)

alterations were transient. Early changes were seen in step length, peak vertical force, peak breaking force, and peak lateral force, but all parameters returned to control levels within 4 weeks of the repair.

Recently, a mouse model of rotator cuff repair has been developed. Surgical detachment and repair of the mouse supraspinatus tendon led to similar changes in biomechanical, histologic, and gene expression properties seen in rat supraspinatus injury models.[24] Because mice can be genetically manipulated, this model of supraspinatus repair will allow for better understanding of the cellular and molecular mechanisms in rotator cuff healing.

Chronic Tears

Chronic rotator cuff tears are associated with degenerative changes and atrophy. Tendon biopsy samples from patients with a supraspinatus tear revealed loss of fiber structure, rounded tenocytes, increased cellularity, increased vascularity, and decreased collagen staining compared with samples from unruptured shoulders.[25] These biopsies were sampled from the middle portion of the supraspinatus tendon, indicating that degeneration occurs throughout and not only at the torn end. Novel infrared imaging can distinguish the chemical and structural properties of tendon biopsy samples from different-size rotator cuff tears.[26] Torn tendons had decreased collagen I, II, and III content. The changes in small tears primarily involved lipids and some proteoglycans, whereas massive tears had the greatest change in collagen. These results demonstrate an association between degeneration and increased tear size.

Muscle biopsies from patients with a rotator cuff tear revealed distinct differences that depended on the size of the rupture.[27] Fatty infiltration was the most obvious difference. Massive tears had significantly greater lipid accumulation between muscle fibers and within the sarcoplasm of type I muscle fibers in comparison with control muscle samples. Although fatty infiltration is commonly used to describe muscular atrophy and accompanying fatty deposits, the origin of the adipocytes has not been firmly established. Massive tears led to decreased number of myofibrils, increased interfiber connective tissue, increased mitochondrial content in slow muscle fibers, and increased blood supply to the supraspinatus muscle. Fatty infiltration is more common in shoulders with a relatively large tear or a tear in the anterior portion of the supraspinatus tendon.[28] A retrospective analysis revealed that the extent of fatty infiltration is related to patient age, delay between the onset of symptoms and diagnosis, and number of involved tendons.[29] Fatty infiltration appeared more quickly and progressed more rapidly if the tear involved more than one tendon. Multiple regression analysis showed that the amount of retraction, abduction torque, and serum calcifediol (vitamin D) levels were independent predictors of supraspinatus fatty infiltration.[30] Low levels of serum vitamin D were related to increased fatty infiltration. Expression levels of α-skeletal muscle actin and myosin heavy chain polypeptide-1, two contractile molecules, were correlated with increasing supraspinatus fatty infiltration.[31] This increase in muscle gene expression suggests that fatty changes occur because of failure in muscle regeneration rather than muscle degeneration.

Animal models have been used to investigate degenerative changes associated with chronic rotator cuff tears. Historically, it has been difficult to induce fatty infiltration in a rat model. Studies investigating acute transection of the supraspinatus tendon in rats found muscle retraction, sarcomere shortening, muscle atrophy, and tendon degeneration but minimal fatty infiltration.[32,33] Even at an advanced age, rats did not have significant levels of fatty infiltration.[34] Scar formation in rats, unlike humans, reattaches the tendon to the humerus, thereby reestablishing load-bearing capabilities. Muscular changes were transient, but tendon degeneration progressed over time. The detrimental tendon changes seen in the rat after a unilateral infraspinatus-supraspinatus detachment are consistent with human chronic tear biopsies. These changes include increased area, percent relaxation (a viscoelastic property that describes load dissipation), disorganization, cellularity, and rounding of cells.[35] The effects of tendon reattachment decreased with increasing size of injury, thus ensuring that the supraspinatus changes were not transient.

Although tendon transection did not result in fatty infiltration, the addition of suprascapular nerve transection led to fatty infiltration, muscular atrophy of the infraspinatus and supraspinatus, and upregulation of adipogenic and myogenic transcription factors[36] (**Figure 4**). In a rabbit model, subscapularis tendon transection decreased muscle wet mass and muscle fiber cross-sectional area and increased fat content.[37] In contrast with the rat model, the addition of nerve transection did not lead to further fatty infiltration and muscle atrophy.

Effect of Tears on Remaining Shoulder Structures

Recent studies investigated the effects of a torn rotator cuff on the intact rotator cuff tendons, the biceps tendon, and the coracoacromial ligament. A supraspinatus detachment in a rat model led to increased cross-sectional area and decreased modulus of the infraspinatus, subscapularis, and long head of the biceps tendons.[38,39] Two tendon tears were more detrimental than a single tendon tear and led to more pronounced changes over time (**Figure 5**). These damages may result from alterations in the loading environment of the remaining tendons. Further investigation using a supraspinatus-infraspinatus detachment in a rat model found that biceps alterations began in the intra-articular region of the tendon before extending to the extra-articular region.[40] Biopsy specimens from patients with different-size rotator cuff tears contained altered levels of matrix metalloproteinases (MMPs) and vascular

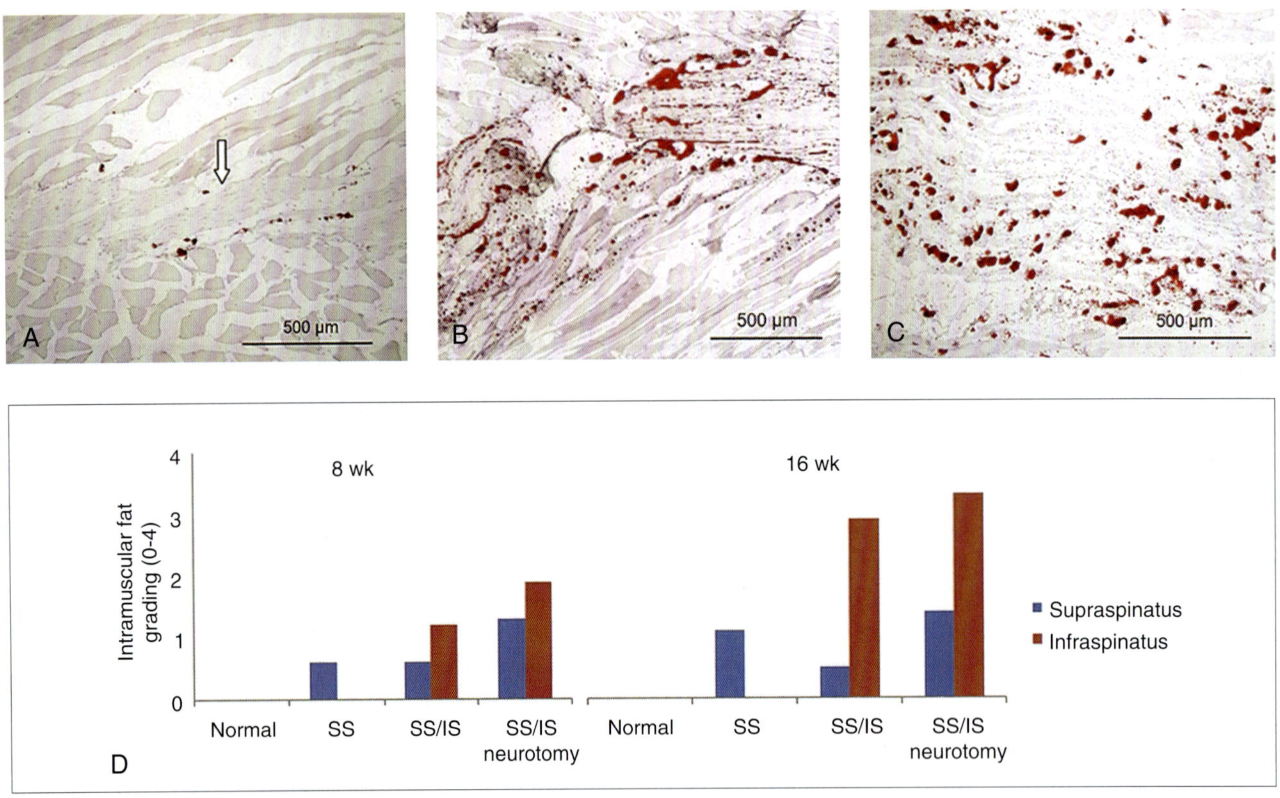

FIGURE 4 **A** through **C**, Oil Red O–stained histology sections from a rat model study. **A**, A normal supraspinatus muscle (longitudinal section in the coronal plane, 10-µm thickness) shows few intramuscular fat deposits and intramyocellular fat droplets. The supraspinatus tendon can be seen at the center of the muscle (arrow), and the muscle fibers can be seen above and below the tendon. **B**, An infraspinatus muscle 16 weeks after tenotomy of the supraspinatus and infraspinatus tendons. Many fat deposits are seen (red staining). **C**, An infraspinatus muscle 16 weeks after tenotomy plus neurotomy shows high levels of intramuscular fat (red staining). **D**, Diagram showing semiquantitative histology grading results for intramuscular fat at 8 and 16 weeks, as seen on Oil Red O–stained histology sections. 0 = no fat deposits, 4 = numerous fat deposits. No fat was seen in normal muscles. The infraspinatus (IS) muscle had more intramuscular fat than the supraspinatus (SS) muscle after tenotomy of the supraspinatus and infraspinatus tendons, with or without neurotomy. The 16-week specimens from each postsurgical group had more intramuscular fat than the 8-week specimens. (Reprinted from *J Shoulder Elbow Surg* 21[7].Kim HM, Galatz LM, Lim C, Havlioglu N, Thomopoulos S: The effect of tear size and nerve injury on rotator cuff muscle fatty degeneration in a rodent animal model, 847-858. Copyright © 2012 Journal of Shoulder and Elbow Surgery Board of Trustees. doi:10.1016/j.jse.2011.05.004.)

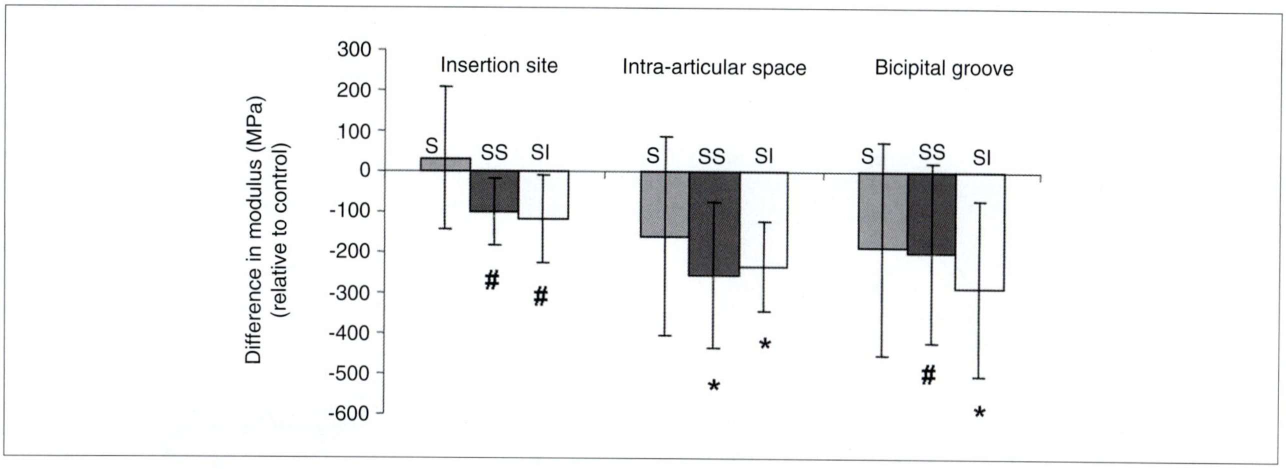

FIGURE 5 Diagram showing the decrease in biceps tendon modulus in a rat model between 4 and 8 weeks after supraspinatus and subscapularis detachment (SS) or supraspinatus and infraspinatus detachment (SI), compared with control rats. * = significant difference from control group, # = trend toward difference from control group, S = supraspinatus detachment. (Reproduced with permission from Peltz CD, Perry SM, Getz CL, Soslowsky LJ: Mechanical properties of the long-head of the biceps tendon are altered in the presence of rotator cuff tears in a rat model. *J Orthop Res* 2009;27[3]:416-420. © Orthopaedic Research Society. Published by Wiley Periodicals, Inc. doi:10.1002/jor.20770.)

endothelial growth factor.[41,42] MMPs are molecules that degrade extracellular matrix proteins, particularly collagen, and vascular endothelial growth factor is associated with angiogenesis. Patients with a rotator cuff tear had increased vascular endothelial growth factor, MMP-1, and MMP-9 expression but decreased MMP-3 expression. There changes were enhanced in articular-side partial tears compared with bursal-side partial tears, but no regional differences were seen with full-thickness tears. Scanning acoustic microscopy revealed an increased coracoacromial ligament elastic modulus in cadaver specimens with a rotator cuff tear or spur compared with control specimens.[43] These findings of altered compositional, histologic, and mechanical properties in shoulder structures with a rotator cuff tear have implications for treatment strategies.

In the presence of a rotator cuff tear, clinicians often recommend long head of the biceps tenotomy to reduce pain and improve function. In a rat model of supraspinatus detachment and overuse activity, biceps tenotomy led to glenohumeral cartilage damage.[44] This finding is likely due to decreased shoulder stability in the absence of the long head of the biceps and highlights the force-couple relationship of the rotator cuff tendons.

Biology and Genetics of Tendon Degeneration

Although the histology of tendon degeneration is well described, the biologic events leading to degeneration have only recently gained attention. Samples collected from patients with rotator cuff disease showed angiogenic and inflammatory imbalances as degeneration progressed.[45] Hypervascularization occurred later in tendinopathy. Although inflammation is not a characteristic of chronic tendon degeneration, it may exist in early stages. Subscapularis tendon biopsies from patients with a torn supraspinatus tendon had increased staining for macrophages, mast cells, and T cells compared with biopsies from the patient's torn supraspinatus tendon or control subscapularis tendons.[46] The larger the supraspinatus tear, the less often the occurrence of inflammatory cell infiltration. The subscapularis tendon in patients with a torn supraspinatus tendon may be a model for early tendinopathy.

The role of apoptosis in rotator cuff disease is debated. Patient biopsies revealed increased numbers of apoptotic cells throughout the torn supraspinatus and paired subscapularis samples.[47] Degenerated supraspinatus tendons from rats and humans had increases in heat shock proteins and caspases, with an imbalance between the antiapoptotic (heat shock protein) and proapoptotic (caspase) genes.[48] However, rats trained on a treadmill for as long as 16 weeks had no apoptosis or neovascularization. These rats did have an increase in insulinlike growth factor-1, which affects proliferation, cell survival, and chondrogenesis.[49] Late-stage rotator cuff disease may develop into calcific tendinopathy, in which the altered expression of genes is related to bone development and resorption.[50] These insights into differences between the stages of rotator cuff disease will lead to improvements in diagnosis and treatment.

Mechanical loading affects tendon degeneration. Altered loading on excised rat supraspinatus tendons changed the expression of MMPs and tissue inhibitors of metalloproteases.[51] One major characteristic of tendinopathy is an imbalance in MMPs and tissue inhibitors of metalloproteases. Overused rat

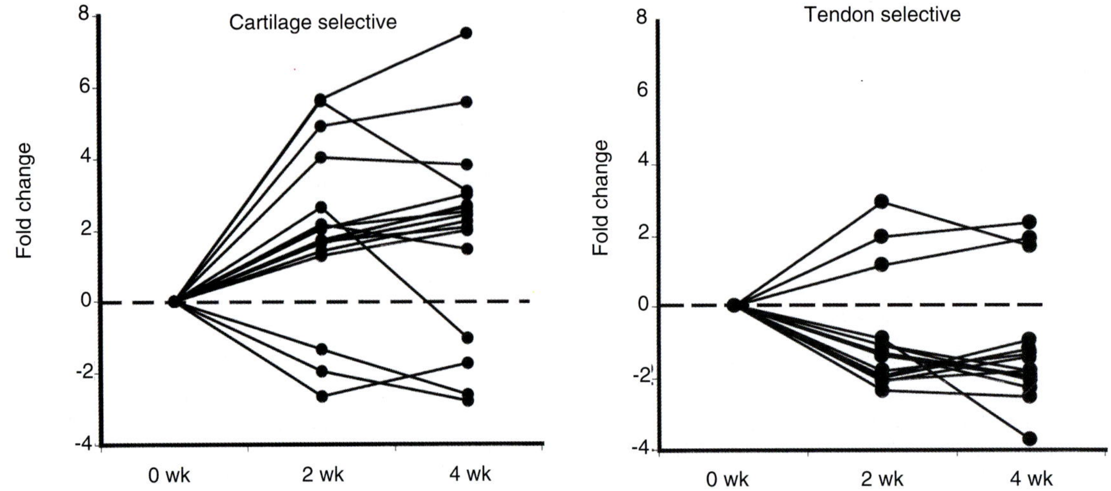

FIGURE 6 Diagram showing the effect of overuse on the supraspinatus tendons of rats that had undergone a treadmill training overuse protocol. Seventeen cartilage-selective (characteristic in cartilage) and 12 tendon-selective (characteristic in tendon) genes were compared with time-zero controls (represented as fold change in gene expression, compared with controls). In general, overuse upregulated cartilage markers and downregulated tendon markers. It appears that overuse causes the supraspinatus tendon to become more like cartilage and less like tendon. (Reproduced with permission from Archambault JM, Jelinsky SA, Lake SP, Hill AA, Glaser DL, Soslowsky LJ: Rat supraspinatus tendon expresses cartilage markers with overuse. *J Orthop Res* 2007;25[5]:617-624. © Orthopaedic Research Society. Published by Wiley Periodicals, Inc. doi:10.1002/jor.20347.)

supraspinatus tendons expressed cartilage markers[52] (**Figure 6**). Proteoglycan and heparin affine regulatory peptide (a chondrogenesis-promoting factor) levels increased with overuse[53] (**Table 1**). These cartilage markers and other genes regulated by short-term overuse returned to near-baseline levels after rest.[54] Tenocytes in rotator cuff tendinopathy may be undergoing a transformation into a chondrocytelike phenotype. Unloading of the supraspinatus can also lead to detrimental changes to the rotator cuff. In a mouse model, supraspinatus muscle paralysis via botulinum toxin A injection leads to decreased mineral organization and strength at the tendon insertion.[55] These changes coincided with insertion-site bone loss, leading to increased injury risk. Although mechanical loading is believed to be the primary source of rotator cuff disease, evidence for a genetic predisposition also exists.[56] Further work is needed to elucidate the complex interactions among mechanics, genetics, and biology in the onset and the progression of rotator cuff degeneration.

Progression of Tendon Degeneration and Tears

Rotator cuff degeneration can lead to a partial-thickness tear, which can progress in both width and thickness into a full-thickness tear. The stages of degeneration are associated with different levels of hypoxia-inducible factor-1α and a trend toward increased apoptosis with increased degeneration.[57] Alterations in hypoxia-inducible factor-1α also were seen in retracted torn rotator cuff tendons.[58] Increasing vessel density is related to the amount of retraction, suggesting that neovascularity may be a useful parameter for tracking tear progression. These degenerated samples also had increased levels of MMP-1 and MMP-9 and decreased levels of MMP-3.[59] Increased MMP-9 expression was correlated with increased retraction. Full-thickness tears had increased proinflammatory cytokines and angiogenic factors in the synovium compared with partial-thickness tears.[60] Supraspinatus tendon biopsies revealed increased tissue remodeling and neovascularization with full-thickness tears. Furthermore, subscapularis biopsies from shoulders with a full-thickness supraspinatus tear showed increased degeneration and remodeling compared with shoulders with a partial-thickness tear. These results suggest that greater tear severity leads to greater synovial inflammation and degeneration of the supraspinatus and subscapularis tendons (**Figure 7**).

Tendon Healing, Repair, and Treatment

Healing

The basic phases of tendon healing are described as inflammatory, proliferative (fibroplasic), and remodeling (maturing). Recent attention has focused on the

Table 1

Genetic and Protein Changes in the Rat Supraspinatus Tendon After a 2- or 4-Week Treadmill Training Overuse Protocol, Compared With Normal Tendon

Molecule	Level of Expression	
	After 2 wk	After 4 wk
Collagen		
1α1 mRNA	–	––
2α1 mRNA	+	+
3α1 mRNA	+	=
6α1 mRNA	++	=
Decorin		
mRNA	+	++
Protein	=	++
Biglycan		
mRNA	++	++
Versican		
mRNA	++	++
Protein	=	++
Aggrecan		
mRNA	++	++
Protein	++	++
SOX9		
mRNA	++	+
Glycosaminoglycans		
Total	=	++
Dermatan sulfate	=	++
Chondroitin sulfate	=	+
Heparan sulfate	=	=
Carbohydrate sulfotransferase-14 (involved in dermatan sulfate synthesis)	++	=
Heparin affine regulatory peptide mRNA	=	=
Protein	+	++

–, decreased expression; ––, further-decreased expression; =, no difference from control expression; +, increased expression; ++, further-increased expression.

Adapted with permission from Attia M, Scott A, Duchesnay A, et al: Alterations of overused supraspinatus tendon: A possible role of glycosaminoglycans and heparin affine regulatory peptide/pleiotrophin in early tendon pathology. *J Orthop Res* 2012;30(1):61-71. © Orthopaedic Research Society. Published by Wiley Periodicals, Inc. doi:10.1002/jor.21479.

preclinical studies of molecular healing, new imaging techniques for healing tendons, and optimal treatment protocols for obtaining the best outcomes during each of the basic phases. To further the understanding of the molecular processes that occur during tendon healing, growth factor concentrations were measured at multiple postoperative time points. Increased expression of growth factors was observed 1 week after surgical detachment and repair of the supraspinatus tendon in a rat model. By 16 weeks, the levels had gradually tapered to control or undetectable levels. The initial increase may be attributable to the inflammatory response, and the midsubstance-specific increase at 8 weeks may be attributable to the increased loading environment as the tendon heals. This finding provides further evidence that loading influences healing[61] (**Table 2**).

Traditional cast or sling immobilization limits gross movement of the shoulder joint. A temporary elimination of motion is suspected to be beneficial in early healing. Rat supraspinatus detachment and repair models were used in two studies to evaluate the effect of total muscle paralysis on insertion site healing. Following supraspinatus surgical repair, injections of botulinum toxin A negatively influenced the mechanical properties of the tendon and its insertion, especially in rats immobilized with a cast.[62] A similar study found not only early decreases in mechanical properties with muscle paralysis but also significantly improved collagen fiber organization at 4 weeks.[63] No significant difference in mechanical properties was seen 24 weeks after surgery.

Contrast-enhanced ultrasonography was used to characterize in vivo vascularity of the supraspinatus tendon in human shoulders 3 months after surgical repair. Tendons with a defect had significantly lower vascular volume and lower resting perfusion at the insertion site.[64] This finding suggests that the quality of vascular supply to the region is an important consideration in surgical repair.

Effects of Repair

Although surgery is generally effective for repairing torn supraspinatus tendons, approximately 25% of repairs are unsuccessful. A significant focus of research has been to investigate and better understand what happens in the body after repair, what factors influence such processes, and how to measure postoperative responses. Multivariate regression was used to analyze factors that may predict functional outcomes following repair. Patient age, long reported to be a determinant of surgical outcome, was not found to be an independent causal factor but merely a correlate of significant factors.[65] These included tear retraction, fatty degeneration, and muscle strength. Preoperative scores for muscle atrophy and fatty infiltration

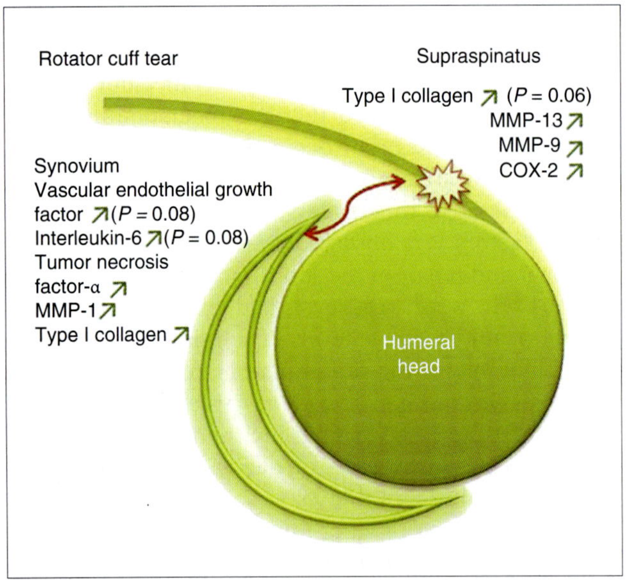

FIGURE 7 Diagram showing the association of a rotator cuff tear with synovial inflammation. Increased tear size is correlated with a greater proinflammatory response in the synovium. Green arrows indicate increase. (Adapted from *J Shoulder Elbow Surg* 20[6]. Shindle MK, Chen CC, Robertson C, et al: Full-thickness supraspinatus tears are associated with more synovial inflammation and tissue degeneration than partial-thickness tears, 917-927. Copyright © 2011 Journal of Shoulder and Elbow Surgery Board of Trustees. doi:10.1016/j.jse.2011.02.015.)

in the supraspinatus and infraspinatus were significant predictors of functional outcome, intercorrelated, and generally worsened with increasing tear size (**Figure 8**). Muscle atrophy and fatty infiltration scores worsened 1 year after surgery if the patient had these conditions at the time of surgery. The progression was worse in shoulders with an unsuccessful repair. Repair should therefore be performed as early as possible to minimize the influences of fatty infiltration and muscle atrophy.[66]

A novel device to measure in vivo shoulder stiffness in anesthetized rats found that stiffness increased if the rat had been immobilized. However, the effect was transient and not significantly different after 8 weeks. The use of a human corollary of this device would be helpful for clinical evaluation. A temporary increase in shoulder stiffness with immobilization may be acceptable, given the benefit to the properties of the repaired insertion site.[67]

Using a rabbit model, researchers found that CT can reveal the strength of a surgically repaired tendon-bone construct.[68] Increased blood flow during healing resulted in lower attenuation, and hypoattenuation increased with time after surgery. Hypoattenuation seen in early images was correlated with a stronger union and a decreased likelihood of failure. Early CT may be useful for predicting surgical success. Another study used roentgen stereophotogrammetric analysis to measure the migration of tendon-embedded markers. Surgeons embedded metal beads into the greater humeral tuberosity and wire sutures into the supraspinatus tendon of patients during open repair of a rotator cuff tear. After 1 year, intact repairs had moved an average of 6.3 mm; the average movement in completely unsuccessful repairs was 23.7 mm. The most movement occurred during the period of active rehabilitation (2 to 3 months after surgery). This timing suggests that the greatest vulnerability to retearing is during this time, possibly as a function of activity levels in physical therapy. Migration was minimal between 3 to 4 months and 1 year after surgery, possibly because the repairs that were intact at the beginning of the period were tolerant of future loading.[69]

Early clinical work suggested that partial repair of a massive tear involving both the infraspinatus and the supraspinatus, in which only the infraspinatus is reattached, may be effective for restoring adequate function. Recent research in a rat model used a two-tendon detachment and quantitative ambulatory measures. Both partial and complete repair improved function compared with no repair, but there were no differences in outcomes observed between partial and complete repair.[70] These findings support the clinical practice of using a partial repair to restore adequate function. A human cadaver study evaluated the influence of type of repair on the interaction between the supraspinatus and infraspinatus tendons. This study found that "transosseous-equivalent arthroscopic techniques" led to decreased interaction at high loads and thereby reduced the ability of the infraspinatus to shield the supraspinatus.[71] This finding highlights the possible risk of a partial repair compared with a traditional open transosseous repair.

Postoperative and Nonsurgical Treatment

The poor outcomes often associated with rotator cuff repair and the treatment of degeneration have stimulated research into treatment techniques. Beyond the specifics of the repair technique, the surgeon can influence patient outcomes through the prescription of rehabilitation protocols. In addition, nontraditional treatment techniques have garnered increasing scientific attention.

A series of experiments using a rat model investigated the effects of immobilization and exercise at multiple time points after repair. Immobilization resulted in improved collagen organization after 4 weeks but not after 16 weeks.[72] Immobilized rats had better mechanical properties after 16 weeks but not after 4 weeks. This finding suggests that long-term immobilization allowed for a more organized repair, which eventually improved mechanical properties. A follow-up study combined immobilization with two distinct passive motion protocols, both of which led to significantly decreased range of motion, likely due to increased subacromial scar formation.[73] A short period of immobilization was followed by either

Table 2

Growth Factor Concentration (Insertion/Midsubstance) in a Rat Model 1 to 16 Weeks After Surgical Detachment and Repair of the Supraspinatus Tendon

Growth Factor	Nonsurgical Control	Postsurgical Week 1	2	4	8	16
Basic fibroblastic growth factor	+/+	+++/+++	++/+++	+/+	++/++	+/–
Bone morphogenetic protein-12	+/+	+++/+++	+/++	+/+	++/++	+/–
Bone morphogenetic protein-13	+/–	++/+++	++/+	++/+	++/+	–/–
Bone morphogenetic protein-14	+/++	++/+++	+/+	+/+	+/++	–/–
Cartilage oligomeric matrix protein	+/+	+++/+++	+/++	++/+	+/+	–/–
Connective tissue growth factor	+/+	+++/++	++/++	+/+	+/++	+/–
Platelet-derived growth factor-β	*/+	*/+++	*/++	*/+	*/+	*/+
Transforming growth factor-β1	+/+	++/++	++/++	–/+	+/++	–/–

Median values of semiquantitative staining intensity: +, low; ++, moderate; +++, high; –, trace; *, undetected.

Adapted from *J Shoulder Elbow Surg* 16[5,suppl]. Würgler-Hauri CC, Dourte LM, Baradet TC, Williams GR, Soslowsky LJ: Temporal expression of 8 growth factors in tendon-to-bone healing in a rat supraspinatus model, S198-S203. Copyright © 2007 Journal of Shoulder and Elbow Surgery Board of Trustees. doi:10.1016/j.jse.2007.04.003.

cage activity or treadmill running. The exercised rats had inferior physical and mechanical properties, suggesting that the tissue was disorganized with increased matrix and scar production.[74]

Clinical studies have sought to determine the relative efficacy of aggressive and limited early passive motion rehabilitation protocols. In one study, patients who underwent aggressive rehabilitation received manual therapy twice a day and were instructed to perform pendulum and stretching exercises three times a day.[75] Those who underwent limited rehabilitation were assisted by a continuous passive motion machine and performed only forward-flexion stretching exercises twice daily. The programs converged after 6 weeks into an active stretching and strengthening protocol. The patients who received aggressive treatment had greater range of motion and better clinical evaluations 3 months after surgery, but these differences were not significant at 1 year. Retearing occurred in 7 of the 30 patients in the aggressive treatment group but only in 3 of the 34 patients in the limited treatment group.

A naturopathic treatment protocol was compared with physical exercise in patients with rotator cuff tendinopathy in the absence of a tear. The naturopathic treatment consisted of anti-inflammatory dietary counseling, the use of a dietary supplement (phlogenzym), and weekly acupuncture. Both groups were provided with a therapeutic doctor-patient relationship, physical therapy, and a pill (placebo for patients in the exercise group). Patients in both groups improved significantly on subjective questionnaires, with those in the naturopathic treatment group improving more than those in the exercise control group. Quantitative measures of range of motion revealed significant improvements in patients in the naturopathic treatment group in comparison both with baseline and with patients in the exercise group. The patients in the exercise group did not improve significantly on the quantitative measures.[76]

SUMMARY

The rotator cuff tendons provide crucial stability and enable the shoulder's unique range of motion, but these structures are prone to degeneration and injury. Research continues to explore the molecular anatomy and healing biology of these structures. Progress has been made in identifying and quantifying important molecules and in describing the insertion site in detail. Modeling the mechanics of the joint has led to an improved understanding of the interactions of related structures. The biology of

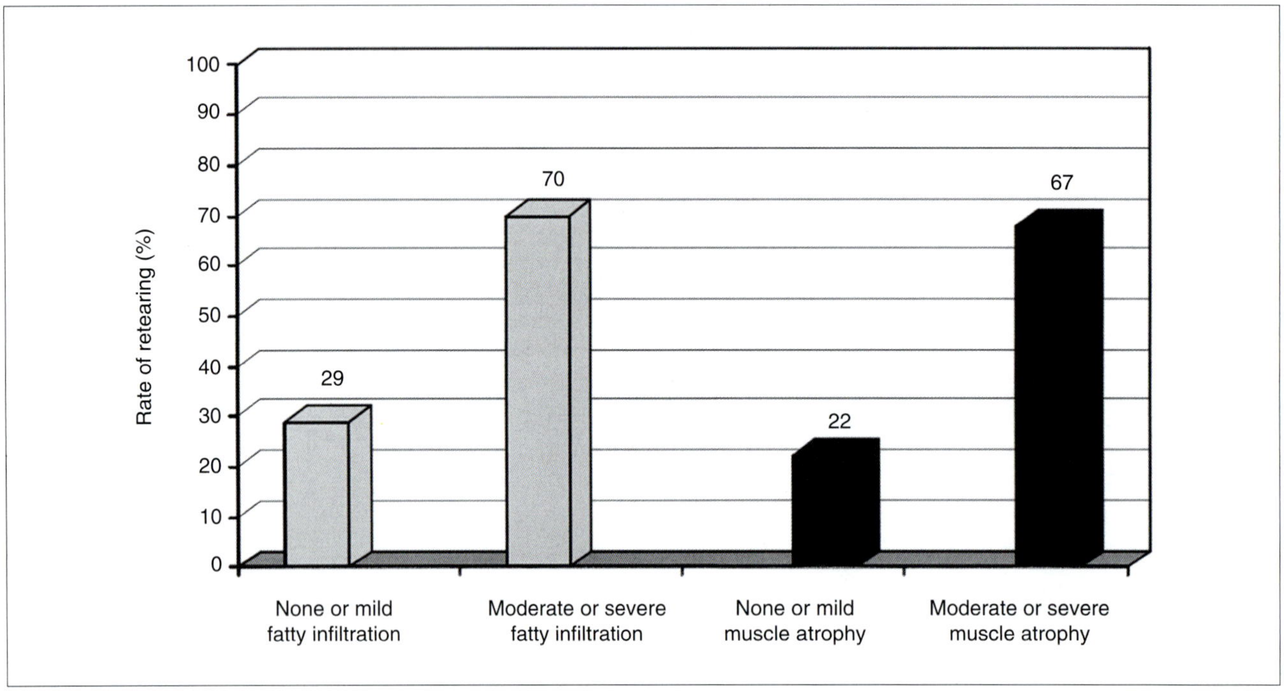

FIGURE 8 Diagram showing the effect of clinically insignificant or significant fatty infiltration or muscle atrophy on the rate of rotator cuff retearing ($P < 0.05$). (Adapted with permission from Gladstone JN, Bishop JY, Lo IK, Flatow EL: Fatty infiltration and atrophy of the rotator cuff do not improve after rotator cuff repair and correlate with poor functional outcome. *Am J Sports Med* 2007;35[5]:719-728. doi:10.1177/0363546506297539.)

tendon pathology progression is being elucidated, and great strides have been made with novel imaging techniques that allow for in vivo measurements. From surgical technique and rehabilitation protocol to genetics and lifestyle, the understanding of the factors that influence degeneration and healing is improving. Future research will continue to explicate these factors through animal, cadaver, and clinical studies. Advances in biologic augmentation and tissue engineering may offer new hope in treating these challenging tendons.

KEY STUDY POINTS

- The supraspinatus tendon has the highest risk of injury because of its complex loading environment, compositional heterogeneity, and interactions with other rotator cuff tendons.
- Animal models have made great strides in understanding the molecular mechanisms behind rotator cuff degeneration, injury, and repair.
- Even small, partial-thickness tears can progress to full-thickness tears and alter the other rotator cuff tendons, leading to muscle and further tendon degeneration.
- Early repair and initiation of rehabilitation are important factors to determine the efficacy of rotator cuff tear treatment.
- Further investigation into in vivo techniques is necessary to provide a better understanding of rotator cuff degeneration, injury, and healing.

Annotated References

1. Matuszewski PE, Chen YL, Szczesny SE, et al: Regional variation in human supraspinatus tendon proteoglycans: Decorin, biglycan, and aggrecan. *Connect Tissue Res* 2012;53(5):343-348.

2. Wopenka B, Kent A, Pasteris JD, Yoon Y, Thomopoulos S: The tendon-to-bone transition of the rotator cuff: A preliminary Raman spectroscopic study documenting the gradual mineralization across the insertion in rat tissue samples. *Appl Spectrosc* 2008;62(12):1285-1294.

3. Cashman PM, Baring T, Reilly P, Emery RJ, Amis AA: Measurement of migration of soft tissue by modified Roentgen stereophotogrammetric analysis (RSA): Validation of a new technique to monitor rotator cuff tears. *J Med Eng Technol* 2010;34(3):159-165.

4. Derwin KA, Milks RA, Davidson I, Iannotti JP, McCarron JA, Bey MJ: Low-dose CT imaging of radio-opaque markers for assessing human rotator cuff repair: Accuracy, repeatability and the effect of arm position. *J Biomech* 2012;45(3):614-618.

5. Bey MJ, Kline SK, Baker AR, McCarron JA, Iannotti JP, Derwin KA: Estimation of dynamic, in vivo soft-tissue deformation: Experimental technique and application in a canine model of tendon injury and repair. *J Orthop Res* 2011;29(6):822-827.

6. Kim YS, Kim JM, Bigliani LU, Kim HJ, Jung HW: In vivo strain analysis of the intact supraspinatus tendon by ultrasound speckles tracking imaging. *J Orthop Res* 2011;29(12):1931-1937.

7. Seki N, Itoi E, Shibuya Y, et al: Mechanical environment of the supraspinatus tendon: Three-dimensional finite element model analysis. *J Orthop Sci* 2008;13(4):348-353.

8. Lake SP, Miller KS, Elliott DM, Soslowsky LJ: Effect of fiber distribution and realignment on the nonlinear and inhomogeneous mechanical properties of human supraspinatus tendon under longitudinal tensile loading. *J Orthop Res* 2009;27(12):1596-1602.

9. Lake SP, Miller KS, Elliott DM, Soslowsky LJ: Tensile properties and fiber alignment of human supraspinatus tendon in the transverse direction demonstrate inhomogeneity, nonlinearity, and regional isotropy. *J Biomech* 2010;43(4):727-732.

10. Chaudhury S, Holland C, Vollrath F, Carr AJ: Comparing normal and torn rotator cuff tendons using dynamic shear analysis. *J Bone Joint Surg Br* 2011;93(7):942-948.

11. Andarawis-Puri N, Ricchetti ET, Soslowsky LJ: Interaction between the supraspinatus and infraspinatus tendons: Effect of anterior supraspinatus tendon full-thickness tears on infraspinatus tendon strain. *Am J Sports Med* 2009;37(9):1831-1839.

12. Andarawis-Puri N, Kuntz AF, Ramsey ML, Soslowsky LJ: Effect of glenohumeral abduction angle on the mechanical interaction between the supraspinatus and infraspinatus tendons for the intact, partial-thickness torn, and repaired supraspinatus tendon conditions. *J Orthop Res* 2010;28(7):846-851.

13. Andarawis-Puri N, Kuntz AF, Kim SY, Soslowsky LJ: Effect of anterior supraspinatus tendon partial-thickness tears on infraspinatus tendon strain through a range of joint rotation angles. *J Shoulder Elbow Surg* 2010;19(4):617-623.

14. Andarawis-Puri N, Kuntz AF, Jawad AF, Soslowsky LJ: Infraspinatus and supraspinatus tendon strain explained using multiple regression models. *Ann Biomed Eng* 2010;38(9):2979-2987.

15. Bonilla KA, Pardes AM, Freedman BR, Soslowsky LJ: Supraspinatus tendons have different mechanical properties across sex. *J Biomech Eng* 2019;141(1):0110021-0110028.

    A study comparing rat supraspinatus tendon properties across sexes found increased stiffness and decreased dynamic modulus in male tendons compared to female tendons.

16. Aagaard KE, Abu-Zidan F, Lunsjo K: High incidence of acute full-thickness rotator cuff tears. *Acta Orthop* 2015;86(5):558-562.

    A prospective study of full-thickness rotator cuff tears found that most of these tears (65%) occurred in male patients. Level of evidence: III.

17. Abboud JA, Kim JS: The effect of hypercholesterolemia on rotator cuff disease. *Clin Orthop Relat Res* 2010;468(6):1493-1497.

18. Beason DP, Abboud JA, Kuntz AF, Bassora R, Soslowsky LJ: Cumulative effects of hypercholesterolemia on tendon biomechanics in a mouse model. *J Orthop Res* 2011;29(3):380-383.

19. Bedi A, Fox AJ, Harris PE, et al: Diabetes mellitus impairs tendon-bone healing after rotator cuff repair. *J Shoulder Elbow Surg* 2010;19(7):978-988.

20. Cadet ER, Vorys GC, Rahman R, et al: Improving bone density at the rotator cuff footprint increases supraspinatus tendon failure stress in a rat model. *J Orthop Res* 2010;28(3):308-314.

21. Ichinose R, Sano H, Kishimoto KN, Sakamoto N, Sato M, Itoi E: Alteration of the material properties of the normal supraspinatus tendon by nicotine treatment in a rat model. *Acta Orthop* 2010;81(5):634-638.

22. Perry SM, Getz CL, Soslowsky LJ: Alterations in function after rotator cuff tears in an animal model. *J Shoulder Elbow Surg* 2009;18(2):296-304.

23. Sarver JJ, Dishowitz MI, Kim SY, Soslowsky LJ: Transient decreases in forelimb gait and ground reaction forces following rotator cuff injury and repair in a rat model. *J Biomech* 2010;43(4):778-782.

24. Lebaschi AH, Deng XH, Camp CL, et al: Biomechanical, histologic, and molecular evaluation of tendon healing in a new murine model of rotator cuff repair. *Arthroscopy* 2018;34(4):1173-1183.

    A mouse model for rotator cuff repair was developed. This model led to reproducible changes in biomechanics, histology, and gene expression patterns similar to those of other animal models of rotator cuff repair.

25. Longo UG, Franceschi F, Ruzzini L, et al: Histopathology of the supraspinatus tendon in rotator cuff tears. *Am J Sports Med* 2008;36(3):533-538.

26. Chaudhury S, Dicko C, Burgess M, Vollrath F, Carr AJ: Fourier transform infrared spectroscopic analysis of normal and torn rotator-cuff tendons. *J Bone Joint Surg Br* 2011;93(3):370-377.

27. Steinbacher P, Tauber M, Kogler S, Stoiber W, Resch H, Sänger AM: Effects of rotator cuff ruptures on the cellular and intracellular composition of the human supraspinatus muscle. *Tissue Cell* 2010;42(1):37-41.

28. Kim HM, Dahiya N, Teefey SA, Keener JD, Galatz LM, Yamaguchi K: Relationship of tear size and location to fatty degeneration of the rotator cuff. *J Bone Joint Surg Am* 2010;92(4):829-839.

29. Melis B, DeFranco MJ, Chuinard C, Walch G: Natural history of fatty infiltration and atrophy of the supraspinatus muscle in rotator cuff tears. *Clin Orthop Relat Res* 2010;468(6):1498-1505.

30. Oh JH, Kim SH, Kim JH, Shin YH, Yoon JP, Oh CH: The level of vitamin D in the serum correlates with fatty degeneration of the muscles of the rotator cuff. *J Bone Joint Surg Br* 2009;91(12):1587-1593.

31. Fuchs B, Zumstein M, Regenfelder F, et al: Upregulation of alpha-skeletal muscle actin and myosin heavy polypeptide gene products in degenerating rotator cuff muscles. *J Orthop Res* 2008;26(7):1007-1011.

32. Ward SR, Sarver JJ, Eng CM, et al: Plasticity of muscle architecture after supraspinatus tears. *J Orthop Sports Phys Ther* 2010;40(11):729-735.

33. Buchmann S, Walz L, Sandmann GH, et al: Rotator cuff changes in a full thickness tear rat model: Verification of the optimal time interval until reconstruction for comparison to the healing process of chronic lesions in humans. *Arch Orthop Trauma Surg* 2011;131(3):429-435.

34. Farshad M, Würgler-Hauri CC, Kohler T, Gerber C, Rothenfluh DA: Effect of age on fatty infiltration of supraspinatus muscle after experimental tendon release in rats. *BMC Res Notes* 2011;4:530.

35. Dourte LM, Perry SM, Getz CL, Soslowsky LJ: Tendon properties remain altered in a chronic rat rotator cuff model. *Clin Orthop Relat Res* 2010;468(6): 1485-1492.

36. Kim HM, Galatz LM, Lim C, Havlioglu N, Thomopoulos S: The effect of tear size and nerve injury on rotator cuff muscle fatty degeneration in a rodent animal model. *J Shoulder Elbow Surg* 2012;21(7):847-858.

37. Rowshan K, Hadley S, Pham K, Caiozzo V, Lee TQ, Gupta R: Development of fatty atrophy after neurologic and rotator cuff injuries in an animal model of rotator cuff pathology. *J Bone Joint Surg Am* 2010;92(13): 2270-2278.

38. Perry SM, Getz CL, Soslowsky LJ: After rotator cuff tears, the remaining (intact) tendons are mechanically altered. *J Shoulder Elbow Surg* 2009;18(1):52-57.

39. Peltz CD, Perry SM, Getz CL, Soslowsky LJ: Mechanical properties of the long-head of the biceps tendon are altered in the presence of rotator cuff tears in a rat model. *J Orthop Res* 2009;27(3):416-420.

40. Peltz CD, Hsu JE, Zgonis MH, Trasolini NA, Glaser DL, Soslowsky LJ: Intra-articular changes precede extra-articular changes in the biceps tendon after rotator cuff tears in a rat model. *J Shoulder Elbow Surg* 2012;21(7):873-881.

41. Lakemeier S, Schwuchow SA, Peterlein CD, et al: Expression of matrix metalloproteinases 1, 3, and 9 in degenerated long head biceps tendon in the presence of rotator cuff tears: An immunohistological study. *BMC Musculoskelet Disord* 2010;11:271.

42. Lakemeier S, Reichelt JJ, Timmesfeld N, Fuchs-Winkelmann S, Paletta JR, Schofer MD: The relevance of long head biceps degeneration in the presence of rotator cuff tears. *BMC Musculoskelet Disord* 2010;11:191.

43. Kijima H, Minagawa H, Saijo Y, et al: Degenerated coracoacromial ligament in shoulders with rotator cuff tears shows higher elastic modulus: Measurement with scanning acoustic microscopy. *J Orthop Sci* 2009;14(1): 62-67.

44. Beach ZM, Tucker JJ, Thomas SJ, et al: Biceps tenotomy in the presence of a supraspinatus tear alters the adjacent intact tendons and glenoid cartilage. *J Biomech* 2017;63:151-157.

    A rat model of supraspinatus detachment and overuse activity ± biceps tenotomy was developed. Biceps tenotomy led to mechanical changes to remaining rotator cuff tendons and glenohumeral cartilage damage.

45. Savitskaya YA, Izaguirre A, Sierra L, et al: Effect of angiogenesis-related cytokines on rotator cuff disease: The search for sensitive biomarkers of early tendon degeneration. *Clin Med Insights Arthritis Musculoskelet Disord* 2011;4:43-53.

46. Millar NL, Hueber AJ, Reilly JH, et al: Inflammation is present in early human tendinopathy. *Am J Sports Med* 2010;38(10):2085-2091.

47. Lundgreen K, Lian OB, Engebretsen L, Scott A: Tenocyte apoptosis in the torn rotator cuff: A primary or secondary pathological event? *Br J Sports Med* 2011;45(13):1035-1039.

48. Millar NL, Wei AQ, Molloy TJ, Bonar F, Murrell GA: Heat shock protein and apoptosis in supraspinatus tendinopathy. *Clin Orthop Relat Res* 2008;466(7): 1569-1576.

49. Scott A, Cook JL, Hart DA, Walker DC, Duronio V, Khan KM: Tenocyte responses to mechanical loading in vivo: A role for local insulin-like growth factor 1 signaling in early tendinosis in rats. *Arthritis Rheum* 2007;56(3):871-881.

50. Oliva F, Barisani D, Grasso A, Maffulli N: Gene expression analysis in calcific tendinopathy of the rotator cuff. *Eur Cell Mater* 2011;21:548-557.

51. Thornton GM, Shao X, Chung M, et al: Changes in mechanical loading lead to tendonspecific alterations in MMP and TIMP expression: Influence of stress deprivation and intermittent cyclic hydrostatic compression on rat supraspinatus and Achilles tendons. *Br J Sports Med* 2010;44(10):698-703.

52. Archambault JM, Jelinsky SA, Lake SP, Hill AA, Glaser DL, Soslowsky LJ: Rat supraspinatus tendon expresses cartilage markers with overuse. *J Orthop Res* 2007;25(5):617-624.

53. Attia M, Scott A, Duchesnay A, et al: Alterations of overused supraspinatus tendon: A possible role of glycosaminoglycans and HARP/pleiotrophin in early tendon pathology. *J Orthop Res* 2012;30(1):61-71.

54. Jelinsky SA, Lake SP, Archambault JM, Soslowsky LJ: Gene expression in rat supraspinatus tendon recovers from overuse with rest. *Clin Orthop Relat Res* 2008;466(7):1612-1617.

55. Deymier AC, Schwartz AG, Cai Z, et al: The multiscale structural and mechanical effects of mouse supraspinatus muscle unloading on the mature enthesis. *Acta Biomater* 2019;83:302-313.

    Mouse supraspinatus muscles were unloaded via botulinum toxin A injection. After 21 days of unloading, tendon enthesis demonstrated decreased organization and strength. Underlying bone showed significant resorption.

56. Tashjian RZ, Farnham JM, Albright FS, Teerlink CC, Cannon-Albright LA: Evidence for an inherited predisposition contributing to the risk for rotator cuff disease. *J Bone Joint Surg Am* 2009;91(5):1136-1142.

57. Benson RT, McDonnell SM, Knowles HJ, Rees JL, Carr AJ, Hulley PA: Tendinopathy and tears of the rotator cuff are associated with hypoxia and apoptosis. *J Bone Joint Surg Br* 2010;92(3):448-453.

58. Lakemeier S, Reichelt JJ, Patzer T, Fuchs-Winkelmann S, Paletta JR, Schofer MD: The association between retraction of the torn rotator cuff and increasing expression of hypoxia inducible factor 1α and vascular endothelial growth factor expression: An immunohistological study. *BMC Musculoskelet Disord* 2010;11:230.

59. Lakemeier S, Braun J, Efe T, et al: Expression of matrix metalloproteinases 1, 3, and 9 in differing extents of tendon retraction in the torn rotator cuff. *Knee Surg Sports Traumatol Arthrosc* 2011;19(10):1760-1765.

60. Shindle MK, Chen CC, Robertson C, et al: Full-thickness supraspinatus tears are associated with more synovial inflammation and tissue degeneration than partial-thickness tears. *J Shoulder Elbow Surg* 2011;20(6):917-927.

61. Wurgler-Hauri CC, Dourte LM, Baradet TC, Williams GR, Soslowsky LJ: Temporal expression of 8 growth factors in tendon-to-bone healing in a rat supraspinatus model. *J Shoulder Elbow Surg* 2007;16(5 suppl):S198-S203.

62. Galatz LM, Charlton N, Das R, Kim HM, Havlioglu N, Thomopoulos S: Complete removal of load is detrimental to rotator cuff healing. *J Shoulder Elbow Surg* 2009;18(5):669-675.

63. Hettrich CM, Rodeo SA, Hannafin JA, Ehteshami J, Shubin Stein BE: The effect of muscle paralysis using Botox on the healing of tendon to bone in a rat model. *J Shoulder Elbow Surg* 2011;20(5):688-697.

64. Gamradt SC, Gallo RA, Adler RS, et al: Vascularity of the supraspinatus tendon three months after repair: Characterization using contrast-enhanced ultrasound. *J Shoulder Elbow Surg* 2010;19(1):73-80.

65. Oh JH, Kim SH, Kang JY, Oh CH, Gong HS: Effect of age on functional and structural outcome after rotator cuff repair. *Am J Sports Med* 2010;38(4):672-678.

66. Gladstone JN, Bishop JY, Lo IK, Flatow EL: Fatty infiltration and atrophy of the rotator cuff do not improve after rotator cuff repair and correlate with poor functional outcome. *Am J Sports Med* 2007;35(5):719-728.

67. Sarver JJ, Peltz CD, Dourte L, Reddy S, Williams GR, Soslowsky LJ: After rotator cuff repair, stiffness – but not the loss in range of motion – increased transiently for immobilized shoulders in a rat model. *J Shoulder Elbow Surg* 2008;17(1 suppl):108S-113S.

68. Trudel G, Ramachandran N, Ryan SE, Rakhra K, Uhthoff HK: Supraspinatus tendon repair into a bony trough in the rabbit: Mechanical restoration and correlative imaging. *J Orthop Res* 2010;28(6):710-715.

69. Baring TK, Cashman PP, Reilly P, Emery RJ, Amis AA: Rotator cuff repair failure in vivo: A radiostereometric measurement study. *J Shoulder Elbow Surg* 2011;20(8):1194-1199.

70. Hsu JE, Reuther KE, Sarver JJ, et al: Restoration of anterior-posterior rotator cuff force balance improves shoulder function in a rat model of chronic massive tears. *J Orthop Res* 2011;29(7):1028-1033.

71. Andarawis-Puri N, Kuntz AF, Ramsey ML, Soslowsky LJ: Effect of supraspinatus tendon repair technique on the infraspinatus tendon. *J Biomech Eng* 2011;133(3):031008.

72. Gimbel JA, Van Kleunen JP, Williams GR, Thomopoulos S, Soslowsky LJ: Long durations of immobilization in the rat result in enhanced mechanical properties of the healing supraspinatus tendon insertion site. *J Biomech Eng* 2007;129(3):400-404.

73. Peltz CD, Dourte LM, Kuntz AF, et al: The effect of postoperative passive motion on rotator cuff healing in a rat model. *J Bone Joint Surg Am* 2009;91(10):2421-2429.

74. Peltz CD, Sarver JJ, Dourte LM, Würgler-Hauri CC, Williams GR, Soslowsky LJ: Exercise following a short immobilization period is detrimental to tendon properties and joint mechanics in a rat rotator cuff injury model. *J Orthop Res* 2010;28(7):841-845.

75. Lee BG, Cho NS, Rhee YG: Effect of two rehabilitation protocols on range of motion and healing rates after arthroscopic rotator cuff repair: Aggressive versus limited early passive exercises. *Arthroscopy* 2012;28(1):34-42.

76. Szczurko O, Cooley K, Mills EJ, Zhou Q, Perri D, Seely D: Naturopathic treatment of rotator cuff tendinitis among Canadian postal workers: A randomized controlled trial. *Arthritis Rheum* 2009;61(8):1037-1045.

Chapter 3

Kinematics and Biomechanics of Reverse Shoulder Arthroplasty

William R. Aibinder, MD • Christopher P. Roche, MSBE, MBA • Shawn M. Gargac, MSBE • George S. Athwal, MD, FRCSC

ABSTRACT

The glenohumeral joint relies on a functioning and balanced rotator cuff for stability. When the rotator cuff fails, a typical pattern of subluxation and degeneration known as cuff tear arthropathy may develop that is effectively treated with a reverse shoulder arthroplasty. Early reverse designs failed because of poor glenoid fixation. The Grammont prosthesis provided more reliable outcomes by medializing the center of rotation and lengthening the humerus to lengthen the abductor moment arms and improve the length-tension relationship of the deltoid. However, this design is associated with less predictable improvements in internal and external rotation and has a high rate of scapular notching. Newer techniques and prosthesis designs focus on improving shoulder rotation and decreasing scapular notching, while maintaining the mechanical advantage of the deltoid without compromising implant survivability.

Mr. Roche or an immediate family member serves as a paid consultant to or is an employee of Exactech, Inc. and has stock or stock options held in Exactech, Inc. Mr. Gargac or an immediate family member serves as a paid consultant to or is an employee of Wright Medical, Inc. Dr. Athwal or an immediate family member has received royalties from Wright Medical Technology, Inc., CONMED Linvatec, Exactech, Inc., Imascap, and Orthospace – Inspace; serves as a paid consultant to or is an employee of Wright Medical, DePuy, a Johnson & Johnson Company, and Stryker; has stock or stock options held in PrecisionOS and Wright Medical Technology, Inc.; has received research or institutional support from Smith & Nephew and Wright Medical Technology, Inc.; and serves as a board member, owner, officer, or committee member of the American Shoulder and Elbow Surgeons. Neither Dr. Aibinder nor any immediate family member has received anything of value from or has stock or stock options held in a commercial company or institution related directly or indirectly to the subject of this chapter.

Keywords: cuff tear arthropathy; deltoid; humeral lateralization; moment arms; reverse shoulder arthroplasty

Introduction

The use of reverse total shoulder arthroplasty has been increasing exponentially worldwide to treat various shoulder pathologies. Following the introduction of the Grammont reverse prothesis in 1987 which has been shown to effective restore forward elevation in the cuff deficient shoulder, various implant designs have evolved with the purpose of decreasing complications and improving clinical and functional outcome as it relates to shoulder rotation. A thorough understanding of the complex biomechanics about the shoulder related to various reverse shoulder prosthetic designs can improve further technological advancement while also allowing the surgeon to optimize patient outcomes. The purpose of this chapter is to describe the various in vitro biomechanical factors associated with different reverse shoulder designs as well as their theoretical and known in vivo clinical effects.

Glenohumeral Joint Anatomy

The glenohumeral joint is the most mobile joint in the human body, but its nonconforming articular curvature and lack of osseous constraint make it inherently unstable. The motion patterns of the glenohumeral joint have been described as spinning (rotation), sliding (translation), and rolling (rotation and translation).[1,2] The stability of the glenohumeral joint is assisted throughout its range of motion by the coordinated action of muscle contractions and is controlled by ligament and capsular tightening. The muscles of the shoulder are required for both mobility and stability.[3]

The deltoid is the largest muscle in the shoulder girdle. This primary mover in the shoulder generates forward elevation in the scapular plane. The three distinct heads of the deltoid are the anterior (the anterior acromion and the clavicle), the middle (the lateral margin of the acromion), and the posterior (scapular spine) deltoid. Together, the three deltoid heads account for approximately 20% of the

This chapter is adapted from Roche CP, Crosby L: Kinematics and biomechanics of reverse shoulder arthroplasty, in Nicholson GP, ed: *Orthopaedic Knowledge Update: Shoulder and Elbow*, ed 4. Rosemont, IL, American Academy of Orthopaedic Surgeons, 2013, pp 45-54.

mass of the shoulder muscles.[4] At low levels of abduction, the wrapping of the middle deltoid around the greater tuberosity of the humeral head generates a stabilizing compressive force; however, this compressive force is small relative to the humeral head compression generated by the rotator cuff.[5,6]

The rotator cuff muscles generate the torque necessary for rotation of the humerus about the glenoid fossa, while they compress the humeral head into the glenoid concavity.[7] The rotator cuff muscles are aligned around the proximal humerus for effective joint compression at all glenohumeral joint positions, allowing the rotator cuff to dynamically balance the joint, thereby compensating for the lack of osseous constraint in the glenohumeral joint.[8-10] Specifically, the anatomic arrangement of the anterior (subscapularis) and posterior (infraspinatus and teres minor) rotator cuff muscles creates a transverse force couple that in all joint positions approximately centers the humeral head on the glenoid fossa in the anterior and posterior directions.[11-13]

Rotator Cuff Tear Arthropathy

Disruption of rotator cuff integrity, most commonly by a tear in the rotator cuff muscle tendons, can have devastating consequences on glenohumeral joint stability. As the rotator cuff fails to compress the humeral head against the glenoid and balance the forces of the other muscles in the shoulder (primarily the deltoid), the humeral head tends to migrate superiorly and contact the undersurface of the acromion. This contact can lead to further tearing of the rotator cuff, which is associated with fatty infiltration of the cuff muscles and secondary arthritic degradation. Continued tearing propagates further compression and results in superior glenoid, acromion, and coracoid erosion.[14,15] The term cuff tear arthropathy has been used to describe this arthritic and eroded or collapsed condition of the glenohumeral joint after prolonged, progressive subacromial compression resulting from massive full-thickness rotator cuff tearing.[14]

The Philosophy and Design History of Reverse Shoulder Arthroplasty

The reverse shoulder prosthesis was devised in the early 1970s for treating patients with cuff tear arthropathy. The use of this device was intended to relieve pain and prevent progressive acromial, coracoid, and glenoid erosion by resisting superior migration of the humeral head.[16] The reverse shoulder inverts the anatomic concavities to create a fixed fulcrum to prevent superior head migration, by which the glenoid articular component is made convex, and the humeral articular component is made concave. Because these articulations are conforming, the motion of a reverse shoulder implant is limited to spinning. Several reverse shoulder designs were developed, including the Fenlin, Reeves-Leeds, Kessel, and Neer-Averill prostheses.[17-22] Each of these prostheses had a constrained and conforming articulation whose center of rotation was lateral to the glenoid fossa. These design features generated excessive torque on the glenoid bone-implant interface that compromised fixation and caused loosening and mechanical failure. As a result, these early designs were removed from the US market.[16,22]

In 1987, the Grammont reverse shoulder design was introduced, consisting of a 42-mm convex glenoid component whose thickness formed approximately two-thirds of a sphere and a concave humeral component whose depth was approximately one-third of a sphere. This initial design was also associated with glenoid failure, and it was redesigned for noncemented fixation with a fixed central peg to include divergent locking and compression screws. In addition, the thickness of the convex glenoid was decreased to half the diameter of the sphere so that the joint center of rotation would be placed medially on the glenoid fossa.[16,23-25]

The Grammont reverse shoulder prosthesis medially shifts the joint center of rotation toward the glenoid to minimize the torque on the glenoid bone-implant interface and increase the moment arm lengths of the abductor muscles to improve deltoid efficiency. With these advancements, the Grammont reverse shoulder prosthesis can restore stability and also improve active abduction and forward flexion in the cuff-deficient shoulder. Such positive clinical experiences have led to a substantial expansion of utilization in reverse shoulder arthroplasty worldwide, including a proliferation of new reverse shoulder prosthesis designs. Although each of these new reverse shoulder designs uses its own unique design configurations, each design also leverages fundamental principles of the Grammont design.[25,26] Positioning the glenoid component along the inferior glenoid rim, with or without an inferior tilt, can minimize impingement between the humeral liner and scapular neck to avoid the complication of scapular notching and has the additional benefit of inferiorly shifting the joint center of rotation, further elongating the deltoid to improve its resting tone and tension.[27] The Grammont humeral prosthesis was inlayed in the proximal humerus and used a 155° neck-shaft inclination angle, which medialized the humerus and shortened the rotator cuff muscles.[28,29] This associated rotator cuff muscle shortening is believed to be why the Grammont prosthesis is less effective in restoring active internal and external rotation in patients with a deficient rotator cuff and a functioning deltoid.[30-32] In a 2009 study, lateralization of the center of rotation and lateralization of the humeral component were proposed to mitigate the risk of scapular notching while also improving rotator cuff muscle tensioning; such design modifications are demonstrating improvements in clinical outcomes without compromising implant survivability.[33]

The Biomechanics and Kinematics of Reverse Shoulder Arthroplasty

Relevant Muscle Physiology

Muscles generate straight-line forces that are converted to torque in proportion to the perpendicular distance between the joint center of rotation and the muscle's line of action.[3,34] This perpendicular distance is called the muscle moment arm; thus, a 50% larger moment arm implies that a 50% lower force is required by a muscle to induce a specific torque or motion. The location of the moment arm relative to the joint center of rotation determines the type of motion the muscle will create. In the shoulder, the motions are abduction-adduction (in the scapular, coronal, and/or transverse planes), internal-external rotation (of the long axis of the humerus), and flexion-extension (in the sagittal plane). Muscles can induce force only in tension, which can be generated either by contraction (muscle shortening) or by stretching beyond resting length (muscle lengthening). Motion thus can result from muscle shortening, muscle lengthening, or no change in muscle length. Motion with no change in muscle length occurs when the line of action coincides with the joint center of rotation.[34] In other words, contraction of a muscle can either cause or stabilize motion, depending on the muscle's line of action relative to the center of rotation. Some muscles can function as an agonist (causing motion), antagonist (stabilizing motion), or both (biphasic functioning as both agonist and antagonist, depending on the specific joint position during a range of motion).[3,34] The greater the muscle's moment arm, the greater the capacity of the muscle to generate the torque required for motion and support external loads. The trade-off for a larger moment arm is that the muscle requires a greater excursion (more muscle shortening is required to generate a given amount of motion). A muscle's moment arm is only one component of its ability to generate torque; the other components include the muscle's physiologic cross-sectional area, architecture, neural activity, and length-tension relationship.[3]

Kinetics and Biomechanics of the Grammont Design

Inverting the anatomic concavities and the resulting inferior and medial shift of the center of rotation with the Grammont reverse shoulder prosthesis dramatically alters the relationship of each shoulder muscle to its normal physiologic function. Inferomedially shifting the center of rotation both elongates the deltoid and increases the length of the abduction moment arms of the anterior, middle, and posterior heads of the deltoid, allowing them to contribute more toward abduction.[5,35-38] These larger abductor moment arms enhance the capacity of the deltoid to elevate the arm in the scapular and coronal planes, compensating for the impaired function of the supraspinatus and the superior portions of the subscapularis and infraspinatus rotator cuff muscles, which typically are involved in the pathology. Translating the humerus medially shortens the rotator cuff muscles and leads to impingement of the humerus when the scapular neck is at low elevation (scapular notching).[29,39,40]

Several studies have assessed the medial shift in the center of rotation relative to the normal shoulder, with variable results ranging between 17 and 31 mm of medialization[5,25,29,35,38,41,42] (**Table 1**). This apparent discrepancy primarily reflects differences in measurement techniques; studies that found smaller medial shifts in general measured joint center of rotation directly from preoperative and postoperative patient radiographs, and the studies that found larger differences used computer models and simulations. Although measurements acquired directly from patients take into account the natural anatomic variation of the proximal humerus (such as humeral head diameter, neck angle, offset, and thickness), the data may be confounded by the collapsed condition of the humeral head often associated with cuff tear arthropathy and by variations in methods of surgical preparation and implantation (such as differences in humeral neck cuts, stem positioning, and glenoid reaming).[40] Additionally, implant design and intraoperative positioning of the implant in the scapula and the humerus can affect how the joint center of rotation changes relative to the normal shoulder. Several studies reported that the Grammont device is associated with an 18-mm medial shift in the joint center of rotation, but other studies reported a 28-mm medial shift.[5,25,29,42]

Patient-specific morphology and deformities can also influence kinematics after reverse shoulder arthroplasty. Abnormal glenoid wear patterns can affect the joint center of rotation, muscle moment arms, muscle lengths, and muscle lines of action and also reduce range of motion. Placement of a prosthesis in a patient with a medially eroded glenoid results in a more medialized joint line, which has been demonstrated to reduce deltoid wrapping around the greater tuberosity and shorten the rotator cuff relative to its usage in a noneroded glenoid. With a sufficient amount of glenoid wear, the humerus can become so medialized that the deltoid generates a distraction force that can result in instability.[43] More recently, the use of glenoid bone graft and/or augmented glenoid baseplates has offered the potential to minimize scapular impingement and better restore the joint line to improve stability and muscle tension in reverse total shoulder arthroplasty patients with eroded glenoids.[44,45]

Section 1: Basic Science

Table 1

Studies on the Joint Center of Rotation in Shoulders With a Reverse Prosthesis

Study (Year)	Reverse Shoulder Prosthesis	Shift in Center of Rotation (Relative to Normal Shoulder) Medial (mm)	Inferior (mm)
Boileau et al[25] (2005)	36-mm Grammont (DePuy)	19.0 ± 9.9	Not reported
Henninger et al[41] (2012)	36-mm Grammont (Tornier)	17.3 ± 1.8	9.7 ± 3.5
Saltzman et al[42] (2010)	36-mm Grammont (DePuy)	28.3	11.1
	Reverse (DJO Medical)	17.2	15.3
Jobin et al[35] (2012)	Grammont (DePuy and Tornier) and Zimmer	18 ± 7	Not reported
Ackland et al[38] (2010)	Zimmer	20.9 ± 3.9	9.5 ± 4.1
Roche et al[29] (2013)	36-mm Grammont, 0° glenosphere tilt, 20° humeral retroversion	28.3	8.0
	36-mm Grammont, 15° tilt, 20° humeral retroversion	31.0	7.7
	36-mm Grammont, 0° tilt, 0° humeral retroversion	28.3	8.0
	36-mm Grammont, 0° tilt, 40° humeral retroversion	28.3	8.0
	36-mm Grammont, 0° tilt, 0° humeral retroversion, 10-mm glenoid bone graft	19.2	8.0
	36-mm Grammont, 0° tilt, 20° humeral retroversion, 10-mm glenoid bone graft	19.2	8.0
	36-mm Grammont, 0° tilt, 40° humeral retroversion, 10-mm glenoid bone graft	19.2	8.0
	36-mm Grammont, 15° tilt, 20° humeral retroversion, 10-mm glenoid bone graft	21.9	10.2
	32-mm DJO, 0° tilt, 20° humeral retroversion	20.0	6.9
	38-mm Equinoxe, 0° tilt, 20° humeral retroversion	27.1	4.5
De Wilde et al[5] (2004)	Grammont (DePuy)	28.6	Not reported
	Reverse (DJO Medical)	16.5	Not reported

Effect of Humeral Lengthening

Inferiorly shifting the humerus when positioning it under the glenosphere with reverse shoulder arthroplasty elongates the deltoid in comparison with a normal shoulder. Elongating the deltoid 10% to 20% improves its resting tone and tension and may increase its strength and improve the overall stability of the joint. With the arm at 0° of abduction, different reverse shoulder implant designs were found to elongate the deltoid between 13% and 17% (compared with the normal shoulder).[5,35] Optimal tension was found to be based on humeral lengthening; arm lengthening of more than 2.5 cm was recommended as the surgical objective because it was associated with greater active elevation.[28,46] In contrast, shortening of the humerus was associated with increased risk of dislocation.

However, humeral lengthening carries potential deleterious effects. Increased deltoid elongation modifies the normal deltoid contour, which decreases its wrapping angle around the greater tuberosity and thus reduces stability. In addition, deltoid elongation creates cosmetic concerns.[5,6,39] Increased humeral lengthening may lead to an acromial stress fracture and brachial plexopathy.[41,47] Restoring the lateral position of the humeral tuberosities is important for tensioning the remaining rotator cuff muscles in a relatively natural physiologic manner to restore rotational strength.[29,39,40] The anterior and posterior rotator cuff muscles can be shortened by up to 45% with implantation of a Grammont design.[29] Although overtensioning these muscles can improve resting tone and tension, it may increase the difficulty of repair after subscapularis tenotomy. Inferiorly shifting the humerus also alters the point at which

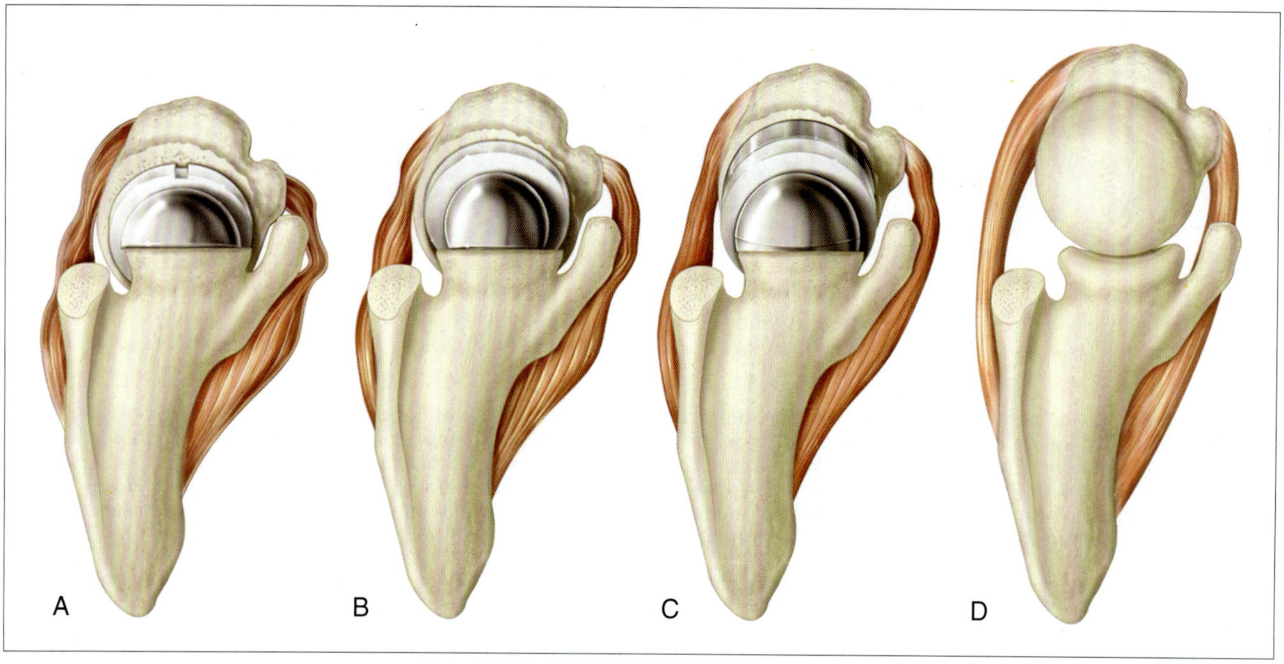

FIGURE 1 Drawings comparing the tension of the subscapularis and infraspinatus tendons and the relative humeral positioning in three different reverse shoulder prostheses (**A** through **C**) and also the normal native shoulder for relative comparison (**D**). **A**, The 36-mm Grammont (DePuy; medialized center of rotation and medialized humeral component). **B**, The 32-mm Reverse (DJO Medical; lateralized center of rotation and medialized humeral component). **C**, The 38-mm Equinoxe (Exactech; medialized center of rotation and lateralized humeral component). **D**, Normal native shoulder.

the native subscapularis and the infraspinatus muscles convert from adductors at low elevation to abductors at high elevation. In the normal shoulder, the subscapularis and infraspinatus tendons span the center of rotation. As the humerus is distalized with reverse shoulder arthroplasty, the subscapularis tendon and infraspinatus tendon become positioned below the joint center of rotation; as a result, the muscles act largely as adductors throughout arm elevation (**Figure 1**). In some patients, these muscles may altogether lose their biphasic function, with important implications for both mobility and stability.[36,39,48]

Lateralization of Center of Rotation

The center of rotation with reverse shoulder arthroplasty is determined by the difference between the glenosphere thickness and the glenosphere articular radius. The Grammont reverse shoulder prosthesis used a glenosphere geometry that had an equivalent radius and thickness; this resulted in a center of rotation of 0 mm. Lateralizing the joint center of rotation relative to the Grammont design has been proposed as a method for improving active internal and external rotation, strength in rotation, and stability.[39] By lateralizing the joint center of rotation, typically by increasing the thickness of the glenosphere relative to a fixed articular radius, the humerus is lateralized by the added thickness of the glenosphere, the remaining rotator cuff muscles are better tensioned, and impingement of the humeral component along the inferior scapular neck is minimized. An alternative method to achieve lateralization through the glenoid is placement of bone graft behind the baseplate; after incorporation of the bone graft, the aforementioned biomechanical effect is equivalent to that of a thicker glenosphere. The authors of a 2013 three-dimensional modeling study demonstrated that lateralizing the glenosphere 8 mm maintained the length and moment arms of the subscapularis and teres minor muscles.[49] Lateralizing the joint center of rotation also increases the torque on the glenoid bone-implant interface and decreases the lengths of the deltoid abductor moment arms.[5,41,50] Specifically, the joint contact forces are increased in compression and shear with progressive lateralization, with an increased bending moment arm at the implant interface.[49] Altering glenosphere diameter and thickness has also been evaluated.[51] The authors of a 2015 study analyzed a prosthesis with a 155° humeral neck-shaft angle while comparing a 38-mm glenosphere and a 42-mm glenosphere at neutral position and 10 mm of lateralization.[51] They reported an increased joint load with glenosphere lateralization, as well as an increased deltoid force required to generate abduction. The clinical significance of the modest increase in joint load, which was between 5% and 10%, is uncertain. Because the deltoid abductor moment arms are decreased as the center of rotation is lateralized, the deltoid becomes less effective as an abductor, and a greater force

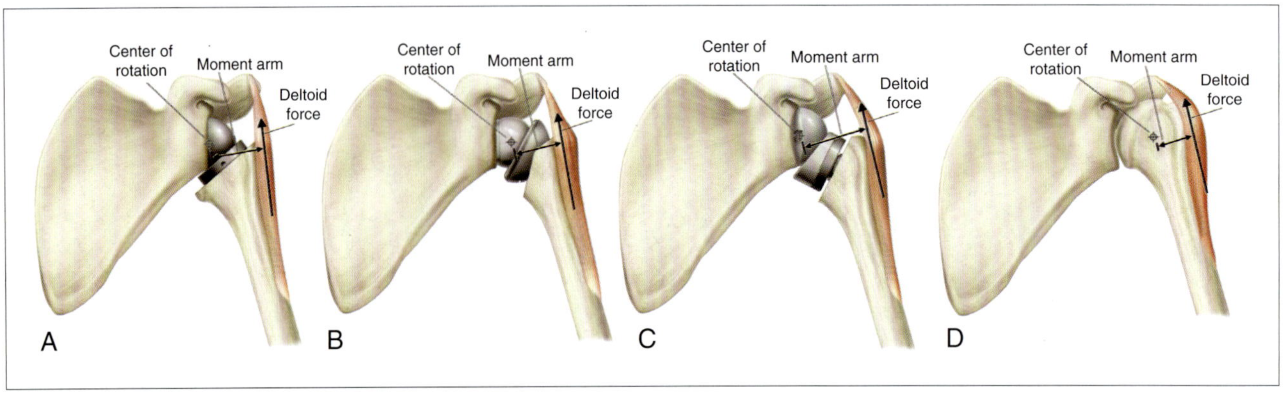

FIGURE 2 Drawings comparing the center of rotation, deltoid moment arm, amount of deltoid wrapping around the greater tuberosity, and humeral position in three reverse shoulder prostheses (**A** through **C**) positioned along the inferior glenoid rim at 0° tilt and also in a normal native shoulder (**D**) for relative comparison. All drawings show abduction to 15° in the scapular plane. **A**, The 36-mm Grammont (DePuy; medialized center of rotation and medialized humeral component). **B**, The 32-mm Reverse (DJO Medical; lateralized center of rotation and medialized humeral component). **C**, The 38-mm Equinoxe (Exactech; medialized center of rotation and lateralized humeral component). **D**, Normal native shoulder.

is required to elevate the arm in the scapular or coronal planes.[41,50] These elevated loads, torques, and forces can have negative implications for prosthesis fixation, patient rehabilitation, muscle fatigue, and stress fracture. Conversely, the increased compressive forces also lead to improved stability of reverse shoulder arthroplasty with higher dislocation forces with increased glenosphere lateralization.[52]

Humeral Lateralization

Lateralizing the humerus relative to the Grammont design has also been proposed as a method for improving active internal and external rotation, strength in rotation, and stability. **Figure 2** illustrates the effect of reverse shoulder arthroplasty design on humeral positioning by depicting a normal shoulder relative to three commercially available prostheses. The humerus can be lateralized without lateralizing the joint center of rotation through the use of an onlay humeral component. Lateralization through the humerus can be accomplished by decreasing the humeral neck angle from the Grammont design humeral neck angle of 155°, decreasing the humeral liner constraint, and/or increasing the medial offset of the humeral liner-humeral stem.[33] Humeral lateralization places the tuberosities in a more anatomic position while minimizing humeral polyimpingement along the inferior scapular neck.[29,33] Doing so has the advantage of restoring the anatomic rotator cuff muscle length and tension while maintaining the Grammont design abductor moment arm lengths and minimizing the torque on the glenoid-bone interface.[53,54] By restoring the rotator cuff length-tension relationship and moment arms of the anterior and posterior rotator cuff, the torque generated by the rotators in various positions of abduction is improved with humeral lateralization.[54] The authors of a 2015 study demonstrated that a lateralized humeral design not only leads to an increased deltoid moment arm to generate abduction but also optimizes the rotational moment arms of the subscapularis and infraspinatus, as well as the external rotation moment arm of the posterior deltoid.[53] Furthermore, the authors of another 2015 study used a biomechanical model to analyze the effect of glenosphere lateralization, polyethylene thickness, and humeral lateralization in 27 various configurations.[55] Lateralization of the humerus was independently evaluated by changing humeral component offset and was associated with a decreased deltoid force required for abduction in this particular simulated design, whereas the other factors increased this force and the joint loads. The larger deltoid moment arms and decreased deltoid forces associated with reverse shoulder prostheses having a medialized glenoid and a lateralized humerus and the shorter deltoid moment arms and increased deltoid forces associated with prostheses having a lateralized glenoid are the most likely explanations for the findings of a recent meta-analysis, which quantified the acromial and scapular spine fracture rates by prosthesis design style.[56] Specifically, it was found that the medial glenoid/lateral humerus reverse shoulder prostheses were associated with the lowest acromial and scapular spine fracture rate and the lateral glenoid reverse shoulder prostheses were associated with the highest fracture rate in the literature.[56]

Subscapularis Integrity and Significance With Reverse Shoulder Arthroplasty

Although increased stability can be achieved by the compensatory action of muscles with smaller moment arms or by the combined force generated by two opposing muscle lines of action positioned about a joint, each of these methods increases the overall joint reaction force.[57] For these reasons, the repair of the subscapularis-lesser tuberosity in reverse shoulder arthroplasty is controversial. When the subscapularis functions as an adductor, its line of action opposes the deltoid at low humeral and midhumeral elevation in the scapular and coronal planes, and this opposing force requires the deltoid to generate a larger force to achieve a given motion.[36,38,58] These opposing forces increase joint stability and perhaps counteract the deltoid's induced torque on the glenoid bone-implant interface. The question of subscapularis-lesser tuberosity repair is even more relevant if the patient has weak external rotators. A 2015 study using a shoulder controller found a subscapularis release required less force to be generated by the deltoid and the posterior rotator cuff in abduction.[58] With repair of the subscapularis-lesser tuberosity, the joint reaction force increased by 28%, the required deltoid force increased by 14% with the largest effect in the posterior deltoid requiring an increase of 32%, and the required posterior rotator cuff force increased by 34%. These increased forces are problematic because in many patients, the posterior rotator cuff is compromised by tearing or fatty infiltration and it may not be able to support elevated loads. Some recommend repairing the subscapularis-lesser tuberosity if possible because the repair was associated with a lower dislocation rate when the Grammont prosthesis was used.[59] A 2019 meta-analysis demonstrated that a subscapularis repair decreased the risk of prosthetic dislocation in both medialized and lateralized designs.[60] However, when the subscapularis was not repaired, a lateralized center of rotation design resulted in a lower dislocation rate regardless of the humeral design used. Based on these data, the subscapularis-lesser tuberosity repair should be performed if feasible, but in instances where it is not, prosthetic considerations should be optimized to enhance the stability of the construct.

Biomechanical Considerations for the External Rotation–Deficient Shoulder

A loss of external rotation and excessive internal rotation impair the patient's ability to maintain the arm in neutral rotation when the arm is elevated (a positive hornblower's sign). The patient is unable to perform numerous activities of daily living, such as drinking, eating, hair washing, and hand shaking.[30-32] The internal rotator muscles predominate in a normally functioning shoulder. There are four internal rotators (subscapularis, teres major, pectoralis major, and latissimus dorsi) and only two external rotators (infraspinatus and teres minor). External rotation deficiency therefore is more debilitating to a patient's activities of daily living than internal rotation deficiency, particularly when the arm is elevated.[30,31] The posterior deltoid alone is insufficient to restore active external rotation, even with a lateralized reverse shoulder design. Therefore, muscle transfers often are recommended in reverse shoulder arthroplasty if the patient has an external rotation deficiency.

In general, one or more of the internal rotation muscles, which attach to the anterior side of the humerus, are transferred across the joint center of rotation to the posterior side of the humerus, where their contraction will now cause external rotation. The latissimus dorsi is the muscle most commonly transferred in reverse shoulder arthroplasty. It is detached from the anterior shaft of the humerus and reattached to the greater tuberosity.[61] Another common muscle transfer method is a modification of the L'Episcopo method, in which both the latissimus dorsi and the teres major are transferred to the greater tuberosity. Although muscle transfers have been shown to restore active external rotation, they should not be performed if the teres minor is functional.[30,31] In addition, it should be recognized that such procedures limit active internal rotation and further alter the relationship of each shoulder muscle relative to its normal physiologic function.

Biomechanical Considerations for the Internal Rotation–Deficient Shoulder

A loss of internal rotation and excessive external rotation can impair a patient's ability to perform several tasks, including self-hygiene. There is a paucity of biomechanical and clinical data to guide surgeons in addressing this deficiency in the setting of a reverse shoulder arthroplasty. Several surgical techniques and concepts should be considered, however.

First, repair of the subscapularis tendon may serve two functions. It may counteract the intact external rotators to provide a more balanced shoulder. Additionally, even in the setting of subscapularis fatty infiltration, tendon repair may serve as an anterior checkrein and decrease the potential for periprosthetic instability and dislocation. Second, to avoid exacerbating the imbalance between the internal and external rotators, care should be taken during exposure to avoid release of the latissimus dorsi tendon. If there remains an excessive imbalance or concern for anterior instability, a pectoralis major tendon transfer for glenohumeral internal rotation may be considered. There is a lack of data regarding this procedure in the setting of a reverse shoulder arthroplasty.

Implant position may also help optimize function in the internal rotation–deficient shoulder. Relative humeral anteversion can tension the remaining internal rotators while relaxing the more prominent external rotators.[29] Additionally, this can permit a greater range of impingement-free internal rotation.

Kinematic Function After Reverse Shoulder Arthroplasty

Reverse shoulder arthroplasty is often performed in the setting of a dysfunctional or absent rotator cuff. Although the deltoid muscle is the primary generator of abduction and motion of the arm following this procedure, the relative contribution of the scapulothoracic articulation to overall motion is increased.[62] In the normal shoulder, the approximate scapulohumeral rhythm is 3:1 with the glenohumeral joint being the primary motion center. Using software to three-dimensionally analyze live fluoroscopic imaging of 28 patients performing abduction following implantation of three different reverse prosthesis designs, one study demonstrated that the scapulothoracic articulation becomes a more predominant contributor to motion with a scapulohumeral rhythm of 1.3:1.[62] This kinematic finding could have significant clinical implications in regard to postoperative rehabilitation following reverse shoulder arthroplasty.

SUMMARY

Reverse shoulder arthroplasty is effective for relieving pain and restoring active abduction and forward flexion in patients with a deficient rotator cuff and a functioning deltoid. The inversion of the anatomic concavities restores stability to the unstable shoulder, and the inferior and medial shift in the joint center of rotation (compared with a normal shoulder) lengthens the abductor moment arms and elongates the deltoid to facilitate improvements in function and mobility. Shoulder rotation can be improved by better tensioning the remaining rotator cuff through lateralization, which can be accomplished by use of thicker glenospheres that position the center of rotation lateral to the glenoid fossa or by use of lateralized humeral components. When achieving lateralization through the glenosphere, consideration should be given to the increased joint forces resulting from the shortened deltoid abductor moment arms. Reverse shoulder kinematics can be affected by prosthesis design parameters, prosthesis positioning on the scapula, and abnormal scapular morphology–glenoid wear patterns. Future work should continue to focus on methods that optimize these kinematic parameters, thereby increasing the overall function of the shoulder and facilitating the patient's ability to conduct activities of daily living.

KEY STUDY POINTS

- Reverse shoulder arthroplasty provides a fixed fulcrum around which the humerus can rotate given an appropriate length-tension relationship of the deltoid muscle as a force generator.
- The Grammont design relies on a medialized center of rotation and humeral lengthening to tension the deltoid muscle to generate abduction but provides limits in internal and external rotation.
- Glenosphere lateralization results in increased joint compressive and shear forces and increased deltoid force necessary to generate abduction, but increased glenohumeral implant stability and reduced scapular notching.
- Humeral lateralization can tension the anterior and posterior rotator cuff muscles to facilitate internal and external rotation with improved torque, while decreasing the deltoid forces due to the larger abductor moment arms.
- Subscapularis repair may increase the joint contact loads and decrease the mechanical advantage of the deltoid, but does provide improved stability.

Annotated References

1. Morrey BF: *The Shoulder*, ed 2. Philadelphia, PA, W.B. Saunders, 1998, pp 233-276.

2. Yu J, McGarry MH, Lee YS, Duong LV, Lee TQ: Biomechanical effects of supraspinatus repair on the glenohumeral joint. *J Shoulder Elbow Surg* 2005;14(1 suppl S):S65-S71.

3. Kuechle DK, Newman SR, Itoi E, Morrey BF, An KN: Shoulder muscle moment arms during horizontal flexion and elevation. *J Shoulder Elbow Surg* 1997;6(5):429-439.

4. Lee SB, An KN: Dynamic glenohumeral stability provided by three heads of the deltoid muscle. *Clin Orthop Relat Res* 2002;400:40-47.

5. De Wilde LF, Audenaert EA, Berghs BM: Shoulder prostheses treating cuff tear arthropathy: A comparative biomechanical study. *J Orthop Res* 2004;22(6):1222-1230.

6. Lemieux PO, Hagemeister N, Tetreault P, Nuno N: Influence of the medial offset of the proximal humerus on the glenohumeral destabilising forces during arm elevation: A numerical sensitivity study. *Comput Methods Biomech Biomed Engin* 2013;16(1):103-111.

A computer model study assessed the influence of humeral head medial offset on joint stability. Varying the medial offset influenced the destabilizing action of the middle deltoid, where a larger medial offset increased the middle deltoid wrapping around the tuberosity.

7. Lippitt SB, Vanderhooft JE, Harris SL, Sidles JA, Harryman DT II, Matsen FA III: Glenohumeral stability from concavity-compression: A quantitative analysis. *J Shoulder Elbow Surg* 1993;2(1):27-35.

8. Sharkey NA, Marder RA: The rotator cuff opposes superior translation of the humeral head. *Am J Sports Med* 1995;23(3):270-275.

9. Parsons IM, Apreleva M, Fu FH, Woo SL: The effect of rotator cuff tears on reaction forces at the glenohumeral joint. *J Orthop Res* 2002;20(3):439-446.

10. Mura N, O'Driscoll SW, Zobitz ME, et al: The effect of infraspinatus disruption on glenohumeral torque and superior migration of the humeral head: A biomechanical study. *J Shoulder Elbow Surg* 2003;12(2):179-184.

11. Burkhart SS, Nottage WM, Ogilvie-Harris DJ, Kohn HS, Pachelli A: Partial repair of irreparable rotator cuff tears. *Arthroscopy* 1994;10(4):363-370.

12. Halder AM, Zhao KD, Odriscoll SW, Morrey BF, An KN: Dynamic contributions to superior shoulder stability. *J Orthop Res* 2001;19(2):206-212.

13. Labriola JE, Lee TQ, Debski RE, McMahon PJ: Stability and instability of the glenohumeral joint: The role of shoulder muscles. *J Shoulder Elbow Surg* 2005;14(1 suppl S):S32-S38.

14. Neer CS II, Craig EV, Fukuda H: Cuff-tear arthropathy. *J Bone Joint Surg Am* 1983;65(9):1232-1244.

15. Visotsky JL, Basamania C, Seebauer L, Rockwood CA, Jensen KL: Cuff tear arthropathy: Pathogenesis, classification, and algorithm for treatment. *J Bone Joint Surg Am* 2004;86-A(suppl 2):35-40.

16. Flatow EL, Harrison AK: A history of reverse total shoulder arthroplasty. *Clin Orthop Relat Res* 2011;469(9):2432-2439.

17. Fenlin JM Jr: Semi-constrained prosthesis for the rotator cuff deficient patient. *Orthop Trans* 1985;9:55.

18. Redfern TR, Wallace WA: *Joint Replacement in the Shoulder and Elbow.* Oxford, United Kingdom, Butterworth and Heinemann, 1998, pp 6-16.

19. Reeves B, Jobbins B, Dowson D, Wright V: A total shoulder endoprosthesis. *Eng Med* 1974;1:64-67.

20. Brostrom LA, Wallensten R, Olsson E, Anderson D: The Kessel prosthesis in total shoulder arthroplasty. A five-year experience. *Clin Orthop Relat Res* 1992;277: 155-160.

21. Wretenberg PF, Wallensten R: The Kessel total shoulder arthroplasty. A 13- to 16-year retrospective followup. *Clin Orthop Relat Res* 1999;365:100-103.

22. Neer CS II: *Shoulder Reconstruction.* Philadelphia, PA, W.B. Saunders, 1990.

23. Grammont P, Trouillod P, Laffay JP, Deries X: Etude et Realisation D'une Novelle Prosthese D'Paule. *Rhumatologie* 1987;39:17-22.

24. Grammont PM, Baulot E: Delta shoulder prosthesis for rotator cuff rupture. *Orthopedics* 1993;16(1):65-68.

25. Boileau P, Watkinson DJ, Hatzidakis AM, Balg F: Grammont reverse prosthesis: Design, rationale, and biomechanics. *J Shoulder Elbow Surg* 2005;14(1 suppl S):S147-S161.

26. Werthel JD, Walch G, Vegehan E, Deransart P, Sanchez-Sotelo J, Valenti P: Lateralization in reverse shoulder arthroplasty: A descriptive analysis of different implants in current practice. *Int Orthop* 2019;43(10):2349-2360.

This article presents a descriptive analysis of 22 different implants with 28 different configurations demonstrating that the lateralization offered by different designs is varied, and thus surgeons should adapt to their surgical technique based on the implant used and the amount of offset offered on the glenoid and/or humeral sides. Level of evidence: IV.

27. Nyffeler RW, Werner CM, Gerber C: Biomechanical relevance of glenoid component positioning in the reverse Delta III total shoulder prosthesis. *J Shoulder Elbow Surg* 2005;14(5):524-528.

28. Ladermann A, Williams MD, Melis B, Hoffmeyer P, Walch G: Objective evaluation of lengthening in reverse shoulder arthroplasty. *J Shoulder Elbow Surg* 2009;18(4):588-595.

29. Roche CP, Diep P, Hamilton M, et al: Impact of inferior glenoid tilt, humeral retroversion, bone grafting, and design parameters on muscle length and deltoid wrapping in reverse shoulder arthroplasty. *Bull Hosp Jt Dis (2013)* 2013;71(4):284-293.

A computer modeling simulation study compared the native shoulder and three various implant designs of reverse total shoulder arthroplasties. Although all implants resulted in a medially and inferiorly shifted center of rotation compared with the native shoulder and lengthened the deltoid while shortening the internal and external rotators, implants that lateralized the humerus resulted in better deltoid wrapping and more native tensioning of the anterior and posterior rotator cuff musculature.

30. Boileau P, Chuinard C, Roussanne Y, Bicknell RT, Rochet N, Trojani C: Reverse shoulder arthroplasty combined with a modified latissimus dorsi and teres major tendon transfer for shoulder pseudoparalysis associated with dropping arm. *Clin Orthop Relat Res* 2008;466(3): 584-593.

Section 1: Basic Science

31. Boileau P, Rumian AP, Zumstein MA: Reversed shoulder arthroplasty with modified L'Episcopo for combined loss of active elevation and external rotation. *J Shoulder Elbow Surg* 2010;19(2 suppl):20-30.

32. Favre P, Loeb MD, Helmy N, Gerber C: Latissimus dorsi transfer to restore external rotation with reverse shoulder arthroplasty: A biomechanical study. *J Shoulder Elbow Surg* 2008;17(4):650-658.

33. Roche C, Flurin PH, Wright T, Crosby LA, Mauldin M, Zuckerman JD: An evaluation of the relationships between reverse shoulder design parameters and range of motion, impingement, and stability. *J Shoulder Elbow Surg* 2009;18(5):734-741.

34. Otis JC, Jiang CC, Wickiewicz TL, Peterson MG, Warren RF, Santner TJ: Changes in the moment arms of the rotator cuff and deltoid muscles with abduction and rotation. *J Bone Joint Surg Am* 1994;76(5):667-676.

35. Jobin CM, Brown GD, Bahu MJ, et al: Reverse total shoulder arthroplasty for cuff tear arthropathy: The clinical effect of deltoid lengthening and center of rotation medialization. *J Shoulder Elbow Surg* 2012;21(10):1269-1277.

36. Kontaxis A, Johnson GR: The biomechanics of reverse anatomy shoulder replacement – A modelling study. *Clin Biomech (Bristol, Avon)* 2009;24(3):254-260.

37. Terrier A, Reist A, Merlini F, Farron A: Simulated joint and muscle forces in reversed and anatomic shoulder prostheses. *J Bone Joint Surg Br* 2008;90(6):751-756.

38. Ackland DC, Roshan-Zamir S, Richardson M, Pandy MG: Moment arms of the shoulder musculature after reverse total shoulder arthroplasty. *J Bone Joint Surg Am* 2010;92(5):1221-1230.

39. Frankle M, Siegal S, Pupello D, Saleem A, Mighell M, Vasey M: The reverse shoulder prosthesis for glenohumeral arthritis associated with severe rotator cuff deficiency. A minimum two-year follow-up study of sixty patients. *J Bone Joint Surg Am* 2005;87(8):1697-1705.

40. Herrmann S, Konig C, Heller M, Perka C, Greiner S: Reverse shoulder arthroplasty leads to significant biomechanical changes in the remaining rotator cuff. *J Orthop Surg Res* 2011;6:42.

41. Henninger HB, Barg A, Anderson AE, Bachus KN, Burks RT, Tashjian RZ: Effect of lateral offset center of rotation in reverse total shoulder arthroplasty: A biomechanical study. *J Shoulder Elbow Surg* 2012;21(9):1128-1135.

42. Saltzman MD, Mercer DM, Warme WJ, Bertelsen AL, Matsen FA III: A method for documenting the change in center of rotation with reverse total shoulder arthroplasty and its application to a consecutive series of 68 shoulders having reconstruction with one of two different reverse prostheses. *J Shoulder Elbow Surg* 2010;19(7):1028-1033.

43. Norris TR, Kelly JD: Management of glenoid bone defects in revision shoulder arthroplasty: A new application of the reverse total shoulder prosthesis. *Tech Shoulder Elbow Surg* 2007;8(1):37-46.

44. Boileau P, Morin-Salvo N, Gauci MO, et al: Angled BIO-RSA (bony-increased offset-reverse shoulder arthroplasty): a solution for the management of glenoid bone loss and erosion. J Shoulder Elbow Surg 2017;26(12):2133-2142.

    A case series of 54 patients at a mean follow-up 36 months who underwent reverse shoulder arthroplasty with the use of a trapezoidal autograft from the humeral head to compensate for residual glenoid bone loss/erosion which demonstrated 94% graft incorporation with the ability to correct glenoid deformity while providing lateralization of the glenosphere. Level of evidence: IV.

45. Virk M, Yip M, Liuzza L, et al: Clinical and radiographic outcomes with a posteriorly augmented glenoid for Walch B2, B3, and C glenoids in reverse total shoulder arthroplasty. J Shoulder Elbow Surg 2019;29(5):e19 6-e204.

    A case series of 67 primary reverse shoulder arthroplasties at a mean follow-up of 40 months treated with an augmented glenoid baseplate to treat posterior glenoid wear demonstrating a 4.5% complication rate, no aseptic glenoid loosening, and a total of 90% of patients exceeding the minimally clinically important difference for various clinical outcome metrics and range of motion. Level of evidence: IV.

46. Ladermann A, Walch G, Lubbeke A, et al: Influence of arm lengthening in reverse shoulder arthroplasty. *J Shoulder Elbow Surg* 2012;21(3):336-341.

47. Gallo RA, Gamradt SC, Mattern CJ, et al: Instability after reverse total shoulder replacement. *J Shoulder Elbow Surg* 2011;20(4):584-590.

48. Werner BS, Ascione F, Bugelli G, Walch G: Does arm lengthening affect the functional outcome in onlay reverse shoulder arthroplasty? *J Shoulder Elbow Surg* 2017;26(12):2152-2157.

    In this retrospective study, 56 patients were reviewed after an onlay reverse shoulder arthroplasty demonstrating that arm lengthening of 1 to 2.5 cm is the best compromise for function with shoulder range of motion. Beyond 2.5 cm of arm lengthening, there was a decrease in forward elevation. Level of evidence: IV.

49. Greiner S, Schmidt C, Konig C, Perka C, Herrmann S: Lateralized reverse shoulder arthroplasty maintains rotational function of the remaining rotator cuff. *Clin Orthop Relat Res* 2013;471(3):940-946.

    A cadaver biomechanical study assessed a lateralized reverse shoulder arthroplasty design using an 8-mm resin block and determined that lateralization maintained the muscle length and rotation moment arms of the subscapularis and teres minor while also increasing the flexion forces required, thereby decreasing the abduction capacity.

50. Costantini O, Choi DS, Kontaxis A, Gulotta LV: The effects of progressive lateralization of the joint center of rotation of reverse total shoulder implants. *J Shoulder Elbow Surg* 2015;24(7):1120-1128.

    A three-dimensional virtual modeling study demonstrated that lateralization results in increased joint contact forces, particularly in compression but also in shear and bending moments. The deltoid moment arm decreases with progressive lateralization. This study may have implications on implant survivability.

51. Langohr GD, Giles JW, Athwal GS, Johnson JA: The effect of glenosphere diameter in reverse shoulder arthroplasty on muscle force, joint load, and range of motion. *J Shoulder Elbow Surg* 2015;24(6):972-979.

    A shoulder motion simulator model with a custom reverse shoulder arthroplasty implant was used to assess the effect of glenosphere diameter and lateralization on muscle force, joint load, and range of motion. This study demonstrated that increasing glenosphere diameter led to increased joint load and deltoid force, and a decrease in internal rotation.

52. Ferle M, Pastor MF, Hagenah J, Hurschler C, Smith T: Effect of the humeral neck-shaft angle and glenosphere lateralization on stability of reverse shoulder arthroplasty: A cadaveric study. *J Shoulder Elbow Surg* 2019;28(5):966-973.

    A cadaver biomechanical study of 19 specimens demonstrated that glenosphere lateralization leads to increased stability in the setting of reverse total shoulder arthroplasty. A lower neck-shaft angle (135°) demonstrated the need for a higher dislocation force when compared with a 145° and 155° humeral component. However, the effect of the neck-shaft angle was less profound than glenosphere lateralization. Neither parameter influences passive external rotation range of motion.

53. Hamilton MA, Diep P, Roche C, et al: Effect of reverse shoulder design philosophy on muscle moment arms. *J Orthop Res* 2015;33(4):605-613.

    A computer digital three-dimensional modeling study demonstrated that a lateralized humeral design increased the external rotation moment arm of the posterior deltoid, suggesting that humeral offset may impact external rotation and implant stability.

54. Chan K, Langohr GDG, Mahaffy M, Johnson JA, Athwal GS: Does humeral component lateralization in reverse shoulder arthroplasty affect rotator cuff torque? Evaluation in a cadaver model. *Clin Orthop Relat Res* 2017;475(10):2564-2571.

    A cadaver study demonstrated that humeral component lateralization improves anterior and posterior rotator cuff torque in multiple positions of glenohumeral abduction.

55. Giles JW, Langohr GD, Johnson JA, Athwal GS: Implant design variations in reverse total shoulder arthroplasty influence the required deltoid force and resultant joint load. *Clin Orthop Relat Res* 2015;473(11):3615-3626.

    A cadaver study using a custom reverse shoulder arthroplasty implant that could vary humeral lateralization, polyethylene thickness, and glenosphere lateralization demonstrated that humeral lateralization improved joint and muscle loading, whereas glenosphere lateralization increased these loads.

56. King JJ, Dalton SS, Gulotta LV, Wright TW, Schoch BS: How common are acromial and scapular spine fractures after reverse shoulder arthroplasty?: A systematic review. *Bone Joint J* 2019;101-B(6):627-634.

    In this systematic review, the authors demonstrated a 2.8% acromial and scapular spine fracture rate following reverse shoulder arthroplasty with a higher rate of fracture associated with a lateralized glenoid design. Level of evidence: IV.

57. Bergmann G, Graichen F, Bender A, Kaab M, Rohlmann A, Westerhoff P: In vivo glenohumeral contact forces – Measurements in the first patient 7 months postoperatively. *J Biomech* 2007;40(10):2139-2149.

58. Hansen ML, Nayak A, Narayanan MS, et al: Role of subscapularis repair on muscle force requirements with reverse shoulder arthroplasty. *Bull Hosp Jt Dis (2013)* 2015;73(suppl 1):S21-S27.

    In this cadaver biomechanical study the authors demonstrated that repair of the subscapularis tendon increases the force required by the deltoid and posterior rotator cuff to generate shoulder motion. Additionally, the joint reaction force was significantly increased compared with when the subscapularis tendon was not repaired.

59. Edwards TB, Williams MD, Labriola JE, Elkousy HA, Gartsman GM, O'Connor DP: Subscapularis insufficiency and the risk of shoulder dislocation after reverse shoulder arthroplasty. *J Shoulder Elbow Surg* 2009;18(6):892-896.

60. Matthewson G, Kooner S, Kwapisz A, Leiter J, Old J, MacDonald P: The effect of subscapularis repair on dislocation rates in reverse shoulder arthroplasty: A meta-analysis and systematic review. *J Shoulder Elbow Surg* 2019;28(5):989-997.

    A systematic review and meta-analysis of seven studies assessed the effect of a subscapularis repair on dislocation rates after reverse total shoulder arthroplasty and demonstrated that repair of the subscapularis tendon in medialized and lateralized prosthetic designs led to a decrease in dislocation risk. This study also demonstrated that a lateralized center of rotation design can decrease the risk of dislocation when a subscapularis tendon is not performed. Level of evidence: III.

61. Gerber C, Maquieira G, Espinosa N: Latissimus dorsi transfer for the treatment of irreparable rotator cuff tears. *J Bone Joint Surg Am* 2006;88(1):113-120.

62. Walker D, Matsuki K, Struk AM, Wright TW, Banks SA: Scapulohumeral rhythm in shoulders with reverse shoulder arthroplasty. *J Shoulder Elbow Surg* 2015;24(7):1129-1134.

Scapulohumeral rhythm is lower in shoulders that have undergone reverse total shoulder arthroplasty compared with normal shoulders. This means that after arthroplasty, patients use more scapulothoracic motion and less glenohumeral motion to elevate the arm, which could have implications on rehabilitation protocols.

Chapter 4

Biomechanics of Elbow Arthroplasty

James A. Johnson, PhD, PEng • Graham J.W. King, MD, MSc, FRCSC, FAAOS

ABSTRACT

Over the past decade, several significant advances have been made in the study of radial head implant design and sizing. In particular, important new knowledge has emerged on the anatomic characteristics of radial head arthroplasty, with a focus on articular contact and kinematics at the radiocapitellar joint. Numerous studies on axisymmetric (ie, circular), bipolar, and anatomic designs have demonstrated marked differences in the stability and capitellar articular tracking. Also, attention has been directed toward the importance of the shape of the radial head around the periphery with a focus on the articulation with the ulna at the proximal radioulnar joint. Studies of total elbow arthroplasty implant fixation have emphasized the influence of stem surface conditions, and also the effect of soft-tissue constraint and ulnohumeral hinge linkage status on load transfer. Investigations on distal humeral hemiarthroplasties have indicated the importance of implant shape on the stresses bourne by cartilage.

Keywords: biomechanics; fixation; implant design; joint stability/kinematics; wear

Introduction

It is well established that the elbow may be subjected to forces that exceed body weight and has highly complex kinematics of the various articulations. Hence, research on the biomechanics of elbow arthroplasty has focused on joint motion and stability, and load transfer. These have led to an improved understanding of the biomechanics of radial head arthroplasty, particularly with respect to the shape of the head and placement. The concept of the design of a more anatomically shaped radial head implants, including patient matching and reverse engineering has now been widely explored. With respect to the ulnohumeral articulation (ie, total elbow arthroplasty), stem loosening remains a concern, and hence biomechanics-based investigations on the load carrying capacity of the interfaces have continued. There have also been some advances related to capitellar, coronoid, and distal humeral hemiarthroplasties, and in particular the importance of the shape of the articular surfaces including the concept of patient-matched surfaces using custom devices.

Dr. King or an immediate family member has received royalties from Wright Medical Technology, Inc.; serves as a paid consultant to or is an employee of Wright Medical Technology, Inc.; and serves as a board member, owner, officer, or committee member of the American Shoulder and Elbow Surgeons. Neither Dr. Johnson nor any immediate family member has received anything of value from or has stock or stock options held in a commercial company or institution related directly or indirectly to the subject of this chapter.

Radial Head Replacement

The two principal features of radial head implants from a biomechanical perspective are the articulating region, which replaces the radial head and the stem, which inserts into the canal of the radial neck to achieve fixation to host bone.

Implant Head Morphology, Design, and Biomechanics

Studies have continued on the geometric characteristics of the native radial head dish, with a focus on guiding radial head implant placement design. Clearly, the morphologic features of these implants have important implications with respect to joint kinematics and contact.

The authors of a 2015 study used three-dimensional cartilage and subchondral bone surface models generated from CT scans to obtain cartilage thickness measurements around the periphery of the radial head and within the articular dish.[1] It was found that regional variations within the rim occurred, with the thickest region located anteriorly and the thinnest region laterally. This has implications with regard to radial head arthroplasty, and in particular the design of anatomic implants, because accounting for such subtle contours may restore radiocapitellar concavity-compression stability better.

The authors of a 2017 study examined the morphology of the radial head with special interest in the design of a population-based and patient-specific radial head implants.[2] Using CT-derived models, it was shown that the mismatch for the existing commercially available axisymmetric implants was higher relative to the population-based and patient-specific designs.

There has also been significant effort directed toward determining the biomechanical characteristics of bipolar radial head implants relative to the monopolar systems. The authors of a 2009 study used a bench-top cadaver-based model that showed the monopolar conferred stability (against subluxation) similar to the native case, but that the bipolar device facilitated subluxation, hence likely compromising concavity compression.[3] In a 2012 study, the authors used a somewhat similar experimental model and confirmed the instability with the bipolar design, but also demonstrated advantages with regard to tracking due to head tilting action.[4] They also demonstrated that the radial head with an anatomic shape had similar stability to the intact case and was more stable than the more classic nonanatomic axisymmetric (ie, circular) head. The authors of a 2010 study also demonstrated that the bipolar devices were quite adaptable from the viewpoint of ensuring articular contact was not affected by joint position, but that there was a tendency for abnormal positioning of the implant to occur.[5] The authors of a 2008 study used an experimental model to demonstrate that bipolar implants offer some advantages with respect to self-alignment, which can otherwise be difficult to achieve with rigid implants.[6] This may be particularly important when implant alignment, which is likely not uncommon, is not properly achieved at surgery.

As established in a wide range of previous studies, soft tissues provide an important constraint to both the intact and implant-reconstructed elbow. Although much of the stability of the radiocapitellar joint arises from the concavity compression of the dish of the implant, additional stability from the collateral ligaments, annular ligament and capsule plays a role to varying extents. The authors of a 2011 study, using a bench-top model, showed that soft-tissue restraint was most important when a bipolar implant is used.[7] However, for the native or monopolar radial head, the soft tissues played a diminished role, with the stability being provided chiefly by the concavity compression of the radial dish with the capitellum.

In a 2011 study, the author examined the influence of the depth and radius of curvature of the articular dish of a monopolar design on stability.[8] It was shown that a deeper-dished "anatomic" implant demonstrated stability that matched that of the native head, while the shallow dished axisymmetric implant with a larger radius of curvature did not (**Figure 1**). The authors of a 2015 study used a finite element model to investigate the axisymmetric design and showed that the contact stress was elevated for both the shallowest and deepest models and an optimal implant dish depth for contact mechanics at approximately 2 mm was identified.[9]

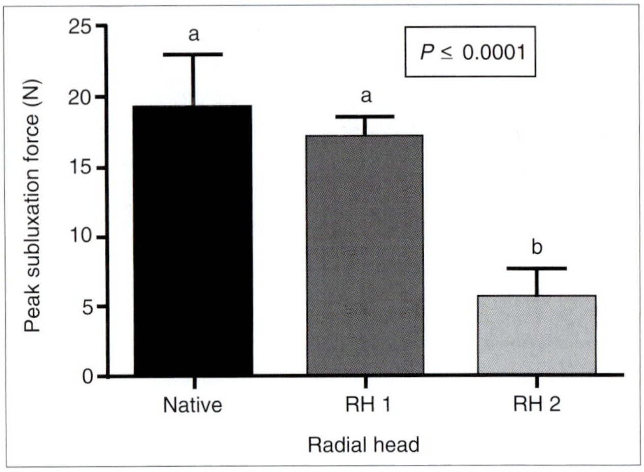

FIGURE 1 Graph comparing mean peak subluxation forces in the native radial head and two radial head prostheses (RH 1 = anatomic radial head, RH 2 = circular radial head). (Reprinted from *J Shoulder Elbow Surg* 20[12]. Chanlalit C, Shukla DR, Fitzsimmons JS, An KN, O'Driscoll SW: Influence of prosthetic design on radiocapitellar concavity-compression stability, 885-890. Copyright © 2011 Journal of Shoulder and Elbow Surgery Board of Trustees. doi:10.1016/j.jse.2011.03.009.)

As noted earlier, it is well established that the radial head has an elliptical shape. Hence, implants are emerging that have an anatomic design with the goal to produce articular tracking similar to the native state. A major focus of biomechanical studies has been the comparison of these designs with the more traditional axisymmetric (ie, axisymmetric) implants.

The authors of a 2015 study conducted a cadaver-based study to compare the kinematics of the radial head relative to the capitellum during forearm rotation.[10] They showed that both anatomic and axisymmetric devices have similar motion profiles and were both different from the native state. The authors of a 2014 study also used a cadaver model to quantify radiocapitellar joint contact distribution under simulated compressive loading[11] (**Figure 2**). For the neutral position of forearm rotation, they reported that the mean contact pressures increased by 29% with an anatomic prosthesis, 230% with a monopolar prosthesis, and 220% with a bipolar prosthesis. They also showed that the anatomically designed radial head prosthesis produced lower and more uniform distributed contact pressures than nonanatomic implants with a shallow articular dish. In a subsequent study using a similar model in 2017, the authors measured radiocapitellar joint contact pressures to determine the effect of subluxation.[12] This was based on the premise that during radiocapitellar subluxation, the use on an anatomically shaped implant would result in contact stresses that more closely mimic those occurring with the native radial head. Testing was conducted for the native radial head, followed by replacement with anatomic, monopolar, and

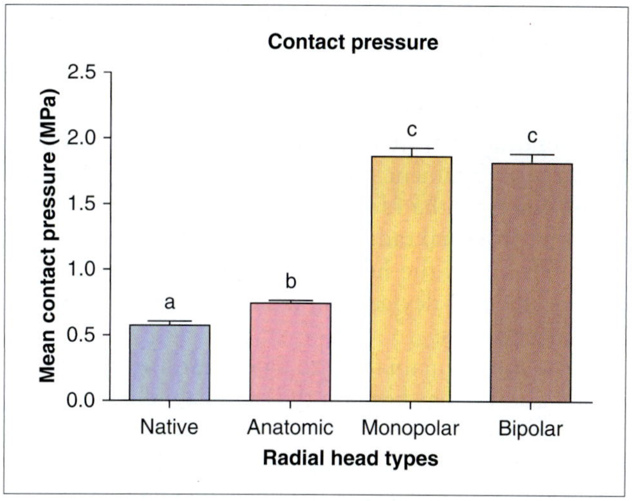

FIGURE 2 Graph showing radial head contact pressure results at 30° of flexion (mean ± standard error of mean). Columns with lowercase letters in common are not significantly different from each other ($P > 0.05$). (Reprinted from *J Shoulder Elbow Surg* 23[4]. Sahu D, Holmes DM, Fitzsimmons JS, et al: Influence of radial head prosthetic design on radiocapitellar joint contact mechanics, 456-462. Copyright © 2014 Journal of Shoulder and Elbow Surgery Board of Trustees. doi:10.1016/j.jse.2013.11.028.)

bipolar axisymmetric prostheses at various magnitudes of subluxation. It was found that joint contact pressures increased with radial head subluxation for all cases. The contact pressures characteristics with the anatomic prosthesis were similar to those produced with the native radial head. The two axisymmetric prostheses had higher contact pressures that were sustained for all levels of subluxation; however, these implants had a shallower dish depth than the more anatomically shaped design. These findings reinforce the importance of radial head articular surface shape and dish depth on joint contact pressures with subluxation. The authors of a 2015 study confirmed that the anatomic implants were more favorable to the axisymmetric implants when tested in neutral rotation and that adjusting the design of the anatomical head can produce more favorable stresses, including those generated against the lateral trochlear ridge.[13]

The authors of a 2015 study used a finite element study to quantify the contact mechanics for the native and both axisymmetric and nonaxisymmetric (ie, anatomic) radial head hemiarthroplasties throughout forearm rotation.[14] Both implants produced markedly elevated stresses and lower contact area when compared with the native state. As expected, the axisymmetric contact characteristics were constant throughout rotation. Although the nonaxisymmetric head provides improved contact mechanics to the axisymmetric devices at certain forearm rotations and flexions, there are also orientations where the contact mechanics were in fact worsened and exceeded the stresses of the axisymmetric device (**Figure 3**). This investigation illustrates the importance of considering the rotation of the radial head on its influence on joint contact mechanics, particularly with the nonaxisymmetric head against the capitellum, which is also known to be nonspherical.

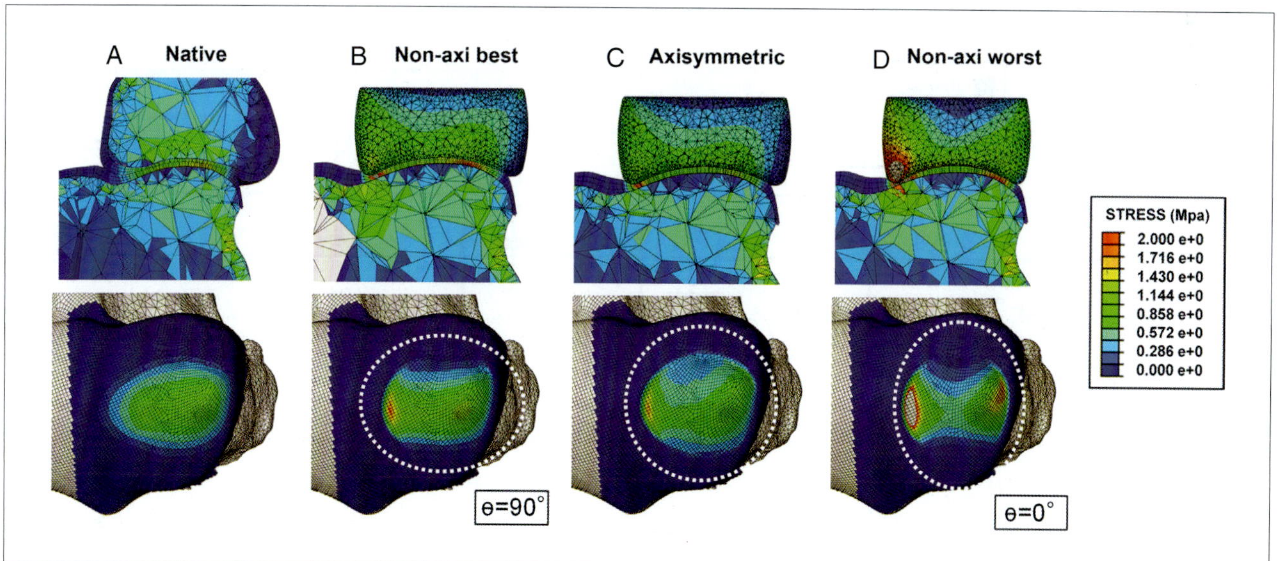

FIGURE 3 Representative cross-sectional contact stress profiles (top) and contact stress maps (bottom) at a 90° flexion angle for (**A**) native, (**B**) best nonaxisymmetric (non-axi), (**C**) axisymmetric, and (**D**) worst non-axi radial head (RH) scenarios. (Reprinted from *J Shoulder Elb Surg* 24[5]. Langohr GDG, Willing RT, Medley JB, King GJW, Johnson JA: Contact analysis of the native radiocapitellar joint compared with axisymmetric and nonaxisymmetric radial head hemiarthroplasty, 787-795. Copyright © 2015 Journal of Shoulder and Elbow Surgery Board of Trustees. doi:10.1016/j.jse.2014.12.011.

An exact restoration both of articular congruity and axial height are difficult to achieve with conventional surgical techniques. Clearly, when the implant height is less than the native structure, joint laxity will increase. Conversely, when the implant height is greater, some overstuffing of the joint will occur, reducing laxity, and likely causing a detrimental increase in joint contact stress and capitellar wear, and also alterations in the congruity of the ulnohumeral articulation. The difficulty in diagnosing overlengthening of a radial head implant was reported by the authors of a 2009 study.[15] They used a cadaver model with muscle loading and plain radiographs to evaluate ulnohumeral joint congruity for overlengthening of the radial head implant in increments of 2 mm. The results showed that incongruity was radiographically apparent only after overlengthening by 6 mm or greater (**Figure 4**). Of course, changes in articular contact stress and tracking will likely result for much smaller magnitudes of changes in the articular height; however, these have not been established to date.

The effect of implant position or height on load transfer has also been studied. The authors of a 2019 study used an elbow joint simulator to generate simulated active muscle loading throughout motion, while radial head height was adjusted using a series of spacers incorporated with a load cell mechanism.[16] As expected, radial loads increased with increasing radial length, and this was a linear trend. Overlengthening the radial neck also produced higher compression forces. Interestingly, tension resulted in underlengthening when in the varus position. These findings emphasized the importance of restoring the correct radial length during head replacement. The occurrence of tensile loading on the radial head is also a novel finding. This may be due to a hammock effect of the annular ligament producing a proximally directed thrust force on the radial head and/or a proximal pull from the proximal radioulnar joint (PRUJ) articulation. This tension on the head may explain stem loosening of noncemented devices and in addition dissociation of bipolar implants.

Although the main focus to date regarding radial head implant design has been on the radiocapitellar articulation, interest has recently emerged on the morphological features of the PRUJ, as this very likely has important implications with regard to tracking and wear on the lesser sigmoid (or radial) notch. The authors of a 2019 study performed CT imaging-based anatomic study to examine the anthropometric features of the radial notch.[17] It was shown that the depth consistently decreased from proximal to distal. These findings suggest that, at least based on ulnar anatomy, a radial head implant should perhaps possess a tapered shape from proximal to distal to optimize contact at the PRUJ. The authors of a 2016 study compared the contact profiles of different radial head hemiarthroplasty articular profiles for the PRUJ to the native radial head using a finite element model.[18] The use of an implant reduced PRUJ contact area and increased peak contact stress compared with the native

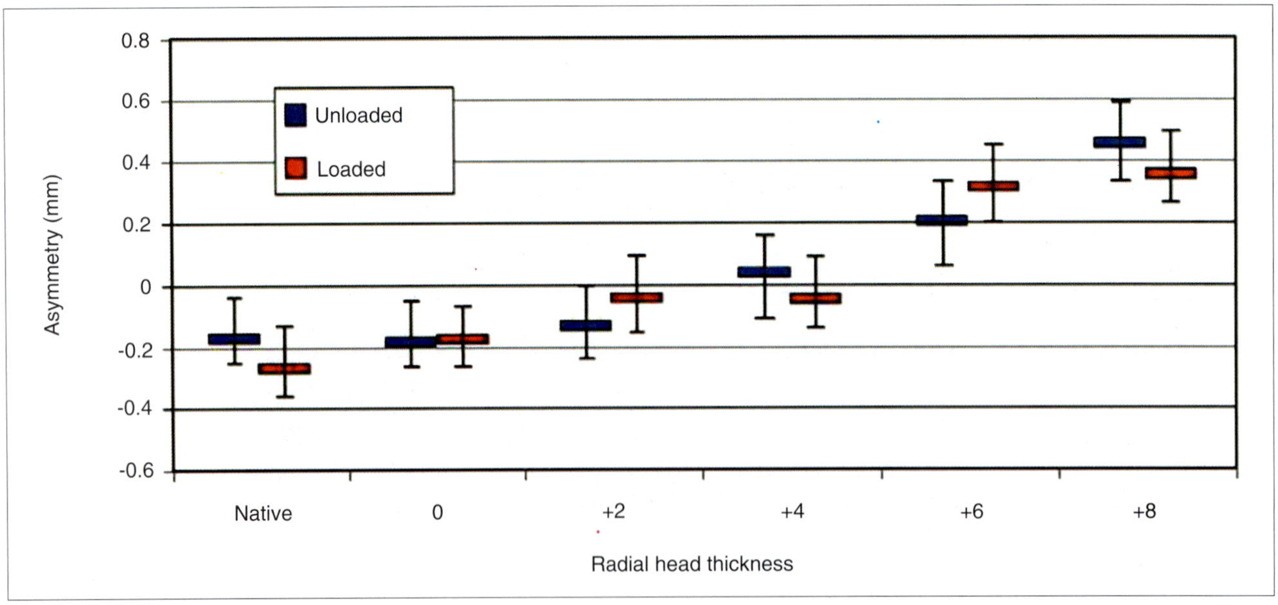

FIGURE 4 Graph showing the increased asymmetry of the medial ulnohumeral joint with progressive increases (overlengthening) in the thickness of the radial head implant. 0 = an implant of the correct size. (Reprinted with permission from Frank SG, Grewal R, Johnson J, Faber KJ, King GJ, Athwal GS: Determination of correct implant size in radial head arthroplasty to avoid overlengthening. *J Bone Joint Surg Am* 2009;91[7]:1738-1746. Copyright © 2009 by The Journal of Bone and Joint Surgery, Incorporated. doi:10.2106/JBJS.H.01161.)

state (**Figure 5**). Decreasing the side radius reduced stresses as the contact migrated toward the center of the ulnar articulation, although radius did not markedly affect contact area. They did not, however, demonstrate that the angle of the side was as important as the radius with regard to stresses.

It is highly likely that work will continue on the development of new and innovative shapes and designs of radial head articular surfaces in an effort to optimize load transfer and reduce capitellar cartilage wear.

Fixation

The optimal technique to fix the stem of radial head implants remains unknown. Stem fixation techniques are highly dependent on the morphology of the head. It is well established from earlier studies that the native radial head is somewhat elliptical and eccentric (to the shaft of the neck). Thus, when using an axisymmetric implant, noncemented fixation permitting toggle of the stem in the canal, or a bipolar concept are commonly used to ensure congruent tracking of the radial dish with the native capitellum. One commercially available implant design attempts to replicate the asymmetric shape of the proximal radius. However, ensuring correct implant orientation to avoid maltracking on the capitellum is necessary, and hence rigid stem fixation is a prerequisite for this design concept. This can be achieved by cementing the stem or porous surfaces with osseointegration.

It is clear that successful ingrowth or ongrowth for noncemented stems requires minimal interface micromotion after implantation. Little is known about this mode of fixation for radial head implants, although it is generally accepted that oversizing of the stem relative to the canal may be advantageous to achieve a solid press-fit. However, similar to intramedullary stem insertion of noncemented devices in other joints such as the femur

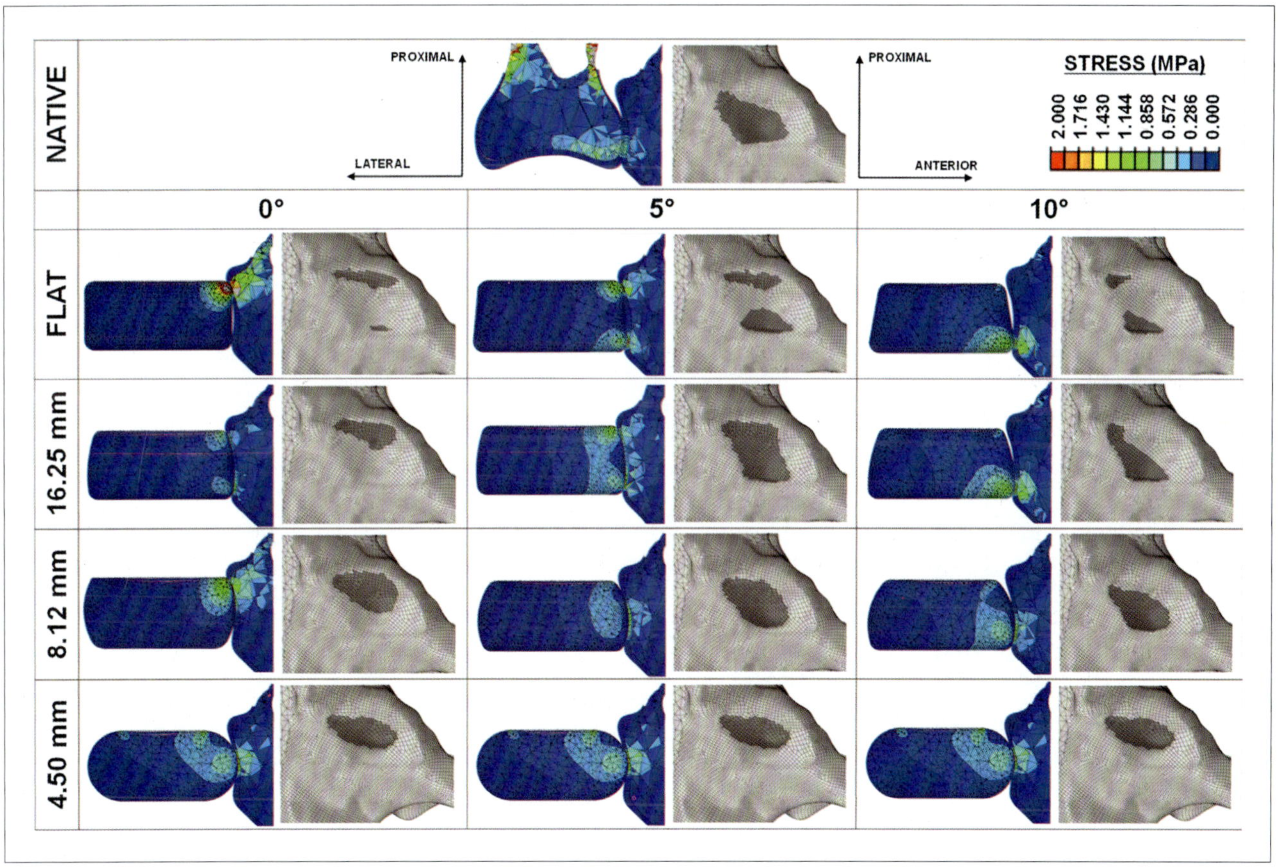

FIGURE 5 Typical stress maps (from one specimen) viewed in the coronal plane (left) and contact area maps (right) for each condition visualized on the lateral ulna articular surface of the native (top) and radial head hemiarthroplasty reconstructed (bottom) proximal radioulnar joint articulations for all side contact radii (flat, 16.25, 8.12, and 4.50 mm; top to bottom) and angles (0, 5, and 10; left to right) investigated. (Reprinted from *J Hand Surg* 41[7]. Langohr GDG, Willing R, Medley JB, King GJW, Johnson JA: The effect of radial head hemiarthroplasty geometry on proximal radioulnar joint contact mechanics, 745-752. Copyright © 2016 by the American Society for Surgery of the Hand. doi:10.1016/j.jhsa.2016.05.001.)

and humerus, fracture is a potential risk. This is of course accentuated by the tapered shape of the stem and/or the host canal.

The authors of a 2011 study examined the effect of stem size on the initial stability using cadaver specimens, with special interest in oversizing and bone fracture due to hoop stresses.[8] The authors concluded that small fractures due to hoop stresses in the cortical shell did not result in excessive micromotion and loss of stability, and hence may be acceptable clinically. In another study, the authors showed that the initial stability of a radial head stem with a partially grit-blasted surface was comparable to the fully frit-blasted device, suggesting that the former may be preferable from the viewpoint of stem removal and stress shielding.[19] The authors of a 2010 study investigated the effect of stem size, length, and shape (straight versus tapered) on the stability of radial head implants when subjected to an eccentric axial load using a cadaver-based model.[20] It was demonstrated that the most important parameter with regard to initial stability is to ensure that canal filling is achieved; stem length and taper did not have a significant effect (**Figure 6**). The authors of a 2009 study also used a bench top model to determine the micromotion of press-fit radial head implant stems, with special interest in rasp size and insertion force.[21] These experiments showed that micromotion was minimized by enlarging the canal and using larger stem diameters.

Canal preparation for stem fixation can also affect implant stability. The authors of a 2013 study conducted a cadaver-based study to compare the stability of rasping versus reaming of the proximal radius for noncemented implant stems in paired specimens.[22] Canal preparation with a reamer allowed for implantation of a 1 mm larger stem relative to rasping while resulting in initial stability similar to that achieved after rasping (**Figure 7**). This suggests that greater accommodation of canal sizes is achievable with reaming.

The authors of a 2014 study[23] also examined the effect of the diameter of grit-blasted titanium stems on initial stability and pull-out strength, using cadaver radii.

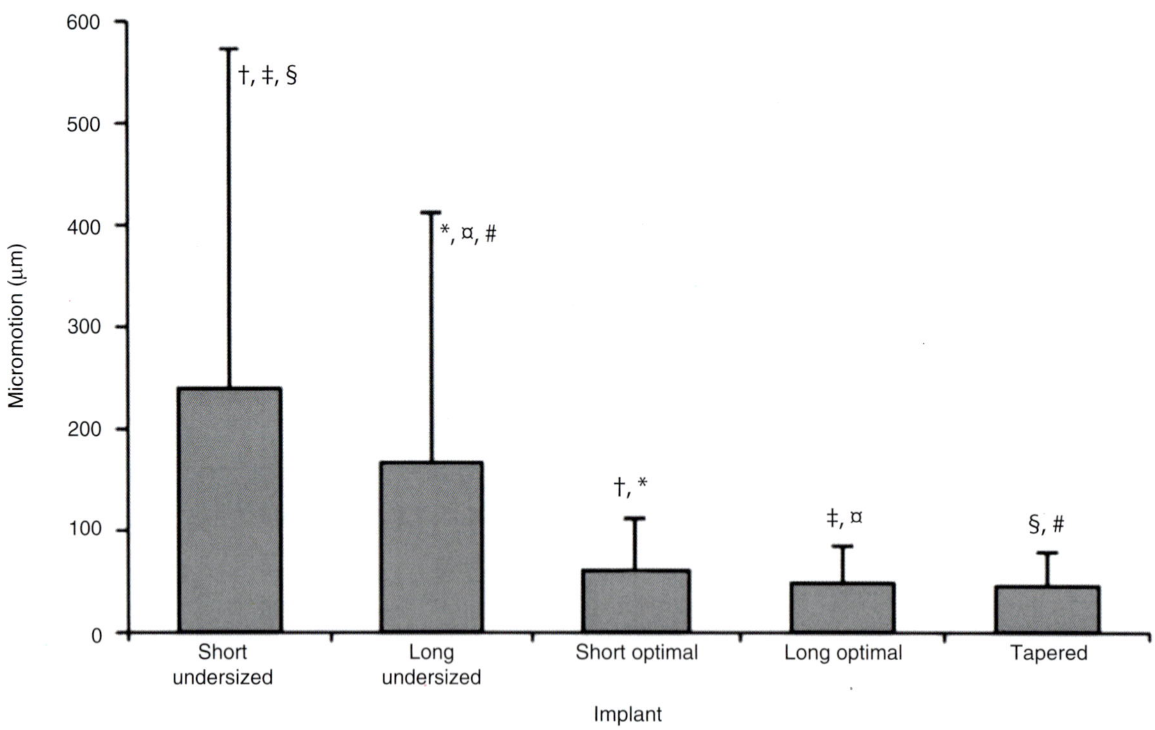

FIGURE 6 Graph showing implant motion for each of the five tested implants (pooled data). Motion significantly increased with the use of an undersized implant ($P < 0.02$). There were no significant differences between the short and long undersized implants or among the short optimal, long optimal, and tapered implants. Matching symbols imply significant difference. (Reprinted from *Clin Biomech* 25[5]. Ferreira LM, Stacpoole RA, Johnson JA, King GJ: Cementless fixation of radial head implants is affected by implant stem geometry: An in vitro study, 422-426. © 2010 Elsevier Ltd. doi:10.1016/j.clinbiomech.2010.02.001.)

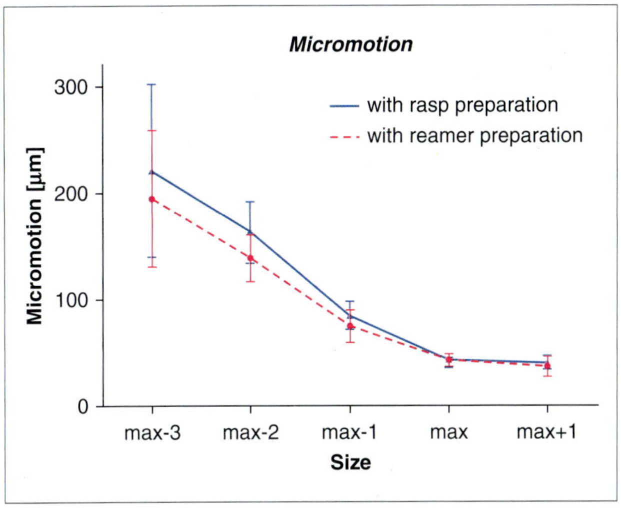

FIGURE 7 Graph showing that micromotion values decreased as the stem size increased. Rasp preparation of the canal did not result in different micromotion values versus reamer preparation of the canal. Data shown are the means standard error of the means (error bars). (Reprinted from *J Shoulder Elbow Surg* 22[11]. Shukla DR, Shao D, Fitzsimmons JS, Thoreson AR, An KN, O'Driscoll SW: Canal preparation for prosthetic radial head replacement: Rasping versus reaming. 1474-1479.Copyright © 2013 Journal of Shoulder and Elbow Surgery Board of Trustees. doi:10.1016/j.jse.2013.06.015.)

The findings demonstrated that the energy required to pull-out a 1 mm suboptimally sized stem was approximately one-third of the optimally sized device. Also, the initial micromotion was less with the optimal size. These findings suggest that the use of an inadequately sized stem decreases fixation stability while increasing the potential for loosening due to pull-out.

Collectively, these studies indicate that initial fixation of an noncemented press-fit radial head implant is perhaps best achieved by employing a stem size that optimizes canal filling, particularly with respect to the cross sectional dimensions. Clinical studies are needed to determine the longer term effect of stem size on implant fixation and performance.

Total Elbow Arthroplasty

The most common causes of failure of total elbow implants (TEAs) continue to be loosening and material wear. Currently, nearly all elbow implants use acrylic bone cement fixation between the implant and the surrounding cortical bone. Loss of fixation at the implant-cement and cement-bone interfaces can be caused by altered motion patterns and loading across the joint. It would appear that the two most significant factors affecting the load and stresses bourne by the implant-cement-bone composite structures of the humerus and ulna are the characteristics of the articulation and alignment.

The Ulnohumeral Articulation

Linked TEAs are often referred to as semiconstrained or sloppy hinge joints, because small secondary motions (such as varus-valgus or internal-external rotation of the ulna) are permitted, along with the primary flexion-extension motion. The amount of secondary motion permitted is considered a design feature, and most linked TEAs incorporate some varus-valgus and rotational laxity. Overconstraint of the linkage mechanism results in higher loads being transferred through the bone-implant interface, which can lead to mechanical loosening, while under-constraint results in elbow instability.

In linked arthroplasty, the constraint between the ulnar and humeral components provides increased stability and prevents dislocation; however it is likely another important source of increased stresses at the implant-cement interface. Although there is a theoretical advantage to unlinked devices designed to decrease loading and wear on the implant, ligament healing has been problematic in some circumstances due to difficulties in achieving an accurate and secure reconstitution of the ligaments.

The authors of a 2019 study tested a series of cadaver specimens in an elbow simulator using active motion control to determine the effect of linking and collateral ligament status.[24] Loading was measured using an instrumented humeral component. Sectioning of the collateral ligaments resulted in greater humeral component loading when unlinked, but not with linking when tested in the valgus position. In the varus position, loading was greater with linking with ligaments intact, but not after ligament sectioning. These findings suggest that ligamentous stability can assist in reducing potentially detrimental hinge loads, and linkage of these convertible devices can increase these loads. These findings have implications with regard to implant wear and fixation.

One experimental study with a companion finite element study examined the bone stresses of the unlinked iBP prosthesis (Biomet, Warsaw, IN).[25] Strain gauges on synthetic humeri and ulnae were used, and measurements were taken before and after replacement. Bone strains adjacent to the implant tip were greatly increased in the humerus and ulna. Epiphyseal cancellous bone strain reductions in the humerus and ulna relative to the intact bones were measured. It was concluded that the unlinked elbow prosthesis may be associated with the risk of bone fatigue failure, particularly in the ulna. Moreover, stress-shielding at the epiphyseal regions may promote bone resorption. It was postulated that this behavior is likely similar in linked prostheses. Modifications of stem shape, length and, materials should be considered to reduce the extent of stress shielding and improve load transfer to bone.

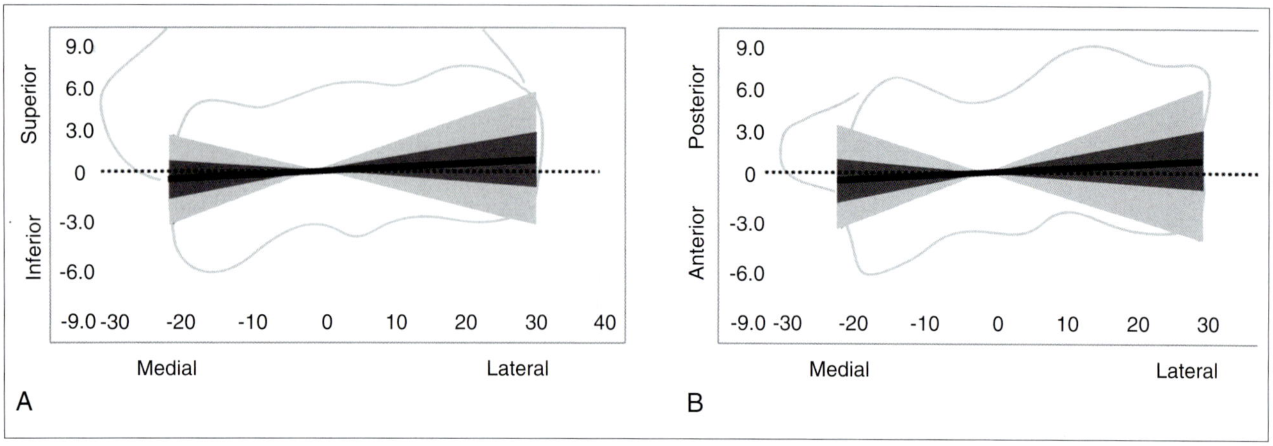

FIGURE 8 Graph showing varus-valgus and internal rotation–external rotation error in flexion-extension axis determination. The varus-valgus (frontal plane) view (**A**) and the internal rotation–external rotation (coronal plane) view (**B**) were generated from unit-vector analysis for all specimens. Dashed line = horizontal axis (0°), solid line = the mean angle (1.5° valgus and 1.6° external rotation), dark gray area = the area within 1 SD of the mean line (4.5° valgus to 1.5° varus, 4.9° external rotation to 1.7° internal rotation), light gray area = remaining values (9.6° valgus to 6.3° varus, 10.2° external rotation to 8.3° internal rotation). Proximal, anterior, and medial were considered positive directions. (Reprinted from *J Shoulder Elbow Surg* 15[4]. Brownhill JR, Furukawa K, Faber KJ, Johnson JA, King GJ: Surgeon accuracy in the selection of the flexion-extension axis of the elbow: An in vitro study, 451-456. Copyright © 2006 Journal of Shoulder and Elbow Surgery Board of Trustees. doi:10.1016/j.jse.2005.09.011.)

Implant Alignment

In patients where alignment of the humeral and ulnar components are not ideal, the additional constraint imposed by the linkage may increase wear rates and stresses at the implant-cement interface, possibly leading to component loosening and mechanical failure The primary cause of changes in kinematics and load transfer is improper joint positioning and alignment. With respect to the ulnohumeral articulation, failure to align the mechanical axis of the component to the anatomic flexion-extension axis changes the normal motion characteristics of the joint. These abnormal motion pathways alter ligament and capsule tension, and muscle moment arms and lines of action. Changes in joint kinematics result in altered forces in the implant and subsequently abnormal forces in the implant-bone structure. The majority of biomechanical studies in total elbow arthroplasty have focussed on the alignment of the ulnohumeral articulation, with special interest is reestablishment of the flexion-extension axis.

Positioning of the humeral stem is based on the alignment of the articulation hinge with the elbow's flexion-extension axis. It is well established that this can be achieved by employing the shapes of the capitellum and trochlea to determine their respective centers which defines the anatomic axis. However, the determination of the flexion-extension axis is difficult to achieve intraoperatively. The authors of a 2006 study demonstrated that the estimation of the orientation of the axis in a series of distal humerii by three subspecialty trained orthopaedic surgeons resulted in alignment errors up to 10° in either direction[26] (**Figure 8**). Improved surgical cutting guides or the use of navigation systems are needed to reduce these errors in humeral component orientation. In a later study in 2009, the authors investigated methods to achieve optimal alignment of the ulnar component.[27] In addition to using the centre and orientation of the ulna's guiding ridge and matching it with the corresponding axis of the ulnar component articulation, the addition of the center of the radial head was shown to be the most accurate predictor of the kinematic derived flexion-extension axis. This suggests when orienting the ulnar component during elbow arthroplasty, the surgeon (or computerized guidance system) should also consider the position and orientation of the radial head when available. Furthermore, ulnar cutting guides should also exploit the radial head to improve the accuracy of ulnar component positioning.

The effect of humeral implant malalignment on loading has also been investigated in a 2012 in vitro biomechanical study.[28] The resultant load of an optimally positioned implant was shown to be significantly lower than for an anterior positioned or malrotated implant (**Figure 9**). These increased loads, and in particular varus-valgus bending and internal-external torsion, will likely result in increased wear on the polyethylene linkage mechanism, and hence potentially increase the likelihood for loosening.

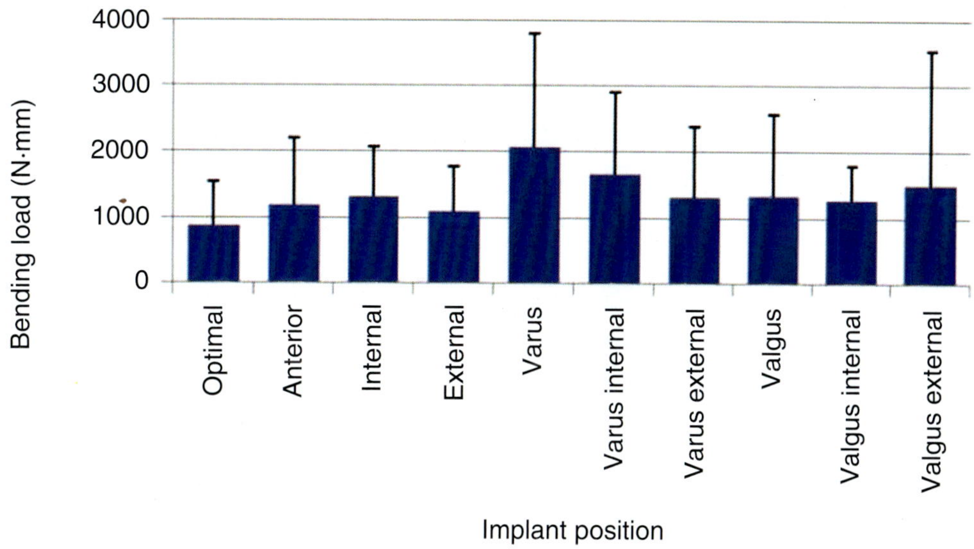

FIGURE 9 Graph showing mean bending load for active-dependent flexion in supination. The resultant bending load (mean + SD) of the entire flexion range is shown for each of the 10 tested implant positions. (Reprinted from *J Shoulder Elbow Surg* 21[8].Brownhill JR, Pollock JW, Ferreira LM, Johnson JA, King GJ: The effect of implant malalignment on joint loading in total elbow arthroplasty: An in vitro study, 1032-1038. Copyright © 2012 Journal of Shoulder and Elbow Surgery Board of Trustees. doi:10.1016/j.jse.2011.05.024.)

Although it appears that reestablishment of the native position of the articulation with the implant is an important precursor to minimizing loading and damage, this may be difficult to achieve for current implant systems due to difficulties in achieving optimal stem placement in the canal. Studies have examined the morphology of the bone and the relationships between joint position and intramedullary canal offset. The authors of a 2007 study used CT scans of the distal humerus to determine the relationship between the medullary canal axis and the flexion-extension axis.[29] The anterior offset and cubital angle between the two axes were also quantified. It was shown that the anterior offset of the flexion-extension axis from canal axis was proportional to the canal length. No relationship was established among the width of the articular surface, cubital angle, and AP and canal curvature. It was thus proposed that the use of modular humeral implants that allow for the variability in the natural anterior bow and articular offset of the distal humerus may better achieve restoration of the flexion-extension axis. In a 2009 study, the same group used 31 scans of the proximal ulna to determine the shape of the medullary canal relative to the articular surface.[27] It was reported that posterior and lateral offsets increased distally from the articulation center. It was concluded that ulnar implants with longer stems may need to be modular to accommodate the variable offsets of the canal to the articular axes.

In the recent years, there has been substantial progress in the exploration of image and computer-assisted procedures for total elbow arthroplasty. This is a logical approach and has the potential to greatly minimize the errors in implant placement that are based on visual landmark identification. Moreover, success at the hip and knee has prompted exploration of these techniques for the upper limb. An initial study, conducted by the authors of a 2007 study, explored the option of using a surface-base registration technique.[30] Using a hand-held laser scanner and conventional paired-point registration methods of the distal articular surfaces of cadaver specimens, registration error ranged between 1 and 2 mm. It was concluded that implementation of surface-based registration should produce a more accurate determination of the target axes than a visual estimation by the surgeon. In a later study in 2008, the authors determined the effect of distal humeral landmark selection and bone loss on the accuracy of image-guided registration using cadaver specimens.[31] It was shown that the anatomic landmarks needed to register surfaces accurately to a preoperative CT-image when not compromised by substantial bone loss was approximately 1 mm in translation and 0.5° in rotation. This study strongly suggests that very good alignment of a CT image with intraoperative surface digitizations can result with only a relatively small portion of the

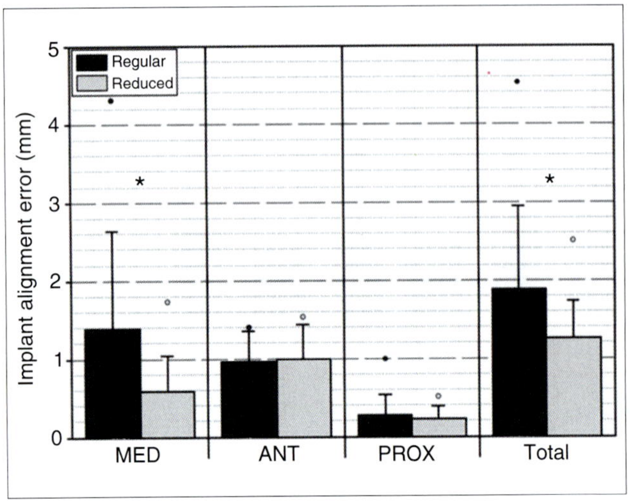

FIGURE 10 Graph showing implant alignment error in translation (mean + 1 SD). For each error, the three directional components (medial-lateral [MED], AP [ANT], and proximal-distal [PROX]) and the total error are provided. Circle = the maximum error for each translational component of error (in mm). * = significance ($P < 0.05$). (Reprinted from *J Shoulder Elbow Surg* 20[6]. McDonald CP, Peters TM, Johnson JA, King GJ: Stem abutment affects alignment of the humeral component in computer-assisted elbow arthroplasty, 891-898. Copyright © 2011 Journal of Shoulder and Elbow Surgery Board of Trustees. doi:10.1016/j.jse.2010.12.012.)

periarticular region of distal humerus available during surgery. Hence, using appropriate tracking technology and imaging, implant alignment can be readily achieved based on imaging of the uncompromised contralateral side. In a subsequent study, these investigators verified that the variations in anatomy of the distal humerus from side to side were in the order of 0.5 mm and 1.0°, and hence in an acceptable range for the concept of image/computer assisted implant reconstruction from the contralateral image.[32] The authors of a 2011 study assessed the accuracy of a computer-assisted implant alignment technique for the humeral stem using a bench top model in a series of cadaver specimens.[33] It was shown that when using an implant with a reduced stem (to minimize medullary canal impingement), the alignment was 1.3 ± 0.5 mm in translation and 1.2° ± 0.4° in rotation. However, when a full (regular) stem was used, the accuracies were 1.9 ± 1.1 mm in translation and 3.6° ± 2.1° in rotation (**Figure 10**). It was concluded that a humeral component with a fixed valgus angulation is difficult to position to accurately restore the alignment of the flexion-extension axis, and hence implant systems offering more variability in valgus angulations may be warranted.

Although it is clear that significant knowledge has been gained on the subject of implant alignment at the ulnohumeral articulation in-vitro, further work is needed to translate these findings into improved prosthesis positioning in patients.

Implant Fixation

The most common causes of failure of total elbow arthroplasties are implant loosening and material wear. Almost all elbow implants are fixed with acrylic bone cement between the implant and the surrounding cortical bone. The characteristics of the articulation and patient activity are the two most significant factors affecting the load and stresses borne by the implant-cement-bone composite structures of the humerus and ulna. Given the wide range of upper limb activities, the loads transferred to the stem-cement interface is complex, including axial, bending, and torsion modes.

Studies have investigated the stem surface conditions and the effect on fixation with cement. The authors of a 2013 study examined the torsional strength of various implant surfaces for cemented applications, with special interest in the humeral and ulnar stem.[34] Using a push-out testing model with cyclic and progressively stepped loading protocol, they showed that implant stems with nonsmooth surfaces were superior in strength, while the plasma spray treatment was superior to the beaded and smooth stem. Also, titanium was shown to have superior interface strength relative to cobalt chrome.

In a subsequent study in 2014 focusing on implant axial stability, the authors compared surface treatment (smooth, beaded, plasma sprayed) and stem substrate material (titanium, cobolt chrome) using a similar loading protocol.[35] In general, the beaded stems were superior with regard to strength and micromotion. With respect to the failure mechanisms, smooth stems debonded at the stem-cement interface, while beaded stems experienced debonding of the beads from the stem. Plasma-spray stems showed loss of frictional force between the surface treatment and cement. These findings suggest that a beaded implant may be preferential to minimize stem pistoning and loosening that has been noted to occur in some series. The weakening of the underlying substrate with bead sintering may make plasma spray a better choice for small diameter implants due to their reported problems with fatigue failure.

Implant wear can also affect stem fixation and potentially fracture. Although not a direct biomechanical study per se, the authors of a 2019 study stressed the importance of bushing design optimization due to excessive wear and osteolysis.[36] Their review of 2,637 primary and revision TEA cases from 1972 to 2016 showed a failure rate of 1.8%. Bushing wear was graded according to percentage loss of polyethylene thickness and metal wear. It was concluded that stem fracture was probably due to fatigue occurring around the junction between the unsupported and well-fixed stem, likely as a result of osteolysis due to bushing wear. Hence, further work on optimizing bushing design is needed.

Other Implant Systems

Recent interest has emerged on the development of implants for capitellar deficiency due to arthritis, fractures, and osteochondritis dissecans. The authors of a 2012 study conducted a CT-based morphologic investigation on 50 specimens.[37] The capitellar surface was quantified in both the sagittal and transverse planes. The sagittal and transverse radii of curvatures were 11.6 ± 1.4 mm and 14.0 ± 3.0 mm (range, 9.6 to 20.9) respectively. These findings indicate that the capitellum is not spherical. It was also noted that there is substantial variability in the various morphological measurements, and hence replication with an off-the-shelf implant may not be optimally achieved. Of course, a significant concern with any hemiarthroplasty is the change in contact mechanics with the native cartilaginous surface. This concept was investigated by the authors of a 2011 study, who compared the joint contact area of spherical and elliptical metal capitellar implants to the native state when articulating against the native radial head in cadaver specimens.[38] The joints were loaded in compression and a specialized impression material was used to quantify the contact area. It was reported that contact areas for the anatomic and spherical hemiarthroplasties were markedly lower at 59% and 51% of the native articulation. In the same study, the contact areas for unicompartmental arthroplasties for two capitellar implant shapes against a ultra high molecular weight polyethylene radial head were similar. This suggests although the native capitellum is elliptical, a spherical capitellar implant should suffice in a clinical implant design. The decrease in contact area is more likely related to the stiffness of the metallic implant; further studies are needed to find alternative materials for joint hemiarthroplasties. In a 2012 investigative study, the authors evaluated the spherical and elliptical implants in cadaver arms for a variety of activities using an elbow simulator.[37] Excision of the capitellum resulted in an increase in varus-valgus laxity of 3.1° and external ulnar rotation of 1.5°, while both implant designs corrected the instability. Collectively these studies support the effectiveness of a spherical implant to manage capitellar deficiency.

The concept of a coronoid implant has also been explored by the authors of a 2012 study.[39] A metal coronoid implant was developed based on detailed anthropometric studies. Using an upper limb joint motion simulator, the varus-valgus laxity was quantified for the intact, coronoid-deficient, and implant-reconstructed states in a series of cadaver specimens. It was shown that both the standard and extended coronoid implant restored joint stability similar to the intact state (**Figure 11**). The extended coronoid implant provided improved stability relative to the standard sized implant in the setting of deficient collateral ligaments—this suggests that coronoid implants, although currently not commercially available, may have an important role in the future management of comminuted unreconstructable coronoid fractures.

Hemiarthroplasty is one treatment option for distal humeral nonunions and comminuted fractures. Owing to the lack of conformity of distal humeral hemiarthroplasty implants, excessive stresses can occur on the cartilaginous surfaces of the radial head and greater sigmoid notch. Hence, cartilage erosion is a concern. There has been some recent interest in the development of new approaches for distal humerus hemiarthroplasty implants.

The authors of a 2014 study conducted a cadaver-based biomechanical study to determine the effect of distal humeral hemiarthroplasty implant size on articular contact.[40] Using an elbow simulator while tracking elbow joint kinematics, three-dimensional reconstructions of bones and cartilage were generated from CT images to determine contact patterns for the native articulation and subsequently optimal, oversized, and undersized implants. Ulnohumeral and radiocapitellar contact area were shown to decrease 44% and 4% following placement of an optimally sized implant, while there was no effect of implant size on contact parameters. The lack of any influence of implant size suggests that implant shape and materials may be more relevant.

In a related study in 2019, the authors used optimization techniques to generate the shape of custom anatomic distal humeral designs with the goal to minimize contact stress on the adjacent ulna and radial head cartilage surfaces.[41] Finite element analyses were conducted to determine cartilage contact mechanics. The results showed that design optimization has promise with respect to improving patient-specific implants. Also, patient-specific implant designs resulted in only slightly improved contact mechanics relative to a population-optimal implant. This may be due to the very large mismatch between cartilage and cobalt-chromium, hence generating larger contact stresses.

Although these novel hemiarthroplasty systems remain in their infancy, it is logical to postulate that

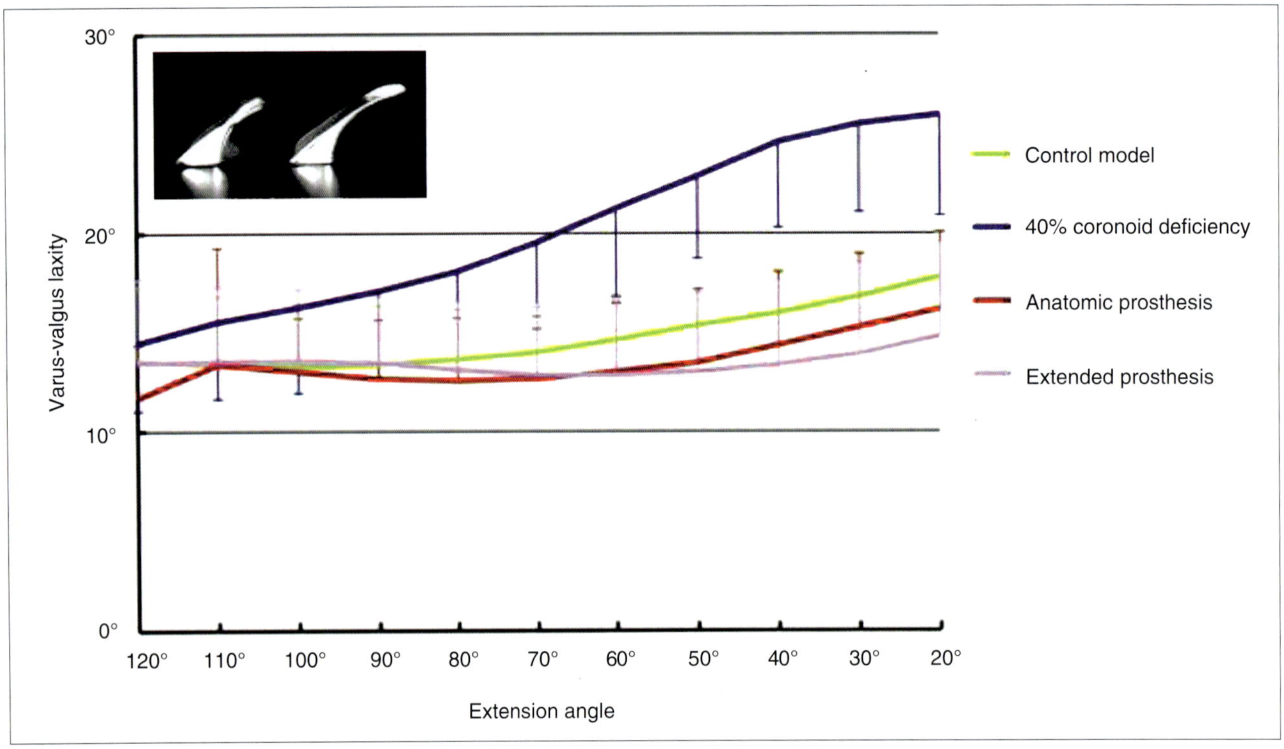

FIGURE 11 Graph showing the effects of simulated passive extension on average varus-valgus laxity in a type II coronoid fracture with the forearm in supination, after repair of collateral ligaments and prosthetic replacement. A 40% coronoid deficiency increases elbow laxity relative to the native coronoid. Prosthetic replacement with an anatomic or extended-length implant creates elbow stability similar to that of the native coronoid. Error bars indicate the SD. Inset: Lateral-view photograph of an anatomic prosthesis (left) and an extended-length prosthesis (right). (Reprinted from *J Shoulder Elbow Surg* 21[7]. Alolabi B, Gray A, Ferreira LM, Johnson JA, Athwal GS, King GJ: Reconstruction of the coronoid using an extended prosthesis: An in vitro biomechanical study, 969-976. Copyright © 2012 Journal of Shoulder and Elbow Surgery Board of Trustees. doi: 10.1016/j.jse.2011.04.014.)

significant advances in their design and development are forthcoming. Moreover, it is likely that other minimally invasive implant materials and designs will emerge.

SUMMARY

This chapter focuses on the biomechanics of radial head and ulnohumeral (or total elbow) arthroplasty that have emerged in the literature over the past decade. With respect to radial head implant design and sizing, significant advances have been made regarding the influence of the anatomic characteristics of the head. Research has focused on articular contact and kinematics at the radiocapitellar joint with an emphasis on axisymmetric (ie, circular), bipolar, and anatomic designs. These have indicating marked differences in capitellar articular tracking and stability among designs. Studies on the influence of soft-tissue constraints on joint stability have also emerged. Most recently, the importance of the shape of the radial head around the periphery, specifically at the articulation with the ulna at the PRUJ, has drawn attention. Findings have demonstrated that both the curvature and angle of the periphery of the implant have important implications regarding PRUJ tracking. Regarding total elbow arthroplasty, studies have demonstrated the influence of stem surface conditions on fixation strength. As well, the effect of the ulnohumeral hinge linkage position and status on load transfer has been reported. Investigations into distal humeral hemiarthroplasties have indicated the importance of implant shape on articular stresses bourne by cartilage.

Acknowledgments

The authors gratefully acknowledge Mr. Jakub Szmit for his assistance in the organization and presentation of this chapter.

KEY STUDY POINTS

- New knowledge has emerged on the anatomic characteristics of radial head arthroplasty, with a focus on articular contact and kinematics at the radiocapitellar joint. Bench-top experimental and computational studies have indicating marked differences in capitellar articular tracking and stability among designs.
- The importance of the shape of the radial head around the periphery with a focus on the articulation with the ulna at the PRUJ has been addressed. Both the curvature and angle of the periphery of the implant have important implications regarding PRUJ tracking.
- Studies of total elbow arthroplasty implant fixation have explored the influence of stem surface conditions and have emphasized the major differences between smooth, plasma sprayed, and beaded implants. Additionally, the effect of the ulnohumeral hinge linkage position has been shown to have a marked influence on implant loading.
- Investigations on distal humeral hemiarthroplasties have indicated the importance of implant shape on the stresses bourne by cartilage and in particular the large changes in contact mechanics that occur relative to the native state.

Annotated References

1. Yeung C, Deluce S, Willing R, Johnson M, King GJW, Athwal GS: Regional variations in cartilage thickness of the radial head: Implications for prosthesis design. *J Hand Surg Am* 2015;40(12):2364-2371.e1. doi:10.1016/j.jhsa.2015.09.005.

This CT-based study quantified cartilage thickness measurements at numerous predetermined landmarks around the periphery of the radial head and within the articular dish. Marked variations within the rim occurred, with the thickest region located anteriorly and thinnest region laterally. This has implications for the design of anatomic implants, particularly with regard to the restoration of radiocapitellar concavity-compression stability. Level of evidence: IV.

2. Lalone EA, Deluce SR, Shannon H, King GJW, Johnson JA: Design of anatomical population-based and patient-specific radial head implants. *J Hand Surg Am* 2017;42(11):924.e1-924.e11. doi:10.1016/j.jhsa.2017.05.028.

This study examined the morphology of the radial head with special interest in the design of population-based and patient-specific radial head implants. Using CT images of normal cadaveric upper extremities, surface models were ellipse-fitted and characterized. An intersurface distance mapping was used to generate these implants, which were compared with the native radial head. The mean mismatch for the existing commercially available axisymmetrical implants was higher relative to the population-based and patient-specific designs. Level of evidence: IV.

3. Moon JG, Berglund LJ, Zachary D, An KN, O'Driscoll SW: Radiocapitellar joint stability with bipolar versus monopolar radial head prostheses. *J Shoulder Elbow Surg* 2009;18(5):779-784. doi:10.1016/j.jse.2009.02.011.

4. Chanlalit C, Shukla DR, Fitzsimmons JS, An KN, O'Driscoll SW: The biomechanical effect of prosthetic design on radiocapitellar stability in a terrible triad model. *J Orthop Trauma* 2012;26(9):539-544. doi:10.1097/BOT.0b013e318238b3a2.

5. Moungondo F, El Kazzi W, van Riet R, Feipel V, Rooze M, Schuind F: Radiocapitellar joint contacts after bipolar radial head arthroplasty. *J Shoulder Elbow Surg* 2010;19(2):230-235. doi:10.1016/j.jse.2009.09.015.

6. Yian E, Steens W, Lingenfelter E, Schneeberger AG: Malpositioning of radial head prostheses: An in vitro study. *J Shoulder Elbow Surg* 2008;17(4):663-670. doi:10.1016/j.jse.2007.12.008.

7. Chanlalit C, Shukla DR, Fitzsimmons JS, Thoreson AR, An KN, O'Driscoll SW: Radiocapitellar stability: The effect of soft tissue integrity on bipolar versus monopolar radial head prostheses. *J Shoulder Elbow Surg* 2011;20(2):219-225. doi:10.1016/j.jse.2010.10.033.

8. Chanlalit C, Shukla DR, Fitzsimmons JS, An KN, O'Driscoll SW: Influence of prosthetic design on radiocapitellar concavity-compression stability. *J Shoulder Elbow Surg* 2011;20(6):885-890. doi:10.1016/j.jse.2011.03.009.

9. Irish SE, Langohr GDG, Willing R, King GJ, Johnson JA: Implications of radial head hemiarthroplasty dish depth on radiocapitellar contact mechanics. *J Hand Surg Am* 2015;40(4):723-729. doi:10.1016/j.jhsa.2015.01.030.

This study investigated the effect of radial head implant dish depth on radiocapitellar joint contact mechanics using finite element modeling. Peak cartilage contact stress was elevated for both the shallowest and deepest models and reached a local minimum. There was an optimal implant dish depth for contact mechanics at approximately 2 mm. Level of evidence: IV.

10. Shannon HL, Deluce SR, Lalone EA, Willing R, King GJW, Johnson JA: Effect of radial head implant shape on joint contact area and location during static loading. *J Hand Surg Am* 2015;40(4):716-722. doi:10.1016/j.jhsa.2014.12.017.

This in vitro cadaver-based study compared radiocapitellar joint kinematics for three radial head implant designs that included axisymmetric, reverse-engineered patient-specific, and population-based quasi-anatomic designs as well as the native head. It was shown that radiocapitellar kinematics were in general similar, and all had different kinematic patterns from the native radial head. Overall, for the different positions of flexion and rotation, patient-specific radial head implants did not prove advantageous relative to conventional implant designs with regard to tracking. Level of evidence: IV.

11. Sahu D, Holmes DM, Fitzsimmons JS, et al: Influence of radial head prosthetic design on radiocapitellar joint contact mechanics. *J Shoulder Elbow Surg* 2014;23(4):456-462. doi:10.1016/j.jse.2013.11.028.

    This experimental study determined the contact pressure for the native radial head, an anatomic implant, a nonanatomic circular monopolar implant, and a bipolar nonanatomic implant. Testing was conducted in pronation, neutral, and supination at different angles of flexion. The mean contact pressures in supination increased by 29% with the anatomic prosthesis, 230% with the monopolar prosthesis, and 220% with the bipolar prosthesis. The anatomically designed radial head prosthesis produced lower and more evenly distributed contact pressures than the nonanatomic implants. Level of evidence: IV.

12. Sahu D, Fitzsimmons JS, Thoreson AR, An KN, O'Driscoll SW: Radiocapitellar contact characteristics during prosthetic radial head subluxation. *J Shoulder Elbow Surg* 2017;26(1):170-177. doi:10.1016/j.jse.2016.07.005.

    This experimental study measured contact pressure of monopolar circular, bipolar circular, and anatomic radial head prostheses undergoing radiocapitellar subluxation. Contact pressures were higher at baseline and did not change significantly during subluxation for the monopolar and bipolar prosthesis, whereas progressive increase in pressure occurred during subluxation of both the native radial head and anatomic prosthesis. This reinforces the importance of articular surface design of radial head prostheses on joint contact pressures for different subluxation positions. Level of evidence: IV.

13. Bachman DR, Thaveepunsan S, Park S, Fitzsimmons JS, An KN, O'Driscoll SW: The effect of prosthetic radial head geometry on the distribution and magnitude of radiocapitellar joint contact pressures. *J Hand Surg Am* 2015;40(2):281-288. doi:10.1016/j.jhsa.2014.11.005.

    This experimental study determined radiocapitellar contact pressures for axisymmetric and different anatomic designs. One anatomic design had similar contact areas and mean pressures as the native radial head, which did not occur with the axisymmetric. The depth of the articular dish affected contact area and pressure. Also, one of the anatomical radial head prototypes tested had improved contact with the lateral trochlear ridge and the sulcus. Level of evidence: IV.

14. Langohr GDG, Willing RT, Medley JB, King GJW, Johnson JA: Contact analysis of the native radiocapitellar joint compared with axisymmetric and nonaxisymmetric radial head hemiarthroplasty. *J Shoulder Elbow Surg* 2015;24(5):787-795. doi:10.1016/j.jse.2014.12.011.

    This finite element study examined the contact mechanics for the native and both axisymmetric and nonaxisymmetric (ie, anatomic) radial head hemiarthroplasties. Both implants produced much higher stresses and lower contact area relative to the native state. As expected, the axisymmetric contact characteristics were constant throughout rotation. The nonaxisymmetric radial head provides improved contact mechanics to the axisymmetric devices at certain forearm rotations, although some positions produced elevated stresses. Level of evidence: IV.

15. Frank SG, Grewal R, Johnson J, Faber KJ, King GJW, Athwal GS: Determination of correct implant size in radial head arthroplasty to avoid overlengthening. *J Bone Joint Surg Am* 2009;91(7):1738-1746. doi:10.2106/JBJS.H.01161.

16. Berkmortel CJ, Gladwell MS, Ng J, et al: Effect of radial neck length on joint loading. *J Shoulder Elbow Arthroplast* 2019;3:1-7. doi:10.1177/2471549219829964.

    This study used a load cell in the neck of cadaveric proximal radial during simulated motion to determine the effects of radial neck length and arm position. Radial loads increased with increasing length. Interestingly, underlengthening produced tensile forces in the varus position. These findings suggest that restoration of correct radial length during radial head replacement is very important. The occurrence of tensile loading on the radial head may explain stem loosening of noncemented devices and head dissociation. Level of evidence: IV.

17. Wegmann K, Knowles N, Lalone E, Müller LP, Athwal GS, King GJW: Computed tomography analysis of the radial notch of the ulna. *J Hand Surg Am* 2019;44(9):794.e1-794.e8. doi:10.1016/j.jhsa.2018.10.010.

    This imaging-based anatomic study focused on the anthropometric features of the morphology of the radial notch, with special interest in implant design. With regard to orientation, the notch was rotated externally relative to the transverse plane of the ulna. The average depth of the notch at its deepest point was 2.2 mm and this depth decreased from proximal to distal. These findings suggest that a radial head implant with a taper from proximal to distal may improve PRUJ contact. Level of evidence: IV.

18. Langohr GDG, Willing R, Medley JB, King GJW, Johnson JA: The effect of radial head hemiarthroplasty geometry on proximal radioulnar joint contact mechanics. *J Hand Surg Am* 2016;41(7):745-752. doi:10.1016/j.jhsa.2016.05.001.

    This study compares the contact profiles of different radial head hemiarthroplasty articular profiles for the proximal radioulnar joint (PRUJ) with those of the native radial head using a finite element model. The use of an implant reduced PRUJ contact area and increased peak contact stress compared with the native state. Decreasing the side radius reduced stresses as the contact migrated toward the center of the ulnar articulation, although the radius did not markedly affect contact area. Level of evidence: IV.

19. Chanlalit C, Fitzsimmons JS, Moon JG, Berglund LJ, An KN, O'Driscoll SW: Radial head prosthesis micromotion characteristics: Partial versus fully grit-blasted stems. *J Shoulder Elbow Surg* 2011;20(1):27-32. doi:10.1016/j.jse.2010.05.030.

20. Ferreira LM, Stacpoole RA, Johnson JA, King GJW: Cementless fixation of radial head implants is affected by implant stem geometry: An in vitro study. *Clin Biomech* 2010;25(5):422-426. doi:10.1016/j.clinbiomech.2010.02.001.

21. Moon JG, Berglund LJ, Domire Z, An KN, O'Driscoll SW: Stem diameter and micromotion of press fit radial head prosthesis: A biomechanical study. *J Shoulder Elbow Surg* 2009;18(5):785-790. doi:10.1016/j.jse.2009.02.014.

22. Shukla DR, Shao D, Fitzsimmons JS, Thoreson AR, An KN, O'Driscoll SW: Canal preparation for prosthetic radial head replacement: Rasping versus reaming. *J Shoulder Elbow Surg* 2013;22(11):1474-1479. doi:10.1016/j.jse.2013.06.015.

    This study reported on a simple overlay device to measure radial head implant length. A series of cadavers were implanted with progressively longer implants, adjusted by neck length of 0, 2, 4, and 8 mm. Fluoroscopic images were obtained in four forearm positions: anteroposterior in supination in full extension, anteroposterior in pronation in full extension, supinated in 45° of flexion, and neutral in 45° of flexion. The SOD measurements (made by two observers) were compared with the native original radial head (control) to assess implant length. In addition, gapping of the ulnohumeral joint space was measured for comparison purposes. It was shown that this technique is reliable for simply determining radial head length with radiographs to an accuracy of 2 mm. Level of evidence: IV.

23. Shukla D, Fitzsimmons J, An KN, O'Driscoll S: Prosthetic radial head stem pull-out as a mode of failure: A biomechanical study. *Int Orthop* 2014;38(1):89-93. doi:10.1007/s00264-013-2074-3.

    This in vitro bench-top study employed cadaveric radii to examine the effect of the diameter of grit-blasted stems on initial stability and pull-out strength. The findings demonstrated that the energy required to pull-out a 1 mm sub-optimally sized stem was approximately one-third of the optimally sized device. Also, the initial micromotion was less with the optimal size. These findings suggest that the use of an inadequately sized stem decreases fixation stability while increasing the potential for loosening due to pull-out. Level of evidence: IV.

24. Brownhill JR, Pollock JW, Ferreira LM, Johnson JA, King GJ: The effect of implant linking and ligament integrity on humeral loading of a convertible total elbow arthroplasty. *Shoulder Elbow* 2019;11(1):45-52. doi:10.1177/1758573217728292.

    This experimental study aimed to evaluate the effect of collateral ligament integrity and implant linkage on wear-inducing loads in a convertible total elbow arthroplasty (TEA). Collateral ligament integrity reduces wear-inducing loads for both linked and unlinked TEA, whereas linkage of a convertible TEA increases humeral loading. Level of evidence: I.

25. Completo A, Pereira J, Fonseca F, Ramos A, Relvas C, Simões J: Biomechanical analysis of total elbow replacement with unlinked iBP prosthesis: An in vitro and finite element analysis. *Clin Biomech* 2011;26(10):990-997. doi:10.1016/j.clinbiomech.2011.06.008.

26. Brownhill JR, Furukawa K, Faber KJ, Johnson JA, King GJ: Surgeon accuracy in the selection of the flexion-extension axis of the elbow: An in vitro study. *J Shoulder Elbow Surg* 2006;15(4):451-456. doi:10.1016/j.jse.2005.09.011.

27. Brownhill JR, Mozzon JB, Ferreira LM, Johnson JA, King GJW: Morphologic analysis of the proximal ulna with special interest in elbow implant sizing and alignment. *J Shoulder Elbow Surg* 2009;18(1):27-32. doi:10.1016/j.jse.2008.03.008.

28. Brownhill JR, Pollock JW, Ferreira LM, Johnson JA, King GJW: The effect of implant malalignment on joint loading in total elbow arthroplasty: An in vitro study. *J Shoulder Elbow Surg* 2012;21(8):1032-1038. doi:10.1016/j.jse.2011.05.024.

29. Nguyen D, Ferreira LM, Brownhill JR, Faber KJ, Johnson JA: Design and development of a computer assisted glenoid implantation technique for shoulder replacement surgery. *Comput Aided Surg* 2007;12(3):152-159. doi:10.3109/10929080701374315.

30. McDonald CP, Brownhill JR, King GJ, Johnson JA, Peters TM: A comparison of registration techniques for computer- and image-assisted elbow surgery. *Comput Aided Surg* 2007;12(4):208-214. doi:10.3109/10929080701517459.

31. McDonald CP, Beaton BJ, King GJ, Peters TM, Johnson JA: The effect of anatomic landmark selection of the distal humerus on registration accuracy in computer-assisted elbow surgery. *J Shoulder Elbow Surg* 2008;17(5):833-843. doi:10.1016/j.jse.2008.02.007.

32. McDonald CP, Peters TM, King GJ, Johnson JA: Computer assisted surgery of the distal humerus can employ contralateral images for pre-operative planning, registration, and surgical intervention. *J Shoulder Elbow Surg* 2009;18(3):469-477. doi:10.1016/j.jse.2009.01.028.

33. McDonald CP, Peters TM, Johnson JA, King GJW: Stem abutment affects alignment of the humeral component in computer-assisted elbow arthroplasty. *J Shoulder Elbow Surg* 2011;20(6):891-898. doi:10.1016/j.jse.2010.12.012.

34. Hosein YK, King GJW, Dunning CE: The effect of stem surface treatment and material onpistoning of ulnar components in linked cemented elbow prostheses. *J Shoulder Elbow Surg* 2013;22(9):1248-1255. doi:10.1016/j.jse.2013.03.007.

This study investigated the role of surface treatment (smooth, beaded, plasma sprayed) and stem substrate material (titanium, cobalt chrome) on implant axial stability, during cyclic pushout testing. In general, the beaded stems were superior with regard to strength and micromotion. Smooth stems debonded at the stem-cement interface, whereas beaded stems experienced debonding of the beads from the stem. Plasma-spray stems showed loss of frictional force between the surface treatment and cement. Level of evidence: IV.

35. Hosein YK, King GJW, Dunning CE: The effect of stem material and surface treatment on the torsional stability at the metal-cement interface of upper limb joint replacement systems. *J Biomed Mater Res B Appl Biomater* 2014;102(6):1217-1222. doi:10.1002/jbm.b.33105.

This study examined the torsional strength of various implant surfaces for cemented applications, with special interest in upper limb implants. The findings showed that implant stems with nonsmooth surfaces were superior in strength, and the plasma-spray treatment was superior to the beaded and smooth stem. Also, titanium had superior torsional interface strength relative to cobalt chrome. Level of evidence: IV.

36. Lee H, Vaichinger AM, O'Driscoll SW: Component fracture after total elbow arthroplasty. *J Shoulder Elbow Surg* 2019;28(8):1449-1456. doi:10.1016/j.jse.2019.02.021.

Although not a biomechanical study per se, this review of 2637 primary and revision TEA cases from 1972 to 2016 showed a failure rate of 1.8%. Bushing wear was graded based on polyethylene thickness and metal wear. The findings suggested that stem fracture was probably due to fatigue occurring around the junction between the unsupported and well-fixed stem, likely as a result of osteolysis due to bushing wear. Level of evidence: III.

37. Sabo MT, Shannon HL, Deluce S, et al: Capitellar excision and hemiarthroplasty affects elbow kinematics and stability. *J Shoulder Elbow Surg* 2012;21(8):1024-1031.e4. doi:10.1016/j.jse.2011.04.019.

38. Sabo MT, Shannon H, Ng J, Ferreira LM, Johnson JA, King GJW: The impact of capitellar arthroplasty on elbow contact mechanics: Implications for implant design. *Clin Biomech* 2011;26(5):458-463. doi:10.1016/j.clinbiomech.2011.01.007.

39. Alolabi B, Gray A, Ferreira LM, Johnson JA, Athwal GS, King GJW: Reconstruction of the coronoid using an extended prosthesis: An in vitro biomechanical study. *J Shoulder Elbow Surg* 2012;21(7):969-976. doi:10.1016/j.jse.2011.04.014.

40. Lapner M, Willing R, Johnson JA, King GJW: The effect of distal humeral hemiarthroplasty on articular contact of the elbow. *Clin Biomech* 2014;29(5):537-544. doi:10.1016/j.clinbiomech.2014.03.010.

This cadaver-based biomechanical study determined the effect of distal humeral hemiarthroplasty and implant size on elbow articular contact. Using an elbow simulator while tracking motion, three-dimensional reconstructions of bones and cartilage were generated from CT images to determine contact patterns for the native articulation and sequentially optimal, oversized, and undersized implants. Ulnohumeral and radiocapitellar contact area decreased 44% and 4% following placement of an optimally sized implant, but there was no effect of implant size on contact parameters. It was concluded that the lack of influence of implant size suggests that implant shape and materials may be more relevant than implant sizing. Level of evidence: IV.

41. Willing R: Design optimisation improves the performance of custom distal humeral hemiarthroplasty implants. *Comput Methods Biomech Biomed Eng Imaging Vis* 2019;7(1):108-115. doi:10.1080/21681163.2018.1446054.

This finite element study used optimization techniques to re-create the shape of custom anatomic distal humeral hemiarthroplasty implants. The distal humerus cartilage surface was replaced by either a rigid surface in the shape of the subchondral bone or various optimized patient-specific or population-specific implants. No differences were observed in terms of resulting contact areas or stresses for the optimized shapes. A trade-off resulted when developing a design to minimize peak stresses of both the ulna and radius. Level of evidence: IV.

Section 2

Instability and Athletic Injuries

SECTION EDITOR:
CAPT MATTHEW T. PROVENCHER, MD, MC, USN

Chapter 5

Clinical Assessment, Imaging, and Classification of Glenohumeral Instability

Taylor J. Wiley, MD • Brett D. Owens, MD

ABSTRACT

The evaluation of patients with shoulder instability begins with a thorough history and physical examination. Pertinent aspects of the patient's history will include the mechanism of injury, arm position during instability, number of instability events, presence of low-energy/sleep symptoms, and sport position and season. In addition to range of motion, strength, and neurovascular evaluation, the physical examination should include special testing for anterior, posterior, and multidirectional instability (such as load and shift, apprehension, jerk, Kim, and sulcus testing). Imaging evaluation begins with plain radiographs to confirm concentric reduction as well as an initial assessment for a bony Bankart and/or Hill-Sachs lesion. MRI, with or without intra-articular gadolinium, is used to evaluate for capsulolabral injury patterns like Bankart, anterior labral periosteal sleeve avulsion, and humeral avulsion of the glenohumeral ligament lesions. CT, particularly with three-dimensional reconstruction, is the current benchmark for evaluation of glenoid bone loss in recurrent shoulder instability. The recognition of bipolar bone loss is essential as it has been increasingly linked to risk of recurrent instability and can be used to direct treatment. The glenoid track concept provides a useful framework within which to consider bipolar bone loss. In addition to bone loss, native glenoid width and version become relevant factors in the evaluation of posterior glenohumeral instability. A multitude of classification systems for shoulder instability exist, from the broad characterization by directionality to more prognostic systems such as the instability severity index score.

Dr. Owens or an immediate family member has received royalties from Linvatec; serves as a paid consultant to or is an employee of Linvatec, Mitek, Musculoskeletal Transplant Foundation, and Vericel; and serves as a board member, owner, officer, or committee member of the American Orthopaedic Society for Sports Medicine. Neither Dr. Wiley nor any immediate family member has received anything of value from or has stock or stock options held in a commercial company or institution related directly or indirectly to the subject of this chapter.

Keywords: bipolar bone loss; glenoid track; imaging; shoulder instability

Introduction

Glenohumeral instability is common among athletes and young, active patients. Its incidence is second only to that of acromioclavicular injury among athletes, and it leads to more severe disability and a greater likelihood of surgical intervention than other shoulder injuries.[1-3] In a patient younger than 25 years with glenohumeral symptoms, the default diagnosis should be instability, until another diagnosis is proven.

The treatment of shoulder instability hinges on proper classification and patient risk profiling. The identification of instability requires a subjective sense that the glenohumeral joint is moving beyond its physiologic limits, whereas laxity is an objective measurement of the amount of motion, as identified by the examiner. Symptomatic instability, physiologic and/or pathologic laxity, and imaging findings are key to ensuring appropriate treatment.

Clinical Assessment

Patient History

Obtaining a high-quality patient history is critical to evaluating a patient with suspected shoulder instability. Complete glenohumeral dislocation is easier to diagnose than subluxation because most patients will have undergone a manual reduction maneuver. Reduction in an emergency department is typical, and as a result, prereduction and postreduction radiographs often are available for assessment. Reduction outside of an emergency department also is common, such as by an athletic trainer, and communication with the person who provided the reduction can yield information on the injury and ease of reduction. Patients with chronic instability may report self-reduction.

There may be more variability in reports of subluxation because a manual reduction maneuver is not required. Patients typically describe their shoulder as "slipping out, and then going back in." These events may include a dislocation that spontaneously reduces (called a transient luxation event).[4] At the opposite end of the instability spectrum, microinstability may be similarly described by a patient who is a throwing or other overhead athlete. Therefore, it is critical to assess the patient's injury mechanism and sports activity in as much detail as can be obtained. Patients with both anterior and posterior instability events may report a fall onto an outstretched arm; posterior events often occur with the arm at 90° of forward flexion, and anterior events often occur as the arm moves rapidly into a position of extreme forward flexion and/or abduction.

If the patient has chronic, recurrent instability, an attempt should be made to determine the number of earlier events. A history of multiple events should alert the clinician to the possibility of bone loss. Determining the activities associated with these events also can provide insight. The presence of voluntary instability may suggest significant capsular laxity.[5] Instability during sleep may be associated with glenohumeral bone loss or soft-tissue deficiency.

Before revision surgery, a complete surgical history should be obtained including surgical reports and any available arthroscopic images. The earlier use of a thermal probe for capsulorrhaphy should alert the surgeon to the possibility that soft-tissue deficiency will be encountered during surgery and that capsular augmentation may be needed.

The patient history should include the patient's athletic goals. A young athlete who is planning to return to an intercollegiate contact sport is at a significantly higher risk of recurrence than a less active patient. The patient should be appropriately counseled on the risk of recurrence as well as the surgical treatment options.

Physical Examination

The patient history may guide the examiner to focus on specific aspects of the physical examination, but a general upper extremity examination is important to avoid missing a contributing pathology that is absent from the history. The physical examination for shoulder instability follows the routine of a thorough musculoskeletal examination and includes inspection, palpation, range of motion assessment, testing of motor strength, neurovascular examination, and specialized tests. The examination should be conducted with both shoulders completely exposed. Each phase of the examination should begin with the asymptomatic shoulder to provide an understanding of the patient's normal laxity and to build the patient's trust in the examiner.

During inspection of the shoulder girdle, the muscular contour should be evaluated for any asymmetry indicating atrophy of the deltoid, supraspinatus, or infraspinatus. Squaring of the lateral shoulder border with a prominent acromion may represent deltoid atrophy from an axillary nerve injury. The scapular body position should be assessed for scapular winging. The skin around the shoulder should be inspected for evidence of previous surgical incisions, thin atrophic skin, or excessive scar widening that may indicate a collagen disorder. Palpation of the entire shoulder girdle can be helpful to rule out concomitant pathology and determine the need for specialized testing and imaging.

Range of Motion

After sites of tenderness are recorded, the shoulder is taken through a full active range of motion. It is helpful to record maximal active forward flexion, internal rotation in adduction and 90° of abduction, and external rotation in adduction and 90° of abduction. Internal rotation in adduction is recorded relative to the nearest vertebral level. Throwing athletes commonly have an increased ability to externally rotate their dominant extremity, with a concomitant loss of internal rotation that leaves the total arc of motion symmetric to that of the contralateral extremity. A glenohumeral internal rotation deficit may exist if the total arc of motion is more than 25° less than that of the contralateral shoulder, and it may predispose the patient to internal impingement or labral pathology.

The examiner should determine whether a patient with an active motion deficit has full passive motion. Importantly, a patient with a locked posterior shoulder dislocation has a loss of external rotation actively and passively on the affected side. A large rotator cuff tear initially may appear as a loss of active external rotation while full passive motion is maintained. The patient is observed from behind during forward flexion and abduction to detect scapular asymmetry or winging during motion. Medial or lateral scapular winging may be attributable to long thoracic or cranial nerve XI palsy but also can be caused by scapular dyskinesis in a patient who is a throwing athlete or has multidirectional instability.

Muscular Strength Testing

During active motion testing, it is important to record general muscle strength in shoulder abduction, elbow flexion and extension, and wrist flexion and extension. The strength of the hand intrinsic muscles also should be recorded. Muscle strength grading is imperfect, because the examination is subjective and measures only static muscle strength, but it is important to provide a baseline reference, usually in comparison with the contralateral extremity.

The rotator cuff muscles should be specifically assessed for strength. The Jobe empty can test isolates the supraspinatus muscle. The test is performed with the arm flexed to 90° in the scapular plane and the thumb pointed downward while the examiner applies a downward force. Pain or weakness as the downward pressure is resisted may indicate pathology in the supraspinatus muscle-tendon unit. Resisted external rotation at the side and in 90° of abduction tests the strength of the posterior rotator cuff.

Independent assessment of subscapularis function is critical in a patient with instability, especially a patient with a history of open surgery. In the lift-off test, the patient lifts the hand away from its position over the lumbar spine. The examiner can perform this test as a lag test by passively lifting the hand away from the back and asking the patient to hold the position. An inability to hold the position suggests subscapularis dysfunction. The examination may be difficult if pain in internal rotation prevents the patient from comfortably placing the hand over the lumbar spine. A false-negative test may result if the patient uses the triceps muscle to move the hand away from the back. The belly-press test is used if the patient is unable to perform the liftoff test because of internal rotation contracture. In the belly-press test, the hand is on the abdomen with the wrist in neutral position and the elbow in the plane of the body. If the subscapularis is intact, the patient is able to apply pressure to the abdomen with internal rotation of the shoulder. A patient with subscapularis dysfunction is unable to internally rotate the shoulder and will instead flex the wrist or move the elbow posteriorly to press on the abdomen. The belly-off test is similar, with the examiner passively holding the affected arm at the elbow in slight flexion and internal rotation and using the other hand to passively place the patient's hand onto the abdomen. The examiner instructs the patient to hold the maximally internally rotated position and releases the hand. In a positive test for subscapularis dysfunction, the hand rises off the patient's abdomen when released. The bear-hug test is performed with the arm in 90° of forward flexion. The elbow is flexed and held as far anterior to the body as possible, and the hand is placed on the contralateral shoulder. The examiner attempts to lift the hand away from the shoulder while the patient resists. An electromyographic evaluation study revealed that all portions of the subscapularis are tested when the bear-hug, lift-off, and belly-press tests are used.[6]

Neurovascular Examination

Neurologic injuries are common in a shoulder dislocation, and it is important to document the initial neurologic examination. A 2012 study found a 13.5% incidence of neurologic deficit in 3,633 patients with dislocation.[7] The axillary nerve can be assessed in terms of sensation over the lateral shoulder. Axillary nerve motor function can be tested by resisted shoulder abduction and by watching and feeling the deltoid fire. Although axillary nerve injury is most common after shoulder dislocation, a neurologic examination of the median, ulnar, radial, and musculocutaneous nerves should be documented.

The vascular examination should begin with a simple inspection of the extremity to note skin pallor, trophic skin changes, venous engorgement, or hair loss. Palpation of the radial and ulnar pulses and observation of capillary refill should be compared in the affected and contralateral extremities.

Anterior Instability

Traumatic anterior instability is most common in young athletes, but it does not always occur in isolation. Combined instability patterns therefore are important to discover. The most commonly used test for elucidating anterior instability is the apprehension test, typically performed with the patient seated or supine with the scapula supported by the edge of the bed.[8] The arm is placed in 90° of abduction, and the elbow is flexed and held by the examiner's right hand for a right shoulder examination. The arm is externally rotated, and an anteriorly directed force is applied when the examiner's left thumb presses the posterior aspect of the humeral head. Pain or apprehension with this maneuver is associated with an injury to the anterior labrum. The augmentation test can be applied if anterior instability is suspected despite the patient's equivocal response to the apprehension test. The augmentation test is performed in the same position of apprehension, abduction, and maximal external rotation, with the examiner placing an anteriorly directed force on the proximal humerus. The relocation test is performed with the patient in the same position, with the arm in the position of apprehension; a posteriorly directed force is applied to the proximal humerus, and relief of apprehension or pain is a positive test result.[9] Relief of shoulder pain with the relocation test has been associated with a superior labrum anterior to posterior (SLAP) lesion.

The release (or surprise) test is performed after the relocation test by removing the posteriorly directed force on the proximal humerus.[10] A positive test result is the return of pain and apprehension in the shoulder. The load-and-shift test is the preferred test for determining passive translation of the humeral head on the glenoid. The test can be done with the patient seated or supine and with the arm abducted 20° and held in slight flexion in the plane of the scapula. To examine the right shoulder, the examiner grasps the patient's right forearm with the right hand and applies a compressive force to center the humeral head on the glenoid. The examiner grasps the proximal humerus with the left thumb and index finger around the humeral head and applies an anteriorly directed force. The force then should be applied posteriorly and inferiorly. The load-and-shift translation test is graded based on the amount of humeral head translation, using the modified Hawkins scale: Grade I is minimal translation along the glenoid fossa, grade II is translation to or over the glenoid rim with reduction once the force is removed, and grade III is translation over the glenoid rim that remains dislocated once the force is removed.[11]

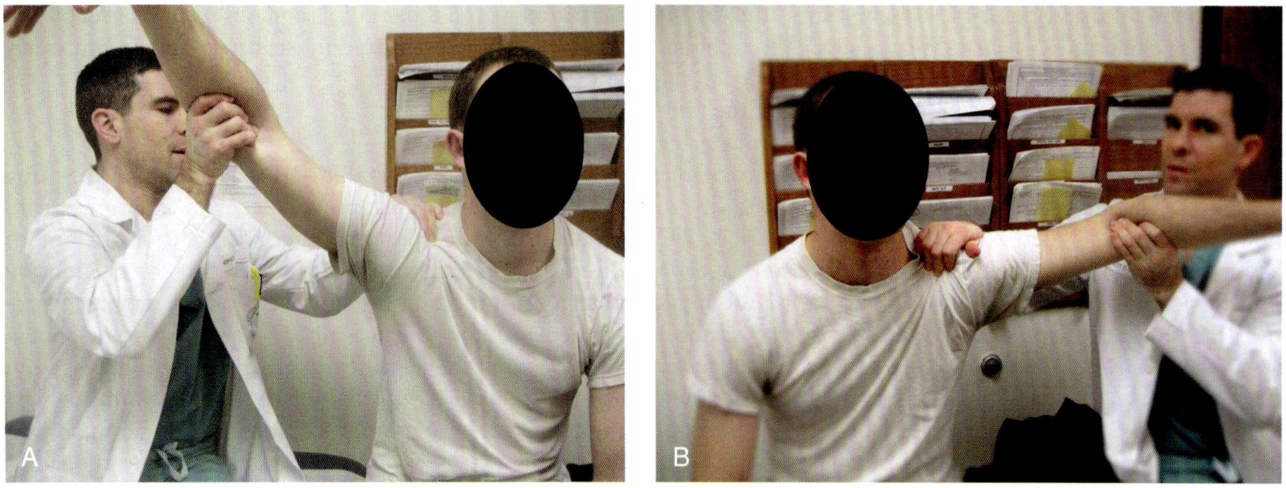

FIGURE 1 Clinical photographs of a 20-year-old man with anterior-inferior instability. A positive Gagey test on the right side (**A**) is compared with the normal left side (**B**). A humeral avulsion of the glenohumeral ligament was detected on MRI.

The Gagey hyperabduction test assesses the integrity of the inferior glenohumeral ligament.[12] The test is performed with the patient seated and the examiner positioned behind the patient. The elbow is positioned at 90°, and the arm is in neutral rotation. One hand of the examiner pushes down on the shoulder girdle, and the other hand lifts the relaxed upper extremity. Passive abduction of more than 105° indicates laxity of the inferior glenohumeral ligament (**Figure 1**). In the initial report of the maneuver, 85% of patients with shoulder instability had passive abduction of more than 105°; abduction was limited by apprehension and pain in the remaining 15% of patients.[12]

Posterior Instability

The posterior load-and-shift test is performed with the patient's arm placed in the plane of the scapula, abducted to 45°, and in neutral rotation. The examiner stands to the side of the seated or supine patient. One hand controls the arm by grasping the elbow and gently loads the humerus into the glenoid while the other hand grasps the humerus near the deltoid insertion and applies a posterior force. The arm is moved into progressive internal rotation to increase the tension of the posterior capsuloligamentous structures and decrease translation. The scoring system is the same as for the load-and-shift translation test. As much as 50% displacement of the humeral head can be considered normal, but the result always should be compared with that of the contralateral shoulder to detect asymmetric increases in translation.

The posterior stress (or posterior apprehension) test is performed with the patient seated or supine; the arm is forward flexed to 90° and maximally internally rotated.[10] The examiner places a posteriorly directed force through the elbow, with the other hand held posterior to the shoulder to palpate a subluxation of the humeral head. The test is positive with palpable subluxation or dislocation, apprehension of a pending dislocation, or pain that reproduces the patient's symptoms. The jerk test is performed with the patient seated on the examination table. The patient's arm is forward flexed to 90° and placed in maximal adduction and internal rotation. The examiner applies a posterior directed force through the elbow. A dislocated or subluxated arm in this position indicates posterior instability. While maintaining the posteriorly directed force, the examiner slowly takes the arm out of adduction; a "clunk" or "jerk" is seen and/or felt as the humeral head reduces into the glenoid. The Kim test is an additional test for posteroinferior instability in which the arm is abducted 90° while the patient is sitting. The examiner then elevates the arm an additional 45°, applying an axial load through the elbow while the examiner's hand on the humerus applies a downward and posterior force. A positive test is indicated by the presence of posterior subluxation with pain.[13]

Inferior and Multidirectional Instability

To quantify inferior laxity, the sulcus sign is elicited with the patient seated and the arms relaxed by the side in neutral rotation. The examiner places a downward distraction force onto the distal humerus while monitoring the lateral acromial edge. Inferior instability allows formation of a sulcus, which can be measured in centimeters, in the deltoid muscle inferior to the lateral acromion. The test is repeated in maximal external rotation, which places the anterior capsule and rotator cuff interval under tension. A sulcus sign that persists in external rotation may indicate incompetence of the rotator cuff interval.

A patient with multidirectional instability may have any of the physical examination findings for instability. Many such patients have signs of ligamentous laxity in multiple joints, including the contralateral shoulder. General articular mobility can be assessed using the Beighton scoring system, in which a score higher than 3 or 4 on a scale of 0 to 9 is associated with general hypermobility in a skeletally mature adult.[14] One point is assigned if the patient is able to perform each of nine maneuvers: metacarpophalangeal hyperextension beyond 90° in the left and/or right small finger, touching of the left and/or right thumb to the volar forearm, hyperextension of the left and/or right elbow more than 10°, hyperextension of the left and/or right knee beyond 10°, and placing of the palms of the hands flat on the floor with the knees fully extended. A score of 4 or higher is associated with a diagnosis of general ligamentous laxity. In addition, a score of 2 or higher is associated with a history of glenohumeral instability.[15]

Biceps and Superior Labrum Anterior to Posterior Lesions

Superior labral detachment may be associated with glenohumeral instability and often is associated with another intra-articular pathology. A comprehensive shoulder evaluation should include testing of the superior labrum. In the active compression test, the examiner stands behind the patient while the patient forward flexes the arm to 90°, adducts the arm 15° across the body, and maximally internally rotates the shoulder to point the thumb toward the floor.[16] The patient resists a downward force applied by the examiner and reports the location of pain. The examination is repeated in maximal supination. Relief of deep pain inside the shoulder when the palm faces upward is a positive test for superior labral pathology. The active compression test has been shown to be the most sensitive test for SLAP lesions (at 47%).[17] Pain on top of the shoulder probably represents acromioclavicular joint pathology or impingement syndrome. The so-called SLAPprehension test also uses traction on the biceps insertion and is performed with cross-chest adduction of the affected shoulder, with the elbow extended and forearm pronated. A positive test result occurs with pain in the bicipital groove, an audible or palpable click, or apprehension. The crank test is performed with the arm elevated to 160° in the scapular plane, axial compression applied by the examiner, and the shoulder passively rotated through full internal and external rotation. This examination is of uncertain usefulness in a patient with previous glenohumeral dislocation because of its similarity to the apprehension position. The anterior slide test is performed with the patient's hands on the hips with the thumbs posterior. The examiner stands behind the patient and places one hand on the patient's superior shoulder and the other hand on the elbow. The examiner places a slightly anterosuperior force on the shoulder to load the biceps anchor.[18] A positive test result consists of pain in the anterior shoulder, a palpable click in the anterior shoulder region, or a reproduction of the symptoms that occur with overhead activities. The anterior slide test has been shown to be the most specific test for an SLAP lesion (at 84%).[17] A patient with an SLAP tear also may have pain with a classic biceps provocation maneuver such as the Speed or Yergason test. In the Speed test, the patient forward flexes the arm with the elbow at 30° of flexion and the forearm supinated. In the Yergason test, the patient performs resisted supination with the elbow flexed to 90°. In both examinations, pain in the bicipital groove is a positive test result.

Imaging

Plain Radiography

Imaging studies are critical for the optimal management of shoulder instability (**Table 1**). The evaluation typically begins with plain orthogonal radiographs. The standard AP and axillary are two typical views of the shoulder useful for evaluating osseous injury or bone loss. The loss of more than 5 mm of the sclerotic subchondral stripe inferiorly on the glenoid on a true AP, or Grashey view, is suggestive of anterior-inferior bone loss.[19] The West Point axillary view can be used to improve the ability to see the anterior-inferior glenoid rim and assess bony avulsions[20] (**Figure 2**). An AP view in internal rotation or a Stryker notch view can improve the ability to see a Hill-Sachs lesion (**Figure 3**). The Bernageau view can facilitate appreciation of glenoid bone loss.[21] A modified Bernageau view can be obtained with the patient lying on the affected shoulder in an abducted position with their head resting on their hand, the so-called TV watching position, and the radiograph beam angled approximately 15° caudally and out of the plane of the contralateral scapula.[22]

Magnetic Resonance Imaging

MRI is indicated for all patients with shoulder instability as the benchmark test to evaluate for the presence and extent of labral injury. The quality of MRI studies can vary among facilities, and indirect or direct gadolinium enhancement may facilitate the assessment of labral and capsular injury patterns as well as capsular volume. The necessity of obtaining MRI as an arthrogram can be debated, but it is the preferred approach of most authors. A Bankart lesion is present in a high proportion of young athletes with traumatic glenohumeral dislocation or subluxation. This pathology often is best seen on axial and

Table 1

Plain Radiographic Views for the Detection of Shoulder Lesions

Shoulder Lesion	Radiographic View(s) for Best Visualization	Imaging Technique
Bony Bankart	West Point axillary	Patient prone with arm abducted to 90° in neutral rotation, cassette placed superior to shoulder, beam directed from axilla with a 25° cephalad tilt (**Figure 2**)
	Bernageau	Patient standing with arm abducted and hand on head, cassette placed over axilla, beam directed at posterior shoulder with a 30° caudal tilt
	Garth	Patient standing, cassette placed behind shoulder, beam directed with a 45° caudal tilt
Glenohumeral dislocation	Axillary lateral	Patient supine with arm abducted, cassette placed superior to shoulder, beam directed into axilla
Hill-Sachs	AP internal rotation	Patient standing or supine with arm internally rotated, cassette placed posterior to shoulder, beam directed posteriorly from front of shoulder
	Garth	Patient standing, cassette placed behind shoulder, beam directed with a 45° caudal tilt
	Stryker notch	Patient supine with hand placed on head and elbow pointing superior, cassette placed posterior to shoulder, beam directed 10° cephalad and aiming at coracoids (**Figure 3**)

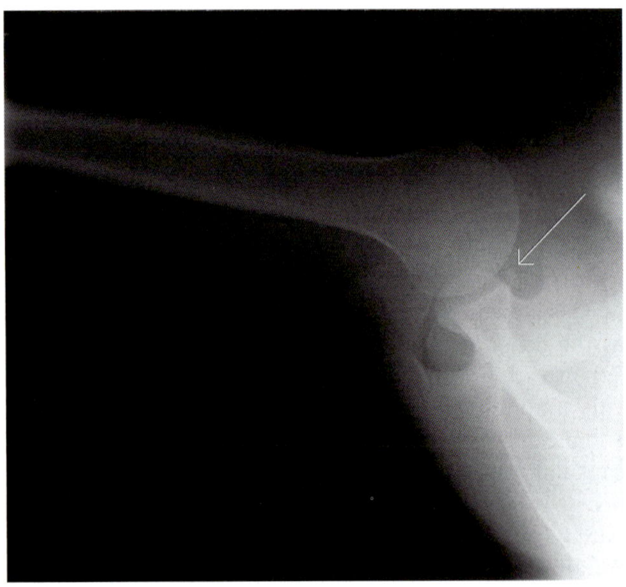

FIGURE 2 A bony Bankart lesion (arrow), as seen on a West Point axillary radiograph.

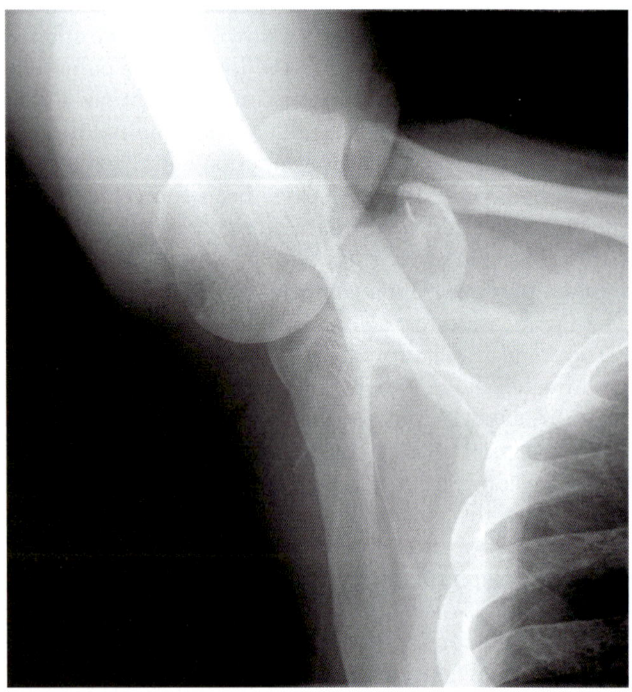

FIGURE 3 A Hill-Sachs lesion, as seen on a Stryker notch radiograph.

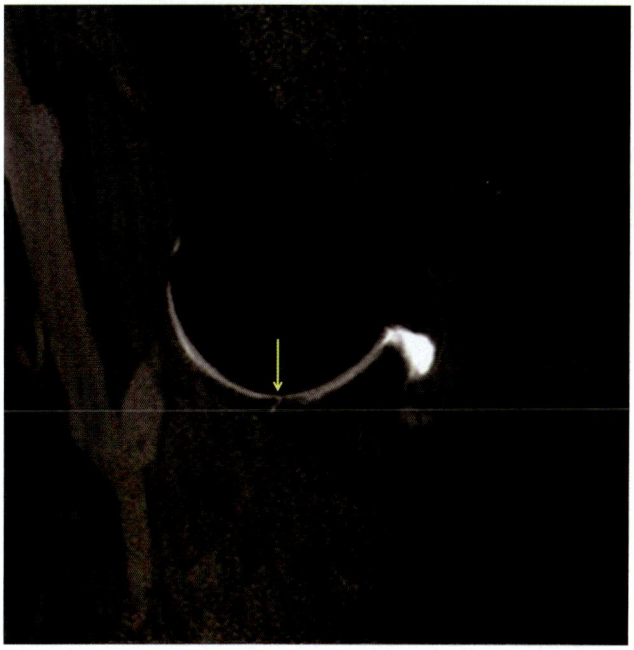

FIGURE 4 Magnetic resonance arthrogram of the shoulder of a 21-year-old collegiate football player with recurrent subluxation events. No labral pathology was noted on axial or coronal views, but a nondisplaced tear in the anterior-inferior labrum (arrow) is visible in the abduction-external rotation view. This finding was corroborated by arthroscopic examination.

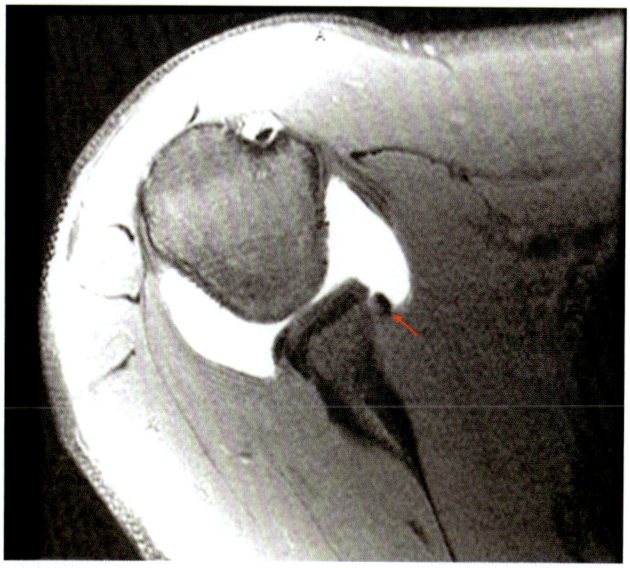

FIGURE 5 Magnetic resonance arthrogram axial cut image with arrow indicating anterior labral periosteal sleeve avulsion (ALPSA) lesion in a patient with recurrent anterior instability.

coronal views but also can be seen in abduction-external rotation views[4,23] (**Figure 4**). MRI can identify an anterior labral periosteal sleeve avulsion (ALPSA) lesion, an injury variant in which the anterior-inferior labrum with an attached periosteal sleeve displaces medially onto the scapular neck (**Figure 5**). This recognition is important as ALPSA lesions have been linked to chronic recurrent instability and inferior outcomes of surgical repair.[24,25] The degree of glenoid bone loss should be assessed carefully when an ALPSA lesion is present, as they have been associated with nearly twice the amount of bone loss compared with Bankart lesions.[26]

A humeral avulsion of the glenohumeral ligament (HAGL) lesion is best seen with gadolinium enhancement and on coronal views (**Figure 6**). HAGL lesions can be difficult to classify based on imaging alone, but it is important to determine whether the anterior or posterior bands of the inferior glenohumeral ligament are intact or torn because this factor can influence the choice of repair technique.[27] HAGL lesions are becoming increasingly identified and have been documented in 25% of young women with instability.[28]

Computed Tomography

Although bone loss can be seen on MRI, most surgeons recommend CT if bone loss is suspected or revision surgery is being considered. The current methods of measuring bone loss incorporate three-dimensional CT reconstruction, with humeral head subtraction for glenoid assessment. The authors of a 2003 study demonstrated the superiority of CT scans over axillary or West Point radiographs for assessing glenoid bone loss.[29] Several subsequent studies have highlighted the accuracy of 3D CT scans for quantification of bone loss, leading to its

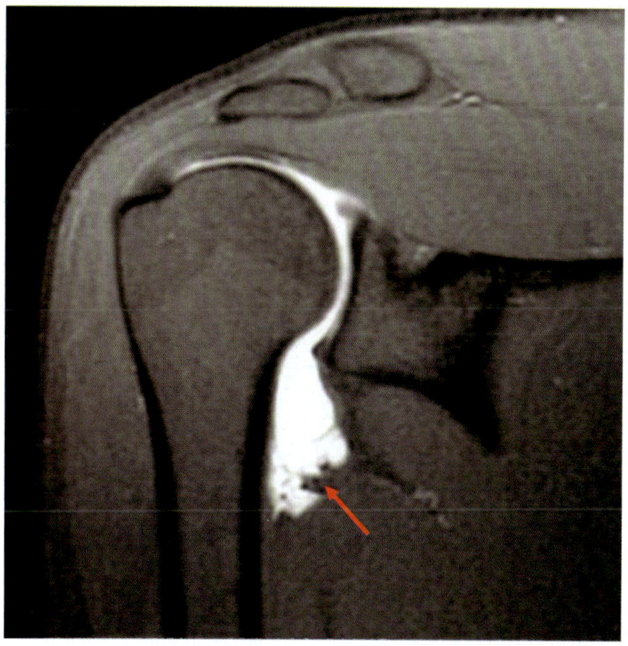

FIGURE 6 Magnetic resonance arthrogram coronal image with arrow indicating humeral avulsion of the glenohumeral ligament (HAGL).

emergence as the benchmark imaging modality.[30,31] The authors of a 2017 study found that 3D reconstructions of both 1.5 and 3 T MRI correlate well to 3D CT scan data and actual defect size in cadaveric models.[32]

Glenoid Bone Loss

Glenoid bone loss increasingly is appreciated as a factor in shoulder instability. The presence of bone loss is associated with a high rate of recurrence after arthroscopic repair alone.[33] Bone loss can be present even in a patient who reports only subluxation events (**Figure 7**). Bone loss may be attritional or involve a bony Bankart lesion. A 2011 study found some level of bone loss in 72% of patients with instability who underwent stabilization, with severe bone loss (more than 20%) in 7.5%.[34] The amount of bone loss that necessitates a bone augmentation procedure is debatable. Traditionally, glenoid bone loss of zero to 15% was felt to be acceptable, while loss of 20% to 30% is considered significant and necessitating a bone augmentation procedure.[35] Recent evaluation of this so-called subcritical bone loss (approximately 13%) suggests that even these small amounts may impact outcomes and recurrence.[36,37] A prospective analysis of first-time anterior instability cohort showed an average of 7% bone loss following initial dislocation or subluxation event.[38]

One challenge of radiographically measuring glenoid bone loss is the absence of clear data as to the normal size of the glenoid. Some researchers recommend comparison imaging of the contralateral shoulder.[39] Glenoid bone loss can be measured on the ipsilateral 3D CT reconstruction en face view by using a best-fit circle overlay.[40] With specialized computer software, researchers were able to digitally establish the area of the defect and to calculate the percentage of loss. Other reported methods of measuring bone loss also involve the use of 3D CT with humeral head subtraction and a superimposed circle over the lower glenoid in the en face view, as shown in **Figure 8**.[35] In one measurement technique, the length of the lesion is directly compared with the radius of the lower glenoid. When the length of the lesion is longer than that of the radius, the resistance to dislocation is less than 70% of that of the intact joint.[41] Another method developed using MRI of both shoulders and the relationship between glenoid height and width produced the following formula for males, $W = 1/3H + 15$ mm, to estimate native glenoid width from MRI of the injured shoulder alone.[42] An overview of a multitude of measurement techniques is provided in **Table 2**.

Neither the optimal method of measurement nor the critical amount of bone loss has been determined. The threshold should be low for obtaining CT to evaluate bone loss preoperatively. If the measured bone loss is more than 20%, the surgeon should consider an alternative

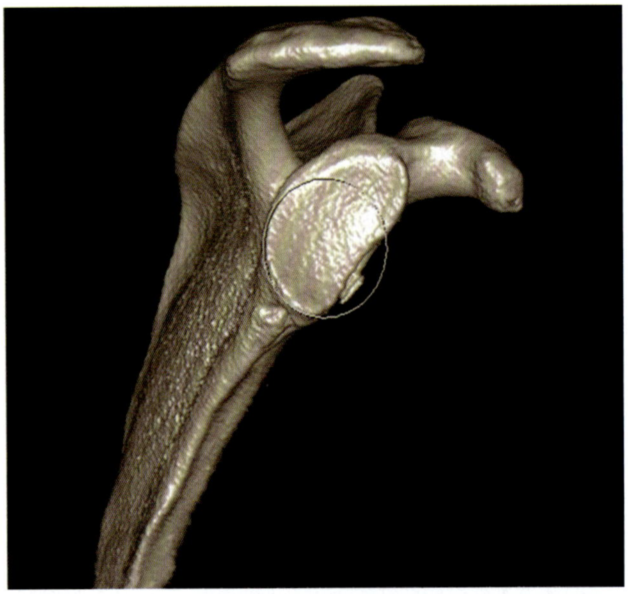

FIGURE 7 Three-dimensional CT reconstruction with the humeral head subtracted (en face view) showing glenoid bone loss (circled) in a 23-year-old patient. The patient had no history of dislocation but reported having experienced many subluxation events.

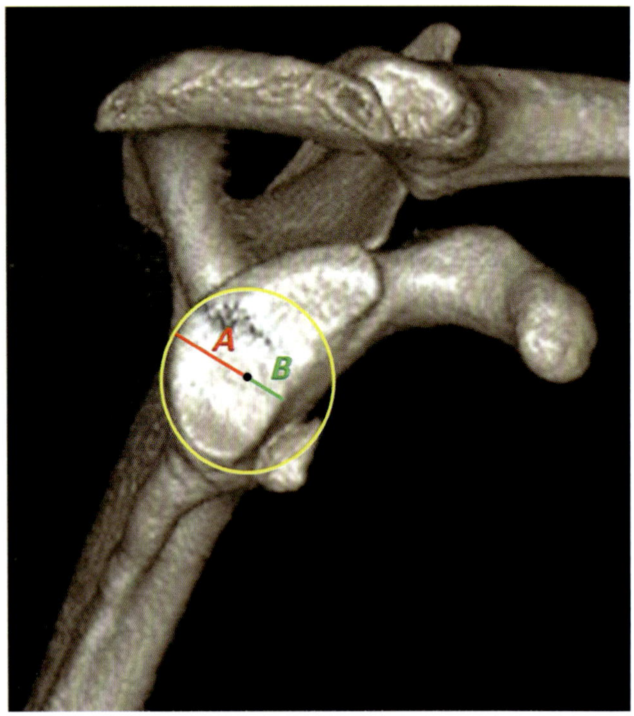

FIGURE 8 Three-dimensional CT reconstruction showing the AP distance method of measuring glenoid bone loss from the bare area (dot) to the edge of defect (*A*) and from the posterior rim to the bare area (*B*). The amount of bone loss is calculated as $(B - A)/2B \times 100\%$.

Table 2

Summary of Radiographic Bone Loss Evaluation

Location	Imaging Method	Measurement Type
Glenoid	CT (two-dimensional sagittal oblique reconstruction or three-dimensional reconstruction en face view of glenoid with humeral head subtraction)	Best-fit circle: Perfect circle is fit to inferior 2/3rd glenoid. Surface area of anterior glenoid defect outlined by circle measured digitally and divided by total circle surface area to obtain percentage
Glenoid	CT (as above)	Ratio method: Percentage calculated from ratio of distance from center of best-fit circle to anterior glenoid and the radius of the circle
Glenoid	CT (three-dimensional reconstruction en face views of both glenoids)	Glenoid index: Ratio of inferior 2/3rd glenoid maximal diameter of injured side compared with uninjured side. Bone block reconstruction recommended for ratio <0.75
Glenoid	CT (two-dimensional CT sagittal oblique en face views of both glenoids)	Pico method: Best-fit circle drawn on uninjured side, with identical circle drawn on injured side and defect size measured as area percentage
Humeral head	Radiographs (AP internal rotation and Bernageau views)	Defect volume = maximum defect width on AP × maximum width on Bernageau × maximum depth on either view
Humeral head	CT	Kodali-maximal H-S defect side selected on axial/sagittal/coronal CT reconstruction, best-fit circle drawn around humeral head, defect dimensions measured in each plane

to an arthroscopic Bankart repair or an augmentative procedure and should counsel the patient about the risk of recurrence.

Humeral Head Bone Loss

Humeral head bone loss can be of concern whether it occurs in isolation (unipolar) or in conjunction with glenoid bone loss (bipolar). The Hall measurement technique remains an excellent way to estimate the percentage of bone loss. Although plain radiographs were originally used for the Hall technique, axial MRI or CT is now used. The angle formed by the defect is measured and divided by the total 180° arc of the articular surface.[43] The Hill-Sachs quotient is another method to quantify humeral bone loss, obtained by multiplying the width by depth by length measurements of the lesion. The authors of a 2012 study described the use of a ratio of humeral defect notch depth to humeral head radius (D/R ratio), finding poor results with a ratio greater than 15% on an AP internal rotation radiograph.[44] Multiple authors have shown good reliability with the use of two-dimensional CT scan to measure width and depth of Hill-Sachs lesions.[45,46] Recently, the authors of a 2018 study demonstrated excellent reliability and moderate accuracy of 3-D CT scans for quantification of Hill-Sachs lesions.[47] In addition to lesion size, the concept of engagement is important. An isolated Hill-Sachs defect as large as 25% may not require treatment if it does not engage.[48,49] An engaging Hill-Sachs lesion comes into contact with the anterior-inferior glenoid during a physiologic range of motion and has been shown to lead to failure of an arthroscopic soft-tissue repair.[33] Although an engaging Hill-Sachs lesion is best appreciated during an arthroscopic examination, radiographic techniques to predict Hill-Sachs engagement have developed, allowing the formulation of a more complete preoperative plan. The authors of a 2013 study utilized CT scans to demonstrate that the location of the medial margin of a Hill-Sachs lesion is more predictive of engagement than the overall lesion width.[50]

The Glenoid Track Concept and Bipolar Bone Loss

The concept of the glenoid track was first described by the authors of a 2007 study.[51] The glenoid track represents the zone of contact between the glenoid and humeral head through an arc of arm abduction to the apprehension position. The authors of a 2007 study, and later those of a 2014 study, calculated the glenoid track to be 84% and 83%, respectively, of the glenoid width.[51,52] The authors of a 2014 study subsequently proposed a treatment algorithm based on the glenoid track concept and whether lesions were considered "on-track" or "off-track" as determined by measurements made on CT scan.[53] The glenoid track serves as an excellent framework by which to consider bipolar bone loss, or bone loss involving both the glenoid and the humeral head. The glenoid track width is narrowed by any anterior-inferior glenoid bone loss. On the humeral side, the Hill-Sachs interval is calculated by measuring the width of the Hill-Sachs lesion from the rotator cuff insertion to the medial margin of the lesion. Based on these measurements, a determination of whether the Hill-Sachs lesion is "off-track" (ie, engaging) or "on-track" can be made. To begin, the glenoid track (GT) width is calculated by subtracting any measured anterior glenoid bone loss (d) from 83% of the intact glenoid diameter D (GT = [0.83D] – d) (**Figure 9**). The Hill-Sachs interval is then measured as described above and compared with the glenoid track. If the HSI is greater than the glenoid track, the lesion is considered "off-track" or engaging as it will contact the anterior glenoid[53] (**Figure 10**).

The clinical significance of this was highlighted in a study by the authors of a 2015 study in which bipolar lesions recreated in cadaveric specimens led to decreased load to translation when small Hill-Sachs lesions were combined with 16% glenoid bone loss and medium lesions were combined with as little as 8% glenoid bone loss despite robust Bankart repairs.[54] Although CT scan remains the most commonly utilized method to assess bipolar bone loss, the authors of a 2015 study demonstrated that MRI can also be used to accurately assess bipolar bone loss utilizing the glenoid track method.[55]

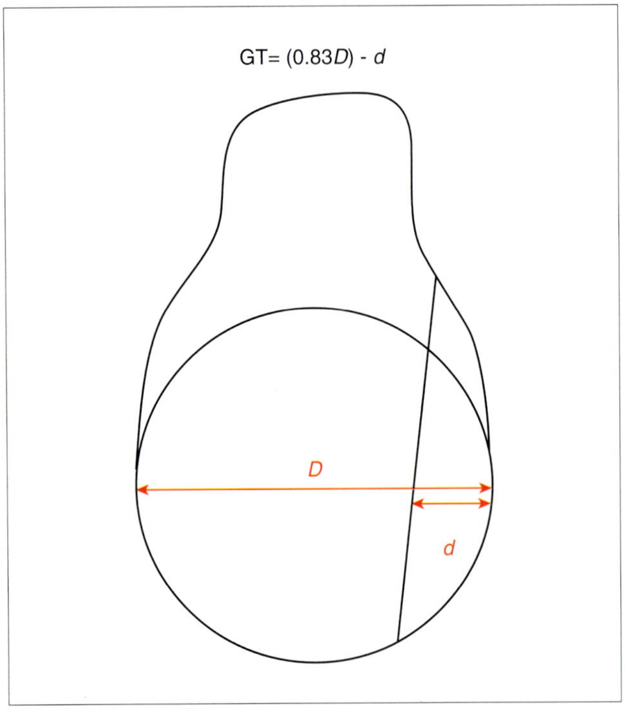

FIGURE 9 Schematic drawing of a glenoid en face view demonstrating the glenoid track calculation, with D measuring the native glenoid diameter and d measuring the anterior glenoid bone loss.

Posterior Instability Imaging

When considering imaging for posterior instability, a few differences should be highlighted. Preoperative imaging should be assessed for glenoid hypoplasia, glenoid bone loss, glenoid retroversion, humeral head defects (reverse Hill-Sachs), and increased humeral head retrotorsion, all of which have been investigated as potential risk factors for posterior shoulder instability. The authors of a 2016 study demonstrated higher mean glenoid retroversion in patients with symptomatic unidirectional posterior instability compared with population normative values, while patients with greater glenoid width measurements had better outcomes following posterior capsulolabral repair[56] (**Figure 11**). In a series of 297 posterior labral repairs, the authors of a 2018 study later found smaller glenoid bone width to be a significant risk factor for revision surgery, while glenoid labral, chondral, and bone version were not risk factors for future revision.[57]

The authors of a 2018 study found that posterior glenoid bone loss is more common than bone loss in anterior-inferior instability, with 69% of their study population having measurable posterior glenoid bone loss and 22% having bone loss greater than the 13.5% subcritical bone loss threshold based on best-fit circle measurement on MRI.[58] A recent cadaver study by Nacca identified 20% posterior glenoid bone loss as a critical defect size, which significantly lowered peak force required for posterior translation despite reverse Bankart repair, suggesting the need for a bony restoration procedure in this scenario.[59]

Classification

Many classification systems for shoulder instability have been proposed, but there is no universally accepted system. Most systems incorporate similar characteristics: direction, the distinction between traumatic and atraumatic instability, and ligamentous laxity.

Direction was among the earliest means of differentiating shoulder instability, with most dislocations classified as anterior. In early research, posterior instability was found to constitute only 4% of all dislocations.[60] Classification by direction has been consistent over time, with a relatively recent prospective cohort study finding that 5% of dislocations in young athletes were posterior in direction.[61] Complete instability events (dislocations) in the posterior direction are rare, but posterior subluxation events are more common, constituting 11% of all subluxation events.[61]

The most commonly used dichotomy in both dislocation and subluxation instability events is related to mechanism of injury. When dislocations were first classified as traumatic or atraumatic, a higher recurrence rate was

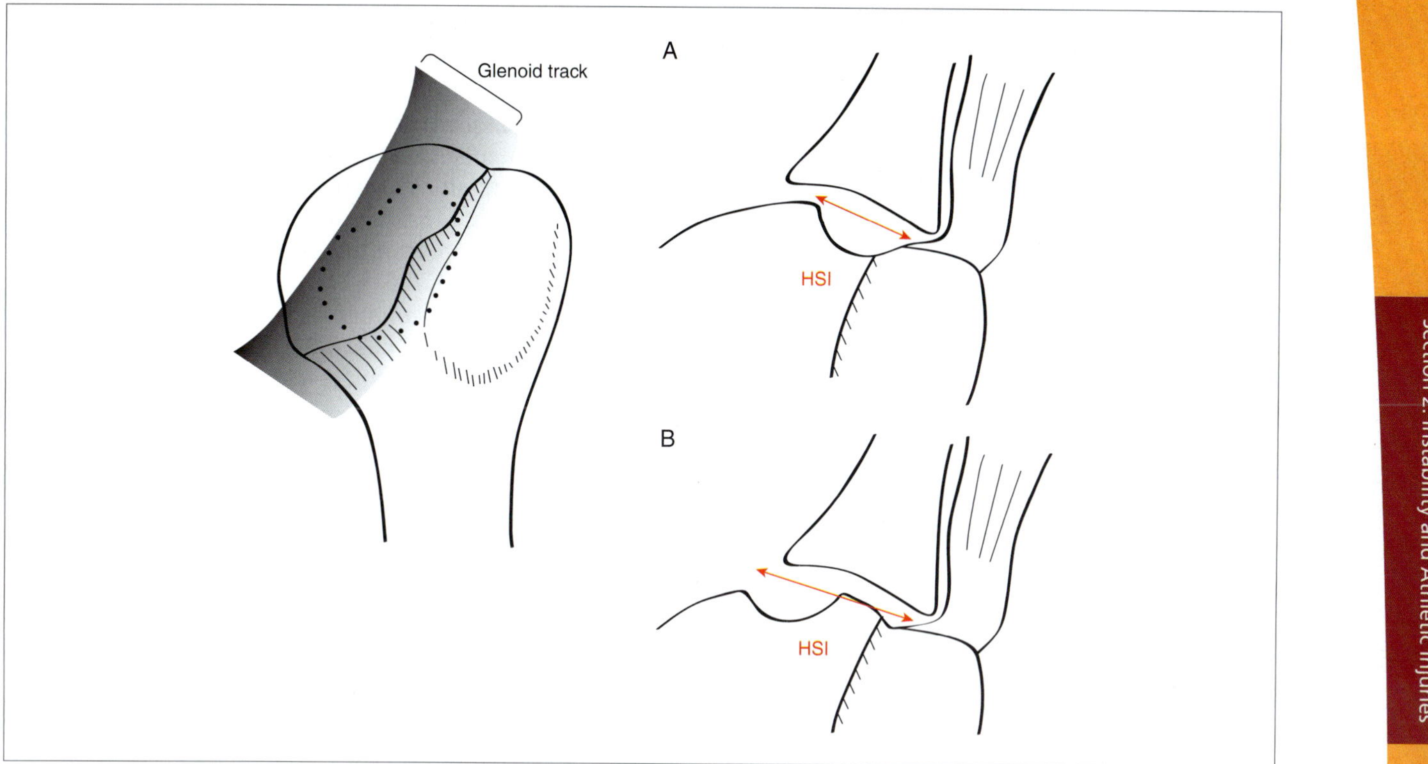

FIGURE 10 Illustrations demonstrating the glenoid track (GT) zone of contact along the humeral head. **A**, An illustration of Hill-Sachs interval (HSI) measurement from the medial margin of the rotator cuff footprint to the medial margin of the Hill-Sachs lesion for an "on-track" lesion (HSI < GT). **B**, Demonstrates the HSI measurement for an "off-track" lesion (HSI > GT). (Adapted from J Shoulder Elbow Surg 16[15]. Yamamoto N, Itoi E, Abe H, et al: Contact between the glenoid and the humeral head in abduction, external rotation, and horizontal extension: a new concept of glenoid track, 649-656. Copyright © 2007 Journal of Shoulder and Elbow Surgery Board of Trustees. doi:10.1016/j.jse.2006.12.012.)

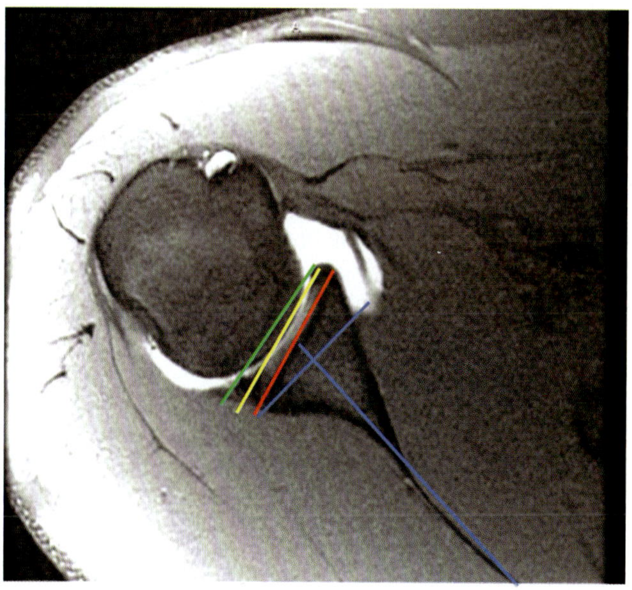

FIGURE 11 Magnetic resonance arthrogram axial image demonstrating the measurement of glenoid version in a patient with symptomatic posterior instability, a posterior labral tear, and glenoid retroversion. The dark blue lines delineate the axis of the scapula and a perpendicular reference line. The red, yellow, and green lines represent measurements of the glenoid bony, chondral, and labral version, respectively.

found in patients with atraumatic dislocation.[62] A classification of subluxations as traumatic, atraumatic, or voluntary found good results when atraumatic or voluntary instability was nonsurgically managed.[63,64] In the most widely used system, two shoulder instability categories broadly define diagnosis and management. Atraumatic, multidirectional, bilateral shoulder instability (the AMBRI category) initially is treated with rehabilitation or an inferior capsular shift. The second broad category (TUBS) includes patients with traumatic dislocation, unilateral direction, and, commonly, a Bankart lesion requiring surgery. The AMBRI and TUBS categories accurately describe two ends of the instability spectrum but not the gradations between them.[65]

Another classification is based on whether shoulder instability is static, dynamic, or voluntary.[41] The static category is subdivided by directionality, and the dynamic category is subdivided based on the presence or absence of ligamentous laxity. A 2010 system takes a scientific approach to the classification of instability.[66] Its four components include frequency within a 1-year period (one, two to five, or more than five occurrences), etiology (traumatic or atraumatic), direction (anterior, inferior, or posterior), and severity (subluxation or dislocation)—FEDS system. This comprehensive FEDS system appears to encompass all possible instability patterns within its 36 possible classes and was shown to be reproducible at one institution.[67]

These classification systems may become important research tools, but they do little to help the surgeon make an appropriate treatment decision. One previous study used published recurrence data for a decision analysis of treatment after an initial anterior dislocation event and may be useful for surgeons in counseling patients on expected risks.[68] The instability severity index score takes several patient variables into consideration, including age, activity level, and pathologic changes, with a score assigned to six specific risk factors. A score of 6 or lower predicts a 10% recurrence risk after arthroscopic stabilization, compared with a 70% recurrence rate in patients with a score of 7 or higher[69] (**Table 3**).

Table 3

The Instability Severity Index Score[a]

Prognostic Factor	Points
Age	
Younger than 20 yr	2
Older than 20 yr	0
Preoperative level of sports participation	
Competitive	2
Recreational or none	0
Preoperative type of sport	
Contact or forced overhead	1
Other	0
Shoulder hyperlaxity	
Anterior or inferior hyperlaxity	1
Normal laxity	0
Hill-Sachs lesion on AP radiograph	
Visible in external rotation	2
Not visible in external rotation	0
Glenoid contour on AP radiograph	
Loss of contour	2
No loss of contour	0
Total	10

[a]Risk of recurrence after arthroscopic repair = 10% if total score is ≤6, 70% if total score is ≥7.

Adapted with permission from British Editorial Society of Bone & Joint Surgery, from Balg F, Boileau P: The instability severity index score: A simple pre-operative score to select patients for arthroscopic or open shoulder stabilization. *J Bone Joint Surg Br* 2007;89(11):1470-1477.

KEY STUDY POINTS

- Patient history should be carefully reviewed for red flags suggestive of glenoid bone loss, such as innumerable instability events, dislocations during sleep, and midrange instability.
- Although MRI remains valuable for evaluating soft-tissue injuries, including Bankart and HAGL lesions, 3D CT has become the test of choice for quantifying glenohumeral bone loss.
- The GT concept has become a useful guide in evaluating anterior shoulder instability and is calculated by subtracting the amount of anterior glenoid bone loss (d) from 83% of the glenoid diameter (D), or GT = $(0.83D) - d$.
- For posterior glenohumeral instability, special attention should be paid to native glenoid width and version, in addition to posterior glenoid bone loss.

SUMMARY

Shoulder instability is common among young athletes. In such patients, shoulder symptoms should be considered to represent instability until proven otherwise. The diagnosis hinges on a combination of a thorough history, a physical examination, and imaging. Plain radiographs and MRI are routinely used to identify the labral and osteochondral lesions commonly seen with both complete dislocation and subluxation events. CT should be obtained if there is any concern about glenoid bone loss, which has been linked to inferior outcomes after arthroscopic soft-tissue stabilization alone. Instability can be classified in many ways, but an understanding of its etiology, direction, severity, and degree of bone loss can be useful in risk stratification and planning of the optimal surgical stabilization technique.

Annotated References

1. Zacchilli MA, Owens BD: Epidemiology of shoulder dislocations presenting to emergency departments in the United States. *J Bone Joint Surg Am* 2010;92(3):542-549.
2. Kaplan LD, Flanigan DC, Norwig J, Jost P, Bradley J: Prevalence and variance of shoulder injuries in elite collegiate football players. *Am J Sports Med* 2005;33(8):1142-1146.
3. Headey J, Brooks JH, Kemp SP: The epidemiology of shoulder injuries in English professional rugby union. *Am J Sports Med* 2007;35(9):1537-1543.

4. Owens BD, Nelson BJ, Duffey ML, et al: Pathoanatomy of first-time, traumatic, anterior glenohumeral subluxation events. *J Bone Joint Surg Am* 2010;92(7):1605-1611.

5. Neer CS II, Foster CR: Inferior capsular shift for involuntary inferior and multidirectional instability of the shoulder: A preliminary report. *J Bone Joint Surg Am* 1980;62(6):897-908.

6. Pennock AT, Pennington WW, Torry MR, et al: The influence of arm and shoulder position on the bearhug, belly-press, and lift-off tests: An electromyographic study. *Am J Sports Med* 2011;39(11):2338-2346.

7. Robinson CM, Shur N, Sharpe T, Ray A, Murray IR: Injuries associated with traumatic anterior glenohumeral dislocations. *J Bone Joint Surg Am* 2012;94(1):18-26.

8. Rowe CR, Zarins B: Recurrent transient subluxation of the shoulder. *J Bone Joint Surg Am* 1981;63(6):863-872.

9. Jobe FW, Kvitne RS, Giangarra CE: Shoulder pain in the overhand or throwing athlete: The relationship of anterior instability and rotator cuff impingement. *Orthop Rev* 1989;18(9):963-975.

10. Silliman JF, Hawkins RJ: Classification and physical diagnosis of instability of the shoulder. *Clin Orthop Relat Res* 1993;291:7-19.

11. McFarland EG, Tanaka MJ, Papp DF: Examination of the shoulder in the overhead and throwing athlete. *Clin Sports Med* 2008;27(4):553-578.

12. Gagey OJ, Gagey N: The hyperabduction test. *J Bone Joint Surg Br* 2001;83(1):69-74.

13. Kim SH, Park JS, Jeong WK, Shin SK: The Kim test: A novel test for posteroinferior labral lesion of the shoulder – A comparison to the Jerk test. *Am J Sports Med* 2005;33(8):1188-1192.

14. Moriatis Wolf J, Cameron KL, Owens BD: Impact of joint laxity and hypermobility on the musculoskeletal system. *J Am Acad Orthop Surg* 2011;19(8):463-471.

15. Cameron KL, Duffey ML, DeBerardino TM, Stoneman PD, Jones CJ, Owens BD: Association of generalized joint hypermobility with a history of glenohumeral joint instability. *J Athl Train* 2010;45(3):253-258.

16. O'Brien SJ, Pagnani MJ, Fealy S, McGlynn SR, Wilson JB: The active compression test: A new and effective test for diagnosing labral tears and acromioclavicular joint abnormality. *Am J Sports Med* 1998;26(5):610-613.

17. McFarland EG, Kim TK, Savino RM: Clinical assessment of three common tests for superior labral anterior-posterior lesions. *Am J Sports Med* 2002;30(6):810-815.

18. Kibler WB, McMullen J: Scapular dyskinesis and its relation to shoulder pain. *J Am Acad Orthop Surg* 2003;11(2):142-151.

19. Jankauskas L, Rudiger HA, Pfirrmann CW, Jost B, Gerber C: Loss of the sclerotic line of the glenoid on anteroposterior radiographs of the shoulder: A diagnostic sign for an osseous defect of the anterior glenoid rim. *J Shoulder Elbow Surg* 2010;19(1):151-156.

20. Rokous JR, Feagin JA, Abbott HG: Modified axillary roentgenogram: A useful adjunct in the diagnosis of recurrent instability of the shoulder. *Clin Orthop Relat Res* 1972;82:84-86.

21. Bernageau J, Patte D, Debeyre J, Ferrane J: Intérêt du profil glénoïdien dans les luxations récidivantes de l'épaule. *Rev Chir Orthop Reparatrice Appar Mot* 1976;62(2 suppl):142-147.

22. Sugaya H: Techniques to evaluate glenoid bone loss. *Curr Rev Musculoskelet Med* 2014;7(1):1-5.

A comprehensive review of glenoid imaging techniques is presented. Level of evidence: V.

23. Taylor DC, Arciero RA: Pathologic changes associated with shoulder dislocations: Arthroscopic and physical examination findings in first-time, traumatic anterior dislocations. *Am J Sports Med* 1997;25(3):306-311.

24. Ozbaydar M, Elhassan B, Diller D, Massimini D, Higgins LD, Warner JJ: Results of arthroscopic capsulolabral repair: Bankart lesion versus anterior labroligamentous periosteal sleeve avulsion lesion. *Arthroscopy* 2008;24(11):1277-1283.

25. Kim DS, Yoon YS, Yi CH: Prevalence comparison of accompanying lesions between primary and recurrent anterior dislocation in the shoulder. *Am J Sports Med* 2010;38(10):2071-2076.

26. Bernhardson AS, Bailey JR, Solomon DJ, Stanley M, Provencher MT: Glenoid bone loss in the setting of an anterior labroligamentous periosteal sleeve avulsion tear. *Am J Sports Med* 2014;42(9):2136-2140.

The authors present a retrospective review of 83 patients with anterior instability: those with an anterior labroligamentous periosteal sleeve avulsion lesion had almost twice the amount of glenoid bone loss and statistically more preoperative instability events. Level of evidence: III.

27. Bui-Mansfield LT, Banks KP, Taylor DC: Humeral avulsion of the glenohumeral ligaments: The HAGL lesion. *Am J Sports Med* 2007;35(11):1960-1966.

28. Patzkowski JC, Dickens JF, Cameron KL, Bokshan SL, Garcia EJ, Owens BD: Pathoanatomy of shoulder instability in collegiate female athletes. *Am J Sports Med* 2019;47(8):1909-1914.

In a retrospective case series of 36 NCAA D1 female athletes undergoing surgical treatment for shoulder instability, soft-tissue Bankart lesions were found at the expected rate (72%), whereas bony Bankart lesions were less common and combined anterior-posterior labral tears and humeral avulsions of the glenohumeral ligament were more common than previously reported. Level of evidence: IV.

29. Itoi E, Lee SB, Amrami KK, Wenger DE, An KN: Quantitative assessment of classic anteroinferior bony Bankart lesions by radiography and computed tomography. *Am J Sports Med* 2003;31(1):112-118.

30. Rerko MA, Pan X, Donaldson C, Jones GL, Bishop JY: Comparison of various imaging techniques to quantify glenoid bone loss in shoulder instability. *J Shoulder Elbow Surg* 2013;22:528-534.

    The authors performed an imaging study in which four blinded independent evaluators estimated glenoid bone loss from radiographs, MRI, CT, and three-dimensional CT of seven cadaver shoulders with varying degrees of glenoid bone loss. Three-dimensional CT was the most accurate modality. Level of evidence: III.

31. Bishop JY, Jones GL, Rerko MA, Donaldson C, MOON Shoulder Group: 3-D CT is the most reliable imaging modality when quantifying glenoid bone loss. *Clin Orthop Relat Res* 2013;471:1251-1256.

    The authors performed an imaging study in which 12 blinded independent evaluators estimated glenoid bone loss from radiographs, MRI, CT, and three-dimensional CT of 7 cadaver shoulders with varying degrees of glenoid bone loss. Three-dimensional CT was the most reliable modality. Standard CT was the second most reliable and reproducible modality. Level of evidence: III.

32. Yanke AB, Shin JJ, Pearson ID, et al: Three-dimensional magnetic resonance imaging quantification of glenoid bone loss is equivalent to 3-dimensional computed tomography quantification: Cadaveric study. *Arthroscopy* 2017;33(4):709-715.

    The authors performed an imaging study in which evaluators measured glenoid bone loss from CT, 1.5T MRI, 3T MRI, and three-dimensional (3D) MRI of six cadaver shoulders with varying degrees of glenoid bone loss. The 1.5T- and 3T-based 3D MRI measurements correlated well with 3D CT and actual defect size measurements. Level of evidence: III.

33. Burkhart SS, De Beer JF: Traumatic glenohumeral bone defects and their relationship to failure of arthroscopic Bankart repairs: Significance of the inverted pear glenoid and the humeral engaging Hill-Sachs lesion. *Arthroscopy* 2000;16(7):677-694.

34. Milano G, Grasso A, Russo A, et al: Analysis of risk factors for glenoid bone defect in anterior shoulder instability. *Am J Sports Med* 2011;39(9):1870-1876.

35. Piasecki DP, Verma NN, Romeo AA, Levine WN, Bach BR Jr, Provencher MT: Glenoid bone deficiency in recurrent anterior shoulder instability: Diagnosis and management. *J Am Acad Orthop Surg* 2009;17(8):482-493.

36. Shaha JS, Cook JB, Song DJ, et al: Redefining "critical" bone loss in shoulder instability: Functional outcomes worsen with "subcritical" bone loss. *Am J Sports Med* 2015;43(7):1719-1725.

    A consecutive series of 72 patients with anterior instability treated with arthroscopic isolated Bankart repair were divided into quartiles based on glenoid bone loss and evaluated for recurrence rates and Western Ontario Shoulder Instability Index scores: bone loss above 13.5% led to a clinically significant decrease in these scores even in the absence of recurrent dislocation. Level of evidence: III.

37. Dickens JF, Owens BD, Cameron KL, et al: The effect of subcritical bone loss and exposure on recurrent instability after arthroscopic bankart repair in intercollegiate American football. *Am J Sports Med* 2017;45(8):1769-1775.

    In a consecutive series of 50 intercollegiate football players undergoing primary arthroscopic stabilization of anterior shoulder instability evaluated for return to sport and recurrent instability, all 3 shoulders with >13.5% glenoid bone loss experienced recurrent instability while none of the 47 shoulders with <13.5% bone loss did. Level of evidence: III.

38. Dickens JF, Slaven SE, Cameron KL, et al: Prospective evaluation of glenoid bone loss after first-time and recurrent anterior glenohumeral instability events. *Am J Sports Med* 2019;47(5):1082-1089.

    A prospective cohort of 714 athletes was followed for shoulder instability events over 4 years. Glenoid bone loss averaging 6.8% was observed after a first-time anterior instability event, whereas in recurrent instability events the total calculated glenoid bone loss was 22.8% with a high prevalence of bony Bankart lesions. Level of evidence: II.

39. Baudi P, Righi P, Bolognesi D, et al: How to identify and calculate glenoid bone deficit. *Chir Organi Mov* 2005;90(2):145-152.

40. Sugaya H, Moriishi J, Dohi M, Kon Y, Tsuchiya A: Glenoid rim morphology in recurrent anterior glenohumeral instability. *J Bone Joint Surg Am* 2003;85(5):878-884.

41. Gerber C, Nyffeler RW: Classification of glenohumeral joint instability. *Clin Orthop Relat Res* 2002;400:65-76.

42. Owens BD, Burns TC, Campbell SE, Svoboda SJ, Cameron KL: Simple method of glenoid bone loss calculation using ipsilateral magnetic resonance imaging. *Am J Sports Med* 2013;41(3):622-624.

    The authors performed a cross-sectional study in which MRI studies of 1,264 shoulders were evaluated and measured to calculate a formula for estimating glenoid width based on glenoid height and patient sex. Level of evidence: III.

43. Hall RH, Isaac F, Booth CR: Dislocations of the shoulder with special reference to accompanying small fractures. *J Bone Joint Surg Am* 1959;41(3):489-494.

44. Hardy P, Lopes R, Bauer T, Conso C, Gaudin P, Sanghavi S: New quantitative measurement of the Hill–Sachs lesion: A prognostic factor for clinical results of arthroscopic glenohumeral stabilization. *Eur J Orthop Surg Traumatol* 2012;22(7):541-547.

45. Kodali P, Jones M, Polster J, Miniaci A, Fening S: Accuracy of measurement of Hill-Sachs lesions with computed tomography. *J Shoulder Elbow Surg* 2011;20(8):1328-1334.

46. Cho SH, Cho NS, Rhee YG: Preoperative analysis of the Hill-Sachs lesion in anterior shoulder instability: How to predict engagement of the lesion. *Am J Sports Med* 2011;39(11):2389-2395.

47. Ho A, Kurdziel MD, Koueiter DM, Wiater JM: Three-dimensional computed tomography measurement accuracy of varying Hill–Sachs lesion size. *J Shoulder Elbow Surg* 2018;27:350-356.

   An imaging study evaluating reliability of CT and three-dimensional CT in determining Hill-Sachs lesion size on 9 humeral head models measured by 6 evaluators showed that three-dimensional CT is effective and reproducible in determining lesion size. Level of evidence: III.

48. Sekiya JK, Jolly J, Debski RE: The effect of a Hill-Sachs defect on glenohumeral translations, in situ capsular forces, and bony contact forces. *Am J Sports Med* 2012;40(2):388-394.

49. Skendzel JG, Sekiya JK: Diagnosis and management of humeral head bone loss in shoulder instability. *Am J Sports Med* 2012;40(11):2633-2644.

50. Kurokawa D, Yamamoto N, Nagamoto H, et al: The prevalence of a large Hill-Sachs lesion that needs to be treated. *J Shoulder Elbow Surg* 2013;22(9):1285-1289.

   The authors evaluated a consecutive series of 100 patients with unilateral recurrent anterior shoulder dislocations with CT and found a 7% incidence of engaging Hill-Sachs lesions. Level of evidence: III.

51. Yamamoto N, Itoi E, Abe H, et al: Contact between the glenoid and the humeral head in abduction, external rotation, and horizontal extension: A new concept of glenoid track. *J Shoulder Elbow Surg* 2007;16(5):649-656.

52. Omori Y, Yamamoto N, Koishi H, et al: Measurement of the glenoid track in vivo as investigated by 3-dimensional motion analysis using open MRI. *Am J Sports Med* 2014;42(6):1290-1295.

   In this descriptive laboratory study, the existence and widths of the glenoid track were confirmed in vivo using three-dimensional motion analysis created from MRI scans of 30 right shoulders of healthy volunteers.

53. Di Giacomo G, Itoi E, Burkhart SS: Evolving concept of bipolar bone loss and the Hill-Sachs lesion: From "engaging/non-engaging" lesion to "on-track/off-track" lesion. *Arthroscopy* 2014;30(1):90-98.

   The authors present a description of the glenoid track concept to determine whether a Hill-Sachs lesion will engage (off track) or not (on track). Level of evidence: V.

54. Arciero RA, Parrino A, Bernhardson AS, et al: The effect of a combined glenoid and Hill-Sachs defect on glenohumeral stability: A biomechanical cadaveric study using 3-dimensional modeling of 142 patients. *Am J Sports Med* 2015;43(6):1422-1429.

   In this controlled laboratory study, 21 cadaver shoulders were tested in varying combinations of glenoid bone loss and Hill-Sachs lesion size with and without soft-tissue Bankart repair. Combined glenoid and humeral head defects demonstrated an additive and negative effect on glenohumeral stability. As little as a 2-mm glenoid defect with a medium-sized Hill-Sachs lesion demonstrated a compromise in soft-tissue Bankart repair, whereas small-sized Hill-Sachs lesions showed compromise of soft-tissue repair with ≥4-mm glenoid bone loss.

55. Gyftopoulos S, Beltran LS, Bookman J, Rokito A: MRI evaluation of bipolar bone loss using the on-track off-track method: A feasibility study. *AJR Am J Roentgenol* 2015;205(4):848-852.

   Two blinded independent evaluators assessed the MRI studies of 75 patients with anterior instability and used the glenoid track concept to predict Hill-Sachs lesion engagement with a sensitivity of 72.2% and a specificity of 87.9%. Level of evidence: III

56. Mauro CS, McClincy MP, Bradley JP: Effect of glenoid version and width on outcomes of arthroscopic posterior shoulder stabilization. *Am J Sports Med* 2016;44(4):941-947.

   The authors reviewed 118 magnetic resonance arthrograms of athletes with unidirectional recurrent posterior shoulder instability treated with an arthroscopic posterior capsulolabral repair and measured for glenoid labral, chondral, and bone version as well as labral and bone width. Higher glenoid retroversion was noted in this population but it did not affect outcome. Increased glenoid width correlated with better outcome. Level of evidence: III.

57. Bradley JP, Arner JW, Jayakumar S, Vyas D: Risk factors and outcomes of revision arthroscopic posterior shoulder capsulolabral repair. *Am J Sports Med* 2018;46(10):2457-2465.

   A retrospective review of 297 shoulders after arthroscopic posterior labral repair at minimum 2-year follow-up is presented. Revision rate was 6.4% and these patients experienced poorer outcomes and return to sport. Risk factors included dominant arm, female sex, concomitant rotator cuff injury, three or fewer anchors, and smaller glenoid. Level of evidence: III.

58. Hines A, Cook JB, Shaha JS, et al: Glenoid bone loss in posterior shoulder instability: Prevalence and outcomes in arthroscopic treatment. *Am J Sports Med* 2018;46(5):1053-1057.

A retrospective review of 43 consecutive patients undergoing arthroscopic isolated posterior labral repair with posterior bone loss determined by preoperative MRI is presented. Posterior glenoid bone loss was present in 69%, and 22% had posterior glenoid bone loss >13.5%. Level of evidence: III.

59. Nacca C, Gil JA, Badida R, Crisco JJ, Owens BD: Critical glenoid bone loss in posterior shoulder instability. *Am J Sports Med* 2018;46(5):1058-1063.

In this controlled laboratory study, 11 cadaver shoulders with various conditions of the posterior labrum and posterior glenoid bone loss were tested. Shoulders with posterior glenoid bone loss of 20% or greater remained unstable after isolated posterior labral repair.

60. McLaughlin HL, MacLellan DI: Recurrent anterior dislocation of the shoulder: II. A comparative study. *J Trauma* 1967;7(2):191-201.

61. Owens BD, Duffey ML, Nelson BJ, DeBerardino TM, Taylor DC, Mountcastle SB: The incidence and characteristics of shoulder instability at the United States Military Academy. *Am J Sports Med* 2007;35(7):1168-1173.

62. Rowe CR: Prognosis in dislocations of the shoulder. *J Bone Joint Surg Am* 1956;38-A(5):957-977.

63. Rockwood CA Jr: Subluxation of the shoulder: The classification, diagnosis, and treatment. *Orthop Trans* 1979;3:306.

64. Burkhead WZ Jr, Rockwood CA Jr: Treatment of instability of the shoulder with an exercise program. *J Bone Joint Surg Am* 1992;74(6):890-896.

65. Thomas SC, Matsen FA III: An approach to the repair of avulsion of the glenohumeral ligaments in the management of traumatic anterior glenohumeral instability. *J Bone Joint Surg Am* 1989;71(4):506-513.

66. Kuhn JE: A new classification system for shoulder instability. *Br J Sports Med* 2010;44(5):341-346.

67. Kuhn JE, Helmer TT, Dunn WR, Throckmorton VTW: Development and reliability testing of the frequency, etiology, direction, and severity (FEDS) system for classifying glenohumeral instability. *J Shoulder Elbow Surg* 2011;20(4):548-556.

68. Mather RC III, Orlando LA, Henderson RA, Lawrence JT, Taylor DC: A predictive model of shoulder instability after a first-time anterior shoulder dislocation. *J Shoulder Elbow Surg* 2011;20(2):259-266.

69. Balg F, Boileau P: The instability severity index score: A simple pre-operative score to select patients for arthroscopic or open shoulder stabilisation. *J Bone Joint Surg Br* 2007;89(11):1470-1477.

Chapter 6

Management Decisions for Acute Versus Chronic Shoulder Instability

Rolando Izquierdo, MD • Geoffrey S. Van Thiel, MD, MBA • Scott Trenhaile, MD • CAPT Matthew T. Provencher, MD, MC, USNR • Anthony Romeo, MD

ABSTRACT

Shoulder instability is both common and complex. There are many imaging studies, physical examination findings, and surgical techniques to address the problem; however, recurrence rates remain relatively high. The direction of instability, soft-tissue and bony lesions, and whether pathology is unipolar or bipolar (humeral side, glenoid, or both) are critical in management decisions. The ultimate goal of surgical intervention is to restore glenohumeral stability by addressing soft-tissue and bony deficiencies and reduce the risk of recurrence.

Keywords: glenohumeral bone loss; glenohumeral instability; labral tear; shoulder dislocation; shoulder instability

Introduction

The incidence of shoulder instability in the United States is approximately 23.9 per 100,000 people.[1] More than 90% of traumatic dislocations occur in the anterior inferior direction,[2] and the recurrence rate can approach 90% in young patients.[3–5] Male gender and age younger than 29 years are the most important risk factors for injury.

History, clinical examination, and imaging studies are critical for accurate diagnosis in both acute and chronic instability. The default diagnosis in patients younger than 25 years with glenohumeral symptoms should be instability until proven otherwise. The direction of instability, soft-tissue and bony lesions, and

Dr. Izquierdo or an immediate family member has received royalties from Lima Corporate; serves as a paid consultant to or is an employee of Lima; has stock or stock options held in Catalyst; and serves as a board member, owner, officer, or committee member of the American Shoulder and Elbow Surgeons. Dr. Van Thiel or an immediate family member has received royalties from Zimmer; is a member of a speakers' bureau or has made paid presentations on behalf of Smith & Nephew, Vericel, and Zimmer; serves as a paid consultant to or is an employee of Smith & Nephew, Trainer Rx, Vericel, and Zimmer; and has stock or stock options held in Trainer Rx. Dr. Trenhaile or an immediate family member has received royalties from Smith & Nephew; is a member of a speakers' bureau or has made paid presentations on behalf of Exactech, Inc., Lake Effect Medical, and Smith & Nephew; serves as a paid consultant to or is an employee of Exactech, Inc., Lake Effect Medical, MinInvasive Ltd, Smith & Nephew, and Xiro, Inc.; has stock or stock options held in Smith & Nephew; has received research or institutional support from OrthoSpace and Smith & Nephew; and serves as a board member, owner, officer, or committee member of the Arthroscopy Association of North America. Dr. Provencher or an immediate family member has received royalties from Arthrex, Inc.; is a member of a speakers' bureau or has made paid presentations on behalf of Arthrex, Inc.; serves as a paid consultant to or is an employee of Arthrex, Inc. and Joint Restoration Foundation (Allosource); and serves as a board member, owner, officer, or committee member of the American Academy of Orthopaedic Surgeons, the American Orthopaedic Society for Sports Medicine, the American Shoulder and Elbow Surgeons, the Arthroscopy Association of North America, the International Society of Arthroscopy, Knee Surgery, and Orthopaedic Sports Medicine, the San Diego Shoulder Institute, and the Society of Military Orthopaedic Surgeons. Dr. Romeo or an immediate family member has received royalties from Arthrex, Inc.; is a member of a speakers' bureau or has made paid presentations on behalf of Arthrex, Inc.; serves as a paid consultant to or is an employee of Arthrex, Inc.; has stock or stock options held in Paragen Technologies, Columbus, OH; has received research or institutional support from Arthrex, Inc., Paragen Technologies; has received nonincome support (such as equipment or services), commercially derived honoraria, or other non–research-related funding (such as paid travel) from AANA, Arthrex, Inc., and MLB; and serves as a board member, owner, officer, or committee member of the American Shoulder and Elbow Surgeons and the Orthopedics Today.

This chapter is adapted from Van Thiel GS, Heard W, Romeo AA, Provencher MT: Acute and chronic shoulder dislocations, in Nicholson GP, ed: *Orthopaedic Knowledge Update: Shoulder and Elbow*, ed 4. Rosemont, IL, American Academy of Orthopaedic Surgeons, 2013, pp 77-91.

whether pathology is unipolar or bipolar (humeral side, glenoid, or both) are critical in management decisions (**Figure 1**).

The ultimate goal of surgical intervention is to restore glenohumeral stability by addressing soft-tissue and bony deficiencies and reduce the risk of recurrence.

Acute Anterior Instability

Anterior dislocation is the most common form of glenohumeral instability. The essential lesion of traumatic anterior dislocation was described as the disruption of the anterior inferior glenohumeral ligament by detachment of

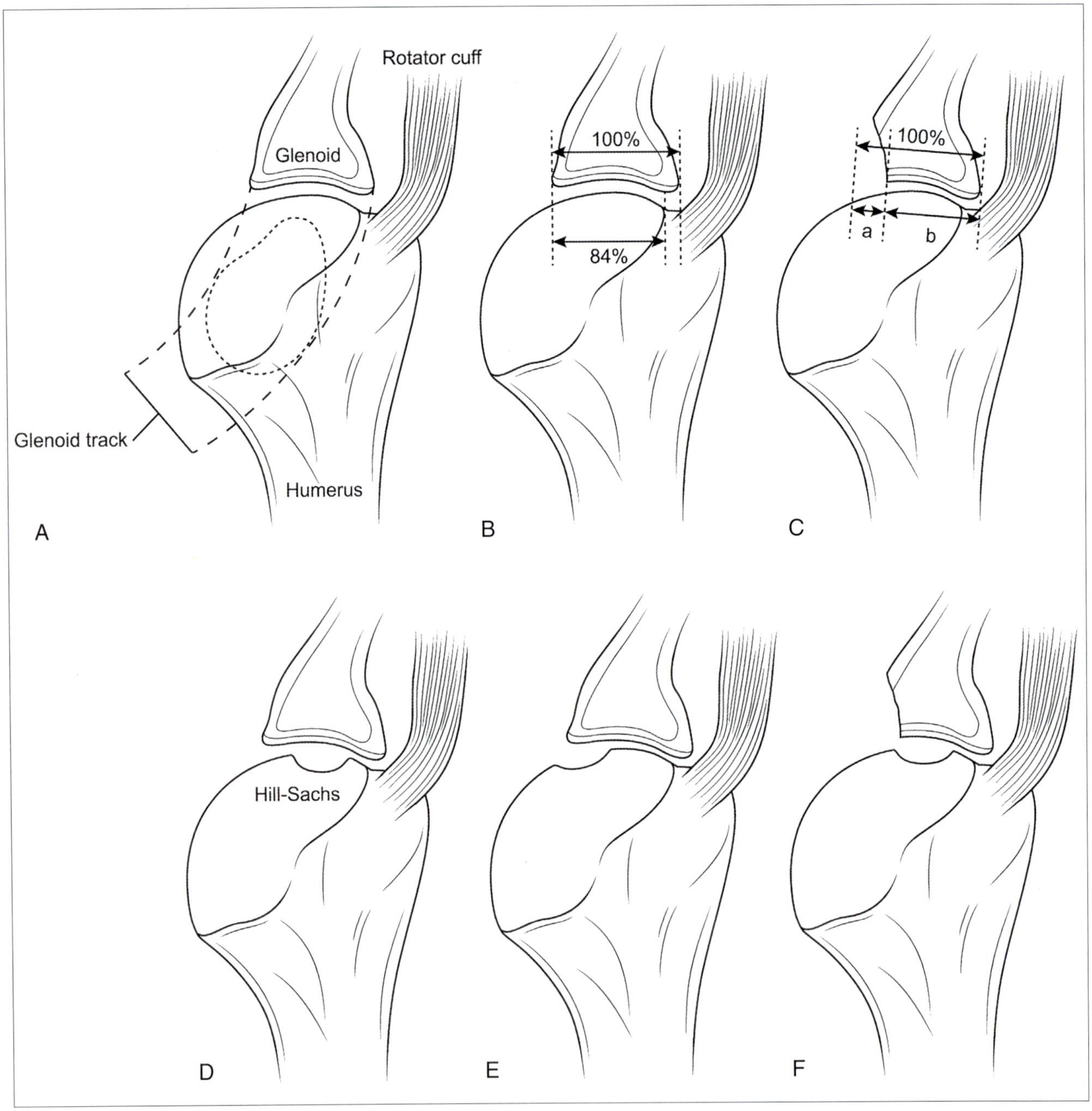

FIGURE 1 Illustrations depicting the glenoid track concept. In external rotation and abduction (**A**), the glenoid displaces the rotator cuff tendon, creating a glenoid track of approximately 84% of the glenoid width (**B**). In the presence of a glenoid rim defect, the defect width is subtracted from the 84% to estimate the actual glenoid track width (**C**). A Hill-Sachs lesion may be contained within the glenoid track and therefore considered an on-track lesion (**D**), or it may be large or medial enough to cause the humeral head to engage the glenoid in an off-track manner (**E**). An otherwise stable humeral lesion may become unstable in the presence of glenoid bone loss (**F**).[6] (Reprinted with permission from Willemot LB, Elhassan BT, Verborgt O: Bony Reconstruction of the Anterior Glenoid Rim. *JAAOS* 2018; 26[10]:e207-e218. © American Academy of Orthopaedic Surgeons. doi:10.5435/JAAOS-D-16-00649.)

its insertion at the glenoid labrum.[7] Once the diagnosis of anterior instability is confirmed by history, physical examination, and imaging studies, the primary goal is to achieve early stability with a reduction, and sling immobilization for comfort followed by early mobilization. Immobilization in external rotation was initially thought to reduce the risk of recurrence. However, a follow-up Level I study in 2011 failed to support this theory.[8]

A rotator cuff tear was identified in 49% of patients older than 60 years following anterior dislocation.[9] This may be a posterior superior rotator cuff tear, greater tuberosity fracture, or a subscapularis avulsion.

During clinical assessment, the status of the axillary nerve must be confirmed. The extension lag sign may be helpful in confirming deltoid function. Imaging studies including radiographic evaluation, MRI (with or without arthrogram component), and CT scan may be necessary to appropriately assess soft-tissue and bony pathology.

In-season dislocations can be treated conservatively. An in-season athlete with no significant bony deficiency on radiographic studies may return to sport in a shoulder brace restricting abduction and external rotation once they regain functional range of motion and symmetric strength. If necessary, surgical stabilization can be performed in the off-season. If the athlete continues to have episodes of instability during return to play with the brace, early surgical stabilization should be considered.

The authors of a 2017 study looked at 83 NFL players who had sustained an in-season shoulder instability event. Seventy-two players sustained a dislocation injury and 11 had subluxation. In those treated nonsurgically, return to play occurred on average at 0 weeks following subluxation and 3 weeks following dislocation. Regardless of treatment, 93% of the NFL players were able to return to play. Twenty-six players (31%) were treated surgically after the index instability event and 57 players (69%) were treated nonsurgically. However, 46% of those who returned to play experienced a recurrent instability event. There was a 26.1% recurrence rate in the surgical group versus 54.6% in the nonsurgical cohort. Players treated surgically were less likely to sustain an instability event and played for a longer interval before recurrence of instability.[10] The authors of a 2019 study[11] further supported the concept that athletes can return in a short period after an instability event. However, they noted that those with a subluxation compared with a dislocation were three times less likely to experience a recurrence.

The recurrence rate of anterior instability is high without surgical management.[3-5] A 25-year follow-up study on nonsurgical management of anterior shoulder instability reported a recurrence rate of 72% in patients between the ages of 12 to 22 years, 56% in patients between 23 and 29 years, and 27% in patients aged 30 years or older.[12] A prospective study comparing arthroscopic and nonsurgical management of acute anterior shoulder dislocations in young patients confirmed better outcomes after surgical treatment. The rate of recurrent instability in the nonsurgical group was 94.5% within the first 18 months.[13]

The most common surgical technique to manage anterior shoulder instability is an arthroscopic Bankart repair (anterior inferior labrum). **Figure 2, A** and **B** shows an anterior bony Bankart with a repair. The techniques for arthroscopic Bankart repair have evolved over time with short-term recurrence rate of 8% to 11%.[14] Long-term failure recurrence rates range between 23% and 35%.[15,16] The authors of a 2019 study reported a 22% recurrence

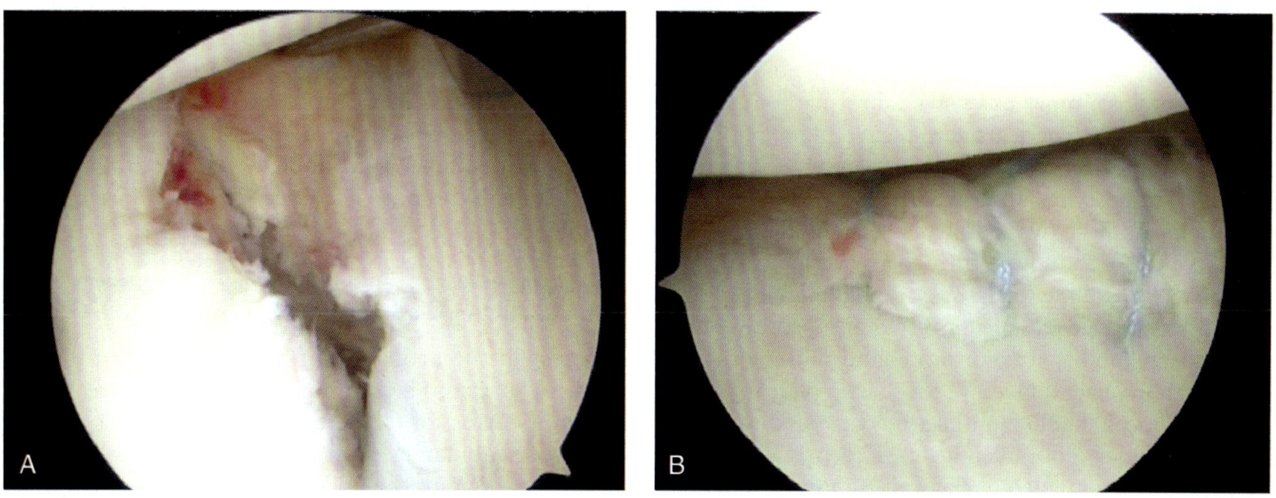

FIGURE 2 **A**, Arthroscopic view showing bony bankart of the anterior shoulder. **B**, Arthroscopic view showing repair of the bony Bankart.

rate in 122 patients treated with arthroscopic Bankart repair (knotless anchors) with an average follow-up of 6.3 years. Interestingly, 64% of the failures occurred in the first 2 years.[17]

In 2017, a meta-analysis comparing open versus arthroscopic stabilization for anterior shoulder dislocations divided outcomes between two separate decades. In studies published between 1995 and 2004, the recurrence rate favored open surgery. However, in studies published between 2005 and 2015, there were no significant differences in recurrence rates when comparing open and arthroscopic techniques. Despite advancements in arthroscopic techniques during the last 20 years, the recurrence rate has only marginally decreased from 16.8% to 14.2%. The author acknowledges the continued difficulty of defining recurrence in the published literature. Some studies consider only recurrent dislocations as failures and exclude subluxations and a positive clinical examination.[14,18]

In a 2017 study, the long-term outcomes following open Bankart repair were published. This included 127 patients with average follow-up of 17.1 years following open Bankart repair using suture anchors. There was one recurrent dislocation (0.8%) and one recurrent subluxation (0.8%). There was a statistically significant difference in external rotation in abduction and internal rotation when compared with the normal shoulder. However, patients did not complain of functional loss. Ninety-one patients underwent radiographic assessment and 48 had normal findings. Thirty-four had mild arthrosis and nine had moderate arthrosis of the glenohumeral joint. The mean ASES score was 93.53 and 125 patients were satisfied and would elect to have the procedure again.[19] **Figure 3** provides a management diagram.

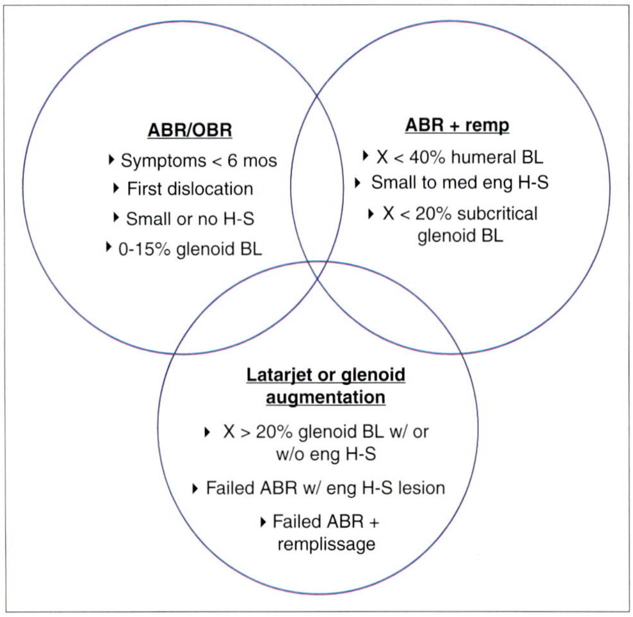

FIGURE 3 Diagram for the management of shoulder instability. ABR = arthroscopic Bankart repair, BL = bone loss, eng = engaging, H-S = Hill-Sachs lesion, med = medium, OBR = open Bankart repair, remp = remplissage

Recurrent Anterior Instability

Recent evidence suggests an increase in glenoid and humeral bone loss, more extensive labral pathology, and capsular injuries in patients with recurrent instability. In a 2015 study, an increase in bipolar bone lesions from 33% with primary instability to 61.8% in shoulders with recurrent instability was confirmed.[20-22] In addition, the authors of a 2018 study confirmed an overall recurrence rate of 18.8% following arthroscopic Bankart repair.[23] They divided their patients into two groups: those with recurrent instability (two or more) and those with only one instability event. Overall, those who were managed surgically more than 6 months after the first dislocation were 5.62 times more likely to have recurrent instability than those managed in the first 6 months. Furthermore, patients who experienced two or more dislocations before surgical intervention were 8.77 times more likely to have a recurrent episode of instability. Ultimately, patients who present with two preoperative dislocations and a duration of instability symptoms of more than 6 months as well as an off-track Hill-Sachs lesion may not be ideal candidates for arthroscopic instability repair. Perhaps delaying surgery after the first dislocation is not the ideal approach and earlier surgical intervention should be considered.[24]

We have learned historically that certain pathologic changes occur in the glenohumeral joint after instability events. As patients have more episodes of instability, there is an increase in number and size of bony Bankart lesions with more attritional glenoid bone loss and development of an inverted pear glenoid.[21,25-27] There is also increased prevalence of Hill-Sachs defects (HSDs) with higher likelihood of having an engaging or off-track Hill-Sachs lesion[21,23,28,29] and more bipolar lesions.[19]

Humeral Head Lesions (Hill-Sachs)

A defect in the articular surface of the humeral head (Hill-Sachs lesion) is common in patients with recurrent instability. Most of the defects are small and do not require surgical management. The HSD occurs as the soft cancellous bone of the posterior superior humeral head engages the hard, cortical bone of the anterior inferior glenoid during an anterior dislocation. A HSD that engages the anterior inferior glenoid rim with abduction and external rotation is referred to as an engaging Hill-Sachs lesion or off-track lesion. This is significant because an engaging or off-track lesion will increase the likelihood of failure if only a glenoid-based soft-tissue procedure is performed.[21,30]

In small or moderate size on-track Hill-Sachs lesions with no substantial glenoid bone loss, managing the anterior soft tissues is probably sufficient. In a larger (greater than 30%)[31] or engaging Hill-Sachs lesion without glenoid bone loss, addressing the anterior glenoid–based soft-tissue injury (Bankart lesion) as well the humeral head defect itself is critical. Several options exist to address the humeral head defect including autograft or allograft, remplissage, disimpaction of the fracture, and prosthetic replacement.

An open transfer of the infraspinatus with a portion of the greater tuberosity into the humeral head defect has been described. This technique converted an intra-articular lesion into extra-articular lesion.[32] An arthroscopic posterior capsulodesis and infraspinatus tenodesis into the humeral head defect has also been described.[33] This has been termed remplissage, which is French for filling. This procedure successfully converts a bony intra-articular defect into an extra-articular defect using soft-tissue coverage with the goal of preventing engagement. There have been concerns of loss of external rotation following remplissage because of a potential soft-tissue mechanical block.[34]

A systematic review was performed to assess the recurrence rate of instability after remplissage (**Figure 4, A** and **B**) in patients with subcritical glenoid bone loss. There were 22 studies that met the inclusion criteria, which included 694 patients with a mean age of 28 years and mean follow-up of 32.5 months. The overall recurrence rate of instability ranged from zero to 20%. There was a negligible loss of external rotation in both abduction and adduction when compared with an isolated arthroscopic Bankart repair. Glenoid bone loss ranged from 5.4% to 16.4% and the reported humeral bone loss ranged from 6.8% to 45.8%. A total of six patients required revision to Latarjet. The author suggests that arthroscopic labral repair and remplissage for engaging Hill-Sachs lesion measuring between 20% and 40% in volume with subcritical glenoid bone loss reduces the odds of re-dislocation compared with isolated Bankart repair.[35]

The amount of glenoid bone loss that warrants a bone augmentation is debatable. There is a consensus that zero to 15% of glenoid bone loss is acceptable, but a loss of >20% is significant and a bone augmentation procedure is recommended.[27,36,37]

Glenoid Deficiency and Bony Augmentation

Glenohumeral instability in the presence of glenoid bone loss is difficult to manage and important to recognize. The stability of the glenohumeral joint changes as the amount of glenoid bone loss approaches 15% to 20% of the articular surface.[36,37] Current techniques for managing anterior glenoid bone deficiency include coracoid transfer (Latarjet, Bristow), fresh distal tibia osteochondral allograft, and iliac crest autograft.[38–40]

In the published clinical outcomes of a prospective cohort of 118 patients with recurrent anterior instability treated with a Bristow-Latarjet procedure at a mean 15.2-year follow-up, re-dislocation occurred in 3.4% of patients and subluxation in 10%.[41] In another study the results of 319 shoulders following Bristow-Latarjet were reported.[42] The procedure yielded consistently good results with bony fusion in 83%. The authors noted

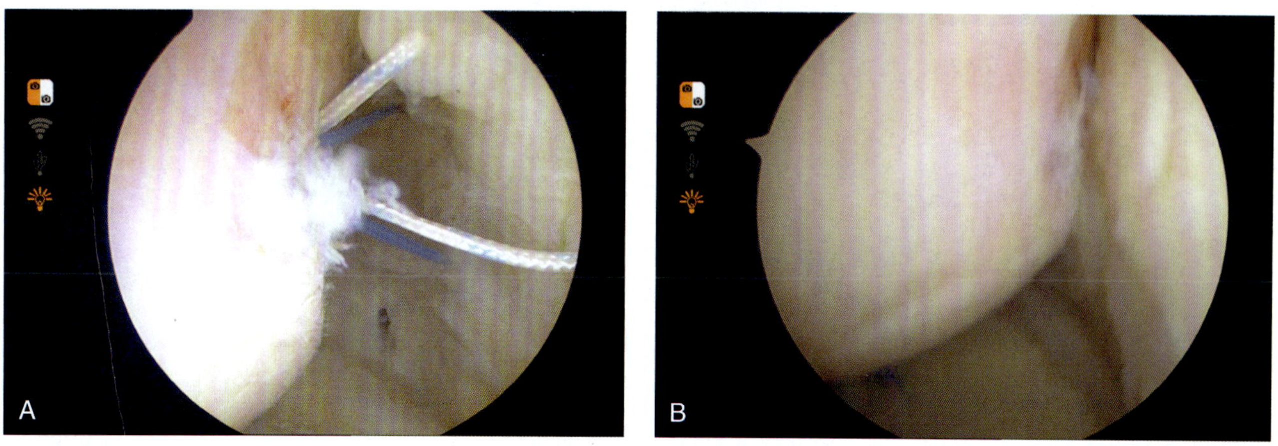

FIGURE 4 **A**, Arthroscopic view showing Hill-Sachs lesion with an anchor placed into the defect. **B**, Arthroscopic view showing repair of the posterior cuff into the defect to create a remplissage.

recurrent instability was more likely if the coracoid graft was placed >1 cm or more medial to the rim. The addition of a horizontal capsular shift improved the recurrence rate and subjective results. Although not statistically significant, glenohumeral arthropathy occurred more frequently in patients whose grafts were placed at or lateral to the glenoid rim.[40]

Historically, the Latarjet procedure has been considered a good option to manage glenoid deficiency with a recurrent dislocation rate of zero to 8% and recurrent subluxation rate of 2% to 15%.[42] **Figure 5, A through E** illustrates the procedure for a Latarjet procedure. The results of the Latarjet procedure versus iliac crest bone graft for the treatment of anterior instability with glenoid bone loss were compared in a level I prospective, randomized, controlled study with 30 patients in each group. All patients were followed up for 2 years showing no significant difference in recurrence, validated scores, or radiologic outcomes when comparing both groups. The iliac crest bone graft group had a 26.7% rate of sensory disturbance around the donor site. There was a statistically significant difference of internal rotation reported when comparing both groups. The average Latarjet internal rotation was T9 compared with T7 for the iliac crest bone graft cohort. Range of motion was otherwise comparable in both groups. There were no recurrent dislocations in either group. There was one reported subluxation in the Latarjet group and two in the bone graft group.[43]

There remains a role for the open capsular shift.[44] This procedure may be helpful in patients with a large humeral avulsion of the glenohumeral ligament (HAGL) that cannot be addressed arthroscopically, patients in whom arthroscopic Bankart repairs have failed with less than 15% glenoid bone loss, and patients with multidirectional instability in whom arthroscopic stabilization had failed.

Acute Posterior Instability

Traumatic posterior shoulder dislocation was first described by Sir Astley Cooper in 1838.[45] Traumatic posterior instability accounts for 2% to 5% of all shoulder dislocations.[46,47] Seizures, high-energy trauma, and electrocutions are associated with posterior instability. The diagnosis is missed or delayed in up to 79% of patients.[46-48] Routine use of axillary images or Velpeau axillary views may reduce the delay in diagnosis. The clinician should have a high index of suspicion for posterior dislocation when there is overlap of the humeral head and the glenoid on the AP image or lightbulb sign. CT scan can confirm the diagnosis.

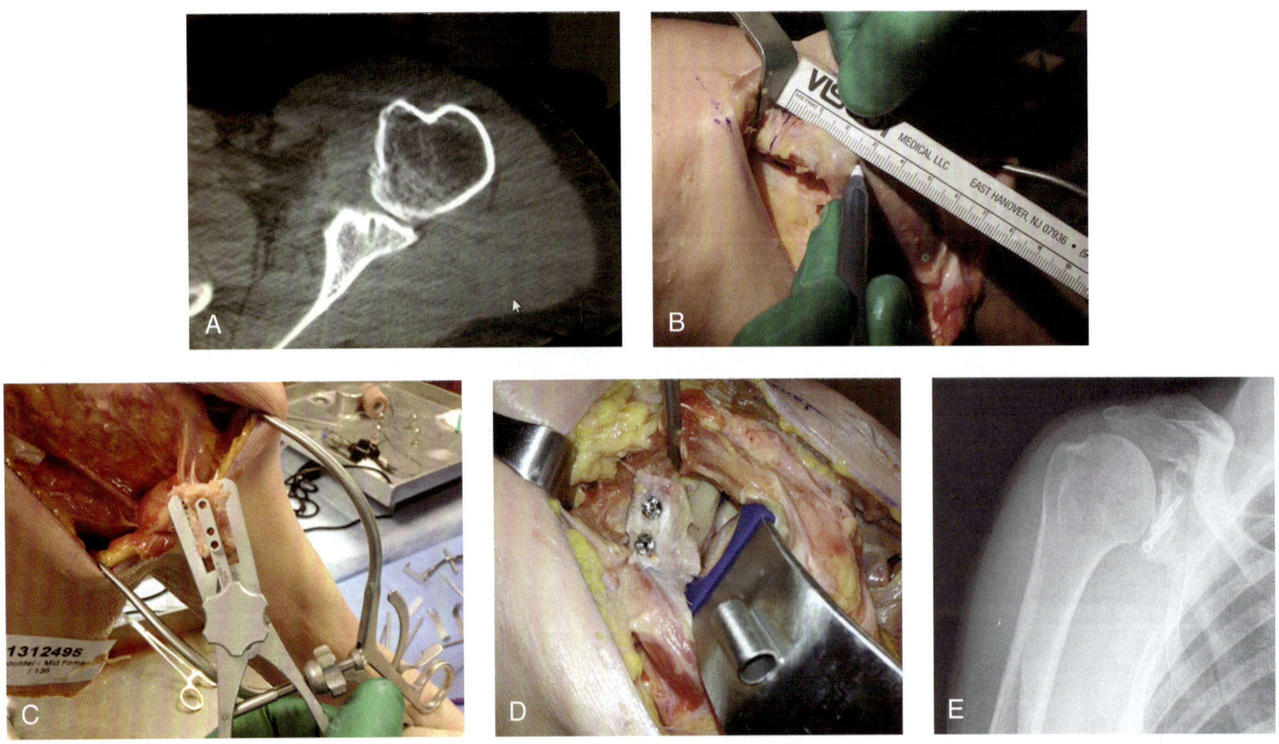

FIGURE 5 **A,** CT scan showing glenoid bone deficiency. **B,** Intraoperative photograph showing coracoid graft for a Latarjet. **C,** Intraoperative photograph showing preparation of the coracoid graft. **D,** Intraoperative photograph showing placement and fixation of the coracoid graft on the anterior glenoid. **E,** AP radiograph showing the screw fixation of the graft.

Closed reduction can be attempted in the setting of an acute dislocation with reverse Hill-Sachs lesion measuring <20%. Recurrent posterior instability and failed closed reduction are both indications for surgical intervention. Management considerations depend on humeral and glenoid bone loss. Reverse Hills-Sachs lesions or humeral bone loss is substantially more common than glenoid bone loss in posterior instability (**Figures 6** and 7).

In a literature review on arthroscopic and posterior shoulder dislocation, 26 open studies and 27 arthroscopic studies published between 1946 and 2014 were analyzed. The analysis consisted of 321 patients treated with an open procedure and 817 patients treated with an arthroscopic procedure. The recurrence rate in the open group was 19.4% ± 4.1%. The average recurrence rate in the arthroscopic group was 8.1% ± 3.8%. Based on current, best available clinical evidence, the preference is an arthroscopic stabilization in patients with <20% humeral or glenoid bone loss.[49]

Currently, there is a paucity of literature to guide practioners in the setting of posterior glenoid bone loss. There is a plethora of data on recognizing and treating anterior glenoid bone loss and the consequences of unrecognized and untreated bony deficiency. Using data from the anterior instability group, it is reasonable to consider patients with >20% glenoid bone loss may benefit from bony augmentation. Posterior bony augmentation can be autograft or allograft. More commonly, humeral defects can affect treatment decisions in posterior instability.

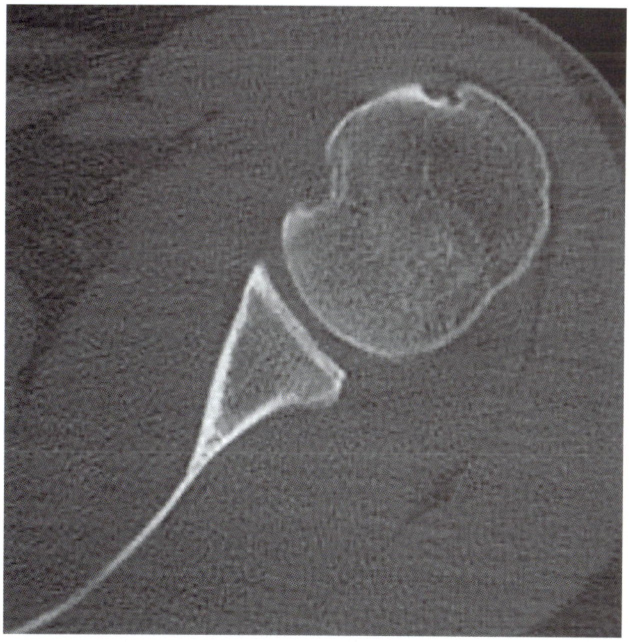

FIGURE 6 CT scan showing reverse Hill-Sachs lesion.

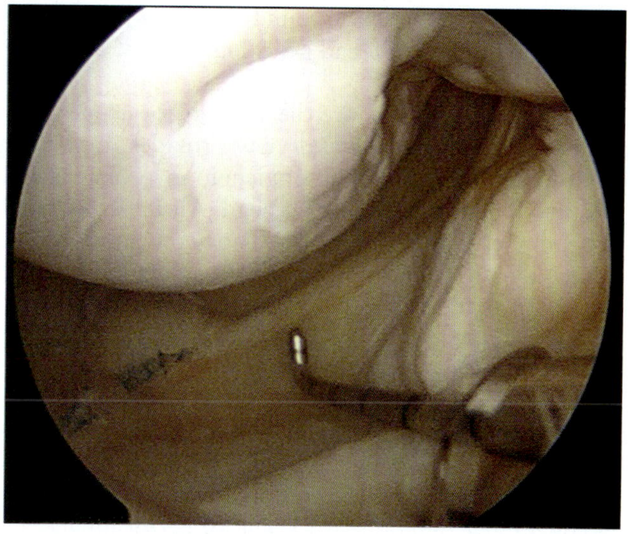

FIGURE 7 Arthroscopic view showing reverse Hill-Sachs lesion.

Patients with reverse Hill-Sachs lesions >20% can be treated with arthroscopic labral repair and a modified McLaughlin procedure (lesser tuberosity osteotomy and transfer into defect) (**Figure 8**). Lesions with a humeral head lesion of >40% may require allograft reconstruction or consideration of arthroplasty options.

Chronic Dislocation

Researchers have used different time points to define chronic dislocation, ranging from 24 hours to 6 weeks. The recommended definition is 3 weeks after initial dislocation.[50] Unrecognized glenohumeral dislocation leading to chronic dislocation is relatively uncommon. A review

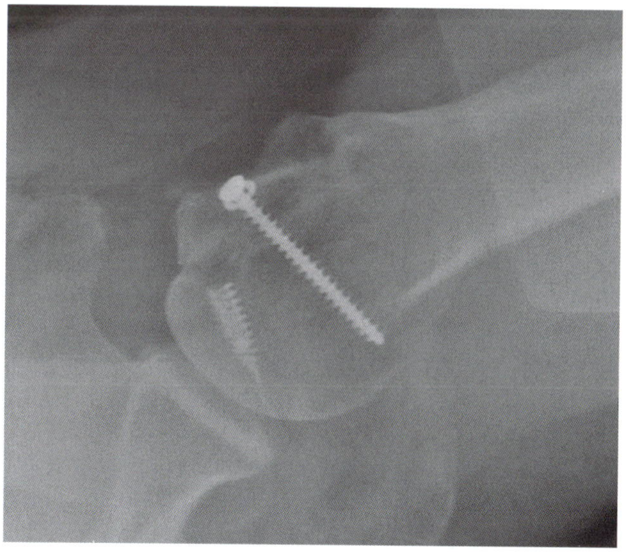

FIGURE 8 Postoperative radiograph following lesser tuberosity transfer into osseous defect of the humeral head.

of 61 chronic dislocations found that 50% had an associated fracture, 33% had neurologic injury, and 28% were posterior.[51]

The imaging studies are the same as for acute dislocations. The axillary lateral view provides important information on the amount of glenoid involvement and any impaction of the humeral head. All images should be examined to detect fracture. If osseous involvement is detected, CT is recommended to evaluate the amount and location of bony destruction.

Management

Despite the anatomic deformity and severe loss of glenohumeral rotation, a chronic posterior dislocation can be surprisingly well tolerated, especially in a patient who is older than 70 years or debilitated. Such a patient may regain a range of motion sufficient for performing activities of daily living with minimal pain. It is important to balance the surgical morbidity with the expected outcomes. Nonsurgical management should be considered for a patient who has uncontrolled seizures, a patient who will be unable or unwilling to undergo postoperative rehabilitation, or a patient who is free of pain and has low functional demands. For these patients, the risks of surgery exceed the potential benefit of an improved outcome (**Figure 9**).

Closed Reduction

Closed reduction can be done if the dislocation is less than 3 weeks old, the humeral head impaction is less than 25%, and there are no other humeral fractures. In one study, reduction was successful in 19 of 30 dislocations no more than 4 weeks old, but it was successful only in 1 of 10 dislocations older than 4 weeks.[51]

Surgical Options

Disimpaction and bone grafting of the humeral head defect can be considered if the patient has a relatively acute injury, less than 50% humeral head involvement, and viable articular cartilage.[52] The procedure requires an access window for elevation of the articular segment and support with autograft or allograft.

Transfer of the subscapularis tendon, which leaves the subscapularis attached to its lesser tuberosity insertion, can be considered if the patient has a relatively small humeral defect (less than 40%).[53] Allograft reconstruction is the preferred method of treating a defect in a viable humeral head, especially in a relatively young patient. A size-matched fresh-frozen humeral or femoral head allograft is required for the reconstruction. Good outcomes were reported at a mean 54-month follow-up in 13 patients with a defect of 25% to 50%.[52]

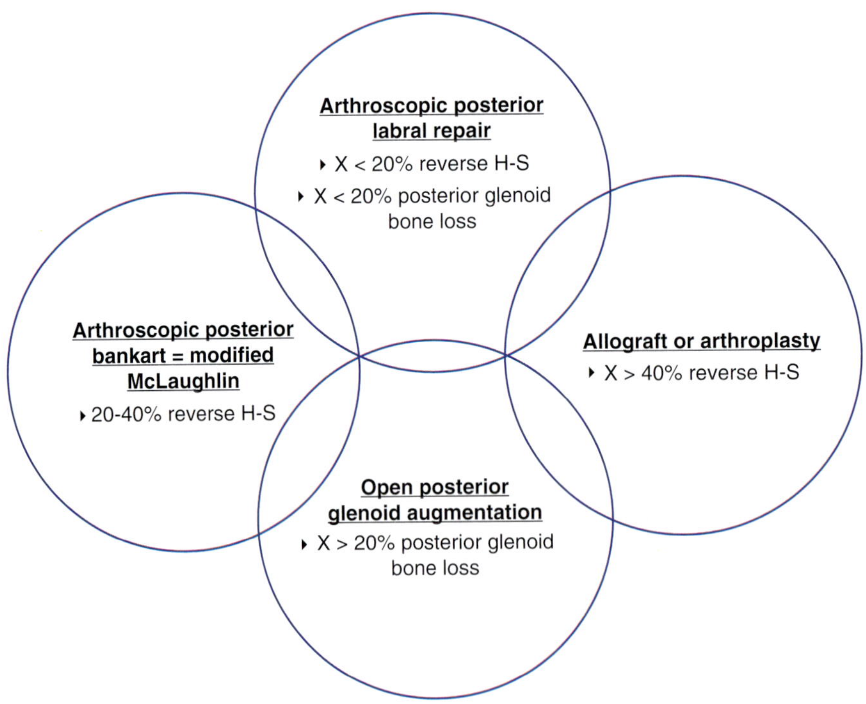

FIGURE 9 Diagram for the management of posterior instability. H-S = Hill-Sachs lesion

The indications for shoulder arthroplasty include a defect of more than 50% of the humeral head, severe articular damage, and significant osteopenia. The choice among hemiarthroplasty, total shoulder arthroplasty, and surface replacement can be difficult and must be made on a case-by-case basis. A study of 12 shoulders with a chronic locked posterior dislocation managed with shoulder arthroplasty found that 11 patients had improved range of motion after surgery but with an average Constant shoulder score of 59.4.[54]

As with a posterior dislocation, several factors influence the indications for surgery in chronic anterior dislocation, including the presence of a bone defect. In contrast to posterior dislocations, in which the glenoid commonly maintains its structural integrity, a chronic anterior dislocation often is associated with anterior-inferior glenoid bone loss. An acute fracture can occur at the time of the dislocation, or progressive attritional bone loss can occur later. The anterior capsular structures often are torn, and reattachment is required to achieve a stable shoulder.

Surgical Management

The neurovascular structures must be carefully evaluated during any surgical approach for a chronic anterior dislocation. Often these structures are adhering to the scar tissue, making the dissection difficult. The axillary nerve should be identified and protected, and a vascular surgeon should be available in case axillary artery injury develops. As for a chronic posterior dislocation, multiple treatment options are available.

Labral repair almost always is a focus in managing an acute anterior dislocation and can be an important component in managing a chronic anterior dislocation. Unreduced chronic shoulder dislocations with a Hill-Sachs lesion of less than 40% were evaluated in eight patients with an average of 10 weeks after the injury.[55] All patients were treated with open reduction and labral repair using transglenoid suturing. At final follow-up, the average Rowe-Zarin score was 86, and the average losses in forward flexion and external rotation were 18° and 17.5°, respectively. A similar case report completed the same repair arthroscopically with good results reported.[6]

Similar to acute anterior instability, if in the chronic setting the glenoid bone loss is less than 20%, a Bankart repair can be completed, with or without bony augmentation. However, a bony augmentation should be used if the glenoid bone loss is greater than 20%. An autograft, allograft, or coracoid transfer can be used.[56]

A lesion involving less than 25% of the humeral head often does not require treatment after reduction, if the shoulder remains stable. A defect larger than 25% should be treated, however. Disimpaction of the defect can be considered if the lesion is smaller than 50%, the articular cartilage remains viable, and the bone stock is good. If the articular segment is not viable, an allograft reconstruction can be considered. In a dislocation of more than 6 months' duration, the bone quality often is poor, and arthroplasty should be considered. A large exposure is required for an allograft reconstruction of a posterolateral humeral head defect from an anterior approach. The subscapularis must be completely detached, and maintenance of the anterior humeral circumflex artery to the humeral head is essential.

Any dislocation of more than 6 months' duration may involve irreversible damage to the articular surface. Thus, arthroplasty should be considered if a patient with such a dislocation has a humeral head defect larger than 50%, poor bone quality, or low functional demands.

SUMMARY

The management of shoulder instability is an evolving concept. Appropriate preoperative assessment needs to be matched with the correct procedure to achieve high rates of success. This can include managing both soft-tissue injuries and bone defects on the glenoid and the humerus.

KEY STUDY POINTS

- The appropriate management for a first-time dislocation is changing with a focus on prevention of recurrence.
- Glenoid bone deficiency must be fully evaluated and managed in all instability cases.
- Management of Hill-Sachs defects is evolving with the growth in the remplissage procedure and the evaluation of humeral and glenoid bone loss.

Annotated References

1. Zacchilli MA, Owens BD: Epidemiology of shoulder dislocations presenting to emergency departments in the United States. *J Bone Joint Surg Am* 2010;92(3):542-549.

2. Goss TP: Anterior glenohumeral instability. *Orthopedics* 1998;11:879.

3. Arciero RA, Wheeler JH, Ryan JB, McBride JB: Arthroscopic Bankart repair versus nonoperative treatment for acute, initial anterior shoulder dislocations. *Am J Sports Med* 1994;22:589-595.

4. Kralinger FS, Gosler K, Wischatta R, Wambacher M, Sperner G: Predicting recurrence after primary anterior shoulder dislocation. *Am J Sports Med* 2002;30:116-120.

5. Rhee YG, Cho NS, Cho SH: Traumatic anterior dislocation of the shoulder: Factors affecting the progress of the traumatic anterior dislocation. *Clin Orthop Surg* 2009;1:188-193.

6. Galano GJ, Dieter AA, Moradi NE, Ahmad CS: Arthroscopic management of a chronic primary anterior shoulder dislocation. *Am J Orthop (Belle Mead NJ)* 2010;39(7):351-355.

7. Bankart ASB: Recurrent or habitual dislocation of the shoulder joint. *Br Med J* 1923;2:1132-1133.

8. Liavaag S, Brox JI, Pripp AH, Enger M, Soldal LA, Svenningsen S: Immobilization in external rotation after primary shoulder dislocation did not reduce the risk of recurrence: A randomized controlled trial. *J Bone Joint Surg Am* 2011;93(10):897-904.

9. Shin SJ, Yun YH, Kim DJ, Yoo JD: Treatment of traumatic anterior shoulder dislocation in patients older than 60 years. *Am J Sports Med* 2012;40(4):822-827.

10. Okoroha KR, Taylor KA, Marshall NE, et al: Return to play after shoulder instability in National Football League athletes. *J Shoulder Elbow Surg* 2017;27:17-22.

    There is a high rate of return to play after shoulder instability events in NFL players. Players who sustain shoulder subluxations return to play faster but are more likely to experience recurrent instability than those with shoulder dislocations. Surgical stabilization of the shoulder after an instability event decreases the chances of a second instability event and affords a player a greater interval between the initial injury and a recurrent event. Level of evidence: III.

11. Shanley E, Thigpen C, Brooks J, et al: Return to sport as an outcome measure for shoulder instability: Surprising findings in nonoperative management in a high school athlete population. *Am J Sports Med* 2019;47(5):1062-1067.

    A high percentage of athletes with shoulder instability achieved successful return to sport without missing any additional time for shoulder injury. Those with subluxations were at almost three times the odds of a successful return compared with those sustaining a dislocation. Level of evidence: II.

12. Hovelius L, Olofsson A, Sandstrom B, et al: Nonoperative treatment of primary anterior shoulder dislocation in patients forty years of age and younger: A prospective twenty five year follow up. *J Bone Joint Surg Am* 2008;90(5):945-952.

13. Larrain MV, Botto GJ, Montenegro HJ, Mauas DM: Arthroscopic repair of acute traumatic anterior shoulder dislocation in young athletes. *Arthroscopy* 2001;17(4):373-377.

14. Hohmann E, Tetsworth K, Glatt V: Open versus arthroscopic surgical treatment for anterior shoulder dislocation: A comparative systematic review and meta-analysis over the past 20 years. *J Shoulder Elbow Surg* 2017;26:1873-1880.

    Despite advances in surgical techniques and devices during the past 20 years, either open or arthroscopic surgical management of anterior shoulder dislocation results in similar clinical outcomes. The recurrence rate for arthroscopic surgical stabilization has only marginally decreased, from 16.8% to 14.2%. However, during the earlier decade from 1995 through 2004, patients treated with arthroscopic surgery had twice the risk of recurrence compared with an open procedure. Level of evidence: IV.

15. Castagna A, Markopoulos N, Conti M, et al: Arthroscopic Bankart suture anchor repair: Radiological and clinical outcome at minimum10 years of follow up. *Am J Sports Med* 2010;38:2012-2016.

16. Van der Linde JA, Van Kampen DA, Terwee CB, et al: Long term results after arthroscopic shoulder stabilization using suture anchors: An 8-10 year follow up. *Am J Sports Med* 2011;39:2396-2403.

17. Vermeulen AE, Landmand EBM, Egbert EJD, et al: Long term clinical outcome of arthroscopic Bankart repair with suture anchors. *J Shoulder Elbow Surg* 2019;28:e137-e143.

    The authors found an overall recurrent instability rate of 22% (dislocation or subluxation). Good long-term results were observed after arthroscopic Bankart repair in patients older than 20 years with three or more suture anchors used. Level of evidence: IV.

18. Harris J, Gupta AK, Mall NA, et al: Long term outcomes after shoulder stabilization. *Arthroscopy* 2013;29:920-933.

    Surgical treatment of anterior shoulder instability using arthroscopic suture anchor and open Bankart techniques yields similar long-term clinical outcomes, with no significant difference in the rate of recurrent instability, clinical outcome scores, or rate of return to sport. Level of evidence: IV.

19. Neviaser RJ, Benke MT, Neviaser MD: Mid-term to long-term outcome of the open Bankart repair for recurrent traumatic anterior dislocation of the shoulder. *J Shoulder Elbow Surg* 2017;26:1943-1947.

    Of 107 patients who participated in sports, 98 returned to the sport; 7 of the remaining 9 discontinued for reasons other than the shoulder. There were 91 patients who agreed to radiography; 48 had normal findings, 34 had mild arthrosis, 9 had moderate arthrosis, and none had severe arthrosis. Mean postoperative outcome scores were as follows: American Shoulder and Elbow Surgeons, 93.53; Rowe, 91.41; and Western Ontario Shoulder Instability Index, 327.7. There were 125 patients who were satisfied and would undergo the procedure again. The open Bankart procedure remains the standard by which other techniques can be measured for management of recurrent, traumatic anterior dislocation of the shoulder. Level of evidence: IV.

20. Nakagawa S, Ozaki R, Take Y, Luchi R, Mae T: Relationship between glenoid defects and Hill-Sachs lesions in shoulders with traumatic anterior instability. *Am J Sports Med* 2015;43:2763-2773.

The prevalence of bipolar lesions was approximately 60%. As glenoid defects became larger, Hill-Sachs lesions also enlarged, but there was no strong correlation. Bipolar lesions were frequent in patients with recurrent instability, patients with repetitive dislocation/subluxation, and those playing collision/contact sports. Instability showed a high recurrence rate in shoulders with bipolar lesions. Level of evidence: III.

21. Burkart SS, De Beer JF: Traumatic glenohumeral bone defects and their relationship to failure of arthroscopic Bankart repairs: Significance of the inverted-pear glenoid and the humeral engaging Hill-Sachs lesion. *Arthroscopy* 2000;16:677-694.

22. Ahmed I, Ashton F, Robinson CM: Arthroscopic Bankart repair and capsular shift for recurrent anterior shoulder instability: Functional outcomes and identification of risk factors for recurrence. *J Bone Joint Surg Am* 2012;94: 1308-1315.

23. Lee SH, Lim KH, Kim JW: Risk factors for recurrence of anterior-inferior instability of the shoulder after arthroscopic Bankart repair in patients younger than 30 years. *Arthroscopy* 2018;34(9):2530-2536.

    The overall results suggest that surgery within 6 months of the first dislocation should be considered, with meticulous attention in patients with a high number of preoperative dislocations or off-track Hill-Sachs lesions. Level of evidence: III.

24. Provencher MT: Is it time to take a stand? When arthroscopic Bankart repair is no longer a viable option for anterior shoulder instability. *Arthroscopy* 2018;34(9):2537-2540.

    Patients who present with 2 preoperative dislocations and a duration of instability symptoms of more than 6 months, as well as off-track Hill-Sachs lesions, may not be ideal candidates for arthroscopic instability repair. There is a "cost" to waiting on surgery after a first dislocation. Level of evidence: IV.

25. Kim DS, Yoon YS, Yi CH: Prevalence comparison of accompanying lesions between primary and recurrent anterior dislocation in the shoulder. *Am J Sports Med* 2010;38:2071-2076.

26. Mologne TS, Provencher MT, Menzel KA, Vachon TA, Dewing CB: Arthroscopic stabilization in patients with an inverted pear glenoid: Results in patients with bone loss of the anterior glenoid. *Am J Sports Med* 2007;35:1276-1283.

27. Piasecki DP, Verma NN, Romeo AA, Levine WN, Bach BR Jr, Provencher MT: Glenoid bone deficiency in recurrent anterior shoulder instability: Diagnosis and management. *J Am Acad Orthop Surg* 2009;17:482-493.

28. Di Giacomo G, de Gasperis N, Scarso P: Bipolar bone defect in the shoulder anterior dislocation. *Knee Surg Sports Traumatol Arthrosc* 2016;24:479-488.

    In the anterior shoulder instability with glenoid bone loss among 25% or more of the inferior glenoid diameter (inverted-pear glenoid), the consensus of recent authors is that glenoid bone grafting (Latarjet procedure) should be performed. Level of evidence: IV.

29. Omori Y, Yamamoto N, Koishi H, et al: Measurement of glenoid track in vivo as investigated by a 3-dimensional motion analysis using open MRI. *Am J Sports Med* 2014;42:1290-1295.

    The existence and widths of the glenoid track were confirmed in vivo. Level of evidence: III.

30. Cetik O, Uslu M, Ozsar BK: The relationship between Hill-Sachs lesion and recurrent anterior shoulder dislocation. *Acta Orthop Belg* 2007;73(2):175-178.

31. Flatow EL, Warner JI: Instability of the shoulder: Complex problems and failed repairs. Part I: Relevant biomechanics, multidirectional instability, and severe glenoid bone loss. *Instr Course Lect* 1998;47:97-112.

32. Connolly JF: Humeral head defects associated with shoulder dislocation: Their diagnostic and surgical significance. *Instr Course Lect* 1972;21:42-54.

33. Wolf EM, Pollock ME, Smalley CC: Hill-Sachs "remplissage": An arthroscopic solution for the engaging Hill-Sachs lesion. *Arthroscopy* 2007;23(6):e1-e2.

34. Deutsch AA, Kroll DG: Decreased range of motion following arthroscopic remplissage. *Orthopedics* 2008; 31:492.

35. Liu JN, Gowd AK, Garcia GH, Cvetanovich GL, Cabarcas BC, Verma NN: Recurrence rate of instability after remplissage for treatment of traumatic anterior shoulder instability: A systematic review in treatment of subcritical glenoid bone loss. *Arthroscopy* 2018;34(10): 2894-2907.

    Arthroscopic remplissage combined with Bankart repair is an effective procedure in the treatment of patients with engaging Hill-Sachs lesions and minimal glenoid bone loss. Patients can expect favorable rates of recurrent instability with a negligible loss of external rotation when compared with isolated Bankart repair. Treatment algorithms may be updated to include this procedure for engaging Hill-Sachs lesions, measuring between 20% and 40% in volume, with subcritical (<20%) glenoid bone loss. Level of evidence: IV.

36. Itoi E, Lee SB, Berglund LJ, Berge LL, An KN: The effect of a glenoid defect on anteroinferior stability of the shoulder after Bankart repair: A cadaveric study. *J Bone Joint Surg Am* 2000;82(1):35-46.

37. Bigliani LU, Newton PM, Steinmann SP, Connor PM, Mcllveen SJ: Glenoid rim lesions associated with recurrent anterior dislocation of the shoulder. *Am J Sports Med* 1998;26(1):41-45.

38. Provencher MT, Ghodadra N, LeClere L, Solomon DJ, Romeo AA: Anatomic osteochondral glenoid reconstruction for recurrent glenohumeral instability with glenoid deficiency using a distal tibia allograft. *Arthroscopy* 2009;25(4):446-452.

39. Warner JJ, Gill TJ, O'Hollerhan JD, Pathare N, Millett PJ: Anatomical glenoid reconstruction for recurrent anterior glenohumeral instability with glenoid deficiency using an autogenous tricortical iliac crest bone graft. *Am J Sports Med* 2006;34(2):205-212.

40. Hovelius L, Sandström B, Olofsson A, Svensson O, Rahme H: The effect of capsular repair, bone block healing, and position on the results of the Bristow-Latarjet procedure (study III): Long-term follow-up in 319 shoulders. *J Shoulder Elbow Surg* 2012;21(5):647-660.

41. Hovelius L, Sandstrom BC, Sundgren K, Saebo M: One hundred eighteen Bristow-Latarjet repairs for recurrent anterior dislocation of the shoulder prospectively followed for fifteen years: Study I-clinical results. *J Shoulder Elbow Surg* 2004;13:509-516.

42. Hovelius L, Vikerfors O, Olofsson A, Svensson O, Rahme H: Bristow-Latarjet and Bankart: A comparative study of shoulder stabilization in 185 shoulders during a seventeen-year follow-up. *J Shoulder Elbow Surg* 2011;20(7):1095-1101.

43. Moroder P, Schulz E, Wierer G, et al: Neer Award 2019: Latarjet vs. iliac crest bone graft transfer for treatment of anterior shoulder instability with glenoid bone loss. A prospective randomized trial. *J Shoulder Elbow Surg* 2019;28(7):1298-1307.

The Latarjet and iliac crest bone graft transfer (ICBGT) procedures for the management of anterior shoulder instability with glenoid bone loss showed no difference in clinical and radiologic outcomes except for significantly worse internal rotation capacity in the Latarjet group and frequently noted donor-site sensory disturbances in the ICBGT group. Level of evidence: I.

44. Neer CS, Foster CR: Inferior capsular shift for involuntary inferior and multidirectional instability of the shoulder. A preliminary report. *J Bone Joint Surg Am* 1980;62(6):897-908.

45. Kowalsky MS, Levine WN: Traumatic posterior glenohumeral dislocation: Classification, pathoanatomy, diagnosis, and treatment. *Orthop Clin North Am* 2008;39:519-533, viii.

46. McLaughlin HL: Posterior dislocation of the shoulder. *J Bone Joint Surg Am* 1952;24(3):584-590.

47. Hatzis N, Kaar TK, Wirth MA, Rockwood CA Jr: The often overlooked posterior dislocation of the shoulder. *Tex Med* 2001;97(11):62-67.

48. Rowe CR, Zarins B: Chronic unreduced dislocations of the shoulder. *J Bone Joint Surg Am* 1982;64(4):494-505.

The literature suggests that patients treated arthroscopically have superior outcomes compared with patients who undergo open procedures with respect to stability, recurrence of instability, patient satisfaction, return to sport, and return to previous level of play. Level of evidence: V.

49. DeLong JM, Jiang K, Bradley JP: Posterior instability of the shoulder: A systemic review and meta-analysis of clinical outcomes. *Am J Sports Med* 2015;43(7):1805-1817.

50. Griggs SM, Holloway B, Williams GR Jr, Iannotti JP: *Disorders of the Shoulder Diagnosis and Management*. Philadelphia, PA, Lippincott, Williams & Wilkins, 2006, pp 461-486.

51. Schulz TJ, Jacobs B, Patterson RL Jr: Unrecognized dislocations of the shoulder. *J Trauma* 1969;9(12):1009-1023.

52. Diklic ID, Ganic ZD, Blagojevic ZD, Nho SJ, Romeo AA: Treatment of locked chronic posterior dislocation of the shoulder by reconstruction of the defect in the humeral head with an allograft. *J Bone Joint Surg Br* 2010.92(1):71-76.

53. Delcogliano A, Caporaso A, Chiossi S, Menghi A, Cillo M, Delcogliano M: Surgical management of chronic, unreduced posterior dislocation of the shoulder. *Knee Surg Sports Traumatol Arthrosc* 2005;13(2):151-155.

54. Gavrilidis I, Magosch P, Lichtenberg S, Habermeyer P, Kircher J: Chronic locked posterior shoulder dislocation with severe head involvement. *Int Orthop* 2010;34(1):79-84.

55. Rouhani A, Navali A: Treatment of chronic anterior shoulder dislocation by open reduction and simultaneous Bankart lesion repair. *Sports Med Arthrosc Rehabil Ther Technol* 2010;2:15.

56. Willemot LB, Elhassan BT, Verborgt O: Bony reconstruction of the anterior glenoid rim. *J Ortho Surg* 2018;26(10):e207-e218.

Recurrent anterior shoulder instability is associated with glenohumeral bone loss. Level of evidence: VII.

Chapter 7

Recurrent Anterior Shoulder Instability

Maj. Travis J. Dekker, MD, MC, USAF • Liam A. Peebles, BA • Peter J. Millett, MD, MSc • CAPT Matthew T. Provencher, MD, MC, USNR

ABSTRACT

Several factors commonly contribute to recurrent anterior shoulder instability. As with most orthopaedic conditions, a complete history and physical examination provide the keys to a correct diagnosis. Advanced imaging studies are desirable for every patient with recurrent instability. Magnetic resonance arthrography can be useful to delineate a superior labrum anterior to posterior lesion or more extensive or subtle labral pathology. If glenoid bone loss or a significant Hill-Sachs lesion is suspected, three-dimensional CT is the preferred imaging modality. Bone loss in the glenoid and/or humeral head is present in almost all patients with recurrent instability, and it must be recognized and appropriately treated to minimize further injury to the joint. Proper diagnosis leads to appropriate patient counseling and the selection of the ideal technique. This chapter is intended to serve as a guide to assessing and addressing various soft-tissue and bony pathologies commonly associated with recurrent anterior glenohumeral joint instability to better tailor both surgical and nonsurgical treatments to a patient's unique condition and provide them with the best possible outcomes.

Keywords: anterior glenohumeral instability; glenoid bone loss; Hill-Sachs lesion; recurrent anterior shoulder instability

The views expressed in this chapter are those of the authors and do not reflect the official policy or position of the Department of the Navy, Department of Defense, or United States Government.

Dr. Millett or an immediate family member has received royalties from Arthrex, Inc. and Medbridge; serves as a paid consultant to or is an employee of Arthrex, Inc.; has stock or stock options held in VuMedi; and has received research or institutional support from Arthrex, Inc., Ossur, Siemens, and Smith & Nephew. Dr. Provencher or an immediate family member has received royalties from Arthrex, Inc.; is a member of a speakers' bureau or has made paid presentations on behalf of Arthrex, Inc.; serves as a paid consultant to or is an employee of Arthrex, Inc. and Joint Restoration Foundation (Allosource); and serves as a board member, owner, officer, or committee member of the American Academy of Orthopaedic Surgeons, the American Orthopaedic Society for Sports Medicine, the American Shoulder and Elbow Surgeons, the Arthroscopy Association of North America, the International Society of Arthroscopy, Knee Surgery, and Orthopaedic Sports Medicine, the San Diego Shoulder Institute, and the Society of Military Orthopaedic Surgeons. Neither of the following authors nor any immediate family member has received anything of value from or has stock or stock options held in a commercial company or institution related directly or indirectly to the subject of this chapter: Dr. Dekker and Mr. Peebles.

Introduction

The glenohumeral joint is the most commonly dislocated joint in the body. The limited bony constraints of the glenohumeral joint allow a wide range of shoulder motion at the inherent risk of instability. The static and dynamic restraints of the glenohumeral joint provide stability through complex musculoskeletal interactions, and injury to one or more of these restraints tilts the delicate balance of shoulder stability toward instability. Many patients who sustain a first anterior shoulder dislocation regain shoulder stability and do not experience another instability event.[1] However, some patients go on to develop recurrent anterior shoulder instability; young male contact athletes are the most susceptible subset of patients.

The critical role of bipolar bone loss and the concept of the glenoid track in recurrent instability has been elucidated and popularized in recent years. This chapter discusses the pathophysiology, the evaluation, and the management of recurrent anterior shoulder instability,

This chapter is adapted from Dierckman BD, Ghodadra N, Solomon DJ, Stanley MD, McNeil JW II, Provencher MT: Recurrent anterior shoulder instability, in Nicholson GP, ed: *Orthopaedic Knowledge Update: Shoulder and Elbow*, ed 4. Rosemont, IL, American Academy of Orthopaedic Surgeons, 2013, pp 93-107.

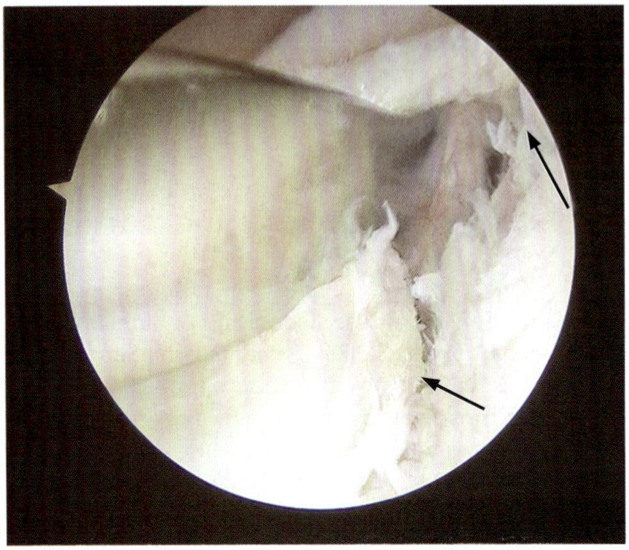

FIGURE 1 Arthroscopic image of a right shoulder from the anterosuperior portal, with the patient in the lateral decubitus position, showing a typical Bankart (anterior labral) tear (arrows), from approximately the 6-o'clock position inferiorly to the 3-o'clock position anteriorly.

with a focus on glenoid and humeral bone loss. The exact roles of glenoid and/or humeral bone loss in recurrent instability are still being defined.

Pathophysiology

With first-time anterior shoulder dislocation, the most common anatomic injury is an avulsion of the anterior-inferior labrum and the capsular attachments from the glenoid rim (a Bankart lesion)[2] (**Figure 1**). Critical evaluation on advanced imaging should evaluate for glenoid bone loss (GBL) as it has been shown that on average, the first-time dislocator suffers 6.8% of GBL and that recurrent dislocators have an average of 22.8% of GBL. Concurrently, most patients have a compression fracture of the posterosuperolateral aspect of the humeral head (a Hill-Sachs lesion) as the head forcibly collides with the harder bone of the anterior-inferior glenoid rim.[3,4] However, most initial Hill-Sachs lesions are small, shallow, and not clinically significant (**Figure 2**).

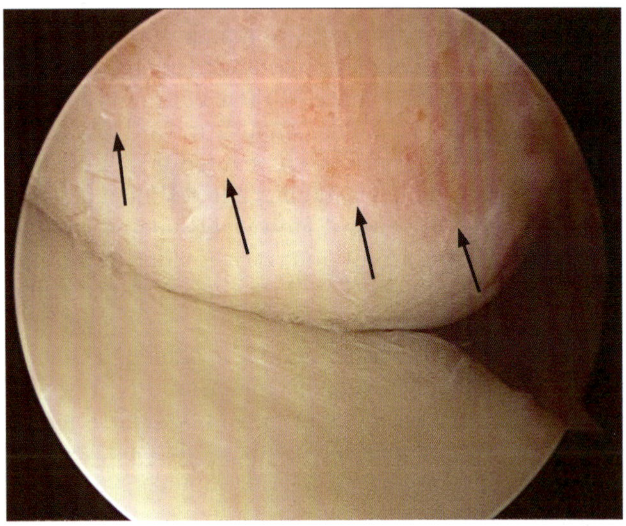

FIGURE 2 Arthroscopic image of a right shoulder from the posterior portal, with the patient in the beach chair position, showing a Hill-Sachs lesion (arrows) that is moderate in size and engages the glenoid with anterior translation and approximately 30° of external rotation.

In recurrent instability, the further compromise of the static and dynamic stabilizers of the shoulder contributes to a downward spiral of bone and cartilage loss, often leading to degenerative changes. Several factors in addition to the typical Bankart lesion contribute to recurrent instability, to a varying extent. Glenoid and humeral head bone loss have been recognized as key pathologic features in most patients with recurrent instability. In each dislocation, the humeral head collides with the anterior glenoid, leading to attritional bone loss in the glenoid as well as enlargement of the Hill-Sachs lesion. The inferior glenohumeral ligament (IGHL) complex is further stretched and attenuated, leading to plastic deformation and further weakening of the shoulder's static restraints.[5] Although subluxation events were once thought to not cause significant changes to the glenohumeral joint, recent findings have demonstrated similar intraarticular concomitant pathology after multiple subluxations and dislocations.[6]

Certain uncommon anatomic findings are seen with relative frequency during imaging evaluation or arthroscopic visualization of patients with recurrent anterior shoulder instability. These include an anterior labral periosteal sleeve avulsion (ALPSA) lesion, a humeral avulsion of the glenohumeral ligament (HAGL), a circumferential or extensive labral tear, and a glenoid labral articular damage (GLAD) lesion.

Anterior Labral Periosteal Sleeve Avulsion Lesions

As the humeral head dislocates anteriorly, the capsulolabral complex is stripped away from the anterior-inferior glenoid. In a typical Bankart lesion, the capsulolabral complex detaches from the surrounding periosteum, but in an ALPSA lesion, the capsulolabral complex remains attached to the periosteum, and the entire sleeve of tissue is peeled back medially along the neck of the glenoid. The injured soft tissues heal in a more medial position along the glenoid neck[7] (**Figure 3**).

ALPSA lesions are uncommon with an initial dislocation. One study found that 78% of the patients with an acute dislocation had a Bankart lesion, and 97% of the patients with recurrent dislocation had either a Bankart or an ALPSA lesion.[8] Only patients with recurrent dislocation had an ALPSA lesion.

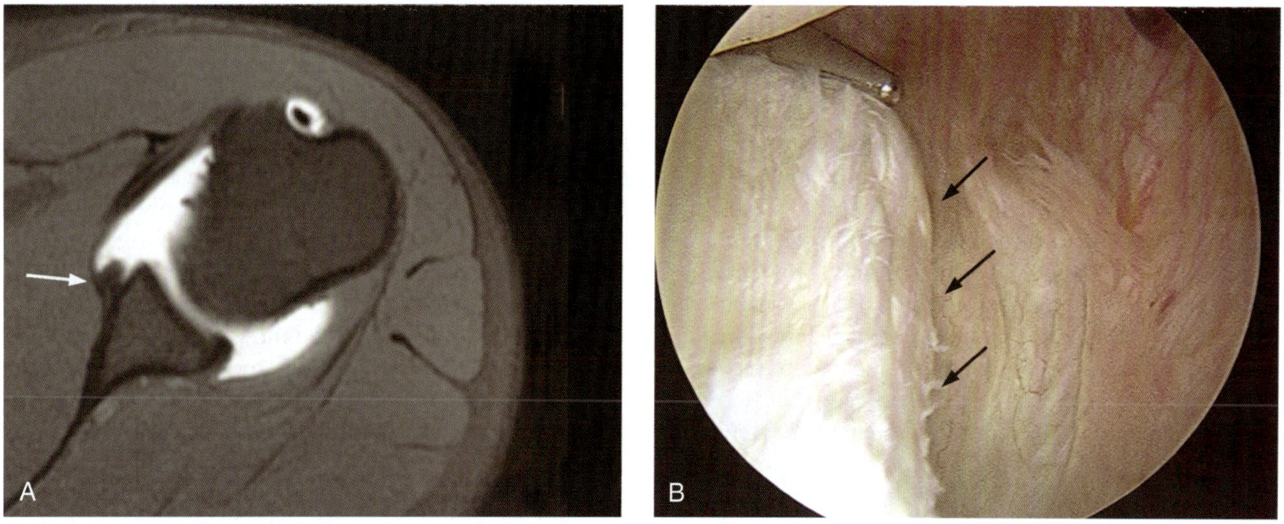

FIGURE 3 Axial magnetic resonance arthrography (**A**) and an arthroscopic image from the anterosuperior portal (**B**) showing the same anterior labral periosteal sleeve avulsion lesion (arrows).

Humeral Avulsion of the Glenohumeral Ligament Lesions

The IGHL and the labrum detach from the glenoid as a capsulolabral complex in almost all anterior shoulder dislocations. Uncommonly, the IGHL instead avulses from its attachment onto the humeral neck.[9] The HAGL lesion often is missed and therefore is not appropriately treated. Furthermore, this pathologic finding has been recently found to be more prevalent in collegiate female athletes than once thought and thus requires critical evaluation in this unique patient population.[10] This pattern was recognized as a relatively common cause of arthroscopic stabilization surgery failure (**Figure 4**).

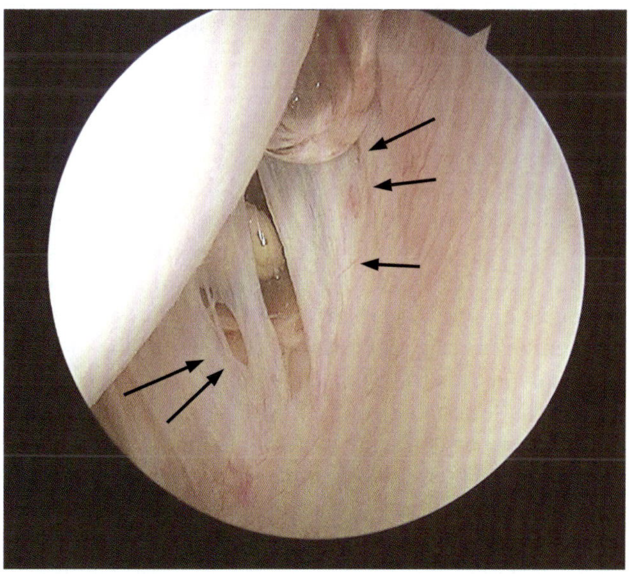

FIGURE 4 Arthroscopic image of a right shoulder, with the patient in the lateral decubitus position, showing a humeral avulsion of the glenohumeral ligament ear of the anterior-inferior capsule (arrows).

Extensive Labral Tears

Recurrent anterior dislocation can cause extensive labral tears as the tear propagates around the glenoid from repetitive trauma.[11] Uncommonly, these extensive lesions result from both anterior and posterior instability events. Initial posterior instability also can lead to circumferential labral tearing. These tears may even propagate around the glenoid to eventually involve the superior labrum, or a superior labrum anterior to posterior (SLAP) lesion may occur at the time of initial injury (**Figure 5**).

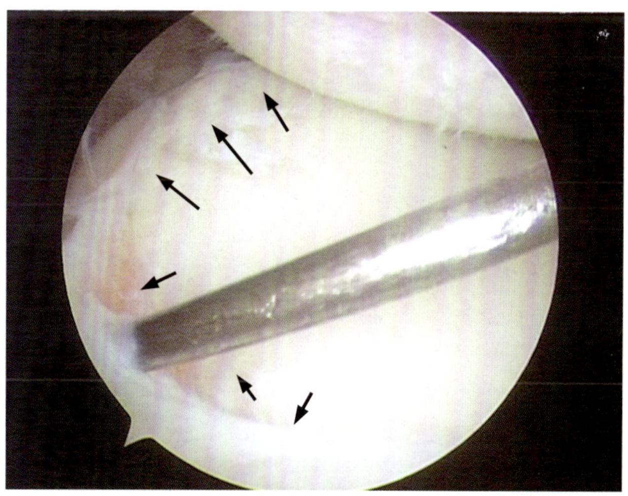

FIGURE 5 Arthroscopic image of a right shoulder from the posterior portal showing an extensive 180° labral tear denoted by the black arrows. In this image, the anterior labrum is located superior to the freer and the posterior labrum is inferior.

Glenoid Labral Articular Damage Lesions

Some surgeons believe GLAD lesions form early in the spectrum of osteochondral injuries to the anterior-inferior glenoid. If a sufficient adduction force is present when the humeral head dislocates anteriorly, the humeral head is compressed into the glenoid, leading to a glenoid rim fracture. A GLAD lesion involves a shear force more than a compressive force to the chondrolabral junction, and the result is cartilage loss rather than a bony fracture (**Figure 6**). The original description of GLAD lesions was that of an anterior labral articular cartilage injury without associated anterior instability. It is important to recognize that a capsulorrhaphy should be avoided if the shoulder otherwise is stable; anterior labral repair with treatment of chondral pathology is preferable. GLAD lesions are an independent risk factor for arthroscopic failure and their presence may suggest underlying changes to the glenoid articular congruency and version.[12]

Bone Loss

A patient with recurrent shoulder instability almost always has osseous injury to the glenoid and/or the humeral head. Understanding and appropriately treating irregularities in the osseous architecture of the glenohumeral joint are critical to the overall success of surgical treatment of glenohumeral instability. Bone loss in recurrent anterior instability must be considered a bipolar phenomenon because most patients have varying bone loss in both the glenoid and the humeral head.

Glenoid Bone Loss

The integrity of the glenoid osseous architecture is one of the most critical factors affecting the outcome of shoulder instability surgery. Regardless of size, the orientation of the bone deficit remains constant as a vertical vector parallel to the long axis of the glenoid. Anterior-inferior GBL decreases the contact area between the humeral head and the glenoid, diminishing the ability of the glenoid to resist humeral head shear forces.[13,14] Anterior bone loss also reduces the concave morphology of the glenoid, further diminishing the stabilizing forces of concavity-compression as well as the buttress effect of the glenoid.[13,15]

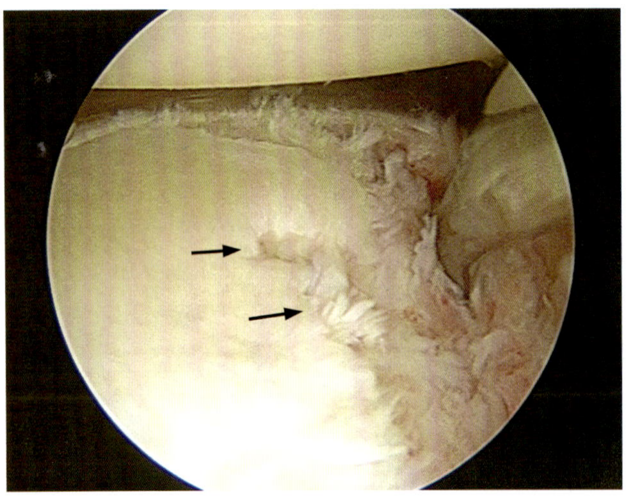

FIGURE 6 Arthroscopic image of a right shoulder from the anterosuperior portal, with the patient in the lateral decubitus position, showing a glenoid labral articular damage lesion (arrows).

Several different glenoid injury patterns have been reported, and no distinct GBL model has been established. Acute glenoid injury can range from a large fracture resulting from a significant axial loading injury to a small bony avulsion occurring as the labroligamentous complex displaces from the glenoid during a rotational shear injury. Chronic, attritional bone loss also occurs in different ways, from blunting or smoothing of the anterior rim after a compression injury to repetitive shearing and erosion of the anterior edge of the glenoid. One study reported that more than 50% of the patients had erosive GBL without visible bone fragments only 15 months after an initial dislocation.[16]

Regardless of the mechanism of injury, recurrent dislocation compromises the already-limited bony constraints of the shoulder. Several studies have found that GBL is the most common cause of failure in arthroscopic shoulder stabilization.[13,17] This finding serves to emphasize the importance of recognizing GBL in developing and executing an appropriate surgical plan. Repetitive injury can lead to flattening or even reversal of the shape of the glenoid cavity and the creation of an inverted pear appearance of the glenoid (**Figure 7**). One study reported a significant increase in the failure rate of arthroscopic repair in patients who had an inverted pear glenoid.[13] The rate was 89% in a subgroup of young contact athletes.

Hill-Sachs Lesions

Hill-Sachs lesions occur as the relatively soft cancellous bone of the posterosuperolateral humeral head contacts the hard cortical bone of the anterior-inferior glenoid during an anterior instability event. The Hill-Sachs lesion is common in recurrent anterior shoulder dislocation; in one study, it was found in 100% of the patients.[2] Most Hill-Sachs lesions are not clinically problematic, but a limited number will contribute to instability. Lesion size and engagement are widely considered the two most important factors in the treatment of Hill-Sachs lesions.[13] Deep and/or broad lesions are most likely to require treatment.[3] Lesion location and orientation also should be considered (**Figure 8**). Several classification systems have been described, but none has been validated or recognized as the most clinically relevant (**Table 1**).

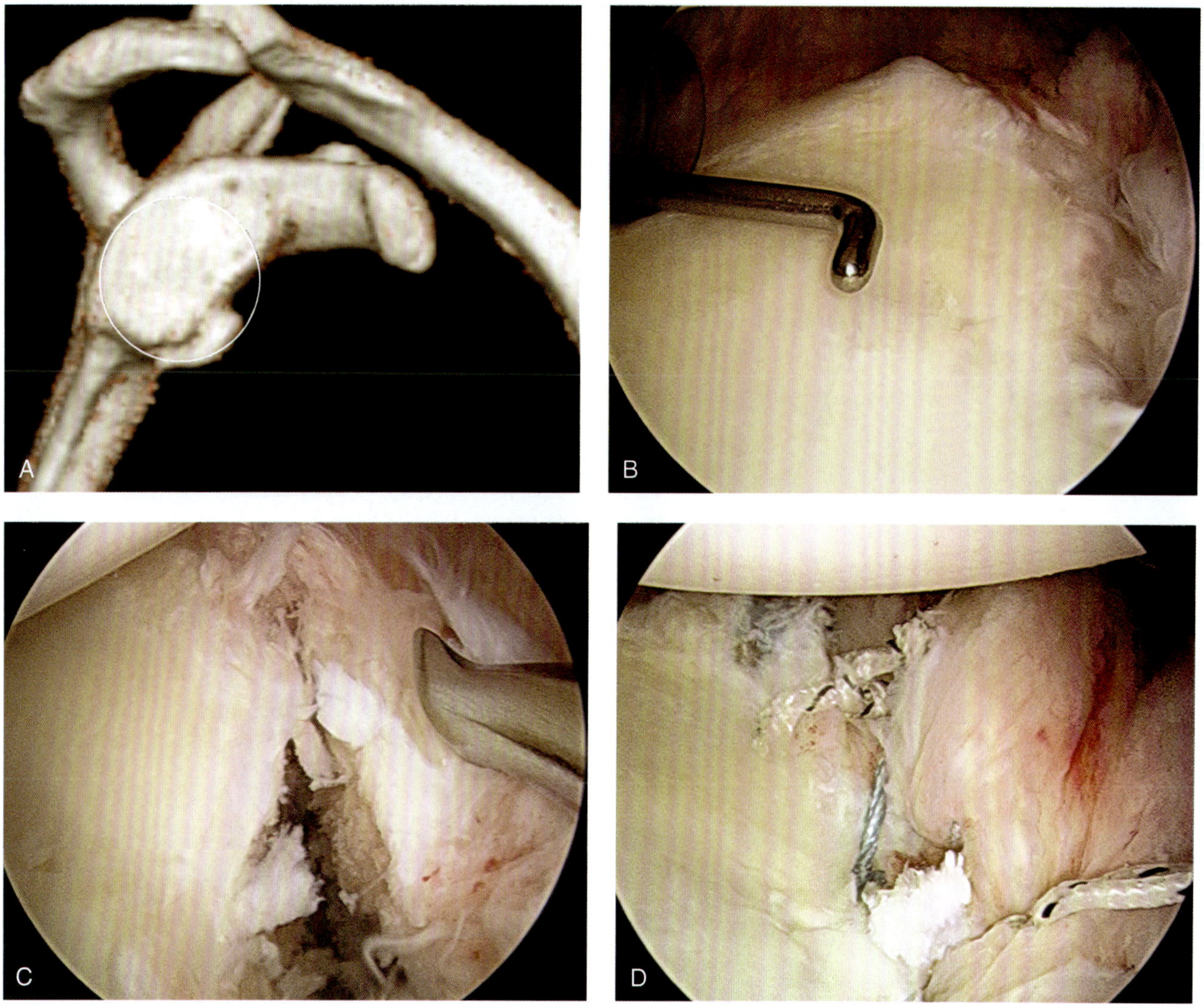

FIGURE 7 **A**, Three-dimensional CT with the humeral head digitally subtracted, showing glenoid bone loss of approximately 20% (circled). Arthroscopic images showing the corresponding tear (**B**), preparation of the tear by ensuring the capsule is completely elevated off the glenoid so the subscapularis can be seen (**C**), and the repair (**D**). A bony fragment is incorporated into the repair.

The concept of the glenoid track was introduced in 2007.[24] In a cadaver model, the contact area between the humeral head and the glenoid was measured at different degrees of abduction and external rotation. Based on the results, the researchers described an area on the humeral head that contacts the glenoid during abduction and external rotation maneuvers. If the Hill-Sachs lesion lies within this glenoid track, it will contact the glenoid and not engage. With GBL, the glenoid track decreases in size and the Hill-Sachs lesion is more likely to be outside the track and at increased risk of engagement, leading to instability (**Figure 9**). A 2016 study evaluating a military population was able to identify the glenoid track as being significantly superior to predict postoperative stability compared with GBL alone, and thus, the authors recommend the utilization of the glenoid track as a routine part of recurrent shoulder instability workup.[25]

Clinical Evaluation of Recurrent Anterior Instability

A thorough patient history is critical for characterizing the etiology of instability and selecting the ideal treatment. Clues are provided as to the anatomic cause of the instability by the type and the magnitude of the initial injury (eg, a football injury or a ground level fall) and subsequent instability events, the trend of these events

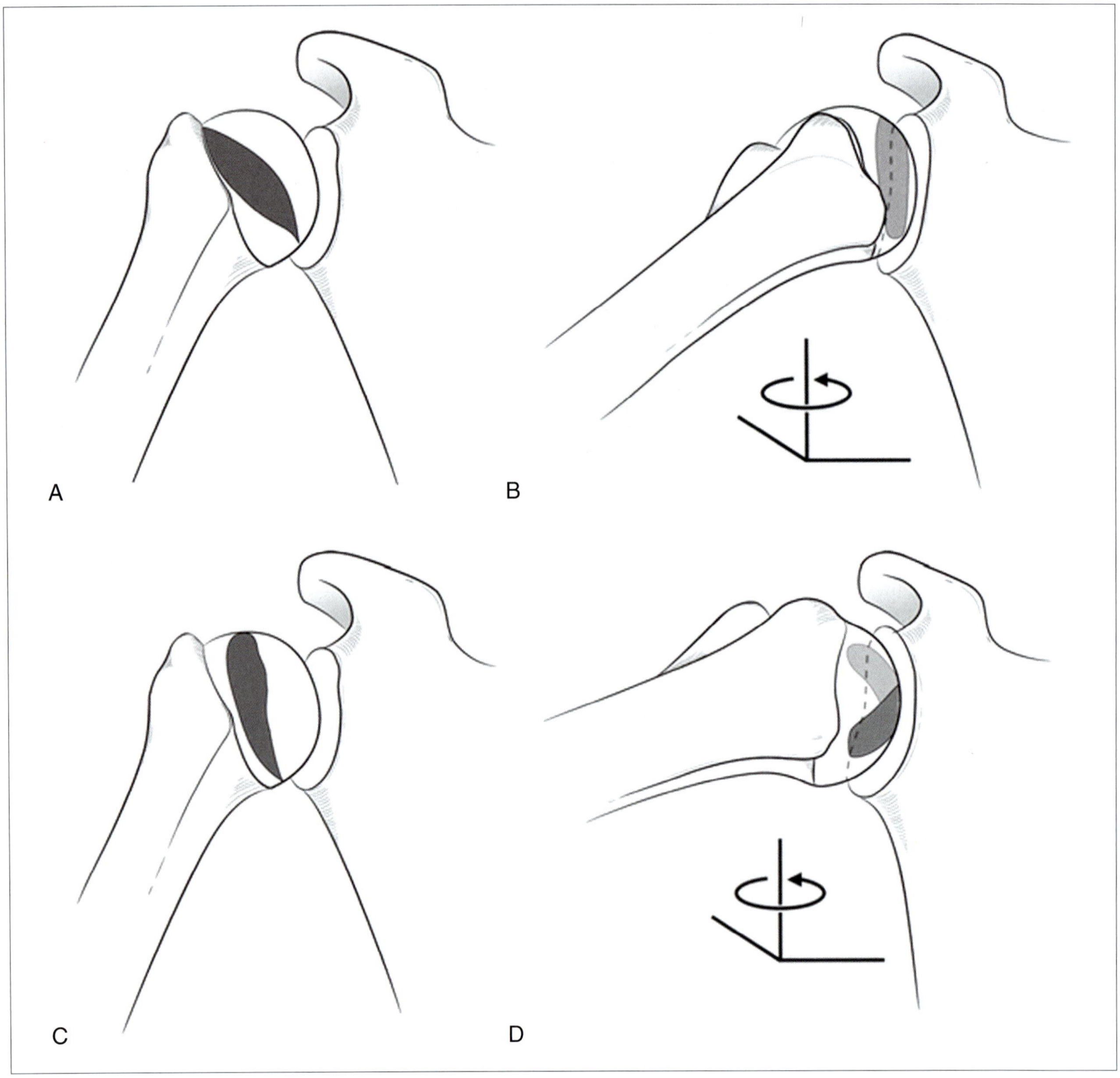

FIGURE 8 Schematic drawings showing an engaging Hill-Sachs lesion (**A**); a lesion oriented parallel to the anterior glenoid with the shoulder in a position of function or in abduction and external rotation, thus engaging it (**B**); a nonengaging lesion, which is created in a nonfunctional position (**C**); and a lesion oriented not parallel to the glenoid with the shoulder in abduction and external rotation, thus not engaging it (**D**). Dark gray = anterior-facing lesion, light gray = posterior-facing lesion, solid lines = axes and plane of rotation

(are they becoming more frequent or initiated by a lower energy mechanism?), the position of the arm at the time of injury, and the ease of relocation (is self-reduction possible or is emergency department reduction required?). A patient whose shoulder initially was dislocated during football playing but now dislocates during sleep or a patient who has instability symptoms during midranges of motion is likely to have significant glenoid and/or humeral bone loss.

History

Relatively young age is a significant risk factor for recurrence. Patients younger than 30 years have a much higher rate of subsequent dislocation than older patients.[26] A 55.7% recurrence rate within the first 2 years of an initial dislocation was reported in a study of 252 patients aged 15 to 35 years, and boys at age 15 years had an 86% probability of recurrence.[27] A study of 105 patients found that 64% of the patients younger than 20 years but only

Table 1

Classification Systems for Hill-Sachs Lesions

System	Visualization	Description
Rowe et al[18]	Axillary radiograph	Mild: 2 cm long, ≤0.3 cm deep Moderate: 2-4 cm long, 0.3-1 cm deep Severe: 4 cm long, ≥1 cm deep
Calandra et al[19]	Direct	Grade I: Confined to articular cartilage Grade II: Extension into subchondral bone Grade III: Large subchondral defect
Franceschi et al[20]	Direct	Grade I: Cartilaginous Grade II: Bony scuffing Grade III: Hatchet fracture
Flatow and Warner[21]	Direct	Grade I: Clinically insignificant, <20% Grade II: Variably significant, 20%-40% Grade III: Clinically significant, >40%
Hall et al[22]	Stryker notch radiograph	Extent of 180° articular arc involvement (percentage)
Richards et al[23]	Axillary MRI	Extent of axillary degree involvement (anterior articular margin = 0°)

6% of the patients older than 40 years had a redislocation within 6 years.[28] In 2011, a Markov decision model was used to predict shoulder stability after an initial anterior shoulder dislocation.[29] The model was internally and externally validated against high-level clinical studies and was found to predict that an 18-year-old man has a 77% chance of developing recurrent instability within 1 year and a 32% chance of stability at 10 years. Patients who underwent surgical intervention were included in the model.

Certain activities substantially increase the risk of shoulder dislocation, including contact sports such as football, rugby, basketball, lacrosse, and martial arts; military training such as hand-to-hand drills and obstacle course training; climbing; whitewater kayaking; and other sports or activities during which the patient's arm may be forcibly abducted and externally rotated.[30] Population studies have reported annual incidence rates widely ranging from 8.2 per 100,000 to 28.3 per 100,000 person-years. The overall incidence of dislocation in a select group of young, active individuals (active-duty US military personnel) was 1.69 per 1,000 person-years.[26] The incidence in men was 1.82 compared with 0.90 for women. An earlier study of US Military Academy cadets found that the incidence of instability events (subluxations and dislocations) was 28.3 per 1,000 person-years.[31] All initial anterior shoulder dislocations were recorded over a 10-year period in a more heterogeneous population composed of the residents of Olmstead County, Minnesota.[32] The overall incidence was 8.2 per 100,000 person-years.

Physical Examination

A standard shoulder examination for laxity and instability should be performed. Specific attention should be given to findings that suggest significant instability and bone loss, including midrange apprehension (at 45° abduction with initiation of external rotation), apprehension at lower degrees of abduction with external rotation beyond 30°, a shoulder that is easily dislocated but requires reduction force during examination under anesthesia, a palpable clunk or catching sensation (suggesting Hill-Sachs lesion engagement), or a shoulder with more than 90° of external rotation with the arm at the side (usually bilateral and often associated with generalized ligamentous laxity).

Scapular dynamics should be carefully evaluated because many patients have poor scapular control after repetitive shoulder injury. If scapular mechanics are not restored, surgical repair will be futile. Positional or volitional dislocation also must be identified because surgical repair of a lesion is unlikely to withstand the substantive muscular forces, leading to instability in such a patient.

Shoulder instability may develop in a patient with greater than normal shoulder laxity, often resulting from a trivial injury. These patients have a relatively high risk of recurrence after an initial dislocation.[17] The surgeon should suspect and evaluate for hyperlaxity (often bilateral) in a patient whose initial dislocation occurred with minimal trauma.[17] Before surgery is considered, the patient should undergo appropriate rehabilitation that focuses on strengthening the dynamic stabilizers, including the rotator cuff and the periscapular musculature. The

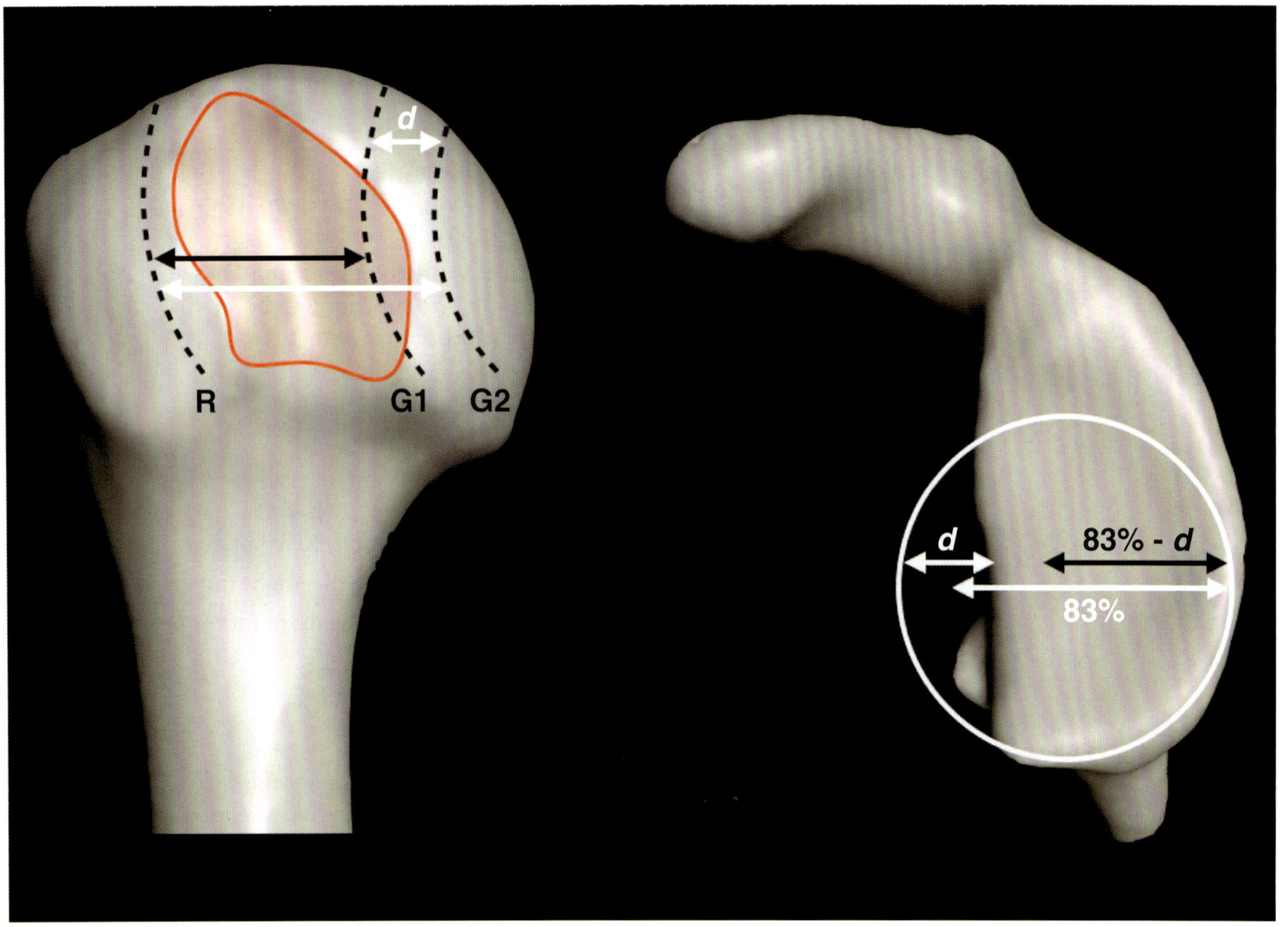

FIGURE 9 Three-dimensional CT reconstructions of a glenoid with significant bone loss (right) and a humeral head with medium-sized Hill-Sachs lesion (left). Using the contralateral glenoid as a reference (100%), 83% of the glenoid width is calculated. The defect width (*d*) is subtracted from this 83% length to obtain the glenoid track width (black double-headed arrow). Dashed line (R) denotes the medial margin of the rotator cuff attachment. Dashed line G1 represents the medial margin of the glenoid track. In the absence of any glenoid bone loss, the medial margin of the glenoid track would have been dashed line G2. This figure shows a Hill-Sachs lesion that extends medially beyond the medial margin of the glenoid track (dashed line G1), thus demonstrating an off-track lesion. (Reprinted from Arthroscopy 30[1]. Di Giacomo G, Itoi E, Burkhart SS: Evolving Concept of Bipolar Bone Loss and the Hill-Sachs Lesion: From "Engaging/Non-Engaging" Lesion to "On-Track/Off-Track" Lesion, 90-98. © 2014 Arthroscopy Association of North America. doi:10.1016/j.arthro.2013.10.004.)

surgeon may consider using the Gagey hyperabduction assessment, which suggests inferior capsular attenuation from recurrent dislocations.[33]

Imaging

Bone loss of the glenoid and/or the humeral head almost always is seen in a patient with recurrent shoulder instability and is the most common cause of failure in arthroscopic stabilization procedures. Radiologic and arthroscopic methods of measuring GBL have been reported. It is preferable to assess the amount of GBL before surgery, using radiography as well as advanced imaging modalities, to allow appropriate preoperative planning and coordination of care. If significant bone loss is detected, the planned surgery is likely to be changed to a bone-restorative procedure (such as a Latarjet, a distal tibial allograft, or an iliac crest allograft procedure).

Radiographs

Standard radiographs (AP, axillary, and scapular Y views) should be obtained for every patient. The West Point and Stryker notch views also may be helpful. The West Point view improves visualization of the anterior-inferior glenoid. Some surgeons believe that radiographs are sufficient to screen for GBL.[30] Any abnormalities should be further evaluated with advanced studies, however. Humeral bone loss also can be assessed with radiographs, specifically with an AP external rotation view of the shoulder.[17] The Stryker notch view provides improved visualization of a Hill-Sachs lesion (**Figure 10**).

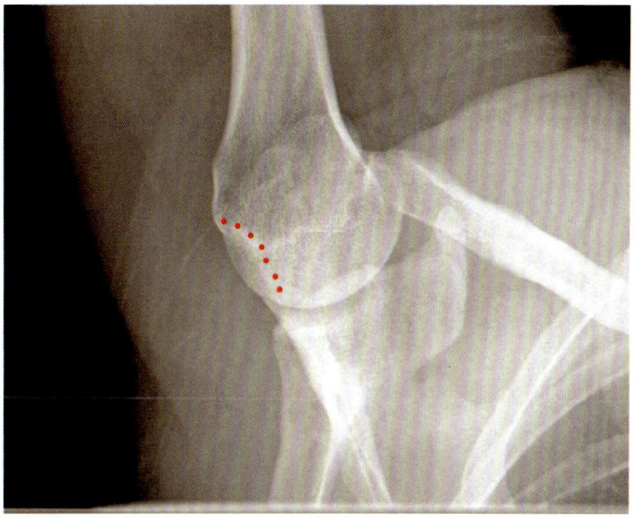

FIGURE 10 Stryker notch radiograph showing a Hill-Sachs lesion (dotted line).

Magnetic Resonance Imaging

High-quality MRI, with or without magnetic resonance arthrography (MRA), is helpful for imaging the capsule, the labrum, and the rotator cuff. Specific lesions of the capsule, including HAGL lesions and capsular redundancy, also can be identified. MRA is especially beneficial if a SLAP lesion or an extensive labral tear is suspected or after an unsuccessful stabilization procedure or recurrence of dislocation (**Figure 11**). Glenoid and humeral head bone loss can be seen on MRI but is more accurately assessed with CT.[34]

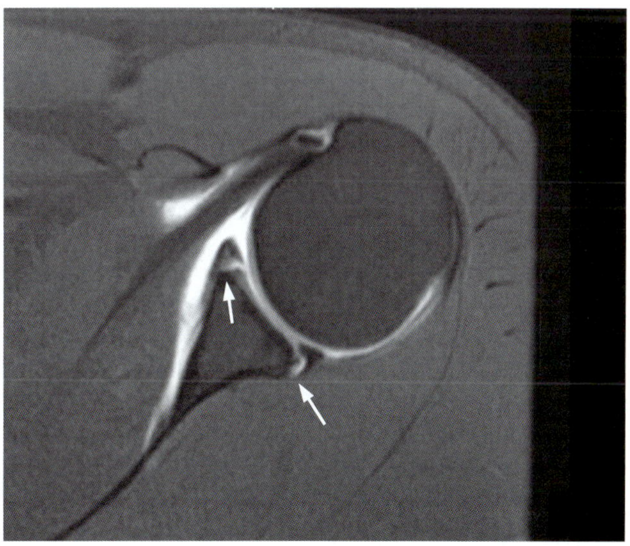

FIGURE 11 Axial magnetic resonance arthrography showing anterior and posterior labral tears (arrows).

Computed Tomography

CT with three-dimensional reconstruction and humeral head subtraction is the benchmark imaging study for evaluating GBL.[35] MRI and MRA may not provide optimal differentiation between labrum and bone, leading to underestimation of the amount of bone loss. CT also allows more accurate evaluation of glenoid version and dysplasia, which are uncommon causes of shoulder instability but should be screened for in a patient who has undergone an unsuccessful procedure or has bilateral instability. In addition, patients with recurrent anterior shoulder instability with a bone fragment present need to be critically evaluated as the bone fragment undergoes rapid attritional bone loss which will prevent the bone that is present to reconstitute the glenoid bone stock.[36]

Several methods of assessing GBL on CT and with arthroscopy have been published, but no method has been widely accepted over others. It is important to understand the limitations of these methods. The use of arthroscopic assessment of bone loss prevents precise preoperative planning because the surgeon must be prepared to immediately treat the pathology with the appropriate arthroscopic or open technique. A 2015 study has shown that arthroscopic evaluation of GBL significantly

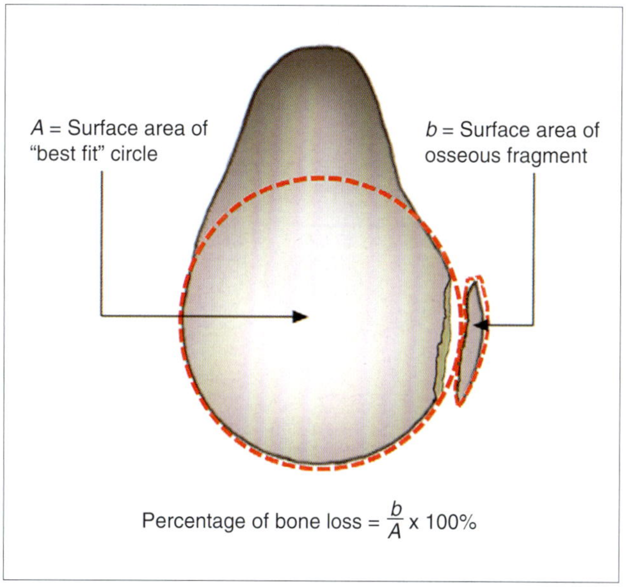

FIGURE 12 Schematic diagram showing the estimation of glenoid bone loss based on surface area. On an en face radiograph of the glenoid, digital measurements are made of the surface areas of the osseous defect (*b*) and a best fit circle superimposed on the inferior two thirds of the glenoid (*A*). The percentage of bone loss is quantified as mentioned in the diagram. (Reproduced with permission from Provencher MT, Bhatia S, Ghodadra NS, et al: Recurrent shoulder instability. Current concepts for evaluation and management of glenoid bone loss. *J Bone Joint Surg Am* 2010;92[suppl 2]:133-151. doi:10.2106/JBJS.J.00906.)

overestimates the total percent of bone loss and calls into question its utility in management; therefore, the authors suggest utilization of a three-dimensional CT to more accurately and precisely identify GBL which may alter treatment plans.[37]

A cadaver study found that the inferior two-thirds of the glenoid has the shape of a true circle, and subsequent methods of bone loss measurement have been based on this model.[38] The center of the circle is roughly correlated with the anatomic bare spot. The most precise method for determining the percentage of GBL is based on surface area measurements[39] (**Figure 12**). Using digital imaging software, the area of the osseous defect is divided by the total surface area of the true circle. Although accurate, this method is not commonly used. Most surgeons (including the authors of this chapter) prefer to use the glenoid rim measurement method for CT and arthroscopic measurement[40] (**Figure 13**). The distances from the bare spot to the anterior rim and the posterior rim are measured, and the anterior-rim distance is subtracted from the posterior-rim distance. This figure is divided by the diameter of the circle to determine the percentage of bone loss. A 2006 work has shown that the bare spot is slightly anterior to the exact center of the true circle, so this method may overestimate bone loss.[41] The secant chord theory was described as a more accurate arthroscopic measurement for assessing GBL but requires additional mathematical steps to ascertain the exact amount of bone loss present[42] (**Figures 14** and **15**).

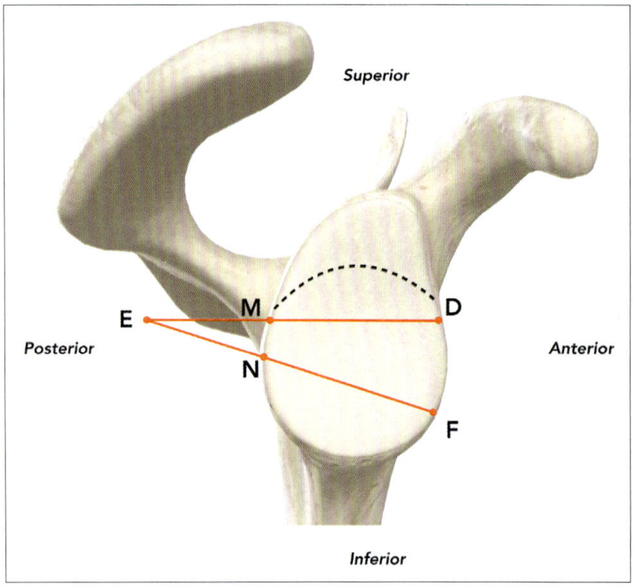

FIGURE 14 Schematic diagram showing secant chord theory method of calculating bone loss. According to the geometric theorem, FN = (DE × ME/NE) – NE. (Adapted from Arthroscopy 25[11]. Detterline AJ, Provencher MT, Ghodadra N, et al: A New Arthroscopic Technique to Determine Anterior-Inferior Glenoid Bone Loss: Validation of the Secant Chord Theory in a Cadaveric Model, 1249-1256. Copyright © 2009 Arthroscopy Association of North America. doi:10.1016/j.arthro.2009.05.019.)

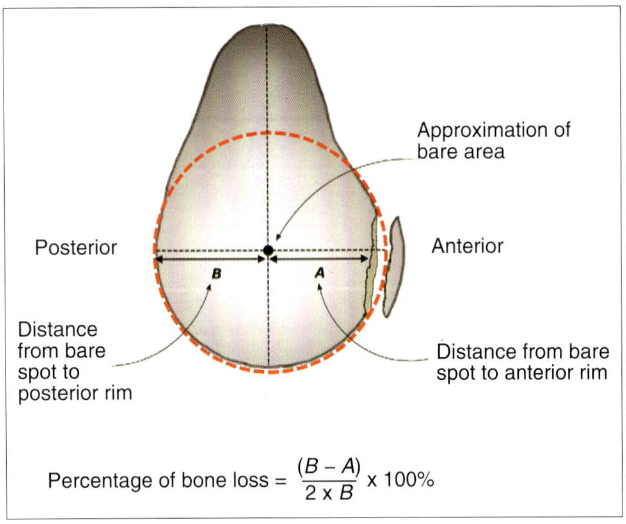

FIGURE 13 Schematic diagram showing the estimation of glenoid bone loss based on glenoid rim distances. On an en face CT view, the bare spot is approximated on the glenoid fossa as the intersection of the longitudinal axis and the widest anterior-posterior diameter of the glenoid. A best fit circle centered on the bare spot approximation is drawn about the inferior two thirds of the glenoid. The distance from the bare spot to the anterior rim (*A*) and the distance from the bare spot to the posterior rim (*B*) are measured, and the percentage of bone loss is calculated as mentioned in the diagram. (Reproduced with permission from Provencher MT, Bhatia S, Ghodadra NS, et al: Recurrent shoulder instability. Current concepts for evaluation and management of glenoid bone loss. *J Bone Joint Surg Am* 2010;92[suppl 2]:133-151. doi:10.2106/JBJS.J.00906.)

The measurement and the classification of humeral head defects have been less thoroughly investigated. The most commonly used system grades the severity of the lesion based on the percentage of articular surface involved.[21] A grade I lesion involves less than 20%, a grade II lesion involves 20% to 40%, and a grade III lesion involves more than 40% of the articular surface.

Management and Outcomes

The ultimate goal of surgery is to provide the patient with a stable and functional shoulder, with minimal risk of arthropathy and a safe return to desired activities. The patient's age, anticipated postoperative activity level, and extent of glenoid and/or humeral bone loss are three of the most important factors to consider when developing a patient-specific treatment plan.

Nonsurgical Management

Nonsurgical management is of limited benefit for most patients with recurrent instability. Nonetheless, surgery

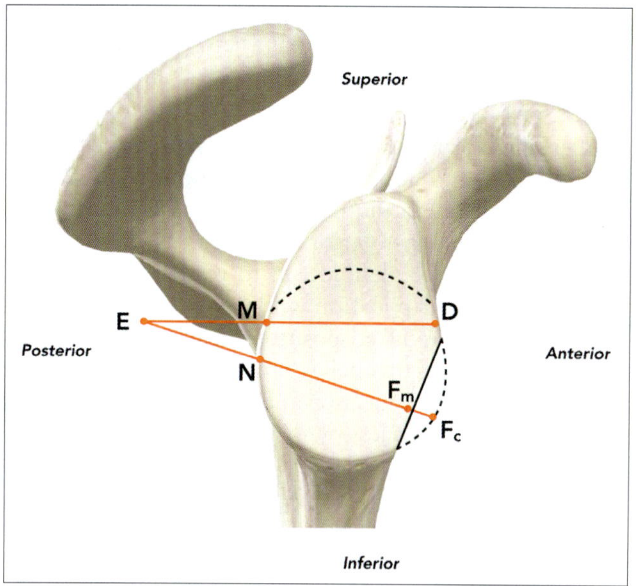

FIGURE 15 Schematic diagram showing that in the presence of anterior-inferior glenoid bone loss, the measured chord FN (F_MN) will be less than the calculated value of FN (F_cN) because the inferior portion of the glenoid is no longer circular. Percent bone loss is equal to ($F_cN - F_mN$)/(F_cN). (Adapted from Arthroscopy 25[11]. Detterline AJ, Provencher MT, Ghodadra N, et al: A New Arthroscopic Technique to Determine Anterior-Inferior Glenoid Bone Loss: Validation of the Secant Chord Theory in a Cadaveric Model, 1249-1256. Copyright © 2009 Arthroscopy Association of North America. doi:10.1016/j.arthro.2009.05.019.)

may not be the preferred treatment in a patient who is older than approximately 50 years and has low physical demands, has a significant medical comorbidity such as uncontrolled seizures, or will be unable to complete the tedious postoperative rehabilitation process. Also, it is important to evaluate for a rotator cuff tear in any patient older than 40 years who has shoulder instability. The most common site of rotator cuff tear in a patient with recurrent instability and older than 40 years occurs at the anterior border of the supraspinatus and is most often classified as a partial articular sided tear of the supraspinatus.[43] Nonsurgical treatment should focus on strengthening the dynamic stabilizers of the shoulder, including the rotator cuff and the periscapular muscles.

In-season athletes are a unique and challenging group of patients. These patients often desire to return to competitive play as quickly as possible and are willing to risk redislocation. They can be successfully treated with a brace to limit at-risk external rotation positions, with surgery delayed until the off-season.[44] Furthermore, a recent observational study found that competitive high school football players sustaining an in season instability event (either subluxation or dislocation) were able to return to sport in season without missing additional time nearly 80% of the time.[45]

Surgical Management

No clear algorithm has been developed to treat the wide range of pathology in recurrent dislocation, but general guidelines aid in selecting specific treatment based on the patient's unique history, examination, and imaging findings. Instability resulting from bone loss of the glenoid and the humeral head should be considered as a continuum because these conditions commonly occur in combination and not as isolated lesions. One patient may have a small, shallow Hill-Sachs lesion combined with 30% attritional GBL; another patient may have only minimal GBL but a large, engaging Hill-Sachs lesion; and a third patient may have 20% GBL with a medium-size engaging Hill-Sachs lesion. Each patient with recurrent anterior shoulder instability must be carefully and individually assessed to determine the cause of the instability, and the clues will help in formulating a patient specific surgical plan. This approach can optimize patient outcomes while avoiding overtreatment or undertreatment, which can result if a nonspecific algorithm is followed. Every patient should receive a thorough and detailed examination under anesthesia. The ease and the direction of humeral head translation should be carefully assessed in the anterior, inferior, and posterior directions.

Most surgeons prefer to use an arthroscopic rather than an open approach for most patients.[46-48] Arthroscopy allows better visualization and more complete capsular plication and shifting in a posterior-to-anterior direction. Arthroscopy also avoids the complications and other issues associated with open surgical dissection. Multiple studies have found that recurrence rates after arthroscopy are equivalent to or lower than those after traditional open surgery.[46-48] It is important to note that most arthroscopic studies excluded patients with significant bone loss. It is well established that arthroscopic treatment of these patients carries a considerable risk of failure.

Some surgeons recommend using the Instability Severity Index Score to help determine whether an open repair should be considered in lieu of an arthroscopic repair.[30] The Instability Severity Index Score was developed based on prospective identification of several patient risk factors for recurrent anterior instability: age younger than 20 years at the time of surgery, participation in a competitive or a contact sport or a sport involving forced overhead activity, shoulder hyperlaxity, and the presence of a Hill-Sachs lesion and/or loss of the sclerotic inferior glenoid contour on an AP radiograph of the shoulder in external rotation. These factors were integrated into a 10-point score that was retrospectively tested in the same population. Patients with a preoperative score higher than 6 points had an unacceptable 70% recurrence risk ($P < 0.001$). Although studies have helped validate this

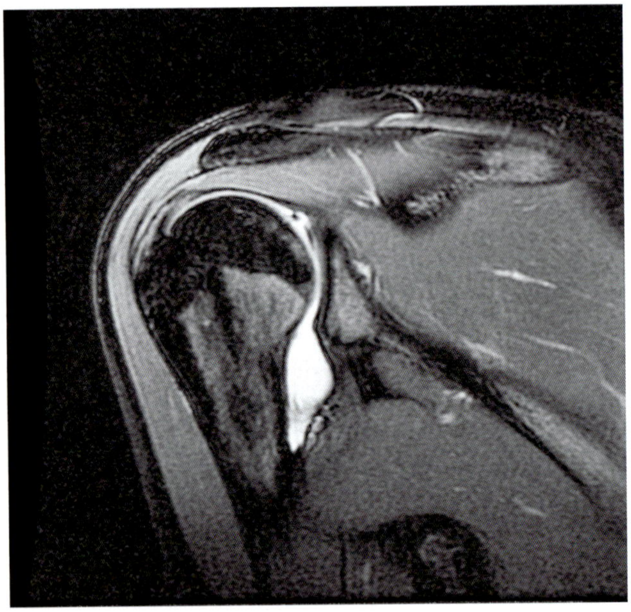

FIGURE 16 Coronal magnetic resonance arthrography showing intra-articular gadolinium leakage inferiorly down the humeral shaft, indicating a humeral avulsion of the glenohumeral ligament tear.

scoring system, other unique populations have found no validity in the scoring system and thus, it continues to be a chief recommendation to treat the individual patient to their respective needs based on demand and use of their shoulder.[49,50] Recent studies advocating for the use of ISIS have now dropped their critical value to determine bone augmentation procedures to a score of two to safely eliminate risk of recurrence.[51,52]

Revision Surgery

An arthroscopic stabilization procedure can fail for a variety of reasons, and the treating surgeon must identify the cause to decide on an appropriate revision treatment. Bone loss, whether glenoid or humeral head, is the primary reason arthroscopic stabilization procedures fail. The presence of an off-track lesion, age less than 22 years and signs of hyperlaxity have recently been found to be independent risk factors for failure of arthroscopic revision shoulder stabilization.[53] Additional factors include forced overhead activity and the use of three or fewer anchors during the repair.[17,30,54]

If the patient has an isolated engaging Hill-Sachs lesion, a revision arthroscopic Bankart repair combined with arthroscopic remplissage may be adequate.[55] Some surgeons believe that an open glenoid bone restorative procedure will restore the functional arc and shoulder stability in such patients without directly treating the humeral head defect.[56] No clearly defined algorithms are available. The surgeon should carefully define all pathology and choose the safest, most effective available procedure.

Specific Lesions

Proper identification of an ALPSA lesion is the key to its treatment. No examination findings specifically distinguish an ALPSA lesion from a Bankart lesion. On imaging studies, the labrum may not be well visualized because it is medialized and adhering to the glenoid neck. During arthroscopy, the labrum must be located (it is best seen through the anterosuperior portal) and carefully mobilized back to the glenoid rim to restore its anatomic location. Capsular plication while leaving the labrum in a medialized, unreduced position creates a high risk of failure. Some surgeons believe that ALPSA lesions are a result of recurrent dislocation and that arthroscopic repair of an ALPSA lesion is less predictably successful than that of a standard Bankart lesion.[57]

A HAGL lesion similarly cannot be reliably distinguished from a Bankart lesion on the basis of the patient history or examination. MRI and especially MRA can be helpful in identifying a HAGL lesion. The most reliable imaging finding is the absence of the teardrop shape of the capsule and the IGHL on coronal MRI studies (**Figure 16**). To treat a HAGL lesion, the patient is best placed in the lateral decubitus position with balanced traction to provide access to the inferior glenohumeral joint. A HAGL lesion can be challenging to treat arthroscopically, and the surgeon should be prepared for an open HAGL repair if arthroscopic repair is not feasible.

The GLAD lesion is of unclear significance, but most experts believe that efforts should be made to sufficiently mobilize the labrum to cover exposed bone or create fibrocartilage along the deficient area of the glenoid with microfracture.

Recurrent anterior dislocation can cause extensive labral tearing as the tear propagates around the glenoid. Patients often describe numerous low-energy dislocation events as well as significant pain, which is uncommon with more isolated labral tears. Provocative testing is likely to reveal both posterior and anterior apprehension or instability and may suggest the presence of a SLAP lesion. MRA can increase diagnostic specificity, especially in evaluating for a SLAP lesion, which can be critical for optimal planning before surgical intervention. Given the need for circumferential access to the glenoid, lateral positioning of the patient is preferred. This challenging surgery must be carefully planned, with an appropriate number of anchors and tools to allow for a circumferential labral repair.[11,58]

Bone Loss

In recurrent anterior instability, bone loss must be considered as a bipolar phenomenon. Treating one lesion without considering the other can lead to surgical failure. Nonetheless, most patients with both glenoid and humeral head bone loss are successfully treated when only the GBL is directly treated. By restoring the relatively normal morphology of the anterior glenoid, the glenoid arc is effectively lengthened, and engagement of the Hill-Sachs lesion is prevented.[5]

Glenoid Bone Loss

GBL in the setting of recurrent instability can be surgically treated with several well-described techniques. Several factors must be considered when selecting the appropriate bone restorative procedure. Although no algorithm for clinical decision making has been validated, a comprehensive review of GBL in recurrent anterior shoulder instability has provided general guidelines that depend on the amount of bone loss.[34] Based on other researchers' biomechanical and clinical research, the review concluded that anterior GBL of more than 25% to 30% significantly increases the risk of instability events.[13,59-61] Although lesions smaller than 15% were rarely thought to be insignificant historically, more recent literature has defined lesions under 13.5% to be "subcritical" with regard to outcomes.[25] In a case-control study, 13.5% as a critical cut-off for arthroscopic stabilization demonstrated reliable outcomes and low risk of recurrence in an American football population.[62]

Coracoid Transfer (Latarjet Procedure)

Coracoid transfer is the most common procedure to restore glenoid bone stock. In the United States, it is typically performed if a patient has more than 25% GBL or after unsuccessful arthroscopic stabilization in a patient with less than 25% bone loss. With both glenoid and humeral head bone deficiency, some surgeons still believe that the humeral head defect will no longer engage when the glenoid bony morphology is reestablished.[56] Several clinical studies found that the Latarjet procedure has excellent results in the setting of combined glenoid and humeral head bone loss.[63-65] One study even suggested that the Latarjet procedure will lead to a stable shoulder in patients with a large, engaging Hill-Sachs lesion without GBL.[56] Preoperative planning can help determine the arc restoration of the coracoid process by determining the degree of bone restoration that will make an off-track and on-track lesion after successful completion of a Latarjet procedure.[66] These researchers stated that the block of bone extends the glenoid arc to the point that the humeral head cannot externally rotate and anteriorly translate sufficiently for the Hill-Sachs lesion to engage over the front of the bone block. Once thought controversial, the Latarjet procedure in older patients (older than 40 years) reliably restores stability and increased satisfaction.[67,68]

Coracoid transfer procedures are invasive and not free of complications.[63] If the graft is malpositioned, further chondral injury can occur.[65] The most common long-term negative effect are radiographic arthritic changes in up to 38% of patients; however, when considering recurrent instability as the primary outcome, instability events were only seen in 8.5% of patients at greater than 16 years of follow-up.[69] Arthroscopic coracoid transfer procedures are challenging and require extensive initial laboratory experience.[70,71] New clinical studies have shown equivalent results between the arthroscopic and open techniques for Latarjet but advocate for the use of arthroscopic Latarjets in high volume centers only due to the steep learning curve.[72,73]

Alternative sources of bone graft for glenoid deficiency have been investigated because a coracoid transfer does not completely re-create the normal anatomy and contour of the anterior glenoid. These glenoid bone graft options include autograft or allograft iliac crest, allograft glenoid, and, distal tibial allograft[74] (**Figure 17**). Studies have shown equivalent clinical results with less overall graft resorption when comparing distal tibial allograft to the open Latarjet procedure. Arthroscopic advances now allow for bone augmentation to be performed to adequately restore the anterior glenoid showing good short- to midterm results with the use of iliac crest.[75-77]

Humeral Head Bone Loss (Hill-Sachs Lesions)

Most Hill-Sachs lesions are small (less than 20% of the articular surface), shallow, and not clinically significant.

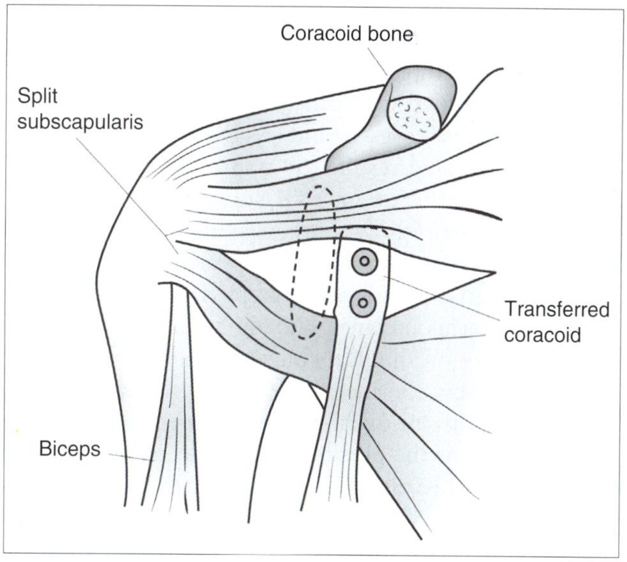

FIGURE 17 Schematic diagram showing that the Latarjet procedure involves a transfer of the coracoid process to the medial glenoid via a split of the subscapularis. The coracoid provides for glenohumeral stability by augmenting the anterior glenoid rim, whereas the conjoined tendon acts as a stabilizer with the arm abducted and externally rotated. (Reproduced from Burns JP, Snyder SJ: Shoulder instability, in Fischgrund JS, ed: *Orthopaedic Knowledge Update*, ed 9. Rosemont, IL, American Academy of Orthopaedic Surgeons, 2008, pp 301-311.)

A lesion larger than 40% of the articular surface almost always is clinically significant and must be directly treated. The challenge is to decide whether a lesion between 20% and 40% of the articular surface is clinically significant enough to treat directly or whether it can be rendered insignificant by appropriate treatment of GBL.

The treatment should be aimed at restoring a stable arc of motion. In many patients, restoration of the glenoid side alone may be sufficient because it restores the normal glenoid track and reduces the risk of Hill-Sachs lesion engagement. It is especially important in this setting to understand that bone loss is a bipolar phenomenon; GBL can potentiate a medium-size Hill-Sachs lesion and increase the risk of instability. Without GBL, the Hill-Sachs lesion may not engage on the anterior glenoid. With GBL, less anterior translation or external rotation is needed for the humeral head lesion to engage. Several techniques have been described to treat the humeral head defect, each of which has a role.

Remplissage

Arthroscopic remplissage (translated from French as "filling") was developed as a means of filling the humeral head defect to render the lesion extra-articular and therefore nonengaging. The open version of this technique, known as the Connolly procedure, was described in 1972 and involves transferring part of the greater tuberosity into the defect, along with the infraspinatus tendon.[78] The arthroscopic technique, described in 2008, involves a posterior capsulodesis and an infraspinatus tenodesis.[79] Although the exact indications for remplissage have yet to be defined, it may be best used in patients with a medium-size or large, shallow, engaging Hill-Sachs lesion and less than 20% GBL.

Early promising results for arthroscopic remplissage have been published, with 98% stability reported in one study.[20,55] In the setting of an engaging Hill-Sachs lesion without an inverted pear glenoid appearance, arthroscopic Bankart repair combine with remplissage has shown excellent long-term outcomes with low recurrence rates with minimal effect on shoulder range of motion.[80,81] Furthermore, this is now considered a viable approach for adolescents with recurrent instability to help optimize shoulder stability without the possible risks of decreased range of motion and arthropathy changes seen with Latarjet.[82] It is important to note that the patients were carefully selected and had limited GBL and a large Hill-Sachs lesion. Remplissage alone probably would be insufficient in patients with more than 25% GBL, and strong consideration should be given to a glenoid-based bony procedure for these patients. The new treatment algorithm advocated in a recent study suggests utilization of the Remplissage technique with Bankart repair for engaging Hill-Sachs lesions measuring between 20% and 40% in volume with less than 20% GBL.[83]

Bone Grafting

Bone grafting procedures have been used in an attempt to restore the bony architecture of the humeral head to prevent lesion engagement. Bone grafting typically is indicated in the uncommon setting of a large Hill-Sachs lesion (more than 40% of the articular surface) with minimal GBL. Filling the defect and restoring normal anatomy reestablishes the articular arc of the humeral head, thus preventing lesion engagement. Both autograft and allograft bone plug techniques have been described, and fresh-frozen osteoarticular allografts also have been used.[5,84] These procedures are technically challenging, and the risk of disease transmission with allograft use must be considered.

Disimpaction of a Hill-Sachs compression fracture is a relatively new procedure with little available clinical or biomechanical data.[5] Several different techniques have been reported, all of which involve elevating the compression fracture and applying bone graft to support the elevated bone. The clinical application of this procedure has not been defined, but it may be best suited for an acute lesion involving less than 40% of the articular surface.

Resurfacing

Partial resurfacing, complete resurfacing, and hemiarthroplasty are used to restore a more normal articular arc to the humeral head. These procedures should be used cautiously in young, active patients because of the risks of hardware loosening and glenoid wear. The indications are unclear, but the use of implants is best suited for patients who are older, have lower physical demands, or have a lesion larger than 40% of the articular surface. One definitive surgery typically is preferred for a patient older than approximately 50 to 60 years, and therefore hemiarthroplasty or total shoulder arthroplasty may be chosen over a resurfacing procedure.

SUMMARY

Several factors commonly contribute to recurrent anterior shoulder instability. As with most orthopaedic conditions, a complete history and physical examination provide the keys to a correct diagnosis. Advanced imaging studies are desirable for every patient with recurrent instability. MRA can be useful to delineate a SLAP lesion or more extensive or subtle labral pathology. If GBL or a significant Hill-Sachs lesion is suspected, three-dimensional CT is the preferred imaging modality. Bone loss in the glenoid and/or humeral head is present in almost all patients with recurrent instability, and it must be recognized and appropriately treated to minimize further injury to the joint. Proper diagnosis leads to appropriate patient counseling and the selection of the ideal technique.

KEY STUDY POINTS

- Certain activities substantially increase the risk of shoulder dislocation, including contact sports such as football, rugby, basketball, lacrosse, and martial arts; military training such as hand-to-hand drills and obstacle course training; climbing; and other sports or activities during which the patient's arm may be forcibly abducted and externally rotated.
- Certain uncommon anatomic findings are seen with relative frequency during imaging evaluation or arthroscopic visualization of patients with recurrent anterior shoulder instability. These include an ALPSA lesion, a HAGL, a circumferential or extensive labral tear, and a GLAD lesion.
- Bone loss in the glenoid and/or humeral head is present in almost all patients with recurrent instability, and it must be recognized and appropriately treated to minimize further injury to the joint. Proper diagnosis leads to appropriate patient counseling and the selection of the ideal technique.
- The ultimate goal of surgery is to provide the patient with a stable and functional shoulder, with minimal risk of failure and a safe return to desired activities. The patient's age, anticipated postoperative activity level, and extent of glenoid and/or humeral bone loss are three of the most important factors to consider when developing a patient-specific treatment plan.
- Glenoid and humeral head bone loss in the setting of recurrent anterior shoulder instability can be surgically treated with several well-described techniques. Several factors must be considered when selecting the appropriate bone restorative procedure.

Annotated References

1. Hovelius L, Augustini BG, Fredin H, Johansson O, Norlin R, Thorling J: Primary anterior dislocation of the shoulder in young patients. A ten-year prospective study. *J Bone Joint Surg Am* 1996;78(11):1677-1684.

2. Taylor DC, Arciero RA: Pathologic changes associated with shoulder dislocations. Arthroscopic and physical examination findings in first-time, traumatic anterior dislocations. *Am J Sports Med* 1997;25(3):306-311.

3. Armitage MS, Faber KJ, Drosdowech DS, Litchfield RB, Athwal GS: Humeral head bone defects: Remplissage, allograft, and arthroplasty. *Orthop Clin North Am* 2010;41(3):417-425.

4. Dickens JF, Slaven SE, Cameron KL, et al: Prospective evaluation of glenoid bone loss after first-time and recurrent anterior glenohumeral instability events. *Am J Sports Med* 2019;47(5):1082-1089.

   A military cohort study of 714 patients demonstrates 6.8% bone loss after a first-time instability event and average of 22.8% with recurrent instability. In addition, patients with a history of instability present with average of 10.8% bone loss regardless of symptoms on presentation. This study advocates for early stabilization in the young and active patient after a first-time dislocation. Level of evidence: II.

5. Provencher MT, Frank RM, Leclere LE, et al: The Hill-Sachs lesion: Diagnosis, classification, and management. *J Am Acad Orthop Surg* 2012;20(4):242-252.

6. Shin SJ, Ko YW, Jeon YS, Lee J, Kim RG, Baek H: Comparison of intra-articular findings and clinical features between patients with symptomatic anterior instability after recurrent shoulder subluxation and dislocation. *Arthroscopy* 2017;33(3):527-533.

   This case control study compares patients with symptomatic subluxation of the glenohumeral joint with those with frank dislocation instability. Despite different degrees of instability, both groups were found to have similar rates of SLAP lesions, ALPSA lesions, and bony Bankart lesions. The subluxation group had significantly fewer Hill-Sachs lesions. The clinical importance of symptomatic recurrent subluxation should be considered comparable with that of recurrent dislocation. Level of evidence: IV.

7. Neviaser TJ: The anterior labroligamentous periosteal sleeve avulsion lesion: A cause of anterior instability of the shoulder. *Arthroscopy* 1993;9(1):17-21.

8. Yiannakopoulos CK, Mataragas E, Antonogiannakis E: A comparison of the spectrum of intra-articular lesions in acute and chronic anterior shoulder instability. *Arthroscopy* 2007;23(9):985-990.

9. Wolf EM, Cheng JC, Dickson K: Humeral avulsion of glenohumeral ligaments as a cause of anterior shoulder instability. *Arthroscopy* 1995;11(5):600-607.

10. Patzkowski JC, Dickens JF, Cameron KL, Bokshan SL, Garcia EJ, Owens BD: Pathoanatomy of shoulder instability in collegiate female athletes. *Am J Sports Med* 2019;47(8):1909-1914.

    In a case series of 36 female military patients with shoulder instability, female patients most often present with a history of multiple subluxation events. In addition, patients presented with higher rates of HAGL lesions (25%) and combined anterior and posterior labral tears (19%) while having fewer bony Bankart lesions (2.8%) compared with prior reports. Level of evidence: IV.

11. Tokish JM, McBratney CM, Solomon DJ, Leclere L, Dewing CB, Provencher MT: Arthroscopic repair of circumferential lesions of the glenoid labrum. *J Bone Joint Surg Am* 2009;91(12):2795-2802.

12. Pogorzelski J, Fritz EM, Horan MP, Katthagen JC, Provencher MT, Millett PJ: Failure following arthroscopic Bankart repair for traumatic anteroinferior instability of the shoulder: Is a glenoid labral articular disruption (GLAD) lesion a risk factor for recurrent instability? *J Shoulder Elbow Surg* 2018;27(8):e235-e242.

    In a series of 72 patients with minimum 2-year follow-up, the presence of a GLAD lesion portended to a worse clinical outcome and higher risk of failure compared with those being treated for an isolated Bankart lesion. Level of evidence: IV.

13. Burkhart SS, De Beer JF: Traumatic glenohumeral bone defects and their relationship to failure of arthroscopic Bankart repairs: Significance of the inverted-pear glenoid and the humeral engaging Hill-Sachs lesion. *Arthroscopy* 2000;16(7):677-694.

14. Bockmann B, Venjakob AJ, Reichwein F, Hagenacker M, Nebelung W: Mapping of glenoid bone loss in recurrent anterior shoulder instability: Is there a particular deficit pattern? *J Shoulder Elbow Surg* 2017;26(9):1676-1680

    In this imaging study, 44 consecutive patients treated for recurrent anterior shoulder instability were evaluated for morphology of bone loss. Regardless of size of lesion, the orientation of the bone loss was vertical in nature. Level of evidence: IV.

15. Lazarus MD, Sidles JA, Harryman DT II, Matsen FA III: Effect of a chondral-labral defect on glenoid concavity and glenohumeral stability. A cadaveric model. *J Bone Joint Surg Am* 1996;78(1):94-102.

16. Mologne TS, Provencher MT, Menzel KA, Vachon TA, Dewing CB: Arthroscopic stabilization in patients with an inverted pear glenoid: Results in patients with bone loss of the anterior glenoid. *Am J Sports Med* 2007;35(8):1276-1283.

17. Boileau P, Villalba M, Hery JY, Balg F, Ahrens P, Neyton L: Risk factors for recurrence of shoulder instability after arthroscopic Bankart repair. *J Bone Joint Surg Am* 2006;88(8):1755-1763.

18. Rowe CR, Zarins B, Ciullo JV: Recurrent anterior dislocation of the shoulder after surgical repair. Apparent causes of failure and treatment. *J Bone Joint Surg Am* 1984;66(2):159-168.

19. Calandra JJ, Baker CL, Uribe J: The incidence of Hill-Sachs lesions in initial anterior shoulder dislocations. *Arthroscopy* 1989;5(4):254-257.

20. Franceschi F, Papalia R, Rizzello G, et al: Remplissage repair—New frontiers in the prevention of recurrent shoulder instability: A 2-year follow-up comparative study. *Am J Sports Med* 2012;40(11):2462-2469.

21. Flatow EL, Warner JI: Instability of the shoulder: Complex problems and failed repairs: Part I. Relevant biomechanics, multidirectional instability, and severe glenoid loss. *Instr Course Lect* 1998;47:97-112.

22. Hall RH, Isaac F, Booth CR: Dislocations of the shoulder with special reference to accompanying small fractures. *J Bone Joint Surg Am* 1959;41-A(3):489-494.

23. Richards RD, Sartoris DJ, Pathria MN, Resnick D: Hill-Sachs lesion and normal humeral groove: MR imaging features allowing their differentiation. *Radiology* 1994;190(3):665-668.

24. Yamamoto N, Itoi E, Abe H, et al: Contact between the glenoid and the humeral head in abduction, external rotation, and horizontal extension: A new concept of glenoid track. *J Shoulder Elbow Surg* 2007;16(5):649-656.

25. Shaha JS, Cook JB, Rowles DJ, Bottoni CR, Shaha SH, Tokish JM: Clinical validation of the glenoid track concept in anterior glenohumeral instability. *J Bone Joint Surg Am* 2016;98(22):1918-1923.

    Over a 2-year period, all patients evaluated in this cohort were evaluated for their glenoid track, which proved to be more accurate in predicting postoperative stability compared with glenoid bone loss. Level of evidence: III.

26. Owens BD, Dawson L, Burks R, Cameron KL: Incidence of shoulder dislocation in the United States military: Demographic considerations from a high-risk population. *J Bone Joint Surg Am* 2009;91(4):791-796.

27. Robinson CM, Howes J, Murdoch H, Will E, Graham C: Functional outcome and risk of recurrent instability after primary traumatic anterior shoulder dislocation in young patients. *J Bone Joint Surg Am* 2006;88(11): 2326-2336.

28. te Slaa RL, Wijffels MP, Brand R, Marti RK: The prognosis following acute primary glenohumeral dislocation. *J Bone Joint Surg Br* 2004;86(1):58-64.

29. Mather RC III, Orlando LA, Henderson RA, Lawrence JT, Taylor DC: A predictive model of shoulder instability after a first-time anterior shoulder dislocation. *J Shoulder Elbow Surg* 2011;20(2):259-266.

30. Balg F, Boileau P: The instability severity index score. A simple pre-operative score to select patients for arthroscopic or open shoulder stabilisation. *J Bone Joint Surg Br* 2007;89(11):1470-1477.

31. Owens BD, Duffey ML, Nelson BJ, DeBerardino TM, Taylor DC, Mountcastle SB: The incidence and characteristics of shoulder instability at the United States Military Academy. *Am J Sports Med* 2007;35(7):1168-1173.

32. Simonet WT, Melton LJ III, Cofield RH, Ilstrup DM: Incidence of anterior shoulder dislocation in Olmsted County, Minnesota. *Clin Orthop Relat Res* 1984;186:186-191.

33. Gagey OJ, Gagey N: The hyperabduction test. *J Bone Joint Surg Br* 2001;83(1):69-74.

34. Piasecki DP, Verma NN, Romeo AA, Levine WN, Bach BR Jr, Provencher MT: Glenoid bone deficiency in recurrent anterior shoulder instability: Diagnosis and management. *J Am Acad Orthop Surg* 2009;17(8):482-493.

35. Rerko MA, Pan X, Donaldson C, Jones GL, Bishop JY: Comparison of various imaging techniques to quantify glenoid bone loss in shoulder instability. *J Shoulder Elbow Surg* 2013;22(4):528-534.

    In this critical imaging study, evaluation of cadaveric specimens was performed to compare 2D and 3D CT scans, radiographs, and magnetic resonance images to evaluate glenoid bone loss. 3D CT scans were most predictive of accurate glenoid bone loss evaluation and most consistent among all evaluators. Level of evidence: III.

36. McNeil JW, Beaulieu-Jones BR, Bernhardson AS, et al: Classification and analysis of attritional glenoid bone loss in recurrent anterior shoulder instability. *Am J Sports Med* 2017;45(4):767-774.

    In the setting of recurrent instability and if a residual bone fragment persists, the bone fragment undergoes extensive remodeling and cannot restore native glenoid bone stock. In addition, patients with longer durations of instability undergo greater amounts of attritional bone loss, and thus symptom duration should be an essential part of any history during examination. Level of evidence: III.

37. Bakshi NK, Patel I, Jacobson JA, Debski RE, Sekiya JK: Comparison of 3-dimensional computed tomography-based measurement of glenoid bone loss with arthroscopic defect size estimation in patients with anterior shoulder instability. *Arthroscopy* 2015;31(10):1880-1885.

    Twenty patients with recurrent anterior shoulder instability had comparisons of evaluation of bone loss with 3D CT and arthroscopy. 3D CT was found to be more reliable and more accurate and is a necessary imaging modality before further treatment. Level of evidence: IV.

38. Huysmans PE, Haen PS, Kidd M, Dhert WJ, Willems JW: The shape of the inferior part of the glenoid: A cadaveric study. *J Shoulder Elbow Surg* 2006;15(6):759-763.

39. Sugaya H, Moriishi J, Dohi M, Kon Y, Tsuchiya A: Glenoid rim morphology in recurrent anterior glenohumeral instability. *J Bone Joint Surg Am* 2003;85(5):878-884.

40. Sugaya H, Kon Y, Tsuchiya A: Arthroscopic repair of glenoid fractures using suture anchors. *Arthroscopy* 2005;21(5):635.

41. Kralinger F, Aigner F, Longato S, Rieger M, Wambacher M: Is the bare spot a consistent landmark for shoulder arthroscopy? A study of 20 embalmed glenoids with 3-dimensional computed tomographic reconstruction. *Arthroscopy* 2006;22(4):428-432.

42. Detterline AJ, Provencher MT, Ghodadra N, Bach BR Jr, Romeo AA, Verma NN: A new arthroscopic technique to determine anterior-inferior glenoid bone loss: Validation of the secant chord theory in a cadaveric model. *Arthroscopy* 2009;25(11):1249-1256.

43. Ueda Y, Sugaya H, Takahashi N, et al: Prevalence and site of rotator cuff lesions in shoulders with recurrent anterior instability in a young population. *Orthop J Sports Med* 2019;7(6):2325967119849876.

    In patients aged 40 years or younger, there is a 7% incidence of partial rotator cuff tears, with most being PASTA lesions involving the anterior border of the supraspinatus. Level of evidence: IV.

44. Buss DD, Lynch GP, Meyer CP, Huber SM, Freehill MQ: Nonoperative management for in-season athletes with anterior shoulder instability. *Am J Sports Med* 2004;32(6):1430-1433.

45. Shanley E, Thigpen C, Brooks J, et al: Return to sport as an outcome measure for shoulder instability: Surprising findings in nonoperative management in a high school athlete population. *Am J Sports Med* 2019;47(5):1062-1067.

    A consecutive series of high school athletes with anterior shoulder instability treated with surgery versus nonsurgical management were compared. There was no difference between groups in patients returning to sport the following season without recurrence. Patients presenting with subluxation versus dislocation were more likely to undergo successful nonsurgical treatment. Level of evidence: II.

46. Zaffagnini S, Marcheggiani Muccioli GM, Giordano G, et al: Long-term outcomes after repair of recurrent post-traumatic anterior shoulder instability: Comparison of arthroscopic transglenoid suture and open Bankart reconstruction. *Knee Surg Sports Traumatol Arthrosc* 2012;20(5):816-821.

47. Petrera M, Patella V, Patella S, Theodoropoulos J: A meta-analysis of open versus arthroscopic Bankart repair using suture anchors. *Knee Surg Sports Traumatol Arthrosc* 2010;18(12):1742-1747.

48. Archetti Netto N, Tamaoki MJ, Lenza M, et al: Treatment of Bankart lesions in traumatic anterior instability of the shoulder: A randomized controlled trial comparing arthroscopy and open techniques. *Arthroscopy* 2012;28(7):900-908.

49. Bouliane M, Saliken D, Beaupre LA, Silveira A, Saraswat MK, Sheps DM: Evaluation of the Instability Severity Index Score and the Western Ontario Shoulder Instability Index as predictors of failure following arthroscopic Bankart repair. *Bone Joint J* 2014;96-B(12):1688-1692.

    At minimum 2 years follow-up, preoperative assessment with both the ISIS score and WOSI was not predictive of recurrent anterior shoulder instability after arthroscopic Bankart repair. Level of evidence: IV.

50. Chan AG, Kilcoyne KG, Chan S, Dickens JF, Waterman BR: Evaluation of the Instability Severity Index score in predicting failure following arthroscopic Bankart surgery in an active military population. *J Shoulder Elbow Surg* 2019;28(5):e156-e163.

    Neither composite ISIS preoperative score nor any of its individual factors were predictive of recurrent shoulder instability in an active and at-risk population at minimum 2-year follow-up.

51. Loppini M, Delle Rose G, Borroni M, et al: Is the Instability Severity Index Score a valid tool for predicting failure after primary arthroscopic stabilization for anterior glenohumeral instability? *Arthroscopy* 2019;35(2):361-366.

    The authors determined a significant increased risk of anterior shoulder instability recurrence with composite ISIS scores greater than 3. Level of evidence: III.

52. Thomazeau H, Langlais T, Hardy A, et al: Long-term, prospective, multicenter study of isolated Bankart repair for a patient selection method based on the Instability Severity Index Score. *Am J Sports Med* 2019;47(5): 1057-1061.

    In patients with isolated anterior shoulder pathology in the setting of instability, a score of 2 or less out of 10 leads to acceptable recurrence rates (10%). Level of evidence: II.

53. Su F, Kowalczuk M, Ikpe S, Lee H, Sabzevari S, Lin A: Risk factors for failure of arthroscopic revision anterior shoulder stabilization. *J Bone Joint Surg Am* 2018;100(15):1319-1325.

    Revision Bankart repairs have unacceptably high rates of recurrence (19%) if they have additional risk factors of being less than 22 years of age, an off-track lesion, and ligamentous laxity. Level of evidence: IV.

54. Calvo E, Granizo JJ, Fernandez-Yruegas D: Criteria for arthroscopic treatment of anterior instability of the shoulder: A prospective study. *J Bone Joint Surg Br* 2005;87(5):677-683.

55. Boileau P, O'Shea K, Vargas P, Pinedo M, Old J, Zumstein M: Anatomical and functional results after arthroscopic Hill-Sachs remplissage. *J Bone Joint Surg Am* 2012;94(7):618-626.

56. Burkhart SS, De Beer JF, Barth JR, Cresswell T, Roberts C, Richards DP: Results of modified Latarjet reconstruction in patients with anteroinferior instability and significant bone loss. *Arthroscopy* 2007;23(10):1033-1041.

57. Ozbaydar M, Elhassan B, Diller D, Massimini D, Higgins LD, Warner JJ: Results of arthroscopic capsulolabral repair: Bankart lesion versus anterior labroligamentous periosteal sleeve avulsion lesion. *Arthroscopy* 2008;24(11):1277-1283.

58. Lo IK, Burkhart SS: Triple labral lesions: Pathology and surgical repair technique—report of seven cases. *Arthroscopy* 2005;21(2):186-193.

59. Lo IK, Parten PM, Burkhart SS: The inverted pear glenoid: An indicator of significant glenoid bone loss. *Arthroscopy* 2004;20(2):169-174.

60. Itoi E, Lee SB, Berglund LJ, Berge LL, An KN: The effect of a glenoid defect on anteroinferior stability of the shoulder after Bankart repair: A cadaveric study. *J Bone Joint Surg Am* 2000;82(1):35-46.

61. Greis PE, Scuderi MG, Mohr A, Bachus KN, Burks RT: Glenohumeral articular contact areas and pressures following labral and osseous injury to the anteroinferior quadrant of the glenoid. *J Shoulder Elbow Surg* 2002;11(5):442-451.

62. Dickens JF, Owens BD, Cameron KL, et al: The effect of subcritical bone loss and exposure on recurrent instability after arthroscopic Bankart repair in intercollegiate American football. *Am J Sports Med* 2017;45(8):1769-1775.

    When critically evaluating glenoid bone loss in the professional American football athlete, patients with <13.5% glenoid bone loss had zero recurrence for mean 1.5 seasons of follow-up. Level of evidence: III.

63. Shah AA, Butler RB, Romanowski J, Goel D, Karadagli D, Warner JJ: Short-term complications of the Latarjet procedure. *J Bone Joint Surg Am* 2012;94(6):495-501.

64. Hovelius L, Vikerfors O, Olofsson A, Svensson O, Rahme H: Bristow-Latarjet and Bankart: A comparative study of shoulder stabilization in 185 shoulders during a seventeen-year follow-up. *J Shoulder Elbow Surg* 2011;20(7):1095-1101.

65. Ghodadra N, Gupta A, Romeo AA, et al: Normalization of glenohumeral articular contact pressures after Latarjet or iliac crest bone-grafting. *J Bone Joint Surg Am* 2010;92(6):1478-1489.

66. Mook WR, Petri M, Greenspoon JA, Horan MP, Dornan GJ, Millett PJ: Clinical and anatomic predictors of outcomes after the Latarjet procedure for the treatment of anterior glenohumeral instability with combined glenoid and humeral bone defects. *Am J Sports Med* 2016;44(6):1407-1416.

    The width of the coracoid can be used preoperatively to determine if a shoulder with combined glenoid and humeral head pathology will be on-track or off-track after undergoing a Latarjet procedure. Level of evidence: IV.

67. Moroder P, Stefanitsch V, Auffarth A, Matis N, Resch H, Plachel F: Treatment of recurrent anterior shoulder instability with the Latarjet or Bristow procedure in older patients. *J Shoulder Elbow Surg* 2018;27(5):824-830.

    Twenty-seven patients older than 40 years were treated for shoulder instability in the setting of glenoid deficits. Although nine patients required revision surgery at mean follow-up of 9 years, patients demonstrated improvement in clinical outcomes, and thus the Bristow-Latarjet is a viable joint-preserving option in this unique older patient population.

68. Ernstbrunner L, Wartmann L, Zimmermann SM, Schenk P, Gerber C, Wieser K: Long-term results of the open Latarjet procedure for recurrent anterior shoulder instability in patients older than 40 years. *Am J Sports Med* 2019;47(13):3057-3064.

    Patients older than 40 years were treated with a Bristow-Latarjet procedure for recurrent anterior shoulder instability. Although clinical outcome scores improved along with maintained stability, a substantial rate of dislocation arthropathy persists. Level of evidence: IV.

69. Hurley ET, Jamal MS, Ali ZS, Montgomery C, Pauzenberger L, Mullett H: Long-term outcomes of the Latarjet procedure for anterior shoulder instability: A systematic review of studies at 10-year follow-up. *J Shoulder Elbow Surg* 2019;28(2):e33-e39.

This systematic review with greater than 10 years follow-up after Latarjet procedures for recurrent anterior shoulder instability found excellent restoration of joint stability, increase in long-term functional outcomes, and a high return rate to sporting activities. Level of evidence: IV.

70. Lafosse L, Boyle S, Gutierrez-Aramberri M, Shah A, Meller R: Arthroscopic Latarjet procedure. *Orthop Clin North Am* 2010;41(3):393-405.

71. Boileau P, Mercier N, Roussanne Y, Thelu CE, Old J: Arthroscopic Bankart-Bristow-Latarjet procedure: The development and early results of a safe and reproducible technique. *Arthroscopy* 2010;26(11): 1434-1450.

72. Zhu Y, Jiang C, Song G: Arthroscopic versus open Latarjet in the treatment of recurrent anterior shoulder dislocation with marked glenoid bone loss: A prospective comparative study. *Am J Sports Med* 2017;45(7):1645-1653.

Outcomes of arthroscopic and open Latarjet were compared with minimum 2-year follow-up. The open group had better placement in the superior-inferior direction. At 1 year after surgery, patients in the arthroscopic Latarjet group showed notably less graft resorption compared with patients in the open Latarjet group. Level of evidence: III.

73. Hurley ET, Lim Fat D, Farrington SK, Mullett H: Open versus arthroscopic Latarjet procedure for anterior shoulder instability: A systematic review and meta-analysis. *Am J Sports Med* 2019;47(5):1248-1253.

Both open and arthroscopic Latarjet procedures result in improvements in patient function and outcome scores with similar complication rates. Level of evidence: III.

74. Provencher MT, Bhatia S, Ghodadra NS, et al: Recurrent shoulder instability: Current concepts for evaluation and management of glenoid bone loss. *J Bone Joint Surg Am* 2010;92(suppl 2):133-151.

75. Provencher MT, Frank RM, Golijanin P, et al: Distal tibia allograft glenoid reconstruction in recurrent anterior shoulder instability: Clinical and radiographic outcomes. *Arthroscopy* 2017;33(5):891-897.

At average follow-up of 45 months, distal tibia allograft resulted in excellent clinical outcomes along with an 89% graft healing rate as determined by 2D CT scans. Level of evidence: IV.

76. Frank RM, Romeo AA, Richardson C, et al: Outcomes of Latarjet versus distal tibia allograft for anterior shoulder instability repair: A matched cohort analysis. *Am J Sports Med* 2018;46(5):1030-1038.

Latarjet and distal tibia allograft reconstruction procedures for anterior shoulder instability in the setting of glenoid bone loss resulted in equivalent clinical outcomes and stability at minimum 2-year follow-up with similar complication rates (10%) between the two groups. Level of Evidence: III.

77. Ernstbrunner L, Plachel F, Heuberer P, et al: Arthroscopic versus open iliac crest bone grafting in recurrent anterior shoulder instability with glenoid bone loss: A computed tomography-based quantitative assessment. *Arthroscopy* 2018;34(2):352-359.

Arthroscopic and open iliac crest bone grafting for glenoid bone loss have similar elements of positioning except for the significantly increased impaction angle in the arthroscopic procedure. Level of evidence: III.

78. Connolly JF. Humeral head defects associated with shoulder dislocations—their diagnostic and surgical significance. *Instr Course Lect* 1972;21:42-54.

79. Purchase RJ, Wolf EM, Hobgood ER, Pollock ME, Smalley CC: Hill-Sachs "remplissage": An arthroscopic solution for the engaging Hill-Sachs lesion. *Arthroscopy* 2008;24(6):723-726.

80. Brilakis E, Mataragas E, Deligeorgis A, Maniatis V, Antonogiannakis E: Midterm outcomes of arthroscopic remplissage for the management of recurrent anterior shoulder instability. *Knee Surg Sports Traumatol Arthrosc* 2016;24(2):593-600.

In the setting of an engaging Hill-Sachs lesion, an arthroscopic Remplissage and Bankart repair results in low risk of recurrent instability (6.3%) and increase in clinical outcome scores. In addition, there was no documentation of decreased or altered range of motion after a Remplissage was performed. Level of evidence: IV.

81. Brilakis E, Avramidis G, Malahias MA, et al: Long-term outcome of arthroscopic remplissage in addition to the classic Bankart repair for the management of recurrent anterior shoulder instability with engaging Hill-Sachs lesions. *Knee Surg Sports Traumatol Arthrosc* 2019;27(1):305-313.

In the setting of an engaging Hill-Sachs lesion, an arthroscopic Remplissage and Bankart repair results in low risk of recurrent instability (5.6%) (mean follow-up of 8.1 years) and increase in clinical outcome scores. In addition, there was no documentation of decreased or altered range of motion after a Remplissage was performed. Level of evidence: IV.

82. Hughes JL, Bastrom T, Pennock AT, Edmonds EW: Arthroscopic Bankart repairs with and without remplissage in recurrent adolescent anterior shoulder instability with Hill-Sachs deformity. *Orthop J Sports Med* 2018;6(12):2325967118813981.

When glenoid bone loss and an engaging Hill-Sachs lesion present in an adolescent patient population, a Bankart repair with Remplissage leads to improvement in clinical outcomes and low risk of recurrence compared to an isolated Bankart repair alone. Level of evidence: III.

83. Liu JN, Gowd AK, Garcia GH, Cvetanovich GL, Cabarcas BC, Verma NN: Recurrence rate of instability after remplissage for treatment of traumatic anterior shoulder instability: A systematic review in treatment of subcritical glenoid bone loss. *Arthroscopy* 2018;34(10):2894-2907.e2.

    Arthroscopic remplissage combined with Bankart repair is an effective procedure in the treatment of patients with engaging Hill-Sachs lesions and minimal glenoid bone loss. Minimal loss of external rotation compared with Bankart repair alone was demonstrated. As a result, the authors recommend performing remplissage in the setting of minimal bone loss (<20%) and Hill-Sachs lesions between 20 and 40%. Level of evidence: IV.

84. Diklic ID, Ganic ZD, Blagojevic ZD, Nho SJ, Romeo AA: Treatment of locked chronic posterior dislocation of the shoulder by reconstruction of the defect in the humeral head with an allograft. *J Bone Joint Surg Br* 2010;92(1):71-76.

Chapter 8

Multidirectional and Posterior Shoulder Instability

Fotios Paul Tjoumakaris, MD • James P. Bradley, MD

ABSTRACT

Posterior and multidirectional instability of the shoulder may be overlapping or isolated diagnoses. Although these instability patterns can commonly occur in the overhead or throwing athlete, a high index of suspicion is warranted for any patient presenting with deep-seated shoulder pain that is exacerbated with activity. Diagnosis is typically made with a detailed history and physical examination, and often confirmed with magnetic resonance arthrography. Initial treatment consists of rest, physical therapy, and slow return to athletic play. For patients in whom a trial of nonsurgical management fails, either open surgical reconstruction (for bone loss or other mitigating factors) or arthroscopic repair has demonstrated good short-term and long-term results.

Keywords: multidirectional instability; posterior shoulder instability; recurrent posterior subluxation; shoulder instability

Introduction

Posterior instability and multidirectional instability of the shoulder are overlapping conditions. Most patients have ill-defined symptoms, and the diagnosis is challenging. The management of patients with posterior or multidirectional instability of the shoulder has evolved considerably in the past decade. With advanced imaging and arthroscopic techniques, surgical management has greatly improved, and better patient outcomes are being reported.

Dr. Tjoumakaris or an immediate family member has stock or stock options held in Franklin/Keystone Biosciences, LLC and Trice Medical, Inc. and serves as a board member, owner, officer, or committee member of the American Academy of Orthopaedic Surgeons, the American Board of Orthopaedic Surgery, Inc., and the American Orthopaedic Society for Sports Medicine. Dr. Bradley or an immediate family member has received royalties from Arthrex, Inc. and serves as a board member, owner, officer, or committee member of the American Orthopaedic Society for Sports Medicine and the Arthroscopy Association of North America.

Clinical Evaluation

Patient History

Patients with posterior or multidirectional instability of the shoulder seldom report traumatic dislocation. Posterior shoulder dislocation classically occurs in patients who have experienced electrocution, seizure, or a posteriorly directed blow to the shoulder (typically in a contact sport or a motor vehicle crash). These patients report pain with attempted range of motion, have difficulty externally rotating the arm, and require emergency closed reduction of the humeral head within the glenoid fossa. Frequently, these patients are most comfortable with the arm resting in a sling in internal rotation.

In contrast, patients with posterior instability report less severe symptoms than patients with a posterior dislocation and have difficulty correlating their symptoms with a particular event or injury. In these patients, certain arm positions or motions, such as crossbody adduction or overhead throwing, can precipitate pain or other symptoms. In many of these patients, the probable cause is recurrent posterior subluxation; patients may report pain, fatigue in the shoulder, or loss of velocity when throwing. Furthermore, many will frequently present with complaints of pain with provocative activities such as bench press, pushups, and other pressing movements, especially when the shoulder is in flexion and internal rotation. When the symptoms become pervasive, the patient may report numbness in the upper extremity or the feeling that the arm is going dead. Patients with multidirectional instability also report pain in the shoulder, may have difficulty using the arm during activities of daily living, and often report bilateral symptoms. Identifying a particular arc of motion or a causative mechanism can be challenging because the patient's symptoms often are vague and may mimic those of rotator cuff impingement (**Table 1**).

Physical Examination

The clinician should carefully assess the cervical spine and its contribution to shoulder and upper extremity pain. The cervical spine assessment includes palpation, range of motion, and provocative testing (Spurling test) to

Table 1

Common Symptoms of Patients With Recurrent Posterior Subluxation

Pain with shoulder in flexion and internal rotation
Fatigue
Loss of throwing velocity
Weakness (dead arm)
Numbness, paresthesias

evaluate for radiculopathy that could be contributing to pain around the shoulder and scapula. A thorough shoulder examination is required in all patients with shoulder pain and dysfunction. Strength testing and assessment for atrophy, passive and active range of motion, and scapular rhythm and synchronization should be an integral part of the examination and may be useful in detecting concomitant pathology. Provocative maneuvers, such as the jerk and Kim tests, can help to elicit instability and pain as the humeral head glides over the posterior glenoid rim.[1,2]

The jerk test is a true test of posterior instability and is performed while the patient is seated. The scapula is stabilized, and the arm is taken horizontally across the body from a position of abduction and internal rotation while a posteriorly directed force is applied to the affected arm. A clunking sound can be heard and the shoulder is seen to subluxate posteriorly off the glenoid. A second clunking sound can be elicited when the shoulder is taken back across the body as the humeral head reduces within the glenoid fossa.

The Kim test is performed with the patient seated and the arm in 90° of abduction. The examiner holds the proximal arm and applies an axial and posteriorly directed force while elevating the arm upward by 45°. Pain with this maneuver indicates a posteroinferior labral lesion, which can contribute to posterior instability (**Figure 1**).

Load-and-shift testing can help to define the extent of shoulder joint laxity, and an apprehension sign can be elicited to evaluate for subjective instability anteriorly. Alleviation of the apprehension sign with a relocation test can further define the direction of instability. In patients undergoing shoulder surgery, the ability to subluxate the shoulder over the glenoid rim was found to be common, and only higher degrees of laxity were correlated with clinical instability of the shoulder.[3] The hyperabduction test or Gagey test can assess for excessive laxity in the inferior glenohumeral ligament and capsule. In this test, passive abduction of the shoulder beyond 105° is associated with laxity and lengthening of the inferior glenohumeral ligament.[4] Ligamentous laxity should be generally assessed by evaluating elbow and knee hyperextension, patellar mobility, metacarpophalangeal joint hyperextension, and the sulcus sign at the anterolateral edge of the acromion with an inferiorly applied force. A sulcus sign that is greater than 2 cm and does not diminish in external rotation is regarded as pathologic in a patient with symptoms and may imply rotator cuff interval laxity. In a 2011 cross-sectional study, the presence of the sulcus sign was correlated with a history of shoulder instability in healthy patients.[5] A thorough neurovascular examination of both upper extremities is performed to evaluate for differences in pulse or nerve function that might suggest thoracic outlet syndrome or a brachial plexopathy.

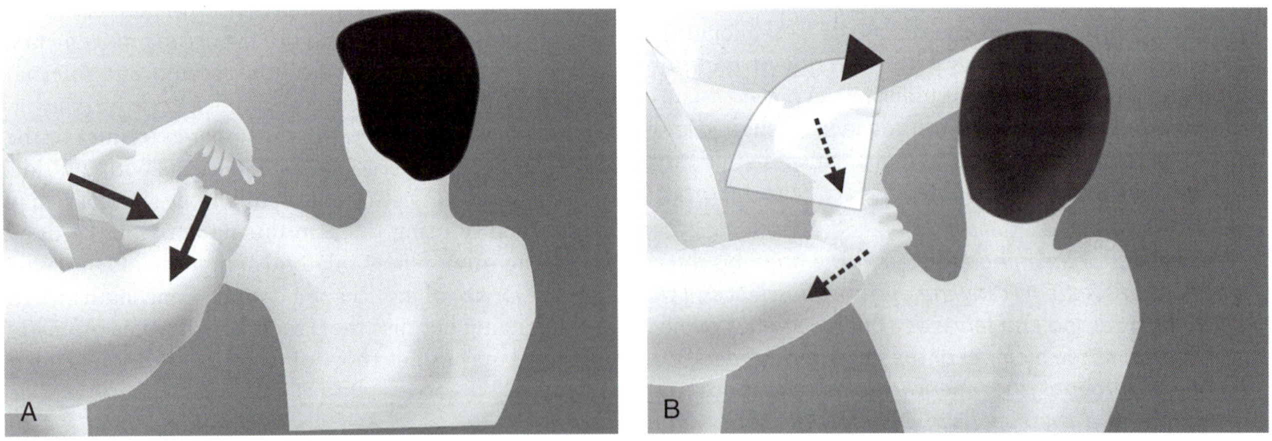

FIGURE 1 Drawings showing the Kim test. **A**, With the arm in 90° of abduction, the examiner applies an axial and downward force to the proximal arm (arrows). **B**, With the abducted arm elevated 45°, the examiner applies a posterior force with axial compression (arrows) while the arm is adducted across the body (arrowhead). If pain is elicited with this maneuver, the test is considered positive and highly suggestive of a posteroinferior labral lesion. (Reprinted with permission from Kim SH, Park JS, Jeong WK, Shin SK: The Kim test: A novel test for posteroinferior labral lesion of the shoulder—A comparison to the jerk test. *Am J Sports Med* 2005;33[8]:1188-1192. doi:10.1177/0363546504272687.)

Patients with multidirectional instability of the shoulder may have increased translation with load-and-shift testing, a positive sulcus sign, a positive apprehension sign, and positive jerk and Kim tests. Positive results on multiple tests indicate capsular laxity that is more global in nature. The Beighton hypermobility score has been used to more objectively quantify patients with joint laxity and can be used to make comparisons among patients presenting with shoulder laxity and instability (**Table 2**). A high score could indicate an underlying soft-tissue or connective tissue disorder and should be further investigated.[6] Patients with posterior instability are most likely to have pain or laxity when the posterior capsule and labrum are stressed (by the posterior load-and-shift, jerk, or Kim tests), indicating an isolated spectrum of injury. Substantial overlap may exist, however, and this factor makes optimal management of these patients challenging.

Epidemiology

Posterior shoulder instability represents 5% of all incidences of shoulder instability, although with better history, examination, and imaging techniques, this prevalence is increasing.[7] Approximately 50% of the patients with posterior instability may have a traumatic etiology. In most patients with dislocation, the reported cause is trauma; in the remaining patients, the cause is a seizure disorder or electrical shock. The reported incidence of posterior dislocation is 1.1 per 100,000 population per year, with peaks in males aged 20 to 49 years and in males and females older than 70 years. Young age at initial dislocation, the presence of a seizure disorder, and the presence of a large reverse Hill-Sachs lesion are correlated with recurrence. Almost 20% of patients have a recurrence during the first year after a posterior shoulder dislocation.[8]

Multidirectional instability occurs more often in patients in the second or third decade of life and may be most prevalent in athletes who engage in overhead repetitive arm use, as in volleyball, swimming, or gymnastics.[9] Instability patterns in two planes are required for a diagnosis of multidirectional instability. The diagnosis often is challenging, and a misdiagnosis of unidirectional instability may lead to failure of the initial treatment. The epidemiologic characteristics of these patients are difficult to quantify because precise diagnostic criteria do not exist in the orthopaedic literature. Whether to include patients who have had unidirectional dislocation but exhibit signs of laxity in other planes is a source of ongoing debate. Patients with collagen disorders or generalized ligamentous laxity are at increased risk for the development of multidirectional instability. Patients with Ehlers-Danlos syndrome and related disorders are among the most difficult patients to treat, and more recent studies have demonstrated good results with open capsular shift techniques.[10]

Table 2

Beighton Hypermobility Score[a]

Joint	Findings	Points
Left fifth finger	Passive DF > 90°	1
Right fifth finger	Passive DF > 90°	1
Left thumb	Passive DF to flexor forearm	1
Right thumb	Passive DF to flexor forearm	1
Left elbow	Hyperextension > 10°	1
Right elbow	Hyperextension > 10°	1
Left knee	Hyperextension > 10°	1
Right knee	Hyperextension > 10°	1
Trunk mobility	Palms and hands can rest on floor with forward flexion of trunk/knees extended	1

DF = dorsiflexion.
[a]Scoring: 0-3 (normal); 4-9 (ligamentous laxity).

Anatomic Considerations

The glenohumeral joint relies on static restraints to stability (the capsule, labrum, and glenoid or chondrolabral version) as well as dynamic stabilizers (the rotator cuff, scapular and thoracic musculature, and neuromuscular control; **Table 3**). In a patient with posterior dislocation from trauma or a seizure disorder, the bony architecture of the humeral head or glenoid may be compromised, resulting in a posterior glenoid fracture or deficiency or an impaction fracture of the anterior humeral head (a reverse Hill-Sachs lesion). In such a patient, the extent of bone loss may substantially contribute to the recurrence of instability. Because the humeral head is internally rotated, the lesion can engage and cause a recurrence of subluxation or dislocation. Relative glenoid or chondrolabral retroversion may be a risk factor or the result of recurrent instability and recurrent posterior subluxation. Labral injury from repetitive posterior loading or instability can range from a posterior labral crack to a Kim lesion (an incomplete, concealed avulsion of the posteroinferior labrum) to a reverse Bankart lesion. Capsular tearing, posterior labrocapsular periosteal sleeve avulsion, or humeral avulsion of the posteroinferior glenohumeral ligament also can occur and contribute to recurrence

Table 3

Anatomic Determinants of Posterior or Multidirectional Instability of the Shoulder

Anatomic Determinant	Pathology
Static Restraint	
Humeral head	Reverse Hill-Sachs lesion
	Increased humeral retroversion
Glenoid	Posterior glenoid fracture or deficiency
	Increased glenoid retroversion
Labrum	Labral tear
	Increased chondrolabral retroversion
	Kim lesion
	Posterior labrocapsular periosteal sleeve avulsion
Capsule	Capsular tear
	Capsular insufficiency or laxity
	Posterior avulsion of the inferior glenohumeral ligament and reverse humeral avulsion of the glenohumeral ligament
Dynamic Restraint	
Muscular control	Rotator cuff tear
	Weakness of scapular stabilizing muscles (rhomboid, pectoralis minor, serratus anterior)
Neuromuscular control	Forceful internal rotation from seizure disorder or electrocution

of posterior instability.[11-15] Altered scapular kinematics, including reduced serratus activation, increased trapezius activity, and short resting length of the pectoralis minor, have been shown to alter the stability of the glenohumeral joint; cadaver studies found that posterior instability increases when posterior scapular tilt is increased more than 15°.[16,17] The rotator cuff also plays a critical role in dynamic joint stability and can be torn in patients who sustain a posterior dislocation at any age. The subscapularis is of particular importance in posterior shoulder instability. Loss of concavity compression and recurrence of instability may occur despite normal bone and ligamentous architecture. In patients with recurrent posterior subluxation, there may be associated rotator cuff pathology from abnormal glenohumeral joint translations. A high level of suspicion on the part of the treating clinician, with careful scrutiny of advanced imaging, is important for an accurate diagnosis and treatment plan.

Imaging

Routine radiographs may be diagnostic in the setting of trauma or a suspected acute dislocation. Plain radiographs typically are obtained in three views (AP, scapular Y, and axillary). In a patient with a posterior dislocation, obtaining an axillary radiograph may be challenging because of the characteristic inability to externally rotate the arm. In such a patient, the AP radiograph may reveal a lightbulb sign, in which the glenoid fossa is relatively empty and the proximal humerus has the shape of a lightbulb secondary to internal rotation (**Figure 2**). A Velpeau axillary view sometimes is helpful if a traditional axillary view cannot be obtained. The radiographs are inspected for a bone defect of the posterior glenoid rim as well as a reverse Hill-Sachs lesion on the anterior humeral head. The radiographs also should be reviewed for associated fractures of the tuberosities, surgical neck, or humeral head, any of which may affect surgical treatment.[18] CT may be helpful for further defining the osseous injury pattern, especially if the plain radiographs are nondiagnostic. CT is beneficial for determining the size of an associated Hill-Sachs lesion, the extent of bone deficiency of the posterior glenoid rim, and the degree of glenoid retroversion, which may contribute to recurrent instability. Most of the research quantifying bone loss using CT measurements (eg, bare spot, best-fit circle placement) has been performed in patients with anterior shoulder instability. As such, there is no currently accepted critical size defect of either

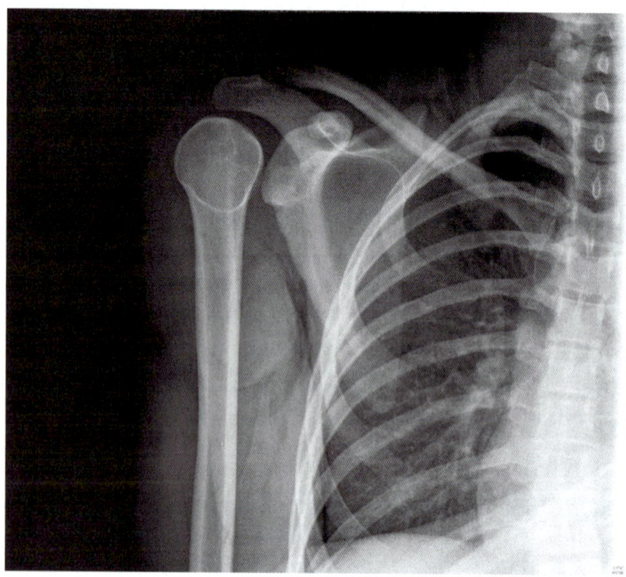

FIGURE 2 AP radiograph of the right shoulder of a patient who sustained a posterior shoulder dislocation while playing rugby. The empty glenoid sign and the lightbulb sign can be clearly seen, indicating dislocation of the glenohumeral joint.

humeral or glenoid bone loss that could compromise surgical efforts when treating posterior glenohumeral instability.[19]

Magnetic resonance arthrography (MRA) and MRI are the best imaging modalities for identifying lesions within the posterior capsulolabral complex. Axial images may reveal posterior translation of the humeral head relative to the glenoid, a posterior labrocapsular avulsion, a posterior labral tear with paralabral cyst formation, or humeral avulsion of the posteroinferior glenohumeral ligament complex.[20] A concealed lesion (Kim lesion or incomplete to near-complete labral crack), a posterior periosteal sleeve avulsion, or increased chondrolabral retroversion also can be seen and quantified on axial MRI or MRA studies (**Figure 3**). A rotator cuff tear, bone edema, an impaction fracture, and an articular cartilage abnormality can be further evaluated with MRI and may be seen in a large number of patients. A 2010 study found that positioning the arm in flexion, adduction, and internal rotation during MRA further defined the injury to the posteroinferior labrum in patients for whom more subtle abnormalities to the posterior capsule and the labrum were identified.[21] Patients with multidirectional instability typically do not have specific labral pathology, but they may have characteristic morphologic osseous changes of instability, such as increased chondrolabral retroversion and a patulous posterior capsule.[22]

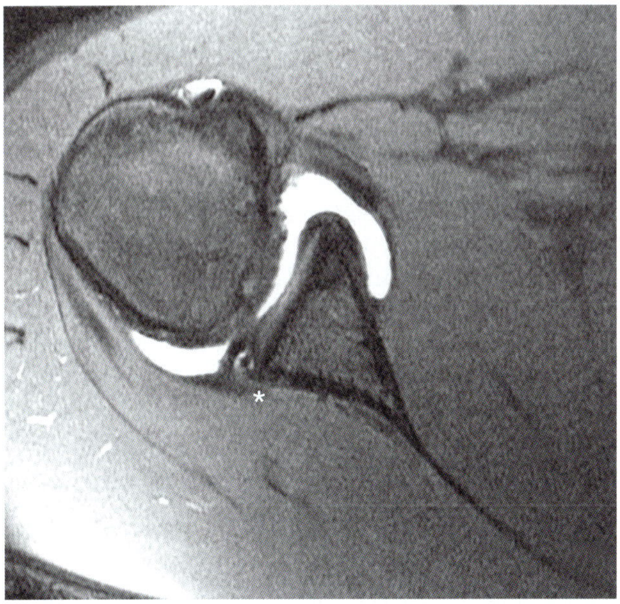

FIGURE 3 Axial T2-weighted magnetic resonance angiographic image showing a posterior labral crack with an associated Kim lesion. The patient's symptoms were consistent with recurrent posterior subluxation. * = area of labral crack

Treatment Considerations

Nonsurgical Treatment

The treatment of patients with posterior or multidirectional instability of the shoulder has evolved considerably in the past decade. For patients with acute dislocation and fracture contributing to instability, closed reduction and fracture fixation often are necessary to restore stability to the glenohumeral joint. In patients with recurrent posterior subluxation or signs of multidirectional instability, physical therapy is the preferred first-line treatment. Despite aggressive therapy and strengthening, nonsurgical treatment is unsuccessful for many patients, and surgical intervention is required.[23] A 2010 study of patients with multidirectional instability found that a combination of capsular shift and physical therapy was superior to physical therapy alone in restoring normal kinematics and muscle activation of the glenohumeral joint.[24] This finding underscores the difficulty of nonsurgical treatment of patients with instability. Nonetheless, many patients, especially those who do not have optimal function of the periscapular musculature, benefit from an initial nonsurgical approach with a particular focus on scapular mechanics and may be able to avoid surgical intervention.

Surgical Treatment

Arthroscopic surgery has become the benchmark for patients who require surgical treatment for posterior or multidirectional instability of the shoulder without associated osseous defects (**Figure 4**). Historically, many patients with posterior instability were treated with an open posterior stabilization procedure, with recurrence rates ranging from zero to 40%. Few patients returned to their previous level of activity or sport following open posterior repairs.[25-31] High recurrence rates as well as patient dissatisfaction with open surgery increased interest in arthroscopic management of the condition. With the use of current arthroscopic techniques, the average recurrence rate is close to 5%, with a range of zero to 10% in most recent studies. A high percentage of patients return to their previous level of activity or sport.[32] A comparative study of arthroscopic and open techniques found that arthroscopically treated patients had superior functional outcomes.[33] A cadaver biomechanics study found that open bone block procedures overcorrected posterior translation and did not restore inferior stability as effectively as arthroscopic posterior Bankart repair.[34] The failure rates in high-demand throwing athletes have remained relatively low (5% to 10%) when modern arthroscopic techniques are used.[35-40] In these retrospective studies, failure to plicate the posterior capsule with suture anchors may have been a factor in the relatively few unsuccessful procedures.[41]

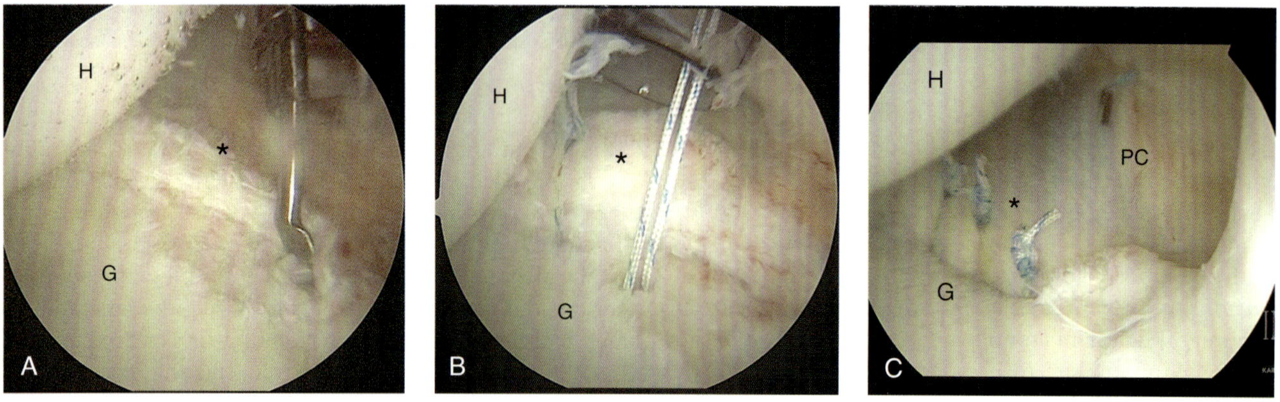

FIGURE 4 Arthroscopic images showing a posterior labral repair from the anterior portal. The patient is in the lateral decubitus position. **A**, The posterior labrum is detached from the posterior glenoid margin, with loss of articular cartilage on the glenoid from recurrent posterior subluxation. **B**, Anchor placement to secure the posterior labrum and capsule back to the glenoid margin. **C**, The final repair. The posterior portal has been repaired to prevent capsular insufficiency through the defect. * = labrum, G = glenoid, H = humeral head, PC = posterior capsule

Open capsular shift has provided solid long-term results for most patients with multidirectional instability. However, in some studies, arthroscopic techniques have had equal rates of success, with a trend toward better rates of return to sport in patients treated arthroscopically.[42] A cadaver study found that capsular volume was reduced more with arthroscopic plication than with a traditional open technique, further validating the shift toward an arthroscopic approach to treatment.[43] A study of high-demand athletes with multidirectional instability found that 91% of the patients had full or satisfactory range of motion, and 86% were able to return to their previous level of competition.[44] The advantages of an arthroscopic technique over traditional open methods include the ability to treat concomitant pathology (such as a superior labrum anterior to posterior tear, global capsular laxity, or a rotator cuff tear) and anterior and posterior capsular laxity, as well as a reduction in the morbidity of an open approach.[45] In challenging cases of multidirectional instability with concomitant bone loss or revision surgery (eg, failed Latarjet procedure), the use of allograft (distal tibia, iliac crest) reconstruction for the glenoid, T-capsular shift of the capsule, and open plication of the rotator interval may be necessary to achieve a satisfactory outcome.[46,47]

In patients with an osseous defect from a locked posterior dislocation, pathologic glenoid retroversion, or bone deficiency or avulsion of the glenohumeral ligaments from the humerus, open surgery may be the preferred method of treatment. For a patient with a large humeral head defect from a reverse Hill-Sachs lesion, the preferred option may be an osteoarticular allograft reconstruction, a humeral head arthroplasty, or a lesser tuberosity transfer (the McLaughlin procedure).[45] For patients with increased glenoid or humeral retroversion, glenoid osteotomy and humeral osteotomy can provide stability, but these procedures have fallen out of favor in recent years.

Arthroscopic Surgery for Posterior Instability

In most patients with posterior instability or recurrent posterior subluxation, arthroscopic surgery with posterior labral or capsular repair can achieve an excellent outcome with low rates of recurrence and complications. The recommended technique described here may be varied as indicated and still achieve a favorable outcome. Lateral decubitus patient positioning typically is used, with a beanbag to avoid pressure injury and interscalene block and general anesthesia to achieve complete muscle relaxation. The affected arm is placed in balanced arm traction in 45° of abduction and slight forward flexion using 10 to 15 lb of weight.

A single posterior portal is preferred for anchor placement and suture management and is created first, in line with the lateral edge of the acromion. This portal should allow for an anchor placement trajectory of 45° relative to the glenoid face (**Figure 5**). If the trajectory of the posterior portal is not optimal for inferior anchor placement, an accessory lateral portal may provide better access to the 7-o'clock position of the glenoid. The anterior portal is made in the rotator cuff interval just inferior to the biceps tendon. A 5.75-mm clear cannula is placed anteriorly for arthroscopic visualization, and an 8.25-mm clear cannula is placed posteriorly for use as the working portal. After identification of the labral and capsular pathology, the labrum is elevated off the posterior glenoid margin with a periosteal elevator. The posterior rim of the glenoid is débrided with a motorized burr or a shaver device (**Figure 6**). Often, it is more useful

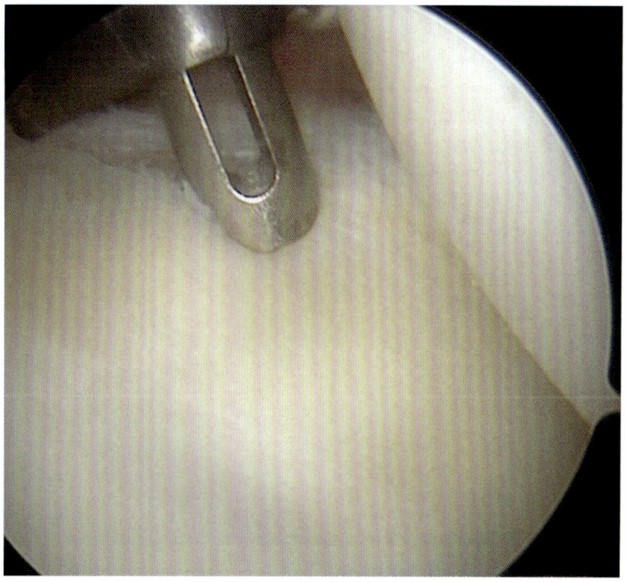

FIGURE 5 Arthroscopic image showing the posterior portal created in line with the lateral edge of the acromion. This placement facilitates anchor placement through a single posterior portal by allowing a 45° trajectory of the anchor drill guide.

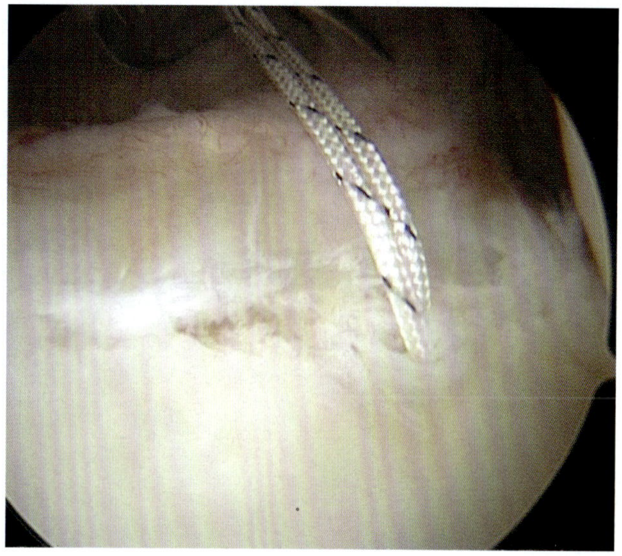

FIGURE 7 Arthroscopic image showing placement of the first anchor inferiorly along the posterior glenoid surface.

to introduce the elevator and the shaver from the anterior portal than to work exclusively from the posterior portal. The arthroscope then can be placed in the anterior portal for anchor placement and suture management. A 70° arthroscope in the anterior portal can be useful for visualization of the posterior and inferior glenoid rim. A knotless repair or knot-tying technique can be used, depending on surgeon preference. One potential advantage of a knotless technique is that there is less risk of knot-stack abrasion against the humeral head and posterior/superior rotator cuff and capsule during shoulder range of motion. For the knot-tying technique, anchors typically are placed along the posterior glenoid margin, starting inferiorly and progressing superiorly, as needed (**Figure 7**). Biocomposite anchors with a 2- to 2.4-mm diameter are recommended; they should be spaced 3 to 5 mm apart to avoid fragmentation of the posterior glenoid bone and prevent later glenoid fracture (**Figure 8**). The posterior suture limb of the anchor (most distant from the glenoid) is shuttled around the labrum and capsule slightly inferior and lateral to the anchor to achieve capsular plication. In a patient for whom plication should be avoided (eg, a high-level throwing

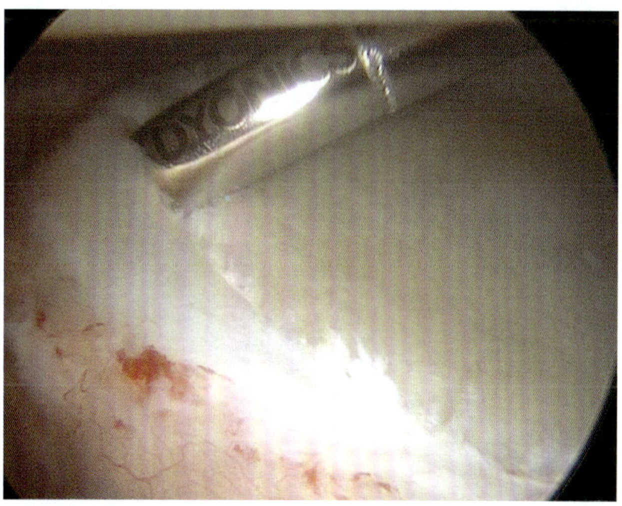

FIGURE 6 Arthroscopic image showing a motorized shaver used to débride the posterior glenoid and the labrum. The shaver has been brought in from the anterior portal and is used to create an optimal healing environment.

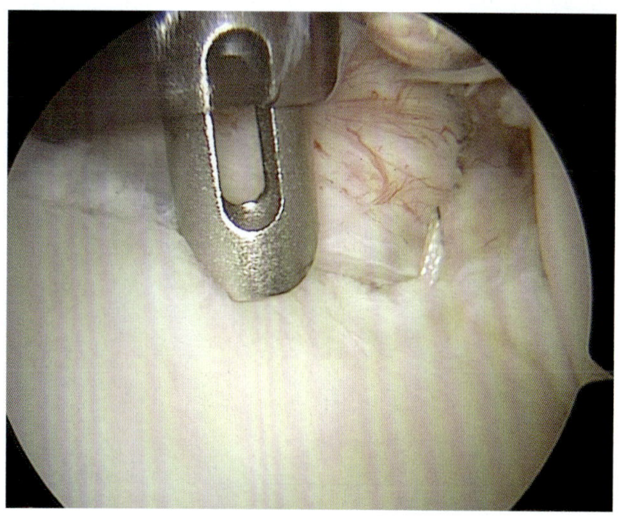

FIGURE 8 Arthroscopic image showing typical anchor spacing (3-5 mm apart) to avoid fragmentation of the posterior glenoid bone.

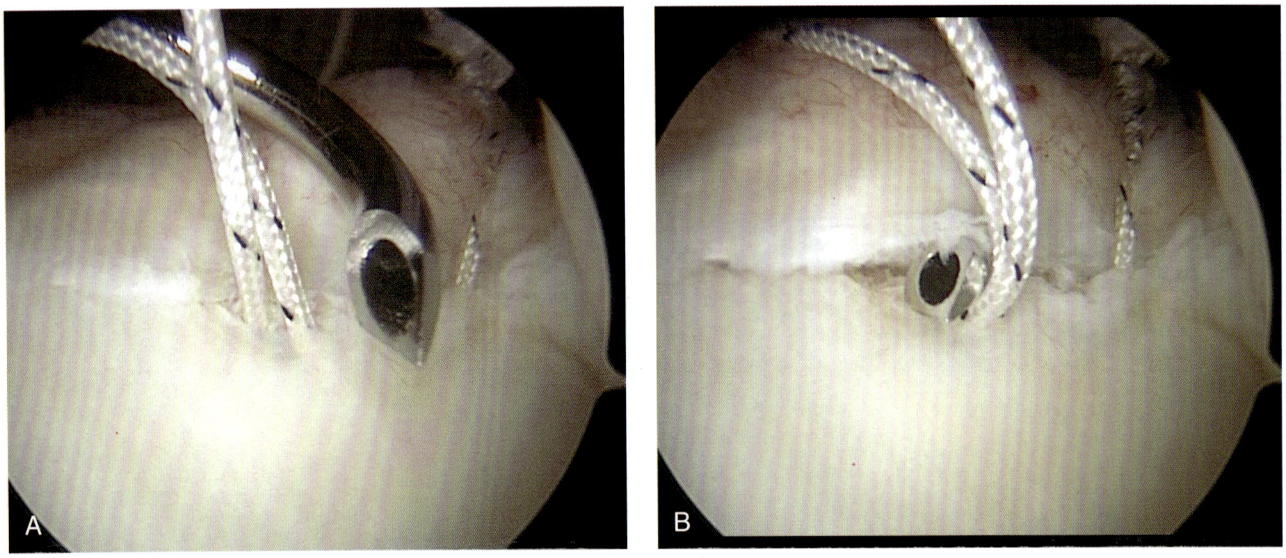

FIGURE 9 Arthroscopic images showing the use of a suture hook to shuttle sutures through the posterior labrum and capsule complex, as seen from the anterior viewing portal. **A**, A short curved suture hook is brought in through the posterior portal. **B**, The suture hook is passed around the labrum and capsule complex at the level of the anchor, or slightly inferior to the anchor if a capsular plication is performed.

athlete), the suture can be shuttled around the labrum at the location of anchor placement to prevent excessive tightening of the posterior capsule. A suture hook is used to assist with suture passage, and the sutures are tied in an inferior-to-superior direction (**Figure 9**). When shuttling sutures through a single posterior cannula, it is important to retrieve the suture limb and the shuttling suture (typically PDS; Ethicon, Somerville, NJ) at the same time to avoid crossing the sutures (**Figure 10**). The sutures are then tied; to allow the knot to be placed away from the glenohumeral joint, the suture that has been passed through the capsule and labrum (most distant from the glenoid) is used as the post limb (**Figure 11**). For a labral tear that extends to the superior labrum, 2-mm anchors loaded with No. 1 suture can be used, or a knotless 2.9-mm anchor can be used to avoid abrasion of the knot against the posterosuperior rotator cuff during glenohumeral motion. When all of the anchors have been

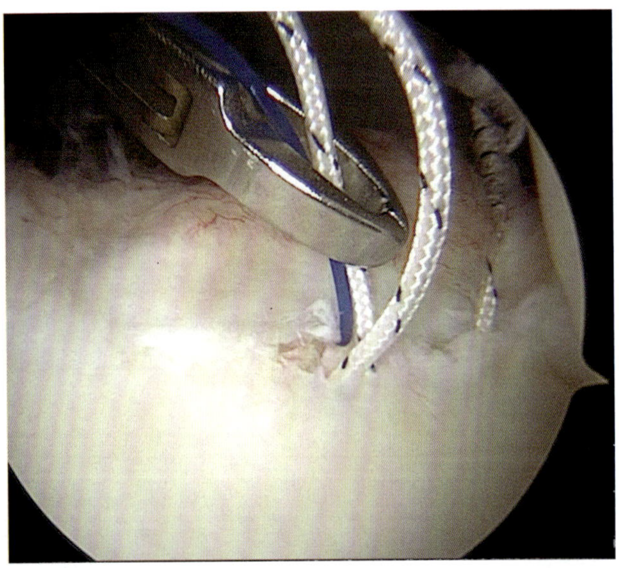

FIGURE 10 Arthroscopic image showing the suture shuttle and suture from the anchor grasped together to avoid suture entanglement. When a single posterior portal is used, this step facilitates passage and prevents early knot formation.

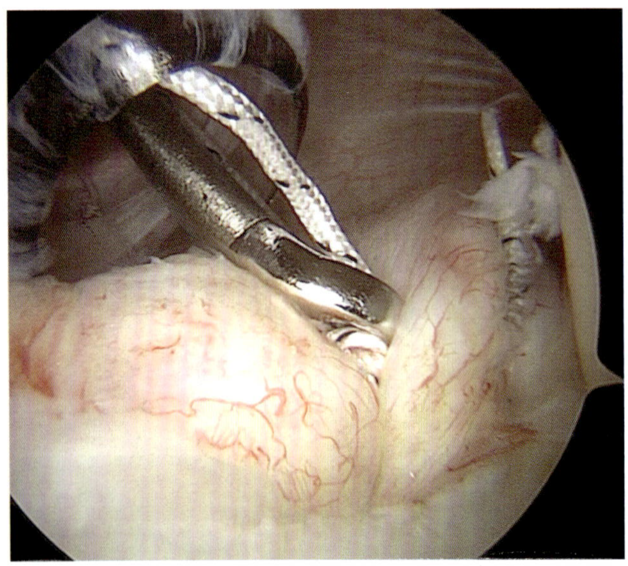

FIGURE 11 Arthroscopic image showing the shuttled suture limb used as the post limb during knot tying to place the knot away from the glenohumeral joint and prevent impingement.

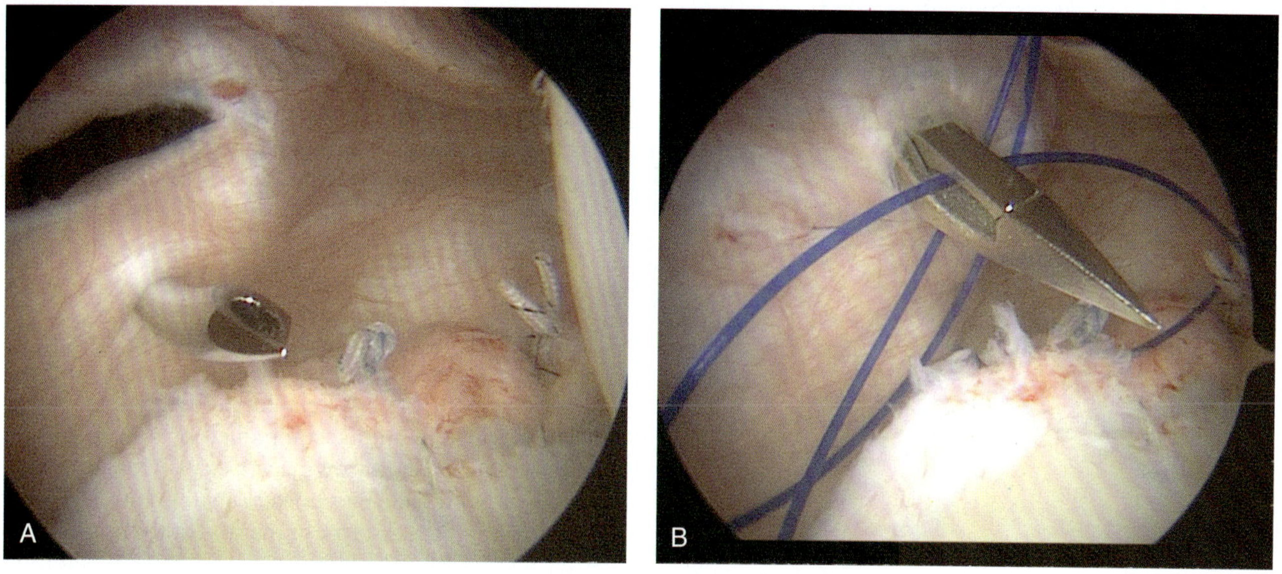

FIGURE 12 Arthroscopic images showing the closure of the posterior portal after completion of the labral repair. **A**, The posterior cannula is backed up just posterior to the posterior portal. On one side of the portal, a crescent suture hook is used to penetrate the posterior capsule. **B**, A penetrating grasper is used to grasp the shuttled blue suture on the opposite side of the posterior portal arthrotomy to allow closure.

placed, the posterior portal typically is closed to prevent stress-riser formation within the posterior capsule. Closure of the capsule also allows the surgeon to titrate the repair after the labrum has been anatomically restored to the glenoid rim. The posterior cannula is withdrawn to a level just posterior to the capsule. A crescent suture hook loaded with suture is used to penetrate one side of the portal incision, and the suture is retrieved from the opposite side with a penetrating grasper (**Figure 12**). The suture then can be tied just beyond the posterior capsule (**Figure 13**). Varying the distance of the suture from the portal incision allows additional tension to be applied to the posterior capsule. The repair is complete when all of the sutures have been tied and the posterior portal is closed, preventing pathologic posterior glenohumeral translation (**Figure 14**).

For the knotless technique, the labrum is prepared in similar fashion, and a suture tape (1.3 mm) is first passed around the labrum in a luggage tag or cinch stitch configuration. As is the case with a traditional knot-tying

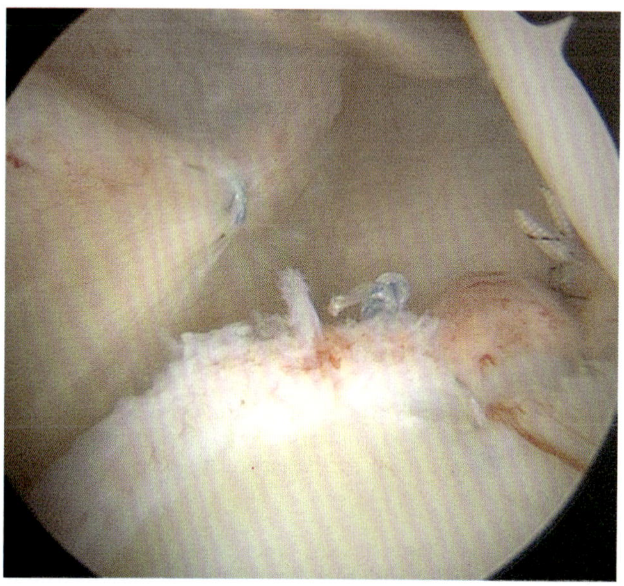

FIGURE 13 Arthroscopic image showing the repair as assessed after closure of the posterior portal.

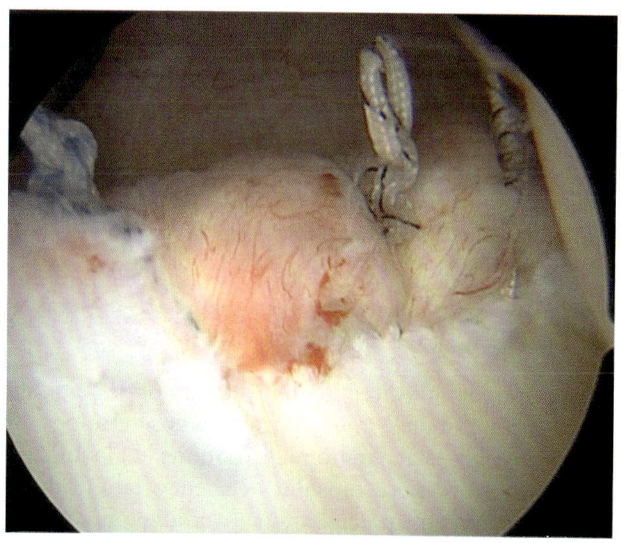

FIGURE 14 Arthroscopic image showing the posterior labrum and capsule anatomically restored to the posterior glenoid rim.

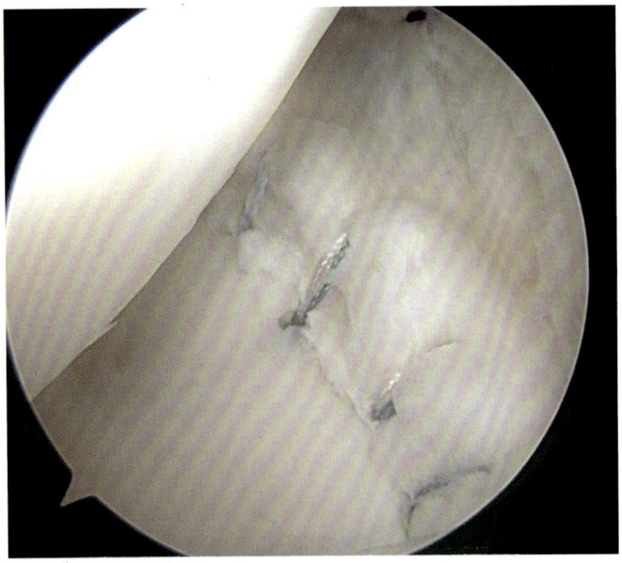

FIGURE 15 Arthroscopic image of a posterior labrum repair completed with an all-knotless technique.

technique, the suture is shuttled around the labrum in a manner that is consistent with the pathology being treated. The tails of each suture are then placed through an anchor eyelet and impacted into the glenoid after predrilling of the glenoid bone. Again, short biocomposite anchors with a 1.9- to 2.4-mm diameter are recommended and should be spaced 3 to 5 mm apart (**Figure 15**).

An abduction sling is used postoperatively, and passive range-of-motion exercises can begin the day after surgery. Neutral external rotation and 90° of forward elevation are allowed by 4 weeks after surgery. At 6 weeks, sling use can be discontinued, and the patient begins active-assisted range-of-motion exercises with a slow progression to active motion without motion constraints. At 4 months, the shoulder often is pain free and has a near-normal range of motion. Rotator cuff strengthening and conditioning are started at this stage. At 5 months, isokinetic and isotonic exercises are advanced. Patients are assessed for return to play at 6 months, depending on the particular sport or activity. An overhead or throwing athlete may begin a throwing program at this stage of rehabilitation.

SUMMARY

Posterior and multidirectional instability of the shoulder represent a complex injury pattern whose etiology often is multifactorial. Anatomic variations in glenoid and humeral retroversion, capsular deficiency, labral injury, osseous defects from acute injury, and dynamic muscle control can contribute to the instability pattern. MRI and MRA have improved the sensitivity and the specificity available for the diagnosis of these conditions. Imaging findings should be correlated with physical examination findings for a tailored treatment approach. If nonsurgical management is unsuccessful, arthroscopic surgery often is the first-line surgical treatment and can be used to treat a variety of pathologies, with low rates of recurrence and high rates of patient satisfaction.

KEY STUDY POINTS

- Most patients with posterior shoulder instability present with activity-related shoulder pain. Athletes may note pain accompanied by a decrease in performance (eg, throwing velocity). Most patients present with recurrent posterior subluxation (RPS) rather than frank glenohumeral instability.
- Patients with multidirectional instability should be screened for generalized hypermobility because these patients may require a more aggressive surgical approach (eg, open capsular plication).
- CT can be helpful to delineate osseous pathology in cases of dislocation, but MRA is likely more useful as a diagnostic tool in the majority of cases.
- Nonsurgical management will be unsuccessful in most patients who present with posterior shoulder instability and multidirectional instability; arthroscopic (preferred) or open shoulder stabilization will be required.
- Most studies evaluating arthroscopic versus open shoulder stabilization for posterior shoulder instability with labrum tear demonstrate superior outcomes with an arthroscopic approach. Studies conducted on patients with multidirectional instability show equivalent outcomes between arthroscopic and open capsular plication.

Annotated References

1. Kim SH, Park JC, Park JS, Oh I: Painful jerk test: A predictor of success in nonoperative treatment of posteroinferior instability of the shoulder. *Am J Sports Med* 2004;32(8):1849-1855.

2. Kim SH, Park JS, Jeong WK, Shin SK: The Kim test: A novel test for posteroinferior labral lesion of the shoulder. A comparison to the jerk test. *Am J Sports Med* 2005;33(8):1188-1192.

3. Jia X, Ji JH, Petersen SA, Freehill MT, McFarland EG: An analysis of shoulder laxity in patients undergoing shoulder surgery. *J Bone Joint Surg Am* 2009;91(9):2144-2150.

4. Gagey OJ, Gagey N: The hyperabduction test. *J Bone Joint Surg Br* 2001;83(1):69-74.

5. Owens BD, Duffey ML, Deberardino TM, Cameron KL: Physical examination findings in young athletes correlate with history of shoulder instability. *Orthopedics* 2011;34(6):460-464.

6. Beighton PH, Horan F: Orthopedic aspects of the Ehlers-Danlos syndrome. *J Bone Joint Surg Br* 1969;51:444-453.

7. Robinson CM, Aderinto J: Recurrent posterior shoulder instability. *J Bone Joint Surg Am* 2005;87(4):883-892.

8. Robinson CM, Seah M, Akhtar MA: The epidemiology, risk of recurrence, and functional outcome after an acute traumatic posterior dislocation of the shoulder. *J Bone Joint Surg Am* 2011;93(17):1605-1613.

9. Gaskill TR, Taylor DC, Millett PJ: Management of multidirectional instability of the shoulder. *J Am Acad Orthop Surg* 2011;19(12):758-767.

10. Vavken P, Tepolt FA, Kocher MS: Open inferior capsular shift for multidirectional shoulder instability in adolescents with generalized ligamentous hyperlaxity or Ehlers-Danlos syndrome. *J Shoulder Elbow Surg* 2016;25(6):907-912.

    This is a review of 15 adolescent patients who underwent open capsular shift in the setting of connective tissue laxity. At a mean follow-up of 7.5 years, 87% of patients reported improved pain and stability, whereas 64% of patients were able to resume sports. Level of evidence: IV.

11. Kim SH, Noh KC, Park JS, Ryu BD, Oh I: Loss of chondrolabral containment of the glenohumeral joint in atraumatic posteroinferior multidirectional instability. *J Bone Joint Surg Am* 2005;87(1):92-98.

12. Kim SH, Ha KI, Yoo JC, Noh KC: Kim's lesion: An incomplete and concealed avulsion of the posteroinferior labrum in posterior or multidirectional posteroinferior instability of the shoulder. *Arthroscopy* 2004;20(7):712-720.

13. Safran O, Defranco MJ, Hatem S, Iannotti JP: Posterior humeral avulsion of the glenohumeral ligament as a cause of posterior shoulder instability: A case report. *J Bone Joint Surg Am* 2004;86-A(12):2732-2736.

14. Shah AA, Butler RB, Fowler R, Higgins LD: Posterior capsular rupture causing posterior shoulder instability: A case report. *Arthroscopy* 2011;27(9):1304-1307.

15. Bokor DJ, Fritsch BA: Posterior shoulder instability secondary to reverse humeral avulsion of the glenohumeral ligament. *J Shoulder Elbow Surg* 2010;19(6):853-858.

16. Ludewig PM, Reynolds JF: The association of scapular kinematics and glenohumeral joint pathologies. *J Orthop Sports Phys Ther* 2009;39(2):90-104.

17. Kikuchi K, Itoi E, Yamamoto N, et al: Scapular inclination and glenohumeral joint stability: A cadaveric study. *J Orthop Sci* 2008;13(1):72-77.

18. Robinson CM, Akhtar A, Mitchell M, Beavis C: Complex posterior fracture-dislocation of the shoulder: Epidemiology, injury patterns, and results of operative treatment. *J Bone Joint Surg Am* 2007;89(7):1454-1466.

19. Longo UG, Rizzello G, Locher J, et al: Bone loss in patients with posterior gleno-humeral instability: A systematic review. *Knee Surg Sports Traumatol Arthrosc* 2016;24(2):612-617.

    In this systematic review of 19 articles (321 patients), 10% of patients sustained a redislocation. Of these, a small number (10% glenoid; 11% humeral) were sustained by patients with bone defects. Level of evidence: IV.

20. Tung GA, Hou DD: MR arthrography of the posterior labrocapsular complex: Relationship with glenohumeral joint alignment and clinical posterior instability. *AJR Am J Roentgenol* 2003;180(2):369-375.

21. Chiavaras MM, Harish S, Burr J: MR arthrographic assessment of suspected posteroinferior labral lesions using flexion, adduction, and internal rotation positioning of the arm: Preliminary experience. *Skeletal Radiol* 2010;39(5):481-488.

22. Jana M, Gamanagatti S: Magnetic resonance imaging in glenohumeral instability. *World J Radiol* 2011;3(9):224-232.

23. Misamore GW, Sallay PI, Didelot W: A longitudinal study of patients with multidirectional instability of the shoulder with seven- to ten-year follow-up. *J Shoulder Elbow Surg* 2005;14(5):466-470.

24. Nyiri P, Illyés A, Kiss R, Kiss J: Intermediate biomechanical analysis of the effect of physiotherapy only compared with capsular shift and physiotherapy in multidirectional shoulder instability. *J Shoulder Elbow Surg* 2010;19(6):802-813.

25. Tibone JE, Bradley JP: The treatment of posterior subluxation in athletes. *Clin Orthop Relat Res* 1993;291:124-137.

26. Hawkins RJ, Janda DH: Posterior instability of the glenohumeral joint: A technique of repair. *Am J Sports Med* 1996;24(3):275-278.

27. Bigliani LU, Pollock RG, McIlveen SJ, Endrizzi DP, Flatow EL: Shift of the posteroinferior aspect of the capsule for recurrent posterior glenohumeral instability. *J Bone Joint Surg Am* 1995;77(7):1011-1020.

28. Fronek J, Warren RF, Bowen M: Posterior subluxation of the glenohumeral joint. *J Bone Joint Surg Am* 1989;71(2):205-216.

29. Misamore GW, Facibene WA: Posterior capsulorrhaphy for the treatment of traumatic recurrent posterior subluxations of the shoulder in athletes. *J Shoulder Elbow Surg* 2000;9(5):403-408.

30. Meuffels DE, Schuit H, van Biezen FC, Reijman M, Verhaar JA: The posterior bone block procedure in posterior shoulder instability: A long-term follow-up study. *J Bone Joint Surg Br* 2010;92(5):651-655.

31. Rhee YG, Lee DH, Lim CT: Posterior capsulolabral reconstruction in posterior shoulder instability: Deltoid saving. *J Shoulder Elbow Surg* 2005;14(4):355-360.

32. Bahk MS, Karzel RP, Snyder SJ: Arthroscopic posterior stabilization and anterior capsular plication for recurrent posterior glenohumeral instability. *Arthroscopy* 2010;26(9):1172-1180.

33. Bottoni CR, Franks BR, Moore JH, DeBerardino TM, Taylor DC, Arciero RA: Operative stabilization of posterior shoulder instability. *Am J Sports Med* 2005;33(7):996-1002.

34. Wellmann M, Bobrowitsch E, Khan N, et al: Biomechanical effectiveness of an arthroscopic posterior Bankart repair versus an open bone block procedure for posterior shoulder instability. *Am J Sports Med* 2011;39(4):796-803.

35. Williams RJ III, Strickland S, Cohen M, Altchek DW, Warren RF: Arthroscopic repair for traumatic posterior shoulder instability. *Am J Sports Med* 2003;31(2):203-209.

36. Mair SD, Zarzour RH, Speer KP: Posterior labral injury in contact athletes. *Am J Sports Med* 1998;26(6):753-758.

37. Radkowski CA, Chhabra A, Baker CL III, Tejwani SG, Bradley JP: Arthroscopic capsulolabral repair for posterior shoulder instability in throwing athletes compared with nonthrowing athletes. *Am J Sports Med* 2008;36(4):693-699.

38. Seroyer S, Tejwani SG, Bradley JP: Arthroscopic capsulolabral reconstruction of the type VIII superior labrum anterior posterior lesion: Mean 2-year follow-up on 13 shoulders. *Am J Sports Med* 2007;35(9):1477-1483.

39. Bradley JP, Baker CL III, Kline AJ, Armfield DR, Chhabra A: Arthroscopic capsulolabral reconstruction for posterior instability of the shoulder: A prospective study of 100 shoulders. *Am J Sports Med* 2006;34(7):1061-1071.

40. Kercher JS, Runner RP, McCarthy TP, Duralde XA: Posterior labral repairs of the shoulder among baseball players: Results and outcomes with minimum 2 year follow-up. *Am J Sports Med* 2019;47(7):1687-1693.

    A retrospective review analyzed 32 male baseball players after arthroscopic management of posterior labrum tears. 94% of patients returned to sport, with 64% of patients returning to their previous level of play. Level of evidence: IV.

41. Tjoumakaris FP, Bradley JP: The rationale for an arthroscopic approach to shoulder stabilization. *Arthroscopy* 2011;27(10):1422-1433.

42. Jacobson ME, Riggenbach M, Wooldridge AN, Bishop JY: Open capsular shift and arthroscopic capsular plication for treatment of multidirectional instability. *Arthroscopy* 2012;28(7):1010-1017.

43. Sekiya JK, Willobee JA, Miller MD, Hickman AJ, Willobee A: Arthroscopic multi-pleated capsular plication compared with open inferior capsular shift for reduction of shoulder volume in a cadaveric model. *Arthroscopy* 2007;23(11):1145-1151.

44. Baker CL III, Mascarenhas R, Kline AJ, Chhabra A, Pombo MW, Bradley JP: Arthroscopic treatment of multidirectional shoulder instability in athletes: A retrospective analysis of 2- to 5-year clinical outcomes. *Am J Sports Med* 2009;37(9):1712-1720.

45. Hawkins RJ, Neer CS II, Pianta RM, Mendoza FX: Locked posterior dislocation of the shoulder. *J Bone Joint Surg Am* 1987;69(1):9-18.

46. Peelbes LA, Aman ZS, Preuss FR, et al: Multidirectional shoulder instability with bone loss and prior failed Latarjet procedure: Treatment with fresh distal tibial allograft and modified T-plasty open capsular shift. *Arthrosc Tech* 2019;8(5):e459-e464.

    In this technical note, the authors describe a novel technique of treating a patient with a connective tissue disorder and prior failed Latarjet procedure. Level of evidence: V.

47. Chen D, Goldberg J, Herald J, Critchley I, Barmare A: Effects of surgical management on multidirectional instability of the shoulder: A meta-analysis. *Knee Surg Sports Traumatol Arthrosc* 2016;24(2):630-639.

    In a systematic review of level II and IV studies, the authors found that arthroscopic capsular shift and open capsular shift provided equal outcomes with less stiffness in the arthroscopic cohort of patients. The authors additionally concluded that thermal capsular shift should be avoided in this patient population. Level of evidence: IV.

Chapter 9

Arthroscopic Reconstruction for Recurrent Shoulder Instability

Daniel F. O'Brien, MD • Robert A. Arciero, MD, FAAOS

ABSTRACT

Shoulder instability is a pathologic state characterized by abnormal translation of the humeral head on or over the glenoid, leading to pain, functional impairment, or even frank dislocation. The most common direction of instability is anterior-inferior. It can result from trauma, repetitive microtrauma, or atraumatic. Age is the most important predictor of recurrence rates after an initial dislocation. Multiple studies have reported that early surgical reconstruction for primary dislocation decreases the risk of recurrence. Surgical treatment options include arthroscopic or open stabilization or coracoid transfer. Arthroscopic stabilization for collision athletes and patients with osseous Bankart lesions is controversial. Contraindications to arthroscopic stabilization include a large Hill-Sachs lesion (the engaging or off-track Hill-Sachs) and bony deficiencies of the glenoid that represent more than 20%. High rates of return to sport are documented for arthroscopic treatment. Multiple early, short-term studies using a suture anchor technique similar to the open method have documented clinical success, with recurrent instability rates of 4% to 10%. Risk factors for failure include young age, male sex, collision athlete, time from dislocation until surgery, glenoid compression fracture, large Hill-Sachs lesion, and inferior shoulder hyperlaxity.

Dr. Arciero or an immediate family member has stock or stock options held in Biorez and Soft Tissue Regeneration; has received research or institutional support from Arthrex and DJ Orthopaedics; serves as a board member, owner, officer, or committee member of the American Orthopaedic Society for Sports Medicine and the American Shoulder and Elbow Surgeons. Neither Dr. O'Brien nor any immediate family member has received anything of value from or has stock or stock options held in a commercial company or institution related directly or indirectly to the subject of this chapter.

Keywords: arthroscopic; bankart repair; shoulder stabilization

Introduction

The glenohumeral joint is one of the least constrained joints, and its stability depends on a delicate balance of dynamic and static constraints. Injury to any of the constraints can lead to an array of conditions, from frank dislocation to repetitive microinstability or atraumatic instability. Glenohumeral dislocation affects approximately 2% of the general population.[1] Most shoulder instability is anterior, and early appropriate treatment often is necessary to avoid recurrence. Advances in understanding pathology, imaging, and surgical techniques have led to the success of arthroscopic reconstruction in managing instability.

Clinical Evaluation

History

A thorough patient history should be obtained for preoperative and intraoperative decision-making (**Table 1**). The patient's age, sex, hand dominance, medical conditions (such as seizures, hyperlaxity, or alcohol use), occupation, activity level, and expectations after surgery should be included. Age at initial dislocation should be included because a relatively young age is associated with an increased risk for recurrence.[2] Older patients have much lower redislocation rates (14%).[3] The exact etiology should be defined by investigating the patient's history of trauma, microtrauma, or hyperlaxity as well as the extent of trauma; each of these will affect preoperative planning. For defining the direction of instability, the exact position of the arm at the time of the dislocation or the subluxation should be determined, as should the arm position that re-creates the symptoms. The patient should be asked about the frequency of instability symptoms, the ease of re-creating symptoms, any instability during sleep, and whether it is becoming easier to subluxate the shoulder. The answers may provide insight into the severity of the soft-tissue and bony deficiency.

This chapter is adapted from Arciero RA, Reed DN: Arthroscopic reconstruction for recurrent shoulder instability, in Nicholson GP, ed: *Orthopaedic Knowledge Update: Shoulder and Elbow*, ed 4. Rosemont, IL, American Academy of Orthopaedic Surgeons, 2013, pp 121-133.

Table 1

Patient History Findings Relevant to Instability

Finding	Significance
Age at initial dislocation	The risk for recurrence is increased in younger patients (especially those younger than 25 yr).
Medical conditions (eg, seizures or electrical shock)	The risk for posterior dislocation or posterior instability is increased.
Trauma or manual reduction	A significant trauma or a manual reduction suggests a relatively severe soft-tissue injury or possible bony injury of the glenoid or the humeral head.
Activity level (sports participation)	Contact athletes may be at increased risk for recurrence.
Arm position at the time of initial event	Anterior instability is suggested by a position of abduction and external rotation. Posterior instability is suggested by a position of forward flexion, adduction, and internal rotation.
Hyperlaxity	Multidirectional instability should be suspected.
Frequency of instability	Relative frequency may be related to bony deficiency.
Instability during sleep	Bony deficiency should be suspected.
Ease of re-creating symptoms or instability	Symptoms that can be re-created at progressively lower levels of abduction and external rotation suggest worsening bony involvement.

Also important is whether the initial episode required a manual reduction. The need for a manual reduction typically indicates a major soft-tissue injury, possibly with a bony injury. Surgical notes and radiographs related to any earlier treatment should be reviewed for their effect on the surgical plan. Any history of voluntary instability or psychiatric disorder should be documented because an affected patient may be best treated nonsurgically.

Physical Examination

A detailed physical examination should be performed on both shoulders to allow a side-to-side comparison (**Table 2**). The involved and noninvolved shoulders should be inspected both anteriorly and posteriorly to detect any asymmetry or surgical scarring. The passive and active range of motion should be documented as well as rotator cuff strength; weakness has been associated with recurrent anterior instability.[4] If the patient has undergone an open procedure, the integrity of the subscapularis must be documented using the belly press and lift-off tests. The arm position that produces the instability should be noted. Instability in a position of abduction and external rotation suggests anterior instability. The exact degrees of abduction and external rotation should be noted because instability with relatively little abduction and external rotation suggests bony deficiency. Forward flexion, adduction, and internal rotation re-creating pain or instability suggests posterior instability. A sulcus sign with internal or external rotation should be documented and compared with the contralateral side. A detailed neurologic examination should be performed, with particular attention to the axillary nerve.

When the initial examination is complete, provocative testing should be performed. The apprehension and relocation tests should be used to assess anterior instability, and the jerk test should be used to detect posterior instability. The load-and-shift test should be used to detect anterior or posterior instability. Patients with a history of recurrent instability are more likely to have positive apprehension, relocation, and sulcus signs as well as greater posterior translation on the involved side than on the contralateral side.[5] Joint hyperlaxity should be determined by assessing elbow recurvatum, metacarpophalangeal hyperlaxity, and the thumb-to-forearm sign; affected patients may benefit from rehabilitation rather than surgery. A comprehensive shoulder examination should include a full neck evaluation to rule out cervical pathology as a cause of shoulder symptoms.

Imaging

The initial imaging should include standard trauma radiographs, including the true AP, scapular Y, and axillary lateral views. Specialized views that should be obtained include the West Point modified axillary view to detect glenoid bone deficiency and the Stryker notch view to detect a humeral head (Hill-Sachs) lesion[6,7] (**Figure 1**).

MRI is useful for evaluating recurrent instability because of its superiority to other imaging modalities in assessing soft-tissue pathology. In patients with traumatic

Table 2

Physical Examination Findings Relevant to Instability

Finding	Significance
Scars or asymmetry	Surgical scarring can provide information on earlier surgeries or trauma. Asymmetry can provide information on muscular atrophy secondary to muscle or tendon injury or neurologic injury.
Shoulder range of motion	Loss of full range of motion compared with contralateral side can signify adhesive capsulitis or bony or soft-tissue blocks.
Rotator cuff testing	A patient older than 40 yr often has a rotator cuff injury with dislocation. Rotator cuff weakness may occur with recurrent instability. The subscapularis should be evaluated closely.
Arm position that re-creates symptoms or instability	Anterior instability is suggested by a position of abduction and external rotation. Posterior instability is suggested by a position of forward flexion, adduction, and internal rotation.
Provocative testing (apprehension, relocation, jerk tests)	Test results can provide information on the direction of instability.
Neurologic examination	The axillary and musculocutaneous nerves should be checked because of possible injury during earlier surgery or dislocation.
Hyperlaxity (elbow recurvatum, thumb-to-forearm test, sulcus sign)	Hyperlaxity suggests multidirectional instability.
Cervical spine evaluation	A full evaluation can rule out cervical pathology mimicking shoulder pain.

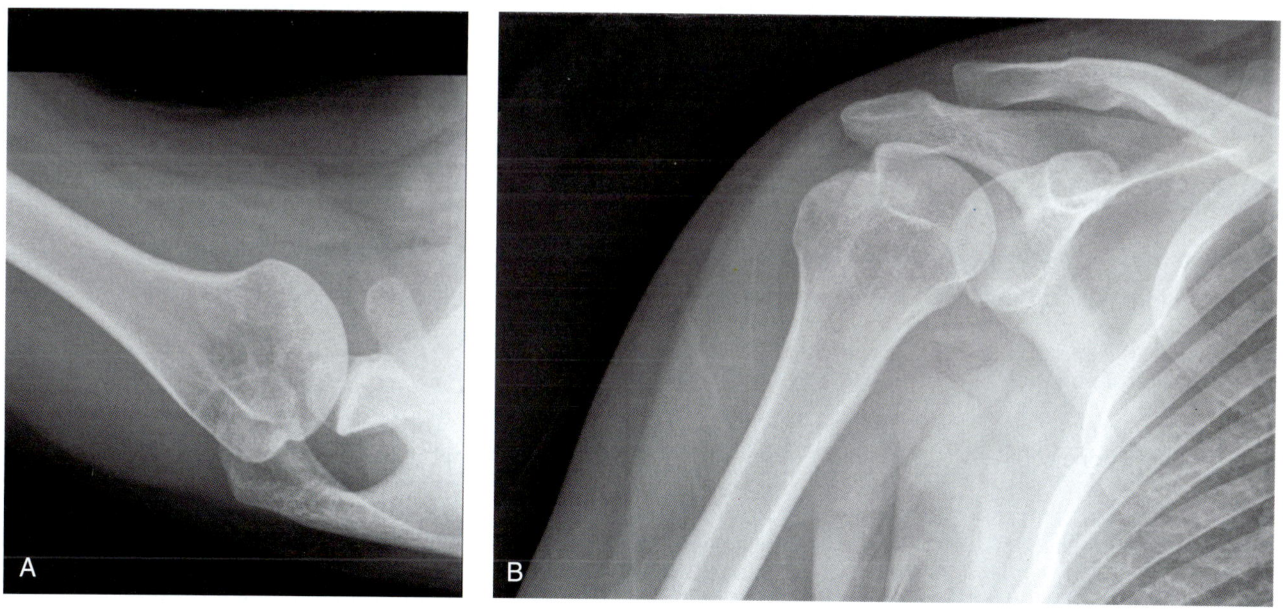

FIGURE 1 **A**, West Point radiograph showing an anterior glenoid rim defect in the shoulder of a patient with recurrent anterior instability. The anterior contour of the glenoid is abnormal compared with the well-defined posterior glenoid rim. **B**, Stryker notch radiograph showing a Hill-Sachs lesion in the right humeral head of a patient with a traumatic dislocation. The abnormal contour of the humeral head can be seen laterally.

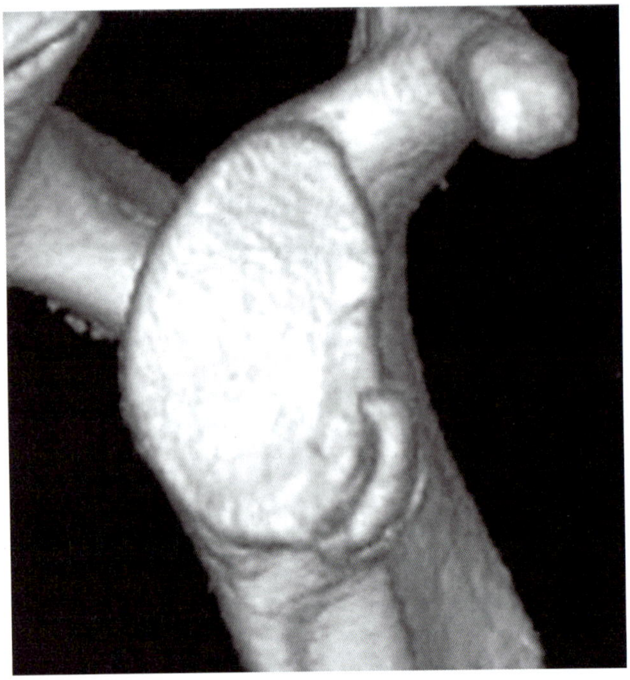

FIGURE 2 Three-dimensional CT of the shoulder in a patient with recurrent instability showing an en face view of the glenoid with rim fracture and bone loss in the anterior-inferior quadrant.

anterior instability, the most frequently diagnosed lesion is the Bankart lesion, which is an anterior-inferior capsulolabral disruption.[8] Patients with recurrent shoulder instability have more posterior labral tears, superior labrum anterior to posterior (SLAP) tears, and rotator cuff pathology than patients with a first dislocation.[9] MRI also allows visualization of a humeral-sided avulsion of the glenohumeral ligaments (HAGL lesion), capsular tearing or attenuation, and bony edema. Preoperative recognition of additional pathology allows the surgeon to be prepared to treat all conditions during surgery and thereby improve the outcome.[10,11]

MRI is less useful than CT for detecting a bony defect. CT allows accurate assessment of bony injuries of both the glenoid and the humeral head. Bony defects are important to recognize and treat appropriately because treating only soft-tissue pathology leads to a high risk that arthroscopic stabilization will fail.[12,13] It is important to understand that as many as 90% of patients with recurrent instability have a glenoid rim defect, and as many as 100% have a Hill-Sachs lesion.[14,15] Three-dimensional CT can allow accurate assessment of a Hill-Sachs lesion or glenoid deficiency by digital subtraction of the humeral head so the glenoid can be viewed en face[16] (**Figure 2**). Many techniques exist for accurately calculating the percentage of bone loss on both the humeral and glenoid sides, and the surgeon should thoroughly understand the use of one of these methods[17-19] (**Table 3; Figure 3**). The threshold should be low for ordering three-dimensional CT before surgical intervention for recurrent instability. Preoperative CT also may be necessary if the patient has significant trauma at the time of initial dislocation, radiographs suggesting bony changes, a history of multiple earlier reductions, increasingly frequent instability, an instability sensation created with decreasing levels of force, instability with minimal abduction and external rotation, instability during sleep, glenoid dysplasia,

Table 3

Common Methods of Evaluating Glenoid Bone Loss

Method	Rationale
Plain radiography, including trauma-series and specialized views (West Point, apical oblique)	Useful for detecting bony abnormalities but not the percentage of bone loss. The West Point view is most precise.
MRI	Useful for evaluating soft-tissue injuries but not the percentage of bone loss.
Three-dimensional CT	Useful for measuring glenoid bone loss. The simplest methods are as follows: • Measure the glenoid bone loss. A measurement of 6 to 8 mm is approximately equivalent to a 25% loss. • Identify the bare area on an en face view of the glenoid. (The bare area is the center of the true circle of the inferior glenoid, and the distance to the anterior and posterior rims should be equal.) Measure from the bare area to the anterior rim of the intact glenoid (*A*) and from the bare area to the posterior glenoid (*B*). The percentage of bone loss is calculated as $([B - A]/2B) \times 100$.
Arthroscopy	Glenoid bone loss should be estimated before arthroscopy but can be calculated intraoperatively by identifying the bare area, measuring from the bare area to the anterior (*A*) and posterior (*B*) glenoid rims, and using the equation $([B - A]/2B) \times 100$.

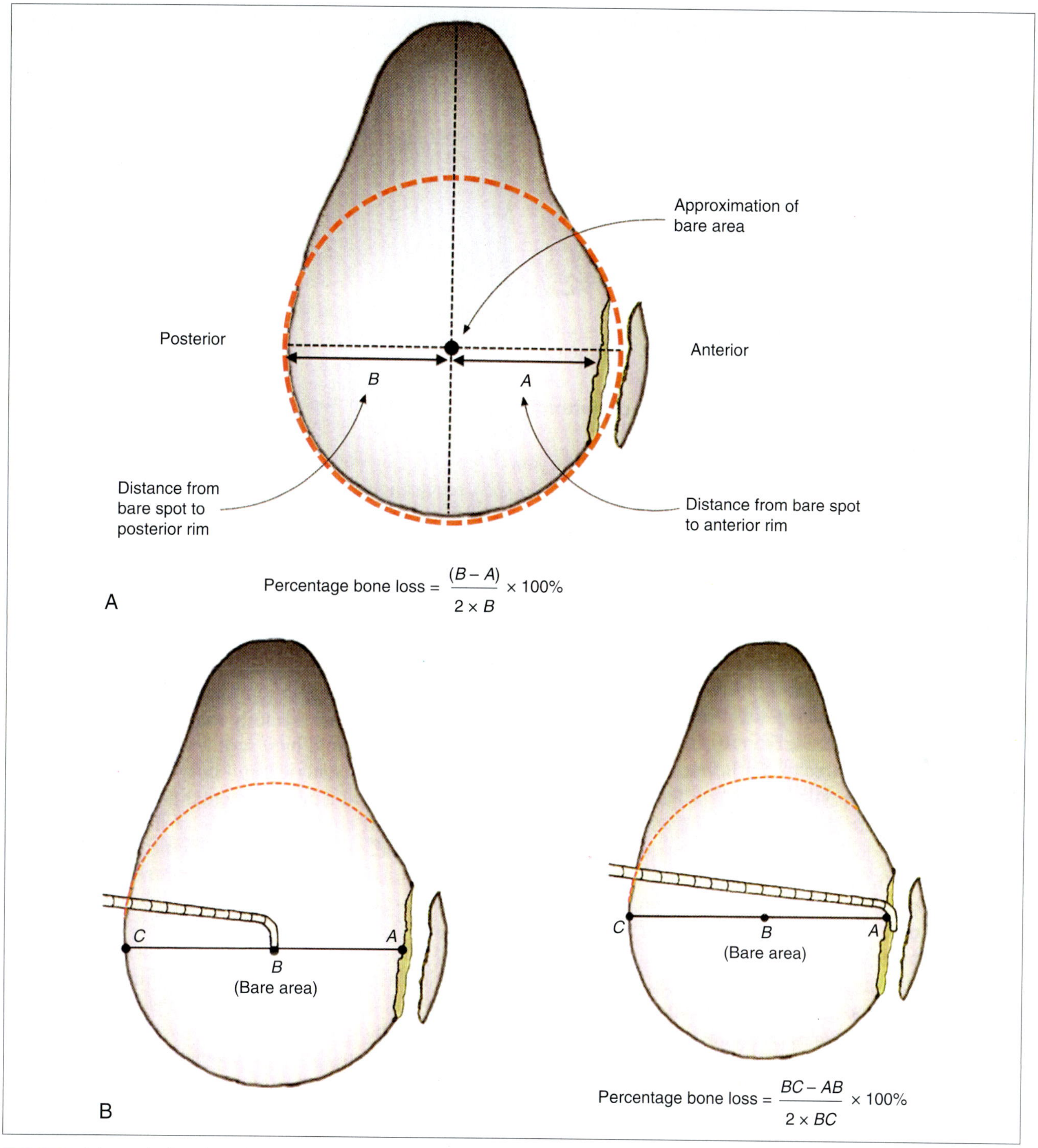

FIGURE 3 Schematic drawings showing the estimation of bone loss based on glenoid rim distances (**A**) and the glenoid bare spot method (**B**). (Reproduced with permission from Provencher MT, Bhatia S, Ghodadra NS, et al: Recurrent shoulder instability: Current concepts for evaluation and management of glenoid bone loss. *J Bone Joint Surg Am* 2010;92[suppl 2]:133-151. Copyright © 2010 by The Journal of Bone and Joint Surgery, Incorporated doi:10.2106/JBJS.J.00906.)

abnormal version, or unsuccessful instability surgery. Recently, the relationship between the Hill-Sachs lesion and the Bankart lesion has become the focus of much research. An engaging or off-track lesion may be a risk factor for recurrent instability as described in a 2007 study.[20] This was demonstrated in a 2015 cadaver study using 3D modeling.[21] This now-validated measurement has been shown to predict failure of arthroscopic repair in off-track lesions.[22,23] MRI can accurately determine if bipolar lesions are on track or off track with 84% accuracy.[24]

Pathoanatomy

Bony Deficiency

Instability surgery is unlikely to succeed if a bony deficiency is not adequately managed.[12,13] The patient's history and physical examination should provide insight into glenoid-side or humeral-side bony deficiency. Both the prevalence and the size of glenoid defects increase with recurrent dislocations. The likelihood of a so-called critical defect (involving more than 20% of the inferior glenoid) is associated with a higher number of dislocations and a younger age at the time of first dislocation.[25] The patient should undergo appropriate preoperative imaging to define the amount of bone loss, which can influence surgical planning.

Labrum and Glenohumeral Ligaments

The labrum is a fibrocartilaginous structure that encircles the glenoid, increasing its surface area and depth and acting as a buttress to translation of the humerus on the glenoid. The inferior glenohumeral ligament (IGHL) complex is a large ligament consisting of an anterior and posterior band connected by a capsular pouch. The IGHL complex is confluent with the labrum and can easily be identified arthroscopically. The IGHL complex resists anterior translation of the humerus on the glenoid when the arm is in 90° of abduction and external rotation. A detachment of the anterior-inferior labrum and the IGHL is called a Bankart lesion. A persistent Bankart lesion can lead to recurrent anterior instability of the shoulder (**Figure 4**). In a patient with recurrent instability, plastic deformation or attenuation of the IGHL occurs. Successful arthroscopic repair requires the labrum to be reattached to the glenoid face and the IGHL complex to have its tension restored.

In patients with recurrent instability, the detached labrum and the IGHL complex can heal in a medial position on the glenoid neck. This condition is called anterior labroligamentous periosteal sleeve avulsion (ALPSA) lesion (**Figure 5**). An ALPSA lesion results in loss of tension of the IGHL complex and loss of the labrum as a bumper, leading to continued instability. Patients with recurrent instability and an ALPSA lesion typically have had more dislocations and are less likely to have successful surgery than patients who have only a Bankart lesion.[26]

Patients with recurrent instability may also have superior extension of labral pathology leading to a SLAP lesion. Patients with a SLAP lesion typically have more dislocations before surgery than patients with only a Bankart lesion. In contrast to patients with an ALPSA lesion, however, those with a SLAP lesion are no different from those with a Bankart lesion with respect to recurrence and function after surgery.[27] A HAGL lesion or a lateral detachment of the IGHL also can be a cause of recurrent instability (**Figure 6**). A HAGL lesion must be recognized before surgery and treated through an open or arthroscopic procedure. Recurrent instability almost always leads to capsular plastic deformation or attenuation. One must be cautious of arthroscopic HAGL repairs and pay careful attention to the axillary nerve. Failure to restore capsular tension can lead to failure of the surgery. Capsular plication of 1 cm in line with the fibers of the anterior band of the IGHL can reduce laxity and restore appropriate tension to the capsule.[28]

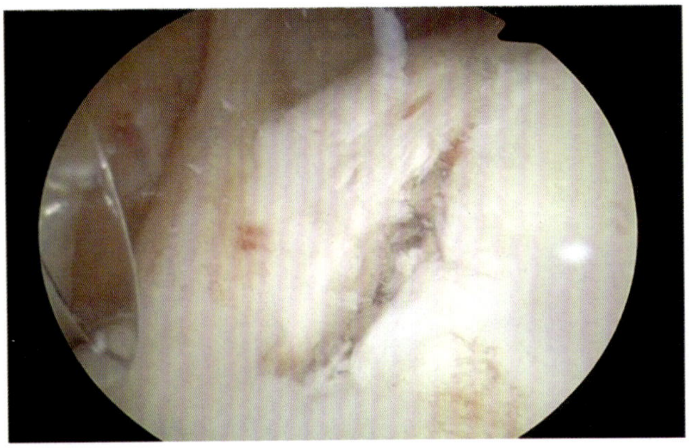

FIGURE 4 Arthroscopic image taken from the anterosuperior portal, showing a bony Bankart lesion in a patient with anterior instability. Detachment of the bony rim with the labrum attached can be seen. The anterior inferior glenohumeral ligament is attached to the labrum.

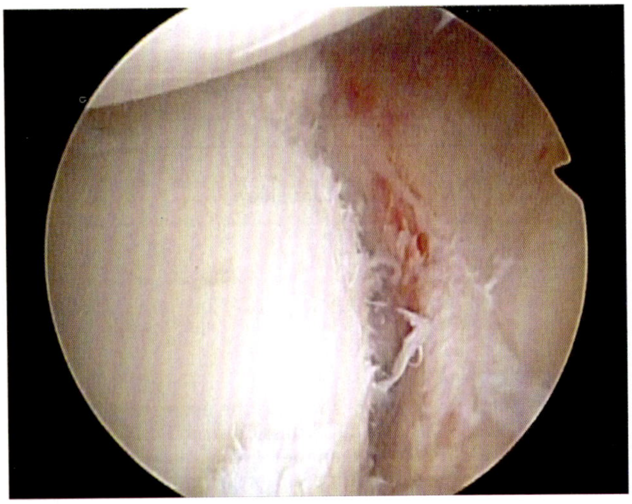

FIGURE 5 Arthroscopic image taken from the anterosuperior portal, showing an anterior labroligamentous periosteal sleeve avulsion lesion in a patient with recurrent instability. The loss of the labrum can be seen at the anterior cartilage rim. The labrum can be seen in a scarred, medialized position on the neck of the glenoid.

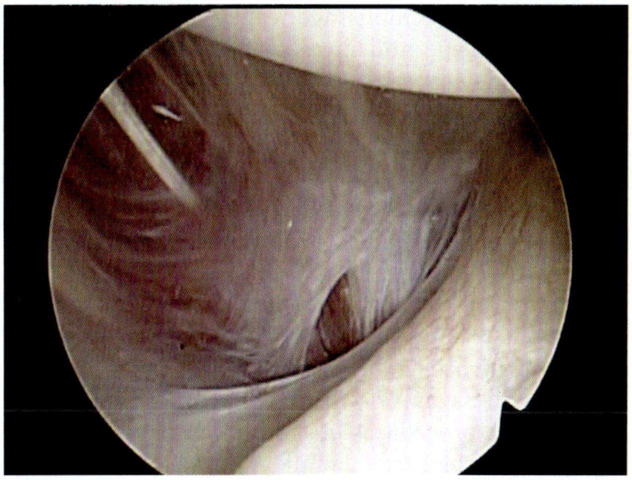

FIGURE 6 Arthroscopic image showing a humeral-sided avulsion of the glenohumeral ligament lesion in a patient with recurrent instability. The retracted inferior glenohumeral ligament complex can be seen, as well as the muscular fibers of the subscapularis adjacent to the humeral head.

The Rotator Cuff Interval

The rotator cuff interval consists of the superior and middle glenohumeral ligaments, the long head of the biceps tendon, the coracohumeral ligament, and the capsule. Controversy surrounds the risks and the benefits of rotator cuff interval closure in patients with anterior instability. Closure can improve anterior stability but result in a loss of external rotation, which can lead to loss of motion and the possible progression of osteoarthritis.[29,30]

The Rotator Cuff

Injury to the rotator cuff is rare in patients with a shoulder dislocation who are younger than 40 years. Patients older than 40 years have an increased risk of rotator cuff injury with shoulder dislocation, and rotator cuff injury should be suspected if the patient continues to have pain and weakness more than 3 weeks after the dislocation.

Treatment Planning

Nonsurgical Treatment

Most patients with recurrent instability require surgical intervention. The exception is the patient with multidirectional instability, who should undergo nonsurgical treatment before surgery is considered. Nonsurgical treatment may also be appropriate for a patient who has a significant medical comorbidity, low physical demands, a seizure disorder, or a psychiatric illness; who voluntarily dislocates for secondary gain; or who is unable or unwilling to complete postsurgical rehabilitation. Nonsurgical treatment typically involves a period of immobilization followed by rotator cuff and periscapular strengthening.

An in-season athlete can be treated nonsurgically with a brief period of immobilization followed by rotator cuff strengthening and the use of a protective brace or harness. However, as many as 37% of such athletes were found to have recurrence, and 50% required surgical intervention.[31] Only 27% of intercollegiate contact athletes were able to complete the season after anterior instability event without subsequent instability.[32] Recurrent instability occurred in most of the patients.

Acute dislocation is managed with sling immobilization. There is controversy regarding the type of sling to be used after an initial acute dislocation. Some studies found that immobilization in external rotation may reduce the risk of recurrent anterior instability after a single dislocation episode, but other studies challenged this finding.[33] However, a subsequent meta-analysis found no benefit to immobilization for longer than 1 week, a greater incidence of recurrence if the patient was younger than 30 years, and no difference in recurrence rates based on whether traditional sling immobilization or immobilization in external rotation was used.[33]

Surgical Management

The role of arthroscopic reconstruction in the management of recurrent shoulder instability continues to evolve. A review of data from the American Board of Orthopaedic Surgery reveals a trend toward arthroscopic stabilization and away from open repair as well as a decreasing number of complications among all-arthroscopically treated patients.[34] Arthroscopic procedures can be as successful as open procedures if the surgeon is able to recognize all underlying soft-tissue and bony deficiency and manage them appropriately using modern techniques and devices.[35] Two meta-analyses confirmed earlier findings that arthroscopic repair of a Bankart lesion using suture anchors is equivalent to open repair.[36,37] However, the open Bankart repair remains a time-tested standard procedure for achieving a stable, well-functioning shoulder joint.[8] The requirements for a successful arthroscopic reconstruction are to recognize and treat bony deficiency, recognize and treat all concomitant soft-tissue pathology, use an appropriate surgical procedure and technique, and determine whether the patient is at high risk for recurrence.

Glenoid Deficiency

The ability to recognize a glenoid defect before surgery and treat it appropriately during an open or an arthroscopic procedure is crucial to surgical success. If glenoid deficiency is missed before surgery, the surgeon can use the bare spot on the glenoid to measure the defect intraoperatively. However, every attempt should be made to identify significant bone loss on the humerus or the glenoid before surgery so that the patient can be adequately counseled as to the options and a definitive plan can be made before surgery. A 6- to 8-mm defect anteriorly rather than posteriorly means that 25% of the glenoid is missing, and the surgical plan must be changed accordingly. Surgical failure rates as high as 80% have been associated with glenoid bone loss in the anterior-inferior region.[12] The extent of bone loss for which an open repair should be performed is debatable, but most experts agree that open repair is required for bone loss greater than 20% to 25%.[38,39] However, all-arthroscopic repair of a bony Bankart lesion with a retained fragment, with incorporation of the bony fragment in the repair, has had acceptable results (failure rates of less than 10%).[40,41] These studies highlight the importance of the glenoid bone stock in glenohumeral stability. If glenoid bone loss is greater than 20% to 25% and there is no bony fragment, an open procedure should be performed to restore the functional arc of the glenoid. Additionally, the engaging or off-track Hill-Sachs lesion is a contraindication for arthroscopic stabilization.[12,42]

Open procedures, such as iliac crest bone grafting, tibial allograft bone grafting, the Bristow procedure (transfer of the tip of the coracoid), and the Latarjet procedure (transfer of the entire coracoid base with the coracoacromial ligament and the conjoined tendon), have yielded good results in terms of recurrence. A 2012 review of the Bristow-Latarjet procedure revealed good and consistent results, with bony fusion in 83% of the patients; recurrence rates were lower when the coracoid was placed less than 1 cm medial to the glenoid rim and a horizontal capsular shift was added to the transfer.[43]

Humeral Head Lesions

A defect in the articular surface of the humeral head (a Hill-Sachs lesion) can be found in almost every patient with recurrent instability. Most defects are small and have little effect on the stability of the shoulder. Surgery for a Hill-Sachs lesion that is associated with glenoid bone loss or engages on the glenoid rim with abduction and external rotation (a so-called engaging Hill-Sachs lesion) is likely to fail if only soft tissue is treated.[12,15] Most such lesions require treatment of only the glenoid defect; doing so increases the arc of rotation and prevents the Hill-Sachs lesion from engaging, which can lead to recurrence. However, large defects of the humeral head (more than 30%) may require managing the humeral head directly.[44] Three-dimensional CT can be useful in quantifying the defect. The arm can be placed in abduction and external rotation intraoperatively to determine whether the Hill-Sachs lesion is engaging; if so, it must be managed.

Arthroscopic remplissage (capsulotenodesis of the posterior capsule and infraspinatus tendon into the Hill-Sachs defect) is an emerging management option that avoids the potential morbidity of an open procedure and may reduce the ability of the humeral head to engage on the glenoid. Several studies have shown that a large or an engaging Hill-Sachs lesion can be treated with arthroscopic Bankart repair and remplissage with no alteration in range of motion; the recurrence rates were similar to those of open procedures.[45-47] However, as many as 33% of patients have experienced posterosuperior pain after remplissage.[48] Open procedures for treating Hill-Sachs lesions are still widely used and reliable. These procedures include elevation of the defect and bone grafting, articular allograft, metal resurfacing, rotational osteotomy, and hemiarthroplasty.

Soft-Tissue Pathology

Arthroscopic reconstruction allows direct visualization of all bony and soft-tissue injures in a patient with recurrent instability. Patients with prolonged recurrent instability typically have extensive soft-tissue injuries, which must be appropriately treated to ensure a successful outcome. The Bankart lesion must be identified and mobilized, and appropriate tension and placement of the labrum and the IGHL complex must be restored on the glenoid face. It is important to carefully visualize the entire labrum and treat any posterior labral tear or SLAP lesion. An ALPSA lesion is best identified from the anterosuperior portal, and it must be mobilized and appropriately tensioned on the face of the glenoid to ensure success. A HAGL lesion typically is identified on preoperative MRI but can be seen arthroscopically. Although experienced surgeons have repaired HAGL lesions arthroscopically, an open subscapularis tendon-sparing approach should be considered. Patients who have capsular deficiency as a result of recurrent instability or earlier surgery are challenging to treat. Allograft reconstruction of anterior capsulolabral structures had promising results at 2-year follow-up and is a viable alternative to arthrodesis in young patients.[49]

The rotator cuff interval structures continue to be a source of controversy in arthroscopic instability surgery. Closure of the rotator cuff interval can improve anterior instability at the cost of external rotation. Rotator cuff interval closure has been suggested for patients with hyperlaxity and recurrent instability, patients with a positive sulcus sign that does not correspond to the contralateral side or cannot be corrected by external rotation with the arm at the side, patients undergoing revision surgery, and athletes in collision sports who consider stability more important than range of motion.[50] Rotator cuff interval closure also has been used for posterior instability; good results have been achieved without closure, however, and the improvement in posterior stability with closure has been called into question.[30]

Patient Selection

To maximize the likelihood of surgical success, an appropriate history and physical examination should be used to select patients for arthroscopic reconstruction. Success is most likely if the patient meets several criteria: no bone defect larger than 20% to 25%, no engaging Hill-Sachs lesion, a well-defined Bankart lesion with good tissue, no other concomitant soft-tissue injuries, no identifiable hyperlaxity, and an initial dislocation. Favorable indicators for an athlete include participation in an overhead sport (or in a noncollision sport if the patient is older than 20 years).

Surgical Technique

The diagnosis and the surgical plan should be established before surgery. Every patient should be examined under anesthesia to confirm the diagnosis and ensure that no abnormalities were missed preoperatively. The patient is positioned according to the surgeon's preference. The lateral decubitus position with longitudinal traction allows excellent visualization and access to the inferior glenoid. Portal placement is important in instability repair. The posterior portal should be placed in line with the glenoid face; this positioning is more lateral than the traditional posterior portal. The anterior portal should be placed using an outside-in technique to ensure appropriate placement and avoid articular injury. The anterosuperior portal should be placed high in the rotator cuff interval, and the anterior-inferior portal should be placed just above the subscapularis. The portals should allow access to the inferior recess.

Visualization of all bony and soft-tissue injuries is critical. All associated injuries must be treated. The Bankart lesion can be seen through the posterior portal, and the anterosuperior portal is used to ensure that an ALPSA lesion is not missed. The Bankart lesion is mobilized in preparation for tensioning and repair. Capsulolabral release is considered adequate when the surgeon can see the muscle fibers of the subscapularis. The glenoid should be prepared by removing all soft tissue from the intended repair site. After mobilization and preparation, the surgeon determines whether anchors or sutures will be placed first. The anchors should be placed at the glenoid face at the level of the articular cartilage and the scapular neck junction. The anchors must not be placed too medial because appropriate tension will not be restored, and they must not be placed too close to the face because of the risk of injury to articular cartilage and subsequent malreduction of the capsulolabral complex.

Proper anchor placement on the glenoid face should begin between the 5-o'clock and 6-o'clock positions with a minimum of three or four anchors.[12,51] The surgeon should ensure that the anchors are adequately seated to avoid postoperative impingement on the humeral head. Multiple studies have evaluated different anchors and sutures, and some studies have found that capsulolabral height can be restored and outcomes are similar regardless of whether the traditional or newer knotless anchor system is used.[52-56] The next step is to restore tension to the IGHL complex. The sutures for tensioning should be placed 5 to 10 mm caudal to the corresponding anchors to allow appropriate tension. For example, an anchor placed in the 5-o'clock position should have a corresponding tension suture placed around 1 cm of capsulolabral and IGHL complex soft tissue at the 6-o'clock position. The soft tissue should be brought to the 5-o'clock anchor, moving all soft tissue within the tension suture cephalad by 5 to 10 mm to create appropriate tensioning (**Figure 7**). Any capsular redundancy noted before or during surgery should be treated to prevent recurrence. This capsular tissue can be included in the repair by placing sutures in the capsule 1 cm lateral to the labrum using the anchor placed for labral repair. Abrasion of the capsule can enhance capsular healing to the labrum.

The repair should be inspected after it is completed to ensure restoration of tension and the bumper effect (**Figure 8**). If needed, a posterior labral anchor can be placed for a posteriorly directed tear, and the rotator cuff interval can be closed if the surgeon decided to do so before surgery. However, rotator cuff interval closure should not be routinely done (**Figure 9**). A summary of tips for successful repair can be found in **Table 4**.

Complications and Controversies

The risk of complications after arthroscopic stabilization, including recurrence, can be minimized by following preoperative and intraoperative recommendations and techniques. Patients such as those with a bone or soft-tissue deficiency should not be treated arthroscopically if their condition is better suited to an open procedure. Complications such as postoperative stiffness can be avoided if only the injured tissue is treated and a strict postoperative rehabilitation regimen is followed. The risk of chondrolysis can be decreased by avoiding thermal ablation and the use of indwelling pain pumps.

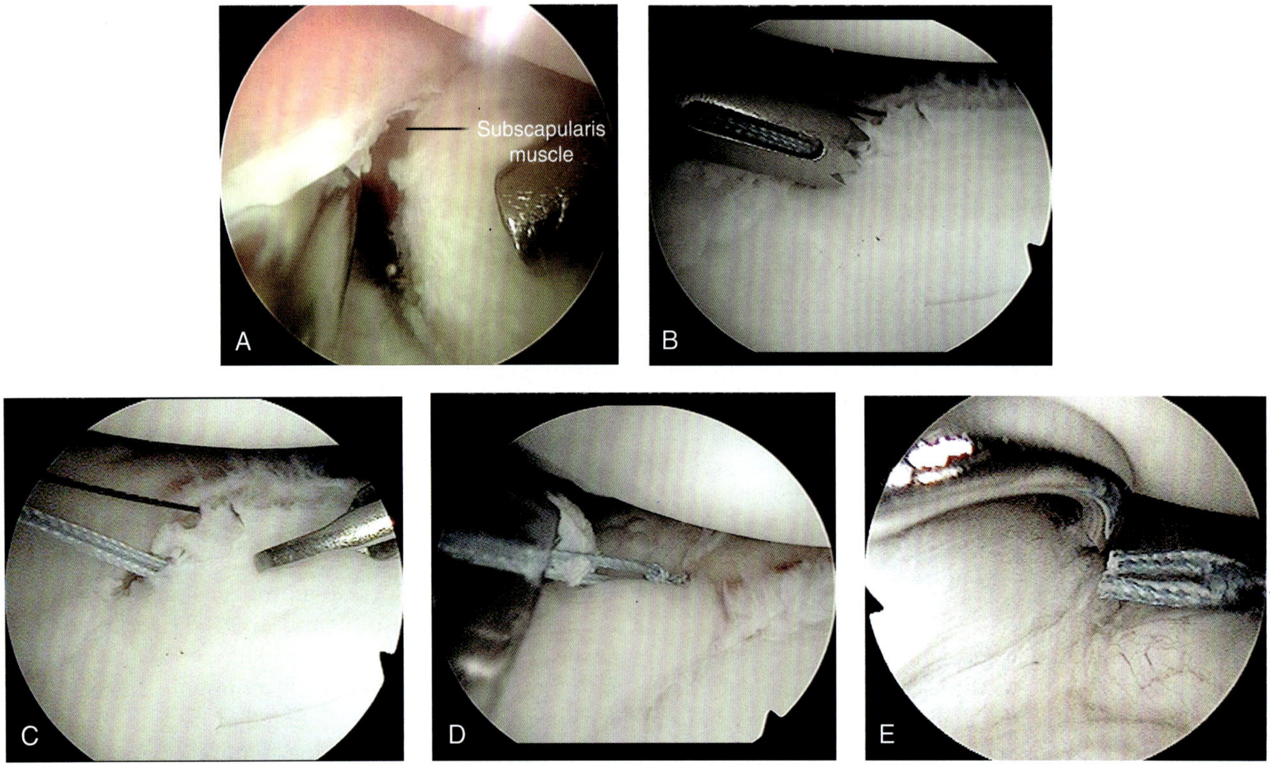

FIGURE 7 Arthroscopic images showing the surgical technique and placement of anchors for the management of anterior instability. **A**, Adequate mobilization is achieved when the muscular fibers of subscapularis are identified. The probe is located between the glenoid rim and the labrum, and the subscapularis muscle belly is identified deep. **B**, Anchors are placed after mobilization is complete. The anchor is in the 5:30 clock-face position on the anterior glenoid face. **C**, The suture-passing shuttle wire exits inferior to the sutures. The entry site for capsule penetration is 1 cm below the exit site to allow adequate retensioning of the inferior glenohumeral ligament (IGHL) complex. **D**, Both suture limbs have been passed and tied in horizontal mattress fashion. The knot is off the articular surface, and the bumper effect and tension on the IGHL complex have been restored with the initial anchor. **E**, The suture has been tied inferiorly, and the crescent hook is being used to grasp tissue for the next anchor, placed above the earlier anchor. The amount of capsulolabral tissue obtained for tensioning can be seen. (Reproduced with permission from Arciero RA, Mazzocca A: Arthroscopic treatment of anterior instability: Surgical technique, in Provencher MT, Romeo AA, eds: *Shoulder Instability: A Comprehensive Approach.* pp 126-146. Copyright 2012 Elsevier.)

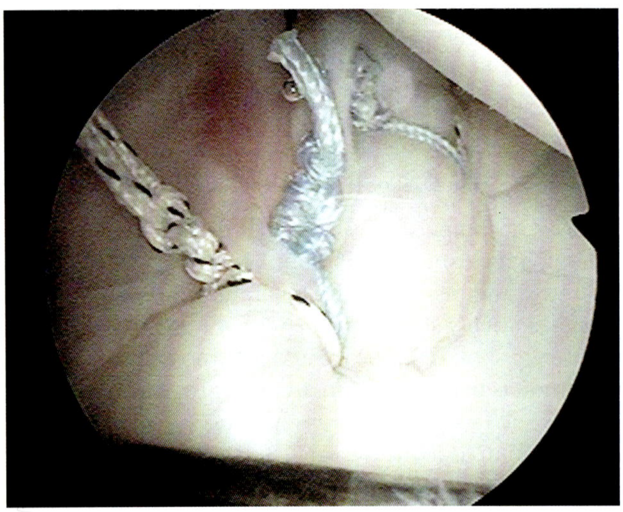

FIGURE 8 Arthroscopic image of a completed Bankart repair, showing the restoration of the bumper effect and tension on the inferior glenohumeral ligament.

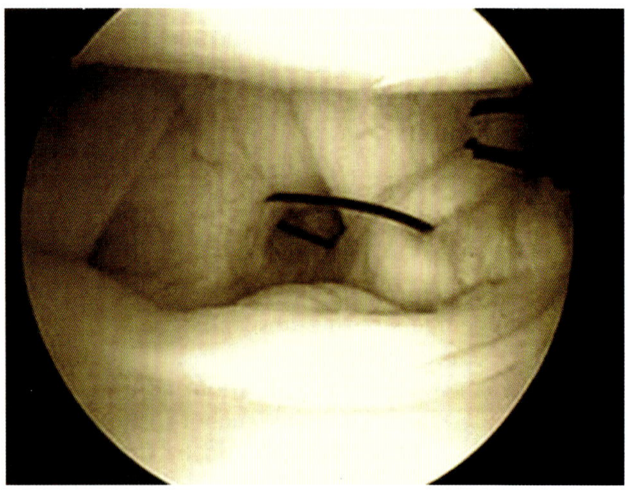

FIGURE 9 Arthroscopic image showing rotator cuff interval closure in a patient with multidirectional instability.

Table 4

Tips for Successful Bankart Repair

Step	Pearls
Positioning	• Lateral decubitus with the aid of bean bag positioner. • Place gel pad just distal to axilla on downside arm to protect radial nerve. • Attach 7 lbs of longitudinal traction and 5 lbs of lateral traction to the balance arm traction device and attach to the arm sleeve. • The arm should be externally rotated with the thumb up and abducted about 25°. • After draping, mark the coracoid process, acromion, acromioclavicular joint, and spine of scapula.
Approach	• The posterior portal is created 2 cm distal to the posterolateral corner of the acromion and slightly lateral to the traditional posterior portal for better visualization of the anterior glenoid rim. • An anterosuperior and an anterior-inferior portal are created under direct visualization using a spinal needle. • The superior portal should be lateral to the coracoid and just distal to the acromion. The trochar should sit just posterior to the biceps tendon. This is the viewing portal. • The inferior portal should be made at the midpoint between the acromioclavicular joint and lateral border of the coracoid. The trochar should pierce the capsule just proximal to the subscapularis tendon and sit flush with the glenoid face. • Inspect the Bankart lesion from the posterior portal first. • Further inspect the lesion from the anterosuperior portal. • Use a small sterile bump in the axilla to distract the joint for better visualization of inferior aspect of lesion.
Repair	• The capsulolabral complex should be mobilized off the scapular neck if scarred down. • Use a rasp from the posterior or anterior-inferior portal to roughen the scapular neck until bleeding occurs to prep the bed for the repair. • Place a double-loaded suture at the 5-o'clock position (left shoulder) or 7-o'clock position (right shoulder). • Pass a zero polydioxanone suture through the capsulolabral complex at the 6-o'clock position. • Use this to shuttle one of the anchor sutures across the capsule and labrum. • Repeat this step to create a mattress suture and tie the suture. • Pass the second suture from the same anchor and tie a simple knot. The labral height has now been established. • Repeat these steps at the 9-o'clock and 10-o'clock positions for the right shoulder or 3-o'clock and 4-o'clock positions for the left shoulder. • Additional anchors can be placed as needed, employing a mattress stitch.

Patients at High Risk

A patient who is at high risk for recurrence must be identified before surgery. A preoperative instability severity index score has been created to help surgeons identify such patients. The system is based on a 10-point scale in which 2 points are assigned if the patient is younger than 20 years, is a competitive athlete, has a Hill-Sachs lesion as noted in external rotation on an AP radiograph, or has any change of the glenoid contour on an AP radiograph; 1 point is assigned if the patient has hyperlaxity or is an athlete in a contact or an overhead sport. Patients with a combined score higher than 6 were found to have a 70% recurrence risk, and those with a score of 6 or less had a 10% risk.[13] Other studies found that male sex, age younger than 22 years, and recurrent instability are risk factors for arthroscopic surgical failure, and such patients also should be closely evaluated.[57,58]

Controversies

There are multiple controversies related to arthroscopic instability surgery. In particular, the treatment of athletes in contact sports continues to be a source of controversy. Some surgeons support open repair for these athletes, and others support arthroscopic repair. Both sides of the controversy are supported by research.[59-62]

SUMMARY

The indications for arthroscopic reconstruction of recurrent instability continue to evolve. Arthroscopic reconstruction can have excellent results in terms of recurrence and function if close attention is paid to all of its preoperative and intraoperative aspects.

KEY STUDY POINTS

- Age is the most important predictor of recurrence rates after an initial dislocation.
- Early surgical reconstruction for primary dislocation decreases the risk of recurrence.
- High rates of return to sport are documented for arthroscopic treatment with low recurrent instability rates.
- Arthroscopic stabilization for collision athletes and patients with osseous Bankart lesions is controversial.
- Contraindications to arthroscopic stabilization include a large Hill-Sachs lesion (the engaging or off-track Hill-Sachs) and bony deficiencies of the glenoid that represent more than 20%.

Annotated References

1. Hovelius L: Incidence of shoulder dislocation in Sweden. *Clin Orthop Relat Res* 1982;(166):127-131.

2. Robinson CM, Howes J, Murdoch H, Will E, Graham C: Functional outcome and risk of recurrent instability after primary traumatic anterior shoulder dislocation in young patients. *J Bone Joint Surg Am* 2006;88(11):2326-2336.

3. Rowe CR, Sakellarides HT: Factors related to recurrences of anterior dislocations of the shoulder. *Clin Orthop* 1961;20:40-48.

4. Edouard P, Degache F, Beguin L, et al: Rotator cuff strength in recurrent anterior shoulder instability. *J Bone Joint Surg Am* 2011;93(8):759-765.

5. Owens BD, Duffey ML, Deberardino TM, Cameron KL: Physical examination findings in young athletes correlate with history of shoulder instability. *Orthopedics* 2011;34(6):460.

6. Itoi E, Hatakeyama Y, Kido T, et al: A new method of immobilization after traumatic anterior dislocation of the shoulder: A preliminary study. *J Shoulder Elbow Surg* 2003;12:413-415.

7. Itoi E, Lee SB, Amrami KK, et al: Quantitative assessment of classic anteroinferior bony Bankart lesions by radiography and computed tomography. *Am J Sports Med* 2003;31(1):112-118.

8. Gill TJ, Micheli LJ, Gebhard F, Binder C: Bankart repair for anterior instability of the shoulder: Long-term outcome. *J Bone Joint Surg Am* 1997;79(6):850-857.

9. Gutierrez V, Monckeberg JE, Pinedo M, Radice F: Arthroscopically determined degree of injury after shoulder dislocation relates to recurrence rate. *Clin Orthop Relat Res* 2012;470(4):961-964.

10. Porcellini G, Paladini P, Campi F, Paganelli M: Shoulder instability and related rotator cuff tears: Arthroscopic findings and treatment in patients aged 40 to 60 years. *Arthroscopy* 2006;22(3):270-276.

11. Rhee YG, Ha JH, Park KJ: Clinical outcome of anterior shoulder instability with capsular midsubstance tear: A comparison of isolated midsubstance tear and midsubstance tear with Bankart lesion. *J Shoulder Elbow Surg* 2006;15(5):586-590.

12. Burkhart SS, De Beer JF: Traumatic glenohumeral bone defects and their relationship to failure of arthroscopic Bankart repairs: Significance of the inverted-pear glenoid and the humeral engaging Hill-Sachs lesion. *Arthroscopy* 2000;16(7):677-694.

13. Balg F, Boileau P: The instability severity index score: A simple pre-operative score to select patients for arthroscopic or open shoulder stabilisation. *J Bone Joint Surg Br* 2007;89(11):1470-1477.

14. Piasecki DP, Verma NN, Romeo AA, Levine WN, Bach BR Jr, Provencher MT: Glenoid bone deficiency in recurrent anterior shoulder instability: Diagnosis and management. *J Am Acad Orthop Surg* 2009;17(8):482-493.

15. Cetik O, Uslu M, Ozsar BK: The relationship between Hill-Sachs lesion and recurrent anterior shoulder dislocation. *Acta Orthop Belg* 2007;73(2):175-178.

16. Provencher MT, Bhatia S, Ghodadra NS, et al: Recurrent shoulder instability: Current concepts for evaluation and management of glenoid bone loss. *J Bone Joint Surg Am* 2010;92(suppl 2):133-151.

17. Sugaya H, Moriishi J, Dohi M, Kon Y, Tsuchiya A: Glenoid rim morphology in recurrent anterior glenohumeral instability. *J Bone Joint Surg Am* 2003;85(5):878-884.

18. Cho SH, Cho NS, Rhee YG: Preoperative analysis of the Hill-Sachs lesion in anterior shoulder instability: How to predict engagement of the lesion. *Am J Sports Med* 2011;39(11):2389-2395.

19. Chuang TY, Adams CR, Burkhart SS: Use of preoperative three-dimensional computed tomography to quantify glenoid bone loss in shoulder instability. *Arthroscopy* 2008;24(4):376-382.

20. Yamamoto N, Itoi E, Abe H, et al: Contact between the glenoid and the humeral head in abduction, external rotation, and horizontal extension: A new concept of glenoid track. *J Shoulder Elbow Surg* 2007;16(5): 649-656.

21. Arciero RA, Parrino A, Bernhardson AS, et al: The effect of a combined glenoid and Hill-Sachs defect on glenohumeral stability: A biomechanical cadaveric study using 3-dimensional modeling of 142 patients. *Am J Sports Med* 2015;43(6):1422-1429.

    This biomechanical study sought to characterize the efficacy of soft tissue Bankart repair on combined bony Bankart and Hill-Sachs lesions. Using cadaveric models, they created these bipolar defects of varying size, performed Bankart repairs on each, and tested load to translation as a marker for instability. They found that bipolar defects have an additive and negative effect on stability. A medium Hill-Sachs lesion with a 2 mm glenoid defect was enough to compromise the Bankart repair. A small Hill-Sachs lesion with a 4 mm glenoid defect also compromised the repair. Level of evidence: IV.

22. Locher J, Wilken F, Beitzel K, et al: Hill-Sachs off-track lesions as risk factor for recurrence of instability after arthroscopic Bankart repair. *Arthroscopy* 2016;32(10):1993-1999.

    This case series reviewed CT or MRI studies from 100 patients who underwent arthroscopic Bankart repair. They found that 33% of patients with an engaging Hill-Sachs lesion underwent revision surgery compared to 6% with a non-engaging Hills-Sachs lesion. Mean follow up was 22.4 months. They concluded that an engaging Hill-Sachs lesion is a significant risk factor for recurrent instability and need for revision surgery after arthroscopic Bankart repair. Level of evidence: IV.

23. Shaha JS, Cook JB, Rowles DJ, et al: Clinical validation of the glenoid track concept in anterior glenohumeral instability. *J Bone Joint Surg Am* 2016;98(22):1918-1923.

    This study looked at 57 shoulders that were treated with arthroscopic Bankart repair. Preoperative MRI was used to identify on-track and off-track lesions. 75% of off-track patients failed their treatment, compared with 8% of on-track patients. The positive predictive value of postoperative stability was 75% for the track measurements, compared with 44% when using the criterion glenoid bone loss >20%. Level of evidence: III.

24. Gyftopoulos S, Beltran LS, Bookman J: MRI evaluation of bipolar bone loss using the on-track off-track method: A feasibility study. *AJR Am J Roentgenol* 2015;205(4):848-852.

    This study assessed whether the on-track off-track method using MRI could predict engaging lesions during arthroscopic evaluation. MRIs from 75 patients were reviewed by two blinded independent reviewers using the on-track off-track method to predict engagement. With high intrareader agreement (correlation coefficient 0.73) their predictions were accurate 84.2% of the time, with a positive predictive value of 65% and negative predictive value of 91.1%. Level of evidence: III.

25. Milano G, Grasso A, Russo A, et al: Analysis of risk factors for glenoid bone defect in anterior shoulder instability. *Am J Sports Med* 2011;39(9):1870-1876.

26. Ozbaydar M, Elhassan B, Diller D, Massimini D, Higgins LD, Warner JJ: Results of arthroscopic capsulolabral repair: Bankart lesion versus anterior labroligamentous periosteal sleeve avulsion lesion. *Arthroscopy* 2008;24(11):1277-1283.

27. Hantes ME, Venouziou AI, Liantsis AK, Dailiana ZH, Malizos KN: Arthroscopic repair for chronic anterior shoulder instability: A comparative study between patients with Bankart lesions and patients with combined Bankart and superior labral anterior posterior lesions. *Am J Sports Med* 2009;37(6):1093-1098.

28. Shapiro TA, Gupta A, McGarry MH, Tibone JE, Lee TQ: Biomechanical effects of arthroscopic capsulorrhaphy in line with the fibers of the anterior band of the inferior glenohumeral ligament. *Am J Sports Med* 2012;40(3):672-680.

29. Randelli P, Arrigoni P, Polli L, Cabitza P, Denti M: Quantification of active ROM after arthroscopic Bankart repair with rotator interval closure. *Orthopedics* 2009;32(6):408.

30. Mologne TS, Zhao K, Hongo M, Romeo AA, An KN, Provencher MT: The addition of rotator interval closure after arthroscopic repair of either anterior or posterior shoulder instability: Effect on glenohumeral translation and range of motion. *Am J Sports Med* 2008;36(6):1123-1131.

31. Buss DD, Lynch GP, Meyer CP, Huber SM, Freehill MQ: Nonoperative management for in-season athletes with anterior shoulder instability. *Am J Sports Med* 2004;32(6):1430-1433.

32. Dickens JF, Owens BD, Cameron KL, et al: Return to play and recurrent instability after in-season anterior shoulder instability: A prospective multicenter study. *Am J Sports Med* 2014;42(12):2842-2850.

    This study prospectively enrolled 45 contact intercollegiate athletes over 2 academic years and assessed their return to play after in-season anterior shoulder instability. Thirty-three players returned to sport after their injury but only 12 (27%) successfully completed

Section 2: Instability and Athletic Injuries

the season without subsequent instability. The remaining 21 had recurrent subluxation or dislocation events. Twenty-two of the 33 completed the season. Level of evidence: II.

33. Paterson WH, Throckmorton TW, Koester M, Azar FM, Kuhn JE: Position and duration of immobilization after primary anterior shoulder dislocation: A systematic review and meta-analysis of the literature. *J Bone Joint Surg Am* 2010;92(18):2924-2933.

34. Owens BD, Harrast JJ, Hurwitz SR, Thompson TL, Wolf JM: Surgical trends in Bankart repair: An analysis of data from the American Board of Orthopaedic Surgery certification examination. *Am J Sports Med* 2011;39(9):1865-1869.

35. Mahiroğulları M, Ozkan H, Akyüz M, Uğraş AA, Güney A, Kuşkucu M: Comparison between the results of open and arthroscopic repair of isolated traumatic anterior instability of the shoulder. *Acta Orthop Traumatol Turc* 2010;44(3):180-185.

36. Petrera M, Patella V, Patella S, Theodoropoulos J: A meta-analysis of open versus arthroscopic Bankart repair using suture anchors. *Knee Surg Sports Traumatol Arthrosc* 2010;18(12):1742-1747.

37. Hobby J, Griffin D, Dunbar M, Boileau P: Is arthroscopic surgery for stabilisation of chronic shoulder instability as effective as open surgery? A systematic review and meta-analysis of 62 studies including 3044 arthroscopic operations. *J Bone Joint Surg Br* 2007;89(9):1188-1196.

38. Yamamoto N, Itoi E, Abe H, et al: Effect of an anterior glenoid defect on anterior shoulder stability: A cadaveric study. *Am J Sports Med* 2009;37(5):949-954.

39. Sugaya H, Moriishi J, Kanisawa I, Tsuchiya A: Arthroscopic osseous Bankart repair for chronic recurrent traumatic anterior glenohumeral instability: Surgical technique. *J Bone Joint Surg Am* 2006;88(suppl 1, pt 2):159-169.

40. Zhu YM, Jiang CY, Lu Y, Xue QY: Clinical results after all arthroscopic reduction and fixation of bony Bankart lesion. *Zhonghua Wai Ke Za Zhi* 2011;49(7):603-606.

41. Ikeda H: "Rotator interval" lesion. Part 1: Clinical study. *Nihon Seikeigeka Gakkai Zasshi* 1986;60(12):1261-1273.

42. Itoi E, Lee SB, Berglund LJ, et al: The effect of a glenoid defect on anteroinferior stability of the shoulder after Bankart repair: A cadaveric study. *J Bone Joint Surg Am* 2000;82(1):35-46.

43. Hovelius L, Sandström B, Olofsson A, Svensson O, Rahme H: The effect of capsular repair, bone block healing, and position on the results of the Bristow-Latarjet procedure (study III): Long-term follow-up in 319 shoulders. *J Shoulder Elbow Surg* 2012;21(5):647-660.

44. Millett PJ, Clavert P, Warner JJ: Open operative treatment for anterior shoulder instability: When and why? *J Bone Joint Surg Am* 2005;87(2):419-432.

45. Park MJ, Tjoumakaris FP, Garcia G, Patel A, Kelly JD IV: Arthroscopic remplissage with Bankart repair for the treatment of glenohumeral instability with Hill-Sachs defects. *Arthroscopy* 2011;27(9):1187-1194.

46. Haviv B, Mayo L, Biggs D: Outcomes of arthroscopic "remplissage": Capsulotenodesis of the engaging large Hill-Sachs lesion. *J Orthop Surg Res* 2011;6:29.

47. Zhu YM, Lu Y, Zhang J, Shen JW, Jiang CY: Arthroscopic Bankart repair combined with remplissage technique for the treatment of anterior shoulder instability with engaging Hill-Sachs lesion: A report of 49 cases with a minimum 2-year follow-up. *Am J Sports Med* 2011;39(8):1640-1647.

48. Nourissat G, Kilinc AS, Werther JR, Doursounian L: A prospective, comparative, radiological, and clinical study of the influence of the "remplissage" procedure on shoulder range of motion after stabilization by arthroscopic Bankart repair. *Am J Sports Med* 2011;39(10):2147-2152.

49. Dewing CB, Horan MP, Millett PJ: Two-year outcomes of open shoulder anterior capsular reconstruction for instability from severe capsular deficiency. *Arthroscopy* 2012;28(1):43-51.

50. Chechik O, Maman E, Dolkart O, Khashan M, Shabtai L, Mozes G: Arthroscopic rotator interval closure in shoulder instability repair: A retrospective study. *J Shoulder Elbow Surg* 2010;19(7):1056-1062.

51. van der Linde JA, van Kampen DA, Terwee CB, Dijksman LM, Kleinjan G, Willems WJ: Long-term results after arthroscopic shoulder stabilization using suture anchors: An 8- to 10-year follow-up. *Am J Sports Med* 2011;39(11):2396-2403.

52. Milano G, Grasso A, Santagada DA, Saccomanno MF, Deriu L, Fabbriciani C: Comparison between metal and biodegradable suture anchors in the arthroscopic treatment of traumatic anterior shoulder instability: A prospective randomized study. *Knee Surg Sports Traumatol Arthrosc* 2010;18(12):1785-1791.

53. Slabaugh MA, Friel NA, Wang VM, Cole BJ: Restoring the labral height for treatment of Bankart lesions: A comparison of suture anchor constructs. *Arthroscopy* 2010;26(5):587-591.

54. Oh JH, Lee HK, Kim JY, Kim SH, Gong HS: Clinical and radiologic outcomes of arthroscopic glenoid labrum repair with the BioKnotless suture anchor. *Am J Sports Med* 2009;37(12):2340-2348.

55. Thal R, Nofziger M, Bridges M, Kim JJ: Arthroscopic Bankart repair using Knotless or BioKnotless suture anchors: 2- to 7-year results. *Arthroscopy* 2007;23(4):367-375.

56. Monteiro GC, Ejnisman B, Andreoli CV, de Castro Pochini A, Cohen M: Absorbable versus nonabsorbable sutures for the arthroscopic treatment of anterior shoulder instability in athletes: A prospective randomized study. *Arthroscopy* 2008;24(6):697-703.

57. Yan H, Cui GQ, Wang JQ, Yin Y, Tian DX, Ao YF: Arthroscopic Bankart repair with suture anchors: Results and risk factors of recurrence of instability. *Zhonghua Wai Ke Za Zhi* 2011;49(7):597-602.

58. Porcellini G, Campi F, Pegreffi F, Castagna A, Paladini P: Predisposing factors for recurrent shoulder dislocation after arthroscopic treatment. *J Bone Joint Surg Am* 2009;91(11):2537-2542.

59. Uhorchak JM, Arciero RA, Huggard D, Taylor DC: Recurrent shoulder instability after open reconstruction in athletes involved in collision and contact sports. *Am J Sports Med* 2000;28(6):794-799.

60. Pagnani MJ, Dome DC: Surgical treatment of traumatic anterior shoulder instability in American football players. *J Bone Joint Surg Am* 2002;84(5):711-715.

61. Ide J, Maeda S, Takagi K: Arthroscopic Bankart repair using suture anchors in athletes: Patient selection and postoperative sports activity. *Am J Sports Med* 2004;32(8):1899-1905.

62. Mazzocca AD, Brown FM, Carreira DS, Hayden J, Romeo AA: Arthroscopic anterior shoulder stabilization of collision and contact athletes. *Am J Sports Med* 2005;33(1):52-60.

Chapter 10

Injuries to the Throwing Shoulder

Kelly Fitzpatrick, DO • John M. Tokish, MD

ABSTRACT

The management of shoulder pathology in the overhead athlete presents many challenges. Obtaining a correct diagnosis, maintaining the high demands of the in-season athlete nonsurgically, using proper and effective surgical techniques, and rehabilitating with efficiency and efficacy are all variables that contribute to the complexity in this particular patient population. This updated review of the disabled overhead athlete will provide insight into the development of the treating surgeon's armamentarium for these particular injuries. The key to treating these patients is having an understanding into the pathogenesis of these injuries.

Keywords: GIRD; internal impingement; overhead athlete; throwing

Introduction

The management of the disabled shoulder in a throwing athlete is a difficult task. The high forces and the kinematic requirements of overhead throwing produce a unique pathophysiology that is most evident in elite throwing athletes. The throwing shoulder exerts a rotational velocity of as much as 7,000°/s, which is reportedly the fastest movement in sports.[1] Throwing shoulders have been found to adapt by increasing external rotation, decreasing internal rotation, increasing humeral and glenoid retroversion, and developing anterior capsular laxity. With each pitch, the soft-tissue envelope surrounding the shoulder is loaded to levels that approach ultimate failure. The combination of the adaptations and the demands on the throwing shoulder means that it is vulnerable to common pathologic conditions such as a partial-thickness rotator cuff tear, anterior capsular laxity or pseudolaxity, posteroinferior capsular contracture, posterior or posterosuperior labral injury, biceps tendon pathology, and scapular dyskinesis.[2]

One of the most difficult challenges in treating a patient with a disabled throwing shoulder is to distinguish a pathologic entity from a normal adaptation. A fix-everything approach can lead to an inability to return to the previous level of throwing. A 2018 study evaluating professional throwing athletes demonstrated a resolution of the pathologic conditions evident on MRI following retirement.[3] This makes a surgical treatment decision very difficult when discussing treatment options with these individuals. It is therefore critical that the surgeon is cautious during the preoperative evaluation when making a decision to pursue surgical intervention.

There are multiple pathologies and etiologies leading to a dysfunctional throwing shoulder. The understanding of contributing pathologies has evolved with improvements over time in diagnostic and surgical technologies. The purpose of this chapter is to review these multiple pathologies and review the recent treatment techniques used to address the symptomatic throwing shoulder.

Biomechanics

A dilemma known as the thrower's paradox ensues as a pitcher pushes for more and more velocity. An extreme range of motion at the highest possible force is required to reach maximum velocity. This maximum velocity is achieved through the transfer of force from the larger muscles in the body (eg, lower extremity, core) to the hand in a process termed the "kinetic chain." During this kinetic chain, the shoulder must retain enough stability to keep itself centered and create a stable fulcrum for the motion. The mechanics of throwing occur in six separate phases (**Figure 1**; **Table 1**). In the first phase, the windup, the body initiates force from the legs, trunk, and core and begins the transfer of energy to the shoulder. Very little stress is placed on the glenohumeral joint during this phase. The early cocking phase ensues with the arm

Dr. Tokish or an immediate family member has received royalties from Arthrex, Inc.; is a member of a speakers' bureau or has made paid presentations on behalf of Arthrex, Inc. and Mitek; serves as a paid consultant to or is an employee of Arthrex, Inc., DePuy, a Johnson & Johnson Company, and Mitek; and serves as a board member, owner, officer, or committee member of the Arthroscopy Association of North America. Neither Dr. Fitzpatrick nor any immediate family member has received anything of value from or has stock or stock options held in a commercial company or institution related directly or indirectly to the subject of this chapter.

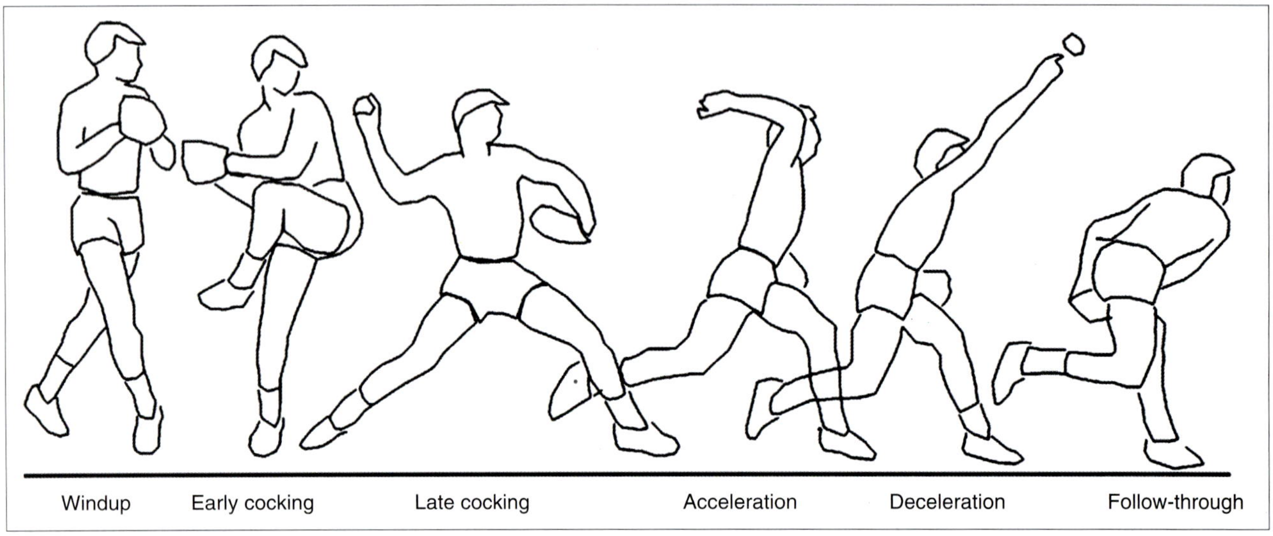

FIGURE 1 Phases of the baseball pitch. (Reproduced from McMahon PJ, Debski RE: Kinematics and kinesiology of the shoulder, in Galatz LM, ed: *Orthopaedic Knowledge Update: Shoulder and Elbow*, ed 3. Rosemont, IL, American Academy of Orthopaedic Surgeons, 2007, p 47.)

in abduction and external rotation. As maximal external rotation is achieved during the late cocking phase and the arm begins to move toward the target, the anterior structures are tensioned and the rotator cuff generates forces as high as 650 N.[4] The acceleration phase is initiated as the arm begins internal rotation, and it ends with the release of the ball. This phase marks the greatest velocity in the upper extremity. Most of the energy is transferred to the ball in this phase, and little stress is imposed on the glenohumeral joint. However, multiple vectors of force are directed within the shoulder and the surrounding tissues during the deceleration phase immediately following release. The shoulder can undergo distraction forces as high as 950 N, compressive forces greater than 1,000 N, and posterior shear forces as high as 400 N.[4,5] During the follow-through phase, the internal forces begin to return to normal, with compression force decreasing to 400 N.

The failure load of the native capsule is 800 to 1,200 N in young individuals. Therefore, it is understandable why throwing athletes are prone to injury and why optimal throwing mechanics are important. A study of young pitchers found that those with proper mechanics had less humeral internal rotation torque, lower elbow valgus load, and more efficiency than pitchers with poor mechanics.[6]

Throwing Adaptation

The extreme motion and force induced through the aforementioned biomechanical process leads the shoulder to undergo adaptive changes. These changes invoke a transformation of the osseous structure, ligamentous tightening and laxity, and overall rotational movement. These changes may lead to better performance when able to achieve more rotational velocity through the kinetic chain. However, certain changes may predispose the overhead athlete to injury (**Table 2**).

An example of this adaptation to the throwing athlete is the ossification of the posterior-inferior structure. In 1959, a posteroinferior glenoid exostosis was described as the inciting pathology for pain in the professional pitcher, secondary to repetitive traction on the posterior capsule and the triceps tendon.[7] This adaptation was termed a Bennett lesion, as it was originally described by George Bennett. This theory later fell out of favor, although more recently the importance of posterior capsular pathology has again been recognized. In 2016, the development of Bennett lesions identified on MRI had a positive correlation to duration of play in the throwing athlete.[8] Treatment of Bennett lesions is a bit controversial given the limited clinical data and the existence of concomitant pathology. There is a small case series of Bennett-plasty (arthroscopic shaving of the osseous overgrowth) with a 68% (11/16) return to play at 1-year follow-up in baseball players.[9]

A more recognized and accepted adaptation to throwing shoulder in elite pitchers is the thickening of the posterior capsule.[10] This contracture is believed to shift the humerus posterosuperiorly, precipitating the contact that leads to pathology in the rotator cuff and the labrum, as seen in the disabled throwing shoulder.[2] The resulting glenohumeral internal rotation deficit (GIRD) is the hallmark of the at-risk throwing shoulder. Other studies have confirmed the high prevalence of GIRD in

Table 1

Phases of a Baseball Pitch (Right-Handed Pitcher)

Phase	Description	Comments
Windup	The hands are together holding the ball. The body is aligned in good balance. The pitcher takes a small, comfortable step back with the left leg, in line with home plate. The right foot is then positioned parallel to the rubber. (Some coaches have the pitcher wedge the foot so that the lateral half is on top of the rubber.) The left lower extremity is picked up in a controlled, active fashion, and the hips remain level while pointing toward home plate. As the hips begin to move forward, a V is formed in which the hips are the apex and the torso and right leg form the two sides. The hips point toward the batter. The right hand comes out of the glove holding the ball.	These are the components of all successful pitches, although a pitcher's windup phase has individual stylistic adaptations that raise the center of gravity. The shoulders are relatively uninvolved. They move slowly, the hands are together, and the muscle activity is low.
Early cocking	The hand stays on top of the ball as it comes out of the glove. The shoulder is then elevated approximately 100° in the scapular plane and is externally rotated to approximately 45°. The V becomes more pronounced as the hips continue to move forward toward home plate. The hips stay level; rotation of the hips is delayed as long as possible. The ball is hidden from the batter, who cannot yet determine the type of pitch to be delivered. The left leg slowly, easily, and comfortably comes down until the foot reaches the mound.	The initial position of the hand helps the shoulder stay in internal rotation, which is a safer position for the glenohumeral joint. The deltoid and the supraspinatus act together to abduct the humerus. The other rotator cuff muscles are not active.
Late cocking	The left foot makes contact with the mound, landing within the width of the right foot and pointing toward home plate. The pitcher's center of gravity has been lowered, releasing energy. The pitcher's weight is evenly distributed between the two legs, and the legs are firm. The torso is balanced between the legs in an upright position. The pitcher delays trunk rotation as long as possible.	The goal is to move the humerus into maximum external rotation. The humerus maintains its level of elevation in the scapular plane and externally rotates from 46° to 170°. Deltoid and supraspinatus activity diminishes, but the other rotator cuff muscles' activity increases for joint stability. The middle portion of the trapezius, rhomboids, levator scapulae, and serratus anterior muscles are active so that the scapula can provide an effective base for the humeral head.
Acceleration	The acceleration phase is initiated when the humerus begins to internally rotate. In approximately 1/20th of a second, the ball is released from the hand at a speed as high as 100 mph. Both feet are on the mound. The acceleration of the arm coincides with the deceleration of the rest of the body, producing efficient transfer of energy to the upper extremity and the ball.	The motion occurs on the very firm base provided by the lower extremities. Synchronous muscular contraction about the glenohumeral joint and scapulothoracic articulation provides both stability and rapid motion of the upper extremity.
Deceleration	The right hip is brought up and over the left leg after the ball is released. The right foot disengages from the mound, and the body goes into a controlled forward fall.	The kinetic energy not transferred to the ball is dissipated by large muscle activity, beginning with the arm.
Follow-through	The arm is brought down.	The forces affecting the arm decrease.

Adapted with permission from McMahon PJ, Tibone JE, Pink MM: Functional anatomy and biomechanics of the shoulder, in Delee JC, Drez D Jr, Miller MD, eds: *Delee and Drez's Orthopaedic Sports Medicine: Principles and Practice*, ed 2. p 850. Copyright Elsevier 2003.

Table 2

Pitching Kinematics and the Nonsurgical Management of Deficits

Point of Breakdown in Kinetic Chain	Result	Treatment
Premature forward motion during windup or stride	Arm lags behind body	Strengthen core muscles
Stride foot landing in closed position	Decreased pelvis-trunk rotation Pitcher must throw across body, decreasing force generation in kinetic chain	Strengthen hip external rotators
Stride foot landing in open position	Premature pelvic rotation Uncoupled kinetic chain Arm lags behind body Shoulder must generate increased forces to maintain velocity	Strengthen hip internal rotators
Throwing from an upright position (diminished forward trunk tilt)	Acceleration forces act on ball over shorter distances Less velocity generated	Strengthen core muscles
Increased lead knee flexion at ball release	Less force generated by torso flexing and rotating over front side	Stretch hamstrings
Diminished internal rotation	Acceleration forces act on ball over shorter distance	Perform sleeper stretch
Scapular dyskinesis	Diminished external rotation in late cocking phase (decreased scapular retraction) Subacromial impingement	Stabilize scapula

throwing shoulders, its association with shoulder pathology, and the resolution of symptoms with the correction of GIRD.[2,11]

There are several definitions of GIRD, including an internal rotation deficit greater than 20° compared with the contralateral side, a loss of internal rotation that exceeds the gain in external rotation, and GIRD in the setting of a loss of total arc of motion. Regardless of the definition applied, the development of GIRD is not necessarily a pathologic process but an adaptive one as it has been found to be present in as many as 40% of asymptomatic throwers.[12] However, GIRD has been demonstrated (although not statistically significant) to be a risk factor in shoulder injuries in professional baseball pitchers.[11] This risk factor (GIRD) is thought to lead to the development of internal impingement in elite throwers. One prevention measure, which has been discussed in detail in a later section, is the use of the sleeper stretch in warm-ups to prevent injury.

Internal impingement is defined as contact between the greater tuberosity and posterior-superior glenoid. The excessive external rotation invoked by those with GIRD may contribute to the development of the pathologic process of internal impingement, which can lead to a culmination of concomitant pathology to include partial-thickness articular-sided rotator cuff tears, posterior labral tears, superior labrum anterior to posterior (SLAP) tears, and biceps pathology. These injuries have multiple etiologies, and concomitant existence in overhead athletes makes this difficult to study because of the heterogeneity in nature. In the early 1990s, this pathologic process was observed with an arthroscopic examination of 16 throwing athletes with internal impingement, and it was found that the rotator cuff impinged in an abducted and externally rotated position, leading to partial-thickness cuff tears and posterior capsular lesions.[13]

The disabled throwing shoulder represents a spectrum of conditions resulting from the adaptations required when an individual's anatomy and physiology are subjected to the extreme demands of throwing an object beyond the individual's physiologic limits.

History and Physical Examination

Patients with a dysfunctional throwing shoulder most often have posterior shoulder pain during the cocking or follow-through phase of the throwing motion. Some patients may describe a loss of control or velocity or a feeling of a dead arm. Physical examination may reveal tenderness to palpation, increased external rotation and decreased internal rotation, instability or laxity, and positive posterior impingement tests, as well as more traditional impingement signs.[14,15]

As described earlier, an internal rotation deficit of more than 20° compared with the contralateral side (measured with the glenohumeral joint abducted to 90°), especially in the setting of a decreased total arc of motion, may signal a pathologic amount of GIRD (**Figure 2**). In such a patient, the examiner must pay particular attention to the core strength of the athlete, the scapula, and any associated shoulder pathology. Another objective measurement of posterior capsular tightness is cross-body adduction. A loss of adduction in comparison to the contralateral shoulder may indicate posterior capsular contracture. This is debatable in the literature as to being a manifestation of the posterior capsule versus posterior deltoid tightness.[16]

Provocative maneuvers such as O'Brien test, Neer sign, and Hawkins sign may be a bit too sensitive and nonspecific to isolate an accurate diagnosis but may provide some insight if they are negative. Jerk test and modified posterior load and shift may be indicative of posterior labral pathology, which can be commonly seen in this particular subset of patients. Anterior instability may be present because of the microtrauma secondary to increased external rotation. This may elicit a positive apprehension sign and pain relief with relocation. Alternatively, in internal impingement, this relocation test may elicit pain. Another internal impingement examination finding is the posterior impingement sign originally described in a 2004 study.[15] This test is similar to the apprehension test with the addition of extension in conjunction with abduction and external rotation. This test is positive if there is pain deep in the posterior aspect of the shoulder.

Scapular dyskinesis usually is seen as static and dynamic scapular malposition that is evident when the patient repeatedly raises and lowers the arms or engages the dynamic stabilizers of the scapula.[17] This asymmetric and uncoordinated movement of the scapula can be evident with the simple movement of forward flexion of the arm and observation of bilateral scapulae. The asymmetric movement may be quite subtle on initial observation. If clinical suspicion is high in these patients, fatigue of the dynamic stabilizers may be necessary either with repetitive forward flexion and abduction or by performing the wall push-up test. Winging of the scapula can often be observed after 5 to 10 push-ups. The clinician may want to consider nerve conduction studies to evaluate for potential neurologic injuries, specifically evaluating the long thoracic nerve (serratus anterior) and the spinal accessory nerve (trapezius) (**Table 3**).

Imaging

Standard radiographs should be included in the workup for a disabled throwing shoulder, but often they are normal. Bennett lesions or glenoid bone loss may be identified on axillary imaging. On axillary view radiographs, a Bennett lesion presents as a curvilinear extra-articular calcification along the posteroinferior rim of the glenoid at or around the attachment of the posterior band of the inferior glenohumeral ligament. If a Bennett lesion is suspected, more advanced imaging, such as MRI, may be indicated to assess the integrity of surrounding soft-tissue structures because

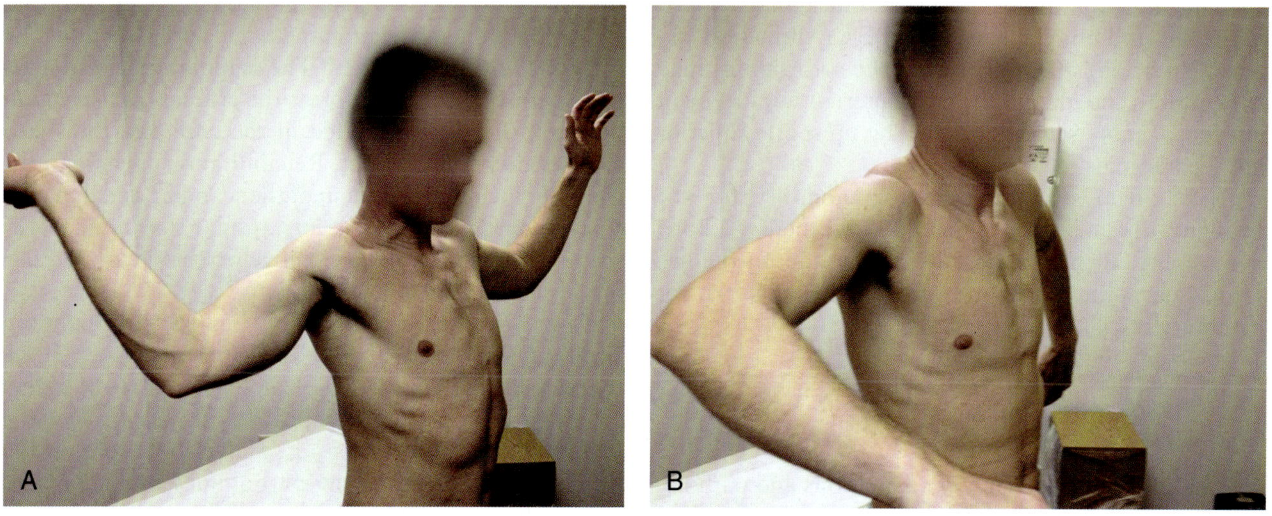

FIGURE 2 Clinical photographs showing glenohumeral internal rotation deficit. **A**, Increased external rotation of the right shoulder as compared with the contralateral shoulder. **B**, Decreased internal rotation on the right shoulder as evident with glenohumeral internal rotation deficit.

Table 3

Comprehensive Management of the Throwing Athlete

Diagnosis	Physical Examination Finding	Nonsurgical Management	Surgical Management
Anterior instability	Apprehension, relief with relocation	Scapular stabilization	Capsular shift/labral repair
Posterior instability	Jerk test, posterior load and shift	Scapular stabilization	Labral repair ± biceps tenodesis
Internal impingement	Pain with relocation, posterior impingement sign[15]	Scapular stabilization Rotator cuff strengthening Sleeper stretch	Rotator cuff débridement (± biceps tenodesis) or repair
SLAP tear	Positive active compression test, O'Brien test	Rest	SLAP débridement, repair or biceps tenodesis
GIRD	Pain with decreased internal rotation	Sleeper stretch	Limited posterior capsular release
Partial-thickness articular-sided rotator cuff tear	Pain or weakness with rotator cuff testing	Rotator cuff strengthening	Débridement or repair
Scapular dyskinesis	Scapular compression test, scapular assistance test	Periscapular strengthening, core strengthening	Addressing underlying cause (ie, above pathologies)

GIRD = glenohumeral internal rotation deficit, SLAP = superior labrum anterior to posterior.

such osseous lesions are commonly associated with posterior labral tears and posterior undersurface rotator cuff tears.

The cornerstone of radiographic evaluation remains MRI or magnetic resonance arthrography, which has greater accuracy for detecting labral pathology, rotator cuff and biceps pathology, capsular thickening, bursal pathology, and bony edema. An ABER (**AB**duction **E**xternal **R**otation) magnetic resonance arthrogram may be helpful in the identification of internal impingement and can be more sensitive in picking up subtle superior labral pathology.

CT is not a standard imaging modality for the throwing athlete but may be indicated if there is a bony abnormality, such as a large Bennett lesion on the initial radiographic evaluation or if there is concern for instability.

Common Pathologic Sequelae and Specific Treatment

Because there is a spectrum of adaptations and pathologies among pitchers, surgical treatment of the throwing shoulder does not lend itself to well-controlled study. Nonsurgical management is successful in preventing the need for surgery in many of these athletes. The throwing action is the culmination of multiple energy transfers from the proximal to the distal kinetic chain. Deficits anywhere along this chain can be translated into a more distal injury. Therefore, successful nonsurgical management of the disabled throwing shoulder must involve all aspects of the kinetic chain, as well as the shoulder itself. Hip and leg strength must be maintained, and core strengthening cannot be overemphasized. The scapular platform must be optimized because it forms the critical transfer point between the power created in the core and the speed generated in the shoulder. Rehabilitation specific to the shoulder includes treatment of the scapular and dynamic stabilizers as well as posterior capsular stretching. SICK scapula syndrome can be effectively treated with retraining of scapular mechanics.[17]

Regardless of etiology, injuries to the throwing shoulder share many final sequelae, including SLAP tears, proximal biceps pathology, partial-thickness rotator cuff tears, and scapular dyskinesis. Over the last few years, multiple studies have shed light on the outcomes of the following pathologic conditions and this updated review should provide proper guidance in treating overhead throwing athletes and their respective injuries.

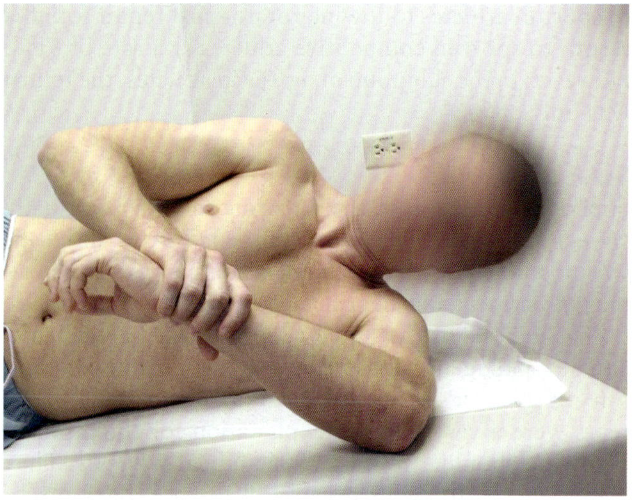

FIGURE 3 Clinical photograph showing the sleeper stretch, in which the patient lies in the lateral position, with the affected side downward, and manually pushes the arm to the floor. For a patient with glenohumeral internal rotation deficit, this movement emphasizes stretching on the posterior capsule.

Glenohumeral Internal Rotational Deficit

As mentioned previously, GIRD is an adaptation and not necessarily a pathologic process. Posterior capsular tightness is among the most detrimental adaptations in the throwing athlete, but resolution of its symptoms can be achieved by using stretching exercises, such as the sleeper stretch (**Figure 3**). Pitchers who participated in an internal rotation stretching program for several years had better internal rotation and total arc of motion than those in shorter structured stretching programs.[18]

In most patients, the disabled throwing shoulder responds to this comprehensive approach. A 2011 report described the researchers' experience with a major league baseball team over 3 years.[11] Many of the pitchers exhibited signs and symptoms of GIRD, but almost all were resolved with a supervised athletic training program. Only 3 of the 40 pitchers with GIRD eventually required surgery. Another study found that nonsurgical management focused on sleeper stretches, and scapulothoracic rehabilitation was 100% effective in returning the shoulders of 96 athletes to throwing.[17]

If a patient has GIRD that has not responded to nonsurgical management, the posterior capsule should be carefully evaluated at arthroscopy for thickening (**Figure 4**). In rare patients, a posterior capsular release may be considered to help restore recalcitrant internal rotation deficit. This release should be done with extreme caution, especially inferiorly, where the axillary nerve is at risk. The use of electrocautery may provide a margin of safety because proximity to the nerve should result in contraction of the deltoid musculature and may provide a warning. An arthroscopic biter also can be cautiously used to perform selective capsular release at the capsulolabral junction. Regardless of the method, the release should be done close to the glenoid because this location offers the best buffer to the axillary nerve. Posterior capsular release for GIRD in throwing athletes has rarely been reported in the peer-reviewed literature. Reliable pain relief with less reliable return to throwing was reported when this approach was used.[19] Eleven of 16 athletes (69%) returned to their preinjury performance level. Only four of these patients had isolated posteroinferior capsular tightness; this finding highlights the complexity of the pathology of the throwing shoulder.[19]

Partial-Thickness Rotator Cuff Tears

Rotator cuff damage is perhaps the most common pathology in the throwing shoulder. Full-thickness tears are uncommon, but partial-thickness articular-sided tears are almost ubiquitous in throwing athletes and are believed to result from acute tension and/or repetitive microtrauma from eccentric failure. These tears have been described as occurring posterosuperiorly at the junction of the infraspinatus and

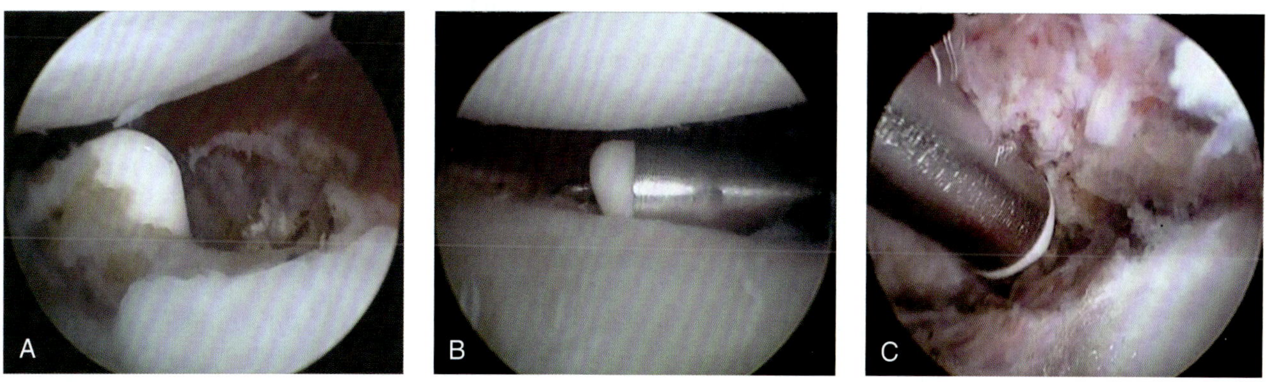

FIGURE 4 Arthroscopic images showing posterior capsule release. **A**, The capsule is released with electrocautery. The characteristic thickened posterior capsule can be seen. **B**, A hook probe can be used for a more precise capsular release. **C**, Release in close proximity to the glenoid is done to avoid injury to the axillary nerve.

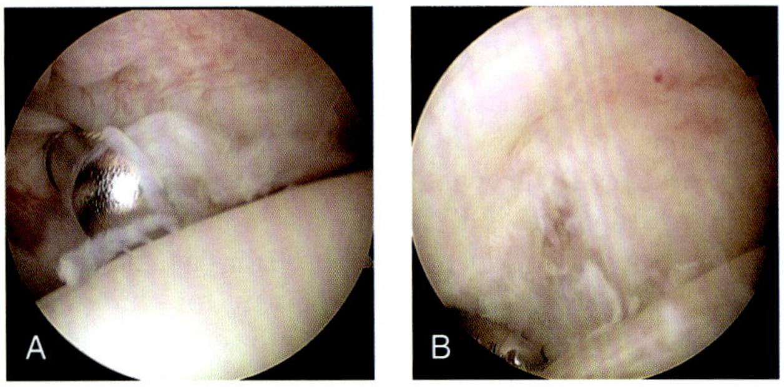

FIGURE 5 Arthroscopic images showing a partial-thickness articular-sided tear with significant fraying before (**A**) and after (**B**) limited débridement intended to avoid interrupting the integrity of the rotator cuff.

supraspinatus insertions, as the result of internal impingement.[13,20] Over the last few years, this topic has not been studied as it was over a decade ago and the treatment is very similar to include limited débridement to diminish the theoretical inflammatory producing torn tissue.

These tears in the throwing athlete are more posterior than a classic rotator cuff tear and can be seen by bringing the arm out of traction and into an abducted, externally rotated position. The treatment most often includes débridement if nonsurgical measures are unsuccessful (**Figure 5**), although a 2001 study reported that in situ repair had good results in returning athletes to throwing.[21] Return-to-throwing rates following débridement or intratendinous repair ranges from 55% to 87% have been reported, with better results after treatment of combined pathology[22-24] (**Table 4**).

The repair of full-thickness tears has not consistently allowed pitchers to return to throwing, and caution should be exercised against overly aggressive débridement or conversion of a partial-thickness to a full-thickness tear repair. A 2019 systematic review looking at return to sport in athletes following rotator cuff repair found a return to sport in competitive athletes at a rate of 61%. However, in the subgroup of overhead athletes, the return was only 38%.[25]

SLAP Tears

Superior labral tears in the throwing shoulder originally were described in 1985, when tensile failure at the biceps was postulated as the mechanism of injury, and the primary treatment was débridement.[22]

The genesis of the SLAP tear is still debated, but it can be a pain generator, create a sense of instability, and affect a thrower's speed and accuracy. Historically, SLAP tears were a very popular explanation for the disabled throwing shoulder in the 1990s and early 2000s. They were believed to occur because of the peel back mechanism in the internal impingement process. This peel back mechanism may be considered to be an adaptation to allow clearance of the posterior-superior labrum and the rotator cuff.

Over the years, we have learned that SLAP tears are difficult to diagnose because they have a low rate of interobserver agreement intraoperatively among surgeons as to what qualifies as a true SLAP tear.[26] Moreover, SLAP repairs have not been as effective in allowing return to play in pitchers as one would hope. Return to play among SLAP repairs is as low as 20% with revision surgery rates up to 40%.[27]

A biceps tenodesis is a surgical treatment alternative for SLAP tears that has gained popularity over the past few years. Its role in the overhead athlete is strongly debated because of the limited data and outcome studies.[28] Its role in the nonthrowing athlete appears to demonstrate good results; however, in the throwing athlete it is unclear as to the ideal treatment of choice.

Table 4

Studies of Rotator Cuff Pathology in Overhead Throwing Athletes

Study (Year)	Patient Description (Number)	Procedure	Outcomes
Reynolds et al[24] (2008)	Competitive baseball pitchers (82)	Débridement of partial-thickness rotator cuff tear	55% returned to previous level of play
Andrews et al[22] (1985)	Throwing athletes (36, including 23 baseball pitchers)	Débridement of partial-thickness articular-sided rotator cuff tear	85% of athletes returned to play; 76% returned to previous level of play
Conway[21] (2001)	Baseball players (9)	Repair of intratendinous rotator cuff tear	89% returned to same or higher level of play
Ferrari et al[23] (1994)	Competitive baseball pitchers (7)	Débridement of rotator cuff tear with or without labrum	85% returned to premorbid activity
Altintas et al[25] (2019)	Recreational and competitive athletes (499)	Rotator cuff repair	38% return to sport in overhead sports

There are limited studies on the management of SLAP with repair or biceps tenodesis in overhead throwing athletes (**Table 5**). An initial study reported a 100% rate of good to excellent results, with 87% of the athletes returning to the previous level of play, but these results were not reproduced in other studies.[29,36] A systematic review evaluated five studies that included baseball throwers and reported a return-to-play rate ranging from 22% to 64% after SLAP repair.[36]

In 2018, two separate studies were published from different authors evaluating the return to sport in baseball players after a biceps tenodesis[28] or SLAP repair.[32]These studies were retrospective and heterogenous in nature but may provide some insight as to proper treatment of the overhead athlete. In the biceps tenodesis study, the return to play was 35% with only 17% of pitchers returning and 80% of field players returning. In the SLAP repair study, there was a 62% rate of return to play with 59% of pitchers returning and 76% of nonpitchers. The biceps tenodesis study was on professional baseball players, whereas the SLAP repair study was on high school to professional players. These two studies, although not comparative, would be suggestive that overhead athletes may have a reasonable return to play with either of the two surgeries. However, pitchers may not fair so well with a biceps tenodesis and a SLAP repair should be considered for this subgroup.

With respect to the recreational overhead athlete, a 2018 study suggests that athletes in their thirties participating in recreational sports have a 100% return to sport with an 80% of overhead athletes returning to their previous level of play after undergoing subpectoral biceps tenodesis for isolated type II SLAP lesions.[35] This study was not comparative nor was it on high-level athletes, making it difficult to conclude this is an effective surgical treatment in young high-level athletes. However, in the recreational cohort, this appears to be a safe and effective treatment method.

In head-to-head comparison, there appears to be similar return to play with a diminished need for revision surgery among the biceps tenodesis studies comparatively to the SLAP repair studies. These comparisons are generated from systematic reviews and not randomized controlled trials.[27,37]

Anterior Capsular Instability

Anterior instability was found to be common in throwing athletes and contributed to internal impingement.[21,38]

Table 5

Studies of Superior Labrum Anterior to Posterior (SLAP) Tear Treatment in Overhead Throwing Athletes

Study (Year)	Patient Description (Number)	Procedure	Outcomes
Morgan et al[29] (1998)	Throwing athletes (102, including 37 baseball pitchers)	SLAP repair	87% returned to previous level of play
Kim et al[30] (2002)	Overhead athletes (18)	SLAP repair	Only 22% returned to previous level of play
Reinold et al[31] (2003)	Overhead athletes (130, including 105 baseball pitchers)	SLAP repair with thermal capsular shrinkage	87% returned to play; the results were better after thermal capsular shrinkage and repair than after repair alone
Ide et al[32] (2005)	Baseball pitchers (19)	SLAP repair	63% returned to previous level of play; the results were worse in pitchers than in other overhead athletes
Neuman et al[33] (2011)	Overhead athletes (30)	SLAP repair	84% returned to preinjury level of play; 93% satisfaction rate
Chalmers et al[28] (2018)	Professional baseball players (17)	Biceps tenodesis	17% return to play in pitchers; 80% return nonpitcher
Gilliam et al[34] (2018)	Baseball players (133)	SLAP repair	59% return to play in pitchers; 76% return nonpitcher
Pogorzelski et al[35] (2018)	Recreational athlete (20)	Biceps tenodesis	100% return to sport; 80% return to previous level in overhead athlete

Laxity continues to be a factor in the disabled throwing shoulder and recently has been implicated as a potential source of vascular compromise.[39] When the effects of throwing on upper extremity arterial blood flow were measured before and after a 50-pitch workout, professional pitchers with laxity had only a 35% increase in blood flow, compared with a 115% increase in pitchers without signs of laxity.

Anterior instability certainly has a spectrum of underlying pathologies, and careful preoperative planning should be used in preparation for surgical repair. With respect to arthroscopic stabilization, a 2019 study out of Korea demonstrated an 80% return to play in professional/elite baseball players and a 57% solid return to play in pitchers following arthroscopic Bankart repair. On average, the recovery process was 7 to 9 months depending on position played.[40]

Posterior Instability

Posterior instability is a well-established pathologic injury in the athletic population leading to pain and diminished performance on the playing field. Unfortunately, there is a paucity of literature for return to play following posterior labral repairs in the athletic population. The literature is suggestive of a high return to play, but the evidence is weak.[41]

One case-matched series among athletes comparing throwers and nonthrowers demonstrated a similar return to play, functional outcomes, and range of motion at long-term follow-up (average 37 months). Pitchers had a poorer return to play as opposed to other throwing athletes. This particular series used heterogenous surgical techniques for the repair. Anchored repairs tended to have a higher rate of return as opposed to all suture plication.[42]

Posterior labral repairs among baseball players have demonstrated a 94% rate of return to play (61% previous level of play) with 2-year follow-up. Again, pitchers had a diminished rate of return (41%) as opposed to the position player (86%). This particular series looked at posterior-superior (32%), 180° posterior (35%), and posterior-inferior (32%) labral repair. Tear size and location did not affect outcomes or return-to-play rates.[43]

Scapular Dyskinesis

As understanding of the mechanics in the shoulder has evolved, glenoid positioning has become an important consideration when evaluating shoulder pain in the throwing athlete. The concept of scapular dyskinesis has been studied clinically and found to play a role in patients with impingement and anterior instability.[44] The term SICK scapula refers to the phenomenon of *s*capular malposition, *i*nferior medial border prominence, *c*oracoid pain and malposition, and dys*k*inesis of scapular movement.[17] Scapular dyskinesis probably results from periscapular muscular imbalance, fatigue, or nerve injury, and several studies have implicated muscular deficits as a risk factor for scapular dyskinesis in the disabled throwing shoulder. Adolescent pitchers with a history of throwing-related pain were found to have a weaker middle trapezius and supraspinatus than their counterparts who did not have pain.[45] Another study found a similar pattern in professional pitchers. Pitchers with preseason weakness of the external rotators and the supraspinatus had a higher risk of in-season throwing-related injury requiring surgical intervention than pitchers without preseason weakness.[46] Pitching itself may contribute to the weakness. A decrease in volitional strength of the external rotators in pitchers was found when a single-performance fatigue model was used.[47] The study concluded that rehabilitation strategies to prevent fatigue and enhance neuromuscular activation may prevent injury in throwing athletes.

Rehabilitation

The postoperative program must be tailored to the surgical procedure for the throwing shoulder. Communication between the surgeon and the physical therapist/athletic trainer is of paramount importance to ensure the soft tissue is protected during early motion and reengagement of muscular rhythm and strength. The athlete's maintenance core-strengthening program should continue unaffected by the surgery. Scapular platform retraining should begin immediately and should include a program of scapular protraction-retraction, elevation-depression, and inward-outward rotation. Table slides are safe and effective in restoring early range of motion and engaging periscapular muscles without damaging the surgical repair.

If the surgical correction did not include repair, the patient is encouraged to move the arm back to full range of active and passive motion as quickly as possible. The motion is supervised to ensure proper stabilization of the scapular musculature. After early motion in the correct rhythm is obtained, the progression of load is started. The objective is to restore the link between the central core and the scapular platform. The progression begins with low resistance at low speed with a stable uniplanar platform. This continues to higher and faster loads in multiple planes that eventually simulate the sport-specific environment. Care should be taken as to not become overly aggressive to resistance training before the restoration of motion. If the shoulder lacks full range of motion, resistance exercises may have a detrimental effect on the recovery process. Once the resistance phase ensues, endurance must not be neglected because fatigue can lead to poor mechanics and is detrimental to return to sport.

When the athlete has regained a solid core, a full range of motion, functional strength, and proper scapular rhythm, a return-to-throwing program is started under the supervision of the athletic training staff. Initially, the athlete must demonstrate the ability to simulate a pitch at slow speed as well as attainment of the proper functional range of motion, core strength, and scapular stability.

The return-to-throwing program embodies the same principles of progression as the earlier phases. Throwing is started at slow speeds with a light ball tossed for short distances. Any deficits in throwing mechanics halt the progression. As the athlete progresses, distance, speed, and the number of repetitions are increased until the ability to perform specific sport mechanics is regained. At this point, the number of repetitions is increased until the athlete is ready to return to competition. This program must be individualized, any labral or rotator cuff repair must be protected until healed, and the necessary restrictions must be accommodated.

SUMMARY

The throwing shoulder remains a therapeutic challenge. Multiple pathologies commonly occur, including labral and rotator cuff tears, pathologic laxity, and posterior capsular tightness. Nonsurgical management is effective for most patients. When surgical treatment is necessary, the surgeon must take care to distinguish between an anatomic adaptation and a pathologic condition. Return to throwing is not accomplished in the operating room alone. It requires a dedicated team to place the repaired shoulder within a properly rehabilitated kinetic chain that can withstand the extreme demands inherent to the throwing shoulder. Return to play in the overhead athlete appears to have a high rate of return to preinjury level following surgical repair. However, pitching in the high-level athlete appears to be a risk factor for a low rate of return with surgical intervention.

KEY STUDY POINTS

- Glenohumeral internal rotational deficit (GIRD) is an adaptive process that predisposes the overhead athlete to the development of pathology. The sleeper stretch is designed to prevent the development of these injuries.
- Rotator cuff repairs have less than favorable results compared with débridement. Full-thickness tears may be a devastating injury to the throwing athlete.
- Internal impingement involves a multifaceted development of partial-thickness rotator cuff tears, posterior-superior labral pathology, and biceps irritation.
- In SLAP tears, biceps tenodesis may be a good alternative to SLAP repair with less need for revision in the nonpitcher.
- Pitching is a risk factor for a low rate of return to play.

Annotated References

1. Andrews JR, Wilk KE: *The Athlete's Shoulder.* New York, NY, Churchill Livingstone, 1994, 748 pp.

2. Burkhart SS, Morgan CD, Kibler WB: The disabled throwing shoulder: Spectrum of pathology. Part I: Pathoanatomy and biomechanics. *Arthroscopy* 2003;19(4):404-420.

3. Schar MO, Dellenbach S, Pfirrmann CW, Raniga S, Jost B, Zumstein MA: Many shoulder MRI findings in elite professional throwing athletes resolve after retirement: A clinical and radiographic study. *Clin Orthop Relat Res* 2018;476(3):620-631.

   A cohort of professional European handball players were identified with bilateral MRI findings during their career. 30 players were identified and 20 wished to participate. Of the 20 players, the throwing shoulder demonstrated 95% (19/20) identification of a diagnosable MRI findings and the nonthrowing shoulder demonstrated a rate of 85% (17/20). Findings included partial-thickness rotator cuff tears, ganglion cysts, and bone cysts. The data suggest that findings of the throwing shoulder such as partial rotator cuff tears, bony cysts, and ganglions do not progress after retirement, and sometimes they resolve. Because of this and because many MRI changes correlate poorly with clinical symptoms, the indication for surgical treatment of these findings should be questioned very carefully. Level of evidence: II.

4. Fleisig GS, Andrews JR, Dillman CJ, Escamilla RF: Kinetics of baseball pitching with implications about injury mechanisms. *Am J Sports Med* 1995;23(2):233-239.

5. Kuhn JE, Lindholm SR, Huston LJ, Soslowsky LJ, Blasier RB: Failure of the biceps superior labral complex: A cadaveric biomechanical investigation comparing the late cocking and early deceleration positions of throwing. *Arthroscopy* 2003;19(4):373-379.

6. Davis JT, Limpisvasti O, Fluhme D, et al: The effect of pitching biomechanics on the upper extremity in youth and adolescent baseball pitchers. *Am J Sports Med* 2009;37(8):1484-1491.

7. Bennett GE: Elbow and shoulder lesions of baseball players. *Am J Surg* 1959;98:484-492.

8. Park JY, Noh YM, Chung SW, et al: Bennett lesions in baseball players detected by magnetic resonance imaging: Assessment of association factors. *J Shoulder Elbow Surg* 2016;25(5):730-738.

   Baseball players with and without Bennett lesions were compared. 388 players were evaluated, and 32.2% (125) of players were identified with Bennett lesions. No significant differences were idenitified among players with respect to demographics, functional outcome scores, physical examination findings, or concomitant diseases. However, players with Bennett lesions had played longer ($P < 0.001$)

Section 2: Instability and Athletic Injuries

compared with those who did not demonstrate this finding. Length of play was thought to be a significant factor in the development of a Bennett lesion. Level of evidence: III.

9. Yoneda M, Nakagawa S, Hayashida K, Fukushima S, Wakitani S: Arthroscopic removal of symptomatic Bennett lesions in the shoulders of baseball players: Arthroscopic Bennett-plasty. *Am J Sports Med* 2002;30(5):728-736.

10. Thomas SJ, Swanik CB, Higginson JS, et al: A bilateral comparison of posterior capsule thickness and its correlation with glenohumeral range of motion and scapular upward rotation in collegiate baseball players. *J Shoulder Elbow Surg* 2011;20(5):708-716.

11. Wilk KE, Macrina LC, Fleisig GS, et al: Correlation of glenohumeral internal rotation deficit and total rotational motion to shoulder injuries in professional baseball pitchers. *Am J Sports Med* 2011;39(2):329-335.

12. Tokish JM, Curtin MS, Kim YK, Hawkins RJ, Torry MR: Glenohumeral internal rotation deficit in the asymptomatic professional pitcher and its relationship to humeral retroversion. *J Sports Sci Med* 2008;7(1):78-83.

13. Walch G, Boileau P, Noel E, Donell ST: Impingement of the deep surface of the supraspinatus tendon on the posterosuperior glenoid rim: An arthroscopic study. *J Shoulder Elbow Surg* 1992;1(5):238-245.

14. Myers JB, Laudner KG, Pasquale MR, Bradley JP, Lephart SM: Glenohumeral range of motion deficits and posterior shoulder tightness in throwers with pathologic internal impingement. *Am J Sports Med* 2006;34(3): 385-391.

15. Meister K, Buckley B, Batts J: The posterior impingement sign: Diagnosis of rotator cuff and posterior labral tears secondary to internal impingement in overhand athletes. *Am J Orthop (Belle Mead NJ)* 2004;33(8): 412-415.

16. Ishigaki T, Ishida T, Samukawa M: Does restriction of glenohumeral horizontal adduction reflect posterior capsule thickening of the throwing shoulder? *J Phys Ther Sci* 2015;27(5):1299-1302.

    Posterior capsular thickness was measured (via ultrasonography) in 39 collegiate baseball players. There was no correlation between posterior capsular thickness and horizontal adduction but capsular thickness did correlate to internal rotation range of motion. This study concluded that posterior capsular thickening relates to internal rotation and restricted horizontal adduction may reflect tightening of other tissues such as the posterior deltoid. Level of evidence: IV.

17. Burkhart SS, Morgan CD, Kibler WB: The disabled throwing shoulder: Spectrum of pathology. Part III: The SICK scapula, scapular dyskinesis, the kinetic chain, and rehabilitation. *Arthroscopy* 2003;19(6): 641-661.

18. Lintner D, Mayol M, Uzodinma O, Jones R, Labossiere D: Glenohumeral internal rotation deficits in professional pitchers enrolled in an internal rotation stretching program. *Am J Sports Med* 2007;35(4):617-621.

19. Yoneda M, Nakagawa S, Mizuno N, et al: Arthroscopic capsular release for painful throwing shoulder with posterior capsular tightness. *Arthroscopy* 2006;22(7): 801.e1-801.e5.

20. Jobe CM: Posterior superior glenoid impingement: Expanded spectrum. *Arthroscopy* 1995;11(5):530-536.

21. Conway JE: Arthroscopic repair of partial-thickness rotator cuff tears and SLAP lesions in professional baseball players. *Orthop Clin North Am* 2001;32(3):443-456.

22. Andrews JR, Broussard TS, Carson WG: Arthroscopy of the shoulder in the management of partial tears of the rotator cuff: A preliminary report. *Arthroscopy* 1985;1(2):117-122.

23. Ferrari JD, Ferrari DA, Coumas J, Pappas AM: Posterior ossification of the shoulder: The Bennett lesion. Etiology, diagnosis, and treatment. *Am J Sports Med* 1994;22(2):171-175; discussion 175-176.

24. Reynolds SB, Dugas JR, Cain EL, McMichael CS, Andrews JR: Debridement of small partial-thickness rotator cuff tears in elite overhead throwers. *Clin Orthop Relat Res* 2008;466(3):614-621.

25. Altintas B, Anderson N, Dornan GJ, Boykin RE, Logan C, Millett PJ: Return to sport after arthroscopic rotator cuff repair: Is there a difference between the recreational and the competitive athlete? *Am J Sports Med* 2019;48(1):252-261.

    A systematic review (15 studies; 499 shoulders) was set out to determine the rate of return to sport after rotator cuff tear. Of the 347 athletes identified in this study, 45 were baseball players. Rate of return to similar level of play was 70.2% with 61.5% of competitive athletes returned. Subgroup analysis of 43 baseball/softball players yielded only a 38% return to previous level of play. Level of evidence: III.

26. Gobezie R, Zurakowski D, Lavery K, Millett PJ, Cole BJ, Warner JJ: Analysis of interobserver and intraobserver variability in the diagnosis and treatment of SLAP tears using the Snyder classification. *Am J Sports Med* 2008;36(7):1373-1379.

27. de Sa D, Arakgi ME, Lian J, Crum RJ, Lin A, Lesniak BP: Labral repair versus biceps tenodesis for primary surgical management of type II superior labrum anterior to posterior tears: A systematic review. *Arthroscopy* 2019;35(6):1927-1938.

    A systematic review (23 studies) evaluated SLAP repair versus biceps tenodesis for the index treatment of type II SLAP tears. A total of 781 patients had a SLAP repair with an average age of 35 years and mean follow-up of

35 months. The biceps tenodesis group had 100 patients with an average age of 44 years with 32 months follow-up. Functional outcome scores were similar for both groups. Rate of return to sport in the SLAP repair group ranged from 20% to 95% versus the biceps tenodesis group ranging from 73% to 100%. The reoperation rate for a SLAP tear ranged from 3% to 40% whereas that of the biceps tenodesis group was zero to 15%. This review demonstrated that biceps tenodesis may be an effective alternative to SLAP repair. Level of evidence: IV.

28. Chalmers PN, Erickson BJ, Verma NN, D'Angelo J, Romeo AA: Incidence and return to play after biceps tenodesis in professional baseball players. *Arthroscopy* 2018;34(3):747-751.

    The return to play (RTP) in professional baseball players (*n* = 17; 12 pitchers) with a minimum of 2 years follow-up after a biceps tenodesis was 35%. Isolated biceps tenodesis demonstrated an RTP of 44%. Pitchers faired worse with an RTP of 17% versus the position player with a rate of 80%. Level of evidence: IV.

29. Morgan CD, Burkhart SS, Palmeri M, Gillespie M: Type II SLAP lesions: Three subtypes and their relationships to superior instability and rotator cuff tears. *Arthroscopy* 1998;14(6):553-565.

30. Kim SH, Ha KI, Kim SH, Choi HJ: Results of arthroscopic treatment of superior labral lesions. *J Bone Joint Surg Am* 2002;84(6):981-985.

31. Reinold MM, Wilk KE, Hooks TR, Dugas JR, Andrews JR: Thermal-assisted capsular shrinkage of the glenohumeral joint in overhead athletes: A 15- to 47-month follow-up. *J Orthop Sports Phys Ther* 2003;33(8):455-467.

32. Ide J, Maeda S, Takagi K: Sports activity after arthroscopic superior labral repair using suture anchors in overhead-throwing athletes. *Am J Sports Med* 2005;33(4):507-514.

33. Neuman BJ, Boisvert CB, Reiter B, Lawson K, Ciccotti MG, Cohen SB: Results of arthroscopic repair of type II superior labral anterior posterior lesions in overhead athletes: Assessment of return to preinjury playing level and satisfaction. *Am J Sports Med* 2011;39(9):1883-1888.

34. Gilliam BD, Douglas L, Fleisig GS, et al: Return to play and outcomes in baseball players after superior labral anterior-posterior repairs. *Am J Sports Med* 2018;46(1):109-115.

    A total of 216 baseball players were identified who had a SLAP repair with or without a partial-thickness rotator cuff débridement. After calling these patients 2 years after surgery, 133 responded to the survey. There was an overall rate of return to play (RTP) of 62%. There were no differences in RTP based on procedure. Pitchers' RTP was 59% compared with 76% in nonpitchers. The authors concluded that SLAP repair should continue to be an option for SLAP tears after conservative treatment measures failed. Level of evidence: IV.

35. Pogorzelski J, Horan MP, Hussain ZB, Vap A, Fritz EM, Millett PJ: Subpectoral biceps tenodesis for treatment of isolated type II SLAP lesions in a young and active population. *Arthroscopy* 2018;34(2):371-376.

    Patients (*n* = 20) with an average age of 38 years with isolated type II SLAP tears had a subpectoral biceps tenodesis. Functional outcome scores were obtained 2 years following the surgery in 16/20 patients. There was significant improvement in functional outcomes (ASES, 66-94 points, *P* = 0.001; QuickDASH, 31-8, *P* = 0.003; SANE, 60-92, *P* = 0.001, SF-12 PCS, 41-52 points, *P* = 0.002), patient satisfaction, and a rate of return to sport of 100% (73% rate of previous level of play). Subgroup analysis demonstrated a rate of 80% previous level of play in overhead atheletes. Level of evidence: IV.

36. Gorantla K, Gill C, Wright RW: The outcome of type II SLAP repair: A systematic review. *Arthroscopy* 2010;26(4):537-545.

37. Abdul-Rassoul H, Defazio M, Curry EJ, Galvin JW, Li X: Return to sport after the surgical treatment of superior labrum anterior to posterior tears: A systematic review. *Orthop J Sports Med* 2019;7(5):2325967119841892.

    A systematic review evaluated the return to sport (RTS) following arthroscopic SLAP repair versus biceps tenodesis. A total of 501 patient-atheletes were evaluated (195 isolated SLAP repair, 222 SLAP repair with rotator cuff débridement, 84 biceps tenodesis). The tenodesis group had an older patient population (mean age 42 years) compared with the isolated SLAP repair (31 years) and the SLAP repair with rotator cuff débridement (22 years). The overall RTS was high in all groups. Biceps tenodesis demonstrated the highest rate of RTS (84.5%) as well as return to preinjury level (78.6%). All surgical treatment options appear to demonstrate an acceptable rate of return, with biceps tenodesis having a slightly higher rate of return in this heterogenous patient-athlete systematic review. Level of evidence: IV.

38. Paley KJ, Jobe FW, Pink MM, Kvitne RS, ElAttrache NS: Arthroscopic findings in the overhand throwing athlete: Evidence for posterior internal impingement of the rotator cuff. *Arthroscopy* 2000;16(1):35-40.

39. Bast SC, Weaver FA, Perese S, Jobe FW, Weaver DC, Vangsness CT Jr: The effects of shoulder laxity on upper extremity blood flow in professional baseball pitchers. *J Shoulder Elbow Surg* 2011;20(3):461-466.

40. Park JY, Lee JH, Oh KS, Chung SW, Lim JJ, Noh YM: Return to play after arthroscopic treatment for shoulder instability in elite and professional baseball players. *J Shoulder Elbow Surg* 2019;28(1):77-81.

    Outcomes among elite and professional baseball players (*n* = 51) were evaluated following arthroscopic Bankart repair. With a follow-up of greater than 2 years, the rate of return to play (RTP) was 82% and solid return to play (sRTP) was 80%. Pitchers appeared to have more difficulty returning with a rate of RTP of 64% and sRTP of

57% compared with catchers (RTP 83%; sRTP 83%) and in-fielders (90% RTP; sRTP 90%). It took on average 8.4 months to RTP after surgery (pitchers took longer). Level of evidence: IV.

41. DeLong JM, Jiang K, Bradley JP: Posterior instability of the shoulder: A systematic review and meta-analysis of clinical outcomes. *Am J Sports Med* 2015;43(7):1805-1817.

    This systematic review evaluated the treatment of posterior instability revealing 53 total articles (27 arthroscopic; 26 open) demonstrating a lack of well-defined outcome measures. Arthroscopic treatment appears to be effective and reliable for unidirectional posterior instability. Throwing athletes appear to be less likely to return to previous level of play following posterior labral repair compared with other athlete subtypes. The use of suture anchors appears to be more effective than that of anchorless repairs. Arthroscopy appears to be superior to open procedures with respect to stability, patient satisfaction, and return to sport. Level of evidence: III.

42. McClincy MP, Arner JW, Bradley JP: Posterior shoulder instability in throwing athletes: A case-matched comparison of throwers and non-throwers. *Arthroscopy* 2015;31(6):1041-1051.

    Overhead athletes (n = 48) were compared with nonthrowing athletes (n = 48) after undergoing an arthroscopic posterior capsulolabral repair. With a mean follow-up of 37 months, no differences were noted with respect to ASES scores, stability, strength, and range of motion between the two groups. Discrete tears and the use of suture anchors were positive predictors of return to play in the throwing athlete (this finding showed no difference in the nonthrower). Pitchers' outcome scores were equivocal when compared with those of other throwing athletes, but they had a lower rate of return to play (50% versus 60%). The authors concluded that the use of suture anchors gives this patient population the best chance for a return to competitive sport. Level of evidence: III.

43. Kercher JS, Runner RP, McCarthy TP, Duralde XA: Posterior labral repairs of the shoulder among baseball players: Results and outcomes with minimum 2-year follow-up. *Am J Sports Med* 2019;47(7):1687-1693.

    Baseball players (n = 32) were evaluated following posterior labral repairs with a minimum 2-year follow-up. Three different tear patterns were identified (32% posterior superior, 35% 180° posterior, 32% posterior-inferior). The most common complaint was pain (78%) and less instability (19%). Functional outcome (ASES score) assessment demonstrated significant improvement with no difference in preoperative and postoperative range of motion. Tear size and number of anchors did not play a role in outcome. There was an overall return to play of 94% with 61% returning to previous level of play. Pitchers struggled to return to previous level (41%) compared with other position players (86%). Level of evidence: III.

44. Warner JJ, Micheli LJ, Arslanian LE, Kennedy J, Kennedy R: Scapulothoracic motion in normal shoulders and shoulders with glenohumeral instability and impingement syndrome. A study using Moiré topographic analysis. *Clin Orthop Relat Res* 1992;(285):191-199.

45. Trakis JE, McHugh MP, Caracciolo PA, Busciacco L, Mullaney M, Nicholas SJ: Muscle strength and range of motion in adolescent pitchers with throwing-related pain: Implications for injury prevention. *Am J Sports Med* 2008;36(11):2173-2178.

46. Byram IR, Bushnell BD, Dugger K, Charron K, Harrell FE Jr, Noonan TJ: Preseason shoulder strength measurements in professional baseball pitchers: Identifying players at risk for injury. *Am J Sports Med* 2010;38(7):1375-1382.

47. Gandhi J, ElAttrache NS, Kaufman KR, Hurd WJ: Voluntary activation deficits of the infraspinatus present as a consequence of pitching-induced fatigue. *J Shoulder Elbow Surg* 2012;21(5):625-630.

Section 3

The Rotator Cuff

Section Editor:

Sumant "Butch" Krishnan, MD

Chapter 11

Anatomy, Pathogenesis, Natural History, and Nonsurgical Management of Rotator Cuff Disorders

Keisuke Matsuki, MD • Hiroyuki Sugaya, MD

ABSTRACT

It is essential to understand the anatomy and function of the shoulder in management of rotator cuff diseases, including rotator cuff tears and tendinitis. A detailed clinical history, imaging studies, and physical examination including assessment of range of motion, posture, and scapular position help to understand patients' pathology. Asymptomatic rotator cuff tears become symptomatic at a certain rate, and the size of tear increases over time in most shoulders. There is no consensus on the best treatment for a rotator cuff tear. Pain management has an important role in nonsurgical management, and injection therapy is commonly used. There is no evidence to suggest a benefit of steroid over local anesthesia injections in the management of rotator cuff–related pain. Subacromial platelet-rich plasma injections can be an alternative to corticosteroid injections, especially in patients with contraindication to corticosteroid administration. Physiotherapy can also be effective treatment for rotator cuff diseases; however, there are no definite indications and protocols. Management options, physiotherapy or surgical management, should be chosen individually with each patient considering various factors such as patient demographics and tear configuration.

Keywords: anatomy; natural history; nonsurgical management; pathogenesis; rotator cuff disorder

Introduction

The term rotator cuff disease includes partial-thickness and full-thickness rotator cuff tears as well as tendinitis. It is not easy to determine whether a rotator cuff disorder itself is responsible for a patient's shoulder pain and disability. MRI and ultrasonography often show an anatomic disorder of the rotator cuff in patients older than 65 to 70 years. Some patients who report shoulder pain have no evidence of an anatomic rotator cuff disorder, and others have no symptoms despite the presence of a rotator cuff tear on imaging studies.[1] The presence or the absence of shoulder symptoms appears to be affected by physiologic and psychologic factors; for example, it is generally believed that the surgical outcomes of patients with a workers' compensation claim tend to be inferior to those of other patients.[2,3]

Surgeons must assess functional as well as anatomic factors. Rotator cuff function, scapular position and mobility, posture, spine mobility and pelvic inclination, and lower extremity function are among the factors that affect shoulder symptoms. The susceptibility of the shoulder to functional disorders is largely attributable to unique features of the shoulder girdle. The rotator cuff connects the scapula and the humeral head as well as the capsule and the biceps tendon. The scapula and upper extremities form a unit that is connected to the trunk and the clavicle only by the acromioclavicular and sternoclavicular joints. In other words, most of the structures connecting the scapula and upper extremity unit to the trunk are periscapular muscles. Scapula position is greatly affected by posture and lower extremity function, and incorrect posture restricts scapular mobility. A functionally deteriorated scapula can easily cause symptoms around the shoulder girdle.[4] Correcting morbid scapulothoracic function is the first-choice nonsurgical management of a patient with shoulder symptoms.[5]

Anatomy of the Rotator Cuff

The anatomy of the shoulder girdle is relatively complex. The scapula is connected to the trunk anteriorly by the serratus anterior and the pectoralis minor and posteriorly by the upper and lower trapezius, rhomboids, levator scapulae, and latissimus dorsi. The muscular tone and flexibility of these structures greatly affect scapular function.[4] The deltoid muscle encases the shoulder. The deltoid originates anteriorly from the medial half of the clavicle and the anterolateral aspect of the acromion, continues posteriorly along the scapular spine, and inserts distally

Dr. Matsuki or an immediate family member has received research or institutional support from Arthrex, Inc. and Exactech, Inc. Dr. Sugaya or an immediate family member is a member of a speakers' bureau or has made paid presentations on behalf of Mitek, Smith & Nephew, and Wright Medical Technology, Inc. and serves as an unpaid consultant to Biomet, Mitek, and Smith & Nephew.

into the proximal third of the humerus at the deltoid tubercle. Thus, the deltoid is the main source of power for shoulder abduction, with the help of rotator cuff function.

Supraspinatus and Infraspinatus

The rotator cuff is formed by the tendinous insertions of the subscapularis, the supraspinatus, the infraspinatus, and the teres minor. The traditional understanding is that the supraspinatus muscle originates from the suprascapular fossa and inserts onto the superior facet of the greater tuberosity, and the infraspinatus muscle originates from the scapular fossa and inserts onto the posterior aspect of the humeral head at the middle facet of the greater tuberosity.[6,7] However, anatomic studies by shoulder surgeons and anatomists have revealed that the supraspinatus inserts onto the limited anteriormost portion of the superior facet and even onto the lesser tuberosity and that the infraspinatus inserts onto the middle facet and almost half of the superior facet[8,9] (**Figure 1**). These studies found that the infraspinatus is divided into two parts: the oblique fibers, which originate from the scapular fossa and insert on the middle and superior facet of the greater tuberosity; and the transverse fibers, which originate from the inferior aspect of the scapula spine and insert onto the tendinous portion of the oblique fibers[10] (**Figure 2**). The glenohumeral capsular insertion has a broad footprint, especially at the tendinous insertion between the infraspinatus and the teres minor[11] (**Figure 3**). Presumably, this thick capsule can function as a tendon along with the tendinous insertion of the infraspinatus and the teres minor, and it may be related to the delamination that is frequently observed during surgery for a large or massive rotator cuff tear.[11]

Subscapularis

The subscapularis is the only anteriorly located rotator cuff muscle, and it has the greatest muscular volume. The development of arthroscopic technology has allowed the importance of subscapularis tendon tears to be recognized. Their prevalence appears to be much greater than earlier reports indicated.[12-14]

Several intramuscular tendons can be observed in the subscapularis muscle. The most cranial tendinous portion was found to be longer and thicker than any other tendinous structure inside the subscapularis.[12] The most proximal insertion of the subscapularis tendon was found to be derived from this long, thick intramuscular tendinous portion. The insertion of this portion was widely located on the most proximal upper limit of the lesser tuberosity. The remainder of the subscapularis tendon inserted onto the anteromedial portion of the lesser tuberosity. The insertion of the subscapularis muscle became narrower in the more distal portion, where the muscle fibers came close to the humeral bone and tendon tissue was very short (**Figure 4**). The most proximal insertion of the subscapularis tendon extended as a thin tendinous slip that attached to the fovea capitis of the humerus. The primary function of this tendinous slip was described as providing a greater insertion area for the subscapularis tendon and the smooth floor of the bicipital groove to stabilize the long head of the biceps tendon and prevent it from dislocating[15] (**Figure 5**). The most cranial part of the tendon insertion was described as the strongest and the clinically most important, and it has the broadest footprint, along with the tendinous slip.[15]

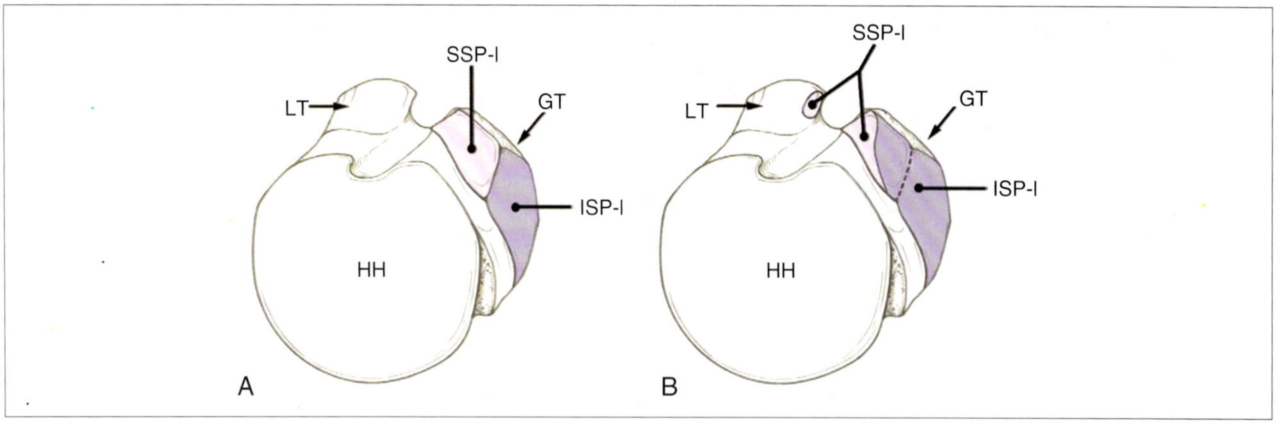

FIGURE 1 Schematic drawings of the superior aspect of the right humerus showing the humeral insertions of the supraspinatus and the infraspinatus. **A**, The generally accepted belief is that the supraspinatus inserts into the highest impression of the greater tuberosity, and the infraspinatus inserts into the middle impression. **B**, Recent research indicates that the insertion area of the infraspinatus occupies approximately half of the highest and all of the middle impression of the greater tuberosity. The insertion area of the supraspinatus is in the anteromedial region of the highest impression and sometimes in the superiormost area on the lesser tuberosity. GT = greater tuberosity, HH = humeral head, ISP-I = insertion area of the infraspinatus, LT = lesser tuberosity, SSP-I = insertion area of the supraspinatus. (Reproduced with permission from Mochizuki T, Sugaya H, Uomizu M, et al: Humeral insertion of the supraspinatus and infraspinatus: New anatomical findings regarding the footprint of the rotator cuff. *J Bone Joint Surg Am* 2008;90[5]:962-969. doi:10.2106/JBJS.G.00427.)

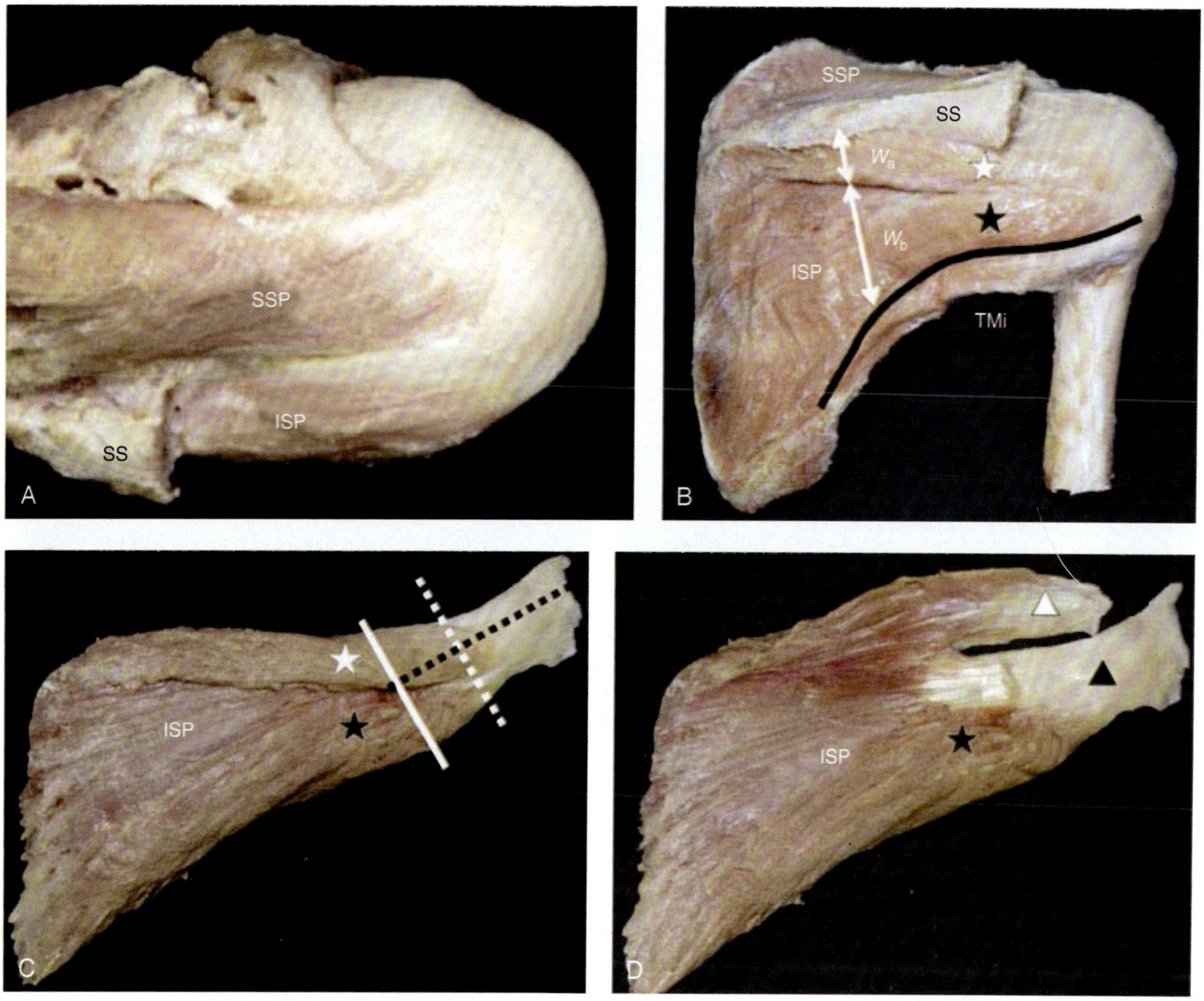

FIGURE 2 Photographs showing the muscular and tendinous geometry of the supraspinatus and the infraspinatus. **A**, The superior aspect of a right shoulder, showing the myotendinous unit of the supraspinatus and the infraspinatus. **B**, The dorsal aspect of a right shoulder, showing the myotendinous unit of the infraspinatus, composed of a transverse part (white star) and an oblique part (black star). The border between the infraspinatus and the teres minor is shown (black line). **C**, The dorsal aspect of the infraspinatus separated from the scapula and the greater tuberosity of the humerus. The transverse (white star) and oblique (black star) parts can easily be seen. Longitudinal (black line) and transverse histologic sections (white lines) are shown. **D**, The dorsal aspect of the infraspinatus muscle, showing the separation of the transverse part (black star) from the oblique part. The transverse part has a long, thick tendinous portion (black triangle) attached to the greater tuberosity. The transverse part has a thin and short tendinous membrane (white triangle) attached only to the tendinous portion of the oblique part and not reaching the tuberosity. ISP = infraspinatus, SS = scapular spine, SSP = supraspinatus, TMi = teres minor, W_a = width of the transverse part at the midpoint of the scapula spine, W_b = width of the oblique part at the midpoint of the scapula spine. (Reprinted by permission from Springer: *Surg Radiol Anat* 34[3]. Kato A, Nimura A, Yamaguchi K, et al: An anatomical study of the transverse part of the infraspinatus muscle that is closely related with the supraspinatus muscle,257-265. Copyright 2012. doi:10.1007/s00276-011-0872-0.)

Some of the intratendinous fibers from the supraspinatus were found to insert onto the lesser tuberosity beyond the long head of the biceps tendon, and these fibers reinforce the most cranial insertion of the subscapularis from above the long head of the biceps tendon.[8,9] The fibers that insert into the lesser tuberosity can be strongly related to the comma sign, which is an important landmark in full-thickness anterosuperior rotator cuff tears.[16] During surgery, footprint reconstruction repair is strongly recommended to increase the initial fixation strength, especially in the cranial portion of a subscapularis tear.

Teres Minor

The teres minor has a smaller volume than the other rotator cuff muscles, and it inserts immediately inferior to the infraspinatus insertion at the greater tuberosity[11] (**Figure 3**). The tendinous insertion of the teres minor

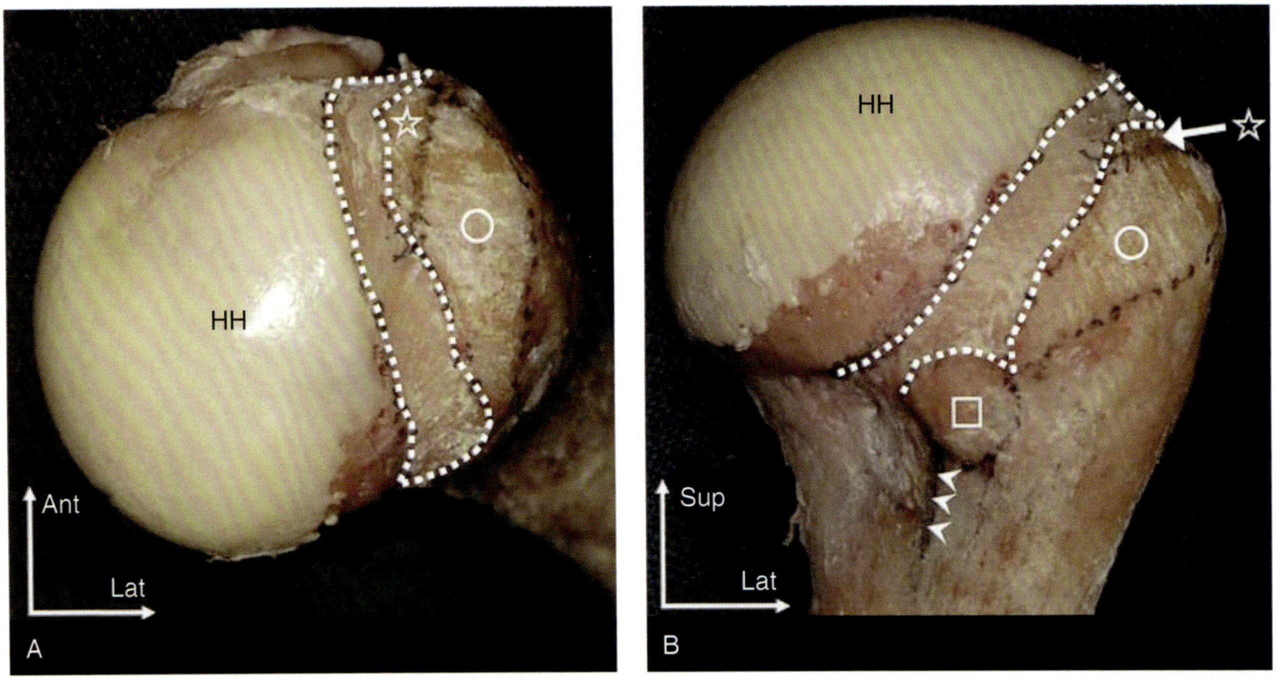

FIGURE 3 Photographs of the superior (**A**) and posterior (**B**) aspects of the humerus, showing the attachment area of the articular capsule (white dashed line). Also shown are the insertion areas of the supraspinatus (star) and infraspinatus (circle) and the tendinous portion (square) and muscular portion of the teres minor (arrowheads). Ant = anterior, HH = humeral head, Lat = lateral, Sup = superior. (Reprinted from *J Shoulder Elbow Surg* 21[7]. Nimura A, Kato A, Yamaguchi K, et al: The superior capsule of the shoulder joint complements the insertion of the rotator cuff, 867-872. Copyright © 2012 Journal of Shoulder and Elbow Surgery Board of Trustees. doi:10.1016/j.jse.2011.04.034.)

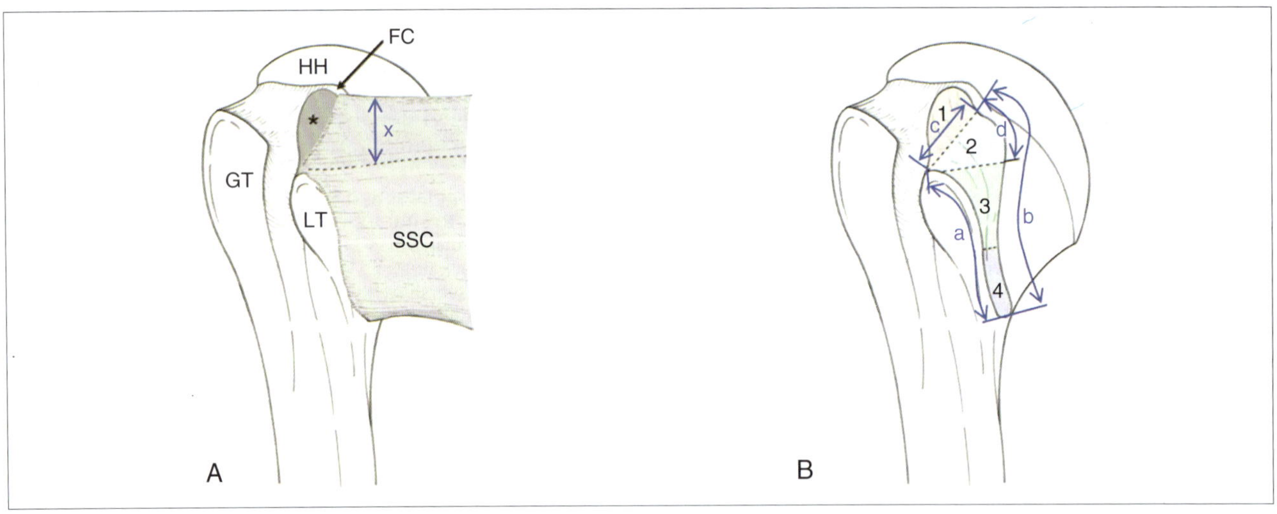

FIGURE 4 Schematic drawings showing the insertion and the footprint of the subscapularis in a right shoulder. **A**, The superiormost part of the intramuscular tendons is inserted into the uppermost margin of the lesser tuberosity, and the remainder of the subscapularis tendon is inserted into the anteromedial portion of the lesser tuberosity. The superiormost insertion—the lateral portion of the cranial part of the intramuscular tendons—and the tendinous slip make up a structure that is in direct contact with the inferior side of the long head of the biceps tendon at its corner portion. The longitudinal diameter (*x*) of the cranial part of intramuscular tendons was found to be long enough to decrease the curvature of the biceps tendon. **B**, The subscapularis footprint is made up of the attaching area of the tendinous slip (1), insertion of the superiormost part of the intramuscular tendon (2), another tendinous insertion (3), and muscular insertion (4). The dimensions of the subscapularis footprint were defined in terms of the lateral margin (a), the medial margin (b), the superiormost lateral margin (c), and the superiormost medial margin (d). The superiormost lateral margin (c) is long enough to support the biceps tendon. FC = fovea capitis of the humerus, GT = greater tuberosity, HH = humeral head, LT = lesser tuberosity, SSC = subscapularis muscle. (Reprinted from *Arthroscopy* 24[9]. Arai R, Sugaya H, Mochizuki T, Nimura A, Moriishi J, Akita K: Subscapularis tendon tear: An anatomic and clinical investigation, 997-1004. Copyright © 2008 Arthroscopy Association of North America. doi:10.1016/j.arthro.2008.04.076.)

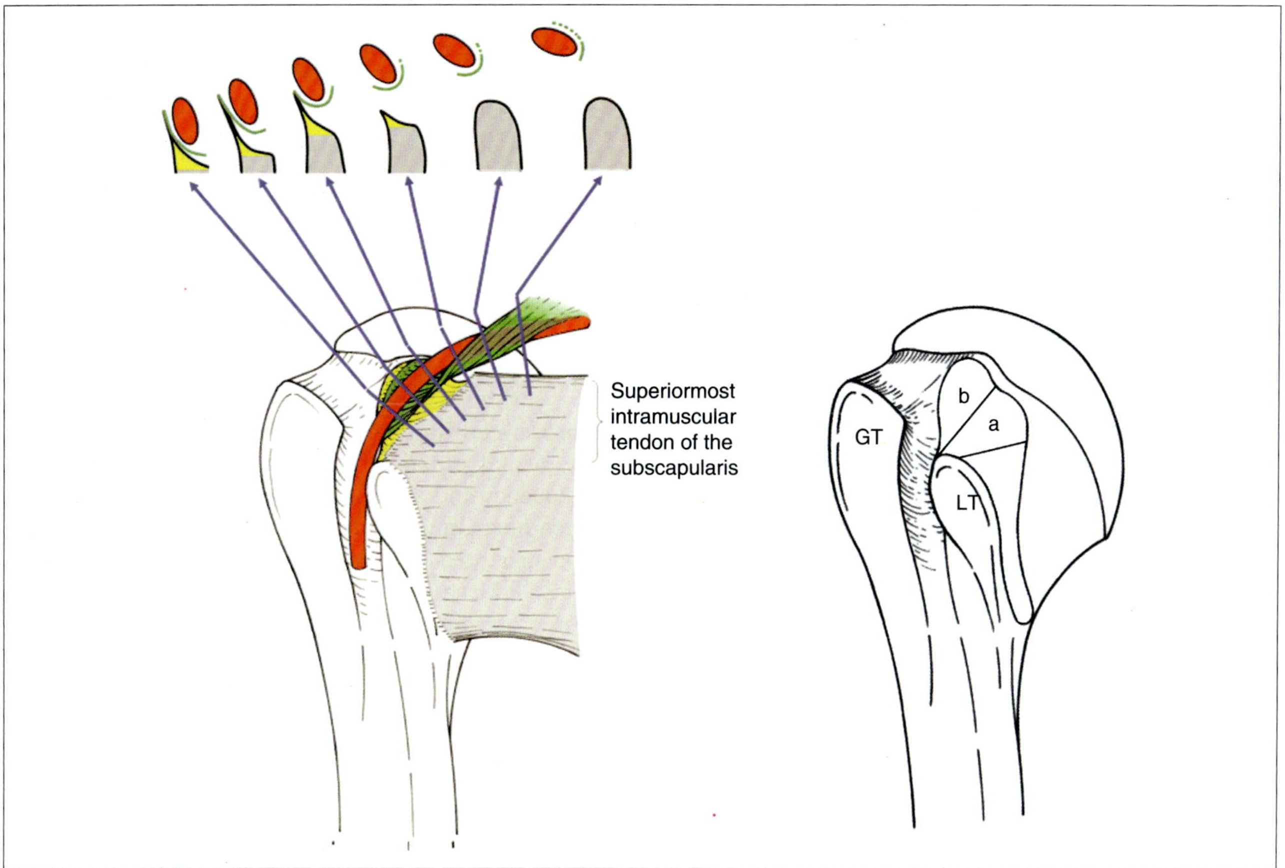

FIGURE 5 Schematic drawings showing two views of the positional relationships among the long head of the biceps (LHB) tendon (red), the superiormost intramuscular tendon of the subscapularis (gray), the superior glenohumeral ligament (SGHL; green), and the tendinous slip of the subscapularis insertion (yellow). The superiormost insertion point of the subscapularis is the wide attachment of the superiormost intramuscular tendon of the subscapularis on the upper margin of the lesser tuberosity (area a). This insertion sends a thin tendinous slip to the fovea capitis of the humerus (area b). The SGHL branches off from the internal wall of the glenohumeral joint near the glenoid in a folded shape, runs laterally to wrap around the LHB in a spiral fashion, and attaches to the tendinous slip of the subscapularis insertion. The area where the SGHL originates is ambiguous. The superiormost insertion of the subscapularis supports the LHB from behind the SGHL. The SGHL and the coracohumeral ligament are continuous, and the tension of the coracohumeral ligament, which covers the whole glenohumeral joint, is considered to be conveyed to the SGHL because the two ligaments form an identical loose connective tissue. This tension may be advantageous for the ability of the SGHL to withstand the dislocation stress of the LHB. GT = greater tuberosity, LT = lesser tuberosity. (Adapted from *J Shoulder Elbow Surg* 19[1]. Arai R, Mochizuki T, Yamaguchi K, et al: Functional anatomy of the superior glenohumeral and coracohumeral ligaments and the subscapularis tendon in view of stabilization of the long head of the biceps tendon, 58-64. Copyright © 2010 Journal of Shoulder and Elbow Surgery Board of Trustees. doi:10.1016/j.jse.2009.04.001.)

usually remains intact, even in a massive three-tendon tear. However, the muscular volume of the teres minor is relevant for surgical decision making because it may predict the prognosis after surgical intervention for a massive rotator cuff tear. The teres minor is innervated by the axillary nerve along with the deltoid muscle. In contrast, the suprascapular nerve passes through the suprascapular notch and innervates the supraspinatus before coursing inferiorly to innervate the infraspinatus.

Physical Examination

A detailed clinical history is particularly important for a precise diagnosis of the cause of shoulder symptoms. The patient should be questioned regarding the onset, duration, and nature of symptoms as well as traumatic episodes, provocative and alleviating factors, earlier treatment, and response to treatment. If pain is an important symptom, it is important to learn whether the pain is present at night and/or with the arm in a resting position. Pain at rest probably results from inflammation of the glenohumeral joint or the subacromial bursa.[17]

Plain radiographs are routinely obtained to help identify rotator cuff tear arthropathy and other shoulder conditions, such as calcific tendinitis, primary osteoarthritis, and simple superior migration of the humeral head. The physical examination should be based on the information obtained through the clinical history and plain radiographs. The physical examination of a patient with rotator cuff disease has four parts: inspection and palpation plus evaluations of strength, scapulothoracic function, and active and passive range of motion with concomitant scapular movement.

To predict scapulothoracic kinematics, postural alignment and scapular position should be assessed by inspection with the patient standing. Scapular malposition, including protraction, anterior tilt, downward rotation, and depression (in comparison with the contralateral side), is a significant indicator of scapular dyskinesis.[4,5] Tenderness at the coracoid process often is prominent in such a shoulder. Assessment of both active and passive range of motion, beginning with the painful arc test, also is done with the patient standing. If the patient cannot fully elevate the affected arm, the clinician must assess whether the restriction of motion is caused by pain, stiffness, or scapular dysfunction. Forward flexion, abduction, external rotation at the side, external and internal rotation at 90° of shoulder abduction, and the highest spine level the thumb can reach are assessed on both sides. Especially during the eccentric phase of lowering the arm from forward flexion or internal rotation at 90° of abduction, the clinician can observe pain provocation and abnormal scapular motion; these are typical in a patient with subacromial pain, regardless of the presence of a rotator cuff tear.

For suspected rotator cuff disease without stiffness, several strength tests are routinely done on both sides with the patient seated or standing, including abduction strength with the shoulder at 30° and 90° of abduction in the scapular plane (Jobe test), forward flexion strength with the shoulder at 90° and 120° of horizontal flexion (Whipple test), and external rotation strength with the arm at the side. Weakness of external rotation and/or an external rotation lag sign are decisive indicators of a large posterosuperior rotator cuff tear. In addition, all patients should be tested for subscapularis strength using the bear hug and belly press tests because subscapularis tears are reported to have a prevalence as high as 27% to 37%.[12-14]

The combined abduction and horizontal flexion test is used to assess scapular dyskinesis with the patient supine.[18] Many provocative maneuvers for specific shoulder conditions have been described, but for the sake of an efficient examination, clinicians must identify the tests they can use most productively.

Pathogenesis of Rotator Cuff Tears

Although tendon fiber failure is the final pathology for all rotator cuff tears, there is no unified theory of the etiology and pathogenesis of atraumatic rotator cuff disease. The causes are multifactorial and generally are divided into intrinsic elements, including age-related tendon degeneration, and extrinsic factors, which are represented by mechanical impingement.[19]

Intrinsic Factors

The rate of both symptomatic and asymptomatic rotator cuff tears increases with age. There is a 50% likelihood that a patient older than 66 years with unilateral shoulder pain has bilateral rotator cuff tears.[20] This fact clearly indicates that tendon degeneration progresses during normal aging. Some histopathologic studies revealed signs of preexisting age-related tendon degeneration.[21,22] Macroscopically intact residual tendon tissue from partial articular-side rotator cuff tears in patients with a mean age of 60 years had moderate histopathologic degeneration.[21] In a study of the medial stumps of torn rotator cuff tendon tissue, the frequency and the distribution of thin and disoriented collagen fibers, myxoid degeneration, and hyaline degeneration suggested early degenerative processes in the torn tendons. The main causes of rotator cuff tears appeared to be microtrauma and preexisting degenerative change in the middle and deep layers of the tendon.[22] Intratendinous vascular patterns were studied in patients with or without a rotator cuff tear, using enhanced ultrasonography after intravenous injection of a contrast agent. Older patients had a significantly decreased blood flow in the intratendinous region compared with younger patients, regardless of the presence of a rotator cuff tear.[23]

Age-related tendon degeneration leads to swelling and thickening of the tendon and thereby narrows the subacromial space, which has already degenerated because of age-related spur formation and bursal tissue thickening. Arm motion can easily cause rotator cuff tearing from the bursal side, especially if scapular mobility is restricted because of scapulothoracic inflexibility. In addition, partial articular-side rotator cuff tearing appears to occur primarily through intrinsic cuff degeneration, without the strong involvement of extrinsic factors.[24] In shoulders with a full-thickness rotator cuff tear, the population of fibroblasts and inflammatory cells decreases as the size of a tear increases; this finding suggests alteration in the healing ability of torn tendons.[25] Also, a progressive decrease in the number of blood vessels and vascularity is observed as the size of the rotator cuff tear increases.[25,26] Cigarette smoking negatively affects the vascularity of the rotator cuff tendons.[27] A dosage-dependent and time-dependent relationship was observed between smoking and rotator cuff tears, which suggests that smoking is an important risk factor for the development of rotator cuff tears.[28]

The development of rotator cuff tendon pathologies and symptoms is partly genetic.[20,29] Familial clustering was found in a study of patients with diagnosed rotator cuff disease and a known genealogy.[30] The risk to both close and distant relatives of patients was significantly elevated. The study findings strongly supported a heritable predisposition to rotator cuff disease. There is increasing evidence to suggest that several gene pathways related to the composition of rotator cuff tendons are altered in rotator cuff disease, affecting the extracellular matrix, vasculature, and intracellular signaling mechanisms.[31] Further studies are required to clarify the genetic and biologic factors involved in rotator cuff tears.

Extrinsic Factors

Extrinsic factors include anatomic variables such as acromial morphologic characteristics, os acromiale, and acromial spurs that compress the rotator cuff by bony impingement or direct pressure from the surrounding soft tissue. Primary subacromial impingement, as originally described by Neer, occurs when the acromiohumeral space is restricted or when a prominent, hooked anterior and lateral acromion or hypertrophied coracoacromial ligament abrades the rotator cuff if the arm is elevated. Constitutional morphologic features seem less likely to cause rotator cuff tearing. In fact, a 2012 study revealed that acromial morphology and the acromion index (a large lateral extension of the acromion proposed as a significant causative factor for full-thickness rotator cuff tearing[32]) were not reliably relevant to rotator cuff disease, but the presence of an acromial spur was highly associated with a full-thickness rotator cuff tear in both symptomatic and asymptomatic patients.[33] A functionally deteriorated scapula caused by scapular dyskinesis is the most likely extrinsic cause of rotator cuff tearing, especially if significant aging-related acromial spur formation is present.[4,5,33] Surgeons should recognize that a dynamic factor, such as loss of complementary scapula motion because of malposition or dyskinesis during arm motion, is an important extrinsic factor for rotator cuff tearing in comparison with static morphologic changes.

Another extrinsically generated cuff pathology results from internal impingement with repetitive microtrauma. This condition is caused by repetitive overhead throwing, which causes articular-sided partial-thickness tearing, especially in the presence of scapular dyskinesis. Although the etiology is still controversial, a patient with internal impingement may have a tight posterior capsule or a loose anterior band of the glenohumeral ligament in association with tight posterior musculature, causing impingement between the medial rotator cuff footprint area of the greater tuberosity and the posterosuperior glenoid during the late cocking and acceleration phases of throwing. The repetitive motion contributes to partial-thickness articular-side tearing of the posterior supraspinatus and the anterior infraspinatus in addition to adjacent posterosuperior glenolabral tearing.

Natural History of Rotator Cuff Tears

Although partial-thickness and small rotator cuff tears may have potential for spontaneous healing, it is generally believed that a tear will progress over time. Some rotator cuff tears do not cause any shoulder-related symptoms, however. This fact suggests that rotator cuff tearing sometimes may be necessary in people older than approximately 65 to 70 years who have functionally altered scapulothoracic articulation resulting from inflexibility and kyphotic deformity of the thoracic spine. It is important for surgeons to understand the natural history of asymptomatic rotator cuff tears when choosing a treatment.

Symptomatic Alteration of an Asymptomatic Tear

The differences between symptomatic and asymptomatic shoulders with a rotator cuff tear are not well understood.[34,35] However, tear progression appears to be one of the factors in symptomatic alteration of full-thickness asymptomatic rotator cuff tears.[36] The longitudinal natural history of asymptomatic rotator cuff tears was studied over 5 years by reviewing consecutive sonograms in 58 patients with unilateral symptoms who had an asymptomatic contralateral rotator cuff tear.[37] Fifty-one percent of the previously asymptomatic shoulders became symptomatic over a mean 2.8 years. Tear size progression was associated with the development of symptoms, including a significant increase in pain and a decrease in the ability to perform activities of daily living. A prospective study also followed 50 patients with initially asymptomatic full-thickness rotator cuff tears over 3 years and found that 18 tears developed symptoms at a mean time of 18 months, which were associated with tear size increase.[38] Bilateral rotator cuff disease, either symptomatic or asymptomatic, was common in patients who initially had unilateral shoulder pain.[20]

Progression of Symptomatic Tears

In a prospective study, patients aged 60 years or younger with a relatively small full-thickness rotator cuff tear were treated nonsurgically.[39] At a mean 29-month follow-up, the size of the tear had increased in 49%, not changed in 43%, and decreased in 8%. There was a correlation between the existence of considerable pain at the time of the follow-up ultrasonography and a clinically significant increase in tear size. A retrospective investigation found that the factors associated with rotator cuff tear progression were age older than 60 years, a full-thickness tear, and fatty infiltration of the rotator cuff muscles.[40] However, small, symptomatic full-thickness tears did not invariably progress over a limited period of time in a study of clinical and structural outcomes in 24 consecutive patients.[41] These patients had declined repair of a symptomatic isolated full-thickness supraspinatus tear. At a median 42-month follow-up after diagnosis, the average tear size had not changed on standardized MRI. The patients had a surprisingly high level of satisfaction.

Tear progression appears to be the most important factor affecting the outcome of nonsurgical management of shoulders with a small, symptomatic rotator cuff tear.[42] The factors related to successful outcome of nonsurgical management were investigated in 123 shoulders with a full-thickness rotator cuff tear diagnosed by high-resolution MRI with a microscopy coil.[43] The integrity of the intramuscular tendon of the supraspinatus was found to be the most significant factor affecting the outcome. In the anatomic footprint of the supraspinatus, the main part of the intramuscular tendon of the supraspinatus inserts into the anteriormost portion of the superior facet; tear progression may be related to whether this portion is disrupted, even in a small tear[8,9,11] (**Figures 1** and **3**). If the anteriormost intramuscular tendon insertion is disrupted, tear progression can occur, and an asymptomatic shoulder eventually becomes symptomatic, or a symptomatic shoulder remains symptomatic.

Fatty Infiltration and Massive Rotator Cuff Tears

Fatty infiltration can progress with an increase in tear size, the number of involved tendons, or the time after the tendon rupture. In a retrospective review of 1,688 patients who underwent surgical repair of a rotator cuff tear, moderate (Goutallier grade 2) supraspinatus fatty infiltration appeared at an average of 3 years after the onset of symptoms, and severe (Goutallier grade 3 or 4) fatty infiltration appeared at an average of 5 years.[44] A positive tangent sign appeared at an average of 4.5 years after the onset of symptoms. In the same patients, infraspinatus fatty infiltration increased significantly with multiple tendon tears and increasing patient age.[45] Goutallier grade 2 fatty infiltration appeared at an average of 2.5 years after symptom onset, and grade 3 or 4 fatty infiltration appeared at an average of 4 years. In the subscapularis, Goutallier grade 2 fatty infiltration appeared at an average of 2.5 years after symptom onset, and grade 3 or 4 appeared at an average of 5 years.[46] It is suggested that surgical repair should be done before moderate (grade 2) fatty infiltration and atrophy (a positive tangent sign) appear, especially if the tear involves multiple tendons.

Some patients with multiple tendon tears remain asymptomatic or moderately symptomatic. Eventually, however, the tear and fatty infiltration progress to the irreparable level. In a study of 19 consecutive patients with a massive rotator cuff tear who underwent nonsurgical treatment, satisfactory shoulder function was maintained for at least 4 years despite significant progression of degenerative structural joint changes, including glenohumeral osteoarthritis and fatty infiltration.[47]

Nonsurgical Management

There is no consensus on the best management for a rotator cuff tear. The management is selected on the basis of the patient's symptoms.[48] A patient with a symptomatic rotator cuff tear may have inflammatory pain and a functional deficit, such as scapular dyskinesis, in addition to a lack of anatomic structural integrity. Successful surgery can resolve only the anatomic issues. Considering the absence of an explicit difference between symptomatic and asymptomatic shoulders with a rotator cuff tear, it is important to attempt to relieve pain and improve functional impairment before surgery is undertaken.

Pain Management

Pain is the initial symptom in most patients. It is important to control the patient's pain early in the management process, especially if inflammatory pain is present, even at rest and at night, regardless of arm position. The use of ice, rest, NSAIDs, injections, and activity modification are considered as the first treatment for the inflammatory pain. Pain associated only with a specific arm motion (a painful arc or an impingement sign) is considered to be mechanical or functional, and the treatment is surgery or physical therapy to correct scapular dyskinesis. Relieving inflammatory pain early in the management process is of particular importance for the effectiveness of physical therapy or surgery to relieve morbidity.

Injections

A steroid injection to the glenohumeral joint or the subacromial bursa is commonly used for management of pain due to rotator cuff diseases and has been reported to be the effective, reliable management.[17,49,50] Several studies and reviews, however, have indicated that there was no evidence to suggest a benefit of steroid over local anesthesia injections in the management of rotator cuff-related pain.[51,52]

Recently, platelet-rich plasma (PRP) has been widely used for management of various musculoskeletal diseases to promote biological regeneration. PRP as a supraphysiological concentration of platelets is an easily producible, low-cost source of several growth factors such as insulinlike growth factor-1.[53] Several studies have reported the effect of subacromial injected PRP on partial rotator cuff tears.[54-56] A prospective randomized control study evaluated 40 shoulders with symptomatic partial rotator cuff tears that had an injection of PRP or corticosteroid and showed earlier better results than corticosteroid injections, though there was no significant difference after 6 months.[54] Another study also reported similar clinical outcomes.[55] Effect of PRP on structural outcomes remains controversial. Several studies have demonstrated no significant improvement of rotator cuff tendon pathology after PRP injection,[54,55] whereas a 2019 study has reported that the size of partial rotator cuff tears significantly decreased after injection.[56] Subacromial PRP injections can be an alternative to corticosteroid injections, especially in patients with contraindication to corticosteroid administration.

Injection of stem cells may be another potential treatment to promote biological healing of torn tendons. Several studies have reported favorable outcomes after stem cell injection for animal models with a rotator cuff tear.[57,58] There have been few clinical studies that assessed efficacy of stem cells on rotator cuff diseases. A recent study investigated the efficacy of intratendinous injection of adipose tissue–derived mesenchymal stem cells for patients with rotator cuff diseases and reported significantly good functional and structural outcomes.[59] Further studies will be needed to prove the potential of stem cells to heal rotator cuff tears.

Physiotherapy

In a middle-aged or older patient with a rotator cuff tear, scapular motion normally is restricted because of the inflexibility of muscles and surrounding structures, along with kyphotic deformity of the thoracic spine.[4,5] Therefore, the most important first step is restoration of scapular and trunk mobility, before proceeding to activation of the remaining rotator cuff function and scapular stabilization. The restoration of normal shoulder girdle mechanics progresses from proper rotator cuff function and scapular stabilization for lifting and reaching to trunk and lower extremity core stabilization for more complex activities.

Appropriate management selection, conservative or surgical management, for rotator cuff tears has been still debated. A prospective study investigated factors at the time of initial clinical presentation that were associated with preferred allocation to surgical or nonsurgical management for full-thickness rotator cuff tears and concluded that patient demographics such as age, body mass index, or duration of symptoms were more predictive of management allocation than the patient-derived outcome scores for activity level and shoulder disability.[60] Recent randomized studies have indicated that there were no or little differences in treatment outcomes between physiotherapy and rotator cuff repair; however, tear size increased in patients with physiotherapy.[61,62] In addition, 20% to 30% of patients failed with physiotherapy and underwent surgery.[62,63] Physiotherapy can be effective in treating shoulders with rotator cuff tears but is not ideal for all patients. As there is no consensus on definite indications and protocols for physiotherapy of rotator cuff diseases, treatment options should be chosen individually with each patient considering various factors such as patient demographics and tear configuration.

SUMMARY

Understanding of the anatomy and function of the shoulder is important for management of rotator cuff disease. There is no consensus on the best treatment for a rotator cuff tear. Management options, conservative or surgical management, should be chosen individually with each patient considering various factors such as patient demographics and tear configuration.

KEY STUDY POINTS

- Understanding of the anatomy is essential for treatment of rotator cuff diseases.
- Approximately, a half of asymptomatic rotator cuff tears become symptomatic over time.
- Tear size and fatty infiltration of the cuff muscle can progress in conservatively treated rotator cuff tears.
- Management options, conservative or surgical management, should be chosen individually with each patient considering various factors such as patient demographics and tear configuration.

Annotated References

1. Yamamoto A, Takagishi K, Kobayashi T, Shitara H, Osawa T: Factors involved in the presence of symptoms associated with rotator cuff tears: A comparison of asymptomatic and symptomatic rotator cuff tears in the general population. *J Shoulder Elbow Surg* 2011;20(7):1133-1137.

2. Holtby R, Razmjou H: Impact of work-related compensation claims on surgical outcome of patients with rotator cuff related pathologies: A matched case-control study. *J Shoulder Elbow Surg* 2010;19(3):452-460.

3. Cuff DJ, Pupello DR: Prospective evaluation of postoperative compliance and outcomes after rotator cuff repair in patients with and without workers' compensation claims. *J Shoulder Elbow Surg* 2012;21(12):1728-1733.

4. Kibler WB, Sciascia A, Wilkes T: Scapular dyskinesis and its relation to shoulder injury. *J Am Acad Orthop Surg* 2012;20(6):364-372.

5. Kibler WB: The scapula in rotator cuff disease. *Med Sport Sci* 2012;57:27-40.

6. Curtis AS, Burbank KM, Tierney JJ, Scheller AD, Curran AR: The insertional footprint of the rotator cuff: An anatomic study. *Arthroscopy* 2006;22(6):609.e1.

7. Dugas JR, Campbell DA, Warren RF, Robie BH, Millett PJ: Anatomy and dimensions of rotator cuff insertions. *J Shoulder Elbow Surg* 2002;11(5):498-503.

8. Mochizuki T, Sugaya H, Uomizu M, et al: Humeral insertion of the supraspinatus and infraspinatus: New anatomical findings regarding the footprint of the rotator cuff. *J Bone Joint Surg Am* 2008;90(5):962-969.

9. Mochizuki T, Sugaya H, Uomizu M, et al: Humeral insertion of the supraspinatus and infraspinatus: New anatomical findings regarding the footprint of the rotator cuff. Surgical technique. *J Bone Joint Surg Am* 2009;91(suppl 2, pt 1):1-7.

10. Kato A, Nimura A, Yamaguchi K, Mochizuki T, Sugaya H, Akita K: An anatomical study of the transverse part of the infraspinatus muscle that is closely related with the supraspinatus muscle. *Surg Radiol Anat* 2012;34(3): 257-265.

11. Nimura A, Kato A, Yamaguchi K, et al: The superior capsule of the shoulder joint complements the insertion of the rotator cuff. *J Shoulder Elbow Surg* 2012;21(7):867-872.

12. Arai R, Sugaya H, Mochizuki T, Nimura A, Moriishi J, Akita K: Subscapularis tendon tear: An anatomic and clinical investigation. *Arthroscopy* 2008;24(9):997-1004.

13. Adams CR, Schoolfield JD, Burkhart SS: Accuracy of preoperative magnetic resonance imaging in predicting a subscapularis tendon tear based on arthroscopy. *Arthroscopy* 2010;26(11):1427-1433.

14. Garavaglia G, Ufenast H, Taverna E: The frequency of subscapularis tears in arthroscopic rotator cuff repairs: A retrospective study comparing magnetic resonance imaging and arthroscopic findings. *Int J Shoulder Surg* 2011;5(4):90-94.

15. Arai R, Mochizuki T, Yamaguchi K, et al: Functional anatomy of the superior glenohumeral and coracohumeral ligaments and the subscapularis tendon in view of stabilization of the long head of the biceps tendon. *J Shoulder Elbow Surg* 2010;19(1):58-64.

16. Lo IK, Burkhart SS: The comma sign: An arthroscopic guide to the torn subscapularis tendon. *Arthroscopy* 2003;19(3):334-337.

17. Gialanella B, Prometti P: Effects of corticosteroids injection in rotator cuff tears. *Pain Med* 2011;12(10):1559-1565.

18. Pappas AM, Zawacki RM, McCarthy CF: Rehabilitation of the pitching shoulder. *Am J Sports Med* 1985;13(4):223-235.

19. Maffulli N, Longo UG, Berton A, Loppini M, Denaro V: Biological factors in the pathogenesis of rotator cuff tears. *Sports Med Arthrosc Rev* 2011;19(3):194-201.

20. Yamaguchi K, Ditsios K, Middleton WD, Hildebolt CF, Galatz LM, Teefey SA: The demographic and morphological features of rotator cuff disease: A comparison of asymptomatic and symptomatic shoulders. *J Bone Joint Surg Am* 2006;88(8):1699-1704.

21. Yamakado K: Histopathology of residual tendon in high-grade articular-sided partial-thickness rotator cuff tears (PASTA lesions). *Arthroscopy* 2012;28(4):474-480.

22. Hashimoto T, Nobuhara K, Hamada T: Pathologic evidence of degeneration as a primary cause of rotator cuff tear. *Clin Orthop Relat Res* 2003;415:111-120.

23. Funakoshi T, Iwasaki N, Kamishima T, et al: In vivo visualization of vascular patterns of rotator cuff tears using contrast-enhanced ultrasound. *Am J Sports Med* 2010;38(12):2464-2471.

24. Modi CS, Smith CD, Drew SJ: Partial-thickness articular surface rotator cuff tears in patients over the age of 35: Etiology and intra-articular associations. *Int J Shoulder Surg* 2012;6(1):15-18.

25. Longo UG, Berton A, Khan WS, Maffulli N, Denaro V: Histopathology of rotator cuff tears. *Sports Med Arthrosc Rev* 2011;19(3):227-236.

26. Hegedus EJ, Cook C, Brennan M, Wyland D, Garrison JC, Driesner D: Vascularity and tendon pathology in the rotator cuff: A review of literature and implications for rehabilitation and surgery. *Br J Sports Med* 2010;44(12): 838-847.

27. Carbone S, Gumina S, Arceri V, Campagna V, Fagnani C, Postacchini F: The impact of preoperative smoking habit on rotator cuff tear: Cigarette smoking influences rotator cuff tear sizes. *J Shoulder Elbow Surg* 2012;21(1): 56-60.

28. Baumgarten KM, Gerlach D, Galatz LM, et al: Cigarette smoking increases the risk for rotator cuff tears. *Clin Orthop Relat Res* 2010;468(6):1534-1541.

29. Gwilym SE, Watkins B, Cooper CD, et al: Genetic influences in the progression of tears of the rotator cuff. *J Bone Joint Surg Br* 2009;91(7):915-917.

30. Tashjian RZ, Farnham JM, Albright FS, Teerlink CC, Cannon-Albright LA: Evidence for an inherited predisposition contributing to the risk for rotator cuff disease. *J Bone Joint Surg Am* 2009;91(5):1136-1142.

31. Chaudhury S, Carr AJ: Lessons we can learn from gene expression patterns in rotator cuff tears and tendinopathies. *J Shoulder Elbow Surg* 2012;21(2):191-199.

32. Nyffeler RW, Werner CM, Sukthankar A, Schmid MR, Gerber C: Association of a large lateral extension of the acromion with rotator cuff tears. *J Bone Joint Surg Am* 2006;88(4):800-805.

33. Hamid N, Omid R, Yamaguchi K, Steger-May K, Stobbs G, Keener JD: Relationship of radiographic acromial characteristics and rotator cuff disease: A prospective investigation of clinical, radiographic, and sonographic findings. *J Shoulder Elbow Surg* 2012;21(10):1289-1298.

34. Keener JD, Steger-May K, Stobbs G, Yamaguchi K: Asymptomatic rotator cuff tears: Patient demographics and baseline shoulder function. *J Shoulder Elbow Surg* 2010;19(8):1191-1198.

35. Moosmayer S, Tariq R, Stiris MG, Smith HJ: MRI of symptomatic and asymptomatic full-thickness rotator cuff tears: A comparison of findings in 100 subjects. *Acta Orthop* 2010;81(3):361-366.

36. Mall NA, Kim HM, Keener JD, et al: Symptomatic progression of asymptomatic rotator cuff tears: A prospective study of clinical and sonographic variables. *J Bone Joint Surg Am* 2010;92(16):2623-2633.

37. Yamaguchi K, Tetro AM, Blam O, Evanoff BA, Teefey SA, Middleton WD: Natural history of asymptomatic rotator cuff tears: A longitudinal analysis of asymptomatic tears detected sonographically. *J Shoulder Elbow Surg* 2001;10(3):199-203.

38. Moosmayer S, Tariq R, Stiris M, Smith HJ: The natural history of asymptomatic rotator cuff tears: A three-year follow-up of fifty cases. *J Bone Joint Surg Am* 2013;95(14):1249-1255.

Eighteen of 50 asymptomatic full-thickness rotator cuff tears developed symptoms at a mean of 18 months. There was a significantly larger increase in the mean tear size in the newly symptomatic group when compared with the still-asymptomatic group. Level of evidence: II.

39. Safran O, Schroeder J, Bloom R, Weil Y, Milgrom C: Natural history of nonoperatively treated symptomatic rotator cuff tears in patients 60 years old or younger. *Am J Sports Med* 2011;39(4):710-714.

40. Maman E, Harris C, White L, Tomlinson G, Shashank M, Boynton E: Outcome of nonoperative treatment of symptomatic rotator cuff tears monitored by magnetic resonance imaging. *J Bone Joint Surg Am* 2009;91(8):1898-1906.

41. Fucentese SF, von Roll AL, Pfirrmann CW, Gerber C, Jost B: Evolution of nonoperatively treated symptomatic isolated full-thickness supraspinatus tears. *J Bone Joint Surg Am* 2012;94(9):801-808.

42. Moosmayer S, Gärtner AV, Tariq R: The natural course of nonoperatively treated rotator cuff tears: An 8.8-year follow-up of tear anatomy and clinical outcome in 49 patients. *J Shoulder Elbow Surg* 2017;26(4):627-634.

Forty-nine small- to medium-sized full-thickness rotator cuff tears that were treated by physiotherapy were retrospectively investigated. Tear size, muscle atrophy, and fatty degeneration progressed in the majority of patients. Level of evidence: II.

43. Tanaka M, Itoi E, Sato K, et al: Factors related to successful outcome of conservative treatment for rotator cuff tears. *Ups J Med Sci* 2010;115(3):193-200.

44. Melis B, DeFranco MJ, Chuinard C, Walch G: Natural history of fatty infiltration and atrophy of the supraspinatus muscle in rotator cuff tears. *Clin Orthop Relat Res* 2010;468(6):1498-1505.

45. Melis B, Wall B, Walch G: Natural history of infraspinatus fatty infiltration in rotator cuff tears. *J Shoulder Elbow Surg* 2010;19(5):757-763.

46. Melis B, Nemoz C, Walch G: Muscle fatty infiltration in rotator cuff tears: Descriptive analysis of 1688 cases. *Orthop Traumatol Surg Res* 2009;95(5):319-324.

47. Zingg PO, Jost B, Sukthankar A, Buhler M, Pfirrmann CW, Gerber C: Clinical and structural outcomes of nonoperative management of massive rotator cuff tears. *J Bone Joint Surg Am* 2007;89(9):1928-1934.

48. Longo UG, Franceschi F, Berton A, Maffulli N, Droena V: Conservative treatment and rotator cuff tear progression. *Med Sport Sci* 2012;57:90-99.

49. Hong JY, Yoon SH, Moon J, Kwack KS, Joen B, Lee HY: Comparison of high- and low-dose corticosteroid in subacromial injection for periarticular shoulder disorder: A randomized, triple-blind, placebo-controlled trial. *Arch Phys Med Rehabil* 2011;92(12):1951-1960.

50. Zufferey P, Revaz S, Degailler X, Balague F, So A: A controlled trial of the benefits of ultrasound-guided steroid injection for shoulder pain. *Joint Bone Spine* 2012;79(2):166-169.

51. Cook T, Minns Lowe C, Maybury M, Lewis JS: Are corticosteroid injections more beneficial than anaesthetic injections alone in the management of rotator cuff-related shoulder pain? A systematic review. *Br J Sports Med* 2018;52(8):497-504.

A systematic review found that corticosteroid injections had a short-term benefit (up to 8 weeks) over local anesthetic injections alone in the management of rotator cuff–related shoulder pain. Beyond 8 weeks, there was no evidence to suggest a benefit of corticosteroid over local anesthetic injections. Level of evidence: I.

52. Alvarez CM, Litchfield R, Jackowski D, Griffin S, Kirkley A: A prospective, double-blind, randomized clinical trial comparing subacromial injection of betamethasone and xylocaine to xylocaine alone in chronic rotator cuff tendinosis. *Am J Sports Med* 2005;33(2):255-262.

53. Pauly S, Klatte-Schulz F, Stahnke K, Schiebel M, Wildemann B: The effect of autologous platelet rich plasma on tenocytes of the human rotator cuff. *BMC Musculoskelet Disord* 2018;19(1):422.

    The possible effect of autologous platelet-rich plasma on rotator cuff tendon cells was assessed. Platelet-rich plasma had an anabolic effect on the human rotator cuff tenocytes of the same individual in vitro by means of cell proliferation and absolute, but not relative, collagen I synthesis. Level of evidence: V.

54. Shams A, El-Sayed M, Gamal O, Ewes W: Subacromial injection of autologous platelet-rich plasma versus corticosteroid for the treatment of symptomatic partial rotator cuff tears. *Eur J Orthop Surg Traumatol* 2016;26(8):837-842.

    A prospective randomized controlled study evaluated the results of subacromial injection of platelet-rich plasma versus corticosteroid injection therapy in 40 patients with symptomatic partial rotator cuff tears. Platelet-rich plasma injections showed earlier better results as compared to corticosteroid injections, although statistically significant better results after 6 months could not be found. Level of evidence: II.

55. von Wehren L, Blanke F, Todorov A, Heisterbach P, Sailer J, Majewski M: The effect of subacromial injections of autologous conditioned plasma versus cortisone for the treatment of symptomatic partial rotator cuff tears. *Knee Surg Sports Traumatol Arthrosc* 2016;24(12):3787-3792.

    The effects of subacromial platelet-rich plasma injections were compared with those of standard cortisone injection therapy in 50 patients with partial rotator cuff tears. Platelet-rich plasma injections showed earlier benefit as compared to cortisone injections although a statistically significant difference after 6 months could not be found. Level of evidence: III.

56. Cai Y, Sun Z, Liao B, Song Z, Xiao T, Zhu P: Sodium hyaluronate and platelet-rich plasma for partial-thickness rotator cuff tears. *Med Sci Sports Exerc* 2019;51(2):227-233.

    A randomized study evaluated the combined use of sodium hyaluronate and platelet-rich plasma in the treatment of partial-thickness rotator cuff tears. The combined sodium hyaluronate and platelet-rich plasma injection yielded better clinical and structural outcomes than sodium hyaluronate or platelet-rich plasma alone. Level of evidence: II.

57. Kwon DR, Park GY, Lee SC: Treatment of full-thickness rotator cuff tendon tear using umbilical cord blood-derived mesenchymal stem cells and polydeoxyribonucleotides in a rabbit model. *Stem Cells Int* 2018;2018:7146384.

    Regenerative effects of injection with human umbilical cord blood–derived mesenchymal stem cells were investigated in a chronic full-thickness rotator cuff tear in a rabbit model. The tear size was significantly smaller in rabbits that received mesenchymal stem cells injection than in control groups. Level of evidence: V.

58. Park GY, Kwon DR, Lee SC: Regeneration of full-thickness rotator cuff tendon tear after ultrasound-guided injection with umbilical cord blood-derived mesenchymal stem cells in a rabbit model. *Stem Cells Transl Med* 2015;4(11):1344-1351.

    The therapeutic effects of human umbilical cord blood–derived mesenchymal stem cell injection were investigated in a full-thickness subscapularis tear in a rabbit model. Mesenchymal stem cells induced regeneration of tendon tear, and the regenerated tissue was predominantly composed of type I collagens. Level of evidence: V.

59. Jo CH, Chai JW, Jeong EC, et al: Intratendinous injection of autologous adipose tissue-derived mesenchymal stem cells for the treatment of rotator cuff disease: A first-in-human trial. *Stem Cells* 2018;36(9):1441-1450.

    A first-in-human trial assessed the safety and efficacy of intratendinous injection of autologous adipose tissue–derived mesenchymal stem cells in patients with rotator cuff disease. Intratendinous injection of autologous mesenchymal stem cells in patients with a partial-thickness rotator cuff tear did not cause adverse events but improved shoulder function and relieved pain through regeneration of rotator cuff tendon. Level of evidence: IV.

60. Kweon C, Gagnier JJ, Robbins CB, Bedi A, Carpenter JE, Miller BS: Surgical versus nonsurgical management of rotator cuff tears: Predictors of treatment allocation. *Am J Sports Med* 2015;43(10):2368-2372.

    A prospective cohort study assessed independent variables at the time of initial clinical presentation that were associated with preferred allocation to surgical versus nonsurgical treatment for patients with known full-thickness rotator cuff tears. Increasing age, higher BMI, and duration of symptoms longer than 1 year were predictive of nonsurgical treatment. Level of evidence: III.

61. Kukkonen J, Joukainen A, Lehtinen J, et al: Treatment of nontraumatic rotator cuff tears: A randomized controlled trial with two years of clinical and imaging follow-up. *J Bone Joint Surg Am* 2015;97(21):1729-1737.

    A randomized controlled study compared the effectiveness of physiotherapy, acromioplasty, and rotator cuff repair for symptomatic, nontraumatic rotator cuff tears. There was no significant difference in clinical outcomes between the three interventions at 2-year follow-up, but tear progression was observed in the nonrepaired treatment groups. Level of evidence: I.

62. Moosmayer S, Lund G, Seljom US, et al: Tendon repair compared with physiotherapy in the treatment of rotator cuff tears: A randomized controlled study in 103 cases with a five-year follow-up. *J Bone Joint Surg Am* 2014;96(18):1504-1514.

    A randomized controlled study compared outcomes of patients treated with primary tendon repair with outcomes of those treated with physiotherapy. Although primary repair of small- and medium-sized rotator cuff tears was associated with better outcome than physiotherapy treatment, the differences were small and may be below clinical importance. In the physiotherapy treatment group, there were increasing tear sizes and inferior outcomes in one-third of patients who did not undergo repair. Level of evidence: I.

63. Dunn WR, Kuhn JE, Sanders R, et al: 2013 Neer Award: Predictors of failure of nonoperative treatment of chronic, symptomatic, full-thickness rotator cuff tears. *J Shoulder Elbow Surg* 2016;25(8):1303-1311.

A prospective, multicenter, cohort study assessed predictors of failure of nonsurgical treatment and identified patient expectations regarding physical therapy as the strongest predictor of surgery. Higher activity level and not smoking were also significant predictors of surgery. Level of evidence: I.

Chapter 12

Partial-Thickness Rotator Cuff Tears

Ian K.Y. Lo, MD, FRCSC • Mustafa S. Rashid, MB, ChB, MSc, PhD

ABSTRACT

Partial-thickness rotator cuff tears challenge even the most experienced surgeons. Although recently there has been a focus on the natural history and management of this ubiquitous pathology, diverse etiologies, management options, and outcomes continue to impede universal approaches. Future studies will focus on biologic approaches to the understanding and management of partial-thickness rotator cuff tears.

Keywords: natural history; partial thickness; repair; rotator cuff

Introduction

Although partial-thickness rotator cuff tears (PTRCTs) are common, their optimal management remains controversial. Most publications on rotator cuff tears have focused on full-thickness rotator cuff tears (FTRCTs), and most available studies of PTRCTs have focused on surgical outcome or technique. Few studies have looked at the etiologic factors or the nonsurgical management of PTRCTs. The relatively poor understanding of the natural history of the disease compounds the debate over optimal management.

Dr. Lo or an immediate family member has received royalties from Arthrex, Inc and Smith & Nephew; is a member of a speakers' bureau or has made paid presentations on behalf of Smith & Nephew; serves as a paid consultant to or is an employee of Smith & Nephew; has received research or institutional support from Smith & Nephew; has received nonincome support (such as equipment or services), commercially derived honoraria, or other non–research-related funding (such as paid travel) from CONMED Linvatec and Smith & Nephew; and serves as a board member, owner, officer, or committee member of the American Shoulder and Elbow Surgeons and the Arthroscopy Association of North America. Neither Dr. Rashid nor any immediate family member has received anything of value from or has stock or stock options held in a commercial company or institution related directly or indirectly to the subject of this chapter.

Relevant Anatomy

The rotator cuff tendon classically is described as a complex coalescence of the supraspinatus, infraspinatus, teres minor, and subscapularis tendons into a multilayered structure that inserts into the humeral head.[1] Several cadaver studies have evaluated the gross anatomy of the rotator cuff tendon insertion. One study measured the medial-to-lateral width and the anterior-to-posterior length of each footprint and found a wide range of widths and lengths for each insertion[2] (**Table 1**). Another study found the supraspinatus tendon to have a mean width of 12.1 mm (range: 9 to 15 mm) and a mean length of 25.0 mm (range: 19 to 27 mm).[3]

A cadaver study led to an alternative interpretation of the rotator cuff tendon insertion[4] (**Figure 1**). A long trapezoid-shaped insertion of the infraspinatus tendon was described, with an anterior curve. The infraspinatus tendon was found to occupy a large portion of the lateral aspect of the superior facet of the greater tuberosity; this area previously was assigned to the supraspinatus tendon. In contrast, the supraspinatus tendon insertion was described as small, triangle-shaped, and on the most anterior aspect of the greater tuberosity; in 21% of the specimens, some fibers inserted into the lesser tuberosity. In a follow-up study, the capsular contribution of the rotator cuff insertion has been previously underestimated and can occupy up to 3.5 to 9.1 mm of footprint of the rotator cuff.[5] This suggests that the actual tendon insertion is a smaller portion of the rotator cuff footprint. These anatomic findings collectively require further investigation as to their clinical relevance. It should be noted, however, that the clinical algorithms for treating a PTRCT (defined as a tear of no more than 50% of tendon thickness) are based on classic descriptions of the rotator cuff tendon insertion.

Incidence, Etiology, and Pathogenesis

Cadaver and imaging studies have found a prevalence of PTRCTs ranging from 13% to 32%.[6-9] An MRI study of asymptomatic individuals found an overall prevalence of 20%.[8] Prevalence was highly age related; 26% of those

Table 1

Medial-to-Lateral Width and Anterior-to-Posterior Length of the Rotator Cuff Tendon Insertions

Rotator Cuff Tendon	Mean Medial-Lateral Width, in mm (Range)	Mean Anterior-Posterior Length, in mm (Range)
Supraspinatus	16 (12-20)	23 (18-33)
Infraspinatus	18 (12-24)	28 (20-45)
Teres minor	21 (10-33)	29 (20-40)
Subscapularis	20 (15-25)	40 (35-55)

Data from Curtis AS, Burbank KM, Tierney JJ, Scheller AD, Curran AR: The insertional footprint of the rotator cuff: An anatomic study. *Arthroscopy* 2006;22(6):603-609. doi:10.1016/j.arthro.2006.04.001.

older than 60 years but only 4% of those younger than 40 years had a PTRCT. Clearly, many PTRCTs are asymptomatic and probably are secondary to age-related degenerative changes. Therefore, it is important to correlate clinical and imaging findings.

Several etiologic factors in isolation or combination can result in the anatomic lesion of a PTRCT. Intrinsic factors include age-related alterations in microscopic anatomy (eg, decreased cellularity, increased apoptosis, fascicular thinning or disruption, or granulation tissue), metabolic anatomy, and vascular anatomy (eg, decreased vascularity or a hypovascular zone). These factors create a predisposition to degenerative tearing or alterations in intratendinous sheer stress. Extrinsic factors include classic subacromial (outlet) impingement, internal impingement, and glenohumeral instability and/or laxity, which can contribute to the development of a PTRCT. Traumatic events, whether single or repetitive (eg, from overhead throwing) can lead to tensile overload and fiber failure.

Although several general etiologic factors have been identified, certain factors are likely to predispose the rotator cuff to particular types of tearing. A PTRCT in an older patient commonly occurs on the articular surface just posterior to the biceps tendon and is secondary to age-related degenerative changes. In contrast, a PTRCT in a young overhead athlete commonly occurs near the confluence of the supraspinatus and infraspinatus tendons. This characteristic suggests a different etiologic factor in young overhead athletes (eg, excessive twisting or torsional stress of the rotator cuff fibers or internal impingement), which leads to a more posterior, articular-surface tear.[10]

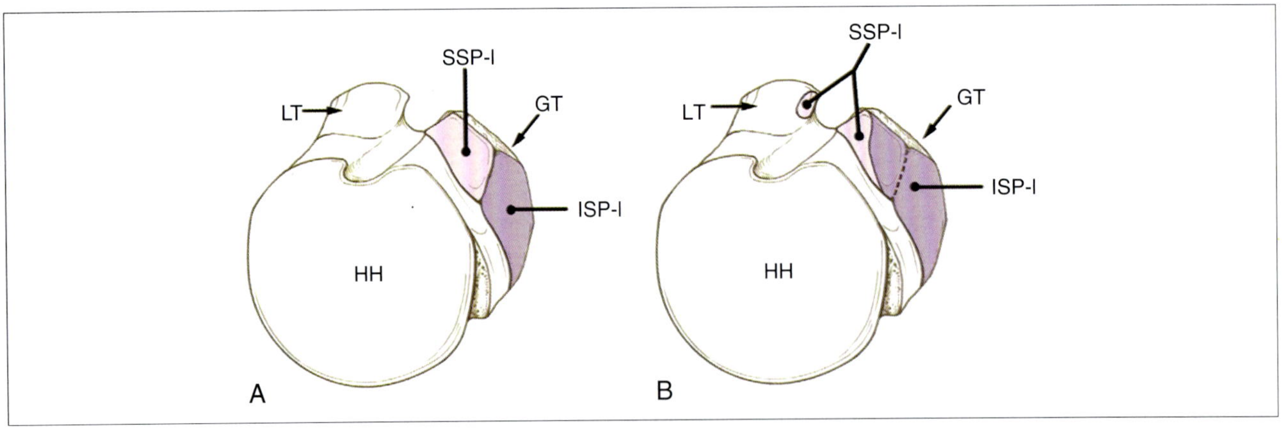

FIGURE 1 Schematic drawings of the superior aspect of the right humerus, showing the humeral insertions of the supraspinatus and the infraspinatus. **A**, The generally accepted concept of the anatomy of humeral insertions, in which the supraspinatus inserts into the highest impression and the infraspinatus inserts into the middle impression of the greater tuberosity. **B**, An alternative concept, in which the insertion area of the infraspinatus occupies approximately half of the highest impression and all of the middle impression of the greater tuberosity. The insertion area of the supraspinatus is in the anteromedial region of the highest impression and sometimes also in the superiormost area of the lesser tuberosity. GT = greater tuberosity, HH = humeral head, ISP-I = insertion area of the infraspinatus, LT = lesser tuberosity, SSP-I = insertion area of the supraspinatus. (Reproduced with permission from Mochizuki T, Sugaya H, Uomizu M, et al: Humeral insertion of the supraspinatus and infraspinatus: New anatomic findings regarding the footprint of the rotator cuff. *J Bone Joint Surg Am* 2008;90:962-969. doi:10.2106/JBJS.G.00427.)

However, once initiated, PTRCTs likely alter the load-carrying properties of the residual rotator cuff tendon during physiologic loading. In simulated articular-surface or bursal-surface tears, biomechanical studies have demonstrated altered strain patterns in the torn and intact rotator cuff tendon and likely mechanically predispose to tear progression.[11,12]

Historically, PTRCTs were thought to have a poor prognosis. In one study, at a mean 1.1-year follow-up, 80% of PTRCTs had increased in size, and 28% of patients had full-thickness progression of their PTRCTs.[13] However, a number of more recent studies have attempted to document the natural history of PTRCTs. Many of these studies are limited because of the diagnostic accuracy of the imaging modality and definition of tear progression. However, in contrast, PTRCTs appear to have a relatively low risk of tear progression when compared with previous studies. In one study of 88 high-grade PTRCTs, in 55% of patients (48 of 88), tear remained stable; 23% of patients (20 of 88) had a reduction in tear size; and 15% of patients (13 of 88) had an increase in tear size at a mean follow-up of 2 years.[14] Similarly, in another study of 37 patients treated nonsurgically, at a mean follow-up of 53 ± 8 months, 65% of tears appeared stable, 11% had improvement in their tear size, and 24% demonstrated evidence of tear progression.[15]

In general, midterm follow-up has revealed that approximately 8% to 53% of partial-thickness tears progress of which 13.3% to 27.5% progress to a full-thickness tear.[13,14,16-19] Factors associated with progression of PTRCTs were older age, time, development of symptoms, and grade of tendinosis.[13,14,17,18] Studies describing the radiologic outcome of nonsurgically managed PTRCTs are summarized in **Table 2**. Some studies have also reported no difference or correlation between symptoms and tear progression, suggesting surveillance monitoring could be considered in high-risk patients.[15,19]

Diagnostic Imaging

The value of ultrasonography for detecting and quantifying PTRCTs and FTRCTs continues to evolve. Ultrasonography has had accuracy similar to that of MRI for detecting FTRCTs, but its use in detecting and quantifying PTRCTs in a community setting is controversial.[21,22] Ultrasonography continues to be limited by its observer-dependent reliability and its limited ability to detect significant glenohumeral pathology. However, its availability particularly in the clinic setting has made it a popular diagnostic modality among surgeons to augment the history and physical examination. Several studies have evaluated the diagnostic performance and learning curve for surgeons learning office ultrasonography for diagnosing rotator cuff tears.[23-25] Most studies have evaluated the detection of full-thickness tears and demonstrated high sensitivity and specificity (sensitivity, 67% to 96.2%; specificity, 88% to 100%).[26] However, there is a reduction in accuracy when attempting to diagnose partial-thickness versus full-thickness tears.[24,25,27] Several studies have documented the sensitivity and specificity of ultrasonography with no significant difference when sonographers and surgeons were compared with radiologists.[28]

Overall, there is no significant difference when comparing ultrasonography and MRI in detecting PTRCTs.[26] However, there has been a wide range of results reported. For ultrasonographic assessment, the sensitivity has been reported to be 52% (95% CI, 33% to 70%) and specificity was 93% (95% CI, 85% to 97%) whereas MRI has been reported to have a sensitivity of 74% (95% CI, 59% to 85%), and specificity was 95% (95% CI, 84% to 97%).[26]

Magnetic resonance angiography (MRA) is considered the imaging modality of choice for evaluating PTRCTs, particularly articular-surface tears. MRA has a range of sensitivity of 62% to 80% and a range of specificity of 47% to 100%, and it is significantly more accurate than ultrasonography or MRI for detecting PTRCTs.[26,28,29] The addition of an abduction-external rotation view can improve the sensitivity of MRA for detecting articular-surface PTRCTs.[30,31] Although still in the investigational stage, 3.0 T MRI has been reported to have higher sensitivities in detecting PTRCTs than 1.5 T MRI; however, the results are not statistically significant.[28]

Classification

PTRCTs can be generally classified by anatomic location (bursal surface, articular surface, or intrasubstance), tendon involvement (supraspinatus, infraspinatus, teres minor, or subscapularis), and/or area of involvement and depth (percentage of the tendon thickness torn).[32,33] The most commonly used classification is based on anatomic location and the depth of tendon tearing[32] (**Table 3**). This classification system fails to recognize several factors, including the extent of sagittal-plane tearing, the area of tearing, tissue quality, and etiology.

The interobserver reliability of rotator cuff classification systems has been questioned. Ten fellowship-trained orthopaedic shoulder surgeons evaluated 27 MRI studies from patients with a surgically confirmed rotator cuff tear.[34] Interobserver agreement was high for distinguishing between FTRCTs and PTRCTs and for identifying the location of a PTRCT (bursal or articular), but it was poor for identifying the grade of PTRCT. In a similar study using videotaped arthroscopy, interobserver agreement also was poor for grading PTRCTs.[35]

Table 2

Natural History of Partial-Thickness Rotator Cuff Tears Managed Nonsurgically

Study (Year)	*n*	Imaging Modality	Follow-up Period	Progression (%)
Kong et al[14] (2018)	81	1.5 T MRI	Mean: 19.9 ± 10.5 mo	13/81 increased in tear size[a] 48/81 unchanged 20/81 decreased in tear size
Lo et al[15] (2018)	37	1.5 T MRI or MRA	Mean: 53 ± 8 mo	9/37 increased in tear size (3/37 progressed to full-thickness tears)[b] 24/37 no change 4/37 decreased in tear size
Kim et al[19] (2017)	88	3.0 T MRI	Mean: 24.4 ± 19.5 mo	23/88 increased in tear size[c] 59/88 no change 6/88 decreased
Yamamoto et al[20] (2017)	83	1.5 T MRI	Mean: 18.6 mo (range: 12-60 mo)	28/83 increased in tear size[d] 49/83 unchanged
Keener et al[16] (2015)	56	USS	Median 5.1 yr (range: 0.3-10.0 yr)	24/56 increased in tear size[e] 30/56 no change
Maman et al[18] (2009)	26	1.5 T MRI	Mean 20 mo (range: 7-58 mo)	2/26 increased in tear size[f] 23/26 unchanged 1/26 decreased
Yamanaka and Matsumoto[13] (1994)	40	Arthrogram	Mean: 412 d	21 increased in tear size (11 of these progressed to FTRCT)[g] 4 unchanged 4 decreased

FTRCT = full-thickness rotator cuff tear, MRA = magnetic resonance arthrography, USS = ultrasound sonography

[a]Defined as increase in tear size: Footprint size ratio >20% as measured on T2 MRI coronal sequences.

[b]Tear size increase was defined as >25% of tendon thickness as measured on T2, fat-suppressed coronal oblique views on MRI or MRA.

[c]Defined as increase >2 mm in maximum medial-lateral (ML) or anterior-posterior (AP) dimensions as measured on T2 MRI sequences.

[d]Defined as increase >2 mm in maximum ML or AP dimensions as measured on T2 MRI sequences.

[e]Defined as >5 mm increase in ML or AP dimension as measured by serial ultrasonography.

[f]Defined as >5 mm increase in ML or AP dimensions as measured by T2 MRI sequences.

[g]Defined as small (<10 mm^2), medium (11-25 mm^2), or large (>26 mm^2) on AP arthrogram.

Nonsurgical Management

PTRCTs can be nonsurgically managed using various modalities, including physical therapy, steroid injection, and anti-inflammatory or pain medication. In addition, the introduction of various biologic modalities (eg, platelet-rich plasma [PRP]) has increased the management options for PTRCTs. Nonsurgical management may be more acceptable for PTRCTs than for FTRCTs because the risk of muscular atrophy, fatty infiltration, or catastrophic tear extension is minimal in PTRCTs. For example, at a mean follow-up of 24 months, only 3% of patients had a decrease in muscle volume and 10% of patients had progression of fatty infiltration in patients with PTRCTs treated nonsurgically.[19]

A 2018 study specifically evaluated the success of nonsurgical management of PTRCTs in 76 consecutive patients.[15] Approximately 50% of the patients initially were successfully treated nonsurgically, and 91% were satisfied with their treatment at a mean 46-month follow-up after initial assessment. Factors associated with success of nonsurgical management were low grade tears (<50% of tendon thickness), of the nondominant extremity with an atrauamatic onset of symptoms.[15]

Traditionally, corticosteroids have been used as a nonsurgical management modality with widespread empirical success. Although few studies have specifically evaluated PTRCTs, the potential effect of corticosteroids on the rotator cuff has recently come under scrutiny. Several recent large database studies have demonstrated negative

Table 3

Classification of Partial-Thickness Rotator Cuff Tears

Location	
Articular	
Bursal	
Intratendinous	
Grade	**Size of tear (percentage of tendon thickness)**
I	<3 mm (<25%)
II	3-6 mm (25%-50%)
III	>6 mm (>50%)

Adapted with permission from Ellman H: Diagnosis and treatment of incomplete rotator cuff tears. *Clin Orthop Relat Res* 1990;254:64-74.

associations between corticosteroid use and postoperative outcomes.[36-41] In one study of over 60,000 patients, those receiving a cortisone injection within 1 month of rotator cuff repair had a significantly higher incidence of postoperative infection.[37] Similarly, in another study of over 22,000 patients, those receiving an injection before rotator cuff repair had an increased likelihood of undergoing subsequent revision rotator cuff repair.[39] In addition, the number of injections and proximity of the injection to repair was also associated with increased rate of revision rotator cuff repair. Further investigations are required to evaluate causation in addition to the multifactorial nature of many of these outcomes.[37] However, these results should be interpreted in light of recent metaanalyses on the use of corticosteroids on rotator cuff disease, which demonstrated only a very small and transient benefit when compared with control patients.[40,41]

Recently, a number of studies have investigated the usage of various biologic agents for the treatment of PTRCTs. Of the cellular therapies, the most widely used is PRP, which involves isolating a centrifuged layer from the patient's own blood, rich in cytokines and growth factors, to administer at the site of pathology. Different systems and techniques are available, leading to a wide variety of preparations. In one case series, a single ultrasound-guided injection of leukocyte-rich PRP (1 mL volume) was administered to 25 patients with intratendinous PTRCTs.[42] At 6 months, 20/25 patients demonstrated a reduction in tear size on MRA. Another study randomized patients to four injection groups including normal saline (control), sodium hyaluronate (SH), PRP, and SH + PRP.[43] There were significant improvements in the American Shoulder and Elbow Surgeons Disability Index, Constant, and visual analog scale (VAS) scores with the greatest improvement demonstrated in patients receiving both SH and PRP. In addition, follow-up MRI at 12 months demonstrated improvements in the SH, PRP, and SH + PRP groups but with the greatest reduction in the anterior-posterior size of the tear in patients receiving both SH and PRP. In contrast, a double-blinded randomized controlled trial of 84 patients investigated the efficacy of two leukocyte-poor PRP injections, 1 month apart, compared with saline injections for intratendinous tears.[44] At 7 months, no differences were seen in the VAS for pain, single assessment numeric evaluation, or Constant scores, and there was no difference in the PTRCT volume as assessed by MRA. However, at final follow-up (mean 19.5 ± 5.3 months), a significantly higher rate of adverse events (frozen shoulder, pain >48 hours, tear extension) was noted in the PRP group (56%) versus the control group (26%). In addition, the authors noted that 7/42 patients in the PRP group underwent surgery versus 2/42 patients in the saline group.[44]

These mixed results may be related to the heterogeneity of the PRP preparations used. In addition, its actual biologic effect in the clinical setting is unclear. In one randomized study, patients who received PRP injections following arthroscopic subacromial decompression demonstrated increased apoptosis, reduced vascularity, and reduced cellularity in tissue biopsies harvested 3 months following surgery.[45] The results further highlight the importance of further high-quality preparation-specific randomized controlled trials to determine the efficacy of PRP either as a primary treatment or as a surgical adjunct.

Surgical Management

Indications

The indication for surgical management of PTRCTs is poorly defined but is based on patient factors (ie, age, activity level, occupation, and sports involvement), clinical factors (ie, traumatic history, severity of pain, weakness, and response to nonsurgical management), and pathologic factors (ie, bursal or articular surface and the percentage of tendon thickness torn). In one study, of patients with PTRCTs, younger patients with a lower functional comorbidity index and a bursal-surface tear were more likely to undergo surgical management.[46] In general, patients with a chronic tear and mild symptoms are initially treated nonsurgically. Surgical management may be considered for younger patients with a traumatic PTRCT involving more than 50% of the tendon or for a patient who has undergone adequate but unsuccessful nonsurgical management. One nonrandomized study has demonstrated no significant difference between immediate surgical intervention versus initial nonsurgical management and delayed repair supporting a trial period of nonsurgical management for PTRCTs.[47]

Rationale for the 50% Rule

The surgical options for treating a PTRCT include débridement or repair, with or without concurrent subacromial decompression. In general, débridement (with or without subacromial decompression) can be used for a patient with a PTRCT involving less than 50% of the tendon. Rotator cuff repair (with or without subacromial decompression) should be considered for a patient with a PTRCT involving more than 50% of the tendon. The rationale for surgically repairing PTRCTs involving more than 50% of the tendon thickness is largely based on a single retrospective study of 65 patients with a PTRCT involving more than 50% of the tendon thickness.[48] Thirty-two patients underwent an arthroscopic acromioplasty, and 33 patients were treated with arthroscopic acromioplasty followed by mini-open rotator cuff repair. At 2- to 7-year follow-up, the mean score on the University of California, Los Angeles (UCLA) Shoulder Rating Scale was 22.7 for patients who underwent arthroscopic acromioplasty and 31.6 for those who underwent arthroscopic acromioplasty and mini-open rotator cuff repair. Although this study had several weaknesses (eg, nonrandomized and retrospective), a recent small long-term study of 18 patients demonstrated that at a mean of 15 years (12 to 17 years) follow-up, patients who received rotator cuff repair had a higher Constant score (89 ± 5) than patients who underwent débridement alone (72 ± 25).[49]

Several biomechanical studies also have supported the so-called 50% rule. In a cadaver study, articular-surface PTRCTs of varying severity were subjected to cyclic load.[11] A significant increase in strain on the residual adjacent rotator cuff fibers occurred only if an articular-surface PTRCT was greater than 50% of the tendon thickness. Repair of the PTRCT returned the strain to its normal state. Another cadaver study created progressively larger bursal-surface PTRCTs in the supraspinatus tendon.[12] The strain in the intact tendon increased when the bursal-surface tear was more than 50% of the tendon thickness. As the depth of the tear increased, the stress on the residual intact tendon increased nonlinearly.

Although the percentage of torn tendon thickness is a factor in determining the surgical procedure, other significant variables (patient, clinical, and pathologic factors) also should be considered before making a decision.

Arthroscopic Débridement and Subacromial Decompression

Arthroscopic débridement commonly is performed for a PTRCT involving less than 50% of the tendon thickness (a grade I or II tear), with good to excellent results as measured using validated shoulder-specific scales.[50-57] The addition of subacromial decompression has not been shown to significantly improve symptoms.[58] Although arthroscopic débridement (with or without acromioplasty) can lead to good results, one study found that certain tears are relatively likely to fail after arthroscopic débridement.[52] At a mean 52-month follow-up, more than 90% of the patients had a good outcome, but the procedure was considered a failure in 8% of the patients, most of whom had a bursal-surface PTRCT. The risk of failure was 29% after arthroscopic débridement and acromioplasty in patients with a bursal-surface PTRCT and 38% in those with more extensive bursal-surface tearing. The study results suggested that repair should be considered for a bursal-surface PTRCT, even if the tear involves less than 50% of the tendon.

The long-term results of arthroscopic débridement or decompression are unclear. At a mean 101-month follow-up, patients had a mean Constant score of 65 for the treated shoulder, which was approximately 20 points lower than the score for the contralateral shoulder.[53] After arthroscopic débridement, only 57% of the patients were able to return without symptoms to their preoperative level of sports; 20% were able to return to sports at a lower level because of ongoing symptoms; and 22% were unable to participate in sports.[51] In even higher-level overhead athletes, there was a 55% return-to-play rate at the same level or higher.[56] In contrast, in the longest reported follow-up at a mean of 22 years (range: 21 to 25 years), the reported relative Constant score was 101 (SD, 22) and the mean Western Ontario Rotator Cuff score was 81% (SD, 20%) in patients with PTRCTs treatment with acromioplasty and débridement.[59]

Anatomically, arthroscopic débridement (with or without decompression) does not appear to heal a PTRCT or prevent its progression. For example, in 46 patients with an articular-surface PTRCT, ultrasonography revealed progression to an FTRCT in 3 patients (6.5%) at a mean 4.2-year follow-up after arthroscopic acromioplasty and débridement.[54] As expected however, with longer follow-up, the rate of tear progression increases. At a mean 8.4-year follow-up after arthroscopic acromioplasty and débridement, 9 of 26 patients (35%) had ultrasonographically detected progression to an FTRCT.[53] Similarly, at a mean follow-up of 21 to 25 years following arthroscopic débridement and acromioplasty, 16/38 patients (42%) with PTRCTs had progressed to an FTRCT.[59] However, only three patients (7%) had evidence of cuff tear arthropathy (Hamada II or more).

Arthroscopic Repair

Several surgical techniques have been described for the repair of PTRCTs, including in situ techniques and conversion of the partial tear to an FTRCT. Conversion to a FTRCT is advantageous because it allows standard arthroscopic techniques to be used for repair. In situ techniques, such as transtendon or all-intra-articular repair, maintain the integrity of at least a portion of the intact rotator cuff. In situ techniques are particularly relevant for articular-surface PTRCTs, in which maintaining the intact lateral rotator cuff can be considered. Maintenance of a viable and robust lateral tendon may allow a more anatomic reconstruction of the rotator cuff footprint.

The biomechanical performance of techniques for repairing a PTRCT has been evaluated in several studies. Transtendon repair was compared with full-thickness conversion followed by double-row repair for 50% articular-surface PTRCTs.[60] Under cyclic loading, gap formation was significantly less, and ultimate failure strength was significantly greater after the transtendon repair. In an ovine model of PTRCT, the footprint contact pressure and the strength of various repair techniques were evaluated.[61] Transtendon repair and double-row repair had similar contact pressures, but transtendon repair had a significantly higher ultimate load to failure.

Although there may be theoretical advantages to maintaining the intact portion of the rotator cuff, nonrandomized clinical studies have not clearly shown a substantial superiority of transtendon repair over conversion to an FTRCT and the subsequent repair[62-85] (**Tables 4 and 5**). Most clinical studies of PTRCT conversion to FTRCT have reported excellent results, with rates of patient satisfaction greater than 90%.[62-65,74] Rotator cuff healing has been shown to occur in most patients after PTRCT conversion to FTRCT. Similarly, transtendon rotator cuff repair has had excellent results, with significant improvement in shoulder-specific scores and patient satisfaction rates greater than 90%[66-70,74,75,79,84] (**Table 4**). In addition, diagnostic imaging studies following transtendon repair have also demonstrated high rates of healing.

Four randomized controlled trials have compared transtendon repair versus completion to a full-thickness tear in articular-sided PTRCTs.[86-88] Three of these studies were included in a meta-analysis of 182 shoulders with

Table 4

Clinical and Anatomic Outcomes in Selected Case Series Using Conversion to Full-Thickness Tear or Transtendon Repair Technique

Study	*n*	Type of Repair	Mean Follow-up (months)	Clinical Outcomes Measure: Preoperative → Postoperative Score	Anatomic Outcome (Imaging Method)
Kamath et al[64] (2009)	42	Conversion	39	ASES: 46.1 → 82.1	21% retear (USS)
Chung et al[80] (2015)	34	Conversion	28.4	VAS: 7.65 → 0.75 UCLA: 18 → 27.12 ASES: 44.45 → 90.58	35% retears (CTA)
Iyengar et al[65] (2011)	22	Conversion	N/A (min 24)	UCLA: 19.1 → 32.9	18% retear (MRI)
Castricini et al[69] (2009)	31	TT repair	33	Constant: 44.4 → 91.6	zero intact (MRI)
Xiao et al[79] (2015)	59	TT repair	37.6	UCLA: 17.3 → 33.3 Constant: 65.3 → 93.9	14% partial retears (MRI)
Ostrander et al[84] (2017)	20	TT repair	32.7	UCLA: N/A → 33.5[a] SST: N/A → 11.5[a] Constant: ? → 86[a]	10% partial retears (USS)
Castricini et al[74] (2019)	153	Conversion: 94 TT repair: 59	73.9	Constant: 47.7 → 84.2	13.7% retear (USS)
Kim[b] et al[81] (2019)	30	Conversion: 16 TT repair: 14	29.4	VAS: 5.8 → 2.5 ASES: 39.8 → 72.8 UCLA: 21.2 → 31.1 Constant: 57.2 → 76	11% retear (MRI/USS)

ASES = American Shoulder and Elbow Surgeons Disability Index, Conversion = conversion to a full-thickness tear, CTA = computed tomography arthrogram, MRA = magnetic resonance imaging arthrogram, N/A = not available, TT repair = transtendon repair, VAS = visual analog scale score, UCLA = University of California, Los Angeles, USS = ultrasound sonography, VAS = visual analog scale score

[a]Only postoperative scores reported.

[b]Only intratendinous tears included.

Table 5

Summary of Outcomes of Transtendon Versus Conversion to Full-Thickness Tear and Repair in Randomized Controlled Trials

Study (Year)	Allocation	Follow-up	Outcomes
Shin[86] (2012)	Conversion: 24 TT repair: 24	31 mo	ASES, Constant, VAS, ROM: • Conversion better at 3 mo • NSD at final F/U MRI (postoperative 6 mo) • TT repair: no retears • Conversion: 2/24 retears
Franceschi et al[87] (2013)	Conversion: 28 TT repair: 32	38 mo	ASES, Constant, ROM: All NSD MRI (final F/U) • Conversion 1/32 retear • TT repair 1/32 retear
Castagna et al[88] (2015)	Conversion: 37 TT repair: 37	>2 yr	Constant, VAS: All NSD at final F/U
Kim et al[89,a] (2015)	Conversion: 45 TT repair: 47	19.1 mo	ASES, Constant, SST, VAS, KSS, ROM: All NSD MRI (6-12 mo postoperative) • Articular tears: NSD in retear rate between groups • Bursal tears: Higher retear rate in conversion TT repair: 1 retear Conversion: 7 retears

ASES = American Shoulder and Elbow Surgeons Disability Index, Constant = Constant-Murley Score, Conversion = conversion to a full-thickness tear, F/U = follow-up, KSS = Korean Shoulder Score, NSD = no significant difference, ROM = range of motion, TT repair = transtendon repair, VAS = visual analog scale score for pain

[a]Included both bursal-surface and articular-surface partial-thickness rotator cuff tears.

a mean age 54 years (range: 21 to 71 years).[90] Overall, the quality of the studies was considered high using the Coleman score. At a mean follow-up of 40.5 months, both groups demonstrated significant improvement following surgery, but there were no significant differences in Constant score, American Shoulder and Elbow Surgeons Disability Index score, VAS score, or range of motion between the transtendon repair versus completion to a full-thickness tear. In addition, two of three studies reported healing rate using MRI with no significant differences noted between surgical groups (transtendon repair group: 98.2% healed versus completion to a full-thickness tear group: 94.2% healed). This study concluded that both techniques therefore were viable options when surgically repairing PTRCTs. In the fourth study, not included in the aforementioned meta-analysis, there was also no clinical difference noted between the two groups.[89] However, when analyzing radiologic outcomes in bursal-sided tears, seven retears were noted in the conversion to FTRCT and repair group compared with no retears in the transtendon group. No difference in retear incidence was noted for articular-sided tears. Another systematic review including lesser quality nonrandomized observational studies concluded that although the clinical outcomes and healing rates were similar, transtendon repair yielded higher rates of postoperative stiffness in the first 3 months and therefore the authors advocated completion to a full-thickness tear.[91] The debate for the optimal surgical management continues, and high quality, well-powered randomized controlled trials are needed to answer the question definitively.

Patch Augmentation

Biological augmentation during massive rotator cuff repair has gained wide attention. Recently, a highly porous, bioinductive bovine collagen graft has been introduced for the treatment of PTRCTs. Two small clinical studies have been published which have evaluated the use of bioinductive grafting of PTRCTs without formal repair.[92,93] In one study, 33 patients demonstrated improvement in the American Shoulder and Elbow Surgeons Disability Index and Constant scores at 12 months postoperatively. In addition, follow-up MRI demonstrated a reduction in tear size in 23 of 32 patients, no defect identifiable on MRI in 8 of 32 patients, and 1 patient remained unchanged. Another study of 13 patients demonstrated incorporation of the graft with induction of new tissue formation and thickening of the tendon by serial MRI.[92] Although still considered investigational, these alternative treatments may have rehabilitation advantages and may herald a new paradigm shift in the surgical management of PTRCTs.

SUMMARY

Despite the number of published studies related to PTRCTs, their optimal management continues to be debated. It is likely that different types of PTRCTs have different etiologic factors, leading to different natural histories and successes after nonsurgical or surgical management. In patients with tears smaller than 50%, arthroscopic débridement with or without subacromial decompression can lead to an excellent short-term result. However, the long-term results of using this technique are unclear. Surgical repair usually is considered for younger, more active patients, with a tear larger than 50%, and it has led to excellent clinical results. Although several repair techniques have been described, the published literature is insufficient for determining whether any single technique is superior to the other. Biologic treatments continue to be developed and require further high-quality long-term studies to determine their efficacy and place in the management of PTRCTs.

KEY STUDY POINTS

- Partial-thickness rotator cuff tears vary in prevalence and increase with age. Many are likely asymptomatic making clinical correlation essential.
- The natural history of PTRCTs has been described showing a moderate risk of tear progression in the midterm.
- Nonsurgical management can be successful in improving symptoms and avoiding surgery in the short term to midterm; however, long-term outcomes are not known. Surgical intervention should be based on individual patients' needs, severity of symptoms, and preferences for treatment.
- Surgery is successful in the majority or patients. No significant clinical or radiologic differences were noted in randomized controlled trials comparing surgical techniques.
- Biologics including cellular therapies and biologic patches have shown promise, but their clinical efficacy has yet to be conclusively proven.

Annotated References

1. Clark JM, Harryman DT II: Tendons, ligaments, and capsule of the rotator cuff. Gross and microscopic anatomy. *J Bone Joint Surg Am* 1992;74(5):713-725.
2. Curtis AS, Burbank KM, Tierney JJ, et al: The insertional footprint of the rotator cuff: An anatomic study. *Arthroscopy* 2006;22(6):609.e1. doi:10.1016/j.arthro.2006.04.001.
3. Ruotolo C, Fow JE, Nottage WM: The supraspinatus footprint: An anatomic study of the supraspinatus insertion. *Arthroscopy* 2004;20(3):246-249. doi:10.1016/j.arthro.2004.01.002.
4. Mochizuki T, Sugaya H, Uomizu M, et al: Humeral insertion of the supraspinatus and infraspinatus. New anatomical findings regarding the footprint of the rotator cuff. Surgical technique. *J Bone Joint Surg Am* 2009;91(suppl 2, pt 1):1-7. doi:10.2106/JBJS.H.01426.
5. Nimura A, Kato A, Yamaguchi K, et al: The superior capsule of the shoulder joint complements the insertion of the rotator cuff. *J Shoulder Elbow Surg* 2012;21(7):867-872. doi:10.1016/j.jse.2011.04.034.
6. Sano H, Ishii H, Trudel G, et al: Histologic evidence of degeneration at the insertion of 3 rotator cuff tendons: A comparative study with human cadaveric shoulders. *J Shoulder Elbow Surg* 1999;8(6):574-579.
7. Fukuda H: Partial-thickness rotator cuff tears: A modern view on Codman's classic. *J Shoulder Elbow Surg* 2000;9(2):163-168. doi:10.1067/mse.2000.101959.
8. Sher J, Uribe J, Posada A, et al: Abnormal findings on magnetic resonance Images of asymptomatic shoulders. *J Bone Joint Surg Am* 1995;77(1):10-15.
9. Lohr J, Uhthoff H: The microvascular pattern of the supraspinatus tendon. *Clin Orthop Relat Res* 1990;254:35-38.
10. Burkhart SS, Morgan CD, Kibler WB: The disabled throwing shoulder: Spectrum of pathology. Part I: Pathoanatomy and biomechanics. *Arthroscopy* 2003;19(4):404-420. doi:10.1053/jars.2003.50128.
11. Mazzocca AD, Rincon LM, O'Connor RW, et al: Intra-articular partial-thickness rotator cuff tears: Analysis of injured and repaired strain behavior. *Am J Sports Med* 2008;36(1):110-116. doi:10.1177/0363546507307502.
12. Yang S, Park HS, Flores S, et al: Biomechanical analysis of bursal-sided partial thickness rotator cuff tears. *J Shoulder Elbow Surg* 2009;18(3):379-385. doi:10.1016/j.jse.2008.12.011.
13. Yamanaka K, Matsumoto T: The joint side tear of the rotator cuff: A followup study by arthrography. *Clin Orthop Relat Res* 1994;304:68-73.

14. Kong BY, Cho M, Lee HR, et al: Structural evolution of nonoperatively treated high-grade partial-thickness tears of the supraspinatus tendon. *Am J Sports Med* 2018;46(1):79-86. doi:10.1177/0363546517729164.

An observational study of 81 of 362 patients diagnosed with high-grade PTRCT who received nonsurgical treatment and minimum follow-up of 12 months (range: 12 to 52 months). Follow-up MRI demonstrated 13 of 81 patients had more than 20% increase in tear size (3 had an FTRCT), 48 of 81 had an unchanged tear size, and 20 of 81 improved in tear size by >20% (10 were considered normal MRI at follow-up). The authors concluded that even high-grade PTRCTs can be monitored and do not progress as often as previously thought. Level of evidence: IV.

15. Lo IK, Denkers MR, More KD, et al: Partial-thickness rotator cuff tears: Clinical and imaging outcomes and prognostic factors of successful nonoperative treatment. *Open Access J Sports Med* 2018;9:191-197. doi:10.2147/OAJSM.S153236.

The nonsurgical management of PTRCTs was reviewed in 74 patients. The success rate was approximately 50%. Patients with an atraumatic onset involving the nondominant extremity and a tear of less than 50% were most likely to have a successful result. Level of evidence: IV.

16. Keener JD, Galatz LM, Teefey SA, et al: A prospective evaluation of survivorship of asymptomatic degenerative rotator cuff tears. *J Bone Joint Surg Am* 2015;97(2):89-98. doi:10.2106/JBJS.N.00099.

A prospective longitudinal clinical and ultrasound study of 224 patients at a median follow-up of 5.1 years demonstrated tear enlargement in 49% of shoulders, which was associated with the development of pain. Level of evidence: II.

17. Mall NA, Kim HM, Keener JD, et al: Symptomatic progression of asymptomatic rotator cuff tears: A prospective study of clinical and sonographic variables. *J Bone Joint Surg Am* 2010;92(16):2623-2633. doi:10.2106/JBJS.I.00506.

18. Maman E, Harris C, White L, et al: Outcome of nonoperative treatment of symptomatic rotator cuff tears monitored by magnetic resonance imaging. *J Bone Joint Surg Am* 2009;91(8):1898-1906. doi:10.2106/jbjs.G.01335.

19. Kim YS, Kim SE, Bae SH, et al: Tear progression of symptomatic full-thickness and partial-thickness rotator cuff tears as measured by repeated MRI. *Knee Surg Sports Traumatol Arthrosc* 2017;25(7):2073-2080. doi:10.1007/s00167-016-4388-3.

In an observational study of RCTs that were treated nonsurgically, 88 patients had PTRCTs. Follow-up MRI demonstrated that FTRCTs (28/34 increased in size) enlarged more often than PTRCTs (23/88 increased in size). Overall, PTRCTs increased in size in 23/88 patients, decreased in size in 6/88 patients, and had no significant change in 59/88 patients. Fatty infiltration progressed in 9 of 88 and muscle volume decreased in 3 of 88. Level of evidence: IV.

20. Yamamoto N, Mineta M, Kawakami J, et al: Risk factors for tear progression in symptomatic rotator cuff tears: A prospective study of 174 shoulders. *Am J Sports Med* 2017;45(11):2524-2531. doi:10.1177/0363546517709780.

Prospective study of 174 shoulders with full-thickness or partial-thickness rotator cuff tears with at least two MRI scans a mean of 19 months demonstrating 47% of shoulder with tear progression and a higher risk of progression in medium-sized tears, full-thickness tears, and smokers. Level of evidence: III.

21. Teefey S, Rubin D, Middleton W, et al: Detection and quantification of rotator cuff tears. Comparison of ultrasonographic, magnetic resonance imaging, and arthroscopic findings in seventy-one consecutive cases. *J Bone Joint Surg Am* 2004;86(4):708-716.

22. Teefey S, Middleton W, Payne W, et al: Detection and measurement of rotator cuff tears with sonography: Analysis of diagnostic errors. *AJR Am J Roentgenol* 2005;184(6):1768-1773.

23. Murphy R, Daines M, Carr A, et al: An independent learning method for orthopaedic surgeons performing shoulder ultrasound to identify full-thickness tears of the rotator cuff. *J Bone Joint Surg Am* 2013;95:266-272. doi:10.2106/JBJS,K.00706.

A training study of orthopaedic surgeons without previous ultrasound experience demonstrated that approximately 50 to 100 scans are required following specific training protocol to demonstrate predictive values comparable to results of experienced radiologists. Level of evidence: I.

24. Moosmayer S, Smith HJ: Diagnostic ultrasound of the shoulder – A method for experts only? Results from an orthopedic surgeon with relative inexpensive compared to operative findings. *Acta Orthop* 2005;76(4):503-508. doi:10.1080/17453670510041484.

25. Ok JH, Kim YS, Kim JM, et al: Learning curve of office-based ultrasonography for rotator cuff tendons tears. *Knee Surg Sports Traumatol Arthrosc* 2013;21(7):1593-1597. doi:10.1007/s00167-012-2105-4.

A diagnostic accuracy study comparing in-office ultrasonography by novice orthopaedic surgeons and MRA with arthroscopy demonstrated similar accuracy for full-thickness tear detection but less accuracy for partial-thickness tears and tear size. Level of evidence: II.

26. Lenza M, Buchbinder R, Takwoingi Y, et al: Magnetic resonance imaging, magnetic resonance arthrography and ultrasonography for assessing rotator cuff tears in people with shoulder pain for whom surgery is being considered. *Cochrane Database Syst Rev* 2013;2013(9):CD009020. doi:10.1002/14651858.CD009020.pub2.

A Cochrane systematic review and meta-analysis demonstrated that for diagnosing PTRCTs the sensitivity of MRI was 74% (95% CI, 59% to 85%) and specificity was 93% (84% to 97%), and the sensitivity for USS was 52% (33% to 70%), which was not statistically significant. All studies were deemed to be at risk of bias because of methodological flaws. Level of evidence: I.

27. Jeyam M, Funk L, Harris J: Are shoulder surgeons any good at diagnosing rotator cuff tears using ultrasound?: A comparative analysis of surgeon vs radiologist. *Int J Shoulder Surg* 2008;2(1):4-6.

28. Roy JS, Braen C, Leblond J, et al: Diagnostic accuracy of ultrasonography, MRI and MR arthrography in the characterisation of rotator cuff disorders: A systematic review and meta-analysis. *Br J Sports Med* 2015;49(20):1316-1328. doi:10.1136/bjsports-2014-094148.

A meta-analysis of imaging studies demonstrated that for PTRCTs the sensitivity for ultrasonography was 0.68; for MRI, 0.67; and for MRA, 0.83, and the specificity for ultrasonography was 0.94; for MRI, 0.94; and for MRA, 0.93. A higher sensitivity and specificity for 3 T magnet versus 1.5 T magnet in MRI were demonstrated although these were found to be not statistically significant. Level of evidence: I.

29. de Jesus JO, Parker L, Frangos AJ, et al: Accuracy of MRI, MR arthrography, and ultrasound in the diagnosis of rotator cuff tears: A meta-analysis. *AJR Am J Roentgenol* 2009;192(6):1701-1707. doi:10.2214/AJR.08.1241.

30. Jung JY, Jee WH, Chun HJ, et al: Magnetic resonance arthrography including ABER view in diagnosing partial-thickness tears of the rotator cuff: Accuracy, and inter- and intra-observer agreements. *Acta Radiol* 2010;51(2):194-201. doi:10.3109/02841850903300298.

31. Herold T, Bachthaler M, Hamer O, et al: Indirect MR arthrography of the shoulder: Use of abduction and external rotation to detect full- and partial-thickness tears of the supraspinatus tendon. *Radiology* 2006;240(1):152-160.

32. Ellman H: Diagnosis and treatment of incomplete rotator cuff tears. *Clin Orthop Relat Res* 1990;254:64-74.

33. Snyder S: *Arthroscopic classification of rotator cuff lesions and surgical decision making*, in *Shoulder Arthroscopy*, 2nd ed. Philadelphia, PA, Lippincott Williams & Wilkins, 2003, pp 201-207.

34. Spencer EE Jr, Dunn WR, Wright RW, et al: Interobserver agreement in the classification of rotator cuff tears using magnetic resonance imaging. *Am J Sports Med* 2008;36(1):99-103. doi:10.1177/0363546507307504.

35. Kuhn JE, Dunn WR, Ma B, et al: Interobserver agreement in the classification of rotator cuff tears. *Am J Sports Med* 2007;35(3):437-441. doi:10.1177/0363546506298108.

36. Kew ME, Cancienne JM, Christensen JE, Werner BC: The timing of corticosteroid injections after arthroscopic shoulder procedures affects postoperative infection risk. *Am J Sports Med* 2019;47(4):915-921.

An insurance database study of 3,946 patients demonstrated that patients who underwent corticosteroid injection within 1 month following rotator cuff repair had a significantly higher rate of infection. Level of evidence: III.

37. Forsythe B, Agarwalla A, Puzzitielleo RN, Sumner S, Romeo AA, Mascarenhas R: The timing of injections prior to arthroscopic rotator cuff repair impacts the risk of surgical site infection. *J Bone Joint Surg Am* 2019;101(8):682-687.

A database study of over 60,000 patients demonstrated multiple factors associated with increased risk of surgical site infection including male sex, obesity, diabetes, smoking status, and preoperative corticosteroid injection within 1 month of arthroscopic rotator cuff repair. Level of evidence: III.

38. Traven SA, Brinton D, Simpson KN, et al: Preoperative shoulder injections are associated with increased risk of revision rotator cuff repair. *Arthroscopy* 2019;35(3):706-713.

An insurance database study of 4,959 patients demonstrated that patients who underwent an injection 6 months before rotator cuff repair were more likely to undergo revision rotator cuff repair within 3 years. Level of evidence: III.

39. Weber AE, Trasolini NA, Mayer EN, et al: Injections prior to rotator cuff repair are associated with increased rotator cuff revision rates. *Arthroscopy* 2019;35(3):717-724.

An insurance database study of approximately 22,000 patients demonstrated correlation between preoperative corticosteroid injections and revision rotator cuff repair, which was frequency-dependent and time-dependent. Level of evidence: III.

40. Mahamadi A, Chan JJ, Claessen MA, Ring D, Chen NC: Corticosteroid injections give small and transient pain relief in rotator cuff tendinosis: A meta-analysis. *Clin Orthop Rel Res* 2017;475:232-243.

A meta-analysis of 11 studies involving 726 patients demonstrated small and transient benefit of corticosteroid injections in patients with rotator cuff tendinosis when compared with placebo controls at 4 and 8 weeks but not at 3 months. Level of evidence: I.

41. Cook T, Minns Lowe C, Maybury M, Lewsi JS: Are corticosteroid injections more beneficial than anaesthetic injections alone in the management of rotator cuff-related shoulder pain? A systematic review. *Br J Sports Med* 2018;52(8):497-504.

A meta-analysis of 13 studies of 1,013 patients demonstrated short-term benefit of corticosteroid injections when compared with local anesthetic injections at 8 weeks but not with longer follow-up. Level of evidence: II.

42. Ladermann A, Zumstein MA, Kolo FC, et al: In vivo clinical and radiological effects of platelet-rich plasma on interstitial supraspinatus lesion: Case series. *Orthop Traumatol Surg Res* 2016;102(8):977-982. doi:10.1016/j.otsr.2016.09.010.

A prospective case series of 25 patients with partial-thickness interstitial tears of the supraspinatus tendon demonstrated a decrease in tear volume and an improvement in clinical outcome scores following ultrasound-guided injection of leukocytes and platelet-rich plasma. Level of evidence: II.

43. Cai YU, Sun Z, Liao B, et al: Sodium hyaluronate and platelet-rich plasma for partial-thickness rotator cuff tears. *Med Sci Sports Exerc* 2019;51(2):227-233. doi:10.1249/MSS.0000000000001781.

A prospective double-blind randomized controlled trial comparing multiple injections of normal saline control, sodium hyaluronate (SH), platelet-rich plasma (PRP), and SH with PRP in 200 patients with partial-thickness rotator cuff tears demonstrated that clinical outcomes improved in patients receiving PRP or SH and PRP with a reduction in tear size. Level of evidence: I.

44. Schwitzguebel AJ, Kolo FC, Tirefort J, et al: Efficacy of platelet-rich plasma for the treatment of interstitial supraspinatus tears: A double-blinded, randomized controlled trial. *Am J Sports Med* 2019;47(8):1885-1892. doi:10.1177/0363546519851097.

A prospective randomized controlled trial compared leukocyte-poor PRP versus saline control in 84 patients with interstitial PTRCTs. At 7 months follow-up, there was no difference in clinical outcome scores or by MRA. At final follow-up, there was a higher adverse event rate (eg, frozen shoulder, persistent pain, and tear extension) in the PRP group and more had undergone surgery. Level of evidence: I.

45. Carr AJ, Murphy R, Dakin SG, et al: Platelet-rich plasma injection with arthroscopic acromioplasty for chronic rotator cuff tendinopathy: A randomized controlled trial. *Am J Sports Med* 2015;43(12):2891-2897. doi:10.1177/0363546515608485.

A prospective randomized trial of 60 patients compared arthroscopic acromioplasty with or without platelet-rich plasma injection. At 2 years follow-up, there was no significant difference in outcome scores between groups; however, tissue biopsies at 12 weeks after surgery demonstrated increased apoptosis and reduced cellularity in patients receiving platelet-rich plasma. Level of evidence: I.

46. Camurcu Y, Ucpunar H, Ari H, et al: Predictors of allocation to surgery in patients older than 50 years with partial-thickness rotator cuff tear. *J Shoulder Elbow Surg* 2019;28(5):828-832. doi:10.1016/j.jse.2018.12.014.

A retrospective study of 272 patients with partial-thickness rotator cuff tears demonstrated by multivariate analysis that patients with a lower functional comorbidity index and bursal-sided tears were more likely to undergo surgery. Level of evidence: II.

47. Kim YS, Lee HJ, Kim JH, et al: When should we repair partial-thickness rotator cuff tears? Outcome comparison between immediate surgical repair versus delayed repair after 6-month period of nonsurgical treatment. *Am J Sports Med* 2018;46(5):1091-1096. doi:10.1177/0363546518757425.

A prospective randomized study of 78 consecutive patients with partial-thickness rotator cuff tears comparing immediate surgical repair versus delayed repair after a 6-month period of nonsurgical treatment demonstrated no significant difference in clinical outcomes or retear rate between groups at final follow-up. Decreased pain and improved American Shoulder and Elbow Surgeons Disability Index score were demonstrated at 6 months in patients with delayed surgical repair. Level of evidence: II.

48. Weber S: Arthroscopic debridement and acromioplasty versus mini-open repair in the treatment of significant partial-thickness rotator cuff tears. *Arthroscopy* 1999;15(2):126-131.

49. Plachel F, Korn G, Traweger A, et al: Long-term results after arthroscopic treatment of symptomatic Ellman grade 2 PASTA lesions. *J Shoulder Elbow Surg* 2019;28(7):1356-1362. doi:10.1016/j.jse.2018.12.002.

This is a long-term retrospective study of 18 patients following arthroscopic rotator cuff repair (11 patients) or arthroscopic débridement and acromioplasty (7 patients) for grade II articular-surface partial-thickness rotator cuff tears. At a mean 15 years follow-up, 94 patients were satisfied with their treatment with a mean Constant score of 78 ± 21 points. Level of evidence: IV.

50. Dwyer T, Razmjou H, Henry P, et al: Short-term outcomes of arthroscopic debridement and selected acromioplasty of bursal- vs articular-sided partial-thickness rotator cuff tears of less than 50. *Orthop J Sports Med* 2018;6(8):2325967118792001. doi:10.1177/2325967118792001.

This is a retrospective analysis of prospectively collected data on 76 patients with bursal-surface (36 patients) or articular-surface (40 patients) rotator cuff tears treated with arthroscopic débridement and selective acromioplasty. At 2 years follow-up, patients demonstrated improvement in clinical outcomes but with no significant difference between the two types of tears. Level of evidence: III.

51. Budoff JE, Rodin D, Ochiai D, et al: Arthroscopic rotator cuff debridement without decompression for the treatment of tendinosis. *Arthroscopy* 2005;21(9):1081-1089. doi:10.1016/j.arthro.2005.05.019.

52. Cordasco F, Backer M, Craig E, et al: The partial-thickness rotator cuff tear: Is acromioplasty without repair sufficient? *Am J Sports Med* 2002;30(2):257-260.

53. Kartus J, Kartus C, Rostgard-Christensen L, et al: Long-term clinical and ultrasound evaluation after arthroscopic acromioplasty in patients with partial rotator cuff tears. *Arthroscopy* 2006;22(1):44-49. doi:10.1016/j.arthro.2005.07.027.

54. Liem D, Alci S, Dedy N, et al: Clinical and structural results of partial supraspinatus tears treated by subacromial decompression without repair. *Knee Surg Sports Traumatol Arthrosc* 2008;16(10):967-972. doi:10.1007/s00167-008-0580-4.

55. Park J, Yoo M, Kim M: Comparison of surgical outcome between bursal and articular partial thickness rotator cuff tears. *Orthopedics* 2003;26(4):387-390.

56. Reynolds SB, Dugas JR, Cain EL, et al: Debridement of small partial-thickness rotator cuff tears in elite overhead throwers. *Clin Orthop Relat Res* 2008;466(3):614-621. doi:10.1007/s11999-007-0107-1.

57. Snyder S, Pachelli A, Del Pizzo W, et al: Partial thickness rotator cuff tears: Results of arthroscopic treatment. *Arthroscopy* 1991;7(1):1-7.

58. Strauss EJ, Salata MJ, Kercher J, et al: Multimedia article. The arthroscopic management of partial-thickness rotator cuff tears: A systematic review of the literature. *Arthroscopy* 2011;27(4):568-580. doi:10.1016/j.arthro.2010.09.019.

59. Ranebo MC, Bjornsson Hallgren HC, Norlin R, et al: Clinical and structural outcome 22 years after acromioplasty without tendon repair in patients with subacromial pain and cuff tears. *J Shoulder Elbow Surg* 2017;26(7):1262-1270. doi:10.1016/j.jse.2016.11.012.

    Retrospective analysis of 69 patients a mean of 22 years following acromioplasty without tendon repair demonstrating in patients with full-thickness tears, 87% of patients had an increase in tear size and 74% of patients had evidence of cuff tear arthropathy on radiography. In patients with partial-thickness rotator cuff tears, 42% had an increase in tear size and 7% had evidence of cuff tear arthropathy on radiography. Level of evidence: IV.

60. Gonzalez-Lomas G, Kippe MA, Brown GD, et al: In situ transtendon repair outperforms tear completion and repair for partial articular-sided supraspinatus tendon tears. *J Shoulder Elbow Surg* 2008;17(5):722-728. doi:10.1016/j.jse.2008.01.148.

61. Peters KS, Lam PH, Murrell GA: Repair of partial-thickness rotator cuff tears: A biomechanical analysis of footprint contact pressure and strength in an ovine model. *Arthroscopy* 2010;26(7):877-884. doi:10.1016/j.arthro.2010.04.007.

62. Porat S, Nottage WM, Fouse MN: Repair of partial thickness rotator cuff tears: A retrospective review with minimum two-year follow-up. *J Shoulder Elbow Surg* 2008;17(5):729-731. doi:10.1016/j.jse.2008.02.019.

63. Deutsch A: Arthroscopic repair of partial-thickness tears of the rotator cuff. *J Shoulder Elbow Surg* 2007;16(2):193-201. doi:10.1016/j.jse.2006.07.001.

64. Kamath G, Galatz LM, Keener JD, et al: Tendon integrity and functional outcome after arthroscopic repair of high-grade partial-thickness supraspinatus tears. *J Bone Joint Surg Am* 2009;91(5):1055-1062. doi:10.2106/JBJS.G.00118.

65. Iyengar JJ, Porat S, Burnett KR, et al: Magnetic resonance imaging tendon integrity assessment after arthroscopic partial-thickness rotator cuff repair. *Arthroscopy* 2011;27(3):306-313. doi:10.1016/j.arthro.2010.08.017.

66. Waibl B, Buess E: Partial-thickness articular surface supraspinatus tears: A new transtendon suture technique. *Arthroscopy* 2005;21(3):376-381. doi:10.1016/j.arthro.2004.11.008.

67. Ide J, Maeda S, Takagi K: Arthroscopic transtendon repair of partial-thickness articular-side tears of the rotator cuff: Anatomical and clinical study. *Am J Sports Med* 2005;33(11):1672-1679. doi:10.1177/0363546505277141.

68. Castagna A, Delle Rose G, Conti M, et al: Predictive factors of subtle residual shoulder symptoms after transtendinous arthroscopic cuff repair: A clinical study. *Am J Sports Med* 2009;37(1):103-108. doi:10.1177/0363546508324178.

69. Castricini R, Panfoli N, Nittoli R, et al: Transtendon arthroscopic repair of partial-thickness, articular surface tears of the supraspinatus: Results at 2 years. *Chir Organi Mov* 2009;93(suppl 1):S49-S54. doi:10.1007/s12306-009-0002-x.

70. Seo YJ, Yoo YS, Kim DY, et al: Trans-tendon arthroscopic repair for partial-thickness articular side tears of the rotator cuff. *Knee Surg Sports Traumatol Arthrosc* 2011;19(10):1755-1759. doi:10.1007/s00167-010-1362-3.

71. Tauber M, Koller H, Resch H: Transosseous arthroscopic repair of partial articular-surface supraspinatus tendon tears. *Knee Surg Sports Traumatol Arthrosc* 2008;16(6):608-613. doi:10.1007/s00167-008-0532-z.

72. Spencer EE Jr: Partial-thickness articular surface rotator cuff tears: An all-inside repair technique. *Clin Orthop Relat Res* 2010;468(6):1514-1520. doi:10.1007/s11999-009-1215-x.

73. Castagna A, Gumina S, Borroni M, et al: Partial articular-sided supraspinatus tear: A comparison between transtendon repair and tear completion and repair, in American Shoulder and Elbow Surgeons , ed. *American Shoulder and Elbow Surgeons Annual Closed Meeting Proceedings.* White Sulpher Springs, VA, American Shoulder and Elbow Surgeons, 2011.

74. Castricini R, La Camera F, De Gori M, et al: Functional outcomes and repair integrity after arthroscopic repair of partial articular supraspinatus tendon avulsion. *Arch Orthop Trauma Surg* 2019;139(3):369-375. doi:10.1007/s00402-018-3044-4.

In a retrospective study of 153 shoulders with articular-surface partial-thickness tears treated with completion of the tear (94 patients) and repair or transtendon repair (59 shoulders) at a mean follow-up of 73.9 months following repair, there were no significant differences between the two repair techniques in clinical outcomes or retear rate. Level of evidence: IV.

75. Ranalletta M, Rossi LA, Bertona AB, et al: Arthroscopic transtendon repair of partial-thickness articular-side rotator cuff tears. *Arthroscopy* 2016;32(8):1523-1528. doi:10.1016/j.arthro.2016.01.027.

A retrospective analysis of 80 patients following transtendon repair of partial-thickness articular-surface rotator cuff tears demonstrated improvements in clinical outcome measure and high patient satisfaction (92.5%). Level of evidence: IV.

76. Rossi LA, Atala NA, Bertona A, et al: Long-term outcomes after in situ arthroscopic repair of partial rotator cuff tears. *Arthroscopy* 2019;35(3):698-702. doi:10.1016/j.arthro.2018.09.026.

A long-term retrospective study of 62 patients at a mean follow-up of 10.4 years following arthroscopic in situ repair of partial-thickness rotator cuff tears demonstrated improved clinical outcomes, low revision rates, most patients returning to sports, and no difference between articular-surface and bursal-surface tears. Level of evidence: IV.

77. Rossi LA, Atala N, Bertona A, et al: Return to sports after in situ arthroscopic repair of partial rotator cuff tears. *Arthroscopy* 2019;35(1):32-37. doi:10.1016/j.arthro.2018.07.037.

A retrospective study of 72 patients at a mean follow-up of 54 months following in situ arthroscopic repair of partial-thickness rotator cuff tears demonstrated that 87% patients (61 patients) were able to return to sport with 80% of patients (56 patients) able to return to their previous level of sport. Level of evidence: IV.

78. Donohue NK, Nickel B, Grindel S: High-grade articular, bursal, and intratendinous partial thickness rotator cuff tears: A retrospective study comparing functional outcomes after completion and repair. *Am J Orthop (Belle Mead NJ)* 2016;45(5):E254-E260.

A retrospective study of 60 patients with partial-thickness rotator cuff tears demonstrated similar outcomes regardless of tear location (ie, bursal, articular, intratendinous). Level of evidence: IV.

79. Xiao J, Cui G: Clinical and structural results of arthroscopic repair of bursal-side partial-thickness rotator cuff tears. *J Shoulder Elbow Surg* 2015;24(2):e41-e46. doi:10.1016/j.jse.2014.07.008.

A retrospective study of 59 patients with bursal-surface rotator cuff tears treated with in situ repair demonstrated improvement in clinical results and 14/49 patients (83.7%) intact on postoperative MRI. Level of evidence: IV.

80. Chung SW, Kim JY, Yoon JP, et al: Arthroscopic repair of partial-thickness and small full-thickness rotator cuff tears: Tendon quality as a prognostic factor for repair integrity. *Am J Sports Med* 2015;43(3):588-596. doi:10.1177/0363546514561004.

A retrospective clinical and imaging study of patients with partial-thickness tears (34 shoulders) and small full-thickness (21 shoulders) following repair demonstrated that partial-thickness tears had a higher tendinosis grade as determined on MRI, which negatively correlated with healing. Level of evidence: III.

81. Kim KC, Lee WY, Shin HD, et al: Repair integrity and functional outcomes of arthroscopic repair for intratendinous partial-thickness rotator cuff tears. *J Orthop Surg (Hong Kong)* 2019;27(2):2309499019847227. doi:10.1177/2309499019847227.

A retrospective study of 29 patients with intratendinous partial-thickness rotator cuff tears demonstrated improved clinical outcomes and partial retearing in 3/28 patients (10.7%) on postoperative imaging. Level of evidence: IV.

82. Aydin N, Karaismailoglu B: High-grade bursal-side partial rotator cuff tears: Comparison of mid- and long-term results following arthroscopic repair after conversion to a full-thickness tear. *J Orthop Surg Res* 2017;12(1):118. doi:10.1186/s13018-017-0619-7.

A retrospective study of 29 patients following arthroscopic repair of partial-thickness rotator cuff tears demonstrated improvement in patient-reported outcomes at 2 and 5 years. Level of evidence: IV.

83. Vap AR, Mannava S, Katthagen JC, et al: Five-year outcomes after arthroscopic repair of partial-thickness supraspinatus tears. *Arthroscopy* 2018;34(1):75-81. doi:10.1016/j.arthro.2017.07.028.

Retrospective study of 20 patients a minimum of 5 years postoperatively demonstrating improved patient-reported outcomes, 76% of patients returning to their previous level of sports participation, and no patient requiring revision surgery. Level of evidence: IV.

84. Ostrander RV, Klauser JM, Menon S, et al: Ultrasound and functional assessment of transtendinous repairs of partial-thickness articular-sided rotator cuff tears. *Orthop J Sports Med* 2017;5(3):2325967117697375. doi:10.1177/2325967117697375.

A clinical and imaging retrospective study of 20 patients following transtendinous repair of articular-surface partial-thickness rotator cuff tears demonstrated excellent clinical outcomes and 18/20 patients with complete healing on MRI. Level of evidence: IV.

85. Woods TC, Carroll MJ, Nelson AA, et al: Transtendon rotator-cuff repair of partial-thickness articular surface tears can lead to medial rotator-cuff failure. *Open Access J Sports Med* 2014;5:151-157. doi:10.2147/OAJSM.S62885.

A small retrospective series of eight patients with transtendon repair of articular-surface partial-thickness rotator cuff tears demonstrated improved clinical outcomes but medial cuff tearing in seven of eight patients on postoperative magnetic resonance arthrogram. Level of evidence: IV.

86. Shin SJ: A comparison of 2 repair techniques for partial-thickness articular-sided rotator cuff tears. *Arthroscopy* 2012;28(1):25-33. doi:10.1016/j.arthro.2011.07.005.

87. Franceschi F, Papalia R, Del Buono A, et al: Articular-sided rotator cuff tears: Which is the best repair? A three-year prospective randomised controlled trial. *Int Orthop* 2013;37(8):1487-1493. doi:10.1007/s00264-013-1882-9.

    Randomized controlled trial comparing surgical repair of 62 high grade (>50%) articular-sided PTRCTs (32 transtendon repairs versus 32 conversion to FTRCT repairs). At a mean 38 months (range: 29 to 49 months), no difference in American Shoulder and Elbow Surgeons Disability Index score, Constant score, or range of motion was noted. On MRI at final follow-up, one retear was found in the transtendon repair group versus five in the conversion to FTRCT repair group. Level of evidence: II.

88. Castagna A, Borroni M, Garofalo R, et al: Deep partial rotator cuff tear: Transtendon repair or tear completion and repair? A randomized clinical trial. *Knee Surg Sports Traumatol Arthrosc* 2015;23(2):460-463. doi:10.1007/s00167-013-2536-6.

    A multicenter randomized controlled trial compared surgical repair techniques in 74 articular-sided PTRCTs (37 transtendon repairs versus 37 conversion to FTRCT repairs). At a minimum follow-up of 2 years, no differences were noted between the groups for VAS or Constant scores. Level of evidence: II.

89. Kim YS, Lee HJ, Bae SH, et al: Outcome comparison between in situ repair versus tear completion repair for partial thickness rotator cuff tears. *Arthroscopy* 2015;31(11):2191-2198. doi:10.1016/j.arthro.2015.05.016.

    This is a prospective randomized study of both bursal and articular PTRCTs. Transtendon repair was performed in 47 patients and conversion to an FTRCT was performed in 45 patients. Both groups improved in outcome measures with no significant differences between groups. In subgroup analysis, more retears were noted in the completion and repair group for bursal-surface tears. Level of evidence: II.

90. Ono Y, Woodmass JM, Bois AJ, et al: Arthroscopic repair of articular surface partial-thickness rotator cuff tears: Transtendon technique versus repair after completion of the tear-A meta-analysis. *Adv Orthop* 2016;2016:7468054. doi:10.1155/2016/7468054.

    A meta-analysis of three prospective randomized studies involving 182 shoulders comparing transtendon versus completion of the tear and repair in partial-thickness rotator cuff tears demonstrated no significant difference in patient-reported outcomes. Level of evidence: II.

91. Jordan RW, Bentick K, Saithna A: Transtendinous repair of partial articular sided supraspinatus tears is associated with higher rates of stiffness and significantly inferior early functional scores than tear completion and repair: A systematic review. *Orthop Traumatol Surg Res* 2018;104(6):829-837. doi:10.1016/j.otsr.2018.06.007.

    A systematic review of 21 studies involving 797 shoulders, comparing transtendinous repair to completion of the tear and repair in partial-thickness rotator cuff tears, demonstrated increased pain and poorer function at 3 months in patients receiving transtendinous repair. Level of evidence: II.

92. Bokor D, Sonnabend D, Deady L, et al: Evidence of healing of partial-thickness rotator cuff tears following arthroscopic augmentation with a collagen implant: A 2-year MRI follow-up. *Muscles Ligaments Tendons J* 2016;19(6):16-25.

    A prospective cohort study of partial-thickness rotator cuff tears in 13 patients treated with a bioinductive implant demonstrated new tissue formation in all patients with complete healing in 7 patients and improvement in tendon quality in 6 patients on postoperative MRI. Level of evidence: IV.

93. Schlegel TF, Abrams JS, Bushnell BD, et al: Radiologic and clinical evaluation of a bioabsorbable collagen implant to treat partial-thickness tears: A prospective multicenter study. *J Shoulder Elbow Surg* 2018;27(2):242-251. doi:10.1016/j.jse.2017.08.023.

    A prospective case series of 33 patients with high-grade PTRCTs treated with subacromial decompression without repair, followed by attachment of a bioinductive implant on the bursal surface of the rotator cuff. At 1-year follow-up, clinical scores improved and mean tendon thickness increased by 2 mm. MRI demonstrated complete healing in 8 patients and a reduction in tear size in 23 patients. Level of evidence: IV.

Chapter 13

Surgical Management of Full-Thickness Rotator Cuff Tears

Raffaele Garofalo, MD • Temilola Majekodunmi, MD • Sumant "Butch" Krishnan, MD

ABSTRACT

Rotator cuff repair is one of the most commonly performed procedures in orthopaedic surgery. The surgical management of full-thickness rotator cuff tears has progressed through the years from open, to mini-open, to arthroscopic. Along with this, surgical evolution has been the advancement in repair methods for rotator cuff tears. An overview of all available techniques and factors to consider in choosing the appropriate surgical method for full-thickness rotator cuff tears is presented.

Keywords: cuff; full-thickness; repair; rotator; surgical

Introduction

Rotator cuff tears represent one of the most common causes of shoulder pain and disability. The spectrum of patients with a rotator cuff lesion ranges from young elite-level overhead athletes with partial-thickness tears to patients of advanced age with massive and irreparable full-thickness tears. One or more tendons may be torn, with a tear of the supraspinatus tendon being the most common. The prevalence of full-thickness rotator cuff tears (FTRCTs) increases with age, with an overall prevalence approaching 50% in individuals aged 50 years or older.[1,2]

Dr. Garofalo or an immediate family member is a member of a speakers' bureau or has made paid presentations on behalf of CONMED Linvatec and serves as a paid consultant to or is an employee of Tornier. Dr. Krishnan or an immediate family member has received royalties from TAG Medical and Wright Medical Technology, Inc. and serves as a board member, owner, officer, or committee member of the Arthroscopy Association of North America and the American Shoulder and Elbow Surgeons. Neither Dr. Majekodunmi nor any immediate family member has received anything of value from or has stock or stock options held in a commercial company or institution related directly or indirectly to the subject of this chapter.

FTRCTs cannot heal spontaneously. Over time, the tear will reach a steady state or enlarge. Furthermore, fatty infiltration and muscle atrophy may also progress over time in the affected muscle-tendon units and may compromise the treatment outcome. The most popular surgical techniques for FTRCTs have evolved from open, to mini-open, to all-arthroscopic. The primary aim of surgical repair is to restore anatomy by reinserting the torn tendons on their proximal humeral footprint.

Unfortunately, not all surgically repaired rotator cuff tears heal. A full understanding of the biologic and biomechanical factors affecting healing of the surgically repaired rotator cuff has not yet been achieved. Because there is no agreement on the most effective methods for repair or postoperative rehabilitation, there are many available surgical treatment options for FTRCTs.

Classification

Rotator cuff tears have been classified by etiology, chronicity, size, shape, number of tendons, and topography or trophicity. Because of the great variability in the characteristics of rotator cuff tears, a standard classification does not exist. Several rotator cuff tear classifications are intended to guide treatment decisions. These classifications often describe the tendon tear in a single dimension either by measuring the greatest width of the tear or by determining the number of torn tendons. A well-informed decision regarding the tear pattern and the preferred repair technique should take into account the three-dimensional information provided by preoperative imaging and subsequent arthroscopy.

A geometric classification using coronal (length) and sagittal (width) dimensions of rotator cuff tears provides guidance for treating a tear and determining the prognosis.[3] A type I tear is crescent shaped (short and wide) and is reparable to the footprint. A type II tear is longitudinal (L- or U-shaped, long and narrow) and usually is reparable to the footprint, with some side-to-side repair. A type III tear is massive and retracted (long and wide); it is often

This chapter is adapted from Krishnan SG, Rudolph GH, Garofalo R: Surgical treatment of full-thickness rotator cuff tears, in Nicholson GP, ed: *Orthopaedic Knowledge Update: Shoulder and Elbow*, ed 4. Rosemont, IL, American Academy of Orthopaedic Surgeons, 2013, pp 187-195.

repaired by margin convergence. A type III tear larger than 2 cm^2 may be partially reparable, but it may require a tendon transfer. A type IV tear occurs with preexisting rotator cuff arthropathy and is associated with loss of the normal acromiohumeral interval and glenohumeral joint space. A type IV tear usually is irreparable and may be treated with arthroplasty.

Associated Lesions

Failure to detect a concomitant shoulder lesion disguised by a rotator cuff tear is a common surgical pitfall. The biceps tendon, glenohumeral joint, acromioclavicular joint, suprascapular nerve, and/or an os acromiale may be involved in the symptom complex of rotator cuff disease. A favorable outcome requires identifying each lesion during the workup phase and treating it appropriately.

Degenerative glenohumeral joint disease is subjectively described as a pain deep inside the shoulder, sometimes with crepitus or night pain. The diagnosis can be made with plain radiography. The presence of advanced glenohumeral degeneration precludes rotator cuff repair because the postoperative immobilization can lead to worsening of existing arthritis. Patients with mild glenohumeral osteoarthritis are at a lower risk for osteoarthritis progression.[4] Acromioclavicular joint arthritis is fairly common among patients with rotator cuff disease, with a prevalence rate directly proportionate to the tear size.[5] Specific findings include radiographic degenerative changes, tenderness to palpation directly over the acromioclavicular joint, and pain at the joint during cross-arm adduction and/or the active compression test. Open or arthroscopic distal clavicle excision can be performed at the time of surgery. An os acromiale is present in approximately 8% of the population and can be identified before surgery on a standard axillary radiograph. Surgical management involves reduction and fixation or excision of the unfused fragment if symptomatic. Suprascapular nerve compression can cause shoulder pain and weakness that mimics a full-thickness supraspinatus and/or infraspinatus tear. This condition can occur in conjunction with a tear that involves supraspinatus retraction of at least 2 cm. An electromyography or nerve conduction velocity study should be performed if a suprascapular nerve lesion is suspected.

Evaluation for an associated symptomatic lesion is crucial to identifying all sources of the patient's pain. A simple injection of 1% lidocaine into an area suspected of being a source of pain can be a powerful tool for diagnosis. This technique requires little time but provides a wealth of information for treatment planning. For planning FTRCT treatment, a classification system that includes tear type and associated pathology has been proposed to summarize all pathologic conditions of the patient before treatment.[6]

Surgical Management

Surgical management of FTRCTs should be individually tailored to the patient, with consideration of the size and pattern of the tears as well as the quality and degree of tendon retraction. FTRCTs can be successfully treated using an open, a mini-open, or an all-arthroscopic technique.[7-9] The goal of all surgical rotator cuff repairs is to obtain secure fixation of tendon to bone at the footprint to allow anatomic healing at the bone-tendon interface. For this purpose, the repair must have high initial fixation strength, minimal gapping at the time of repair, and continued mechanical stability under cyclic loading until healing.

Regardless of the surgical approach for repair of FTRCTs, the coracoacromial arch and the deltoid must be treated with care. The acromion and the coracoacromial ligament function in part to restrain anterosuperior translation of the humeral head. The deltoid is responsible for generating powerful synchronized glenohumeral motion. Deltoid detachment and insufficiency of the coracoacromial arch represent a potentially serious complication after rotator cuff repair that may result in significant disability of the arm. Acromioplasty and subacromial decompression have valid therapeutic roles in rotator cuff surgery. The goal is to reduce pressure and abrasion on the rotator cuff by smoothing the undersurface of the acromion, without disrupting the deltoid origin or destabilizing the coracoacromial arch.[10] However, a level I study found no benefit to subacromial decompression in association with arthroscopic rotator cuff repair in terms of functional results.[10]

Open and Mini-Open Repair

Historically, open repair had been considered the benchmark for rotator cuff repairs.[11] A planned open rotator cuff repair should also include diagnostic arthroscopy. Arthroscopy enables the surgeon to observe and treat concomitant pathology in conjunction with the open rotator cuff repair. As the pathology dictates, the treatment plan can be altered to include arthroscopic glenohumeral joint débridement, management of the long head of the biceps, and/or treatment of the acromioclavicular joint.[12]

After the diagnostic arthroscopy and before the open rotator cuff repair, the arthroscopic portals should be closed and the shoulder should be re-prepped and draped to reduce the risk of postoperative infection. Skin incisions should be carefully planned to allow for potential revision surgery. Planning is particularly important during an open repair of a large or massive tear. An oblique incision from the posterior edge of the acromioclavicular joint to the anterolateral corner of the acromion, extending 2 to 3 cm distally over the raphe between the anterior and middle deltoid, provides excellent visualization for cuff repair. This approach also allows anterosuperior access through the same incision for any future reverse shoulder arthroplasty in cases with failed irreparable tears.

A distal clavicle excision and a two-step acromioplasty improve access to the subacromial space without extending the deltoid split. Subacromial bursectomy improves visualization and is facilitated by rotating the arm. The coracohumeral ligament is palpated in external rotation and adduction and is released if it is tight. The rotator cuff is exposed for evaluation, mobilization, and repair.

Deltoid reattachment to the acromion is a critical component of open rotator cuff repair, and it has specific implications for postoperative rehabilitation. A meticulous and strong repair is essential for avoiding dehiscence during rehabilitation. The longitudinal deltoid split is repaired with nonabsorbable sutures in a simple fashion, and the reattachment to bone is often done using suture around the distal clavicle and through tunnels in the acromion. Overall survivorship (defined as not requiring additional surgery) of 94% and 83% was reported at 5 and 10 years, respectively, after open rotator cuff repair.[13] A repair that did not require surgical intervention within the first 2 years was likely to remain intact at 10 years. Rotator cuff repair survivorship was correlated with the number of tendons repaired.

Mini-open repairs were developed to reduce deltoid morbidity by splitting the deltoid fibers rather than detaching the deltoid origin. The results have been similar to those of open repairs.[14] In a randomized study, outcomes at 3-month follow-up were significantly better after mini-open rotator cuff repair than after open repair. However, between-group differences were not significant at 2-year follow-up.[7] In retrospective cohort studies, mini-open repairs led to approximately twice the risk of revision or arthrofibrosis.[14]

Arthroscopic Repair

Arthroscopic rotator cuff repair is the most commonly practiced approach and currently recognized standard for repair of FTRCTs. Successful and efficient repair requires a methodical stepwise approach. Patient positioning is determined by the surgeon, either modified beach-chair position or lateral decubitus. Multiple portals (ie, posterior, posterolateral, anterolateral, anterosuperior, and/or open juxta-acromial) can be used. The three-dimensional evaluation possible with the arthroscope allows the tear pattern to be recognized, and the surgeon can then formulate an appropriate repair technique and configuration. The pattern and size of the tear can best be seen through the lateral portals, and the posterolateral portal may be preferred for viewing the remaining subacromial space relative to cuff anatomy. A subacromial decompression may be performed first, by removing soft tissues and bony prominences. The coracoacromial ligament should be preserved in a repair of a large or massive tear.

Excellent outcomes after arthroscopic rotator cuff repairs have been demonstrated thanks to improvements in instrumentation and implants. There are currently four widely used arthroscopic repair methods: single-row repair, conventional double-row repair, transosseous-equivalent (TOE) suture-bridge repair, and anchorless transosseous repair.

Arthroscopic Single-Row Repair

Single-row repair has been the standard arthroscopic technique in arthroscopic rotator cuff repairs for the past 2 decades. In the single-row technique, suture anchors are placed in a linear fashion close to the medial or lateral aspect of the tuberosity footprint, depending on tendon mobility and surgeon preference (**Figure 1**). Suture anchors are made from a variety of materials. Claims that any one material is superior to another are not scientifically supported.[15,16] A randomized prospective study in which FTRCTs were treated with metal or biodegradable suture anchors did not find between-group functional differences.[17] The angle of anchor insertion influences fixation stability at the suture-tendon interface. In an experimental rotator cuff

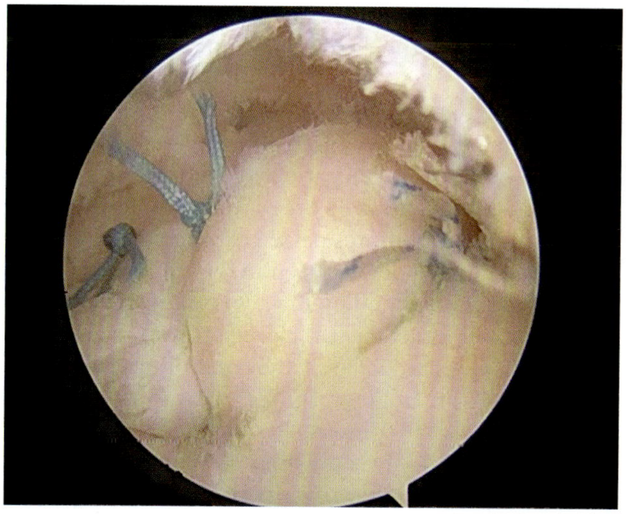

FIGURE 1 Arthroscopic view of a left shoulder via a posterolateral portal showing single-row repair using a triple-loaded suture anchor for a full-thickness rotator cuff tear. (Courtesy of the Shoulder Service, Baylor University Medical Center, Dallas, TX, and the Department of Orthopaedics, Shoulder Service, F. Miulli Hospital, Acquaviva delle Fonti, BA, Italy.)

model, suture anchors placed at 90° to the surface of the footprint provided better soft-tissue fixation irrespective of greater tuberosity decortication, compared with anchors placed at the standard 45° angle.[18,19] Mechanical failure at the bone-anchor interface can lead to suture anchor loosening, migration, and pullout; this complication has been reported in approximately 0.3% of patients.[20]

The most common mode of failure after single-row repair is suture cutout through the tendon. Several strategies have been used to improve tissue grip. Single-row reconstruction with a modified suture configuration has demonstrated improved biomechanical properties relative to a simple suture with results comparable to those of a double-row repair.[21,22] A prospective study compared clinical outcomes between a modified stitch and a simple stitch used for arthroscopic repair of a small- to medium-sized FTRCT. No significant difference was found, but the modified cuff stitch was superior to the simple stitch in maintaining repair integrity on ultrasonographic evaluation.[23]

The use of multiple sutures per anchor has been promoted for improving integrity in a single-row repair. Supporting data on triple-loaded suture use, now the emerging standard of single-row repair, showed excellent outcomes and biomechanical superiority of single-row configuration.[24]

Knotless single-row repair techniques have been developed to provide larger contact area and more uniform pressure distribution when compared with knotted single-row techniques.[25] Although knotless single-row repair techniques are reported to be more suitable for small to medium tears rather than large to massive tears, the use of newer, less aggressive sutures to improve results warrants further studies of this technique.[15,26]

Arthroscopic Double-Row Repair

In the conventional double-row repair technique, anchors are placed at two locations: medially and laterally (**Figure 2**). Medial anchors are placed close to the articular cartilage, and sutures passed through the tendon. A second row of anchors is placed in the lateral portion of the greater tuberosity, allowing a wider coverage area of tendon to bone attachment. This technique appears more suitable for tears reducible at the lateral footprint of the greater tuberosity without significant tension.

There is no clear consensus as to whether single-row or conventional double-row repair of rotator cuff tears is superior.[27,28] Double-row fixation is more costly, time-consuming, and technically more difficult when performed arthroscopically. Some biomechanical studies have found conventional double-row repair to be superior to single-row repair, offering a stronger fixation, better footprint restoration, and decreased gap formation and strain.[21,29-32] However, another bovine study found no biomechanical advantage to double-row versus single-row repair.[27] Several recent prospective randomized studies also did not find a difference in clinical outcomes and range of motion at short-term follow-up after either single-row or double-row repair.[28,33-38] When evaluating relative integrity, one study has similar rates of retearing,[38] whereas other studies suggest that single-row repair is more likely to lead to retear than double-row repair.[35,36]

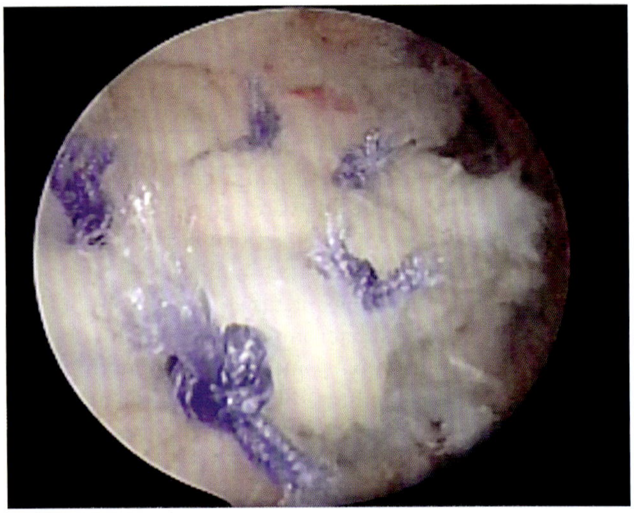

FIGURE 2 Arthroscopic view of a right shoulder via a posterolateral portal showing conventional double-row repair of a full-thickness rotator cuff tear. (Courtesy of the Shoulder Service, Baylor University Medical Center, Dallas, TX, and the Department of Orthopaedics, Shoulder Service, F. Miulli Hospital, Acquaviva delle Fonti, BA, Italy.)

Tear size may be a determining factor in the choice of technique.[37] At 2-year follow-up, patients had higher outcome scores after double-row fixation of tears larger than 3 cm.[39] Another study also reported better outcomes after double-row repair of large tears.[40] At a minimum 2-year follow-up after arthroscopic rotator cuff repair, patients with a tear larger than 3 cm showed greater clinical strength after conventional double-row repair than after a single-row suture anchor repair.[41] However, there was no significant MRI-detected difference in repair integrity at 6- or 24-month follow-up in patients with tears of different sizes. Most published data suggest that double-row fixation may be preferable for a large chronic tear, but single-row fixation is sufficient for a smaller tear (less than 3 cm).[42]

Arthroscopic Transosseous-Equivalent Suture Bridge Repair

The suture bridge configuration (known as a transosseous-equivalent repair or TOE repair) was developed to exploit the mechanical properties of a double-row repair while offering the footprint coverage of a transosseous repair. In this technique, suture anchors are placed medially and the associated sutures are passed in a horizontal mattress fashion through the rotator cuff. Knots are tied medially, and the tails of the suture are brought over the rotator cuff in a bridging fashion, and attached to anchors inserted at the lateral aspect of the greater tuberosity (**Figure 3**). This method preserves tendon vascularity by precluding tendon tissue penetration at the lateral row, and tissue strangulation by the knots.[43] Its favorable pressure properties are attributable to the oblique suture bridge limbs. The suture bridge imparts edge stability by flattening the lateral tendon edge, thereby preventing contact with the acromion-coracoacromial ligament arch, which is believed to lead to failure.[44] TOE rotator cuff repair techniques offer low bone-tendon interface motion, excellent footprint restoration, a high number of cycles to failure, and favorable distribution of stress over the repair in biomechanical and clinical evaluation, particularly in younger patients.[45-49]

A 2010 study has shown that TOE technique and conventional double-row procedures led to comparable patient satisfaction, functional outcomes, and rates of tearing. The only factor that significantly influenced tendon healing was patient age older than 60 years. Two types of retearing were identified: unhealed tendons and medial failures with a healed footprint.[50] In a comparison of the single-row, double-row, and TOE techniques, the TOE technique led to the lowest rate of postoperative retearing. The TOE technique was found to be particularly useful for large or massive tears.[51]

A recent modification to the TOE repair addresses the potential issue of tissue strangulation at the musculotendinous junction with a knotless technique. In knotless TOE, suture tapes with wider surfaces are loaded to the medial row anchors and passed through the medial aspect of the tendon (without tying any knots), crossed over and fixed to the lateral row knotless anchors. By eliminating the medial row knots, this technique reduces tendon strangulation and high suture-tendon surface pressure that could diminish healing potential. Though easier and quicker to perform, knotless TOE may pose biomechanical inferiority compared with knotted medial rows.[52,53] Though intriguing, no clinical study has shown definitive superiority of one technique over the other.[54-58]

Arthroscopic Anchorless Transosseous Repair

Arthroscopic anchorless transosseous repair is a novel technique designed to replicate the original transosseous tunnel repair, without anchors or implants.[11] In this technique, tunnels are created at the medial and lateral aspects of the greater tuberosity rotator cuff footprint. Sutures are placed through the tunnels and through the rotator cuff, mimicking the original benchmark transosseous repair (**Figure 4**). In addition to a greater contact area, the

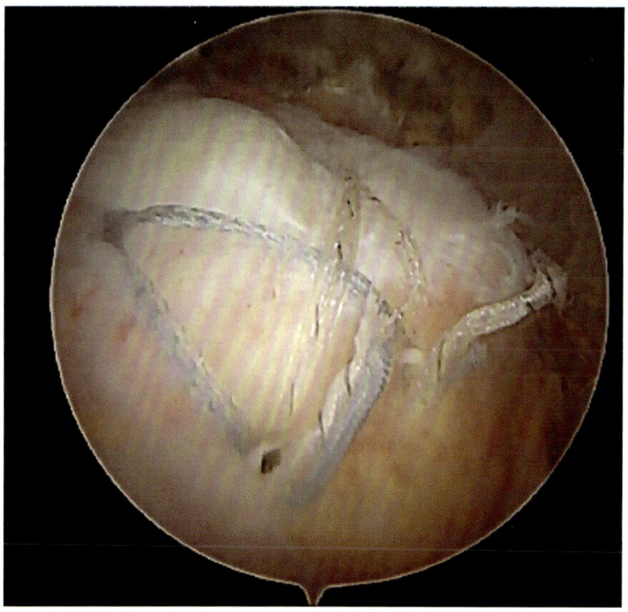

FIGURE 3 Arthroscopic view of a right shoulder via a posterolateral portal showing transosseous-equivalent repair of a full-thickness rotator cuff tear. (Courtesy of the Shoulder Service, Baylor University Medical Center, Dallas, TX, and the Department of Orthopaedics, Shoulder Service, F. Miulli Hospital, Acquaviva delle Fonti, BA, Italy.)

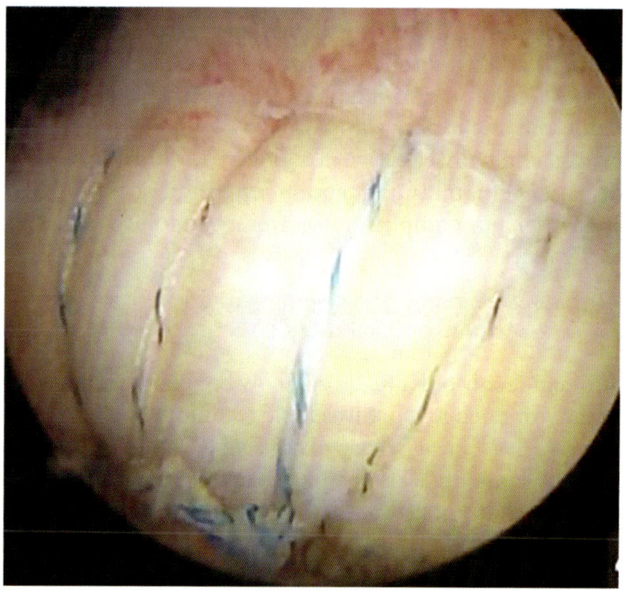

FIGURE 4 Arthroscopic view of a left shoulder posterolateral portal showing anchorless transosseous repair of a full-thickness rotator cuff tear. (Courtesy of the Shoulder Service, Baylor University Medical Center, Dallas, TX, and the Department of Orthopaedics, Shoulder Service, F. Miulli Hospital, Acquaviva delle Fonti, BA, Italy.)

Section 3: The Rotator Cuff

anchorless transosseous technique provides higher mean footprint pressures when compared with single-row and conventional double-row repair. A finite element model was used to examine stress distribution in simulated supraspinatus tendon repairs with 23 common techniques and suture configurations (single-row, double-row, and anchorless transosseous). Stress concentrations in single-row and double-row repairs were located at the anchor insertion sites. During muscle contraction, the highest stress concentrations were shifted to the bursal surface of tendon. With anchorless transosseous repair, stress concentration occurs at the bone-tendon interface, with no stress concentrated in the tendon.[45]

Several techniques have been developed to arthroscopically replicate the original open transosseous repair. An anterior cruciate ligament tibial drill guide has been used to create holes in the greater tuberosity. The sutures are passed through the tunnels and subsequently through the rotator cuff using cannulated needles or suture passers.[59] An arthroscopic giant bone needle has been described to improve the method of suture passage through bone.[37] Other dedicated devices for arthroscopic transosseous tunnel and suture placement have been in use for several years with successful results.[20,60,61]

A recent clinical study demonstrated increased blood supply after anchorless transosseous repairs compared with suture anchor repair.[62] This may theoretically contribute to biologic healing with potential enhancement of tendon integrity. Another comparative short-term clinical and radiologic outcome study of single-row versus anchorless transosseous repair demonstrated greater pain reduction in the anchorless transosseous group, with higher tendon repair integrity at final follow-up.[63,64] Finally, the anchorless transosseous repair technique has proved clinically effective in a long-term study with 66% of patients maintaining tendon repair integrity on MRI with no major complications after mean follow-up of 12 to 18 years.[65,66]

SUMMARY

Surgical repair of FTRCTs can now be accomplished by a variety of open and arthroscopic techniques. There have been many exciting recent advances, such as arthroscopic transosseous and TOE repairs, but the peer-reviewed literature has not established the definitive superiority of any one technique. Surgeons should be familiar with the strengths and weaknesses of each technique to achieve the best potential outcome for each patient. Ongoing studies are intended to improve the success of these mechanical surgical techniques with respect to healing the repaired rotator cuff.

KEY STUDY POINTS

- FTRCTs are prevalent in nature and more pronounced with increasing age.
- There are associated lesions with FTRCTs that must be evaluated when considering surgical treatment.
- Surgical treatment can be divided into open techniques and arthroscopic techniques, of which arthroscopic techniques have evolved and are now the recognized standard for FTRCT repair.
- Arthroscopic technique can be further divided into single-row, double-row, TOE, and anchorless transosseous repair techniques.
- Currently, no in vivo study demonstrates superiority of one arthroscopic technique over the other.

Annotated References

1. Yamaguchi K, Tetro AM, Blam O, Evanoff BA, Teefey SA, Middleton WD: Natural history of asymptomatic rotator cuff tears: A longitudinal analysis of asymptomatic tears detected sonographically. *J Shoulder Elbow Surg* 2001;10(3):199-203. doi:10.1067/mse.2001.113086.

2. Wylie JD, Baran S, Granger EK, Tashjian RZ: A comprehensive evaluation of factors affecting healing, range of motion, strength, and patient-reported outcomes after arthroscopic rotator cuff repair. *Orthop J Sports Med* 2018;6(1):2325967117750104. doi:10.1177/2325967117750104.

   This study of 81 patients evaluated the effect of various patient factors and tendon healing on range of motion, strength, and functional outcomes after arthroscopic rotator cuff repair. Level of evidence: III.

3. Davidson J, Burkhart SS: The geometric classification of rotator cuff tears: A system linking tear pattern to treatment and prognosis. *Arthroscopy* 2010;26(3):417-424. doi:10.1016/j.arthro.2009.07.009.

4. Jeong HY, Jeon YS, Lee DK, Rhee YG: Rotator cuff tear with early osteoarthritis: How does it affect clinical outcome after large to massive rotator cuff repair? *J Shoulder Elbow Surg* 2019;28(2):237-243. doi:10.1016/j.jse.2018.07.022.

   Evaluating the influence glenohumeral osteoarthritis in patients with large to massive tears, the study showed progression of osteoarthritis was significantly higher in patients with retears. Level of evidence: III.

5. Herve A, Thomazeau H, Favard L, et al: Clinical and radiological outcomes of osteoarthritis twenty years after rotator cuff repair. *Orthop Traumatol Surg Res* 2019;105(5):813-818. doi:10.1016/j.otsr.2019.02.013.

A level IV study evaluating the prevalence and clinical impact of osteoarthritis 20 years following rotator cuff repair showed that at long-term follow-up, glenohumeral osteoarthritis would have developed in most shoulders. Level of evidence: IV.

6. Lafosse L, Van Isacker T, Wilson JB, Shi LL: A concise and comprehensive description of shoulder pathology and procedures: The 4D code system. *Adv Orthop* 2012;2012:1-10. doi:10.1155/2012/930543.

7. Mohtadi NG, Hollinshead RM, Sasyniuk TM, Fletcher JA, Chan DS, Li FX: A randomized clinical trial comparing open to arthroscopic acromioplasty with mini-open rotator cuff repair for full-thickness rotator cuff tears: Disease-specific quality of life outcome at an average 2-year follow-up. *Am J Sports Med* 2008;36(6):1043-1051. doi:10.1177/0363546508314409.

8. Zumstein MA, Jost B, Hempel J, Hodler J, Gerber C: The clinical and structural long-term results of open repair of massive tears of the rotator cuff. *J Bone Joint Surg Am* 2008;90(11):2423-2431. doi:10.2106/JBJS.G.00677.

9. Morse K, Davis AD, Afra R, Kaye EK, Schepsis A, Voloshin I: Arthroscopic versus mini-open rotator cuff repair: A comprehensive review and meta-analysis. *Am J Sports Med* 2008;36(9):1824-1828. doi:10.1177/0363546508322903.

10. Milano G, Grasso A, Salvatore M, Zarelli D, Deriu L, Fabbriciani C: Arthroscopic rotator cuff repair with and without subacromial decompression: A prospective randomized study. *Arthroscopy* 2007;23(1):81-88. doi:10.1016/j.arthro.2006.10.011.

11. Ramsey ML, Getz CL, Parsons BO: What's new in shoulder and elbow surgery. *J Bone Joint Surg Am* 2009;91(5):1283-1293. doi:10.2106/JBJS.I.00105.

12. Boileau P, Baqué F, Valerio L, Ahrens P, Chuinard C, Trojani C: Isolated arthroscopic biceps tenotomy or tenodesis improves symptoms in patients with massive irreparable rotator cuff tears. *J Bone Joint Surg Am* 2007;89(4):747-757. doi:10.2106/JBJS.E.01097.

13. Millett PJ, Horan MP, Maland KE, Hawkins RJ: Long-term survivorship and outcomes after surgical repair of full-thickness rotator cuff tears. *J Shoulder Elbow Surg* 2011;20(4):591-597. doi:10.1016/j.jse.2010.11.019.

14. Nho SJ, Shindle MK, Sherman SL, Freedman KB, Lyman S, MacGillivray JD: Systematic review of arthroscopic rotator cuff repair and mini-open rotator cuff repair. *J Bone Joint Surg Am* 2007;89(suppl 3):127-136. doi:10.2106/JBJS.G.00583.

15. Huntington L, Coles-Black J, Richardson M, et al: The use of suture-tape and suture-wire in arthroscopic rotator cuff repair: A comparative biomechanics study. *Injury* 2018;49(11):2047-2052. doi:10.1016/j.injury.2018.09.004.

Suture tape offers greater pressurized tendon-bone contact compared with suture wire in three-anchor suture-bridge repairs, whereas a four-anchor suture-bridge achieves greater mechanical strength. Level of evidence: IV.

16. Thiébat G, Capitani P, de Girolamo L, et al: The effect of three different suture anchors for rotator cuff repair on primary cultures of human bone marrow mesenchymal stem cells. *Joints* 2018;6(2):100-103. doi:10.1055/s-0038-1660789.

The biocompatibility of three different suture anchors was studied in vitro to determine effects on normal cell function in terms of inflammatory reaction and osteogenic differentiation. Level of evidence: IV.

17. Milano G, Grasso A, Salvatore M, Saccomanno MF, Deriu L, Fabbriciani C: Arthroscopic rotator cuff repair with metal and biodegradable suture anchors: A prospective randomized study. *Arthroscopy* 2010;26(9 suppl):S112-S119. doi:10.1016/j.arthro.2010.01.030.

18. Strauss E, Frank D, Kubiak E, Kummer F, Rokito A: The effect of the angle of suture anchor insertion on fixation failure at the tendon-suture interface after rotator cuff repair: Deadman's angle revisited. *Arthroscopy* 2009;25(6):597-602. doi:10.1016/j.arthro.2008.12.021.

19. Hong CK, Hsu KL, Kuan FC, et al: When deadman theory meets footprint decortication: A suture anchor biomechanical study. *J Orthop Surg Res* 2019;14(1):157. doi:10.1186/s13018-019-1209-7.

Inserting suture anchors at 90° is recommended because of the significantly larger ultimate failure load in both decorticated and nondecorticated bones. Level of evidence: IV.

20. Garofalo R, Castagna A, Borroni M, Krishnan SG: Arthroscopic transosseous (anchorless) rotator cuff repair. *Knee Surg Sports Traumatol Arthrosc* 2012;20(6):1031-1035. doi:10.1007/s00167-011-1725-4.

21. Lorbach O, Bachelier F, Vees J, Kohn D, Pape D: Cyclic loading of rotator cuff reconstructions: Single-row repair with modified suture configurations versus double-row repair. *Am J Sports Med* 2008;36(8):1504-1510. doi:10.1177/0363546508314424.

22. Nelson CO, Sileo MJ, Grossman MG, Serra-Hsu F: Single-row modified Mason-Allen versus double-row arthroscopic rotator cuff repair: A biomechanical and surface area comparison. *Arthroscopy* 2008;24(8):941-948. doi:10.1016/j.arthro.2008.03.011.

23. Ko SH, Friedman D, Seo DK, Jun HM, Warner JJP: A prospective therapeutic comparison of simple suture repairs to massive cuff stitch repairs for treatment of small- and medium-sized rotator cuff tears. *Arthroscopy* 2009;25(6):583-589, 589.e1-4. doi:10.1016/j.arthro.2008.11.001.

24. Dierckman BD, Ni JJ, Karzel RP, Getelman MH: Excellent healing rates and patient satisfaction after arthroscopic repair of medium to large rotator cuff tears with a single-row technique augmented with bone marrow vents. *Knee Surg Sports Traumatol Arthrosc* 2018;26(1):136-145. doi:10.1007/s00167-017-4595-6.

    Repair integrity and patient clinical outcomes evaluated with MRI demonstrated intact repair in 91% of cases and excellent clinical outcomes in patients compared with reported results of similar studies in literature. Level of evidence: IV.

25. Simmer Filho J, Voss A, Pauzenberger L, et al: Footprint coverage comparison between knotted and knotless techniques in a single-row rotator cuff repair: Biomechanical analysis. *BMC Musculoskelet Disord* 2019;20(1):123. doi:10.1186/s12891-019-2479-2.

    When comparing footprint coverage in knotted and knotless single-row repair technique, the knotless technique demonstrated significantly higher footprint reconstruction, larger contact area, and a more uniform pressure distribution. No significant difference in mean contact pressure among groups was observed. Level of evidence: IV.

26. Bae KH, Kim JW, Kim TK, et al: Is the arthroscopic modified tension band suture technique suitable for all full-thickness rotator cuff tears? *J Shoulder Elbow Surg* 2016;25(9):1457-1463. doi:10.1016/j.jse.2016.01.004.

    Sixty-three patients were treated and followed up for about 29 months. Postoperative clinical outcomes and MRI showed arthroscopic modified tension band suture technique was a more suitable method for small to medium rotator cuff tears than for large to massive tears. Level of evidence: IV.

27. Mahar A, Tamborlane J, Oka R, Esch J, Pedowitz RA: Single-row suture anchor repair of the rotator cuff is biomechanically equivalent to double-row repair in a bovine model. *Arthroscopy* 2007;23(12):1265-1270. doi:10.1016/j.arthro.2007.07.010.

28. Aydin N, Kocaoglu B, Guven O: Single-row versus double-row arthroscopic rotator cuff repair in small- to medium-sized tears. *J Shoulder Elbow Surg* 2010;19(5):722-725. doi:10.1016/j.jse.2009.11.053.

29. Ahmad CS, Kleweno C, Jacir AM, et al: Biomechanical performance of rotator cuff repairs with humeral rotation: A new rotator cuff repair failure model. *Am J Sports Med* 2008;36(5):888-892. doi:10.1177/0363546508316285.

30. Baums MH, Buchhorn GH, Gilbert F, Spahn G, Schultz W, Klinger HM: Initial load-to-failure and failure analysis in single- and double-row repair techniques for rotator cuff repair. *Arch Orthop Trauma Surg* 2010;130(9):1193-1199. doi:10.1007/s00402-009-1036-0.

31. Baums MH, Spahn G, Steckel H, Fischer A, Schultz W, Klinger HM: Comparative evaluation of the tendon-bone interface contact pressure in different single- versus double-row suture anchor repair techniques. *Knee Surg Sports Traumatol Arthrosc* 2009;17(12):1466-1472. doi:10.1007/s00167-009-0771-7.

32. Milano G, Grasso A, Zarelli D, Deriu L, Cillo M, Fabbriciani C: Comparison between single-row and double-row rotator cuff repair: A biomechanical study. *Knee Surg Sports Traumatol Arthrosc* 2008;16(1):75-80. doi:10.1007/s00167-007-0382-0.

33. Grasso A, Milano G, Salvatore M, Falcone G, Deriu L, Fabbriciani C: Single-row versus double-row arthroscopic rotator cuff repair: A prospective randomized clinical study. *Arthroscopy* 2009;25(1):4-12. doi:10.1016/j.arthro.2008.09.018.

34. Burks RT, Crim J, Brown N, Fink B, Greis PE: A prospective randomized clinical trial comparing arthroscopic single- and double-row rotator cuff repair: Magnetic resonance imaging and early clinical evaluation. *Am J Sports Med* 2009;37(4):674-682. doi:10.1177/0363546508328115.

35. Franceschi F, Ruzzini L, Longo UG, et al: Equivalent clinical results of arthroscopic single-row and double-row suture anchor repair for rotator cuff tears: A randomized controlled trial. *Am J Sports Med* 2007;35(8):1254-1260. doi:10.1177/0363546507302218.

36. Charousset C, Grimberg J, Duranthon LD, Bellaiche L, Petrover D: Can a double-row anchorage technique improve tendon healing in arthroscopic rotator cuff repair? A prospective, nonrandomized, comparative study of double-row and single-row anchorage techniques with computed tomographic arthrography tendon healing assessment. *Am J Sports Med* 2007;35(8):1247-1253. doi:10.1177/0363546507301661.

37. Sugaya H, Maeda K, Matsuki K, Moriishi J: Repair integrity and functional outcome after arthroscopic double-row rotator cuff repair. A prospective outcome study. *J Bone Joint Surg Am* 2007;89(5):953-960. doi:10.2106/JBJS.F.00512.

38. Koh KH, Kang KC, Lim TK, Shon MS, Yoo JC: Prospective randomized clinical trial of single- versus double-row suture anchor repair in 2- to 4-cm rotator cuff tears: Clinical and magnetic resonance imaging results. *Arthroscopy* 2011;27(4):453-462. doi:10.1016/j.arthro.2010.11.059.

39. Park JY, Lhee SH, Choi JH, Park HK, Yu JW, Seo JB: Comparison of the clinical outcomes of single- and double-row repairs in rotator cuff tears. *Am J Sports Med* 2008;36(7):1310-1316. doi:10.1177/0363546508315039.

40. Pennington WT, Gibbons DJ, Bartz BA, et al: Comparative analysis of single-row versus double-row repair of rotator cuff tears. *Arthroscopy* 2010;26(11):1419-1426. doi:10.1016/j.arthro.2010.03.013.

41. Ma HL, Chiang ER, Wu HTH, et al: Clinical outcome and imaging of arthroscopic single-row and double-row rotator cuff repair: A prospective randomized trial. *Arthroscopy* 2012;28(1):16-24. doi:10.1016/j.arthro.2011.07.003.

42. Krishnan SG, Harkins DC, Schiffern SC, Pennington SD, Burkhead WZ: Arthroscopic repair of full-thickness tears of the rotator cuff in patients younger than 40 years. *Arthroscopy* 2008;24(3):324-328. doi:10.1016/j.arthro.2007.09.005.

43. Christoforetti JJ, Krupp RJ, Singleton SB, Kissenberth MJ, Cook C, Hawkins RJ: Arthroscopic suture bridge transosseus equivalent fixation of rotator cuff tendon preserves intratendinous blood flow at the time of initial fixation. *J Shoulder Elbow Surg* 2012;21(4):523-530. doi:10.1016/j.jse.2011.02.012.

44. Park MC, Tibone JE, ElAttrache NS, Ahmad CS, Jun BJ, Lee TQ: Part II: Biomechanical assessment for a footprint-restoring transosseous-equivalent rotator cuff repair technique compared with a double-row repair technique. *J Shoulder Elbow Surg* 2007;16(4):469-476. doi:10.1016/j.jse.2006.09.011.

45. Sano H, Yamashita T, Wakabayashi I, Itoi E: Stress distribution in the supraspinatus tendon after tendon repair: Suture anchors versus transosseous suture fixation. *Am J Sports Med* 2007;35(4):542-546. doi:10.1177/0363546506296310.

46. Zheng N, Harris HW, Andrews JR: Failure analysis of rotator cuff repair: A comparison of three double-row techniques. *J Bone Joint Surg Am* 2008;90(5):1034-1042. doi:10.2106/JBJS.G.00049.

47. Tocci SL, Tashjian RZ, Leventhal E, Spenciner DB, Green A, Fleming BC: Biomechanical comparison of single-row arthroscopic rotator cuff repair technique versus transosseous repair technique. *J Shoulder Elbow Surg* 2008;17(5):808-814. doi:10.1016/j.jse.2008.02.016.

48. Lee SH, Kim JW, Kim TK, et al: Is the arthroscopic suture bridge technique suitable for full-thickness rotator cuff tears of any size? *Knee Surg Sports Traumatol Arthrosc* 2017;25(7):2138-2146. doi:10.1007/s00167-016-4415-4.

    A consecutive series of 128 patients who underwent the modified tension band and suture bridge showed lower retear rates, significant improvements in hypotrophy, and fatty infiltration of the rotator cuff in the suture bridge group, making it a more effective method for the repair of rotator cuff tears of all sizes compared with the modified tension band technique. Level of evidence: III.

49. Hantes ME, Ono Y, Raoulis VA, et al: Arthroscopic single-row versus double-row suture bridge technique for rotator cuff tears in patients younger than 55 years: A prospective comparative study. *Am J Sports Med* 2018;46(1):116-121. doi:10.1177/0363546517728718.

    Radiologic and clinical midterm outcomes were compared between single-row and double-row (suture bridge) fixation techniques for arthroscopic rotator cuff repair in patients younger than 55 years. Double-row repair technique potentially provided superior tendon healing compared with the single-row technique and should be considered in younger patients with medium to large rotator cuff tears. Level of evidence: II.

50. Voigt C, Bosse C, Vosshenrich R, Schulz AP, Lill H: Arthroscopic supraspinatus tendon repair with suture-bridging technique: Functional outcome and magnetic resonance imaging. *Am J Sports Med* 2010;38(5):983-991. doi:10.1177/0363546509359063.

51. Mihata T, Watanabe C, Fukunishi K, et al: Functional and structural outcomes of single-row versus double-row versus combined double-row and suture-bridge repair for rotator cuff tears. *Am J Sports Med* 2011;39(10):2091-2098. doi:10.1177/0363546511415660.

52. Pauly S, Kieser B, Schill A, Gerhardt C, Scheibel M: Biomechanical comparison of 4 double-row suture-bridging rotator cuff repair techniques using different medial-row configurations. *Arthroscopy* 2010;26(10):1281-1288. doi:10.1016/j.arthro.2010.02.013.

53. Wieser K, Farshad M, Vlachopoulos L, Ruffieux K, Gerber C, Meyer DC: Suture slippage in knotless suture anchors as a potential failure mechanism in rotator cuff repair. *Arthroscopy* 2012;28(11):1622-1627. doi:10.1016/j.arthro.2012.04.150.

54. Spang JT, Buchmann S, Brucker PU, et al: A biomechanical comparison of 2 transosseous-equivalent double-row rotator cuff repair techniques using bioabsorbable anchors: Cyclic loading and failure behavior. *Arthroscopy* 2009;25(8):872-879. doi:10.1016/j.arthro.2009.02.023.

55. Burkhart SS, Adams CR, Burkhart SS, Schoolfield JD: A biomechanical comparison of 2 techniques of footprint reconstruction for rotator cuff repair: The SwiveLock-FiberChain construct versus standard double-row repair. *Arthroscopy* 2009;25(3):274-281. doi:10.1016/j.arthro.2008.09.024.

56. Park MC, Peterson AB, McGarry MH, Park CJ, Lee TQ: Knotless transosseous-equivalent rotator cuff repair improves biomechanical self-reinforcement without diminishing footprint contact compared with medial knotted repair. *Arthroscopy* 2017;33(8):1473-1481. doi:10.1016/j.arthro.2017.03.021.

    In a comparison group of knotted and knotless TOE repair, the knotless repair group had significant decreases in contact area, contact force, contact pressure, and peak pressure with increasing abduction angles from 0° to 30° ($P < 0.5$). Medial knots showed an adverse biomechanical effect by inhibiting self-reinforcement, without improving contact characteristics compared with knotless repair at each abduction angle tested. Level of evidence: IV.

57. Millett PJ, Espinoza C, Horan MP, et al: Predictors of outcomes after arthroscopic transosseous equivalent rotator cuff repair in 155 cases: A propensity score weighted analysis of knotted and knotless self-reinforcing repair techniques at a minimum of 2 years. *Arch Orthop Trauma Surg* 2017;137(10):1399-1408. doi:10.1007/s00402-017-2750-7.

    A retrospective comparative study highlighted the outcomes of TOE arthroscopic rotator cuff repair techniques for full-thickness supraspinatus tendon tears using a robust multipredictor model. Level of evidence: III.

58. Rhee YG, Cho NS, Parke CS: Arthroscopic rotator cuff repair using modified Mason-Allen medial row stitch: Knotless versus knot-tying suture bridge technique. *Am J Sports Med* 2012;40(11):2440-2447. doi:10.1177/0363546512459170.

59. Kim KC, Rhee KJ, Shin HD, Kim YM: Arthroscopic transosseous rotator cuff repair. *Orthopedics* 2008;31(4):327-330. Available at: http://www.ncbi.nlm.nih.gov/pubmed/18453167. Accessed September 6, 2019.

60. Flanagin B, Garofalo R, Lo E, et al: Midterm clinical outcomes following arthroscopic transosseous rotator cuff repair. *Int J Shoulder Surg* 2016;10(1):3-9. doi:10.4103/0973-6042.174511.

In the short term, arthroscopic transosseous rotator cuff repair technique showed significant improvement in postoperative range of motion, patient satisfaction, and low complication/failure rates in patients who had medium-sized rotator cuff tears and minimal fatty infiltration. Level of evidence: IV.

61. Liu XN, Yang CJ, Lee GW, Kim SH, Yoon YH, Noh KC: Functional and radiographic outcomes after arthroscopic transosseous suture repair of medium sized rotator cuff tears. *Arthroscopy* 2018;34(1):50-57. doi:10.1016/j.arthro.2017.07.035.

With minimum 2-year follow-up, arthroscopic transosseous rotator cuff repair demonstrated significant clinical improvement. Tear size, acromiohumeral distance, and degree of supraspinatus fatty infiltration were independently associated with cuff repair failure. Level of evidence: III.

62. Urita A, Funakoshi T, Horie T, Nishida M, Iwasaki N: Difference in vascular patterns between transosseous-equivalent and transosseous rotator cuff repair. *J Shoulder Elbow Surg* 2017;26(1):149-156. doi:10.1016/j.jse.2016.06.010.

Vascular patterns within the repaired rotator cuff depends on the suture technique used. Bone tunnels through the footprint may contribute to biologic healing by increasing blood flow in the repaired rotator cuff.

63. Randelli P, Stoppani CA, Zaolino C, Menon A, Randelli F, Cabitza P: Advantages of arthroscopic rotator cuff repair with a transosseous suture technique: A prospective randomized controlled trial. *Am J Sports Med* 2017;45(9):2000-2009. doi:10.1177/0363546517695789.

This level I randomized controlled trial found no significant differences in terms of functional and radiologic results when using the single-row technique versus transosseous hardware-free suture repair. However, postoperative pain decreased more quickly after the transosseous procedure, which portrays a possible improvement in the surgical repair of the rotator cuff. Level of evidence: I.

64. Garofalo R, Calbi R, Castagna A, Cesari E, Budeyri A, Krishnan SG: Is there a difference in clinical outcomes and repair integrity between arthroscopic single-row versus transosseous (anchorless) fixation? A retrospective comparative study. *J Orthop Sci* 2018;23(5):770-776. doi:10.1016/j.jos.2018.05.011.

Arthroscopic rotator cuff repair using single-row and transosseous anchorless techniques yielded successful clinical outcomes. Transosseous technique showed fewer type 3 Sugaya MRI results, suggesting a possible benefit with transosseous repair. Level of evidence: II.

65. Plachel F, Traweger A, Vasvary I, Schanda JE, Resch H, Moroder P: Long-term results after arthroscopic transosseous rotator cuff repair. *J Shoulder Elbow Surg* 2019;28(4):706-714. doi:10.1016/j.jse.2018.09.003.

A single surgeon treated patients with full-thickness rotator cuff tears arthroscopically over a 5-year period using the transosseous rotator cuff repair. The study showed that arthroscopic transosseous rotator cuff repair provided good clinical results 12 to 18 years after surgery when used in the management of full-thickness rotator cuff tears. Level of evidence: IV.

66. Black EM, Austin LS, Narzikul A, Seidl AJ, Martens K, Lazarus MD: Comparison of implant cost and surgical time in arthroscopic transosseous and transosseous equivalent rotator cuff repair. *J Shoulder Elbow Surg* 2016;25(9):1449-1456. doi:10.1016/j.jse.2016.01.003.

Compared with TOE repair, anchorless rotator cuff repair seemed to provide substantial implant-related cost savings, with no significant differences in surgical time for medium and large rotator cuff tears. Case time for TOE was proportional to tear size. Level of evidence: IV.

Chapter 14

Massive Rotator Cuff Tears

Robert Stephen Otte, MD • Lisa G. M. Friedman, MD, MA • Grant E. Garrigues, MD

Section 3: The Rotator Cuff

ABSTRACT

Massive rotator cuff tears are challenging to manage as they have a high retear rate given the often concomitant tendon retraction and fatty infiltration. Whether force couples across the shoulder are balanced often determines whether patients can compensate for these massive rotator cuff tears without surgery. Massive rotator cuff tears tend to progress over time without repair, with worsening rotator cuff arthropathy and decreasing acromiohumeral interval. A thorough clinical examination is mandatory to determine the optimal treatment. This includes imaging and physical examination, to assess for rotator cuff arthropathy, the extent of the tear, associated tendon retraction, fatty infiltration, weakness, stiffness, pseudoparalysis, lag signs, and instability. There are a variety of treatment options available for the massive rotator cuff tear. For poor surgical candidates, a structured deltoid rehabilitation program can provide benefit. Subacromial débridement, biceps tenotomy or tenodesis, tuberoplasty, and partial rotator cuff repair may all provide pain relief and some functional gains when a full rotator cuff repair is not possible. A variety of tendon transfers have been described that can provide strength to compensate for specific deficiencies from massive rotator cuff tears. Graft augmentation, superior capsular reconstruction, and subacromial balloon spacers are newer technologies that may also grant both functional improvements and pain relief. The reverse total shoulder arthroplasty is an operation proven to relieve pain and restore function for patients with massive rotator cuff tears.

Keywords: massive; retear; reverse total shoulder arthroplasty; rotator cuff; shoulder; superior capsular reconstruction; tear; tendon transfer

Dr. Garrigues has received royalties from DJ Orthopaedics and Tornier/Wright; serves as a paid consultant to or is an employee of DJ Orthopaedics, Tornier/Wright, and Mitek; and serves as a board member, owner, officer, or committee member of the American Shoulder and Elbow Surgeons, the Arthroscopy Association of North America, and the American Academy of Orthopaedic Surgeons. Neither of the following authors nor any immediate family member has received anything of value from or has stock or stock options held in a commercial company or institution related directly or indirectly to the subject of this chapter: Dr. Otte and Dr. Friedman.

Introduction

Consensus for the term massive rotator cuff tear has not been definitively delineated, although a variety of definitions and classifications have been proposed. Some classification schemes are based on a tear size of more than 5 cm in maximum dimension, whereas others are based on the complete detachment of two or more tendons.[1,2] For the purposes of this chapter, the former definition has been used. Because of the lack of consistency among definitions, it can be challenging to directly compare studies and patient outcomes. A massive rotator cuff tear can be the result of an acute injury. However, most massive rotator cuff tears occur with retraction as part of the natural history of chronic rotator cuff tears. An acute-on-chronic massive rotator cuff tear occurs when a traumatic event causes enlargement of a preexisting, smaller tear.[3] The prevalence of massive rotator cuff tears ranges from 10% to 40%, with an increasing incidence seen in the aging population.[1]

A chronic rotator cuff tear is often associated with significant fatty infiltration of the rotator cuff muscles and tendon retraction, both of which make a repair more challenging, if a repair is even possible. Not all massive rotator cuff tears are irreparable; however, not all irreparable rotator cuff tears are massive. Most patients with a massive rotator cuff tear have significant, disabling

This chapter is adapted from Hampton DM, Delaney RA, Higgins LD: Massive rotator cuff tears, in Nicholson GP, ed: *Orthopaedic Knowledge Update: Shoulder and Elbow*, ed 4. Rosemont, IL, American Academy of Orthopaedic Surgeons, 2013, pp 197-208.

weakness, particularly with their arms outstretched. As a consequence, younger active patients experience more disability from massive tears than older patients because of greater functional demands. The literature suggests that massive posterosuperior tears involving the supraspinatus and the infraspinatus are more common than anterosuperior tears involving the supraspinatus and the subscapularis.[4]

Biomechanics

The biomechanical function of the rotator cuff is to provide compression of the humeral head into the concave glenoid to keep the humeral head centered in the glenoid during movement.[5] The well-functioning rotator cuff is so adept at this task that the measured center of rotation moves less than 2 mm through a full range of motion.[6] In the setting of a massive rotator cuff tear, the forces across the shoulder can become unbalanced. With a massive rotator cuff tear, the rotator cuff cannot resist the pull of the deltoid and the humeral head begins to ride superiorly into the subacromial bursa and the undersurface of the acromion. However, based on the location of the massive tear, more so than the size of the tear, well-coordinated and balanced force couples still may be able to successfully compensate and lead to reasonable functional outcomes in the absence of repair. Alternatively, when massive rotator cuff tears occur at such a location that the forces became uncoupled, it is difficult for the shoulder to compensate for the grossly abnormal shoulder kinematics.[7]

It is unknown what the tipping point is for the force couples across the shoulder to be irretrievably compromised. In a 2011 cadaver study, the progression of a supraspinatus tear into the infraspinatus marked the critical stage for significant changes in humeral head kinematics. In this study, a tear of the entire supraspinatus without infraspinatus involvement decreased abduction capability at high loads, but humeral head kinematics were not disrupted.[8] These findings suggest that, if the remainder of the rotator cuff is functioning well in an isolated supraspinatus tear, the anterior and posterior forces across the shoulder can maintain balance.

Natural History

Many rotator cuff tears are asymptomatic and, indeed, may be a normal finding seen in the aging shoulder. Cadaver and MRI studies of patients estimate that for patients older than 65 years, 12% to 25% have rotator cuff tears with increasing incidence as patients continue to age.[9-11] Incidence of massive rotator cuff tears is increased in higher risk patients with obesity, diabetes mellitus, tobacco use, hyperlipidemia, and those with cuff muscle with fatty infiltration.

Further knowledge of the natural history of massive rotator cuff tears has been gained by examining the outcomes of both nonsurgical and surgical management. A retrospective review of 19 consecutive patients with massive rotator cuff tears treated conservatively demonstrated, at a mean final follow-up of 4 years with MRI, that the size of the tears increased by a mean of 3.29 cm.[2,3] Fatty infiltration increased on average by one Goutallier grade and the acromiohumeral interval (AHI) decreased by a mean of 2.6 mm to an overall distance of less than 7 mm.[3] In addition, there was a radiographic increase in the stage of glenohumeral osteoarthritis by one to two grades. Importantly, several risk factors for progression were identified: the number of ruptured tendons, tear size, and abduction weakness. These factors correlated with increased severity of glenohumeral arthritis, stage of fatty infiltration, and acromiohumeral distance.[3,8]

The most comprehensive natural history study of large and massive rotator cuff tears treated surgically used ultrasonography to follow these rotator cuff tears following arthroscopic repair. At 1-year follow-up, 17/18 patients had ultrasonography evidence showing a lack of complete healing. Despite this, 13 patients had American Shoulder and Elbow Surgeons (ASES) scores greater than or equal to 90. However, at 2-year follow-up, only 12/18 patients had an ASES score greater than or equal to 80.[12]

Clinical Evaluation

Patients with massive rotator cuff tears usually seek surgical consultation because of persistent pain and weakness. Symptomatic tears often are painful at night and during activities of daily living that are performed with the arm outstretched. Depending on the size and location of the tear, the patient may have pseudoparalysis, which is commonly defined as an inability to actively elevate the arm above 90° in the setting of unrestricted passive range of glenohumeral motion without neurologic impairment.[10] However, the extent of weakness varies, as does the loss of range of motion. It is important to determine whether the pain reported by the patient is indeed the result of symptomatic rotator cuff disease as opposed to other pathologies, such as adhesive capsulitis, subacromial bursitis, cervical spine disease, biceps tendinopathy, and/or acromioclavicular arthritis. The pain from a rotator cuff tear, similar to other disorders of the subacromial space, is typically localized to the lateral proximal humerus and can be referred to the deltoid insertion. Pain will often radiate proximally into the trapezius in patients with significant scapular substitution associated with upper trapezius overactivation. Pain radiating below the elbow to the hand should raise suspicion of cervical radiculopathy or peripheral nerve compression.

The examination always should begin with an inspection of both exposed shoulders. Marked atrophy of the posterior rotator cuff muscles within their fossae often is present with a massive tear and often can be easily seen and palpated. The active and passive range of motion should be recorded and compared with that of the unaffected side. The differences between passive and active motion can provide important clues as to the integrity of the rotator cuff. It is vital to observe scapular kinematics during active motion. Scapular substitution often is present in a patient with a massive tear and should be noted. Strength testing of the rotator cuff muscles should be performed, and lag signs should be evaluated. Anterosuperior tears tend to cause weakness during internal rotation and painful weakness in elevation. Posterosuperior tears cause weakness and/or pain during elevation and external rotation.

Several clinical signs portend a poor prognosis for repair of the massive cuff tear. Static anterosuperior subluxation of the humeral head is a sign of a large, irreparable anterosuperior tear. A tear with dynamic anterosuperior subluxation or anterosuperior escape during resisted abduction also has a poor repair prognosis. Pseudoparalysis and a true drop arm sign—the inability for the patient to lower the arm from an elevated position in a controlled manner—indicate severe disease with fatty infiltration of the infraspinatus classified as Goutallier grade 2 or higher.[13] A positive hornblower's sign—or weakness with active external rotation at 90° of abduction—indicates teres minor dysfunction with likely significant fatty infiltration, and that a repair will not succeed.[14] Other physical examination tests that are specific for large to massive rotator cuff tears include the bear hug, lift-off, and modified lift-off, which test for deficiencies in the subscapularis and the external rotation lag sign, which is a nonspecific test for tears of the posterior rotator cuff.

Imaging

Plain radiographs are the first-line of imaging for a patient with shoulder pain. Radiographs can diagnose glenohumeral arthritis and assess the AHI, the acromioclavicular joint, and acromial morphology. A true AP view of the shoulder (Grashey view), a scapular Y view (outlet view), and an axillary lateral view are standard for evaluating suspected rotator cuff pathology.

On a Grashey view in neutral forearm rotation, proximal migration of the humeral head can be observed and quantified.[1] In a healthy shoulder, the normal range for the AHI is 7 to 14 mm. The AHI is correlated with the size of the rotator cuff tear and repair prognosis. In a study of 112 shoulders with large rotator cuffs that underwent arthroscopic repair, AHI was found to be a significant though not independent risk factor for rotator cuff retear, with an average AHI of 7.5 ± 2.0 in the group that had a retear and 8.2 ± 1.7 in the group that healed.[15] The Hamada classification system for the AHI ranges from grade 1 to grade 5 and quantifies the amount of superior migration of the humeral head.[16] It was modified slightly to divide grade 4 into two subtypes[17] (**Table 1**).

Advanced imaging can be useful for precisely identifying the size of the tear, the number of torn tendons, tendon retraction, tissue quality, bony morphology, and fatty infiltration of the muscle bellies. Noncontrast-enhanced shoulder MRI has become the mainstay of soft-tissue evaluation of the shoulder. A rotator cuff tear can be reliably identified and characterized on MRI. If the patient cannot undergo MRI, CT arthrogram can be used to define both the tear and extent of fatty infiltration.[18] The Goutallier classification of fatty infiltration that was originally described for CT arthrogram was modified for MRI evaluation. This system provides predictive and prognostic information regarding success of an attempted rotator cuff repair (**Table 2**). The sagittal T1 sequence is best for evaluating muscle fat content, given the cuts are sufficiently medial for visualizing the muscle belly[19] (**Figure 1**). Severe muscle retraction can cause bunching of the muscle and can lead to an underestimation of the extent of fatty infiltration.[20] In addition, fatty infiltration of the rotator cuff has been shown to be present in the intact cuff of obese patients, though it is not clear if this etiology imparts the same poor prognosis as fatty infiltration caused by the neurogenic injury of chronic rotator cuff tear.[21]

As the AHI decreases in size—and increases in Hamada grade—the extent of fatty infiltration of the rotator cuff muscles also increases.[18] A 2011 review found that in patients who underwent repair of a grade 1 or 2 massive tear, the retearing rate was higher among those with a grade 2 tear. Although it appears that muscle atrophy and fatty infiltration does not reverse with successful rotator cuff repair, repair was successful in halting the progression of fatty infiltration in that none of the successfully repaired tears advanced past Goutallier grade 3 or higher.[22] The extent of fatty infiltration is an important prognostic indicator for repair. The outcome for a patient with grade 3 or 4 infiltration has been shown to be inferior to that of a patient with grade 1 or 2 fatty infiltration.[12,20] It is not quite clear which patients with large and massive tears will benefit from repair. In a 2007 study, 22 patients with grade 3 or 4 fatty infiltration were followed up and it was found that some patients showed clinical improvement after repair.[23] Despite this finding, most researchers agree that the clinical and radiographic results of surgery are worse with grade 3 to 4 fatty infiltration. Although some patients with this grade of fatty infiltration do appear to

Table 1

The Hamada Classification of the Acromiohumeral Interval, for Superior Migration of the Humeral Head in Rotator Cuff Arthropathy

Grade	Status of the Acromiohumeral Interval
1	Normal (7 to 14 mm)
2	Narrowing
3	Narrowing, with acetabulization of the acromion
4	Narrowing, with acetabulization of the acromion and glenohumeral joint narrowing[a]
5	Narrowing, with acetabulization of the acromion and humeral head collapse

[a]In the Walch classification, 4A = glenohumeral arthritis without subacromial arthritis and 4B = glenohumeral arthritis with subacromial arthritis.

receive some benefit from surgical repair, it is clear that these results are not as good as in patients whose fatty infiltration is grade 2 or less.[24]

Ultrasonography is increasingly being used to evaluate the rotator cuff. The advantages of portable shoulder ultrasonography are its low cost, noninvasive nature, absence of adverse effects, ability to visualize the rotator cuff dynamically during physiologic motion, and the immediate availability of results. Ultrasonography cannot penetrate bone and therefore is inadequate to diagnose large rotator cuff tears when the tendons have retracted medial to the acromion. The accuracy of the evaluation is highly dependent on the experience and the skill of the operator.[25] Some studies have found a positive predictive value of 96% and a negative predictive value of 95% in cases in which the operator was experienced.[26] Experienced ultrasonographers can detect larger tears with greater accuracy.[26] For orthopaedic surgeons, it appears that competence in detecting rotator cuff tears by ultrasonography can be gained quickly. One study demonstrated that, after a few hours of instruction, orthopaedic surgeons could accurately diagnose a full-thickness tear 88% of time.[25]

Table 2

The Goutallier Classification of Fatty Infiltration of the Rotator Cuff

Grade	Extent of Fatty Infiltration
0	Normal muscle
1	Some fatty streaks
2	Less fat than muscle
3	Equal amounts of fat and muscle
4	More fat than muscle

Nonsurgical Management

Massive rotator cuff tears may be amenable to nonsurgical management in certain circumstances. A structured anterior deltoid rehabilitation program is recommended for managing a massive rotator cuff tear in a patient who is medically unable or chooses not to undergo surgery. One study prospectively assessed 17 patients with a massive rotator cuff tear and Goutallier grade 4 fatty infiltration of the supraspinatus and the infraspinatus. They found an improvement in the mean Constant score from 26 to 63 after a structured anterior deltoid rehabilitation program. All components of shoulder motion improved, particularly forward elevation. In these patients, the stabilizing effect of recruiting the anterior deltoid was able to compensate for the massive rotator cuff tear, resulting in adequate improvement in both function and pain. The researchers concluded that structured anterior deltoid rehabilitation, in combination with scheduled anti-inflammatory pain medication, should be the first treatment of a massive rotator cuff tear in a patient of advanced age and/or significant comorbidities.[27]

Another study followed up 19 patients treated nonsurgically for massive rotator cuff tears and found progression in glenohumeral arthritis, a decrease in acromiohumeral distance, and an increase in tear size and fatty infiltration. However, at a mean final follow-up of 4 years, the mean relative Constant score was 83%, the mean Subjective Shoulder Value was 68%, and range of motion was preserved. Of note, 50% of the tears classified as repairable at diagnosis had become irreparable at final follow-up. The researchers concluded that moderately symptomatic patients with a massive rotator cuff tear can maintain satisfactory shoulder function after nonsurgical management despite the progression of structural changes. However, they cautioned that a repairable tear may become symptomatic and irreparable over time. At that point, the surgical treatment options are fewer and may be limited to more technically demanding and less reliable.[3]

Surgical Management

Débridement and Biceps Tenodesis Versus Tenotomy

The goal of surgically relieving pain from a massive, irreparable rotator cuff tear has led to interest in the

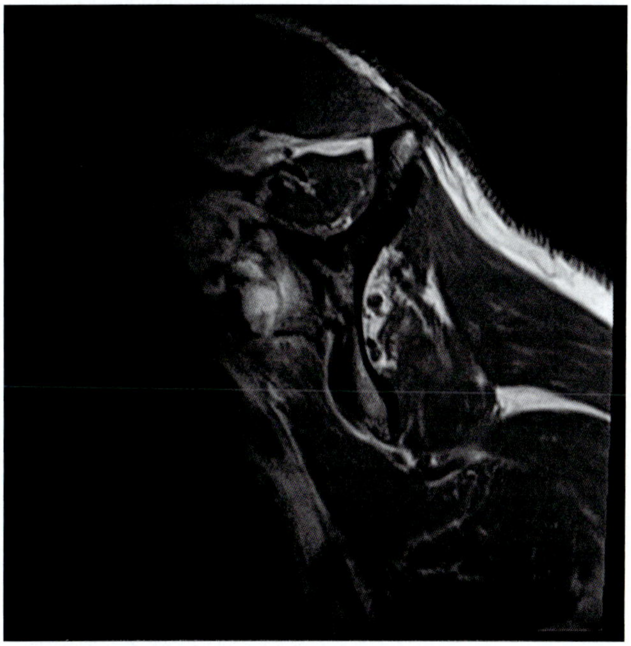

FIGURE 1 T1-weighted sagittal MRI of the scapular Y, showing significant fatty infiltration of the infraspinatus.

débridement of massive tears with or without acromioplasty or subacromial decompression. These techniques may not yield functional benefit in terms of regaining strength or range of motion, but they can provide significant pain relief, particularly for a patient with relatively low physical demands. The patient may have secondary functional gains related to decreased pain, especially if other pain generators, such as the long head of the biceps tendon or the acromioclavicular joint, also are treated.[17]

One study followed up 31 patients (mean age 70.6 years) who underwent arthroscopic débridement of an irreparable rotator cuff tear. Twenty-four of the patients also underwent a biceps tenotomy. To preserve the coracoacromial arch, acromioplasty was not performed. At a mean 47-month follow-up, the mean ASES score had significantly improved from 24.0 to 69.8, and the pain score on visual analog scale had improved from 7.8 to 2.9. However, the Constant score for the surgical shoulder was significantly lower than that of the contralateral shoulder. The result was rated as excellent by 10 patients (32%), good by 7 (22%), average by 9 (29%), and poor by 5 (16%). As with nonsurgical management, radiographic deterioration was evident at follow-up, with glenohumeral osteoarthritis progressing in 10 patients (32%), and the mean acromiohumeral distance decreasing from 8.3 to 7.0 mm. Overall, the patients had significant functional improvement despite radiographic progression of degenerative changes.[28]

The long head biceps tendon runs over the superior aspect of the humerus, and in the setting of a massive rotator cuff tear, some think it might act as a secondary stabilizer to resist superior translation. One longitudinal study evaluated this concept in a study comparing the change in AHI in 307 patients who underwent isolated arthroscopic biceps tenotomy if they had an irreparable rotator cuff tear or if they were unwilling to undergo the rehabilitation required following rotator cuff repair. It was found that although performing a tenotomy does not significantly alter the radiographic changes that occur in long-standing rotator cuff tears, it does provide objective improvement and increased patient satisfaction.[17]

Subacromial Decompression, Tuberoplasty, and Reversed Subacromial Decompression

Anterior-inferior partial acromioplasty has become a common arthroscopic procedure.[4,29] As experiences with this procedure accrued, the importance of the stabilizing effect of the coracoacromial arch also evolved. Superior humeral head migration is now recognized as a potential complication of acromioplasty in the presence of a massive rotator cuff tear. One cadaver study of seven shoulders measured anterosuperior humeral head translation after the sequential application of an anterosuperior 150-N load in five scenarios: the intact coracoacromial ligament, subperiosteal coracoacromial ligament release, standard acromioplasty, coracoacromial reconstruction, and modified Neer acromioplasty. A significant decrease in anterosuperior migration was found after coracoacromial ligament reconstruction compared with anterior acromioplasty or modified Neer acromioplasty. The researchers concluded that an intact or reconstructed coracoacromial ligament provides a stabilizing force in a massive rotator cuff tear to prevent excessive anterosuperior translation and possible anterosuperior escape of the humeral head.[30] In another study of 36 patients undergoing repair of a massive rotator cuff tear, the coracoacromial ligament was repaired with bone sutures to the acromion. Twenty-two of the 24 patients available for follow-up had an excellent or satisfactory result and 20 were able to perform overhead activities, but 2 patients had an unsatisfactory result. Anterosuperior humeral head subluxation did not occur in any patients postoperatively. Although the tears in this study were not irreparable, acromioplasty with coracoacromial ligament preservation or repair was found to maintain some of the passive stabilizing effect of the coracoacromial arch.[31] If an open rotator cuff repair is attempted in the setting of a massive rotator cuff tear, particularly an anterosuperior tear, great care must be taken to preserve or repair the coracoacromial arch.

In 2002, an open procedure was introduced for treating massive, irreparable rotator cuff tears while preserving the coracoacromial ligament. The procedure, described as a tuberoplasty, involves removing exostoses on the humerus and reshaping the greater tuberosity to create a smooth, congruent acromiohumeral articulation. Notably, an acromioplasty is not performed. The acromion and the coracoacromial ligament are left intact until a decision is made about the reparability of the cuff before violation of the coracoacromial arch. In this study, 20 patients treated with this procedure had disabling preoperative pain and an irreparable tear of at least 5 cm involving both the supraspinatus and the infraspinatus. At a minimum 27-month follow-up of 19 patients, the result was excellent in 12 patients, good in 6, and fair in 1. Thirteen patients (68%) were totally pain free, and no patient had night pain after surgery. All patients had residual external rotation weakness. These results clearly show improvement in pain and function using a tuberoplasty technique, but they are inferior to those achieved with acromioplasty and primary repair of the rotator cuff.[32]

This tuberoplasty has also been described as an all-arthroscopic reversed subacromial decompression. This procedure has the goal of creating a more hiplike humeroscapular interface by using an arthroscopic burr to reshape the greater tuberosity. A concomitant glenohumeral joint débridement, thorough subacromial bursectomy and débridement, and if pathologic, biceps tenotomy or tenodesis can also be considered. Similar to a subacromial decompression, the greater tuberosity is reshaped to allow for a smoother articulation with the undersurface of the acromion with preservation of the coracoacromial arch. In one study, authors found a significant improvement in Constant scores from 65.9% to 90.6% in 23 patients undergoing a reversed subacromial decompression. Although 19/23 patients rated their outcome as good or excellent, osteoarthritis continued to progress, and the acromiohumeral distance decreased from 5.1 to 4.5 mm over the mean 40-month follow-up of the study.[33] Whether open or arthroscopic, these procedures should only be considered in shoulders with balanced force couples and preserved active elevation in which pain from subacromial contact is felt to be the main issue.

Débridement of a massive rotator cuff tear and subacromial decompression produce results inferior to repair of the rotator cuff. However, these surgical techniques have a role in patients with low physical demands for whom pain relief is the priority and functional goals are limited. The results do deteriorate over time. A satisfactory result is most likely to be achieved if the patient has an intact posterior rotator cuff before surgery, and preserved deltoid and external rotation strength.

Partial Repair

If complete repair is not possible, the theory behind partial rotator cuff repair is to stabilize the shoulder by balancing the anterior and posterior forces acting on it. This is accomplished by at least securing some of the torn rotator cuff tendon to bone. While a defect may persist superiorly, the partial repair theoretically works through the rotator cable—a thickened fibrous band of fibers that connects the anterior and posterior rotator cuff. It may be effective in providing strength to the shoulder, restoring more normal kinematics, and balancing forces across the shoulder.

In truly immobile tears, an interval slide, in which the supraspinatus is released posteriorly from the infraspinatus, or anteriorly from the rotator interval and the coracohumeral ligament, sometimes allows an additional 1 to 2 cm of lateral excursion of the supraspinatus tendon, thereby permitting a more complete partial repair.[34]

Partial rotator cuff repair has been the subject of interesting clinical research. One study found that partial repair resulted in an initial improvement of symptoms, but that functional outcomes were variable, and results deteriorated over time. Approximately half of the 31 patients in the study were not satisfied at 2-year final follow-up.[35] Other authors found similarly mixed results in their study of 34 patients with a minimum of 5 years follow-up with massive rotator cuff tears (and no evidence of glenohumeral arthritis) treated with partial rotator cuff repair and biceps tenotomy. At final follow-up, patients had no significant change in their motion and 75% of those patients were satisfied with the procedure. However, although patients saw significant improvement in ASES, the Simple Shoulder Test, and visual analog scale scores, 36% had progression in their Hamada classification, and the failure rate was 29%.[36] Although partial repair is an option for treating massive rotator cuff tears, results are not as reliable as full repair.

Margin Convergence and Primary Repair

The term margin convergence describes the progressive, side-to-side closure of a massive, U-shaped rotator cuff tear. This is performed before repairing the tendon directly to bone, if possible. Most massive rotator cuff tears are not retracted but instead are L-shaped with a vertical split from medial to lateral, which assumes a U shape because of the elasticity of the muscle-tendon unit.[37] Repair using a combination of side-to-side, tendon-to-tendon sutures before end-on tendon-to-bone sutures was recommended beginning in the 1940s by McLaughlin. Direct mobilization of these tears without side-to-side margin convergence leads to repair failure because of the tension overload at the apex of the tear at the bone-to-tendon interface. However, side-to-side closure provides a mechanical advantage because of the biomechanical principle of margin convergence. In margin convergence, the free margin of the tear converges toward the greater tuberosity as side-to-side repair progresses (**Figure 2**). As the margin converges, the strain at the free edge of the cuff is significantly reduced, leaving an almost tension-free rotator cuff margin overlying the humeral bone bed. In some circumstances, this allows the tendon to be repaired directly to bone. Side-to-side closure of two-thirds of a U-shaped tear has been shown to reduce the strain at the rotator cuff margin to one-sixth of the strain at the rotator cuff margin before margin convergence. The use of this repair lowers the risk of failure when the rotator cuff tendon is fixated to bone by anchors or transosseous tunnels.

This principle was proven by a cadaver study that examined whether there was a biomechanical rationale for margin convergence in large, retracted rotator cuff tears. The supraspinatus muscle-tendon unit was removed in 20 cadaver shoulders to create a large retracted rotator cuff tear, and margin convergence was performed in an open fashion by placing simple sutures 5 mm apart beginning at the glenoid rim medially and proceeding laterally. Gap area was measured after each suture placement. Each suture produced statistically significant gap closure amounting to 50% after the first suture, 60% after the second, 67% after the third, and 75% after the fourth suture ($P < 0.05$). After suture placement, infraspinatus and subscapularis strain was found to be reduced, as much as 58% at all degrees of rotation at 0° of abduction ($P < 0.05$). The first margin convergence suture caused the greatest increase in intrinsic rotator cuff tension, with each subsequent suture having a similar but less dramatic effect.[38] These results supported the hypothesis that margin convergence decreases the size of the tear gap and reduces strain. As such, the medial margin of a massive, U-shaped tear should not be excessively mobilized from the glenoid or the scapular neck by pulling it over to the humeral bone bed. Such mobilization would lead to large tensile forces in the middle of the repaired rotator cuff margin that would predispose the repair to failure. Margin convergence is a much safer technique that reduces the tensile forces at the repair site and increases the success rate of the operation.

Rotator Cuff Repair With Graft Augmentation

Using allograft, xenograft, or synthetic patches can improve the initial biomechanical strength of a rotator cuff repair and augment the biologic surface area for footprint healing. Typically, the rotator cuff is repaired and the patch is placed over the repair site as an augment for the deficient tissue, though some authors have used these patches (off-label) in a bridge configuration to span massive rotator cuff tear gaps that cannot be reduced to even the medial footprint.[39] Recent meta-analyses have shown that in large to massive rotator cuff tears, addition of a synthetic or biologic patch, in addition to rotator cuff repair, can decrease retear rates and improve ASES scores compared with rotator cuff repair alone.[40,41] Therefore, adding graft augmentation appears to be a helpful technical weapon to increase the chances of healing for the difficult surgical repair of the massive rotator cuff tear.

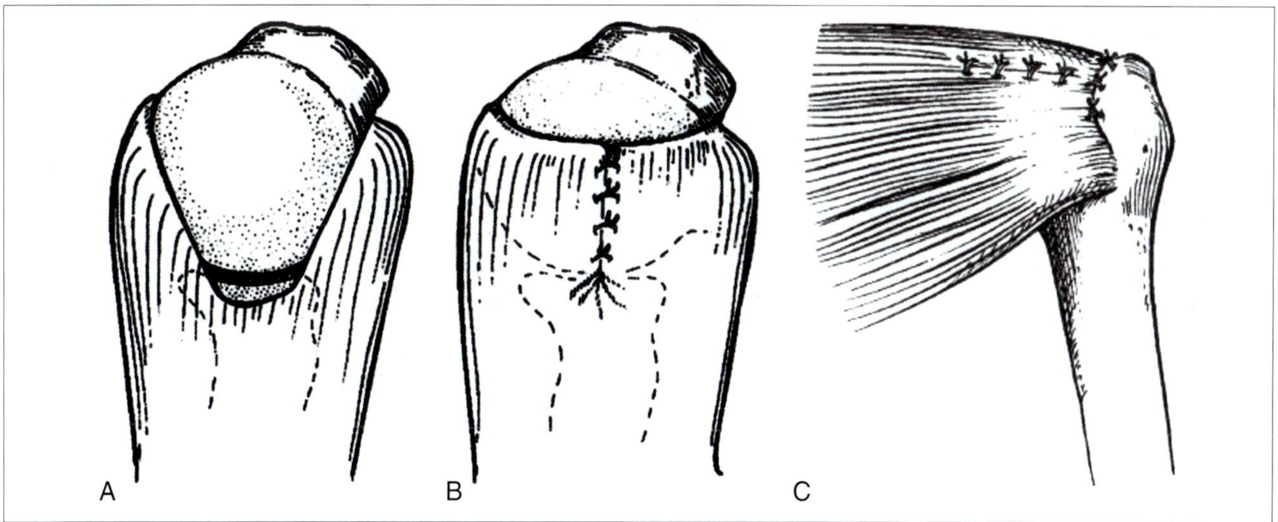

FIGURE 2 Schematic drawings showing a U-shaped rotator cuff tear (**A**), a partial side-to-side repair (**B**), and the placement of side-to-side sutures and repair of the free margin of the cuff to bone with suture anchors (**C**). During the repair, margin convergence of the tear toward the greater tuberosity increases the cross-sectional area and decreases the length of the tear, thereby decreasing strain. (Reproduced with permission from Burkhart SS: Arthroscopic treatment of massive rotator cuff tears. *Clin Orthop Relat Res* 2001;(390):107-118.)

Superior Capsule Reconstruction

Advances in arthroscopic techniques have led to the development of new procedures for addressing the massive rotator cuff tear. First introduced by Mihata in 2013 using fascia lata autograft, the superior capsular reconstruction (SCR) has gained increasing popularity[42] (**Figure 3**). In addition to fascia lata autografts, long head of the biceps tendon autograft has also been described.[43] However, the use of human dermal allograft tissue as a free graft spanning from the superomedial glenoid to the greater tuberosity is most common. In addition, the authors of a 2017 study showed that it is beneficial to perform partial rotator cuff when possible in the setting of SCR as such a repair can help restore the balanced force couples of the shoulder.[44]

Clinical results are beginning to emerge for this relatively novel technique. A recent meta-analysis of six articles on superior capsule reconstruction found that for massive irreparable rotator cuff tears, arthroscopic SCR showed short-term improvements in pain, range of motion, and patient-reported outcomes, with low complications, and few graft failures and revision surgeries.[45] This appears to be a promising new technology to combat the challenging problem of the massive rotator cuff tear that warrants more study to clarify its indications and requires more long-term follow-up.

Subacromial Spacer/Balloon Interposition

Another novel device that has shown promising results in the treatment of massive superior rotator cuff tears is the subacromial balloon spacer (**Figure 4**). This device is a biodegradable balloon placed in the subacromial space and inflated in situ. In the setting of a massive rotator cuff tear, in which the rotator cuff is unable to resist the superior pull of the deltoid, this synthetic spacer can keep the AHI from dynamically compressing.

The balloon, which is made of poly(L-lactide-*co*-ε-caprolactone) (a widely used biodegradable material/polymer), is inserted either fluoroscopically or, more commonly, arthroscopically. The spacer deflates over approximately 8 to 12 weeks and undergoes complete degradation around 12 months postoperatively. Interestingly, patients typically continue to experience relief of symptoms beyond the time period by which the device has degraded. At the set inflation volume, the balloon provides an acromiohumeral distance of 6 mm at the time of implantation. Although currently not FDA approved for use in the United States, 124 patients across

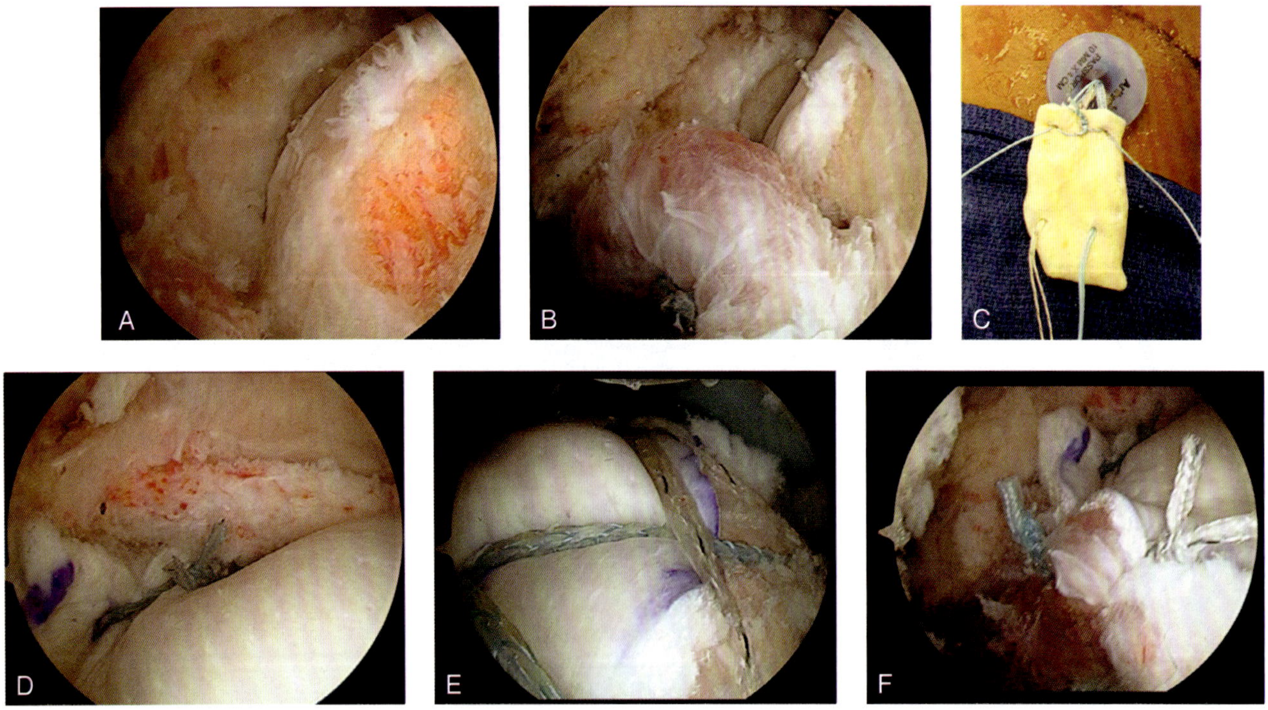

FIGURE 3 Fifty-one-year-old, right-hand dominant male rodeo rider with a massive, irreparable rotator cuff tear. **A**, Arthroscopic view of the right shoulder via posterolateral portal showing massive tear of supraspinatus and upper half of infraspinatus with retraction medial to the glenoid. **B**, Arthroscopic view showing repair of the infraspinatus. **C**, Intraoperative photograph of a dermal graft measured with sutures passed, and ready to be placed through lateral portal. **D**, Arthroscopic view showing placement of the dermal graft with fixation medial on the glenoid. **E**, Arthroscopic view showing fixation of the dermal allograft laterally on the tuberosity. **F**, Arthroscopic view showing fixation of the graft to the infraspinatus with side-to-side sutures. (Courtesy of Grant E. Garrigues, MD.)

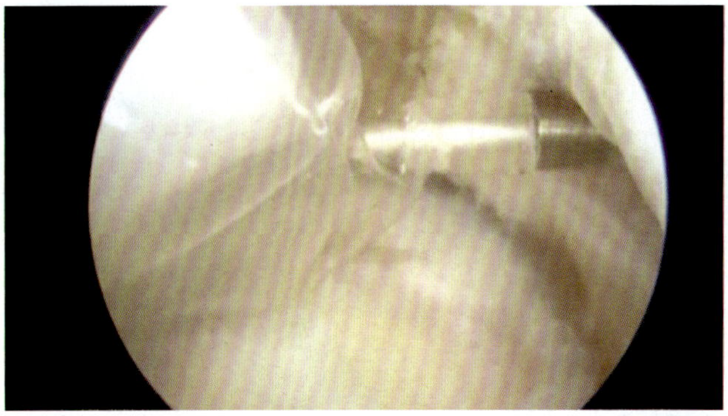

FIGURE 4 Seventy-year-old right-hand dominant man with massive rotator cuff tear. Arthroscopic view of the right shoulder from posterior portal demonstrating spacer (InSpace Balloon; ISB) deploying in subacromial space. (Courtesy of Grant E. Garrigues, MD.)

four studies from Europe showed 80% of patients had a significant improvement in Constant scores. A biomechanical cadaver study showed that peak pressures on the rotator cuff tendon were decreased with the spacer balloon.[46] In clinical studies, patients experienced significant improvements in forward elevation, abduction, and external rotation, as well as improved Constant scores and decreased night pain.[47-49] This technology seems promising in providing symptomatic relief to patients with irreparable, massive rotator cuff tears.

Tendon Transfers

An irreparable tear can be defined as a tear in which direct tendon-to-bone repair and healing are not possible. Tendon transfers have gained increased acceptance as a treatment for such tears by recreating the muscle force that has been lost by the torn rotator cuff muscle by substituting the pull of a different muscle that has been moved to a new location. Historically, local tendon transposition, distant tendon transfer, and deltoid flap transposition have been proposed as methods of reconstructing the rotator cuff. However, more reproducible and long-term success has been achieved by distant tendon transfer in the form of a latissimus dorsi or lower trapezius transfer for massive posterosuperior tears or pectoralis major transfers for less common anterosuperior tears.

Latissimus Dorsi Transfer for Posterosuperior Rotator Cuff Deficiency

Latissimus dorsi transfer was proposed in 1988 for reconstructing tears that involve complete loss of the supraspinatus and the infraspinatus.[50] The transfer of the latissimus dorsi to the superolateral humeral head converts the latissimus dorsi into a humeral head depressor and external rotator by virtue of its insertion relative to the humeral head and its almost-vertical orientation.

Preoperative shoulder function and general strength were found to influence the outcome of a latissimus dorsi transfer. In one study, 14 patients underwent latissimus dorsi transfer for a massive rotator cuff tear and it was found that women with poor preoperative shoulder function and generalized muscle weakness were most likely to have a poor result. It was reported that the most significant predictors of outcome were preoperative active range of motion and strength in forward flexion and external rotation. It was inferred that pseudoparalysis could not be overcome by latissimus dorsi transfer and was established as a relative contraindication.[51] Another study found that latissimus dorsi transfer as a salvage procedure following unsuccessful rotator cuff repair was successful in restoring range of motion and improving pain and function, and that deltoid function was linked to the extent of improvement.[52]

Inferior outcomes after latissimus transfer have been associated with subscapularis dysfunction, severe teres minor fatty infiltration, revision procedures, and patients with arthritic changes of the glenohumeral joint at the time of transfer.[53,54] Additionally, one-third of patients have progression of arthritis following latissimus transfer.[55]

Relatively recent modifications of the latissimus dorsi transfer technique include harvesting of the tendon with a small piece of bone to enable direct transosseous bone-to-bone healing of the transfer, a single-incision technique, and a single-incision technique using a minimally invasive approach that exposes only the humeral tendon insertion and the site of transfer reinsertion.[56,57] Despite the theoretic advantages of these modifications, none of them has led to superior results over other techniques thus far. Latissimus dorsi transfer has waned in popularity likely because of the very limited indications and the modest functional improvements.

Lower Trapezius Transfer

The lower trapezius transfer has become increasingly used for the management of the massive, irreparable posterosuperior rotator cuff tear[58] (**Figure 5**). In one large clinical study, authors followed up 33 patients treated with lower trapezius transfer for irreparable posterosuperior rotator cuff tears with an average age of 53 years. Their technique involved harvest of the lower trapezius tendon and augmenting it with an Achilles tendon allograft before reattaching it at the superolateral proximal humerus. At an average of 37 months follow-up, 32/33 patients had significant improvements in pain and the subjective shoulder value scores. Patients with >60° of preoperative forward flexion showed more significant gains in range of motion, whereas shoulder external rotation improved in all patients regardless of their preoperative motion.

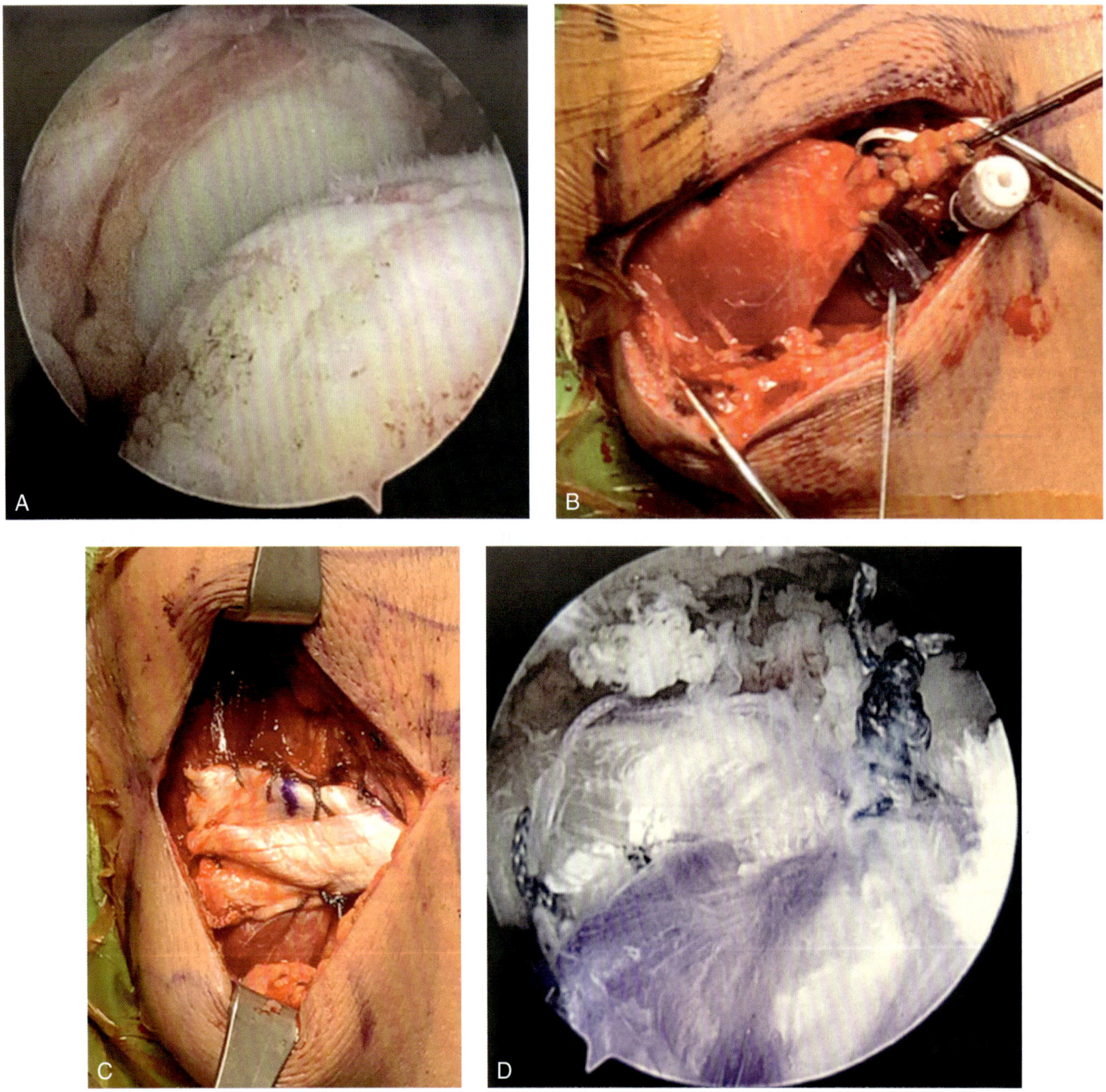

FIGURE 5 Forty-eight-year-old right-hand dominant man with massive rotator cuff tear. **A**, Arthroscopic view of right shoulder via posterolateral portal showing a massive tear of the supraspinatus and infraspinatus retracted medial the glenoid. **B**, Intraoperative photograph showing right shoulder with harvested lower trap from the medial portion of the scapular spine. Note the cannula in place with sutures for shuttling under the deltoid. **C**, Intraoperative photograph showing lower trap with Achilles tendon augmentation after passing under the posterior deltoid. **D**, Arthroscopic view from the posterolateral portal after successful passage and fixation of Achilles tendon allograft. (Courtesy of Grant E. Garrigues, MD.)

In this study, the potential benefit of the lower trapezius transfer is its improved line of pull, closely mimicking that of the infraspinatus. In addition, in contradistinction to the latissimus, the lower trapezius is normally active during abduction and external rotation, so as a natural infraspinatus agonist, it is easier to retrain. A biomechanical study was performed to compare latissimus dorsi transfer with lower trapezius transfer in the treatment of massive posterosuperior rotator cuff tears. Eight cadavers were used to test the shoulder at 0°, 30°, and 60° of shoulder abduction. Four conditions were tested including intact rotator cuff, massive rotator cuff tear, lower trapezius transfer, and latissimus dorsi transfer. This study found that the lower trapezius is superior to latissimus in restoring native glenohumeral joint kinematics and shoulder joint reactive forces.[59]

Pectoralis Major Transfer

A pectoralis major transfer is an option for treating a massive anterosuperior rotator cuff tear. Historically, several techniques have been described. Routing the transferred pectoralis major tendon under the conjoined tendon has a biomechanically preferable line of pull, but the disadvantage of a higher risk of musculocutaneous nerve injury when compared with placing it over the conjoined tendon. However, there is no evidence that the technically less demanding over-the-tendon technique leads to clinically inferior results.[60,61]

One study followed up 12 patients of mean age of 65 years who had an irreparable subscapularis tear and who were treated with a subcoracoid split pectoralis major transfer.[61] The superior one-half to two-thirds of the pectoralis major was used as a substitute for the subscapularis tendon. The split portion of the pectoralis muscle transfer was routed behind the conjoined tendon to the lesser tuberosity to adapt the orientation of the pectoralis major to that of the subscapularis (**Figure 6**). At a mean 28-month follow-up, the outcome was excellent in five patients, good in four, and fair in three. The mean Constant score improved from 26.9 to 67.1, and all patients had healing of the transfer on ultrasonography. There were no complications, including no evidence of injury to neurovascular structures.[61]

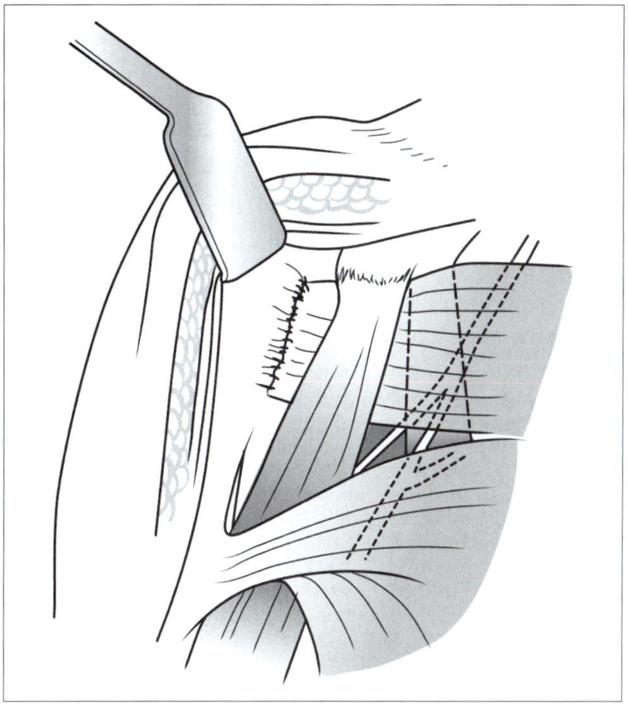

FIGURE 6 Schematic drawing showing the course of the transferred pectoralis major under the conjoined tendon. (Adapted with permission from Resch H, Povacz P, Ritter E, et al: Transfer of the pectoralis major muscle for the treatment of irreparable rupture of the subscapularis tendon. *J Bone Joint Surg Am* 2000;82[3]:372-382.)

More recently, authors followed a series of 27 patients who underwent subcoracoid pectoralis major transfer for irreparable anterosuperior rotator cuff tear with average 10-year follow-up. They found that patients had improved pain and internal rotation, with 77% satisfaction. However, 67% of patients showed progression of rotator cuff arthropathy, and one patient required revision surgery to a reverse shoulder arthroplasty.[62] Both major techniques of placing the transported pectoralis major tendon above or below the conjoint tendon appear to be effective in providing durable pain relief and functional improvement to patients with massive anterosuperior rotator cuff deficiency. Although rotator cuff arthropathy appears to continue to progress despite pectoralis major transfer, this does not seem to have a negative effect on patient satisfaction from the procedure, even with long-term follow-up.

Conversely, another study followed 30 consecutive pectoralis major transfers over the conjoined tendon at average age of 53 years for either isolated tears of the subscapularis or subscapularis tears also associated with tears of the posterior rotator cuff (**Figure 7**). At a mean of 32-month follow-up, the mean relative Constant score improved from 47% before surgery to 70%. The patients with an isolated subscapularis tear or both a subscapularis tear and a repairable supraspinatus tear had a postoperative higher relative Constant score. Patients with a subscapularis tear and an irreparable supraspinatus tear had a clearly inferior clinical outcome and lower relative Constant score at final follow-up.[60]

Latissimus Dorsi and Combined Latissimus and Teres Major Transfer for Subscapularis Insufficiency

For patients with isolated subscapularis deficiency or anterosuperior rotator cuff deficiency, latissimus tendon transfer with or without transfer of the teres major has been described. The theoretical benefits of this are the relative ease of access to the donor tendons, as well as the improved line of pull of the donor tendons. In a feasibility study, researchers described the dimensions of the latissimus and teres major tendons compared with that of the subscapularis. They found a low risk of axillary nerve compression, except in the case in which both the latissimus and teres major tendon transfer was used and were transferred to the proximal third of the subscapularis insertion.[63]

Reverse Total Shoulder Arthroplasty

In situations in which a patient has a massive rotator cuff tear and the patient is considered an arthroplasty candidate, reverse total shoulder arthroplasty (RTSA) is an excellent consideration. Although RTSA was initially

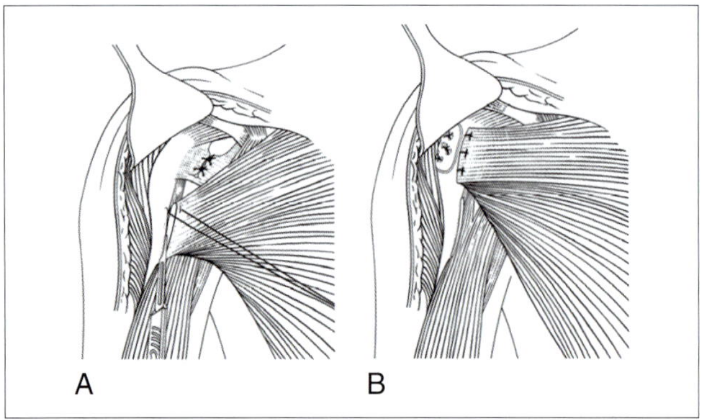

FIGURE 7 Schematic drawings showing the course of the transferred pectoralis major over the conjoined tendon. **A**, The deltoid muscle is retracted. After mobilization of the subscapularis, an attempt is made to repair the remaining tendon, scar, and fascial tissue to the lesser tuberosity. The pectoralis major tendon is then released completely from its insertion. A reinsertion area for the pectoralis major tendon on the medial aspect of the greater tuberosity is then prepared. **B**, The pectoralis major tendon is transferred to the medial aspect of the greater tuberosity over the conjoined tendon. (Reproduced with permission from Jost B, Puskas GJ, Lustenberger A, Gerber C: Outcome of pectoralis major transfer for the treatment of irreparable subscapularis tears. *J Bone Joint Surg Am* 2003;85[10]:1944-1951.)

reserved for elderly patients with rotator cuff tear arthropathy classified as at least Hamada grade 3, its indications have expanded because comfort with the technique and medium-term results have improved.[64] RTSA allows the rotator cuff–deficient shoulder to function by substituting the centering effect of the semiconstrained reverse bearing in place of the deficient rotator cuff. The design of the prosthesis exploits the mechanical advantage of the long fulcrum of the deltoid to abduct and elevate the arm without causing superior translation of the humeral head because of the constraint afforded by the implant.

Although RTSA has proven to be a reliable option for elderly patients with limited functional demands, clinical results are less predictable in other populations. In one study of patients with irreparable rotator cuff tears without arthritis, age younger than 60 years, high preoperative function, and neurologic dysfunction, RTSA was associated with poorer outcomes.[65] Similarly, other studies have shown worse outcomes in younger patient populations with better preoperative range of motion. One study found that, in patients with preoperative forward elevation greater than 90°, there was an overall decrease in postoperative forward elevation and that subgroup had a 27% dissatisfaction rate.[66] Similarly, others studied the long-term results of RTSA for massive rotator cuff tears in patients younger than 65 years, and, although functional scores and ROM improved, there was 37.5% complication rate.[67] Although short-term and medium-term results of RTSA for patients with massive rotator cuff tears and no arthritis have been encouraging, caution is urged in patients with increased preoperative range of motion and function and in younger patients for whom there may be another nonarthroplasty alternative.

Reverse Total Shoulder Arthroplasty With Concomitant Latissimus Dorsi Tendon Transfer

In patients who have a massive rotator cuff tear and combined loss of active elevation and external rotation and who are arthroplasty candidates, an RTSA with combined latissimus dorsi tendon transfer may be indicated. The loss of both active elevation and external rotation is very disabling to one's ability to perform the activities of daily life. This combined procedure can be performed through a single deltopectoral incision. The latissimus tendon, with or without the teres major, is harvested and rerouted around the humerus. It is attached laterally, just posterior to the long head biceps tendon and the insertion of the pectoralis major, which is typically partially transected to facilitate exposure. In a review of 15 consecutive patients who underwent latissimus dorsi tendon transfer, 8 of which were combined with RTSA, authors found that in the patients with combined loss of active elevation and external rotation, the average increase in active external rotation was 28°, and the whole cohort had an average increase in forward elevation of 34.7°. They found that the major contributor to patient satisfaction was the ability to control the spatial positioning of the surgical arm. All but one patient was satisfied or very satisfied.[68]

SUMMARY

Massive rotator cuff tears remain a clinical challenge. A thorough history and physical examination are vital for accurate diagnosis of the patient's condition. A variety of imaging modalities can be used; most commonly plain radiography, CT arthrography, and MRI, to help delineate the extent and severity of the pathology. The natural history is not well understood, but some patients can do well with conservative treatment using physical therapy and pain management. However, most patients experience increasing pain and disability over time and require surgical intervention. The choice of intervention can be unclear as there are many options with overlapping indications. The treatment modality chosen for a massive rotator cuff tear must be tailored to the patient's needs, expectations, and ability to comply with intensive rehabilitation. However, these patients can do remarkably well with an individually tailored approach that matches the patient pathology and functional demands with an appropriately chosen nonsurgical or surgical management.

In a patient with low physical demands, but preserved active elevation, simple débridement of the inflamed subacromial tissue may provide pain relief and some secondary functional improvement if the cuff cannot be repaired. However, the results deteriorate over time, especially as tear size increases. Partial repair using the margin convergence technique decreases the size of the tear gap and reduces strain, with minimal effect on glenohumeral translation and intrinsic tendon strain. For tears with poor tissue, or in young active patients, partial repair with graft augmentation or SCR has been performed with encouraging results. In older patients, with massive, irreparable rotator cuff tears and without glenohumeral arthritis, subacromial spacers and balloon interposition have been used to restore the glenohumeral joint relationship and increase the acromiohumeral distance. Tendon transfers offer a good result for a patient with a massive, irreparable rotator cuff tear who has intact deltoid function and disabling weakness without pseudoparalysis. However, a tendon transfer will not halt the progression of cuff tear arthropathy. Finally, in lower demand patients with massive rotator cuff tears, the reverse shoulder arthroplasty, with or without concomitant tendon transfer, has become a reliable option to eliminate pain and restore motion as it relies on the deltoid for active elevation.

KEY STUDY POINTS

- Massive rotator cuff tears are challenging to treat, tend to progress over time, and have a high degree of retear rate given the often concomitant tendon retraction and fatty infiltration.
- Subacromial débridement, biceps tenotomy or tenodesis, tuberoplasty, reversed subacromial decompression, and partial rotator cuff repair all provide pain relief and some functional gains, perhaps partially mediated through pain relief, when a full rotator cuff repair is not possible.
- Graft augmentation, superior capsular reconstruction, and subacromial spacers are new technologies in which new tissues/devices provide extrinsic stability and robustness to a repair in the shoulder with an irreparable, massive rotator cuff tear, granting functional improvements and pain relief.
- A variety of tendon transfers can provide strength to compensate for specific deficiencies from massive rotator cuff tears.
- Reverse total shoulder arthroplasty is an operation with a reliable track record for relieving pain and increasing function for patients with massive rotator cuff tears, particularly in those with limited functional demands.

Annotated References

1. Bedi A, Dines J, Warren RF, Dines DM: Massive tears of the rotator cuff. *J Bone Joint Surg Am* 2010;92(9):1894-1908. doi:10.2106/JBJS.I.01531.

2. Cofield RH, Parvizi J, Hoffmeyer PJ, Lanzer WL, Ilstrup DM, Rowland CM: Surgical repair of chronic rotator cuff tears. A prospective long-term study. *J Bone Joint Surg Am* 2001;83(1):71-77. doi:10.2106/00004623-200101000-00010.

3. Zingg PO, Jost B, Sukthankar A, Buhler M, Pfirrmann CWA, Gerber C: Clinical and structural outcomes of nonoperative management of massive rotator cuff tears. *J Bone Joint Surg Am* 2007;89(9):1928-1934. doi:10.2106/JBJS.F.01073.

4. Harryman DT, Hettrich CM, Smith KL, Campbell B, Sidles JA, Matsen FA: A prospective multipractice investigation of patients with full-thickness rotator cuff tears: The importance of comorbidities, practice, and other covariables on self-assessed shoulder function and health status. *J Bone Joint Surg Am* 2003;85(4):690-696. doi:10.2106/00004623-200304000-00016.

5. Su WR, Budoff JE, Luo ZP: The effect of anterosuperior rotator cuff tears on glenohumeral translation. *Arthroscopy* 2009;25(3):282-289. doi:10.1016/j.arthro.2008.10.005.

6. Paletta GA, Warner JJP, Warren RF, Deutsch A, Altchek DW: Shoulder kinematics with two-plane x-ray evaluation in patients with anterior instability or rotator cuff tearing. *J Shoulder Elbow Surg* 1997;6(6):516-527. doi:10.1016/S1058-2746(97)90084-7.

7. Burkhart SS: Fluoroscopic comparison of kinematic patterns in massive rotator cuff tears. A suspension bridge model. *Clin Orthop Relat Res* 1992;(284):144-152. doi:10.1097/00003086-199211000-00018.

8. Oh JH, Jun BJ, McGarry MH, Lee TQ: Does a critical rotator cuff tear stage exist? A biomechanical study of rotator cuff tear progression in human cadaver shoulders. *J Bone Joint Surg Am* 2011;93(22):2100-2109. doi:10.2106/JBJS.J.00032.

9. Gerber C, Wirth SH, Farshad M: Treatment options for massive rotator cuff tears. *J Shoulder Elbow Surg* 2011;20(2 suppl):S20-S29. doi:10.1016/j.jse.2010.11.028.

10. Abate M, Schiavone C, Salini V: Sonographic evaluation of the shoulder in asymptomatic elderly subjects with diabetes. *BMC Musculoskelet Disord* 2010;11:278. doi:10.1186/1471-2474-11-278.

11. Yamamoto A, Takagishi K, Osawa T, et al: Prevalence and risk factors of a rotator cuff tear in the general population. *J Shoulder Elbow Surg* 2010;19(1):116-120. doi:10.1016/j.jse.2009.04.006.

12. Galatz LM, Ball CM, Teefey SA, Middleton WD, Yamaguchi K: The outcome and repair integrity of completely arthroscopically repaired large and massive rotator cuff tears. *J Bone Joint Surg Am* 2004;86(2):219-224. doi:10.2106/00004623-200402000-00002.

13. Zumstein MA, Jost B, Hempel J, Hodler J, Gerber C: The clinical and structural long-term results of open repair of massive tears of the rotator cuff. *J Bone Joint Surg Am* 2008;90(11):2423-2431. doi:10.2106/JBJS.G.00677.

14. Nové-Josserand L, Costa P, Liotard JP, Safar JF, Walch G, Zilber S: Results of latissimus dorsi tendon transfer for irreparable cuff tears. *Orthop Traumatol Surg Res* 2009;95(2):108-113. doi:10.1016/j.otsr.2008.10.002.

15. Jeong HY, Kim HJ, Jeon YS, Rhee YG: Factors predictive of healing in large rotator cuff tears: Is it possible to predict retear preoperatively? *Am J Sports Med* 2018;46(7):1693-1700. doi:10.1177/0363546518762386.

    A case-control study of 112 patients determined that preoperative supraspinatus muscle atrophy and fatty infiltration of the infraspinatus were independent predictors of retear following rotator cuff repair. Level of evidence: III.

16. Hamada K, Fukuda H, Mikasa M, Kobayashi Y: Roentgenographic findings in massive rotator cuff tears. A long-term observation. *Clin Orthop Relat Res* 1990;(254):92-96. doi:10.1097/00003086-199005000-00014.

17. Walch G, Edwards TB, Boulahia A, Nové-Josserand L, Neyton L, Szabo I: Arthroscopic tenotomy of the long head of the biceps in the treatment of rotator cuff tears: Clinical and radiographic results of 307 cases. *J Shoulder Elbow Surg* 2005;14(3):238-246. doi:10.1016/j.jse.2004.07.008.

18. Nové-Josserand L, Edwards TB, O'Connor DP, Walch G: The acromiohumeral and coracohumeral intervals are abnormal in rotator cuff tears with muscular fatty degeneration. *Clin Orthop Relat Res* 2005;(433):90-96. doi:10.1097/01.blo.0000151441.05180.0e.

19. Fuchs B, Weishaupt D, Zanetti M, Hodler J, Gerber C: Fatty degeneration of the muscles of the rotator cuff: Assessment by computed tomography versus magnetic resonance imaging. *J Shoulder Elbow Surg* 1999;8(6):599-605. doi:10.1016/S1058-2746(99)90097-6.

20. Lippe J, Spang JT, Leger RR, Arciero RA, Mazzocca AD, Shea KP: Inter-rater agreement of the Goutallier, Patte, and Warner classification scores using preoperative magnetic resonance imaging in patients with rotator cuff tears. *Arthroscopy* 2012;28(2):154-159. doi:10.1016/j.arthro.2011.07.016.

21. Matson AP, Kim C, Bajpai S, Green CL, Hash TW, Garrigues GE: The effect of obesity on fatty infiltration of the rotator cuff musculature in patients without rotator cuff tears. *Shoulder Elbow* 2019;11(1 suppl):30-38. doi:10.1177/1758573217736008.

    Twenty-five patients from each of four different body mass index ranges were randomly selected from consecutive shoulder magnetic resonance scans and assigned Goutallier grades to the rotator cuff and adjacent muscles. This study demonstrated that obesity without rotator cuff tear, as well as old age, and diabetes had more fatty infiltration in rotator cuff muscles. Level of evidence: III.

22. Hamada K, Yamanaka K, Uchiyama Y, Mikasa T, Mikasa M: A radiographic classification of massive rotator cuff tear arthritis. *Clin Orthop Relat Res* 2011;469(9):2452-2460. doi:10.1007/s11999-011-1896-9.

23. Burkhart SS, Barth JRH, Richards DP, Zlatkin MB, Larsen M: Arthroscopic repair of massive rotator cuff tears with stage 3 and 4 fatty degeneration. *Arthroscopy* 2007;23(4):347-354. doi:10.1016/j.arthro.2006.12.012.

24. Yoo JC, Ahn JH, Yang JH, Koh KH, Choi SH, Yoon YC: Correlation of arthroscopic repairability of large to massive rotator cuff tears with preoperative magnetic resonance imaging scans. *Arthroscopy* 2009;25(6):573-582. doi:10.1016/j.arthro.2008.12.015.

25. Iannotti JP, Ciccone J, Buss DD, et al: Accuracy of office-based ultrasonography of the shoulder for the diagnosis of rotator cuff tears. *J Bone Joint Surg Am* 2005;87(6):1305-1311. doi:10.2106/JBJS.D.02100.

26. Al-Shawi A, Badge R, Bunker T: The detection of full thickness rotator cuff tears using ultrasound. *J Bone Joint Surg Br* 2008;87(6):1305-1311. doi:10.1302/0301-620x.90b7.20481.

27. Levy O, Mullett H, Roberts S, Copeland S: The role of anterior deltoid reeducation in patients with massive irreparable degenerative rotator cuff tears. *J Shoulder Elbow Surg* 2008;17(6):863-870. doi:10.1016/j.jse.2008.04.005.

28. Liem D, Lengers N, Dedy N, Poetzl W, Steinbeck J, Marquardt B: Arthroscopic debridement of massive irreparable rotator cuff tears. *Arthroscopy* 2008;24(7):743-748. doi:10.1016/j.arthro.2008.03.007.

29. Neer CS: Anterior acromioplasty for the chronic impingement syndrome in the shoulder. *J Bone Joint Surg Am* 1972;54(1):41-50. doi:10.2106/00004623-197254010-00003.

30. Fagelman M, Sartori M, Freedman KB, Patwardhan AG, Carandang G, Marra G: Biomechanics of coracoacromial arch modification. *J Shoulder Elbow Surg* 2007;16(1):101-106. doi:10.1016/j.jse.2006.01.010.

31. Flatow E, Rodosky M, Yamaguchi K, Self E, Pollock RG, Bigliani LU: Coracoacromial ligament preservation in rotator cuff surgery. *J Shoulder Elbow Surg* 1996;5(2):S78.

32. Fenlin JM, Chase JM, Rushton SA, Frieman BG: Tuberoplasty: Creation of an acromiohumeral articulation—A treatment option for massive, irreparable rotator cuff tears. *J Shoulder Elbow Surg* 2002;11(2):136-142. doi:10.1067/mse.2002.121764.

33. Scheibel M, Lichtenberg S, Habermeyer P: Reversed arthroscopic subacromial decompression for massive rotator cuff tears. *J Shoulder Elbow Surg* 2004;13(3):272-278. doi:10.1016/j.jse.2004.01.007.

34. Tauro JC: Arthroscopic "interval slide" in the repair of large rotator cuff tears. *Arthroscopy* 1999;15(5):527-530. doi:10.1053/ar.1999.v15.0150521.

35. Shon MS, Koh KH, Lim TK, Kim WJ, Kim KC, Yoo JC: Arthroscopic partial repair of irreparable rotator cuff tears: Preoperative factors associated with outcome deterioration over 2 years. *Am J Sports Med* 2015;43(8):1965-1975. doi:10.1177/0363546515585122.

    In this case series of 31 patients who underwent arthroscopic partial rotator cuff repair, results initially improved, before deteriorating over time, with 15 poor responses to treatment. Level of evidence: IV.

36. Cuff DJ, Pupello DR, Santoni BG: Partial rotator cuff repair and biceps tenotomy for the treatment of patients with massive cuff tears and retained overhead elevation: Midterm outcomes with a minimum 5 years of follow-up. *J Shoulder Elbow Surg* 2016;25(11):1803-1809. doi:10.1016/j.jse.2016.04.001.

    In this case series, 34 patients with massive rotator cuff tear and retained forward elevation were treated with partial repair and biceps tenotomy. Patients had 75% satisfaction rate, 36% of patients had progression of the Hamada stage, and in 29% of patients the procedure failed at minimum of 5-year follow-up. Level of evidence: IV.

37. Burkhart SS: Arthroscopic treatment of massive rotator cuff tears. *Clin Orthop Relat Res* 2001;390:107-118. doi:10.1097/00003086-200109000-00013.

38. Mazzocca AD, Bollier M, Fehsenfeld D, et al: Biomechanical evaluation of margin convergence. *Arthroscopy* 2011;27(3):330-338. doi:10.1016/j.arthro.2010.09.003.

39. Neumann JA, Zgonis MH, Rickert KD, et al: Interposition dermal matrix xenografts: A successful alternative to traditional treatment of massive rotator cuff tears. *Am J Sports Med* 2017;45(6):1261-1268. doi:10.1177/0363546516683945.

    In this case series, 61 patients with massive rotator cuff tear were treated with porcine acellular dermal matrix xenograft as an interposition graft. Patients had significant improvement in pain, range of motion, and manual muscle strength; and 91.8% of patients had intact repair at final follow-up. Level of evidence: IV.

40. Bailey JR, Kim C, Alentorn-Geli E, et al: Rotator cuff matrix augmentation and interposition: A systematic review and meta-analysis. *Am J Sports Med* 2019;47(6):1496-1506. doi:10.1177/0363546518774762.

    A systematic review of 1291 shoulders demonstrated that graft augmentation or interposition appeared to provide a lower retear rate and improved ASES scores when compared with rotator cuff repair alone. Level of evidence: IV.

41. Sanchez G, Chahla J, Moatshe G, Ferrari MB, Kennedy NI, Provencher MT: Superior capsular reconstruction with superimposition of rotator cuff repair for massive rotator cuff tear. *Arthrosc Tech* 2017;6(5):e1775-e1779. doi:10.1016/j.eats.2017.06.049.

    This technical note describes superior capsule reconstruction with superimposition of rotator cuff repair in the treatment of massive rotator cuff tears. Level of evidence: V.

42. Mihata T, Lee TQ, Watanabe C, et al: Clinical results of arthroscopic superior capsule reconstruction for irreparable rotator cuff tears. *Arthroscopy* 2013;29(3):459-470. doi:10.1016/j.arthro.2012.10.022.

    In this case series of 24 shoulders with irreparable rotator cuff repair, superior capsule reconstruction was first introduced. These shoulders underwent SCR using fascia lata autograft, which restored superior glenohumeral stability and function of the shoulder joint. Level of evidence: IV.

43. Hermanowicz K, Góralczyk A, Malinowski K, Jancewicz P, Domżalski ME: Long head biceps tendon – Natural patch for massive irreparable rotator cuff tears. *Arthrosc Tech* 2018;7(5):e473-e478. doi:10.1016/j.eats.2017.11.008.

    This technical note describes the utilization of the long head of the biceps tendon as a vascularized graft bridging over a partial rotator cuff repair in the treatment of massive rotator cuff tears. Level of evidence: V.

44. Sutter EG, Godin JA, Garrigues GE: All-arthroscopic superior shoulder capsule reconstruction with partial rotator cuff repair. *Orthopedics* 2017;40(4):e735-e738. doi:10.3928/01477447-20170615-01.

    This technical note describes an arthroscopic superior capsular reconstruction with a dermal allograft with concomitant partial rotator cuff repair. Level of evidence: V.

45. Sochacki KR, McCulloch PC, Lintner DM, Harris JD: Superior capsular reconstruction for massive rotator cuff tear leads to significant improvement in range of motion and clinical outcomes: A systematic review. *Arthroscopy* 2019;35(4):1269-1277. doi:10.1016/j.arthro.2018.10.129.

    A review of six articles analyzed arthroscopic superior capsular reconstruction for massive irreparable rotator cuff tears. Results showed significant improvement in patient-reported outcomes and shoulder range of motion with low graft failure, complication, and revision surgery rates at short-term follow-up. Level of evidence: IV.

46. Chevalier Y, Pietschmann MF, Thorwächter C, et al: Biodegradable spacer reduces the subacromial pressure: A biomechanical cadaver study. *Clin Biomech (Bristol, Avon)* 2018;52:41-48. doi:10.1016/j.clinbiomech.2017.12.008.

This cadaver study investigated the effects of the subacromial spacer on compression pressures over a repaired supraspinatus tendon in passive motion and found the mean and peak pressures in abduction-adduction were significantly reduced after insertion of the subacromial spacer.

47. Yallapragada RK, Apostolopoulos A, Katsougrakis I, Selvan TP: The use of a subacromial spacer-inspace balloon in managing patients with irreparable rotator cuff tears. *J Orthop* 2018;15(3):862-868. doi:10.1016/j.jor.2018.08.004.

A prospective nonrandomized case series of 14 patients established the role of biodegradable subacromial spacer (InSpace) insertion in the treatment of patients with massive irreparable rotator cuff tear. The spacer resulted in a noticeable improvement in pain relief and shoulder function at a mean 12.6 months follow-up. Level of evidence: IV.

48. Holschen M, Brand F, Agneskirchner JD: Subacromial spacer implantation for massive rotator cuff tears: Clinical outcome of arthroscopically treated patients. *Obere Extrem* 2017;12(1):38-45. doi:10.1007/s11678-016-0386-9.

The study retrospectively analyzed the clinical outcome of 11 patients treated with conventional arthroscopy and 12 patients treated with a supplementary subacromial spacer. Preoperative shoulder function was lower in patients treated with a subacromial spacer, and both groups had improved shoulder function and satisfaction showing that subacromial spacer is a feasible treatment option for massive rotator cuff tear. Level of evidence: IV.

49. Senekovic V, Poberaj B, Kovacic L, et al: The biodegradable spacer as a novel treatment modality for massive rotator cuff tears: A prospective study with 5-year follow-up. *Arch Orthop Trauma Surg* 2017;137(1):95-103. doi:10.1007/s00402-016-2603-9.

In this case series, 21 patients with massive repairable or irreparable rotator cuff tears were analyzed to confirm the long-term safety and efficacy of the biodegradable inflatable InSpace system. Results suggested the system as an effective treatment. Level of evidence: IV.

50. Gerber C, Vinh T, Hertel R, Hess CW: Latissimus dorsi transfer for the treatment of massive tears of the rotator cuff. A preliminary report. *Clin Orthop Relat Res* 1988;(232):51-61. doi:10.1097/00003086-198807000-00008.

51. Iannotti JP, Hennigan S, Herzog R, et al: Latissimus dorsi tendon transfer for irreparable posterosuperior rotator cuff tears. Factors affecting outcome. *J Bone Joint Surg Am* 2006;88(2):342-348. doi:10.2106/JBJS.D.02996.

52. Birmingham PM, Neviaser RJ: Outcome of latissimus dorsi transfer as a salvage procedure for failed rotator cuff repair with loss of elevation. *J Shoulder Elbow Surg* 2008;17(6):871-874. doi:10.1016/j.jse.2008.04.007.

53. Namdari S, Voleti P, Baldwin K, Glaser D, Huffman GR: Latissimus dorsi tendon transfer for irreparable rotator cuff tears: A systematic review. *J Bone Joint Surg Am* 2012;94(10):891-898. doi:10.2106/JBJS.K.00841.

54. Gerber C, Rahm SA, Catanzaro S, Farshad M, Moor BK: Latissimus dorsi tendon transfer for treatment of irreparable posterosuperior rotator cuff tears: Long-term results at a minimum follow-up of ten years. *J Bone Joint Surg Am* 2013;95(21):1920-1926. doi:10.2106/JBJS.M.00122.

In this case series, 46 patients who were treated with latissimus dorsi tendon transfer for irreparable posterosuperior rotator cuff tears were followed up. Patients demonstrated substantial and durable improvements in shoulder function and pain relief on final follow-up, which was performed at a mean of 147 months. Level of evidence: IV.

55. Petriccioli D, Bertone C, Marchi G: Recovery of active external rotation and elevation in young active men with irreparable posterosuperior rotator cuff tear using arthroscopically assisted latissimus dorsi transfer. *J Shoulder Elbow Surg* 2016;25(9):e265-e275. doi:10.1016/j.jse.2015.12.011.

In this case series of 33 patients who underwent arthroscopically assisted lattisimus dorsi transfer for irreparable posterosuperior rotator cuff tear, patients, particularly active men under 60 years old with intact subscapularis and low forward elevation did well, but 1/3 had progression of osteoarthritis. Level of evidence: IV.

56. Gerhardt C, Lehmann L, Lichtenberg S, Magosch P, Habermeyer P: Modified l'Episcopo tendon transfers for irreparable rotator cuff tears: 5-year followup. *Clin Orthop Relat Res* 2010;468(6):1572-1577. doi:10.1007/s11999-009-1030-4.

57. Lehmann LJ, Mauerman E, Strube T, Laibacher K, Scharf HP: Modified minimally invasive latissimus dorsi transfer in the treatment of massive rotator cuff tears: A two-year follow-up of 26 consecutive patients. *Int Orthop* 2010;34(3):377-383. doi:10.1007/s00264-009-0782-5.

58. Elhassan BT, Wagner ER, Werthel JD: Outcome of lower trapezius transfer to reconstruct massive irreparable posterior-superior rotator cuff tear. *J Shoulder Elbow Surg* 2016;25(8):1346-1353. doi:10.1016/j.jse.2015.12.006.

In this case series, 33 patients with symptomatic massive irreparable rotator cuff tear and in whom conservative or prior surgical treatment failed underwent reconstruction with lower trapezius transfer augmented by Achilles tendon allograft. Follow-up at an average of 47 months showed that this technique may lead to good outcomes, specifically for those who have preoperative flexion of >60°. Level of evidence: IV.

59. Omid R, Heckmann N, Wang L, McGarry MH, Vangsness CT, Lee TQ: Biomechanical comparison between the trapezius transfer and latissimus transfer for irreparable posterosuperior rotator cuff tears. *J Shoulder Elbow Surg* 2015;24(10):1635-1643. doi:10.1016/j.jse.2015.02.008.

A cadaver study tested shoulders at varying degrees of shoulder abduction to characterize the biomechanical effects of the lower trapezius transfer to compare it with the latissimus dorsi transfer in a massive posterosuperior rotator cuff tear. Results showed that the lower trapezius transfer is superior to the latissimus transfer at restoring native glenohumeral kinematics and joint reaction forces.

60. Jost B, Puskas GJ, Lustenberger A, Gerber C: Outcome of pectoralis major transfer for the treatment of irreparable subscapularis tears. *J Bone Joint Surg Am* 2003;85(10):1944-1951. doi:10.2106/00004623-200310000-00012.

61. Resch H, Povacz P, Ritter E, Matschi W: Transfer of the pectoralis major muscle for the treatment of irreparable rupture of the subscapularis tendon. *J Bone Joint Surg Am* 2000;82(3):372-382. doi:10.2106/00004623-200003000-00008.

62. Moroder P, Schulz E, Mitterer M, Plachel F, Resch H, Lederer S: Long-term outcome after pectoralis major transfer for irreparable anterosuperior rotator cuff tears. *J Bone Joint Surg Am* 2017;99(3):239-245. doi:10.2106/JBJS.16.00485.

In this case series, 27 patients with irreparable anterosuperior rotator cuff tears without advanced cuff arthropathy or advanced humeral head migration were treated with a partial subcoracoid pectoralis major tendon transfer, which resulted in a significant clinical improvement at 10 years after surgery. Level of evidence: IV.

63. Elhassan B, Christensen TJ, Wagner ER: Feasibility of latissimus and teres major transfer to reconstruct irreparable subscapularis tendon tear: An anatomic study. *J Shoulder Elbow Surg* 2014;23(4):492-499. doi:10.1016/j.jse.2013.07.046.

An anatomic study that demonstrates that transfer of the lattisimus dorsi and trapezius muscle to reconstruct irrepairable subscapularis tears is technically feasible.

64. Bacle G, Nové-Josserand L, Garaud P, Walch G: Long-term outcomes of reverse total shoulder arthroplasty: A follow-up of a previous study. *J Bone Joint Surg Am* 2017;99(6):454-461. doi:10.2106/jbjs.16.00223.

In this case series, 84 patients were treated with a Grammot-style reverse total shoulder arthroplasty after a minimum of 10 years. Outcomes showed deterioration when compared with medium-term results, and this decrease was thought to be due to patient aging coupled with bone erosion and/or deltoid impairment over time. Level of evidence: IV.

65. Hartzler RU, Steen BM, Hussey MM, et al: Reverse shoulder arthroplasty for massive rotator cuff tear: Risk factors for poor functional improvement. *J Shoulder Elbow Surg* 2015;24(11):1698-1706. doi:10.1016/j.jse.2015.04.015.

In this study, reverse shoulder arthroplasty for massive rotator cuff tear treatment, reported outcomes, and surgical techniques were reviewed. Reverse shoulder arthroplasty was found to be a successful treatment for cuff tear arthropathy, but management in the absence of arthritis is controversial. Level of evidence: III.

66. Boileau P, Gonzalez JF, Chuinard C, Bicknell R, Walch G: Reverse total shoulder arthroplasty after failed rotator cuff surgery. *J Shoulder Elbow Surg* 2009;18(4):600-606. doi:10.1016/j.jse.2009.03.011.

67. Ek ETH, Neukom L, Catanzaro S, Gerber C: Reverse total shoulder arthroplasty for massive irreparable rotator cuff tears in patients younger than 65 years old: Results after five to fifteen years. *J Shoulder Elbow Surg* 2013;22(9):1199-1208. doi:10.1016/j.jse.2012.11.016.

In this case series, 46 patients younger than 65 years were treated with reverse shoulder arthroplasty for irreparable rotator cuff tear with at least 5-year follow-up. Patients had improved function, but had a high complication rate. Level of evidence: IV.

68. Boileau P, Chuinard C, Roussanne Y, Neyton L, Trojani C: Modified latissimus dorsi and teres major transfer through a single delto-pectoral approach for external rotation deficit of the shoulder: As an isolated procedure or with a reverse arthroplasty. *J Shoulder Elbow Surg* 2007;16(6):671-682. doi:10.1016/j.jse.2007.02.127.

Chapter 15

Factors Affecting the Outcome of Rotator Cuff Surgery

Michael E. Angeline, MD • Joshua Wright-Chisem, MD • Joshua S. Dines, MD

ABSTRACT

Rotator cuff tears are a common cause of disability and pain, with surgical repair accounting for over 75,000 procedures in the United States each year. Despite the clinical success of rotator cuff repairs, the repair site heals with a fibrovascular scar at the tendon-bone interface, leaving it mechanically weaker than the normal tendon insertion. Recent literature has been introduced which supports the notion that patients with fully healed rotator cuff repairs have improved clinical outcomes. As such, there has been increasing interest in the factors that affect outcomes following rotator cuff surgery. These factors include biologic factors, medical comorbidities, tendon integrity, social factors, and physician-determined factors. This chapter provides an overview of factors that contribute to the outcome of rotator cuff repair surgery.

Keywords: cuff; outcome; rotator; surgery

Introduction

Tears of the rotator cuff are a common cause of disability and pain, and surgical repair of the rotator cuff accounts for over 250,000 procedures in the United States each year.[1] All-arthroscopic repairs have good results, with stable functional outcomes after 5 years.[2] Despite the clinical success of rotator cuff repairs, the repair site heals with a fibrovascular scar at the tendon-bone interface. It is important to remember that a rotator cuff repair does not regenerate the native tendon insertion site, which was formed during embryologic development. The construct is mechanically weaker than the normal tendon enthesis and is probably more prone to failure.[3] A 2010 research supported the belief that patients whose rotator cuff fully heals after a repair tend to have better functional outcomes.[4] There has been much interest in the factors that may affect the outcome of rotator cuff surgery, as well as ways to improve healing rates.

The native rotator cuff tendon-to-bone insertion site functions to minimize stress concentration at the junction between the soft tendinous portion of the enthesis and the hard bony portion. The enthesis is composed of four distinct transition zones: tendon, fibrocartilage, mineralized fibrocartilage, and bone (**Figure 1**). The collagen content differs based on the tissue type.[5] The tendinous portion predominantly is composed of types I and III collagen, and the fibrocartilaginous zone is composed of types I, II, and III collagen. The mineralized fibrocartilage zone contains types I, II, and X collagen. The bone portion of the enthesis is composed of type I collagen.[6,7]

Biologic Factors

The prevalence of rotator cuff tears in the general population ranges from 5% to 39%.[8,9] The known risk factors include a history of trauma, injury to the dominant arm, and advancing age. The natural history of symptomatic and asymptomatic rotator cuff tears is suggested by the finding that 39% to 49% of nonsurgically treated tears had increased in size at midrange follow-up.[10,11] Pain development has previously been found to be associated with an increase in tear size and an increased rate of tear progression. However, recent evidence has only demonstrated a correlation between tear size and shoulder function, not pain.[12,13] As a rotator cuff tear progresses and becomes more symptomatic, the decision of whether to operate is based on multiple factors. Biologic factors that can affect the outcome of rotator cuff surgery include the patient's age, genetic influences, medical comorbidities, and rotator cuff integrity.

Dr. Angeline or an immediate family member has stock or stock options held in Baxter International Inc. and serves as a board member, owner, officer, or committee member of the American Academy of Orthopaedic Surgeons, the American Orthopaedic Society for Sports Medicine, and the American Shoulder and Elbow Surgeons. Dr. Dines or an immediate family member has received royalties from Linvatec; is a member of a speakers' bureau or has made paid presentations on behalf of Arthrex, Inc.; serves as a paid consultant to or is an employee of Arthrex, Inc.; has received research or institutional support from Arthrex, Inc.; and serves as a board member, owner, officer, or committee member of the American Shoulder and Elbow Surgeons. Neither Dr. Wright-Chisem nor any immediate family member has received anything of value from or has stock or stock options held in a commercial company or institution related directly or indirectly to the subject of this chapter.

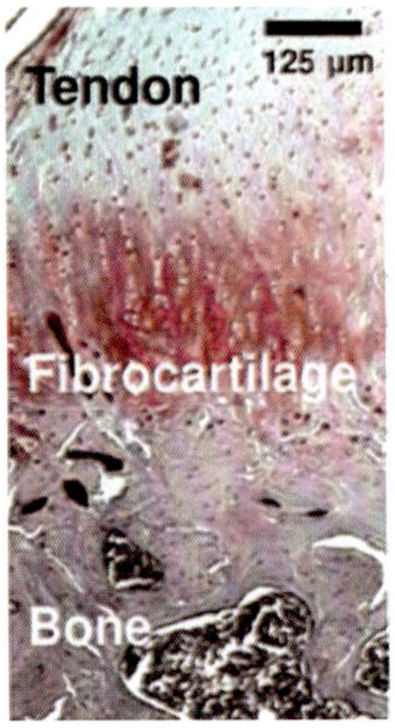

Tissue region	Cell type	Major matrix component
Tendon	Fibroblasts	Collagen types I, III (Diameter: 40-400 nm)
Nonmineralized fibrocartilage	Fibrochondrocytes	Collagen types I, II, III
Mineralized fibrocartilage	Hypertrophic fibrochondrocytes	Collagen types I, II, X
Bone	Osteoblasts Osteocytes Osteoclasts	Collagen type I (Diameter: 34.5-39.5 nm)

FIGURE 1 Illustration showing the structure and composition of the direct tendon-to-bone insertion site. (Reprinted from *J Shoulder Elbow Surg* 21[2]. Zhang X, Bogdanowicz D, Eriksen C, et al: Biomimetic scaffold design for functional and integrative tendon repair, 266-277. doi:10.1016/j.jse.2011.11.016. Copyright © 2012 Journal of Shoulder and Elbow Surgery Board of Trustees.)

Patient Age

With advancing age, the ability of the rotator cuff tendon to heal is adversely affected by reduced bone quality, tendon cellularity, and vascularity. Several case studies examined the outcomes of rotator cuff repair in patients older than 65 years.[14-16] Older patients were found to have improvement in pain, range of motion, and functional status after arthroscopic repair, regardless of whether the study evaluated these patients alone or in comparison with younger patients. These studies suggest that age alone is not associated with poor functional outcomes in older patients. However, most of the studies were at level IV, with only a univariate analysis of age and functional outcomes. In addition, confounding variables may have affected the perceived outcome. For example, the higher physical demands of younger patients may have influenced their perception of the surgical outcome.

In tendon healing, a 2010 research using multivariate analysis found that advanced age was the main biologic limitation at the repair site, even when the biomechanical strength of the repair site was maximized with a double-row repair construct.[17] With advancing age, fatty degeneration of the infraspinatus and tear retraction may become greater and have a further negative influence on anatomic outcomes after a repair. Overall, older patients may have improvement in functional outcome measures after rotator cuff repair, but the repair site has a reduced ability to heal with increasing age.

Genetics

Although no single gene is involved in rotator cuff pathology, the gene pathways are altered in tears and tendinopathies. The resulting changes affect the composition of the rotator cuff tendon in terms of collagen composition, vasculature, and intracellular signaling mechanisms as well as the ability to regenerate the native enthesis after a repair. Within the healing tendon, altered collagen gene expression results in an increase in type III collagen and a decrease in type I collagen, which coincide with a scar-mediated healing pathway. Modulation of the ratio of collagen I to collagen III has the potential for enhancing the structural properties of the healing tendon.

In 2011, there has been interest in the levels of expression of the cytokine transforming growth factor-β (TGF-β1, -β2, and -β3), which is believed to influence cellular proliferation, differentiation, and matrix synthesis within the healing tendon. As the adult tendon heals, levels of TGF-β1 and TGF-β2 are elevated, with resultant scar formation and low levels of expressed TGF-β3. Fetal wound healing is known to have higher levels of TGF-β3 expression and a subsequent lack of scar formation.[18]

In a rat supraspinatus repair model, localized delivery of TGF-β3 was found to improve the repair site strength at 4 weeks postoperatively and increase type I collagen expression, reflecting more mature healing.[19] These results are promising, but further research is necessary to establish the optimal dosing and delivery of TGF-β3.

Matrix metalloproteinases (MMPs) and their tissue inhibitors recently have been studied because changes in their dynamic expression patterns were found to regulate remodeling of the extracellular matrix in rotator cuff tears. Loss of the balance between MMPs and their tissue inhibitors results in increased MMP activity, affecting tendon healing through tendon degradation and possible rupture.[20] Localized delivery of an MMP inhibitor in a rat supraspinatus repair model led to significantly greater collagen organization and decreased collagen degradation.[21] These results show that modulating the MMP activity after a rotator cuff repair augments tendon-to-bone healing at the repair site.

Doxycycline, an antibiotic, has MMP inhibitory effects through a pathway independent of its antimicrobial efficacy. The effects of doxycycline on tendon healing were examined in a follow-up study using a rat model.[20] After acute rotator cuff repair, doxycycline-mediated inhibition of MMP activity was associated with improved biomechanical and histologic healing parameters at the tendon-bone interface. Further research is needed to define the exact mechanism of improved tendon healing through MMP inhibition, but doxycycline may become an adjunct treatment for improving the outcomes of rotator cuff surgery.

Studies also have evaluated the inherited risk of rotator cuff tears or pathology.[22,23] These studies provided evidence of a strong genetic predisposition to rotator cuff disease with increased observed risk among patients' first- and second-degree relatives, and they suggested that individuals having a genetic predisposition may be more affected by age-related tendon degeneration than those without such a predisposition. Unfortunately, the role of genetic inheritance patterns on healing of the tendon-bone unit after a repair was not examined. Future research is required to fully identify the predisposing genes responsible for these observations and understand the exact mechanism of genes associated with rotator cuff disease.

Medical Comorbidities

A patient's medical comorbidities can greatly affect tendon healing. Obesity is a worldwide problem associated with a risk of diabetes, vascular disease, and hypercholesterolemia. These disease states result in decreased vascularity and could affect the tendon-to-bone healing response. Two retrospective case-control studies examined the correlation between obesity and functional outcomes after arthroscopic rotator cuff repair.[24,25] The results were conflicting. One study found a statistically significant correlation between obesity and poor functional outcome, longer hospital stay, and longer surgical time.[24] After controlling for confounding variables, the other study found that body mass index and obesity were not related to outcomes after arthroscopic rotator cuff repair.[25] A more recent retrospective study compared outcomes of normal weight, preobese, and obese patients after arthroscopic and open rotator cuff repair.[26] In this study, obese patients were found to have higher failure rates, with significantly worse DASH and Constant functional outcome scores. It is difficult to directly compare these studies because they were based on different outcome measures and follow-up time points and involved different surgeons. At best, the true correlation between obesity and rotator cuff pathology remains unclear.

Diabetes mellitus can affect tendon healing. It was shown that rats with diabetes had poorer biomechanical properties, less fibrocartilage, and less organized collagen at the tendon-bone interface after rotator cuff repair compared with controls.[27] These findings suggest that sustained hyperglycemia can impair rotator cuff tendon-to-bone healing. A prior retrospective study compared patients with and without diabetes who had undergone arthroscopic rotator cuff repair.[28] Constant scores improved postoperatively in both groups of patients. However, improvement was greater in the patients without diabetes, who demonstrated better scores for forward flexion, external rotation, activities of daily living, and power components. Patients with diabetes had less forward flexion and external rotation as well as a slightly higher incidence of infection. More recently, a retrospective study compared functional outcomes in patients with and without diabetes with one year follow up.[29] Although patients with diabetes had significantly lower Japanese Orthopedic Association and UCLA shoulder scores, there was no significant difference postoperatively between the groups. Range of motion was lower preoperatively in the diabetic cohort but there was no difference between the groups postoperatively. This study notably only included patients with diabetes with good perioperative glycemic control. The findings of preclinical and clinical studies on the effects of diabetes on tendon healing should not be construed as precluding these patients from undergoing arthroscopic rotator cuff repair. Patients with diabetes do have improved pain and function postoperatively, although the expected outcomes may not be as good as those without diabetes.

Tendon Integrity

Although chronicity and size of a rotator cuff tear are significant factors affecting anatomic and functional outcomes after a repair, the quality of the rotator cuff musculature in terms of the extent of atrophy and fatty infiltration may have an even greater influence. Research on a sheep chronic rotator cuff tear model showed that the crucial event in the pathogenesis of infraspinatus fatty infiltration is the change in the pennation angle (the angle at which muscle fibers insert into tendon in pennate skeletal muscles).[30] As the pennation angle increased, the muscle fibers shortened, and fat was allowed to infiltrate. This factor can result in a poor biologic capacity of the tendon to heal at the insertion site and decreased mechanical properties of the muscle-tendon unit. Relatively severe preoperative atrophy and fatty infiltration were associated with an increased rate of repair failure, loss of muscle function, and inferior achievable outcomes during the postoperative period.[31-33] The muscle quality and the extent of fatty infiltration of the infraspinatus are more influential than those of the supraspinatus.

It is believed that poor infraspinatus function can offset the biomechanics of the glenohumeral joint and lead to a poor patient outcome.[31,34]

The natural history and the extent of muscle fatty infiltration in rotator cuff tears can be correlated with tear size, location, time to onset, and patient age.[35,36] For example, a large tear in an older patient with a long delay after tendon rupture will result in more severe fatty infiltration. In all tear types, Goutallier grade 2 fatty infiltration was found to occur in the supraspinatus muscle at an average of 4 years after the onset of symptoms[37] (**Table 1**). The progression was faster in tears that were traumatic or involved more than one tendon. Grade 2 fatty infiltration occurred in the infraspinatus muscle an average of 2.5 years after the onset of symptoms.[38] These fatty changes occurred regardless of whether the tear included an infraspinatus tendon rupture.

With an understanding of the time progression and influencing factors, the clinician should be able to appreciate the extent of atrophy and fatty infiltration before surgery and intervene appropriately (**Figure 2**). Surgical repair ideally should be attempted before grade 2 fatty infiltration appears, in an effort to avoid poor anatomic and functional results.[31,33] It is important to note that no clinical study has found a post repair reversal of grade 2 fatty infiltration and the associated structural changes.[35]

Social Factors

Social factors including cigarette smoking and a workers' compensation-related claim can have a significant role in the outcome of rotator cuff surgery and are important for the surgeon to recognize. Smoking was found to be more prevalent in patients with a rotator cuff tear than in individuals without a tear, and pain from a rotator cuff disorder is second only to back pain as the most common upper extremity symptom among manual workers.[39,40]

Table 1

The Goutallier-Bernageau Classification of Fatty Infiltration

Grade	Description
0	Completely normal muscle with no fatty streaking
1	Muscle containing some fatty streaks
2	More muscle than fat
3	As much fat as muscle
4	More fat than muscle

Nicotine use was found to negatively affect the amount of collagen deposition and repair at surgical wound sites because its potent vasoconstrictive effects decrease the delivery of oxygen to tissues.[39] These effects were correlated using a rat rotator cuff model, in which nicotine delivery through an implanted osmotic pump was found to affect tendon-to-bone healing by delaying scar degradation and remodeling.[41] Several research studies also examined the influence of cigarette smoking on rotator cuff pathology.[39,42] In patients undergoing ultrasonography for unilateral atraumatic shoulder pain, a questionnaire revealed a strong association and possible causation between smoking and rotator cuff disease.[39] The findings were independent of age and were both dosage and time dependent. The dosage-dependent relationship involved rotator cuff tear size and the amount of tobacco use; smokers with greater tobacco use had a correspondingly larger and more severe rotator cuff tear.[34]

Patients with a pending workers' compensation claim also were found to have relatively poor outcomes after a rotator cuff repair.[40,43,44] Two studies used multivariable and matched case-control analysis to find a negative correlation while controlling for cofounding factors.[40,44] One year after a rotator cuff repair, functional measures were worse for the patients with a compensation claim than for other patients, and a compensation claim had a negative effect on recovery. Although these findings are significant, it is important to recognize that a compensation claim does not preclude a patient's receiving surgical management for rotator cuff pathology. Patients with a compensation claim can benefit from surgical intervention and have some improvement on subjective and objective measures.[40]

The potential factors contributing to impairment after a rotator cuff repair in patients with a work-related injury were examined in a 2008 cross-sectional study.[43] At least one definable explanation for continued impairment was found in half of the patients with reported surgical failure. The reasons were anatomic in nature (missed glenohumeral pathology or fixation failure) or were a consequence of the surgery itself (complex regional pain syndrome or failure of deltoid reattachment in an open repair). The clinician must look for identifiable causes of surgical failure in a patient with a work-related injury who has a poor outcome.

Physician-Determined Factors

The orthopaedic surgeon can influence the outcome of rotator cuff surgery through decisions involving surgical timing, surgical procedure, postsurgical rehabilitation, and possibly use of biologic adjuncts to surgery.

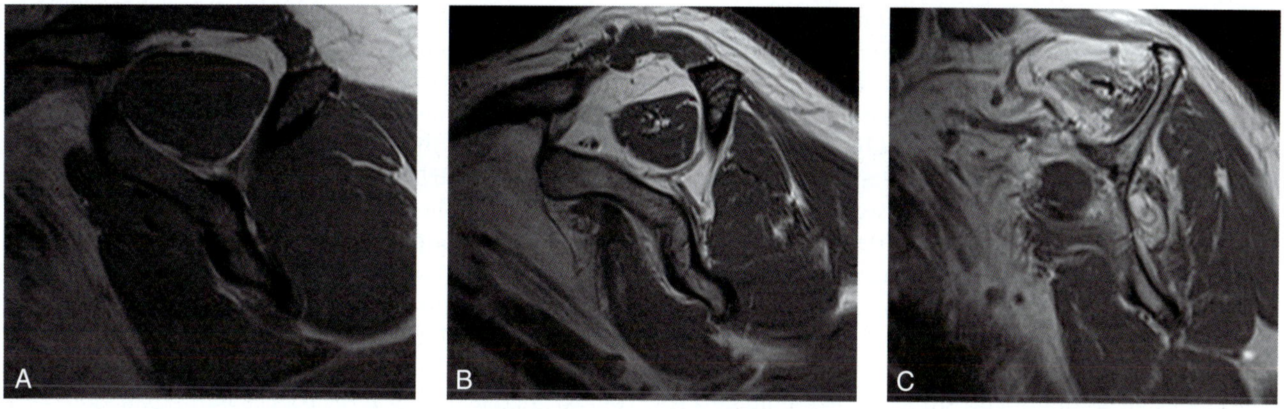

FIGURE 2 Sagittal-view MRI showing fatty infiltration of the supraspinatus muscle: Goutallier grades 0 (**A**), 2 (**B**), and 4 (**C**).

Timing

The decision to operate on a chronic rotator cuff tear should be influenced by the extent of atrophy and fatty infiltration. Surgical repair should preferably be performed before the onset of Goutallier grade 2 fatty infiltration. Fatty degeneration of the infraspinatus muscle has been reported with isolated chronic, degenerative supraspinatus tendon tears.[45] This finding represents a factor that must be considered because muscle quality and extent of fatty infiltration in the infraspinatus can influence the outcome of repair. The surgeon also must be cognizant of surgical timing for an acute rotator cuff tear. Previously, it was believed that a better functional outcome was achieved if an acute rotator cuff tear was repaired within 3 weeks of the time of injury.[46] Two retrospective reviews found that patients who underwent a delayed open repair within 3 to 4 months of injury had a satisfactory functional outcome similar to that of patients who underwent an early open repair.[46] In general, the surgeon can safely delay repair of an acute tear beyond the 3-week window without affecting the functional outcomes.

Surgical Procedures

The choice of repair technique can affect the outcome of rotator cuff repair surgery. Concern over a lack of anatomic healing and/or retearing after a repair has led to a persistent debate as to the optimal surgical technique (specifically, single-row, double-row, or transosseous anchorless repair). Current double-row and transosseous repair techniques enhance the biomechanical strength of the repair and increase the surface area of the repaired tendon on the footprint,[47,48] but their ability to provide superior anatomic and functional outcomes is still controversial.[49,50] The surgeon should perform a risk-reward analysis before deciding on the best repair technique. The patient's size, functional demands, and tear characteristics all need to be incorporated into the decisionmaking process.

Postsurgical Rehabilitation

Stiffness in the shoulder joint before or after surgical repair can occur with any torn rotator cuff tendon. In a rotator cuff model, long periods of immobilization after a repair were found to improve the biomechanical characteristics of the repaired insertion site.[51] However, stiffness may be more likely to develop. Patients with a full-thickness tear or an acute traumatic tear were observed to have substantially more preoperative stiffness.[52] In a rat rotator cuff model, joint stiffness resulting from immobilization after a repair was transient and, in the long term, was not significantly different from that of nonimmobilized repairs.[53] Furthermore, early passive motion possibly was detrimental to shoulder joint mechanics,[54] resulting in a loss of motion after repair of the supraspinatus tendon in comparison with continuously immobilized shoulders.[51] These findings together highlight the potential beneficial effect of postoperative immobilization for tendon healing. A retrospective clinical review supported this concept by finding that 6 weeks of sling immobilization after arthroscopic rotator cuff repair did not affect stiffness or functional outcomes at 1-year follow-up.[55] In addition, there was a trend toward a lower rate of retearing when this conservative postoperative rehabilitation protocol was used. A recent randomized control trial investigated the effect of postoperative immobilization. The study randomized patients into two cohorts: immediate sling for four weeks versus no sling. The no sling cohort demonstrated no difference in postoperative pain at any time point relative to the sling cohort. The no sling cohort also demonstrated significantly higher early active elevation, external rotation and internal rotation as well. Overall, the authors concluded that early sling immobilization was associated decreased range of motion, increased pain, and lower functional scores. No significant differences were noted with respect to tendon size or repair integrity between the cohorts.[56]

Biologic Adjuncts to Surgery

The challenge in rotator cuff surgery is to stimulate a regenerative rather than a reparative healing pathway. None of the patient or physician-determined factors can enable the healing tendon to regenerate the native tendon-bone interface formed during prenatal development. As a result, the use of biologic agents and cell-based therapies is being examined as potential means for augmenting the repair site and improving tendon healing through a scarless process.

Platelet-Derived Growth Factor

During the early inflammatory phase of tendon healing, platelet-derived growth factor (PDGF) helps direct cell chemotaxis, proliferation, differentiation, and matrix synthesis.[5] The cytokine PDGF basic protein family is composed of two subunits (A and B chains) derived from platelets and other cell types, including smooth muscle. Rotator cuff healing results in reactive scar formation rather than a histologically normal insertion site, and it may be possible to augment the repair site biology by adding PDGF.

Recombinant human PDGF (rhPDGF)-BB is the first exogenous growth factor to be tested in a clinical study of rotator cuff repair. A sheep rotator cuff model was used to examine the effects of rhPDGF-BB on rotator cuff healing.[56] Sutures coated with the growth factor were found to enhance histologic properties after rotator cuff repair but did not improve biomechanical properties compared with standard suture repair. Another sheep rotator cuff repair study examined the effects of an interpositional graft composed of rhPDGF-BB and a type I collagen matrix.[57] Twelve weeks after repair, low- and medium-dosage rhPDGF-BB grafts showed improved biomechanical strength and anatomic appearance compared with control or high-dosage grafts. These studies highlight the importance of growth factor-dependent dosage, timing, and delivery methods. PDGF augmentation holds promise for tendon-to-bone healing, and phase I clinical studies are under way using rhPDGF-BB to augment rotator cuff repairs.

Platelet-Rich Plasma

Many growth factors (cytokines) are upregulated within the cascade of events that leads to natural healing of the tendon-to-bone insertion. Combining and increasing the concentration of these factors has potential for enhancing tenocyte, stem cell, and endothelial cell recruitment and proliferation at the healing interface. Platelet-rich plasma (PRP) has become popular for augmenting tendon healing because it is an autologous concentration of platelets and growth factors including PDGF, vascular endothelial growth factor, TGF-β, fibroblast growth factor-2, and insulinlike growth factor-1. Several studies examined the use of PRP augmentation at the rotator cuff repair site.[58-61] In two cohort studies, PRP application during arthroscopic rotator cuff repair did not improve functional outcome measures compared with those of patients in the control group.[60,61] Another level I randomized study had similar findings at the 6-, 12-, and 24-month postoperative time points.[62] However, pain scores were lower during the first postoperative month, and clinical outcomes were improved 3 months after surgery compared with patients in the control group. These results raise the possibility that PRP may have a positive influence on early tendon healing.

The study results conflicted as to whether PRP augmentation improved the structural integrity of the healing rotator cuff repair site. In contrast, animal and clinical studies of Achilles tendon rupture found that application of PRP enhances healing and functional recovery.[63,64] The effects of PRP may depend on the mechanical loading characteristics of the healing tendon. A 2011 study also found a difference in the growth factor concentration in three commercially available PRP separation systems.[65] Further research is needed to fully understand the mechanisms by which PRP improves tendon healing and the significance of different growth factor concentrations.

Mesenchymal Stem Cells

As research on regenerative tendon healing has evolved, it has become evident that therapy based on cytokine growth factors alone may not be sufficient for improving the material properties of the tissue. Combining these factors with undifferentiated cells may lead to enhanced tissue healing. Mesenchymal stem cells (MSCs) are distinguished by their unique ability to self-renew and differentiate into cell lines, including adipocytes, tenocytes, and chondrocytes. Currently, autologous stromal cells can be obtained only by isolating them from the bone marrow, but other harvesting techniques are being developed. Cell-based therapy can influence the repair process through a direct local paracrine effect or through anti-inflammatory effects. In a rat rotator cuff model, the biomechanical or histologic properties of the tendon attachment site were not enhanced by the addition of bone marrow-derived MSCs alone.[66] A combination of MSCs and other factors may be necessary for augmenting the repair site. The optimal combinations ideally will be based on knowledge of the mechanism and signaling events that lead to the formation of the natural enthesis.

Research involving the use of MSCs and the transcription factor scleraxis has highlighted the potential benefits of combined therapy. Scleraxis was found to play an important role in the developing enthesis and tenogenesis in general, and it remains present during the formation of the tendon proper as well as the tendon-to-bone insertion site. By using bone marrow-derived MSCs transduced with adenoviral-mediated scleraxis in a rat rotator cuff model, a recent study found significantly better biomechanical properties after repair compared with those of controls.[67] The rats treated with adenoviral-mediated scleraxis also had more fibrocartilage, which more closely resembled that of the native tendon-to-bone insertion site. Further research is needed to fully understand the complex signaling events necessary to regenerate the tendon-to-bone insertion site as well as the optimal combination, dosing, and delivery vehicles for biologic augmentation.

Biomimetic Scaffolds

Tissue engineering strategies have evolved to include a biomimetic scaffold that has the potential to achieve functional integration with the host environment. The ideal scaffold design would enable restoration of the histologic and the mechanical properties of the native tendon-to-bone interface. Current research is focused on a biphasic scaffold design composed of poly lactic-co-glycolic acid nanofibers and a composite of poly lactic-co-glycolic acid nanofibers and hydroxyapatite nanoparticles.[7] The purpose of this biphasic design is to promote the postrepair regeneration of both the nonmineralized and the mineralized fibrocartilaginous regions of the native enthesis. In a rat rotator cuff repair model, the biphasic scaffold was found to stimulate the formation of a continuous noncalcified and calcified matrix region rather than the fibrovascular scarring observed in the control group.

Although biomimetic scaffolding has promise for augmenting and promoting regenerative healing, research is required to gain an in-depth understanding of the signaling mechanisms that lead to the formation of graded structures in the native enthesis.[7] A thorough understanding of developmental biology at the tendon-to-bone insertion site will directly affect future scaffold designs. Growth factors and other signaling molecules may be incorporated into these structures.

SUMMARY

Both patient- and physician-derived factors influence the outcome of rotator cuff surgery. The patient factors include biologic factors (such as age and genetic factors), medical comorbidities, tendon integrity, and social factors. Patient age alone may not influence the functional outcomes of rotator cuff surgery, but age negatively influences anatomic outcomes. There may be a genetic predisposition to rotator cuff disease, and controlling MMP activity or delivering TGF-β3 to the repair site may lead to better tendon healing. Diabetes mellitus is known to negatively affect tendon healing and the outcomes of rotator cuff surgery, but the true correlation between obesity and rotator cuff pathology is unclear. The extent of atrophy and fatty infiltration of the rotator cuff musculature has a significant effect on anatomic and functional outcomes after a repair. Surgery should ideally be performed before Goutallier grade 2 fatty infiltration occurs. Smoking and the presence of a worker's compensation claim were found to negatively affect the outcomes after a rotator cuff repair.

Physician-determined factors that influence the outcomes of rotator cuff surgery include surgical timing, surgical procedure, postsurgical rehabilitation, and the use of biologic adjuncts. An acute rotator cuff tear can be safely repaired within 3 to 4 months of the injury without negatively affecting the outcome. For a chronic rotator cuff tear, the extent of atrophy and fatty infiltration should be assessed, and the repair should preferably be performed before the onset of Goutallier grade 2 fatty infiltration. Preclinical research in a rat model showed that prolonged immobilization can improve the strength of the repair, but the ideal length of postoperative immobilization remains controversial.

Future directions for augmenting the rotator cuff repair site to improve healing include the use of biologic adjuncts such as PDGF, PRP, MSCs, and biomimetic scaffolds. Used alone, PDGF may improve the biomechanical strength and the anatomic appearance of the repaired rotator cuff. In contrast, the use of PRP or MSCs alone may not significantly enhance the biomechanical or histologic properties of the repair site. Further research must establish the optimal combinations of these growth factors (cytokines) as well as the optimal dosing and delivery methods. The use of a biomimetic scaffold to augment regenerative healing has promise, but research is still required.

Section 3: The Rotator Cuff

KEY STUDY POINTS

- **Biologic factors:** Biologic factors that may influence the outcome of rotator cuff surgery include patient age, genetic influences, medical comorbidities, and rotator cuff integrity.
- **Patient age:** With advanced age, fatty degeneration and tear retraction are more prevalent and portend a negative influence on anatomic outcomes following repair. Regardless, older patients still have been found to have improvements in pain, range of motion, and functional status after repair.
- **Genetics:** Although no single gene is involved in rotator cuff pathology, altered collagen genetic expression can result in an increase in type III collegen and a decrease in type 1 college, coinciding with a scar-mediated healing pathway following rotator cuff tendon repair.
- **Medical comorbidities:** Medical comorbidities play a role in tendon healing as obese patients have been found to have lower function scores. Diabetes mellitus has been associated with lower biomechanical function in animal studies and lower functional outcomes as well.
- **Tendon integrity:** Quality of musculature and the extent of atrophy and fatty infiltration play a larger role play a large role in anatomic and functional outcomes after rotator cuff repair. Animal models have also shown that the change in pennation angle may represent a crucial event in the pathogenesis of infraspinatus fatty infiltration.
- **Social factors:** Social factors play a role in outcomes following rotator cuff repair, as studies have shown that patients who sustain a rotator cuff tear are more likely to have smoked than their noninjured counterparts. Nicotine has also been found to be an independent factor in lower tendon healing rates.
- **Physician-determined factors:** Physician-determined factors play a large role in outcomes following rotator cuff repair, as surgical timing, repair technique, postsurgical rehabilitation protocol, and biologic adjuncts all can affect outcomes after repair.

Annotated References

1. Jain NB, Higgins LD, Losina E, Collins J, Blazar PE, Katz JN: Epidemiology of musculoskeletal upper extremity ambulatory surgery in the United States: *BMC Musculoskelet Disord* 2014;15:4. doi:10.1186/1471-2474-15-4.

An estimated 272,148 (95% confidence intervals [CI] = 218,994, 325,302) rotator cuff repairs, 257,541 (95% CI = 185,268, 329,814) shoulder arthroscopies excluding those for cuff repairs, 576,924 (95% CI = 459,239, 694,609) carpal tunnel releases, and 25,250 (95% CI = 17,304, 33,196) wrist arthroscopies excluding those for carpal tunnel release were performed. Level of evidence: III.

2. Gulotta LV, Nho SJ, Dodson CC, et al: Prospective evaluation of arthroscopic rotator cuff repairs at 5 years: Part I – Functional outcomes and radiographic healing rates. *J Shoulder Elbow Surg* 2011;20(6):934-940.

3. Galatz LM, Sandell LJ, Rothermich SY, et al: Characteristics of the rat supraspinatus tendon during tendon-to-bone healing after acute injury. *J Orthop Res* 2006;24(3):541-550.

4. Slabaugh MA, Nho SJ, Grumet RC, et al: Does the literature confirm superior clinical results in radiographically healed rotator cuffs after rotator cuff repair? *Arthroscopy* 2010;26(3):393-403.

5. Bedi A, Maak T, Walsh C, et al: Cytokines in rotator cuff degeneration and repair. *J Shoulder Elbow Surg* 2012;21(2):218-227.

6. Galatz L, Rothermich S, VanderPloeg K, Petersen B, Sandell L, Thomopoulos S: Development of the supraspinatus tendon-to-bone insertion: Localized expression of extracellular matrix and growth factor genes. *J Orthop Res* 2007;25(12):1621-1628.

7. Zhang X, Bogdanowicz D, Erisken C, Lee NM, Lu HH: Biomimetic scaffold design for functional and integrative tendon repair. *J Shoulder Elbow Surg* 2012;21(2):266-277.

8. Yamamoto A, Takagishi K, Osawa T, et al: Prevalence and risk factors of a rotator cuff tear in the general population. *J Shoulder Elbow Surg* 2010;19(1):116-120.

9. Sambandam SN, Khanna V, Gul A, Mounasamy V: Rotator cuff tears: An evidence based approach. *World J Orthop* 2015;6(11):902-918. doi:10.5312/wjo.v6.i11.902.

Abundant data from across the world has been published on the prevalence of rotator cuff tears. Yamaguchi et al (as cited by Ref. 4 of this article), from Missouri, United States, evaluated 588 patients with unilateral shoulder complaints. Their analysis revealed 199 (33.8%) unilateral and 177 (30.1%) bilateral rotator cuff tears with average ages of 58.7 and 67.8 years, respectively. Level of evidence: III.

10. Safran O, Schroeder J, Bloom R, Weil Y, Milgrom C: Natural history of nonoperatively treated symptomatic rotator cuff tears in patients 60 years old or younger. *Am J Sports Med* 2011;39(4):710-714.

11. Codding JL, Keener JD: Natural history of degenerative rotator cuff tears. *Curr Rev Musculoskelet Med* 2018;11(1):77-85. doi:10.1007/s12178-018-9461-8.

This 2018 research has more closely examined patterns of tear progression for degenerative rotator cuff tears. Regarding tear propagation, 139 asymptomatic tears followed for a median of 6 years were classified based on the integrity of the anterior 3 mm (rotator cable) of the supraspinatus tendon. These rotator cable-intact tears propagated by ultrasound bidirectionally (median of 5 mm anteriorly and 4 mm posteriorly), while cable-disrupted tears propagated a median of 7 mm posteriorly. Level of evidence: III.

12. Mall NA, Kim HM, Keener JD, et al: Symptomatic progression of asymptomatic rotator cuff tears: A prospective study of clinical and sonographic variables. *J Bone Joint Surg Am* 2010;92(16):2623-2633.

13. Wylie JD, Suter T, Potter MQ, Granger EK, Tashjian RZ: Mental health has a stronger association with patient-reported shoulder pain and function than tear size in patients with full-thickness rotator cuff tears. *J Bone Joint Surg* 2016;98(4):251-256. doi:10.2106/JBJS.O.00444.

The SF-36 MCS had the strongest correlation with the visual analog scale for shoulder pain (Pearson correlation coefficient, −0.48; $P < 0.001$). Tear severity only correlated with the visual analog scale for shoulder function. Level of evidence: II.

14. Park JG, Cho NS, Song JH, Baek JH, Jeong HY, Rhee YG: Rotator cuff repair in patients over 75 years of age: Clinical outcome and repair integrity. *Clin Orthop Surg* 2016;8(4):420-427. doi:10.4055/cios.2016.8.4.420.

There were significant improvements in clinical outcomes after RC repair in patients ≥75 years. Structural integrity after cuff repair did not affect the final clinical outcome. Even in elderly patients older than 75 years, healing of repaired RC can be expected in cases of small to medium tears. Although the retear rate was relatively high for large to massive tears, clinical outcomes still showed significant improvement. Level of evidence: III.

15. Charousset C, Bellaïche L, Kalra K, Petrover D: Arthroscopic repair of full-thickness rotator cuff tears: Is there tendon healing in patients aged 65 years or older? *Arthroscopy* 2010;26(3):302-309.

16. Osti L, Papalia R, Del Buono A, Denaro V, Maffulli N: Comparison of arthroscopic rotator cuff repair in healthy patients over and under 65 years of age. *Knee Surg Sports Traumatol Arthrosc* 2010;18(12):1700-1706.

17. Tashjian RZ, Hollins AM, Kim HM, et al: Factors affecting healing rates after arthroscopic double-row rotator cuff repair. *Am J Sports Med* 2010;38(12):2435-2442.

18. Manning CN, Kim HM, Sakiyama-Elbert S, Galatz LM, Havlioglu N, Thomopoulos S: Sustained delivery of transforming growth factor beta three enhances tendon-to-bone healing in a rat model. *J Orthop Res* 2011;29(7):1099-1105.

19. Kovacevic D, Fox AJ, Bedi A, et al: Calcium-phosphate matrix with or without TGF-β3 improves tendon-bone healing after rotator cuff repair. *Am J Sports Med* 2011;39(4):811-819.

20. Bedi A, Fox AJ, Kovacevic D, Deng XH, Warren RF, Rodeo SA: Doxycycline-mediated inhibition of matrix metalloproteinases improves healing after rotator cuff repair. *Am J Sports Med* 2010;38(2):308-317.

21. Bedi A, Kovacevic D, Hettrich C, et al: The effect of matrix metalloproteinase inhibition on tendon-to-bone healing in a rotator cuff repair model. *J Shoulder Elbow Surg* 2010;19(3):384-391.

22. Gwilym SE, Watkins B, Cooper CD, et al: Genetic influences in the progression of tears of the rotator cuff. *J Bone Joint Surg Br* 2009;91(7):915-917.

23. Tashjian RZ, Farnham JM, Albright FS, Teerlink CC, Cannon-Albright LA: Evidence for an inherited predisposition contributing to the risk for rotator cuff disease. *J Bone Joint Surg Am* 2009;91(5):1136-1142.

24. Warrender WJ, Brown OL, Abboud JA: Outcomes of arthroscopic rotator cuff repairs in obese patients. *J Shoulder Elbow Surg* 2011;20(6):961-967.

25. Namdari S, Baldwin K, Glaser D, Green A: Does obesity affect early outcome of rotator cuff repair? *J Shoulder Elbow Surg* 2010;19(8):1250-1255.

26. Ateschrang A, Eggensperger F, Ahrend MD, et al: Obesity causes poorer clinical results and higher re-tear rates in rotator cuff repair. *Arch Orthop Trauma Surg* 2018;138:835-842. doi:10.1007/s00402-018-2921-1.

Both the failure rate and the clinical outcome were significantly worse for obese patients (body mass index >30, $P = 0.007$). The failure rate was 15.8% for the normal-weight patients, 8.2% in the preobese group, and in the obese group 28.6%. Level of evidence: III.

27. Bedi A, Fox AJ, Harris PE, et al: Diabetes mellitus impairs tendon-bone healing after rotator cuff repair. *J Shoulder Elbow Surg* 2010;19(7):978-988.

28. Clement ND, Hallett A, MacDonald D, Howie C, Mc-Birnie J: Does diabetes affect outcome after arthroscopic repair of the rotator cuff? *J Bone Joint Surg Br* 2010;92(8):1112-1117.

29. Miyatake K, Takeda Y, Fujii K, et al: Comparable clinical and structural outcomes after arthroscopic rotator cuff repair in diabetic and non-diabetic patients. *Knee Surg Sports Traumatol Arthrosc* 2018;26(12):3810-3817. doi:10.1007/s00167-018-4994-3.

Preoperative Japanese Orthopedic Association and UCLA scores of patients with diabetes were significantly lower than those without diabetes ($P < 0.001$, and $P = 0.006$, respectively); however, the scores at final follow-up were not different. Range of motion was significantly restricted in patients with diabetes before surgery (forward flexion, abduction, internal rotation: $P < 0.001$, external rotation: $P = 0.035$), but at the final follow-up, there was no significant difference except for internal rotation ($P = 0.005$). The retear rate in patients with diabetes (23.3%) was not significantly different from that in those without diabetes (15.1%). Level of evidence: III.

30. Gerber C, Meyer DC, Frey E, et al: Neer Award 2007: Reversion of structural muscle changes caused by chronic rotator cuff tears using continuous musculotendinous traction. An experimental study in sheep. *J Shoulder Elbow Surg* 2009;18(2):163-171.

31. Gladstone JN, Bishop JY, Lo IK, Flatow EL: Fatty infiltration and atrophy of the rotator cuff do not improve after rotator cuff repair and correlate with poor functional outcome. *Am J Sports Med* 2007;35(5):719-728.

32. Oh JH, Kim SH, Ji HM, Jo KH, Bin SW, Gong HS: Prognostic factors affecting anatomic outcome of rotator cuff repair and correlation with functional outcome. *Arthroscopy* 2009;25(1):30-39.

33. Liem D, Lichtenberg S, Magosch P, Habermeyer P: Magnetic resonance imaging of arthroscopic supraspinatus tendon repair. *J Bone Joint Surg Am* 2007;89(8):1770-1776.

34. Kuzel BR, Grindel S, Papandrea R, Ziegler D: Fatty infiltration and rotator cuff atrophy. *J Am Acad Orthop Surg* 2013;21(10):613-623. doi:10.5435/jaaos-21-10-613.

    Moderate to severe fatty infiltration and rotator cuff atrophy are commonly associated with poor clinical outcomes and failed rotator cuff repair. Level of evidence: III.

35. Melis B, Nemoz C, Walch G: Muscle fatty infiltration in rotator cuff tears: Descriptive analysis of 1688 cases. *Orthop Traumatol Surg Res* 2009;95(5):319-324.

36. Kim HM, Dahiya N, Teefey SA, Keener JD, Galatz LM, Yamaguchi K: Relationship of tear size and location to fatty degeneration of the rotator cuff. *J Bone Joint Surg Am* 2010;92(4):829-839.

37. Goutallier DB, Patte D: L'évaluation par le scanner de la trophicite' des muscles de la coiffe ayant une rupture tendineuse. *Rev Chir Orthop Reparatrice Appar Mot* 1989;75:126-127.

38. Baumgarten KM, Gerlach D, Galatz LM, et al: Cigarette smoking increases the risk for rotator cuff tears. *Clin Orthop Relat Res* 2010;468(6):1534-1541.

39. Holtby R, Razmjou H: Impact of work-related compensation claims on surgical outcome of patients with rotator cuff related pathologies: A matched case control study. *J Shoulder Elbow Surg* 2010;19(3):452-460.

40. Galatz LM, Silva MJ, Rothermich SY, Zaegel MA, Havlioglu N, Thomopoulos S: Nicotine delays tendon-to-bone healing in a rat shoulder model. *J Bone Joint Surg Am* 2006;88(9):2027-2034.

41. Carbone S, Gumina S, Arceri V, Campagna V, Fagnani C, Postacchini F: The impact of preoperative smoking habit on rotator cuff tear: Cigarette smoking influences rotator cuff tear sizes. *J Shoulder Elbow Surg* 2012;21(1):56-60.

42. Razmjou H, Lincoln S, Axelrod T, Holtby R: Factors contributing to failure of rotator cuff surgery in persons with work-related injuries. *Physiother Can* 2008;60(2):125-133.

43. Henn RF III, Kang L, Tashjian RZ, Green A: Patients with workers' compensation claims have worse outcomes after rotator cuff repair. *J Bone Joint Surg Am* 2008;90(10):2105-2113.

44. Kim HM, Dahiya N, Teefey SA, et al: Location and initiation of degenerative rotator cuff tears: An analysis of three hundred and sixty shoulders. *J Bone Joint Surg Am* 2010;92(5):1088-1096.

45. Petersen SA, Murphy TP: The timing of rotator cuff repair for the restoration of function. *J Shoulder Elbow Surg* 2011;20(1):62-68.

46. Burks RT, Crim J, Brown N, Fink B, Greis PE: A prospective randomized clinical trial comparing arthroscopic single- and double-row rotator cuff repair: Magnetic resonance imaging and early clinical evaluation. *Am J Sports Med* 2009;37(4):674-682.

47. Ma HL, Chiang ER, Wu HT, et al: Clinical outcome and imaging of arthroscopic single-row and double-row rotator cuff repair: A prospective randomized trial. *Arthroscopy* 2012;28(1):16-24.

48. Duquin TR, Buyea C, Bisson LJ: Which method of rotator cuff repair leads to the highest rate of structural healing? A systematic review. *Am J Sports Med* 2010;38(4):835-841.

49. Grasso A, Milano G, Salvatore M, Falcone G, Deriu L, Fabbriciani C: Single-row versus double-row arthroscopic rotator cuff repair: A prospective randomized clinical study. *Arthroscopy* 2009;25(1):4-12.

50. Dines JS, Bedi A, ElAttrache NS, Dines DM: Single-row versus double-row rotator cuff repair: Techniques and outcomes. *J Am Acad Orthop Surg* 2010;18(2):83-93.

51. Seo SS, Choi JS, An KC, Kim JH, Kim SB: The factors affecting stiffness occurring with rotator cuff tear. *J Shoulder Elbow Surg* 2012;21(3):304-309.

52. Sarver JJ, Peltz CD, Dourte L, Reddy S, Williams GR, Soslowsky LJ: After rotator cuff repair, stiffness—But not the loss in range of motion—Increased transiently for immobilized shoulders in a rat model. *J Shoulder Elbow Surg* 2008;17(1 suppl):S108-S113.

53. Parsons BO, Gruson KI, Chen DD, Harrison AK, Gladstone J, Flatow EL: Does slower rehabilitation after arthroscopic rotator cuff repair lead to long-term stiffness? *J Shoulder Elbow Surg* 2010;19(7):1034-1039.

54. Peltz CD, Dourte LM, Kuntz AF, et al: The effect of postoperative passive motion on rotator cuff healing in a rat model. *J Bone Joint Surg Am* 2009;91(10):2421-2429.

55. Uggen C, Dines J, McGarry M, Grande D, Lee T, Limpisvasti O: The effect of recombinant human platelet-derived growth factor BB-coated sutures on rotator cuff healing in a sheep model. *Arthroscopy* 2010;26(11):1456-1462.

56. Tirefort J, Schwitzguebel AJ, Collin P, Nowak A, Plomb-Holmes C, Lädermann A: Postoperative mobilization after superior rotator cuff repair: Sling versus No sling: A randomized prospective study. *J Bone Joint Surg Am* 2019;101(6):494-503. doi:10.2106/JBJS.18.00773.

The principal finding of our study was that, compared with sling immobilization during the first 4 weeks after superior rotator cuff repair, no immobilization was significantly associated with reduced pain and improved function at 6 months, independent of adjuvant procedures or patient characteristics. There were no significant differences in VAS pain scores at 10 days. Moreover, no immobilization was significantly associated with a greater early range of motion. Level of evidence: I.

57. Hee CK, Dines JS, Dines DM, et al: Augmentation of a rotator cuff suture repair using rhPDGF-BB and a type I bovine collagen matrix in an ovine model. *Am J Sports Med* 2011;39(8):1630-1639.

58. Jo CH, Kim JE, Yoon KS, et al: Does platelet-rich plasma accelerate recovery after rotator cuff repair? A prospective cohort study. *Am J Sports Med* 2011;39(10):2082-2090.

59. Bergeson AG, Tashjian RZ, Greis PE, Crim J, Stoddard GJ, Burks RT: Effects of platelet-rich fibrin matrix on repair integrity of at-risk rotator cuff tears. *Am J Sports Med* 2012;40(2):286-293.

60. Barber FA, Hrnack SA, Snyder SJ, Hapa O: Rotator cuff repair healing influenced by platelet-rich plasma construct augmentation. *Arthroscopy* 2011;27(8):1029-1035.

61. Castricini R, Longo UG, De Benedetto M, et al: Platelet-rich plasma augmentation for arthroscopic rotator cuff repair: A randomized controlled trial. *Am J Sports Med* 2011;39(2):258-265.

62. Randelli P, Arrigoni P, Ragone V, Aliprandi A, Cabitza P: Platelet rich plasma in arthroscopic rotator cuff repair: A prospective RCT study, 2-year follow-up. *J Shoulder Elbow Surg* 2011;20(4):518-528.

63. Aspenberg P, Virchenko O: Platelet concentrate injection improves Achilles tendon repair in rats. *Acta Orthop Scand* 2004;75(1):93-99.

64. Lyras DN, Kazakos K, Verettas D, et al: The influence of platelet-rich plasma on angiogenesis during the early phase of tendon healing. *Foot Ankle Int* 2009;30(11):1101-1106.

65. Castillo TN, Pouliot MA, Kim HJ, Dragoo JL: Comparison of growth factor and platelet concentration from commercial platelet-rich plasma separation systems. *Am J Sports Med* 2011;39(2):266-271.

66. Gulotta LV, Kovacevic D, Ehteshami JR, Dagher E, Packer JD, Rodeo SA: Application of bone marrow-derived mesenchymal stem cells in a rotator cuff repair model. *Am J Sports Med* 2009;37(11):2126-2133.

67. Gulotta LV, Kovacevic D, Packer JD, Deng XH, Rodeo SA: Bone marrow-derived mesenchymal stem cells transduced with scleraxis improve rotator cuff healing in a rat model. *Am J Sports Med* 2011;39(6):1282-1289.

Section 4

Arthroscopy

SECTION EDITORS:
AUGUSTUS D. MAZZOCCA, MS, MD
RANJAN GUPTA, MD

Chapter 16

Arthroscopic Treatment of Subacromial and Acromioclavicular Pathology

Daniel Aaron, MD • Bradford Parsons, MD • Paul Cagle, MD • Evan Flatow, MD

ABSTRACT

Pathology involving the subacromial space and the acromioclavicular (AC) joint affects a patient's shoulder function and can be a source of pain. The initial management of subacromial impingement syndrome, AC joint arthritis, distal clavicle osteolysis, and most AC joint separations is nonsurgical. Initial management with physical therapy and NSAIDs is supported, and in some cases, additional treatments such as a corticosteroid injection may be beneficial. Surgical management of subacromial impingement syndrome both in isolation and with rotator cuff repair, and surgical management of AC separation pathology will be analyzed.

Keywords: acromioclavicular; acromioplasty; impingement; shoulder arthroscopy

Introduction

Shoulder pain due to pathology involving the subacromial space and the acromioclavicular (AC) joint is common, and those symptoms can substantially affect a patient's quality of life. When nonsurgical measures for treating these conditions fail to resolve the symptoms, surgical intervention often is warranted. As techniques and technology have evolved, arthroscopic surgery has become the standard method of surgical management for many of these conditions. The etiology, evaluation, and treatment of the most common conditions affecting the subacromial space and the AC joint are discussed, with particular attention to arthroscopic technique.

Subacromial Pathology

Anatomy and Etiology

Extrinsic compression or impingement of the rotator cuff is one of the most important proposed mechanisms of rotator cuff disease and tearing. Intrinsic factors also play a critical role. The extent to which mechanical compression of the rotator cuff tendons contributes to symptoms and the development and the progression of tendon pathology is controversial, however.

The anatomy of the subacromial space has been studied with regard to its contribution to rotator cuff disease: from bursitis, to tendinitis, to partial cuff tendon failure, to full-thickness tendon tears. Many theories exist concerning the anatomic features of the subacromial space and their relationship to rotator cuff pathology and symptoms. The subacromial space can be defined by the humeral head inferiorly, the edge and undersurface of the anterior third of the acromion and coracoacromial (CA) ligament anterosuperiorly, and the confines of the subacromial bursa laterally. There is tremendous variability in this anatomic space. If the fine balance that regulates the shoulder kinematics is compromised, the humeral head migrates superiorly and the bursa protecting the rotator cuff, as well as the cuff itself, becomes increasingly compressed against the superior ceiling of acromion and CA ligament.

The author of a 1972 study was the first to describe the anterior acromion as the principal site of impingement on the rotator cuff and the long head of the biceps tendon.[1] A ridge of spurs and excrescences on the undersurface of the anterior acromion, with some cadaver specimens having eburnation of the anterior third, were noted. It was concluded that elevation of the arm in internal or external rotation brought these structures under the anterior acromion, where they were vulnerable to compression, impingement, and, ultimately, mechanical failure.[1] Later anatomic study revealed that the CA ligament at the

Dr. Aaron or an immediate family member serves as a paid consultant to or is an employee of DePuy, A Johnson & Johnson Company. Dr. Parsons or an immediate family member has received royalties from Arthrex, Inc.; is a member of a speakers' bureau or has made paid presentations on behalf of Arthrex, Inc.; serves as a paid consultant to or is an employee of Arthrex, Inc.; and serves as a board member, owner, officer, or committee member of the American Academy of Orthopaedic Surgeons. Dr. Cagle or an immediate family member serves as a paid consultant to or is an employee of Stryker. Dr. Flatow or an immediate family member has received royalties from Innomed and Zimmer; serves as an unpaid consultant to Zimmer; and serves as a board member, owner, officer, or committee member of the Health Association of NY.

anterior margin of the acromion was stretched by passage of the greater tuberosity beneath it, and the tuberosity and the supraspinatus impinged on the CA ligament and the anterior acromion during flexion and internal rotation.[2] In addition, impingement of the biceps occurred at the CA ligament. Another cadaver study found that the acromiohumeral interval decreased in 60° to 120° of elevation, with contact centered at the supraspinatus insertion. Contact was significantly increased with an anterior-hooked acromion.[3] Anterolateral undersurface acromial excrescence was noted to be caused by ossification of the attachment of the coracoacromial ligament. This spur formation was more prevalent with increasing age.[4] The association of the anatomy of the anterior acromion and CA ligament with rotator cuff impingement was supported by the finding that flattening of the anterior third of the acromion was necessary to reduce impingement on the rotator cuff.[5]

With continued investigation and better understanding of the mechanisms of shoulder pain, particularly subacromial space distribution pain, the term impingement syndrome may not be the most accurate. Clearly, the etiology is mutlifactorial and thus rotator cuff disease[6] or subacromial inflammation syndrome would be more accurate. Shoulder impingement clinical symptoms result from an inflammation and degeneration of the anatomic structures in the region of the subacromial space.

Patient Evaluation

The evaluation of subacromial impingement depends on a focused but thorough patient history and physical examination, with adjunct imaging studies. The typical symptom of impingement is anterolateral shoulder and/or arm pain that radiates into the lateral deltoid region, in the distribution of the subacromial bursa.[7] Patients often state that particular positions and activities aggravate the pain. Pain may cause difficulty during overhead activities, such as reaching for an object on a high shelf, or activities requiring terminal internal rotation, such as putting on a coat or fastening a brassiere. Lifting objects with an extended arm also frequently causes symptoms. Night pain and sleep disturbance is a common complaint.

Physical Examination

Subacromial pain is very common in patients with shoulder pain and pathology. This may be a primary problem or a secondary issue due to concomitant pathology. Thus it is critical to assess range-of-motion abnormalities, scapular position and kinetics, pain generators, and strength deficits. The clinician should begin with a visual assessment of the skin, inspect the contour of the glenohumeral joint and the scapula compared with the contralateral side, and check for the presence of any atrophy or deformity. Passive and active range of motion and rotator cuff strength should be measured. Subacromial impingement can be assessed by performing provocative maneuvers, of which the most commonly used are the Neer and Hawkins tests. The principle of these tests is to decrease the subacromial space and increase contact between the rotator cuff and the bony and ligamentous borders, as validated by several studies. An MRI analysis found that the rotator cuff is in closeproximity to the anterior-inferior acromion in abduction and internal rotation (the Hawkins sign position) but not in full forward elevation (the Neer sign position).[8] An arthroscopic study found that a positive Neer test is more likely to be related to rotator cuff contact with the glenoid than with the acromion.[9] Another MRI study found that both tests decreased the distance between the supraspinatus insertion and the bony borders of the subacromial space, although the Hawkins test produced more space reduction and rotator cuff contact.[10] A cadaver study also found rotator cuff contact occurred with both tests. The Neer test produced contact with the medial acromion, and the Hawkins test produced contact with the CA ligament. Both tests produced contact between the articular side of the rotator cuff and the anterosuperior glenoid.[11] In clinical practice, both tests are sensitive but not particularly specific for the diagnosis of subacromial impingement.[12] A subacromial injection of local anesthetic (with or without corticosteroid) into the subacromial bursa can provide therapeutic and important diagnostic information. The primitive pain fibers are in the bursa.[13] If the patient has significant pain relief and improved motion after the injection, this has been termed a positive impingement test. But it also allows the patient and the clinician the ability to assess other potential pain generators in and around the shoulder.

Imaging

In addition to the patient history and the physical examination, imaging studies should be obtained and assessed. The typical set of shoulder radiographs includes AP views in the normal and scapular planes as well as axillary lateral and outlet or scapula Y views. The normal AP projection offers a view of osteophytes about the AC joint, and the scapular plane AP (true AP, Grashey) view best displays the glenohumeral joint and can show cystic change in the greater tuberosity. The axillary view is best for revealing an os acromiale, and the outlet view is best for acromial morphology. A correlation was observed between impingement and acromiohumeral distance as measured on AP radiographs and coronal plane MRI.[14] Radiographic findings may support a diagnosis of rotator cuff disease, that is, impingement, but they must be correlated with the clinical signs and symptoms.[15]

Nonsurgical Management

A treatment strategy must be developed after shoulder impingement syndrome is diagnosed. The presence or the absence of associated pathology, particularly a rotator cuff tear, is crucial to any treatment plan. If the patient has impingement without full-thickness tearing of the rotator cuff, the treatment algorithm typically begins nonsurgically.

Nonsteroidal Anti-inflammatory Drugs

The use of NSAIDs often is recommended to treat inflammation of the subacromial bursa. These agents can be clinically effective. A molecular basis for their effect was found in the downregulation of inflammatory cytokines and mediating receptors in the subacromial bursa.[16] The detrimental systemic and local effects of NSAIDs make their use controversial. Nonselective NSAIDs (cyclooxygenase [COX] inhibitors) increase the risk of upper gastrointestinal complications, such as ulceration and bleeding. COX-2 inhibitors have decreased the gastrointestinal adverse effect profile but are associated with cardiovascular risk.[17] NSAIDs were shown to inhibit tendon-to-bone healing in an animal model, and this finding raises questions about their use in patients after rotator cuff repair.[18]

Physical Therapy

Physical therapy is a commonly used treatment modality. Compared with patients with subacromial impingement who received nonspecific physical therapy, a significantly lower percentage of patients needed surgical intervention after receiving a specific rehabilitation protocol consisting of stretches, eccentric rotator cuff strengthening, and concentric-eccentric scapular stabilizing exercises.[19]

Subacromial Injections

Subacromial injections often are administered for subacromial impingement syndrome. Corticosteroids are the most commonly injected agent. Corticosteroids also have been shown to downregulate inflammatory cytokines in the subacromial bursa.[16] However, a meta-analysis found only weak support for using corticosteroid injections in treating conditions in the spectrum of rotator cuff disease.[20] Corticosteroid use is contraindicated in certain patients because of the risk of an elevation in blood glucose, and further use is contraindicated in patients who have received multiple injections. A transient decrease in rotator cuff tendon strength and histologic changes were reported after a single administration of methylprednisolone in an animal model.[21] Nonetheless, corticosteroid injections are a low-risk intervention in most patients, and they may facilitate participation in physical therapy.

The current American Academy of Orthopaedic Surgeons practice guidelines recommend initial management of subacromial impingement syndrome with physical therapy and NSAIDs but neither support nor refute the use of corticosteroid injections, pulsed electromagnetic fields, iontophoresis, phonophoresis, transcutaneous electrical nerve stimulation, ice, heat, massage, or activity modification.[22]

Surgical Management

If nonsurgical measures are not effective, surgical intervention may be indicated. In the absence of tearing of more than 50% thickness of the rotator cuff, subacromial decompression alone can be effective. This procedure typically consists of removing the subacromial bursa, anterior acromioplasty, and excision of the CA ligament. Flattening of the anterior third of the acromion is adequate to eliminate extrinsic rotator cuff compression.[5] The standard method of decompression is arthroscopic.

Technique

Arthroscopic subacromial decompression (ASD) typically involves the use of two portals. A standard posterior portal is created approximately 2 cm medial and 2 cm distal to the posterolateral corner of the acromion. Palpation of the soft spot of the posterior glenohumeral joint line is recommended to confirm portal placement, although this step can be difficult in a patient with a large deltoid musculature or adipose layer. A No. 11 blade is used to incise the skin. The trocar-cannula assembly is advanced into the subacromial space and can be used to create space for viewing by a sweeping motion along the undersurface of the acromion and the CA ligament. Longitudinal traction on the arm may increase acromiohumeral distance and facilitate entry into the space. The trocar is withdrawn, and the cannula is held in place. When the arthroscope is inserted into the cannula, the camera is aimed superiorly so that the acromion is in view. A standard lateral portal is then created. A spinal needle routinely is used to place this portal so that the anterior acromion and the CA ligament are easily accessible and the angle between the instruments and the acromion will allow an even acromioplasty. The portal is typically located 3 to 4 cm distal to the lateral border of the acromion at the border of the anterior one-third and posterior two-thirds. It must be kept in mind that the axillary nerve crosses this area 5 to 7 cm distal to the lateral acromial edge. After the portal location has been determined, a transverse portal is created, using a No. 11 blade to incise only 5 mm of skin. A clear plastic cannula is advanced into the space to allow simple insertion and the removal of instrumentation. A motorized shaver is inserted first to remove bursal tissue and expand the area that can be visualized. Bleeding areas are immediately cauterized. The bursal surface of the rotator cuff is inspected visually and with a probe to rule out tendon tearing. The electrocautery is used to remove all adherent soft tissue from the acromial undersurface. This process begins with a relaxing incision through the deltoid fascia from the cannula entry site directly medial to the acromion edge; the purpose is to improve instrument access to the anterior acromial edge and the CA ligament. The lateral border of the acromion is defined by incising the deltoid fascia until muscle fibers are seen, and the anterior edge is defined by peeling off the CA ligament until none of its fibers remain attached. The ligament is not fully released if there is a large tear of the rotator cuff because the passive stabilizing effect of the arch must be preserved.[22] The remainder of the acromion undersurface can then be exposed. An anterior acromioplasty is performed with a motorized burr. The goal of this step is simply to flatten the anterior surface. After determining how much bony resection will be required, the surgeon resects that thickness at the anterolateral corner. This step-cut technique in effect creates a template for the more medial resection. When the level of resection is even from lateral to medial, the arthroscope is moved to the lateral portal for viewing the acromion in an orthogonal, cutting-block plane. The burr is inserted into the posterior portal, and the acromion is smoothed to the original step-cut. Throughout the procedure, care must be taken to fully define the bony edges but avoid cutting the deltoid muscle. Meticulous hemostasis with the electrocautery and the use of epinephrine in the irrigant solution (1:300,000) are recommended to minimize bleeding, and a low pump pressure (35 torr) is recommended to avoid swelling.

Results

ASD can effectively relieve symptoms originating from impingement syndrome. The results of ASD are superior to those of open decompression. A 1998 review concluded both open and arthroscopic decompression had high success rates that were not significantly different (90.0% and 89.3%, respectively), but the arthroscopic technique allowed earlier rehabilitation because the deltoid was not detached.[23] The importance of the relatively long learning curve of the arthroscopic technique has been largely obviated as it has become more widely used. A recent meta-analysis found that the two techniques had equivalent clinical outcomes, but patients who underwent ASD returned to work more quickly and spent fewer days in the hospital than those who underwent open decompression.[24] Small full-thickness supraspinatus tears did not progress after ASD without tendon repair.[25] There is also evidence that ASD may reduce the risk of future rotator cuff tearing in patients with subacromial impingement; 18% of patients had a rotator cuff tear 15 years after ASD (4% had a full-thickness tear), compared with approximately 40% in age-matched historic control patients.[26] Despite this, recent data have also brought into question the efficacy of ASD performed in isolation. A recent randomized trial with up to 14 years follow-up of patients randomized to either a bursectomy or a bursectomy combined with acromioplasty demonstrated no difference in clinical outcome when acromioplasty was performed.[27]

Adjunct to Rotator Cuff Repair

There is debate as to whether ASD performed concurrently with arthroscopic repair of a full-thickness rotator cuff tear leads to an improved outcome. In a study of patients with a full-thickness rotator cuff tear who were treated with repair alone or with repair and ASD, researchers have determined that clinical outcome was correlated with several variables, including patient age, tear pattern, tendon quality and retraction, and repair technique.[28] No correlation was found between concurrent ASD and outcome. In a randomized, prospective study of patients with a full-thickness, single-tendon rotator cuff tear, no significant functional differences were found at 1-year follow-up based on whether the patient's rotator cuff repair included ASD (patients with acromial spurs were excluded).[29] In a study of 2,441 patients undergoing rotator cuff repairs, 6% of the patients did not have an acromioplasty at the time of rotator cuff repair, and at 24-month follow-up, no difference in pain or functional scores was appreciated.[30] In a more recent study, 114 patients undergoing an arthroscopic repair of a full-thickness rotator cuff tear were randomized, and the results at 2 years follow-up demonstrated no difference in clinical outcome with or without an acromioplasty.[31] A systematic review including four studies with 354 total patients demonstrated no statistically significant difference in clinical outcomes between patients who did or did not have an acromioplasty.[32] Another study found no significant difference in the clinical outcomes of patients who underwent rotator cuff repair alone or with concurrent ASD, but the revision surgery rate was lower in patients who underwent ASD.[33] A recent meta-analysis reviewing five randomized controlled trials demonstrated no difference in the majority of the outcome scores and retear rates in patients undergoing an acromioplasty.[34] However, a 2012 meta-analysis demonstrated no difference in revision surgery rates or functional outcomes.[35] ASD is routinely performed as an adjunct to repair of a full-thickness rotator cuff tear when clear impingement or spurs are noted arthroscopically.

Acromioclavicular Pathology

Etiology

The AC joint may be affected by a degenerative condition, such as osteoarthritis, or a traumatic condition, such as dislocation or separation. Radiographic degeneration of the AC joint is common, but it is not necessarily symptomatic. AC joint pain can also develop as a result of inflammatory or crystalline arthropathy, trauma, or joint sepsis.[36] AC joint arthritis can exist in isolation or in association with another condition affecting the shoulder. Osteolysis of the distal clavicle also leads to pain and tenderness at the AC joint and is thought to be caused by hypervascularization and bone resorption after repeated small subchondral fractures. An AC separation typically occurs as a result of trauma.

Anatomy

The AC joint is the articulation between the acromion process of the scapula and the distal end of the clavicle. It is the only connection between the upper extremity and the axial skeleton. It is a diarthrodial joint and contains a fibrocartilaginous disk. The width of the joint space typically is 1 to 3 mm.[37] The joint is stabilized by a complex set of ligamentous and muscular restraints. Anterior-posterior translation is primarily limited by the AC ligaments, especially the superior and posterior capsular sections or ligaments. Superior translation of the distal clavicle is primarily limited by the two coracoclavicular (CC) ligaments, with the conoid being the stronger of the two. The deltotrapezial fascia may also contribute to stability, but its exact role has not been well characterized. The insertions of the stabilizing ligaments are important to understand because resection of the insertion sites can lead to iatrogenic instability, and reconstruction of the ligaments may be more effective if done in anatomic fashion.

An anatomic study of the clavicle and the coracoid in both dry osteologic and fresh cadaver specimens found the average distance from the distal end of the clavicle to the center of the trapezoid tuberosity to be 25.4 (±3.7) mm in men, and 22.9 (±3.7) mm in women.[38] The distance to the medial border of the conoid tuberosity was 47.2 (±4.6) mm and 42.8 (±5.6) mm in male and female specimens, respectively. Interestingly, the ratio of these distances to overall clavicle length was consistent between the sexes. Specifically, the ratio of the distance to the trapezoid center to overall clavicle length was 0.17 and to the medial border of the conoid tuberosity was 0.31. In the fresh cadaver specimens, the ratio of the distance to the trapezoid to clavicle length was 0.17 and to the conoid center was 0.24.[38]

Patient Evaluation

Patients having pathology of the AC joint frequently experience pain directly over the joint and in the anterolateral neck, the trapezius-supraspinatus region, and over the coracoid region.[7] It is very uncommon to have lateral deltoid pain (subacromial distribution) in cases of isolated AC symptomology. Physical examination of the AC joint begins with a visual assessment, with attention to prominence of the distal clavicle to detect separation. If separation is suspected, stability of the joint in the anterior-posterior and superoinferior planes should be examined. If the AC separation is obvious, reducibility should be assessed by applying a superiorly directed force onto the humerus at the elbow. If no separation is suspected and the pathology is likely to be chronic in nature, the joint should be palpated and tenderness should be noted. Direct tenderness is reported to be 96% to 97% sensitive as a test for AC pathology.[39,40] This is the best test for direct AC pain and involvement. Also commonly used is the cross-body adduction test, in which pain at the AC joint is elicited by maximally adducting the arm with the shoulder in 90° of elevation. This maneuver has a reported sensitivity of 67%.[40] The O'Brien active compression test also is widely used; the arm is adducted 15° across the body, the shoulder is internally rotated, and the patient actively elevates the arm against resistance. A positive test consists of pain during this maneuver, with substantially less pain when the test is repeated with the shoulder in external rotation. The O'Brien test has reported sensitivity as high as 83%, with 90% specificity.[39,40] In a combined cross-body adduction and O'Brien test, the shoulder is elevated to 90°, the arm is maximally adducted across the body, and the patient actively elevates against resistance with the shoulder in internal rotation.[40] A positive test consists of pain during this maneuver and only slightly less pain with external rotation. The sensitivity of this Bell-van Riet test was reported to be 98%.[40] The sternoclavicular joint should also be examined for tenderness, deformity, and instability.

Imaging of the AC joint begins with standard radiographs. The radiographic views for the AC joint were described as including several AP views: with the beam angled caudad and cephalad by 15°, with the humerus in internal and external rotation, with the arm maximally abducted and in 30° to 35° of cephalad angulation.[37] The most commonly used of these AP radiographs is the so-called Zanca view, in which the beam is angled 15° cephalad (**Figure 1**). A standard AP view often is sufficient (**Figure 2**), but the Zanca view reliably prevents the AC joint from being obscured by the scapular spine and allows detection of erosive changes, osteophyte formation, and joint-space narrowing in the presence of arthritis as well as joint widening and displacement in the setting of trauma.[37,41]

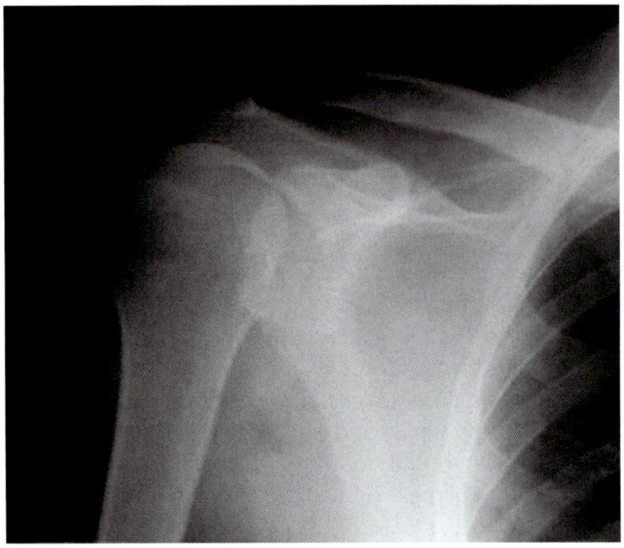

FIGURE 1 Zanca radiograph with no superimposition of the scapular spine over the acromioclavicular joint. The even resection of the distal clavicle can be seen.

MRI has reported sensitivity of 85% for atraumatic AC joint pathologic changes, and it allows ligamentous structures to be seen in patients with AC separation.[39] Nuclear bone scanning also has high accuracy (76%).[39] Ultrasonography has been used to detect AC joint arthritis, but in one study, 65% of the asymptomatic individuals had a positive finding.[42] Intra-articular anesthetic injection is the benchmark for the diagnosis of atraumatic AC joint pathology, although it can be challenging to ensure the anesthetic actually enters the joint.[39]

Management of Acromioclavicular Joint Arthritis and Distal Clavicle Osteolysis

Nonsurgical Management

The management of chronic conditions affecting the AC joint, such as degenerative joint disease and osteolysis, begins nonsurgically with the use of NSAIDs and physical therapy. If these modalities are not effective, intra-articular corticosteroid injections often are used. Recent data suggest that these injections have a low rate of short-term clinical success, but if relief is provided, the benefit is likely to endure.[43] Specifically, only 16 of 58 patients (28%) had adequate relief of pain 1 month after AC joint corticosteroid injection. However, at an average 42-month follow-up, 15 of the 16 patients had relief sufficient to allow them to decline surgery. No complications of corticosteroid injection were noted.[43] Injection of corticosteroid mixed with a local anesthetic can have diagnostic value, and it is a relatively safe and sometimes effective treatment modality.

Surgical Management

The mainstay of surgical management of AC joint arthritis or osteolysis is resection of the distal clavicle. Distal clavicle resection (DCR) can be performed open or arthroscopically, although the arthroscopic approach has become the standard. Regardless of the approach, the success of the procedure depends on resecting an even and adequate amount of distal clavicle bone while avoiding joint destabilization caused by compromise of the supporting ligaments and their bony insertions.

The recommended technique for arthroscopic DCR depends on whether the AC joint pathology is isolated

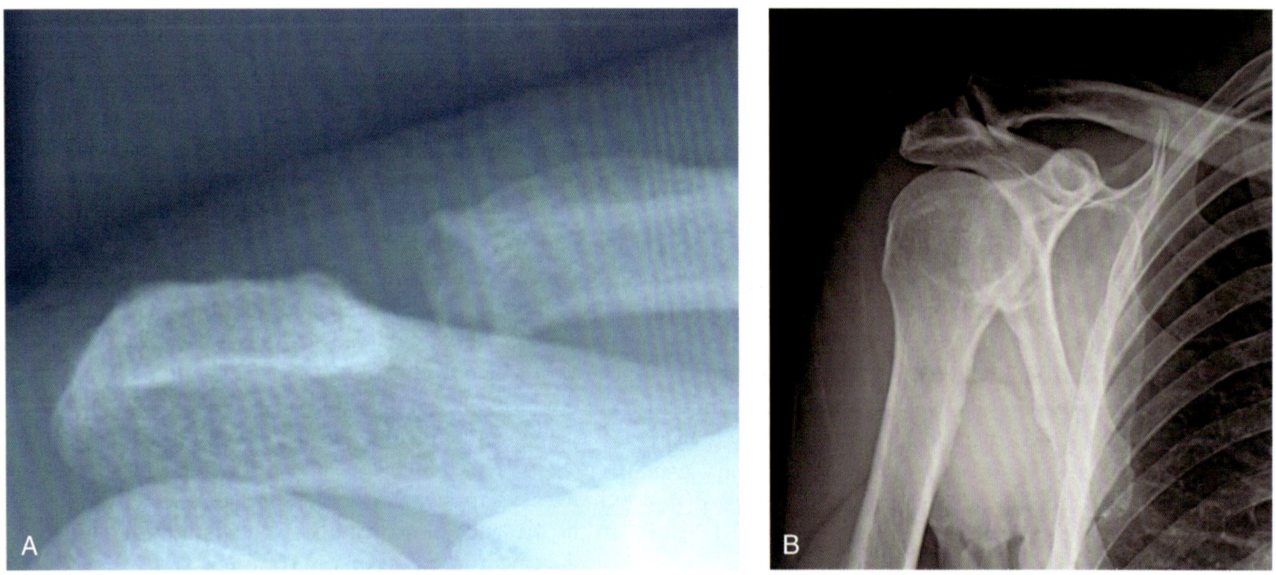

FIGURE 2 Radiographic appearance of distal clavicle osteolysis (**A**) and osteoarthritis with osteophytes (**B**).

or associated with a condition such as subacromial impingement or rotator cuff tearing. When another condition exists, a bursal approach is used in which ASD is performed first. When the subacromial space is decompressed, the scope is placed in the posterior portal and an additional portal is created at the anterior aspect of the AC joint. The joint is palpated from the outside, and a spinal needle is introduced. The needle should be placed exactly at the midline of the anterior joint line (the anterosuperior portal) so that the angle of the instruments will provide access for an even resection. When portal placement is confirmed, a No. 11 blade is used to create a 5-mm portal and is inserted completely into the joint until it can be seen through the arthroscope. The portal is expanded with a blunt trocar, and a motorized shaver is inserted. The inferior AC capsule, the intra-articular disk, and other soft tissues are excised. Blood vessels frequently are encountered and are cauterized with the electrocautery. Great care is taken to obtain a complete exposure of the articular surface of the clavicle so that the evenness of the bony resection can be accurately gauged. Although exposure of the superior aspect of the distal clavicle must be obtained, it is important to avoid detaching the superior AC ligament to avoid anterior-posterior instability. When all soft tissue is removed, the bony resection is performed with a motorized burr. As with ASD, a step-cut technique is used to ensure an even resection. The goal is an 8 to 10 mm resection of distal clavicle. The burr is used to resect the desired amount of bone at the anterior edge of the clavicle. The burr is then advanced posteriorly, and resection to the level of the step-cut is performed. The surgeon carefully examines the bony contour, with particular attention to the posterior and superior aspects, which often are left incompletely resected. Any undesired remaining bone is removed with the burr. The shaver is then reinserted, and any loose debris is removed. Visualization of the AC joint from the posterior portal sometimes is difficult, and if necessary for this purpose, the posterior aspect of the acromial facet is minimally excised. No more bone should be removed than is necessary to ensure adequate visualization of the joint.

In a patient with isolated AC joint disease, a direct approach is used that can be technically more demanding than the bursal approach but does not violate the bursa and thereby minimizes swelling and bleeding.[44] Furthermore, variability in the orientation of the AC joint can be accommodated because portals are placed according to AC joint anatomy only. In the direct approach, concomitant intra-articular pathology can be ruled out by diagnostic glenohumeral arthroscopy through standard posterior and anterior portals. The exact location and orientation of the AC joint are determined by successful entry into the joint using two or three 22-gauge needles, which then are used to describe the orientation of the AC joint. The joint can be insufflated through these needles to create space, and backflow can confirm intra-articular positioning. A 0.5-cm portal is created at the posterior joint line, and a 2.7-mm arthroscope is inserted (**Figure 3**). The needles in the AC joint are visualized. A spinal needle is used to guide placement of an anterior AC joint portal in the same fashion as for the bursal approach. A 0.5-cm portal is created, a 2.0-mm motorized shaver is inserted, and soft tissue is removed. The edges of the AC joint are defined, and a 2.0-mm burr is used to begin the bony resection in step-cut fashion. A standard arthroscope and a larger burr can be used to complete the resection after adequate space has been created. As

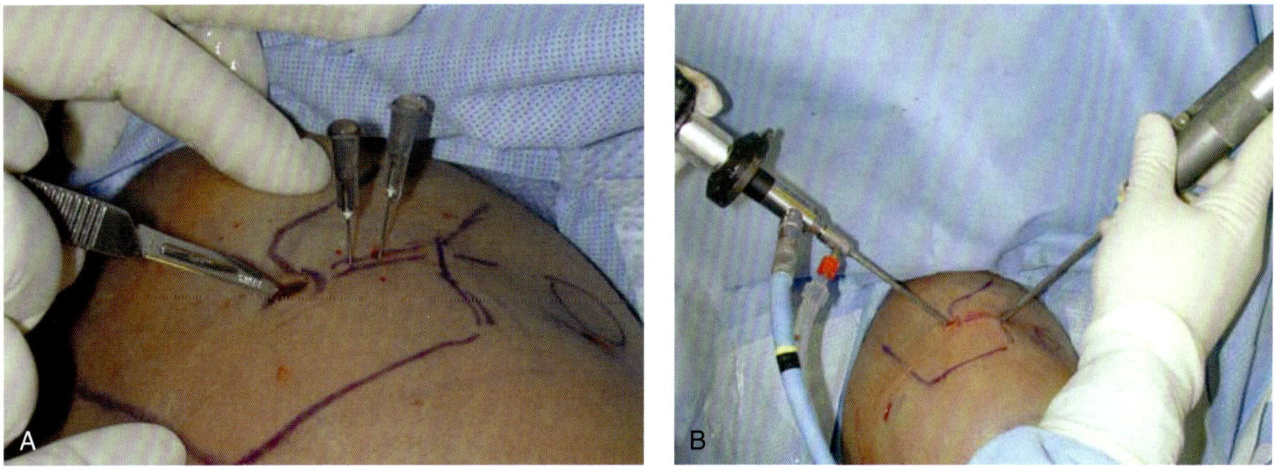

FIGURE 3 Photographs showing acromioclavicular joint localization with needles and the creation of the posterior acromioclavicular portal (**A**) plus instrumentation inserted for a direct arthroscopic approach for distal clavicle resection (**B**).

with the bursal approach, meticulous attention is paid to the depth of resection, the evenness of the joint contour, and the preservation of the superior AC ligament.

In either the bursal or the direct technique, the adequacy of resection can be assessed by inserting an instrument of a known width. Rasps serve this purpose well because they can be used to smooth any remaining rough edges as well as judge the resection. An anatomic study found that the trapezoid insertion lies an average 25.4 mm from the lateral clavicle edge in men and 22.4 mm in women, but a clinical study found that resection of 10 mm can significantly increase anterior translation, even with intact CC and superior and posterior AC ligaments.[38,45] Complete sectioning of the AC capsule significantly increased instability. Therefore, it is recommended that no more than 8 to 10 mm of distal clavicle be resected and that the superior capsuloligamentous structures be preserved.

Arthroscopic DCR has favorable results in comparison with open DCR. Several studies found that patients undergoing open or arthroscopic DCR for AC joint arthritis had predictably good pain relief and low rates of complications or revision surgery.[46-48] One comparison study found significantly less pain in patients treated with arthroscopic DCR than those treated with open DCR. There was no difference between the two patient groups in amount of resection, surgical time, or functional score.[47] Patients who underwent arthroscopic DCR were found to return to work more quickly, particularly if a direct approach was used.[48] A higher revision surgery rate not reaching statistical significance was found when an arthroscopic technique was used.[46] DCR was found to be highly effective for the treatment of osteolysis; 92.6% of patients who underwent arthroscopic DCR for osteolysis of the distal clavicle had a good to excellent result.[49] Treatment for posttraumatic arthropathy was less consistently successful.[49] Arthroscopic DCR is commonly performed concomitantly with rotator cuff repair in patients with symptomatic AC joint arthritis in addition to rotator cuff pathology. DCR at the time of rotator cuff repair may be indicated for asymptomatic AC joint arthritis with inferiorly directed osteophytes; better outcomes at 2-year follow-up and a lower revision surgery rate were noted in patients who underwent DCR in addition to rotator cuff repair.[50]

Acromioclavicular Trauma

Mechanism of Injury

Dislocation or separation of the AC joint typically occurs as a result of a direct impact. The direction and the magnitude of the impact force dictate the direction and the severity of joint displacement (**Figure 4**). The most common mechanism is a fall in which ground impact on the superior aspect of the shoulder forces the acromion inferiorly. Injury is more likely and may be more severe if the shoulder is driven into the ground, as might happen in a collision sport.

Classification

AC separations originally were organized into three grades based on the amount of inferior displacement of the acromion relative to the clavicle.[51] Three additional grades subsequently were added, all of which are indications for surgical management.[52] The advent of MRI led to anatomic correlation with the plain radiographic classification, but the relationship may not be consistent.[53]

Anatomic Reconstruction of the Coracoclavicular Ligaments

Most AC separations are managed nonsurgically, but when surgical management is indicated, the trend is to perform an anatomic reconstruction of the CC ligaments.

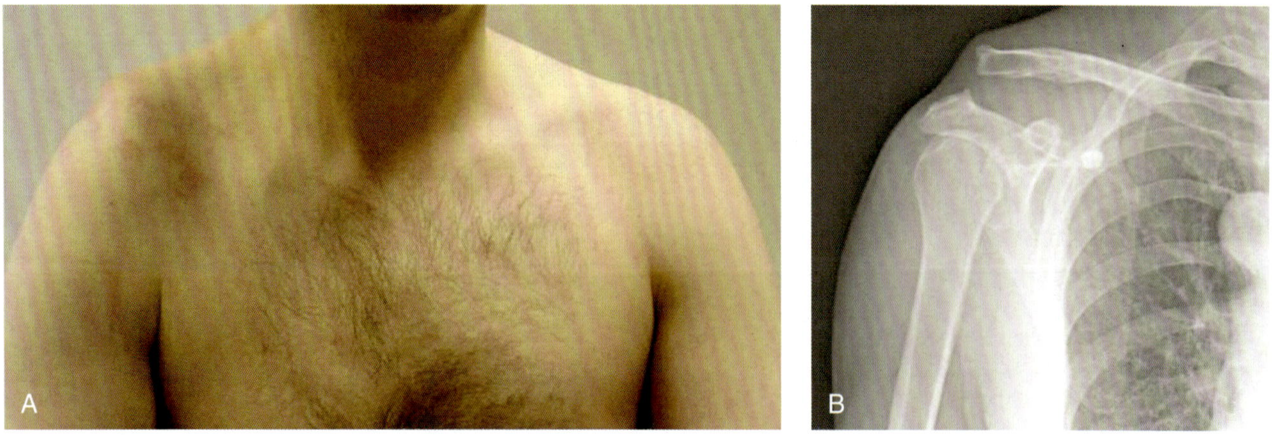

FIGURE 4 Photograph (**A**) and Zanca radiograph (**B**) showing the appearance of complete acromioclavicular joint separation.

Biomechanical studies found that anatomic reconstruction of both CC ligaments is superior to older techniques in which a single construct was used. In testing of the native CC ligament complex in fresh cadaver specimens, the remaining ligamentous tissue was removed after failure, and an anatomic reconstruction was performed with a semitendinosus graft. Each of the two ends of the graft was passed through a medial or a lateral tunnel in the clavicle, and together they were passed through a single coracoid tunnel. The orientation of the graft ends in the coracoid tunnel re-created the individual specimen's native orientation. The same biomechanical testing was performed on the surgical construct. The absence of significant permanent graft elongation after cyclic loading suggests the ability to withstand early rehabilitation.[54] In a comparison of the biomechanics of anatomic reconstruction with the modified Weaver-Dunn procedure in cadaver specimens, the anatomic reconstruction was superior to the modified Weaver-Dunn repair in laxity and both anterior and posterior translation. The anatomic reconstruction was performed with a semitendinosus graft through bone tunnels in the distal clavicle.[55] The tunnel for the conoid ligament was approximately 45 mm medial to the distal end of the clavicle in the posterior half of the shaft. The tunnel for the trapezoid ligament was placed more anteriorly, in the center of the clavicle shaft, and approximately 15 mm lateral to the conoid tunnel (**Figure 5**). The authors concluded that anatomic reconstruction was biomechanically superior and may allow earlier rehabilitation. The biomechanics of anatomic reconstruction depend on the strength of the graft. A recent analysis found that an anatomic reconstruction with the palmaris longus was inadequate and that anatomic reconstruction with the flexor carpi radialis produced a construct superior to that of the modified Weaver-Dunn procedure.[56]

Arthroscopic Coracoclavicular Reconstruction

An early arthroscopic CC reconstruction technique involved arthroscopically guided percutaneous placement of a suture anchor in the coracoid base and percutaneous creation of two bone tunnels in the clavicle. Suture passers were used to pass the suture through the clavicular tunnels, with tying over a titanium plate (**Figure 6**). The anatomic reduction was maintained in 10 of 13 patients, with subluxation in 2 patients and redislocation in 1 patient.[57] Another arthroscopic method involves the use of the TightRope device (Arthrex, Naples, FL) to provide nonrigid fixation between the coracoid and the clavicle. Fixation failure was reported in 2 of 12 patients (16.7%) after this procedure, but 11 of 12 patients were satisfied with the results.[58] Significantly greater strength was reported in both vertical and anterior planes when a double-TightRope construct was used for anatomic reconstruction in a cadaver model, compared with native ligaments[59] (**Figures 7** and **8**). The double-TightRope construct also was used clinically in

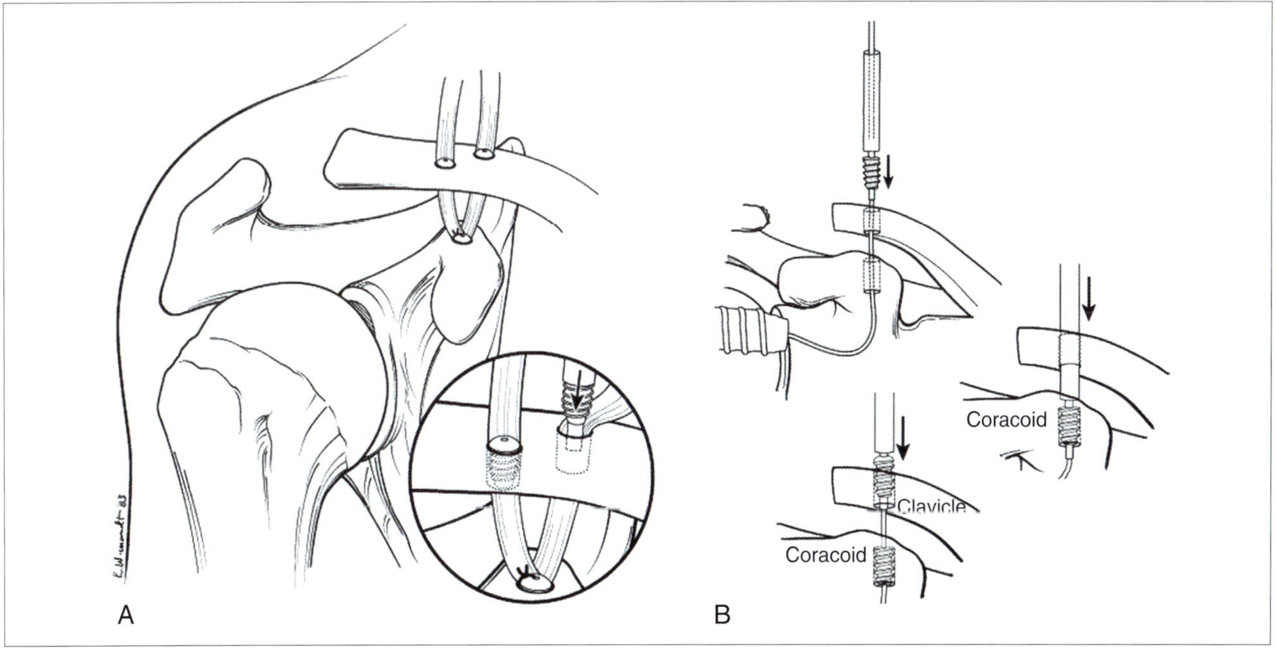

FIGURE 5 Schematic drawings showing an anatomic (**A**) and an arthroscopic (**B**) coracoclavicular reconstruction. (Reproduced with permission from Mazzocca AD, Santangelo SA, Johnson ST, Rios CG, Dumonski ML, Arciero RA: A biomechanical evaluation of an anatomic coracoclavicular ligament reconstruction. *Am J Sports Med* 2006;34[2]:236-246. doi:10.1177/0363546505281795.)

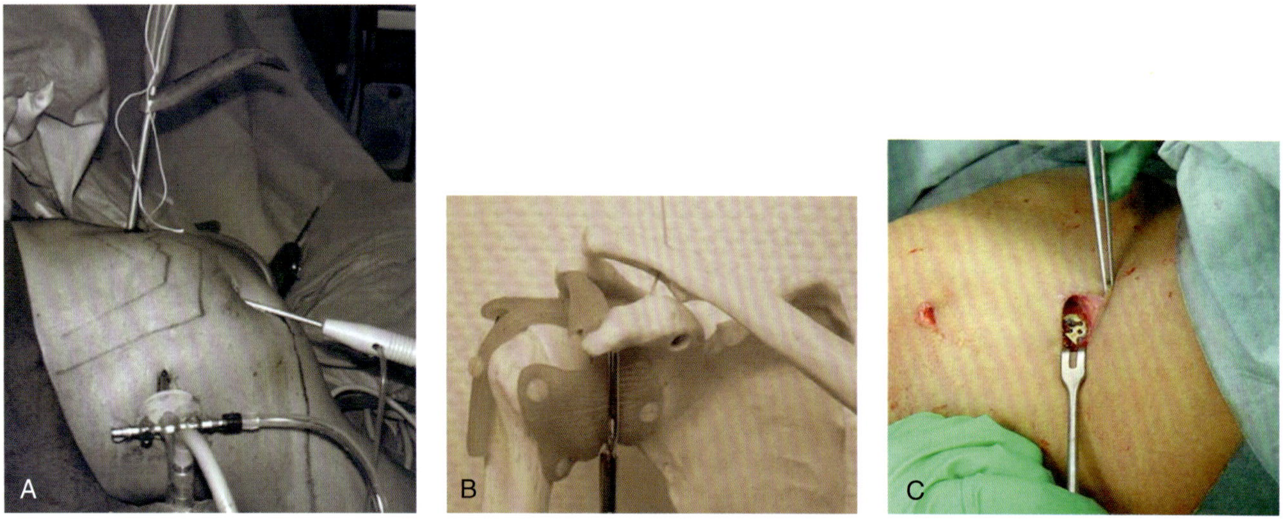

FIGURE 6 Photographs showing arthroscopic coracoclavicular reconstruction. **A**, Arthroscopic setup with the camera in the posterior portal and additional instruments in the lateral and anterior portals. **B**, Suture passage shown on a model. **C**, Knot tying over a titanium plate on the clavicle. (Reprinted by permission from Springer Nature: Chernchujit B, Tischer T, Imhoff AB. Arthroscopic reconstruction of the acromioclavicular joint disruption: Surgical technique and preliminary results. *Arch Orthop Trauma Surg*; 126[9]:575-581. Copyright 2006. doi:10.1007/s00402-005-0073-6.)

an arthroscopic-assisted anatomic reconstruction.[60] At an average 30-month follow-up, 8 of 23 patients had radiographic evidence of loss of reduction that was not correlated with the clinical outcome. In a study of 10 patients, an all-arthroscopic procedure consisting of DCR and a bone-block transfer of the anterior acromion and the CA ligament to the resected surface (the Chuinard modification of the Weaver-Dunn procedure) was augmented by a four-strand CC ligament reconstruction with heavy braided suture over titanium buttons on the coracoid and clavicular surfaces[61] (**Figure 9**). The rationale for this technique was that the suture construct would maintain reduction while the bone-block transfer healed, thereby producing a dynamic construct. The bone blocks completely healed in eight patients and partially healed in two patients. No loss of reduction was noted, and all patients were satisfied with the results. Only one patient had not returned to work at 3 months or to preinjury level of sports at the last follow-up.[61] Although this reconstruction method was not anatomic, the two bundles to some extent mimicked the orientation of the CC ligaments, and living biologic tissue was included. Clinical studies of all-arthroscopic anatomic reconstructions with tendon autograft have yet to be published and have not demonstrated superior or even equivalent results relative to the open technique.

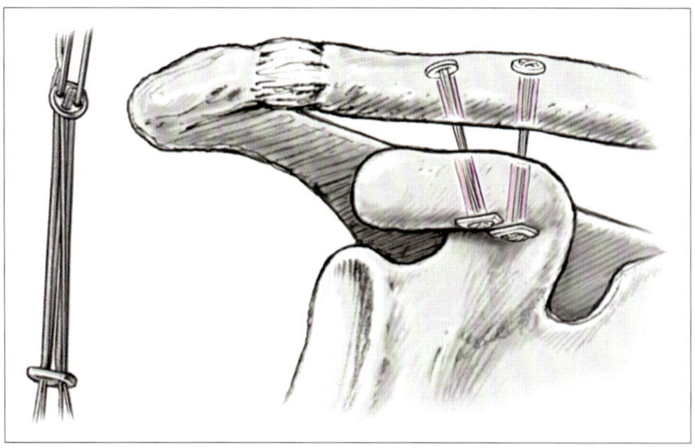

FIGURE 7 Schematic drawing showing anatomic coracoclavicular reconstruction using two TightRope devices. (Reproduced with permission from Walz L, Salzmann GM, Fabbro T, Eichhorn S, Imhoff AB: The anatomic reconstruction of acromioclavicular joint dislocations using 2 TightRope devices: A biomechanical study. *Am J Sports Med* 2008;36[12]:2398-2406. doi:10.1177/0363546508322524.)

Some surgeons resect the distal clavicle at the time of CC ligament reconstruction. In situ CC graft forces were found to be increased with sectioning of the AC joint, but no further increase in force is caused by DCR. The increased graft forces remained much lower than their load to failure, and there was no apparent clinical significance.[62]

Os Acromiale

Os acromiale is a condition in which ossification centers in the acromion process of the scapula remain unfused. Often, os acromiale is an incidental radiographic finding, but it causes pain and rotator cuff impingement in some individuals. The incidence of os acromiale is approximately 8%, and it is most common in men and in individuals of African descent.[63]

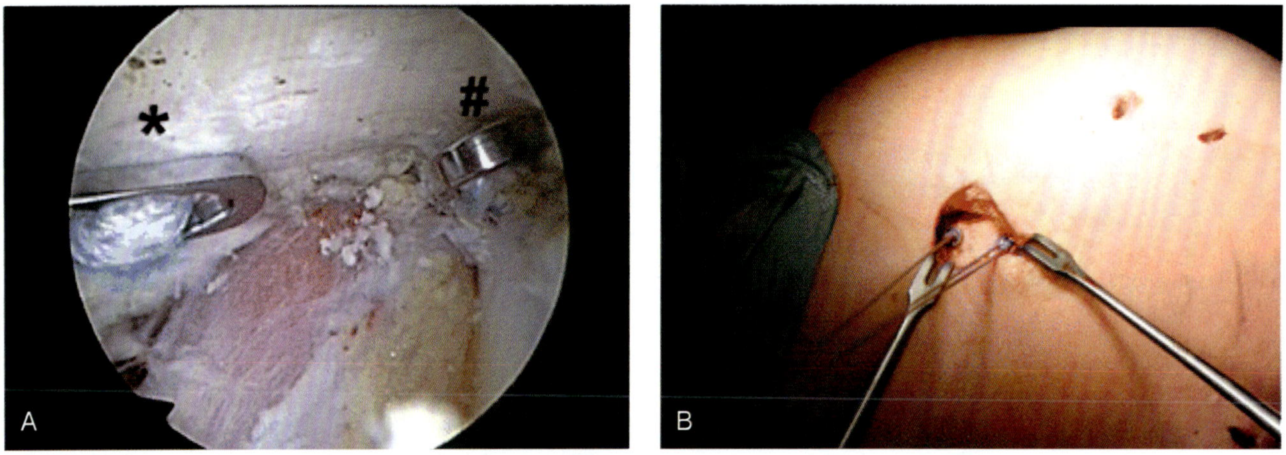

FIGURE 8 Arthroscopically assisted coracoclavicular reconstruction using two TightRope devices. **A**, Arthroscopic view from the anterolateral portal. * = posteromedial portal, conoid ligament; # = anterolateral portal, trapezoid ligament. **B**, Photograph showing two clavicle buttons after AC joint reduction and fixation. (Reproduced with permission from Salzmann GM, Walz L, Buchmann S, Glabgly P, Venjakob A, Imhoff AB: Arthroscopically assisted 2-bundle anatomic reduction of acute acromioclavicular joint separations. *Am J Sports Med* 2010;38[6]:1179-1187. doi:10.1177/0363546509355645.)

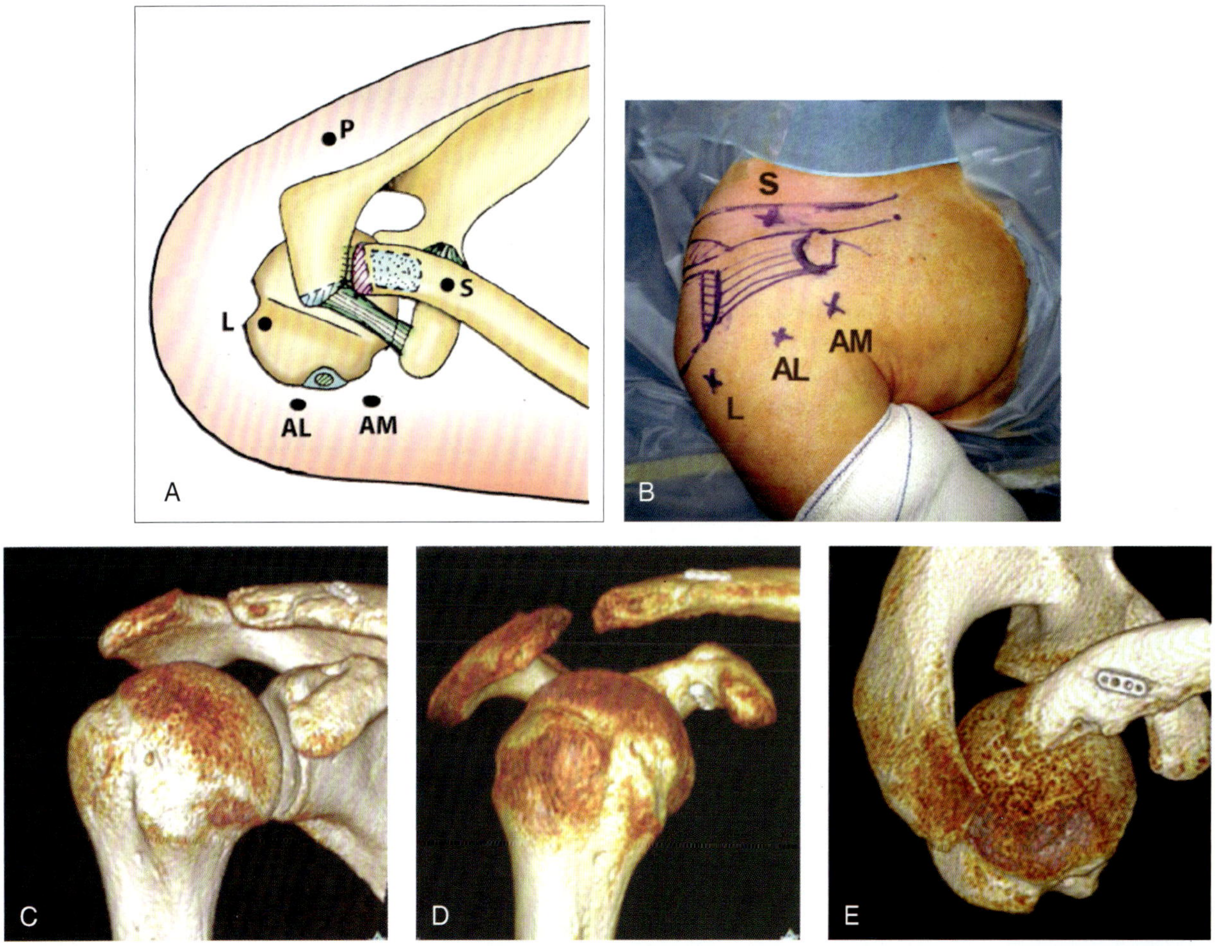

FIGURE 9 All-arthroscopic Weaver-Dunn-Chuinard repair. Schematic drawing (**A**) and photograph (**B**) showing portal placement. AL = anterolateral, AM = anteromedial, L = lateral, P = posterior, S = superior. Three-dimensional CT reconstruction in the coronal (**C**), sagittal (**D**), and axial (**E**) planes showing button placement on the superior aspect of the lateral clavicle and the inferior aspect of the coracoid. (Reprinted from *Arthroscopy* 26[2]. Boileau P, Old J, Gastaud O, Brassart N, Roussanne Y: All-arthroscopic Weaver-Dunn-Chuinard procedure with double-button fixation for chronic acromioclavicular joint dislocation, 149-160. Copyright © 2010 Arthroscopy Association of North America. doi:10.1016/j.arthro.2009.08.008.)

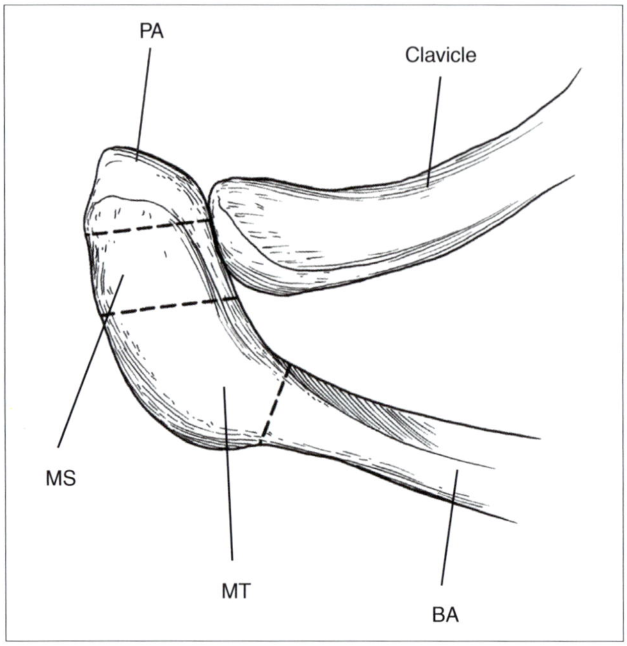

FIGURE 10 Schematic drawing showing the ossification centers of the acromion. BA = basiacromion, MS = mesoacromion, MT = meta-acromion, PA = preacromion. (Reproduced from Kurtz CA, Humble BJ, Rodosky MW, Sekiya JK: Symptomatic os acromiale. *J Am Acad Orthop Surg* 2006;14[1]:12-19.)

The acromion consists of the basiacromion, the meta-acromion, the mesoacromion, and the preacromion (**Figure 10**). The entire acromion may fuse as late in life as age 25 years. The posterior, middle, and anterior deltoid fibers attach to the meta-acromion, the mesoacromion, and the preacromion, respectively. The preacromion also is the anchor of the CA ligament.[63]

Evaluation

Any symptoms of os acromiale typically are characteristic of subacromial impingement, including pain with overhead activities. Physical examination may find positive impingement tests, weakness of the rotator cuff, and tenderness to palpation at the site of the nonunion. Os acromiale can be seen, often incidentally, on plain radiographs, CT, MRI, and bone scans[64] (**Figure 11**).

Management

The initial treatment of symptoms attributable to os acromiale consists of NSAIDs, physical therapy, and corticosteroid injections.[63] If nonsurgical treatment is unsuccessful, several surgical options are available. Open excision of the distal fragment has had variable results, with most poor outcomes resulting from weakening of the deltoid. Open excision is considered only for a small preacromion fragment.[64] Arthroscopic excision may have a lower rate of deltoid weakening with larger fragments, but no comparison studies have been published.[65] Successful open reduction and internal fixation with cannulated screws or a tension-band construct has been reported, but nonunion rates are high and hardware removal often is required.[65,66]

Os acromiale in the setting of subacromial impingement often is treated with simple acromioplasty that leaves only a thin cortical shell and continues the decompression back to the nonunion site. Extreme care is taken not to violate the deltoid attachment to avoid destabilizing the fragment. DCR is avoided for this reason, but usually it is not necessary because of the AC joint decompression achieved by the aggressive acromioplasty.[64] Eleven of 13 patients had a satisfactory result after ASD for unstable symptomatic os acromiale.[67]

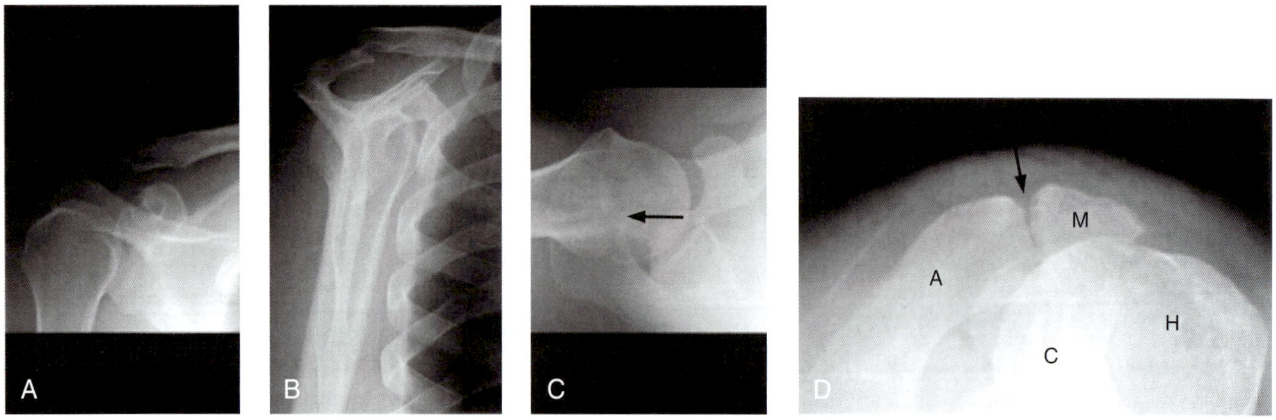

FIGURE 11 AP (**A**), outlet (**B**), axillary lateral (**C**), and acromion profile (**D**) radiographs of the right shoulder showing an os acromiale (arrow) between the meta-acromion and the mesoacromion. A = acromion, C = clavicle, H = humeral head, M = mesoacromion. (Reproduced from Kurtz CA, Humble BJ, Rodosky MW, Sekiya JK: Symptomatic os acromiale. *J Am Acad Orthop Surg* 2006;14[1]:12-19.)

SUMMARY

Arthroscopic management has been found to be safe and effective for many conditions affecting the subacromial space and the AC joint, including subacromial impingement syndrome and rotator cuff disease syndromes, AC joint arthritis, distal clavicle osteolysis, AC joint separation, and os acromiale. The role of arthroscopy is likely to increase as techniques and technology evolve.

KEY STUDY POINTS

- Current practice guidelines support initial management of subacromial impingement syndrome with physical therapy and NSAIDs, but adjuncts such as the use of corticosteroid injections may also be used.
- Surgical treatment of subacromial impingement has efficacy when conservative management has failed. Studies with varying degrees of evidence with newer trials bring into question the role of routine acromioplasty.
- Initial management of AC joint arthritis and pain is nonsurgical with a course of physical therapy and NSAIDs. The surgical treatment of AC joint arthritis or osteolysis is open or arthroscopic resection of the distal clavicle.
- Most AC separations can be managed nonsurgically. When surgery is indicated, anatomic reconstruction of the CC ligaments has been found to be biomechanically superior.

Annotated References

1. Neer CS II: Anterior acromioplasty for the chronic impingement syndrome in the shoulder: A preliminary report. *J Bone Joint Surg Am* 1972;54(1):41-50.

2. Burns WC II, Whipple TL: Anatomic relationships in the shoulder impingement syndrome. *Clin Orthop Relat Res* 1993;294:96-102.

3. Flatow EL, Soslowsky LJ, Ticker JB, et al: Excursion of the rotator cuff under the acromion: Patterns of subacromial contact. *Am J Sports Med* 1994;22(6):779-788.

4. Nicholson GP, Goodman DA, Flatow EL, Bigliani LU: The acromion: Morphology and age-related changes. A study of 420 scapulae. *J Shoulder Elbow Surg* 1996;5(1):1-11.

5. Flatow EL, Colman WW, Kelkar R, et al: The effect of anterior acromioplasty on rotator cuff contact: An experimental and computer simulation. *J Shoulder Elbow Surg* 1995;4:S53-S54.

6. McFarland EG, Maffulli N, Del Buono A, Murrell GA, Garzon-Muvdi J, Petersen SA: Impingement is not impingement: The case for calling it "rotator cuff disease". *Muscles Ligaments Tendons J* 2013;3(3):196-200.

   A review compares the evidence associating impingement and overall shoulder pain. A conceptual shift is suggested moving away from the use of impingement with various underlying shoulder pathologies. Level of evidence: V.

7. Gerber C, Galantay RV, Hersche O: The pattern of pain produced by irritation of the acromioclavicular joint and the subacromial space. *J Shoulder Elbow Surg* 1998;7(4):352-355.

8. Roberts CS, Davila JN, Hushek SG, Tillett ED, Corrigan TM: Magnetic resonance imaging analysis of the subacromial space in the impingement sign positions. *J Shoulder Elbow Surg* 2002;11(6):595-599.

9. Jia X, Ji JH, Pannirselvam V, Petersen SA, McFarland EG: Does a positive Neer impingement sign reflect rotator cuff contact with the acromion? *Clin Orthop Relat Res* 2011;469(3):813-818.

10. Pappas GP, Blemker SS, Beaulieu CF, McAdams TR, Whalen ST, Gold GE: In vivo anatomy of the Neer and Hawkins sign positions for shoulder impingement. *J Shoulder Elbow Surg* 2006;15(1):40-49.

11. Valadie AL III, Jobe CM, Pink MM, Ekman EF, Jobe FW: Anatomy of provocative tests for impingement syndrome of the shoulder. *J Shoulder Elbow Surg* 2000;9(1):36-46.

12. Park HB, Yokota A, Gill HS, El Rassi G, McFarland EG: Diagnostic accuracy of clinical tests for the different degrees of subacromial impingement syndrome. *J Bone Joint Surg Am* 2005;87(7):1446-1455.

13. Vangsness CT, Ennis M, Taylor JG, Atkinson R: Neural anatomy of the glenohumeral ligaments, labrum, and subacromial bursa. *Arthroscopy* 1995;11(2):180-184.

14. Mayerhoefer ME, Breitenseher MJ, Wurnig C, Roposch A: Shoulder impingement: Relationship of clinical symptoms and imaging criteria. *Clin J Sport Med* 2009;19(2):83-89.

15. Harrison AK, Flatow EL: Subacromial impingement syndrome. *J Am Acad Orthop Surg* 2011;19(11):701-708.

16. Kim YS, Bigliani LU, Fujisawa M, et al: Stromal cell-derived factor 1 (SDF-1, CXCL12) is increased in subacromial bursitis and downregulated by steroid and nonsteroidal anti-inflammatory agents. *J Orthop Res* 2006;24(8):1756-1764.

17. Labianca R, Sarzi-Puttini P, Zuccaro SM, Cherubino P, Vellucci R, Fornasari D: Adverse effects associated with non-opioid and opioid treatment in patients with chronic pain. *Clin Drug Investig* 2012;32(suppl 1):53-63.

Section 4: Arthroscopy

18. Cohen DB, Kawamura S, Ehteshami JR, Rodeo SA: Indomethacin and celecoxib impair rotator cuff tendonto-bone healing. *Am J Sports Med* 2006;34(3):362-369.

19. Holmgren T, Björnsson Hallgren H, Öberg B, Adolfsson L, Johansson K: Effect of specific exercise strategy on need for surgery in patients with subacromial impingement syndrome: Randomised controlled study. *BMJ* 2012;344:e787.

20. Buchbinder R, Green S, Youd JM: Corticosteroid injections for shoulder pain. *Cochrane Database Syst Rev* 2003;1:CD004016.

21. Mikolyzk DK, Wei AS, Tonino P, et al: Effect of corticosteroids on the biomechanical strength of rat rotator cuff tendon. *J Bone Joint Surg Am* 2009;91(5):1172-1180.

22. Pedowitz RA, Yamaguchi K, Ahmad CS, et al: American Academy of Orthopaedic Surgeons clinical practice guideline on: Optimizing the management of rotator cuff problems. *J Bone Joint Surg Am* 2012;94(2):163-167.

23. Checroun AJ, Dennis MG, Zuckerman JD: Open versus arthroscopic decompression for subacromial impingement: A comprehensive review of the literature from the last 25 years. *Bull Hosp Jt Dis* 1998;57(3):145-151.

24. Davis AD, Kakar S, Moros C, Kaye EK, Schepsis AA, Voloshin I: Arthroscopic versus open acromioplasty: A meta-analysis. *Am J Sports Med* 2010;38(3):613-618.

25. Norlin R, Adolfsson L: Small full-thickness tears do well ten to thirteen years after arthroscopic subacromial decompression. *J Shoulder Elbow Surg* 2008;17 (1 suppl):S12-S16.

26. Björnsson H, Norlin R, Knutsson A, Adolfsson L: Fewer rotator cuff tears fifteen years after arthroscopic subacromial decompression. *J Shoulder Elbow Surg* 2010;19(1):111-115.

27. Kolk A, Thomassen BJW, Hund H, et al: Does acromioplasty result in favorable clinical and radiologic outcomes in the management of chronic subacromial pain syndrome? A double-blind randomized clinical trial with 9 to 14 years' follow-up. *J Shoulder Elbow Surg* 2017;26(8):1407-1415.

    A double blind randomized clinical trial compared arthroscopic bursectomy to bursectomy and acromioplasty. No relevant difference were appreciated. Level of evidence: II.

28. Milano G, Grasso A, Salvatore M, Zarelli D, Deriu L, Fabbriciani C: Arthroscopic rotator cuff repair with and without subacromial decompression: A prospective randomized study. *Arthroscopy* 2007;23(1):81-88.

29. Gartsman GM, O'Connor DP: Arthroscopic rotator cuff repair with and without arthroscopic subacromial decompression: A prospective, randomized study of one-year outcomes. *J Shoulder Elbow Surg* 2004;13(4):424-426.

30. Bond EC, Maher A, Hunt L, et al: The role of acromioplasty when repairing rotator cuff tear-no difference in pain or functional outcome at 24 months in s a cohort of 2,441 patients. *N Z Med J* 2017;130(1458):13-20.

    A nationwide database was utilized to evaluate patients undergoing a rotator cuff repair with or without an acromioplasty. Overall results demonstrated not difference in functional outcomes. Level of evidence: IV.

31. Abrams GD, Gupta AK, Hussey KE, et al: Arthroscopic repair of full-thickness rotator cuff tears with and without acromioplasty: Randomized prospective trial with 2-year follow-up. *Am J Sports Med* 2014;42(6):1296-1303.

    A randomized trial compares patients undergoing a full thickness rotator cuff tear with and without acromioplasty. No difference in clinical outcomes were appreciated. Level of evidence: II.

32. Familiari F, Gonzalez-Zapata A, Iannò B, Galasso O, Gasparini G, McFarland EG: Is acromioplasty necessary in the setting of full-thickness rotator cuff tears? A systematic review. *J Orthop Traumatol* 2015;16(3):167-174.

    A systematic review compared four trials examining rotator cuff repair with and without acromioplasty. Support for routine acromioplasty was not appreciated. Level of evidence: I and II.

33. MacDonald P, McRae S, Leiter J, Mascarenhas R, Lapner P: Arthroscopic rotator cuff repair with and without acromioplasty in the treatment of full-thickness rotator cuff tears: A multicenter, randomized controlled trial. *J Bone Joint Surg Am* 2011;93(21):1953-1960.

34. Song L, Miao L, Zhang P, Wang WL: Does concomitant acromioplasty facilitate arthroscopic repair of full-thickness rotator cuff tears? A meta-analysis with trial sequential analysis of randomize controlled trials. *Springerplus* 2016;5(1):685.

    A meta-analysis compared five randomized controlled trials examining rotator cuff repair with and without acromioplasty. ASEs scores were increased when associated with acromioplasty. Level of evidence: III.

35. Chahal J, Mall N, MacDonald PB, et al: The role of subacromial decompression in patients undergoing arthroscopic repair of full-thickness tears of the rotator cuff: A systematic review and meta-analysis. *Arthroscopy* 2012;28(5):720-727.

36. Noh KC, Chung KJ, Yu HS, Koh SH, Yoo JH: Arthroscopic treatment of septic arthritis of acromioclavicular joint. *Clin Orthop Surg* 2010;2(3):186-190.

37. Zanca P: Shoulder pain: Involvement of the acromioclavicular joint. (Analysis of 1,000 cases). *Am J Roentgenol Radium Ther Nucl Med* 1971;112(3):493-506.

38. Rios CG, Arciero RA, Mazzocca AD: Anatomy of the clavicle and coracoid process for reconstruction of the coracoclavicular ligaments. *Am J Sports Med* 2007;35(5):811-817.

39. Walton J, Mahajan S, Paxinos A, et al: Diagnostic values of tests for acromioclavicular joint pain. *J Bone Joint Surg Am* 2004;86(4):807-812.

40. van Riet RP, Bell SN: Clinical evaluation of acromioclavicular joint pathology: Sensitivity of a new test. *J Shoulder Elbow Surg* 2011;20(1):73-76.

41. Mazzocca AD, Spang JT, Rodriguez RR, et al: Biomechanical and radiographic analysis of partial coracoclavicular ligament injuries. *Am J Sports Med* 2008;36(7):1397-1402.

42. Girish G, Lobo LG, Jacobson JA, Morag Y, Miller B, Jamadar DA: Ultrasound of the shoulder: Asymptomatic findings in men. *AJR Am J Roentgenol* 2011;197(4): W713-W719.

43. van Riet RP, Goehre T, Bell SN: The long term effect of an intra-articular injection of corticosteroids in the acromioclavicular joint. *J Shoulder Elbow Surg* 2012;21(3):376-379.

44. Flatow EL, Cordasco FA, Bigliani LU: Arthroscopic resection of the outer end of the clavicle from a superior approach: A critical, quantitative, radiographic assessment of bone removal. *Arthroscopy* 1992;8(1):55-64.

45. Beitzel K, Sablan N, Chowaniec DM, et al: Sequential resection of the distal clavicle and its effects on horizontal acromioclavicular joint translation. *Am J Sports Med* 2012;40(3):681-685.

46. Elhassan B, Ozbaydar M, Diller D, Massimini D, Higgins LD, Warner JJ: Open versus arthroscopic acromioclavicular joint resection: A retrospective comparison study. *Arthroscopy* 2009;25(11):1224-1232.

47. Robertson WJ, Griffith MH, Carroll K, O'Donnell T, Gill TJ: Arthroscopic versus open distal clavicle excision: A comparative assessment at intermediate-term follow-up. *Am J Sports Med* 2011;39(11):2415-2420.

48. Pensak M, Grumet RC, Slabaugh MA, Bach BR Jr: Open versus arthroscopic distal clavicle resection. *Arthroscopy* 2010;26(5):697-704.

49. Zawadsky M, Marra G, Wiater JM, et al: Osteolysis of the distal clavicle: Long-term results of arthroscopic resection. *Arthroscopy* 2000;16(6):600-605.

50. Kim J, Chung J, Ok H: Asymptomatic acromioclavicular joint arthritis in arthroscopic rotator cuff tendon repair: A prospective randomized comparison study. *Arch Orthop Trauma Surg* 2011;131(3):363-369.

51. Tossy JD, Mead NC, Sigmond HM: Acromioclavicular separations: Useful and practical classification for treatment. *Clin Orthop Relat Res* 1963;28:111-119.

52. Rockwood CA, Williams GR, Young DC: *Rockwood and Green's Fractures in Adults*, ed 3. Philadelphia, PA, J.B. Lippincott, 1991, pp 1181-1239.

53. Barnes CJ, Higgins LD, Major NM, Basamania CJ: Magnetic resonance imaging of the coracoclavicular ligaments: Its role in defining pathoanatomy at the acromioclavicular joint. *J Surg Orthop Adv* 2004;13(2): 69-75.

54. Costic RS, Labriola JE, Rodosky MW, Debski RE: Biomechanical rationale for development of anatomical reconstructions of coracoclavicular ligaments after complete acromioclavicular joint dislocations. *Am J Sports Med* 2004;32(8):1929-1936.

55. Mazzocca AD, Santangelo SA, Johnson ST, Rios CG, Dumonski ML, Arciero RA: A biomechanical evaluation of an anatomical coracoclavicular ligament reconstruction. *Am J Sports Med* 2006;34(2):236-246.

56. Grutter PW, Petersen SA: Anatomical acromioclavicular ligament reconstruction: A biomechanical comparison of reconstructive techniques of the acromioclavicular joint. *Am J Sports Med* 2005;33(11):1723-1728.

57. Chernchujit B, Tischer T, Imhoff AB: Arthroscopic reconstruction of the acromioclavicular joint disruption: Surgical technique and preliminary results. *Arch Orthop Trauma Surg* 2006;126(9):575-581.

58. Thiel E, Mutnal A, Gilot GJ: Surgical outcome following arthroscopic fixation of acromioclavicular joint disruption with the TightRope device. *Orthopedics* 2011;34(7):e26 7-e274.

59. Walz L, Salzmann GM, Fabbro T, Eichhorn S, Imhoff AB: The anatomic reconstruction of acromioclavicular joint dislocations using 2 TightRope devices: A biomechanical study. *Am J Sports Med* 2008;36(12):2398-2406.

60. Salzmann GM, Walz L, Buchmann S, Glabgly P, Venjakob A, Imhoff AB: Arthroscopically assisted 2-bundle anatomical reduction of acute acromioclavicular joint separations. *Am J Sports Med* 2010;38(6):1179-1187.

61. Boileau P, Old J, Gastaud O, Brassart N, Roussanne Y: All-arthroscopic Weaver-Dunn-Chuinard procedure with double-button fixation for chronic acromioclavicular joint dislocation. *Arthroscopy* 2010;26(2):149-160.

62. Kowalsky MS, Kremenic IJ, Orishimo KF, McHugh MP, Nicholas SJ, Lee SJ: The effect of distal clavicle excision on in situ graft forces in coracoclavicular ligament reconstruction. *Am J Sports Med* 2010;38(11):2313-2319.

63. Kurtz CA, Humble BJ, Rodosky MW, Sekiya JK: Symptomatic os acromiale. *J Am Acad Orthop Surg* 2006;14(1):12-19.

64. Ortiguera CJ, Buss DD: Surgical management of the symptomatic os acromiale. *J Shoulder Elbow Surg* 2002;11(5):521-528.

65. Harris JD, Griesser MJ, Jones GL: Systematic review of the surgical treatment for symptomatic os acromiale. *Int J Shoulder Surg* 2011;5(1):9-16.

66. Warner JJ, Beim GM, Higgins L: The treatment of symptomatic os acromiale. *J Bone Joint Surg Am* 1998;80(9):1320-1326.

67. Wright RW, Heller MA, Quick DC, Buss DD: Arthroscopic decompression for impingement syndrome secondary to an unstable os acromiale. *Arthroscopy* 2000;16(6):595-599.

Chapter 17

Arthroscopic and Open Treatment of the Proximal Biceps Tendon

Lukas N. Muench, MD • Cameron Kia, MD • Knut Beitzel, MD • Augustus D. Mazzocca, MS, MD

Section 4: Arthroscopy

ABSTRACT

Tendinitis and ruptures of the long head of the biceps tendon (LHBT) are well documented; however, the pathology is not yet fully understood. Clinical examination to isolate biceps pathology is difficult because of the low specificity of each test; however, the subpectoral biceps test may be a useful guide to detect LHBT injury. Multiple surgical approaches have been proposed for the management of patients with LHBT-related pain, without an existing consensus regarding treatment. Arthroscopic procedures include simple tenotomy as well as intra-articular and suprapectoral tenodesis. The tendon stump can be fixed using suture anchors or tenodesis screws. An open procedure is preferable for subpectoral tenodesis. The results of tenotomy and tenodesis (whether done arthroscopically or open) have been variable, with none of the techniques showing a clear clinical superiority. Thus, surgical decision making should be adjusted to patient-individual demands, using a technique the surgeon is most comfortable with.

Keywords: biceps tenodesis; LHBT, long head of the biceps tendon; subpectoral; tenotomy

Dr. Beitzel or an immediate family member is a member of a speakers' bureau or has made paid presentations on behalf of Arthrex, Inc. and serves as a paid consultant to or is an employee of Arthrex, Inc. Dr. Mazzocca or an immediate family member serves as a paid consultant to or is an employee of Arthrex, Inc. and has received research or institutional support from Arthrex, Inc. Neither of the following authors nor any immediate family member has received anything of value from or has stock or stock options held in a commercial company or institution related directly or indirectly to the subject of this chapter: Dr. Muench and Dr. Kia.

Introduction

The biceps muscle originates from two proximal tendons: the long head of the biceps tendon (LHBT) and the short head of the biceps tendon. The LHBT is of particular interest because of its intra-articular origin on the supraglenoid tubercle of the glenohumeral joint, with most of the fibers arising from the posterior aspect of the superior labrum.[1,2] The intra-articular portion of the tendon is extrasynovial and has an average length of 34.5 mm (± 4.2 mm). Before entering the intertubercular groove, the tendon is guided by the structures of the pulley system, which consists of the superior glenohumeral ligament (SGHL) and the subscapularis tendon anteriorly and of the coracohumeral ligament and the anterior fibers of the supraspinatus tendon posterolaterally[3] (**Figure 1**). The short head of the biceps tendon originates on the coracoid process of the scapula, remaining completely extra-articular. The biceps muscle crosses both the shoulder and the elbow. At the elbow, the distal biceps primarily acts as a forearm supinator and secondarily as an elbow flexor. The role of the biceps at the shoulder has been a matter of debate.[1,4] The LHBT previously was believed to act as a humeral head depressor; however, recent research suggests that this function is unlikely because of its anterior position relative to the glenohumeral joint. Despite debate over the function of the biceps at the shoulder, there is general agreement among surgeons that the proximal LHBT acts as a pain generator.[1,4]

Pathology of the LHBT includes tendinitis and tendon rupture, which are well documented but not fully understood, probably because of the unique anatomic features of the LHBT. The intra-articular portion of the tendon is subject to compression, shearing, and friction forces, whereas the extra-articular distal segment is primarily under the influence of tensional strain. The vascular anatomy of the LHBT also may play a role in the pathogenesis of disorders. The first 3 cm of the intra-articular portion of the tendon, as measured from

This chapter is adapted from Mazzocca AD, Cote MP, Beitzel K: Arthroscopic and open treatment of the proximal biceps tendon, in Nicholson GP, ed: *Orthopaedic Knowledge Update: Shoulder and Elbow*, ed 4. Rosemont, IL, American Academy of Orthopaedic Surgeons, 2013, pp 265-271.

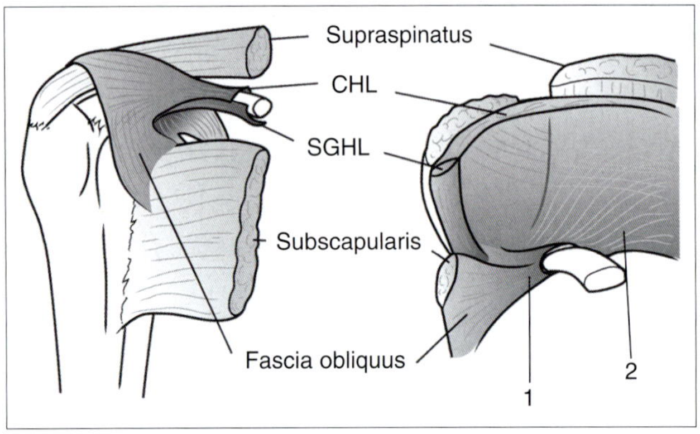

FIGURE 1 Schematic drawing of the structures of the biceps pulley. 1 = insertion of the subscapularis tendon, 2 = insertion of the supraspinatus tendon, CHL = coracohumeral ligament, SGHL = superior glenohumeral ligament.

its insertion on the glenoid, comprises specific areas of hypovascularization, being correlated with the areas of increased mechanical strain.[5] This combination of specific multidirectional force distributions and the segmental blood supply is believed to be the primary contributor to intra-articular degenerative processes of the LHBT.

Etiology

Multiple intra-articular lesions of the shoulder joint may generate a secondary lesion of the LHBT, such as bursitis, rotator cuff tears, superior labrum anterior to posterior (SLAP) lesions, or acromioclavicular joint disorders. Primary tendinitis and rupture of the LHBT also have been observed. Rupture commonly occurs near the insertion or at the proximal intertubercular groove. If the rupture is distal to the insertion, the stump may be pinched in the joint. Tendinitis of the LHBT has been recognized for more than 50 years, but is increasingly reported as an isolated source of shoulder pain or in combination with one or more additional disorders. An hourglass biceps is described as a lesion of the biceps tendon complex in which a hypertrophic portion of the intra-articular segment of the LHBT cannot slide during elevation of the arm, resulting in incarceration of the tendon.[6]

Clinical Evaluation

If the tendon is completely ruptured, physical examination may reveal a Popeye deformity, in which hollowness appears proximally and laterally. Patients often describe an onset of pain in the anterior shoulder before rupture, with pain relief after the injury. If the tendon did not rupture, significant pain during motion, particularly with resisted elbow flexion or forearm supination, is a typical symptom. Tenderness often is noted during palpation of the bicipital groove.

The subpectoral biceps test can be useful for detecting biceps pathology, as anterior palpation of the proximal third of the biceps may be misleading, given the course of the anterior deltoid fibers and a possible medial subluxation of the LHBT in the presence of concomitant subscapularis pathology.[7] The examiner palpates the biceps tendon with the patient contracting in adduction and internal rotation, allowing for identifying the pectoralis tendon insertion into the humerus. The index finger is used to palpate the biceps tendon as it courses under the pectoralis tendon. Pain elicited on palpation of the tendon is considered indicative of proximal biceps disease. To ensure that the pain elicited is representative to true biceps disease, the test should also be performed on the contralateral shoulder.[7] Occasionally, there may be ecchymosis in this area. It is important to examine for concomitant rotator cuff pathology. Range of motion should be assessed, to detect possible incarceration of the biceps tendon stump in the glenohumeral joint (hourglass biceps). The O'Brien test can be used to identify a SLAP lesion. The Yergason and Speed tests can be used to evaluate pathologies occurring more distally to the tendon (within the sulcus). Clinical tests have to be considered as a set, as the specificity for diagnosis of each test alone is limited. The authors of a 2017 study[8] compared the diagnostic value of using a "3-pack" examination (bicipital tunnel palpation, the throwing test, O'Brien sign) and found that together the test had a sensitivity of 73% to 98%; however, specificity ranged from 46% to 79%.

Usually, the diagnosis is made clinically, but may be supplemented by imaging. Ultrasonography is an inexpensive tool for detecting absence of the LHBT in the bicipital groove or at its insertion. MRI with an intra-articular contrast agent may be the only reliable method to clearly distinguish between SLAP and pulley lesions. Although being sufficient for detecting complete dislocation of the LHBT, preoperative imaging is limited to make a reliable diagnosis of LHBT pathology, especially in the setting of rotator cuff tears.[9] Arthroscopic evaluation may be the only approach to objectively prove a diagnosed tendon instability, highlighting the importance of inspecting the entire intra-articular length of the LHBT before treatment. However, arthroscopy is unreliable in diagnosing extra-articular LHBT pathology, and macroscopic appearance of the tendon may not accurately reflect tendinopathy, complicating surgical decision making.[7,10]

Classification

Multiple classifications of disorders of the LHBT have been proposed, without an existing consensus. The classifications primarily focus on secondary lesions of the shoulder combined with LHBT instability. The lesions of the LHBT can be broadly classified into three groups: isolated tendinitis, tendinitis associated with a SLAP lesion or tendon instability, and tendon instability combined with a high-grade lesion of the stabilizing pulley sling and a rotator cuff tear.

The Habermeyer classification identifies four types of pulley lesions of the LHBT.[11] Type I is a lesion of the SGHL resulting in anterior instability of the LHBT; type II, an SGHL lesion combined with a partial rupture of the anterior portion of the supraspinatus tendon; type III, an SGHL lesion combined with a partial rupture of the cranial portion of the subscapularis tendon; and type IV, a lesion of the anterior supraspinatus tendon combined with a lesion of the cranial portion of the subscapularis tendon, which is believed to result from anterior-posterior instability.

The Lafosse arthroscopic classification considers the direction and extent of LHBT instability, macroscopic lesions of the LHBT, and concomitant lesions of the subscapularis and/or supraspinatus tendon.[12]

Management

Both nonsurgical and surgical management approaches have been described; however, few objective data exist to determine which treatment is best.[4,13] Nonsurgical management typically is sufficient for treating a spontaneous rupture. A patient electing nonsurgical care may have a residual cosmetic deformity and report persistent cramping during strenuous activity. Patients generally do well with a home exercise program and rarely have stiffness. Full range of motion, including overhead activity, should be encouraged to allow evaluation for a possibly incarcerated tendon stump.

Some physicians recommend surgical treatment for physically active younger patients, laborers with an injury of the dominant side, athletes, and, in general, patients who require great supination strength or want to avoid a cosmetic deformity. These patients often report aching pain and spasm with repeated activity. It is preferable to perform the surgery within 3 months following injury.

Several terms are used to delineate locations about the shoulder in reference to the tenodesis of the LHBT, with multiple techniques and materials used being described in the literature. The term proximal often refers to an intra-articular arthroscopic tenodesis of the LHBT as part of a rotator cuff repair, or extra-articular tenodesis in the bicipital groove slightly inferior to the articular margin. The term suprapectoral describes an arthroscopic tenodesis of the LHBT below the bicipital groove and above the superior edge of the pectoralis tendon.[14] The term subpectoral describes an open tenodesis of the LHBT below the pectoralis tendon using an incision in the axilla. Both arthroscopic and open tenodesis techniques have been reported to provide satisfactory, comparable outcomes, without clear evidence of one technique being superior to the others.[15]

Arthroscopic Treatment

Tenotomy is currently the most performed arthroscopic treatment.[1] A standard working portal is used to cut the LHBT at its insertion using an arthroscopic scissor or radiofrequency cutter (**Figure 2**). Damage to the superior labrum should be avoided to preserve its function. After detaching the tendon, the surgeon should confirm that the tendon has slipped back into the sulcus. A SLAP lesion in an older adult may be débrided at this time. The available methods for tenodesis of the LHBT can be distinguished using the anatomic regions of fixation of the tendon stump.

Proximal tenodesis usually is performed arthroscopically. The tendon stump can be fixed with sutures, suture anchors, or tenodesis screws.[16,17] A biomechanical comparison of repair techniques concluded that keyhole tenodesis was substantially stronger compared with a classic interference screw fixation, but not stronger than fixation using a bioabsorbable screw.[18] In addition, four fixation techniques have been compared biomechanically: subpectoral bone tunnel (suture fixation in the bone tunnel), arthroscopic interference screw, subpectoral interference screw, and arthroscopic suture anchor. Bone tunnel fixation had substantially more cyclic displacement than the other three methods, all of which had favorable load-to-failure characteristics.[19]

The advantages of arthroscopic techniques are the preservation of tendon length and the ability to perform refixation without an additional skin incision. Usually,

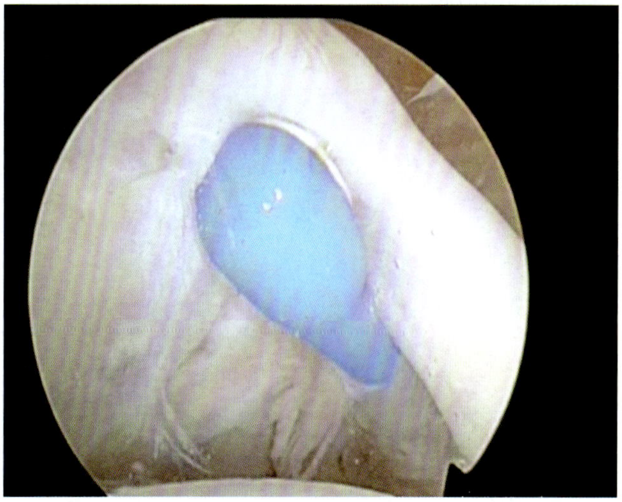

FIGURE 2 Arthroscopic image showing tenotomy using a radiofrequency cutter.

proximal tenodesis is performed before addressing concomitant injuries. A standard posterior portal is used for initial diagnostic evaluation of the joint and the LHBT. A probe may be used to examine the intertubercular portion of the tendon by pulling the tendon into the joint; however, complete visualization of the extra-articular portion of the LHBT may be unfeasible. A needle is used to pierce the tendon for placement of a nonabsorbable shuttle suture. At this point, several methods of fixation may be used. For soft-tissue tenodesis, the tendon is fixed to the rotator cuff interval. Tenodesis also can be performed using a suture anchor, such as the 5.5-mm bioabsorbable Corkscrew FT suture anchor (Arthrex) armed with two No. 2 FiberWire (Arthrex) sutures (**Figure 3**), or a biotenodesis screw, such as the 4.5-mm bioabsorbable SwiveLock anchor (Arthrex). In these techniques, the anchor is placed at the entrance of the bicipital groove after decortication using a motorized burr. The suture anchor allows fixation without pulling the tendon out of the anterior portal. For fixation using a tenodesis screw, the tendon stump is pulled out of the anterior portal and loaded into the screw. The tenotomy is done by transecting the tendon proximal to the sutures and close to its origin (**Figure 4**).

In the preferred arthroscopic technique, a tenodesis screw is used for suprapectoral fixation of the tendon stump within the intertubercular groove. A holding suture is placed through the tendon. The tendon is then cut close to its origin, while preserving the superior labral complex. The arthroscope is moved to the subacromial space using the lateral portal. The falciform ligament of the pectoralis tendon is identified, and the biceps tendon is found underneath. The accessory anterior portal is localized with a spinal needle into the rotator cuff interval. The proximal 20 mm of the tendon are removed to eliminate diseased tendon and re-create an anatomic fit. The proximal 15 mm of the remaining tendon stump are whip-stitched (alternatively, Krackow stitches can be used). The intertubercular groove is located, and a 2-mm guidewire is inserted. The guidewire is reamed over with a 7- or 8-mm cannulated reamer to a depth of 30 mm. The tendon is pulled out of the accessory anterior portal, and one suture is inserted through the tenodesis screw and tightened. Finally, the screw is inserted into the tunnel, and an arthroscopic knot pusher is used to tie suture over the top of the tenodesis screw. The use of a forked tenodesis screw allows direct insertion of the tendon into the hole (**Figure 5**).

Open Treatment

Early surgical techniques for open tenodesis involved transferring the tendon to the coracoid process. As large dissections were necessary using this technique, keyhole tenodesis was proposed as an alternative. In this technique, the bicipital groove is exposed via a deltopectoral approach, and a 1-cm hole is burred with a keyhole inferior and sufficiently narrow to contain the tendon. A knot is created in the biceps tendon and delivered into the keyhole. An immediate improvement in cosmesis and supination strength was reported, following treatment using this technique.[20]

However, procedure of choice remains the subpectoral tenodesis using an interference screw. The subpectoral approach is close to the muscle belly of the biceps.[21] Even if initially ruptured, the biceps tendon generally does not retract beyond the point of fixation. Before tenodesis, arthroscopy is performed to identify concomitant pathologies as well as to tenotomize and débride the bicipital

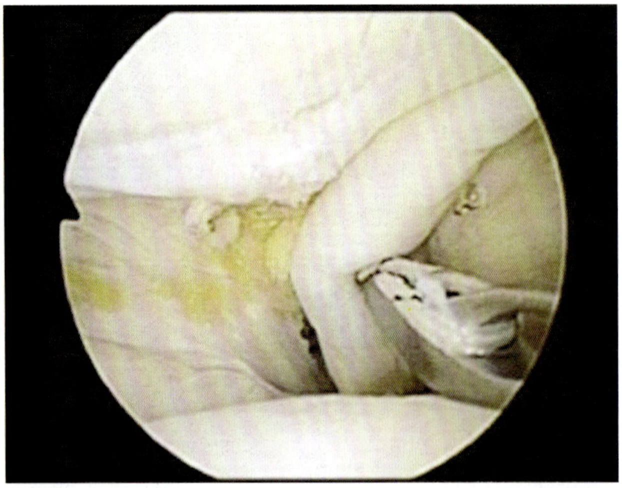

FIGURE 3 Arthroscopic image showing a tenodesis suture inserted through the long head of the biceps tendon using a penetration instrument.

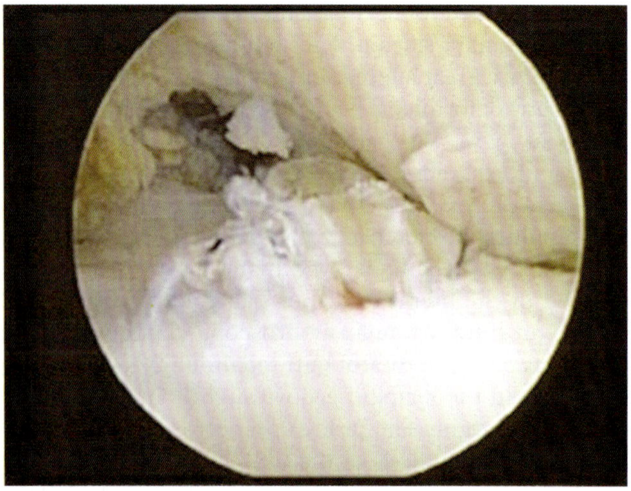

FIGURE 4 Arthroscopic image showing an intra-articularly fixed long head of the biceps tendon after tenodesis using a Corkscrew FT suture anchor.

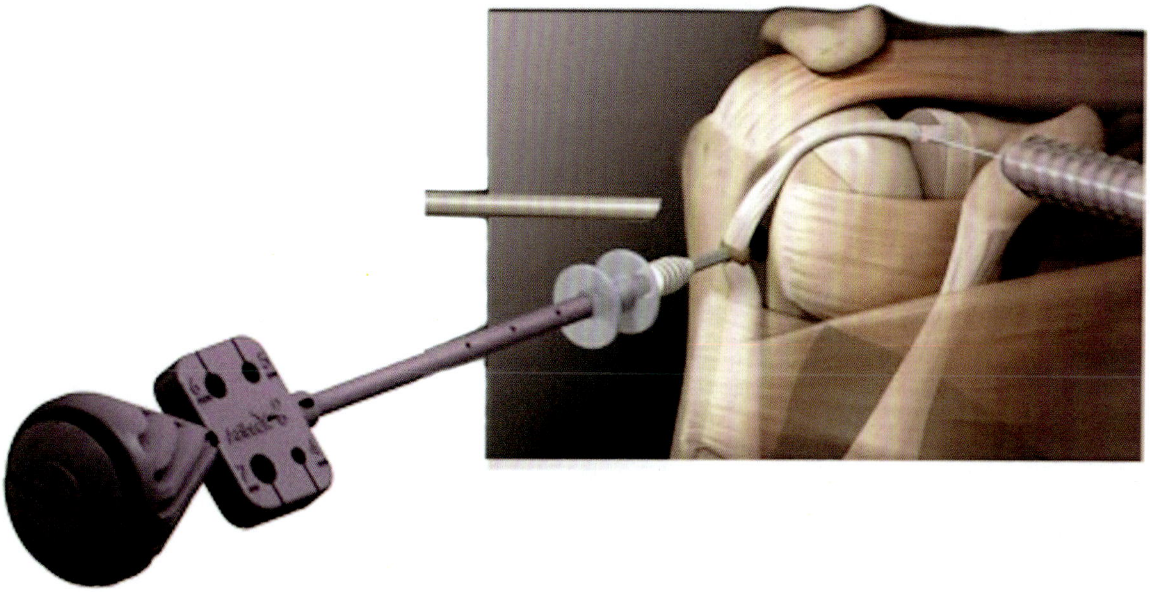

FIGURE 5 Schematic drawing showing arthroscopic suprapectoral tenodesis using a fork-tipped tenodesis screw (SwiveLock, Arthrex) and arthroscopic cannulas.

tendon stump. With the arm abducted and internally rotated, the inferior border of the pectoralis major tendon is palpated. The incision is made from above the inferior border of the pectoralis tendon to 3 cm below the inferior border on the medial aspect of the arm (**Figure 6, A**). A scalpel is used to dissect the subcutaneous tissue, while controlling bleeding with an electrocautery device. A Gelpi or Weitlaner self-retaining retractor may be used for visualization. The adipose tissue is cleared until the fascia, overlying the pectoralis major, coracobrachialis, and biceps, is identified, to avoid performing the dissection too laterally. If the cephalic vein can be seen in the deltopectoral groove, the dissection is too proximal and too lateral. Following identification of the inferior border of the pectoralis major, the fascia overlying the coracobrachialis and biceps is incised in a proximal-to-distal manner (**Figure 6, B**). A pointed Hohmann retractor is placed under the pectoralis major and on the proximal humerus to retract the muscle proximally and laterally. A blunt Chandler retractor is placed in the medial aspect of the humerus to retract the coracobrachialis and the short head of the biceps tendon. Vigorous medial retraction should be avoided to prevent injury to the musculocutaneous nerve. The LHBT musculotendinous junction should be located and then withdrawn from the field. To ensure appropriate tensioning of the LHBT, the proximal portion is resected to leave 20 to 25 mm proximal to the musculotendinous portion of the biceps. One centimeter proximal to the pectoralis major tendon, the periosteum is reflected. A No. 2 nonabsorbable suture, such as FiberWire, is placed onto the tendon, and 12 mm of the tendon is secured to ensure maintaining adequate fixation and placing the musculotendinous portion of the biceps underneath the inferior border of the pectoralis major tendon. This step is critical for proper tensioning of the musculotendinous unit as well as cosmesis.

For most patients, an 8-mm cannulated reamer is of adequate size for securing tendon fixation into the bone tunnel using an 8-mm bioabsorbable interference-fit screw. The calibrated reamer is advanced over the guide pin to the 30-mm mark (**Figure 6, C**). Drilling beyond the posterior cortex of the humerus may increase the risk of complications and is not necessary. With a wire loop passed through the driver, one limb of the suture is pulled through the screw and the screwdriver handle, while holding the other limb loosely. The limb that is passed through the driver is pulled tightly until the end of the tendon is securely placed against the tip of the driver. The tip of the driver is placed at the superior aspect of the bone socket and manually inserted until the tendon reaches the base of the tunnel. The bioabsorbable interference screw is then placed directly over the top of the tendon until the head of the screw is below the cortex (**Figure 6, D**).

Clinical Results of Surgical Management

Studies comparing tenotomy and tenodesis have reported varying results, with no technique showing clear clinical superiority.[4,13,22] Regarding tenodesis, both arthroscopic

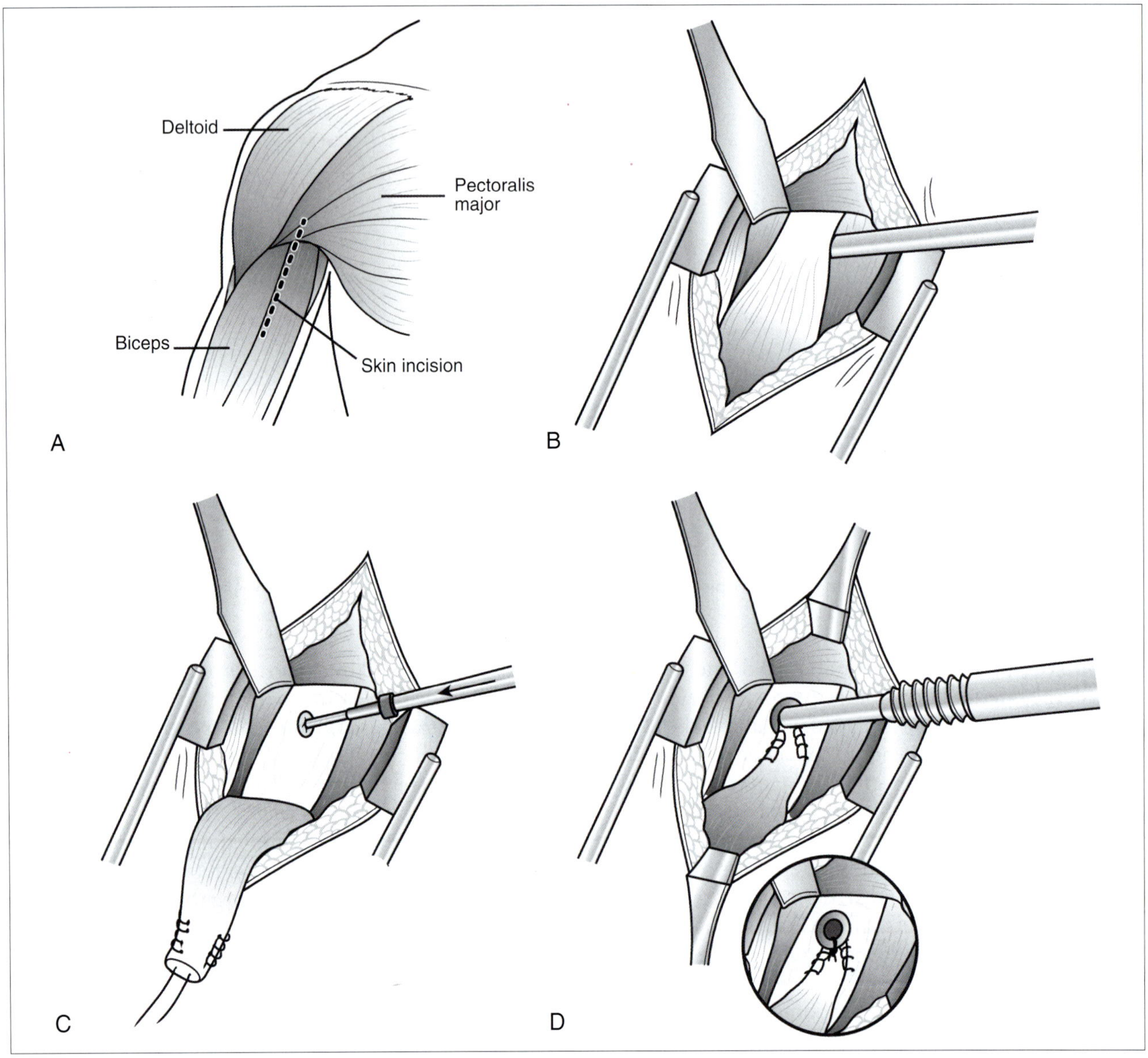

FIGURE 6 Schematic drawings showing an open subpectoral tenodesis. **A**, The skin incision. **B**, The distal tendon exiting the groove under the pectoralis muscle. **C**, Drilling of the socket for tendon fixation, using a tenodesis screw directly under the retracted tendon of the pectoralis muscle. **D**, Insertion of the interference screw, with the completed subpectoral tenodesis (inset).

and open techniques have been reported to achieve similar results.[15,23] As no surgical procedure can be recommended over others, the choice should be made for each patient individually using a technique the surgeon is most comfortable with.[1]

Arthroscopic Treatment

No consensus exists as to whether the LHBT should be treated with tenotomy or tenodesis, as both procedures have shown good clinical results.[13,22] Substantial pain reduction and functional improvement occurred after arthroscopic tenodesis or tenotomy, with a low complication rate.[24,25] A systematic review found comparably favorable results after both tenotomy and tenodesis. The only relevant difference may be that biceps tenotomy led to a higher incidence of cosmetic deformity.[22] Another study showed similar results, with 30% of patients having a cosmetic defect following tenotomy.[26] Cramping and weakness with vigorous activity has also been reported.[1] Tenotomy has been suggested as effective for relief of pain related to LHBT lesions; however, an increased incidence of postoperative stiffness has been reported following arthroscopic tenodesis when compared with an open subpectoral approach.[27] Tenotomy may be primarily useful for treating older patients or patients having severe comorbidities or other contraindications for tenodesis.[22]

Open Treatment

Good results have been reported for open tenodesis of the LHBT.[4,15,28-30] Proximal techniques for tenodesis may lead to persistent tenosynovitis and pain.[31] The risk of this complication may be decreased by performing a subpectoral tenodesis.[28,30,32] Even in patients older than 65 years, subpectoral tenodesis is a successful procedure with similar complication rates compared with patients younger than 65 years.[33] However, no technique has been proven to be superior to others. Thus, clinical studies are needed to provide evidence for decision making in LHBT surgery.

SUMMARY

Although tendonitis or ruptures of the LHBT are well documented, knowledge of the exact pathology is limited. Clinical examination to isolate biceps pathology remains difficult, as each clinical tests only has a low specificity. Thus, it should be considered a test battery, with the subpectoral biceps test being a useful guide for the detection of LHBT pathology. Although multiple surgical approaches have been described for the management of patients with LHBT-related pain, current literature still lacks a definite consensus regarding treatment. All-arthroscopic and open procedures have been described, including simple tenotomy as well as subsequent intra-articular, suprapectoral, or subpectoral tenodesis. The tendon stump can be fixed using suture anchors or tenodesis screws. As both arthroscopic and open tenodesis techniques have been reported to result in similar outcomes without clear clinical superiority of one technique, surgical decision making should be adjusted to patient-individual demands using a technique the surgeon is most comfortable with.

KEY STUDY POINTS

- Pathologies of the LHBT include tendinitis and tendon rupture, which are well documented, but not fully understood.
- Clinical examination has to be considered a test battery because of the low specificity of each test; however, the subpectoral biceps test may be a useful guide to detect LHBT pathology.
- Multiple surgical treatment options have been described, including all-arthroscopic and open techniques, with only tenotomy or subsequent tenodesis of the LHBT at various locations (proximal, suprapectoral, subpectoral).
- As both arthroscopic and open tenodesis techniques have been reported to result in similar outcomes, surgical decision making should be adjusted to patient-individual demands using a technique the surgeon is most comfortable with.

Annotated References

1. Barber A, Field LD, Ryu R: Biceps tendon and superior labrum injuries: Decision-making. *J Bone Joint Surg Am* 2007;89(8):1844-1855.

2. Vangsness CT Jr, Jorgenson SS, Watson T, Johnson DL: The origin of the long head of the biceps from the scapula and glenoid labrum: An anatomical study of 100 shoulders. *J Bone Joint Surg Br* 1994;76(6):951-954.

3. Werner A, Mueller T, Boehm D, Gohlke F: The stabilizing sling for the long head of the biceps tendon in the rotator cuff interval: A histoanatomic study. *Am J Sports Med* 2000;28(1):28-31.

4. Elser F, Braun S, Dewing CB, Giphart JE, Millett PJ: Anatomy, function, injuries, and treatment of the long head of the biceps brachii tendon. *Arthroscopy* 2011;27(4):581-592.

5. Cheng NM, Pan WR, Vally F, Le Roux CM, Richardson MD: The arterial supply of the long head of biceps tendon: Anatomical study with implications for tendon rupture. *Clin Anat* 2010;23(6):683-692.

6. Ahrens PM, Boileau P: The long head of biceps and associated tendinopathy. *J Bone Joint Surg Br* 2007;89(8):1001-1009.

7. Dwyer C, Kia C, Apostolakos JM, et al: Clinical outcomes after biceps tenodesis or tenotomy using subpectoral pain to guide management in patients with rotator cuff tears. *Arthroscopy* 2019;35(7):1992-2000.

   In patients with rotator cuff tears surgically treated with concomitant biceps tenodesis or tenotomy, 94% had resolution of their subpectoral tenderness. A positive SBT was associated with gross pathologic changes of the biceps in 93% of patients. Level of evidence: III.

8. Taylor SA, Newman AM, Dawson C, et al: The "3-pack" examination is critical for comprehensive evaluation of the biceps-labrum complex and the bicipital tunnel: A prospective study. *Arthroscopy* 2017;33(1):28-38.

   The 3-Pack has excellent inter-rater reliability, sensitivity, and negative predictive value and is a critical screening tool for biceps-labrum complex disease in all zones. Hidden extra-articular bicipital tunnel disease can reliably be excluded based on negative tenderness to palpation or a negative O'Brien sign. Level of evidence: III.

9. Rol M, Favard L, Berhouet J: Diagnosis of long head of biceps tendinopathy in rotator cuff tear patients: Correlation of imaging and arthroscopy data. *Int Orthop* 2018;42(6):1347-1355.

   Except for long head of the biceps (LHB) dislocation, pre-operative imaging is not sufficient to make a reliable diagnosis of LHB tendinopathy. Arthroscopy remains the gold standard for the management of LHB tendinopathy, as diagnosed intraoperatively. Level of evidence: IV.

10. Jordan RW, Saithna A: Physical examination tests and imaging studies based on arthroscopic assessment of the long head of biceps tendon are invalid. *Knee Surg Sports Traumatol Arthrosc* 2017;25(10):3229-3236.

    Arthroscopy allows visualisation of only a small part of the extra-articular long head of the biceps (LHB) tendon. This leads to a high rate of missed pathology in the distal part of the tendon. Published figures for sensitivities and specificities of common physical examination and imaging tests for LHB pathology that are based on arthroscopy as the gold standard are therefore invalid. In clinical practice, it is important to note that a "negative" arthroscopic assessment does not exclude a lesion of the LHB tendon as this technique does not allow visualisation of common sites of distal pathology. Level of evidence: IV.

11. Habermeyer P, Magosch P, Pritsch M, Scheibel MT, Lichtenberg S: Anterosuperior impingement of the shoulder as a result of pulley lesions: A prospective arthroscopic study. *J Shoulder Elbow Surg* 2004;13(1):5-12.

12. Lafosse L, Reiland Y, Baier GP, Toussaint B, Jost B: Anterior and posterior instability of the long head of the biceps tendon in rotator cuff tears: A new classification based on arthroscopic observations. *Arthroscopy* 2007;23(1):73-80.

13. Slenker NR, Lawson K, Ciccotti MG, Dodson CC, Cohen SB: Biceps tenotomy versus tenodesis: Clinical outcomes. *Arthroscopy* 2012;28(4):576-582.

14. Lutton DM, Gruson KI, Harrison AK, Gladstone JN, Flatow EL: Where to tenodese the biceps: Proximal or distal? *Clin Orthop Relat Res* 2011;469(4):1050-1055.

15. Abraham VT, Tan BH, Kumar VP: Systematic review of biceps tenodesis: Arthroscopic versus open. *Arthroscopy* 2016;32(2):365-371.

    Both open and arthroscopic biceps tenodesis provided satisfactory outcomes in most patients, and there were no identifiable differences in this review. Level of evidence: IV.

16. Gartsman GM, Hammerman SM: Arthroscopic biceps tenodesis: Operative technique. *Arthroscopy* 2000;16(5):550-552.

17. Geaney LE, Mazzocca AD: Biceps brachii tendon ruptures: A review of diagnosis and treatment of proximal and distal biceps tendon ruptures. *Phys Sportsmed* 2010;38(2):117-125.

18. Jayamoorthy T, Field JR, Costi JJ, Martin DK, Stanley RM, Hearn TC: Biceps tenodesis: A biomechanical study of fixation methods. *J Shoulder Elbow Surg* 2004;13(2):160-164.

19. Mazzocca AD, Bicos J, Santangelo S, Romeo AA, Arciero RA: The biomechanical evaluation of four fixation techniques for proximal biceps tenodesis. *Arthroscopy* 2005;21(11):1296-1306.

20. Froimson AI, Oh I: Keyhole tenodesis of biceps origin at the shoulder. *Clin Orthop Relat Res* 1975;(112):245-249.

21. Mazzocca AD, Rios CG, Romeo AA, Arciero RA: Subpectoral biceps tenodesis with interference screw fixation. *Arthroscopy* 2005;21(7):896.

22. Gurnani N, van Deurzen DF, Janmaat VT, van den Bekerom MP: Tenotomy or tenodesis for pathology of the long head of the biceps brachii: A systematic review and meta-analysis. *Knee Surg Sports Traumatol Arthrosc* 2016;24(12):3765-3771.

    Based on this meta-analysis, no differences in postoperative functional outcome between tenotomy and tenodesis for the treatment of LHB lesions were observed. A Popeye deformity and cramping pain in the bicipital groove are more frequently observed in patients treated with tenotomy. Level of evidence: IV.

23. Gombera MM, Kahlenberg CA, Nair R, Saltzman MD, Terry MA: All-arthroscopic suprapectoral versus open subpectoral tenodesis of the long head of the biceps brachii. *Am J Sports Med* 2015;43(5):1077-1083.

    Patients undergoing an all-arthroscopic suprapectoral tenodesis in the distal aspect or distal to the bicipital groove showed similar pain relief and clinical outcomes as compared with patients undergoing open subpectoral tenodesis. Open subpectoral biceps tenodesis may carry a higher complication risk secondary to a more invasive technique. Level of evidence: III.

24. Brady PC, Narbona P, Adams CR, et al: Arthroscopic proximal biceps tenodesis at the articular margin: Evaluation of outcomes, complications, and revision rate. *Arthroscopy* 2015;31(3):470-476.

    Arthroscopic biceps tenodesis performed at the articular margin results in a low surgical revision rate, a low rate of residual pain, and significant improvement in objective shoulder outcome scores. Level of evidence: IV.

25. Gill TJ, McIrvin E, Mair SD, Hawkins RJ: Results of biceps tenotomy for treatment of pathology of the long head of the biceps brachii. *J Shoulder Elbow Surg* 2001;10(3):247-249.

26. Osbahr DC, Diamond AB, Speer KP: The cosmetic appearance of the biceps muscle after long-head tenotomy versus tenodesis. *Arthroscopy* 2002;18(5):483-487.

27. Werner BC, Pehlivan HC, Hart JM, et al: Increased incidence of postoperative stiffness after arthroscopic compared with open biceps tenodesis. *Arthroscopy* 2014;30(9):1075-1084.

    Results show a notably increased incidence of postoperative stiffness after arthroscopic suprapectoral biceps tenodesis compared with open subpectoral biceps tenodesis. This appears to occur more commonly in female patients and smokers and may have a relation to the position of the tenodesis, with a more superiorly placed tenodesis site being a potential influencing factor. On the basis of this series, this complication most commonly will improve over time and with symptom-based management. Level of evidence: III.

28. Mazzocca AD, Cote MP, Arciero CL, Romeo AA, Arciero RA: Clinical outcomes after subpectoral biceps tenodesis with an interference screw. *Am J Sports Med* 2008;36(10):1922-1929.

29. Millett PJ, Sanders B, Gobezie R, Braun S, Warner JJ: Interference screw vs. suture anchor fixation for open subpectoral biceps tenodesis: Does it matter? *BMC Musculoskelet Disord* 2008;9(1):121.

30. Voss A, Cerciello S, Yang J, Beitzel K, Cote MP, Mazzocca AD: Open subpectoral tenodesis of the proximal biceps. *Clin Sports Med* 2016;35(1):137-152.

A safe and reproducible blunt dissection of the pectoralis major tendon allows access to the biceps directly inferior. It is important to have a sufficient lateral retraction of the pectoralis major muscle-tendonunit and medial retraction of the conjoined tendons to permit access to the bicipital groove. Create an 8 mm bone tunnel by an 8-mm canulated reamer in the center portion of the proximal humerus to prevent fractures. The visual examination and palpation of the tenodesis are a major key point to confirm the screw is flush with the cortex and the tendon is in correct position. Level of evidence: IV.

31. Friedman DJ, Dunn JC, Higgins LD, Warner JJ: Proximal biceps tendon: Injuries and management. *Sports Med Arthrosc Rev* 2008;16(3):162-169.

32. Nho SJ, Reiff SN, Verma NN, Slabaugh MA, Mazzocca AD, Romeo AA: Complications associated with subpectoral biceps tenodesis: Low rates of incidence following surgery. *J Shoulder Elbow Surg* 2010;19(5):764-768.

33. Voss A, Cerciello S, DiVenere J, et al: Open subpectoral biceps tenodesis in patients over 65 does not result in an increased rate of complications. *BMC Musculoskelet Disord* 2017;18(1):430.

This study demonstrates that in patients over the age of 65, biceps tenodesis is a successful procedure when performed for biceps tendinopathy and concomitantly with other surgical procedures of the shoulder, and does not result in an increased rate of complications when compared to a group of patients under the age of 65. Level of evidence: IV.

Chapter 18

Subscapularis Tears and Subcoracoid Impingement

Stephen S. Burkhart, MD • Robert U. Hartzler, MD, MS

ABSTRACT

The advent of the modern era of shoulder arthroscopy brought better visualization and thus increased recognition of subscapularis tendon tears and associated pathologic lesions of the anterior shoulder. Yet, subscapularis tendon tears are still difficult to diagnose. Without a high index of suspicion with careful clinical, imaging, and intraoperative investigation, many subscapularis tears will be missed by the surgeon. Arthroscopic repair can be technically challenging but is possible for the vast majority of subscapularis tears. Excellent midterm to long-term results have been demonstrated in clinical outcomes and structural healing after arthroscopic subscapularis repair.

Keywords: rotator cuff repair; subscapularis tendon; shoulder arthroscopy

Introduction

The subscapularis tendon and closely associated structures are commonly affected in patients with rotator cuff disease. Yet, the surgeon must be diligent to search out these lesions, particularly at the time of diagnostic arthroscopy, since they can easily be missed by common screening tests. Subscapularis tears have a high rate of successful surgical treatment, particularly when modern arthroscopic techniques are employed.

Dr. Burkhart or an immediate family member has received royalties from Arthrex, Inc. and serves as a paid consultant to or is an employee of Arthrex, Inc. Dr. Hartzler or an immediate family member is a member of a speakers' bureau or has made paid presentations on behalf of Arthrex, Inc.; serves as a paid consultant to or is an employee of Arthrex, Inc.; and serves as a board member, owner, officer, or committee member of the Arthroscopy Association of North America.

Anatomy and Function

An understanding of the insertional anatomy of the subscapularis is necessary for the treatment of a subscapularis tear. The footprint of the subscapularis is larger than that of any other rotator cuff tendon.[1] The subscapularis insertion area has been described as trapezoidal; it is widest superiorly and gently tapers as it extends inferiorly.[2,3] The superior-to-inferior tendinous footprint length is approximately 25 mm, and the average width is approximately 17 mm superiorly and 3 mm inferiorly. The subscapularis has a muscular attachment along the humeral neck immediately distal to the upper tendinous insertion, which is similar to the teres minor posteriorly.[4] The entire length of the upper and lower myotendinous insertion averages approximately 40 mm.[3] Approximately 60% of the tendon attaches at the wide superior one-third of the footprint.[2,3] This area has been shown to be the strongest attachment point for the subscapularis as well as the point of greatest load transmission.[5] The tendinous upper insertion has two layers: the deeper structure inserts onto the lesser tuberosity whereas the superficial layer extends across the bicipital grove, encircles the long head of biceps tendon (LHBT), and attaches onto the greater tuberosity.[6] Fibers from the supraspinatus and upper subscapularis blend with the nearby capsular structures (superior glenohumeral, coracohumeral, and middle glenohumeral ligaments) to form the biceps sling (pulley).[7]

Prevalence and Pathology

Shoulder arthroscopy offers the surgeon an enhanced ability to recognize subscapularis pathology. The description of a subscapularis tear usually includes the location and amount of tendon involvement, whether the tear is partial or full thickness, and whether it is degenerative or traumatic. No classification system[8-12] has been universally adopted but that of Lafosse[13] is the most commonly used in modern series. Most subscapularis tears involve

This chapter is adapted from Duey RE, Burkhart SS: Subscapularis tears and subcoracoid impingement, in Nicholson GP, ed: *Orthopaedic Knowledge Update: Shoulder and Elbow*, ed 4. Rosemont, IL, American Academy of Orthopaedic Surgeons, 2013, pp 273-286.

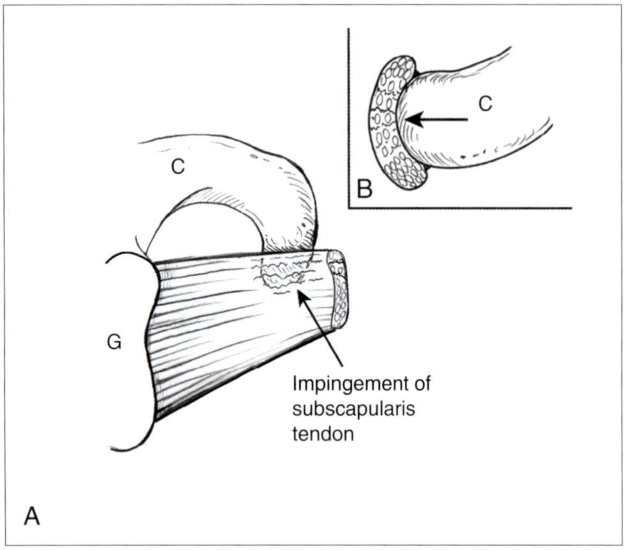

FIGURE 1 Schematic drawings showing subcoracoid impingement. Repetitive compression of the subscapularis tendon fibers by the coracoid tip in the anterior-to-posterior direction causes spreading of the fibers in the superior-to-inferior direction (**A**), with resultant longitudinal splits between subscapularis tendon fiber bundles (**B**). C = coracoid, G = glenoid. (Reproduced with permission from Burkhart SS, Lo IKY, Brady PC, Denard PJ: Subscapularis tendon tears, in *The Cowboy's Companion: A Trail Guide for the Arthroscopic Shoulder Surgeon.* Philadelphia, PA, Lippincott Williams & Wilkins, 2012, pp 101-128.)

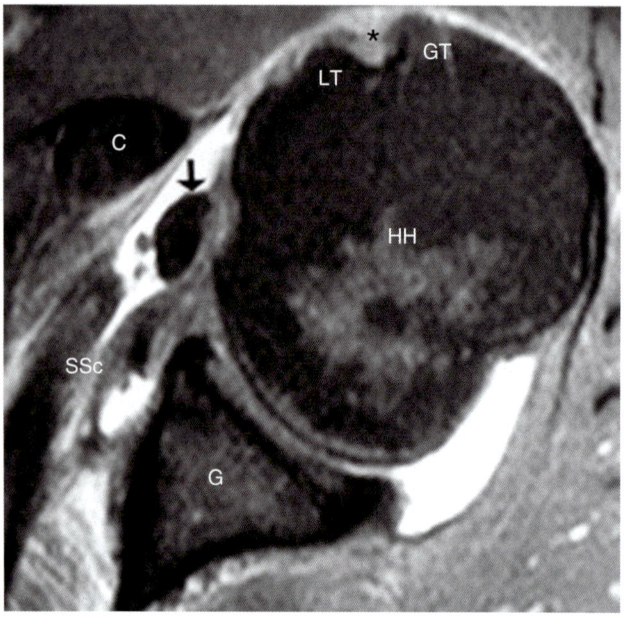

FIGURE 2 Axial MRI of a left shoulder with a medial dislocation of the long head of the biceps tendon (black arrow) into a split tear of the subscapularis tendon (SSc). The empty biceps groove (*) is seen between the lesser tuberosity (LT) and greater tuberosity (GT). C = coracoid, G = glenoid, HH = humeral head.

the upper subscapularis insertion and are articular-sided, partial thickness, and degenerative.[14,15] This tear pattern may be caused by subcoracoid stenosis and impingement (the so-called roller-wringer effect).[16] As the subscapularis moves across the coracoid, increased tensile forces on the articular side of the tendon lead to the development of a tensile undersurface fiber failure lesion. Subcoracoid impingement can also cause longitudinal splits along the deep surface of the tendon (**Figure 1**).

Modern reports indicate that 27% to 69% of all rotator cuff tears involve the subscapularis.[13,15,17-19] The prevalence of subscapularis tears was found to be almost identical to that of infraspinatus tears.[20] Subscapularis tears are very common in massive tears involving two or more rotator cuff tendons,[13,18,20,21] but most isolated subscapularis tendon tears result from traumatic injury.[13,22,23] The reported mechanisms of injury included forced abduction with external rotation, a fall onto an outstretched upper extremity, severe traction, a direct blow, and heavy lifting. One study found that most of the isolated tears were full-thickness lesions involving at least the upper one-third of the tendinous insertion.[13]

Several studies found a strong correlation between subscapularis tendon tears and pathologic changes involving the LHBT.[11,13,15,18,20-22,24] The reported prevalence of LHBT lesions associated with subscapularis tears ranged from 63% to 100%.[13,20-22,24,25] Anterior instability of the LHBT almost always occurs in conjunction with a tear of the subscapularis[11,15,18] (**Figure 2**). The rate of LHBT dislocation also is substantially higher when there is a full-thickness subscapularis tear, particularly if it involves more than one-third of the insertion.[11,15]

The strong association between subscapularis tears and LHBT subluxation or dislocation probably results from loss of the stability the subscapularis normally offers the LHBT. The superior insertion of the subscapularis and associated structures (ligaments and supraspinatus tendon) may be the most important LHBT stabilizer.[7] Anatomic and histologic analysis revealed that the subscapularis forms a buttress that supports the LHBT tendon as it makes its acute turn out of the intertubercular groove before entering the joint.[6,7,15] The wide uppermost insertion of the subscapularis extends as a distinct tendinous slip over the fovea capitis of the humeral head. This tendinous slip at the widest section of the subscapularis tendon insertion comes into direct contact with the LHBT where it turns over the top of the humeral head. The upper subscapularis insertion directly supports the LHBT, and this tendinous slip serves as a secondary attachment point (in addition to the bone insertion) for the superior glenohumeral ligament and the medial head of the coracohumeral ligament as they spiral to form the medial sling of the biceps and stabilize the LHBT.[7]

Clinical Evaluation and Imaging

Clinical tests can be used to evaluate the integrity and function of the subscapularis, and this is generally accomplished by testing internal rotation strength in an internal rotation position of the shoulder, which minimizes the effectiveness of the other internal rotators. Common specific tests for the subscapularis (eg, bear hug, belly press, lift-off, Napoleon) have wide ranging sensitivities (12% to 88%) and are not trustworthy to rule out tears. The specificity of special subscapularis tests is much better, generally in the 80% to 90% range.[26,27] Additionally, many patients are unable to perform special testing of the subscapularis because of pain or stiffness.[13] Therefore, the subscapularis should be routinely examined during diagnostic arthroscopy in patients with positive physical examination findings for the subscapularis.

Plain radiographs are the initial studies obtained for patients with a suspected rotator cuff tear. Although a poor screening test for subscapularis tears, plain radiographs can reveal concomitant pathology, including narrowing of the coracohumeral interval, glenohumeral arthritis, or fracture. Anterosuperior migration or anterior subluxation of the humeral head can also be identified: these conditions may result from a long-standing massive rotator cuff tear or an acute injury involving the subscapularis, with loss of the coronal and transverse plane force couples.

MRI, magnetic resonance arthrography, CT arthrography (CTA), and ultrasonography have been used to evaluate the subscapularis. CTA is most commonly used in Europe, and MRI and magnetic resonance arthrography are more commonly used in North America. Ultrasonography is cost-effective, can be used in the clinical setting, and allows dynamic evaluation of the subscapularis. However, its usefulness depends on the expertise of the sonographer. MRI, magnetic resonance arthrography, and CTA are able to detect labral injury, fatty infiltration, and muscle atrophy, but ultrasonography does not have this ability.

The accuracy of shoulder ultrasonography in detecting subscapularis tears has been investigated by comparison with arthroscopic findings.[17] Analysis of the results determined ultrasonography to have a sensitivity of 30% and a specificity of 100% for detecting subscapularis tears. The positive predictive value was 100%, and the negative predictive value was 78%. Ultrasonography was effective in detecting full-thickness subscapularis tears, with a sensitivity of 86%.[17]

A small prospective study of the results of arthroscopic subscapularis repair also examined the effectiveness of CTA in detecting subscapularis tears in 17 patients with an isolated subscapularis lesion.[13] A sensitivity of 94% was reported for CTA. However, 15 of the tears were full-thickness lesions involving at least one-third of the tendon insertion.

The accuracy of MRI for detecting subscapularis tears has also been evaluated.[20] The preoperative MRI studies were interpreted by radiologists and compared with findings at the time of shoulder arthroscopy. MRI had a low sensitivity (36%) but an excellent specificity (100%). The overall accuracy was 69%.[20]

One study examined the ability of fellowship trained orthopaedic surgeons to accurately detect subscapularis tears using MRI and four specific criteria: in axial images, a tear of the subscapularis tendon off the lesser tuberosity or medial subluxation-dislocation of the LHBT (**Figure 2**); and in sagittal oblique images, a tear from the lesser tuberosity or atrophy of the subscapularis muscle.[18] A subscapularis that met two or more criteria was considered torn. This approach had sensitivity of 73%, specificity of 94%, positive predictive value of 90%, negative predictive value of 84%, and accuracy of 86% for detecting subscapularis tears. Based on these findings, the systematic use of these criteria may improve a surgeon's ability to preoperatively detect a subscapularis tear on MRI.[18]

These studies show that advanced imaging modalities (ultrasonography, MRI, and CTA) are most effective in detecting a large, full-thickness tear of the subscapularis. Smaller, partial-thickness tears frequently are not evident. Like clinical examination tests, advanced imaging studies have much better specificity than sensitivity: negative tests do not effectively rule out tears. Therefore, a high index of suspicion and a thorough arthroscopic examination are required to detect these lesions.

Management

Questions remain as to which subscapularis tears should be managed surgically and which should be managed nonsurgically. An acute, traumatic tear typically is repaired surgically. A small, degenerative tear initially can be managed nonsurgically, particularly if the patient has low demands and is older than approximately 65 years. However, some experts believe that, given the critical role of the subscapularis in shoulder function, most subscapularis tears ultimately lead to substantial disability and should be repaired, particularly if discovered arthroscopically in isolation or in combination with a larger rotator cuff tear.[28,29] Even in the presence of substantial fatty infiltration, some experts believe that the subscapularis can and should be repaired for its tenodesis effect, which stabilizes the glenohumeral joint and provides a stable fulcrum for glenohumeral kinematics.[29-31] In retracted anterosuperior rotator cuff tears, repair of the subscapularis aids subsequent repair of the supraspinatus and reestablishes the anterior attachment of the rotator cable.

The arthroscopic treatment of subscapularis tears and any associated pathology can be challenging, but evolving techniques and instrumentation are making these repairs easier. The subscapularis can be arthroscopically repaired with the patient in the beach-chair or lateral decubitus position. For a multitendon tear, it is advisable to treat the subscapularis first, before swelling further restricts the already limited subcoracoid space. The anterosuperolateral and anterior portals are the standard working portals. The posterior or lateral portal is used for visualization. Often, tears of the subscapularis can be identified by using a 30° arthroscope in the posterior portal. However, the view of the subscapularis footprint can be substantially improved when a 70° arthroscope is used. Some experts believe that the use of a lateral viewing portal with a 30° arthroscope offers the best view of the subscapularis footprint, but others hold that a posterior viewing portal with a 70° arthroscope provides the best view.[13,28,29]

The 70° arthroscope offers the ability to see 2 cm down the intertubercular groove from a posterior portal.[28,32] It is essential to inspect the medial sidewall of the intertubercular groove in this manner when evaluating the subscapularis. Doing so may reveal a rent in the sidewall, which indicates an occult subscapularis tendon tear. This tear may be obstructed from view by the proximal portion of the medial sling. Sling take-down combined with a 70° arthroscopic view may be required to identify such a tear[33] (**Figure 3**).

Proper manipulation of the arm also is useful for visualizing the subscapularis. Bringing the arm into forward flexion and internal rotation can be helpful in examining the tendon insertion. With the patient in the lateral decubitus position, applying a so-called posterior lever push not only increases the anterior working space but also improves visualization of the subscapularis insertion.[21,29]

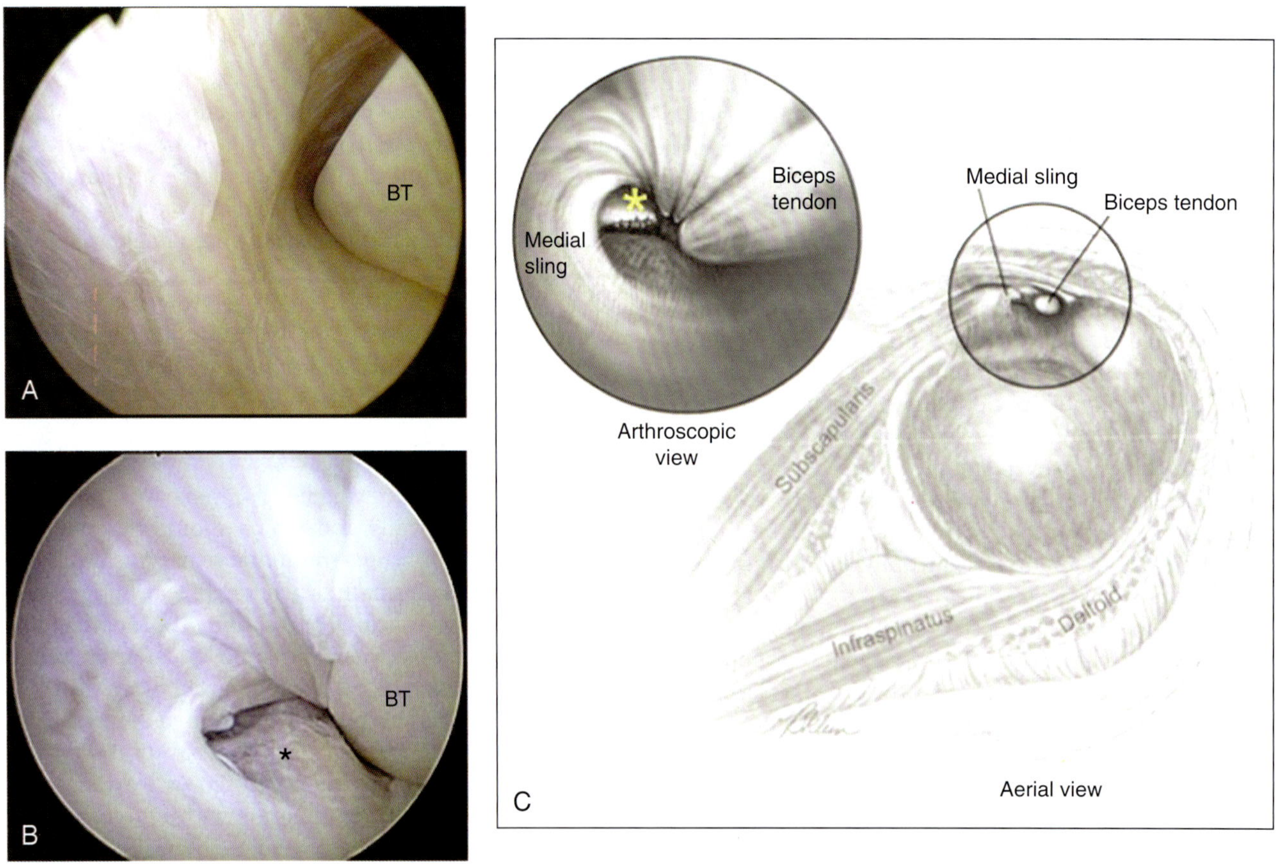

FIGURE 3 **A**, Arthroscopic image of a normal shoulder as seen from a posterior viewing portal with a 70° arthroscope, showing approximately 2 cm of the floor and sidewalls of the bicipital groove. **B**, Arthroscopic image of a shoulder with disruption in the medial sidewall, with a bare lesser tuberosity footprint distally. **C**, Schematic drawings of the shoulder in **B**, showing a mid to distal tendon tear of the subscapularis. * = disrupted medial sidewall, BT = biceps tendon. (Reproduced with permission from Burkhart SS, Lo IKY, Brady PC, Denard PJ: Subscapularis tendon tears, in *The Cowboy's Companion: A Trail Guide for the Arthroscopic Shoulder Surgeon*. Philadelphia, PA, Lippincott Williams & Wilkins, 2012, pp 101-128.)

This maneuver is performed by stabilizing the patient's elbow while slightly internally rotating the arm with one hand and applying a posteriorly directed force to the proximal humerus with the other hand. The posterior lever push has proved useful for visualization from a posterior portal, particularly with a 70° arthroscope. A similar maneuver with the patient in the beach-chair position can be attempted.

A narrowed coracohumeral interval and subscapularis pathology have been significantly correlated.[34,35] Therefore, the subcoracoid space must be dealt along with a tear of the subscapularis. From an intra-articular viewpoint, it is useful to internally and externally rotate the shoulder and to observe whether the coracoid tip (seen as a rolling bulge at the top of the subscapularis tendon) is compressing and impinging on the subscapularis tendon as the shoulder moves back and forth. This finding is a strong indicator that the coracohumeral interval is substantially narrowed. The coracoid and subcoracoid space can be seen from an intra-articular viewpoint by placing the tip of the arthroscope through a window created in the medial aspect of the rotator interval. Care should be taken to preserve the more lateral comma tissue during this step (**Figure 4**). A 30° arthroscope initially is used to identify the tip of the coracoid because the use of a 70° arthroscope may be disorienting and cause a drift too far inferiorly and medially. Many surgeons use a coracohumeral interval of 6 mm or less as an indication for coracoplasty during a subscapularis repair.[24,29,36] The bursa and other soft tissue can be removed from the subcoracoid space by using a combination of electrocautery and shaving. A burr is then used to resect the posterolateral tip of the coracoid in the plane of the conjoined tendon and the subscapularis. The goal is to enlarge the coracohumeral interval to between 7 and 10 mm[21,29] (**Figure 5**). Coracoplasty also can be done through a subacromial approach, depending on the surgeon's preference. Familiarity with the surrounding anatomy is important during a coracoplasty. Surgery about the posterolateral aspect of the coracoid tip is relatively safe because all major neurovascular structures are located at least 28 mm from the tip of the coracoid.[37]

Resection of the coracoid should be limited to less than 10 mm, depending on the size of the patient, to preclude any substantial soft-tissue disruption.[38]

There is a high correlation between LHBT pathology and a subscapularis tendon tear; the LHBT is usually treated at the same time as a subscapularis tear.[11,13,15,18,20-22,24] Many surgeons treat the biceps based on its appearance at the time of arthroscopy.[13,22,24] Others routinely perform either a tenodesis or tenotomy of the LHBT during repair of a subscapularis tear, unless the patient is younger than approximately 35 years or is an overhead throwing athlete.[29] The decision to perform a tenodesis rather than tenotomy is based on the patient factors, including age, activity level, concern about cosmesis, and personal preference. Anatomic studies have highlighted the role of the upper subscapularis tendon in stabilizing the LHBT.[7,15] Routinely treating the biceps may, therefore, protect the subscapularis repair. Clinical outcomes were improved after subscapularis repair with LHBT tenotomy or tenodesis, regardless of the appearance of the LHBT at the time of surgery.[39] Two studies found that some patients with a healed subscapularis after arthroscopic repair had an unsatisfactory clinical outcome related to pathology involving the LHBT, although the biceps had a normal appearance at the time of surgery.[13,24] Instability of the LHBT can recur, however,

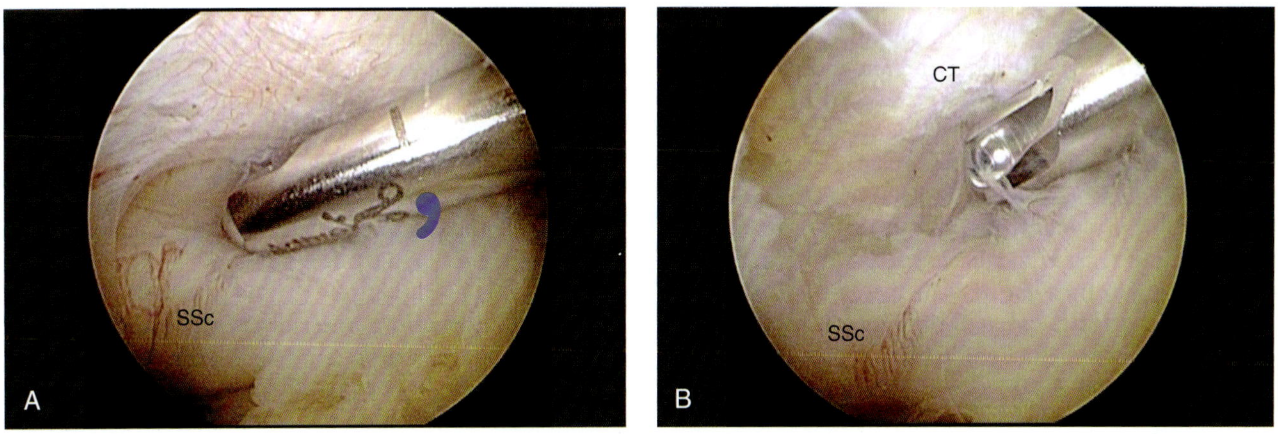

FIGURE 4 Arthroscopic images showing a right shoulder as seen from a posterior viewing portal. **A**, A shaver is used to make a window in the rotator interval medial to the comma tissue (blue symbol). **B**, The coracoid tip is located by palpation with the shaver. CT = coracoid tip, SSc = subscapularis tendon. (Reproduced with permission from Burkhart SS, Lo IKY, Brady PC, Denard PJ: Subscapularis tendon tears, in *The Cowboy's Companion: A Trail Guide for the Arthroscopic Shoulder Surgeon*. Philadelphia, PA, Lippincott Williams & Wilkins, 2012, pp 101-128.)

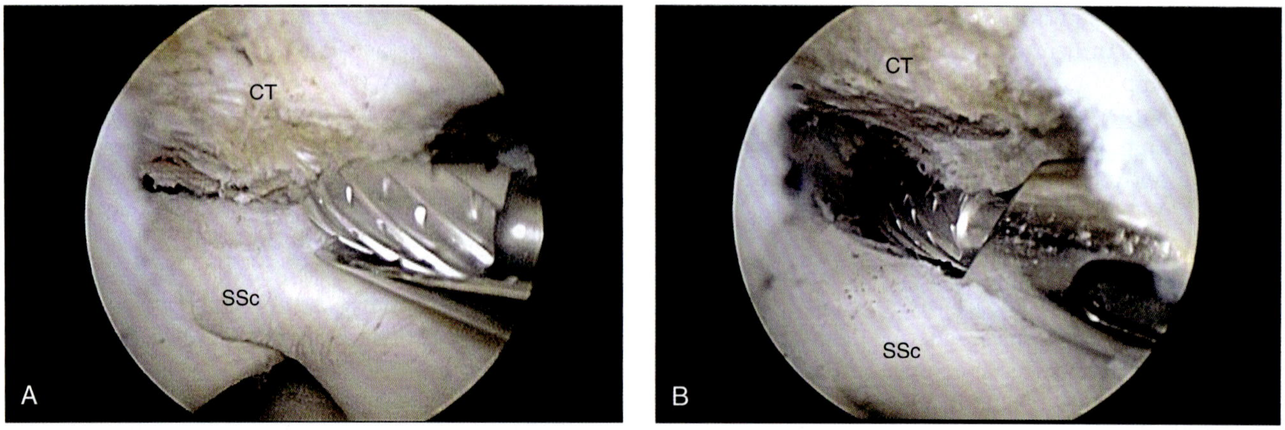

FIGURE 5 Arthroscopic images of a right shoulder as seen from a posterior glenohumeral portal with a 70° arthroscope, showing coracohumeral interval evaluation. **A**, The native coracohumeral interval can be estimated by comparison with the known width of an instrument; here, the width of the interval is less than that of the 5-mm burr. **B**, Coracoplasty has created a coracohumeral interval of at least 7 mm. CT = coracoid tip, SSc = subscapularis tendon. (Reproduced with permission from Burkhart SS, Lo IKY, Brady PC, Denard PJ: Subscapularis tendon tears, in *The Cowboy's Companion: A Trail Guide for the Arthroscopic Shoulder Surgeon*. Philadelphia, PA, Lippincott Williams & Wilkins, 2012, pp 101-128.)

causing failure of the subscapularis repair. Therefore, most experts prefer to use tenotomy or tenodesis to treat the LHBT in the context of a subscapularis tear.[13,22,24,29,39]

Preparation of the bony footprint is important to a successful repair of the subscapularis. All soft tissue is carefully removed from the bone bed using a combination of a cautery, a shaver, a high-speed burr, and ring curets. The goal is a uniform bleeding bone surface to which the subscapularis can heal and form a strong attachment. In a complete chronic tear, reduced tendon excursion may lead to inadequate apposition of the tendon to the native footprint. If necessary, the footprint can be medialized 5 to 7 mm to improve the contact surface area between the tendon and the bone and to reduce the tension on the repair. One study compared two groups of patients after primary arthroscopic repair of a 100% retracted full-thickness subscapularis tear.[40] Patients in one group had a repair to the native footprint, and those in the other group required medialization of the footprint of as much as 7 mm. At a minimum 2-year follow-up, there was no significant between-group difference in functional scores, patient satisfaction, or return to activity.

A chronic tear can leave the subscapularis severely retracted and scarred to adjacent structures. Identifying the tendon margins can be difficult, but the process is facilitated by identification of the comma sign and its attachment to the superolateral corner of the subscapularis tendon insertion.[41] A traction stitch then can be placed in the subscapularis tendon, and the meticulous process of releasing the tendon is begun. The posterolateral coracoid is skeletonized, and anterior adhesions between the subscapularis, the conjoined tendon, and the internal deltoid fascia are resected. Care must be taken to avoid straying too far inferior or medial to the conjoined tendon. Often, there are adhesions between the subscapularis and the inferior neck and base of the coracoid process, and a 30° elevator can be extremely useful in releasing these adhesions. The upper subscapular nerve insertion can be as close as 11 mm to the medial aspect of the base of the coracoid. Therefore, it is important to avoid straying medial to the coracoid during this release. A posterior release of the subscapularis from the anterior glenoid neck also should be done. This plane is relatively avascular, and a 15° elevator can be helpful with this portion of the release. Release of the coracohumeral ligament from the base of the coracoid with preservation of the comma tissue can greatly improve tendon excursion. This portion of the release has been called the anterior interval slide in continuity.[42] Release of inferior adhesions between the subscapularis and the axillary nerve and the brachial plexus has been described.[13,43] This step can be dangerous, and it is unusual to require an inferior release for gaining adequate tendon excursion before repair and therefore is not routinely performed or advocated.[22,24,29]

Suture anchors usually are placed from inferior to superior along the footprint. In general, one anchor per linear centimeter of torn tendon (in the superior-to-inferior dimension) is used. Sutures can be passed antegrade or retrograde through an anterior or anterosuperolateral portal, depending on the surgeon's preference. Inferior sutures are tied before superior sutures. Superior sutures can be brought medial to the comma tissue over the superior margin of the tendon and tied, thereby using the comma tissue as a rip stop to suture cutout.

Most subscapularis tears are repaired using a single-row technique, especially those less than or equal to 50% of the length of the tendinous insertion, and excellent short-term and long-term results have been reported.[13,21,22,24,44,45] However, some surgeons prefer to use a double-row repair if at all possible.[13,29,36,44-46] There is growing evidence that linked, double-row rotator cuff repairs (transosseous equivalent) result in better healing and strength for larger rotator cuff tears. A biomechanical study found that a double-row repair using a suture-bridge technique had substantially higher stiffness and ultimate load for a complete subscapularis tear compared with a single-row repair.[46] Tendon elongation before failure was substantially less in patients with a double-row repair, and the strength of the double-row repair surpassed the predicted loads for everyday activities involving the subscapularis.[36] Despite this, clinical and structural outcomes of single-row and double-row subscapularis repairs seem to be equivalent for full-thickness, isolated tears, as discussed later.[47]

Tears of the subscapularis typically involve the upper portion of the tendon insertion.[14,15] The use of a double-loaded suture anchor has been described for a double inverted mattress repair of the upper subscapularis.[48] This technique improves the compression of the tendon against the footprint, compared with the use of simple sutures. However, there is a risk of cutout in poor-quality tissue. A knotless technique using modern tape suture is an option for repairing an upper subscapularis tear.[49] The tape suture is placed in the superolateral corner of the subscapularis tendon, and both limbs are brought medial to the comma tissue and secured in the superomedial corner of the footprint using a knotless anchor (**Figure 6**). The wide suture tape provides superior compression of the tendon against the footprint as well as better resistance than suture to tendon cut-through. After the two limbs are secured, the tails can be brought anterior to the comma tissue and secured laterally within a biceps tenodesis construct or with a second knotless suture anchor.[45] This technique provides double-row fixation of an upper subscapularis tear in a relatively straightforward and efficient manner.

After surgery, immobilization in a sling with a small abduction pillow is required. Active elbow motion is allowed. Passive external rotation is limited to 0° with the arm at the side. The use of the sling is discontinued at 6 weeks, and progressive, active-assisted range-of-motion exercises are begun. Strengthening exercises are initiated 12 to 16 weeks after surgery, depending on the size of the tear. A return to full activities requires at least 6 months, depending on the size of the tear.

Results

The published literature on isolated subscapularis repair—whether done open or arthroscopically—demonstrates very good improvements in patient outcomes with good rates of structural healing and low complication rates as demonstrated by two systematic reviews (up to 2015).[25,50] In comparing the earlier series of arthroscopic isolated subscapularis repairs with those performed in an open fashion, the authors of a 2012 study found similar reported rates of structural healing (34 of 38, 90% versus 38 of 40, 95%).[50] The overall results in clinical outcomes and complications also appear to be equivalent for open and arthroscopic repairs.[25,50] Single-row and double-row repairs also demonstrate similar outcomes. Modern studies consistently demonstrate excellent healing rates that approach 100% for arthroscopic, single-row repair of full-thickness subscapularis tears.[23,47,51]

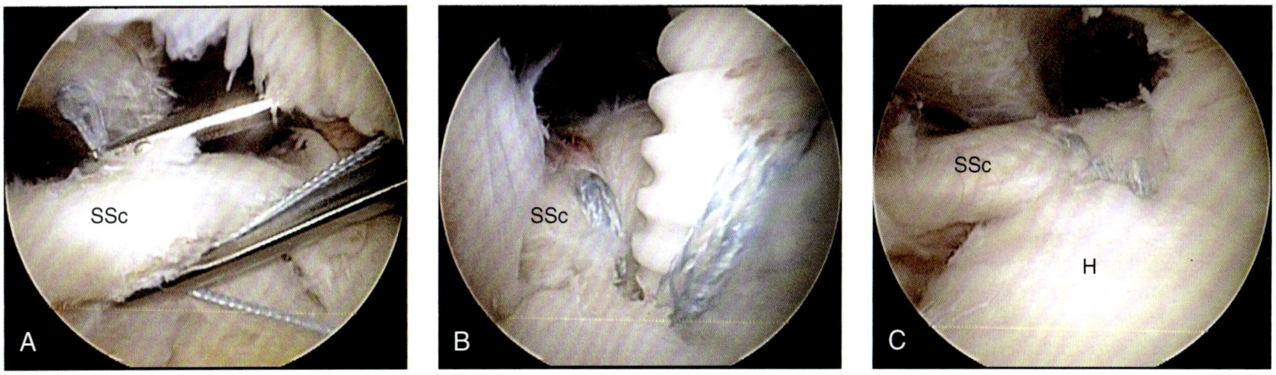

FIGURE 6 Arthroscopic images of a right shoulder as seen from a posterior viewing portal, showing knotless repair of an upper subscapularis tendon tear. **A**, A FiberTape suture is passed antegrade through the upper subscapularis tendon. **B**, The tape is secured to the prepared bone bed with a BioComposite SwiveLock C anchor (Arthrex). **C**, Restoration of the footprint with a low-profile knotless repair. H = humerus, SSc = subscapularis tendon. (Reproduced with permission from Burkhart SS, Lo IKY, Brady PC, Denard PJ: Subscapularis tendon tears, in *The Cowboy's Companion: A Trail Guide for the Arthroscopic Shoulder Surgeon*. Philadelphia, PA, Lippincott Williams & Wilkins, 2012, pp 101-128.)

SUMMARY

The diagnosis and treatment of subscapularis tears and subcoracoid impingement continue to evolve. Arthroscopic shoulder surgery has enabled better recognition and understanding of these clinical entities and has allowed less invasive treatment. Both short-term and long-term outcome studies evaluating these techniques have had encouraging results and support their continued use. Further work is needed to better delineate the tenodesis function of the subscapularis as well as the specific role of subcoracoid impingement in subscapularis pathology. Most subscapularis tears can be repaired arthroscopically using single-row techniques with the expectation of excellent clinical and structural outcomes. Double-row repair techniques may at some point prove clinically advantageous for repairing larger subscapularis tears.

KEY STUDY POINTS

- Subscapularis tears are common but easily missed because physical examination and imaging tests lack sensitivity for diagnosing these lesions.
- Subscapularis tears are often partial or nonretracted, and so the surgeon must be diligent during diagnostic arthroscopy to identify them.
- Owing to their structural and functional importance, all subscapularis tears found intraoperatively to have significant fiber detachment from the lesser tuberosity should be repaired.
- Arthroscopic subscapularis repair carries technical challenges, but excellent clinical results with a high rate of tendon healing with a variety of repair techniques can be expected.

Annotated References

1. Curtis AS, Burbank KM, Tierney JJ, Scheller AD, Curran AR: The insertional footprint of the rotator cuff: An anatomic study. *Arthroscopy* 2006;22(6):609.e1.

2. Richards DP, Burkhart SS, Tehrany AM, Wirth MA: The subscapularis footprint: An anatomic description of its insertion site. *Arthroscopy* 2007;23(3):251-254.

3. Ide J, Tokiyoshi A, Hirose J, Mizuta H: An anatomic study of the subscapularis insertion to the humerus: The subscapularis footprint. *Arthroscopy* 2008;24(7):749-753.

4. Collin P, Lädermann A, Le Bourg M, Walch G: Subscapularis minor – An analogue of the Teres minor? *Orthop Traumatol Surg Res* 2013;99(4 suppl):S255-S258.

   The authors propose that the subscapularis should be thought of as two separate muscles, with the inferior subscapularis analagous to the teres minor. Subscapularis tears extending into the inferior portion cause significantly greater motor dysfunction (80% pseudoparalysis, average forward flexion [FF] 83°) versus those isolated to the superior subscapularis (zero pseudoparalysis, FF 178°). The upper and lower subscapularis muscles have different insertional anatomy (tendinous versus muscular) and innervation and activation patterns. Level of evidence: II.

5. Halder A, Zobitz ME, Schultz E, An KN: Structural properties of the subscapularis tendon. *J Orthop Res* 2000;18(5):829-834.

6. Tebaa E, Tantot J, Isaac-Pinet S, Nové-Josserand L: Histologic characteristics of the subscapularis tendon from muscle to bone: Reference to subscapularis lesions. *J Shoulder Elbow Surg* 2019;28(5):959-965.

   The gross anatomic characteristics and histology of 10 cadaver shoulders were analyzed. The lower third of the subscapularis predominantly has a muscular insertion onto bone, whereas the upper two-thirds have a complex tendinous structure that has two layers. The deeper layer inserts directly onto the lesser tuberosity, whereas the thicker superficial layer splits around and encircles the long head of biceps tendon inserting onto the lesser and greater tuberosities.

7. Arai R, Mochizuki T, Yamaguchi K, et al: Functional anatomy of the superior glenohumeral and coracohumeral ligaments and the subscapularis tendon in view of stabilization of the long head of the biceps tendon. *J Shoulder Elbow Surg* 2010;19(1):58-64.

8. Fox JA, Noerdlinger MA, Romeo AA: Arthroscopic subscapularis repair. *Tech Shoulder Elbow Surg* 2003;4(4):154-168.

9. Yoo JC, Rhee YG, Shin SJ, et al: Subscapularis tendon tear classification based on 3-dimensional anatomic footprint: A cadaveric and prospective clinical observational study. *Arthroscopy* 2015;31(1):19-28.

   A cadaver and clinical study with five tear types proposed based on subscapularis insertion onto four bony facets. Subscapularis tears were diagnosed in 50% of shoulder arthroscopies (821) in 29 months. First facet tears (one-third of the footprint) accounted for 80% of subscapularis lesions. Level of evidence: II.

10. Pfirrmann CW, Zanetti M, Weishaupt D, Gerber C, Hodler J: Subscapularis tendon tears: Detection and grading at MR arthrography. *Radiology* 1999;213(3):709-714.

11. Lafosse L, Reiland Y, Baier GP, Toussaint B, Jost B: Anterior and posterior instability of the long head of the biceps tendon in rotator cuff tears: A new classification based on arthroscopic observations. *Arthroscopy* 2007;23(1):73-80.

12. Toussaint B, Barth J, Charousset C, et al: New endoscopic classification for subscapularis lesions. *Orthop Traumatol Surg Res* 2012;98(8 suppl):S186-S192.

13. Lafosse L, Jost B, Reiland Y, Audebert S, Toussaint B, Gobezie R: Structural integrity and clinical outcomes after arthroscopic repair of isolated subscapularis tears. *J Bone Joint Surg Am* 2007;89(6):1184-1193.

14. Sakurai G, Ozaki J, Tomita Y, Kondo T, Tamai S: Incomplete tears of the subscapularis tendon associated with tears of the supraspinatus tendon: Cadaveric and clinical studies. *J Shoulder Elbow Surg* 1998;7(5):510-515.

15. Arai R, Sugaya H, Mochizuki T, Nimura A, Moriishi J, Akita K: Subscapularis tendon tear: An anatomic and clinical investigation. *Arthroscopy* 2008;24(9):997-1004.

16. Lo IK, Burkhart SS: The etiology and assessment of subscapularis tendon tears: A case for subcoracoid impingement, the roller-wringer effect, and TUFF lesions of the subscapularis. *Arthroscopy* 2003;19(10):1142-1150.

17. Singisetti K, Hinsche A: Shoulder ultrasonography versus arthroscopy for the detection of rotator cuff tears: Analysis of errors. *J Orthop Surg (Hong Kong)* 2011;19(1):76-79.

18. Adams CR, Brady PC, Koo SS, et al: A systematic approach for diagnosing subscapularis tendon tears with preoperative magnetic resonance imaging scans. *Arthroscopy* 2012;28(11):1592-1600.

19. Furukawa R, Morihara T, Arai Y, et al: Diagnostic accuracy of magnetic resonance imaging for subscapularis tendon tears using radial-slice magnetic resonance images. *J Shoulder Elbow Surg* 2014;23(11):e283-e290.

    Fifty-five shoulders with rotator cuff tears diagnosed by arthroscopy were studied. Sixty-nine percent had subscapularis tears. The sensitivity of radial magnetic resonance images for subscapularis tears was 95%. Level of evidence: III.

20. Adams CR, Schoolfield JD, Burkhart SS: Accuracy of preoperative magnetic resonance imaging in predicting a subscapularis tendon tear based on arthroscopy. *Arthroscopy* 2010;26(11):1427-1433.

21. Adams CR, Schoolfield JD, Burkhart SS: The results of arthroscopic subscapularis tendon repairs. *Arthroscopy* 2008;24(12):1381-1389.

22. Bartl C, Salzmann GM, Seppel G, et al: Subscapularis function and structural integrity after arthroscopic repair of isolated subscapularis tears. *Am J Sports Med* 2011;39(6):1255-1262.

23. Hasler A, Boyce G, Schallberger A, Jost B, Catanzaro S, Gerber C: Arthroscopic repair of isolated subscapularis tears: Clinical outcome and structural integrity with a minimum follow-up of 4.6 years. *J Shoulder Elbow Surg* 2019;28(11):2171-2180.

    Thirty-six isolated subscapularis repairs were performed arthroscopically using a single-row technique. Despite a complication rate of 16%, including one retear, one deep infection, and four cases of adhesive capsulitis, clinical and structural outcomes were excellent. Advanced imaging was obtained in all patients and demonstrated a 97% rate of complete tendon healing. No deterioration in fatty infiltration or clinical outcomes occurred between midterm and long-term follow-up. Subjective shoulder value averaged 85% and relative total Constant score was 87 points at the latest reported follow-up. Level of evidence: IV.

24. Ide J, Tokiyoshi A, Hirose J, Mizuta H: Arthroscopic repair of traumatic combined rotator cuff tears involving the subscapularis tendon. *J Bone Joint Surg Am* 2007;89(11):2378-2388.

25. Saltzman BM, Collins MJ, Leroux T, et al: Arthroscopic repair of isolated subscapularis tears: A systematic review of technique-specific outcomes. *Arthroscopy* 2017;33(4):849-860.

    Eight level IV studies on arthroscopically performed isolated subscapularis repairs with short-term follow-up (range 12 to 49 months) and 115 total patients were reviewed. The vast majority (97%) were complete tears. Single-row versus double-row repair technique was reported inconsistently; the majority of patients had concomitant biceps tenotomy or tenodesis. Constant total scores were consistently reported and demonstrated excellent improvements ranging from 20 to 50 points with final postoperative scores generally between 80 and 90 points. The majority of studies (63%) reported no complications or revision surgeries. Five reruptures (4%) were reported overall with an overall trend of a lower rate for double-row repairs. Level of evidence: IV.

26. Hartzler RU, Burkhart SS: Management of subscapularis tendon tears. *Oper Tech Sports Med* 2018;26(1):10-23.

    The diagnostic utility of six special tests (bear-hug, belly-press, lift-off, internal rotation lag sign, Napoleon test, internal rotation resistance) for subscapularis tendon tears in six clinical studies was summarized. The sensitivity of the tests varied widely (12% to 88%) indicating poor reliability as a screening test for ruling out tears. The specificity of the tests was more consistent and higher (69% to 100%) and generally in the 80% to 90% range. Level of evidence: V.

27. Bartsch M, Greiner S, Haas NP, Scheibel M: Diagnostic values of clinical tests for subscapularis lesions. *Knee Surg Sports Traumatol Arthrosc* 2010;18(12):1712-1717.

28. Koo SS, Burkhart SS: Subscapularis tendon tears: Identifying mid to distal footprint disruptions. *Arthroscopy* 2010;26(8):1130-1134.

29. Denard PJ, Lädermann A, Burkhart SS: Arthroscopic management of subscapularis tears. *Sports Med Arthrosc Rev* 2011;19(4):333-341.

30. Burkhart SS, Tehrany AM: Arthroscopic subscapularis tendon repair: Technique and preliminary results. *Arthroscopy* 2002;18(5):454-463.

31. Ticker JB, Burkhart SS: Why repair the subscapularis? A logical rationale. *Arthroscopy* 2011;27(8):1123-1128.

32. Sheean AJ, Hartzler RU, Denard PJ, Lädermann A, Hanypsiak BT, Burkhart SS: A 70° arthroscope significantly improves visualization of the bicipital groove in the lateral decubitus position. *Arthroscopy* 2016;32(9):1745-1749.

    In 10 cadaver specimens and 11 patients, the visible length of the bicipital groove was measured using 30° and 70° arthroscopes. The 70° scope allows better visualization, generally 2 cm or greater of the length of the groove. Level of evidence: III.

33. Hartzler RU, Burkhart SS: Medial biceps sling takedown may be necessary to expose an occult subscapularis tendon tear. *Arthrosc Tech* 2014;3(6):e719-e722.

    Occult subscapularis tears are defined as those that require more than intraoperative inspection of the tendon insertion. One subtype of occult tear may require incision of the capsuloligamentous medial biceps sling for diagnosis. A combination of physical examination and intraoperative findings (subcoracoid stenosis, longitudinal tendon splitting, medial sidewall of biceps groove tearing) should lead to suspicion of this tear type. If the biceps sling is taken town, tenodesis of the biceps should follow. Level of evidence: V.

34. Nové-Josserand L, Edwards TB, O'Connor DP, Walch G: The acromiohumeral and coracohumeral intervals are abnormal in rotator cuff tears with muscular fatty degeneration. *Clin Orthop Relat Res* 2005;(433):90-96.

35. Richards DP, Burkhart SS, Campbell SE: Relation between narrowed coracohumeral distance and subscapularis tears. *Arthroscopy* 2005;21(10):1223-1228.

36. Park JY, Park JS, Jung JK, Kumar P, Oh KS: Suture-bridge subscapularis tendon repair technique using low anterior portals. *Knee Surg Sports Traumatol Arthrosc* 2011;19(2):303-306.

37. Lo IK, Burkhart SS, Parten PM: Surgery about the coracoid: Neurovascular structures at risk. *Arthroscopy* 2004;20(6):591-595.

38. Kleist KD, Freehill MQ, Hamilton L, Buss DD, Fritts H: Computed tomography analysis of the coracoid process and anatomic structures of the shoulder after arthroscopic coracoid decompression: A cadaveric study. *J Shoulder Elbow Surg* 2007;16(2):245-250.

39. Edwards TB, Walch G, Sirveaux F, et al: Repair of tears of the subscapularis. *J Bone Joint Surg Am* 2005;87(4):725-730.

40. Denard PJ, Burkhart SS: Medialization of the subscapularis footprint does not affect functional outcome of arthroscopic repair. *Arthroscopy* 2012;28(11):1608-1614.

41. Lo IK, Burkhart SS: The comma sign: An arthroscopic guide to the torn subscapularis tendon. *Arthroscopy* 2003;19(3):334-337.

42. Lo IK, Burkhart SS: The interval slide in continuity: A method of mobilizing the anterosuperior rotator cuff without disrupting the tear margins. *Arthroscopy* 2004;20(4):435-441.

43. Denard PJ, Jiwani AZ, Lädermann A, Burkhart SS: Long-term outcome of a consecutive series of subscapularis tendon tears repaired arthroscopically. *Arthroscopy* 2012;28(11):1587-1591.

44. Lafosse L, Lanz U, Saintmard B, Campens C: Arthroscopic repair of subscapularis tear: Surgical technique and results. *Orthop Traumatol Surg Res* 2010;96(8 suppl):S99-S108.

45. Denard PJ, Lädermann A, Burkhart SS: Double-row fixation of upper subscapularis tears with a single suture anchor. *Arthroscopy* 2011;27(8):1142-1149.

46. Wellmann M, Wiebringhaus P, Lodde I, et al: Biomechanical evaluation of a single-row versus double-row repair for complete subscapularis tears. *Knee Surg Sports Traumatol Arthrosc* 2009;17(12):1477-1484.

47. Yoon JS, Kim SJ, Choi YR, Kim SH, Chun YM: Arthroscopic repair of the isolated subscapularis full-thickness tear: Single- versus double-row suture-bridge technique. *Am J Sports Med* 2019;47(6):1427-1433.

    A level III study compared the short-term outcomes of isolated arthroscopic repair of full-thickness subscapularis tears using single-row versus double-row techniques. The 31 patients with a single-row repair had equivalent outcomes in pain, subjective shoulder value, and American Shoulder and Elbow Surgeons scores compared with the 25 patients with a double-row repair. Structural healing rates were also similar (87% versus 88%). Level of evidence: III.

48. Yoo JC, Kim JH, Lee YS, Park JH, Kang HJ: Arthroscopic double mattress repair in incomplete subscapularis tears. *Orthopedics* 2008;31(9):851-854.

49. Denard PJ, Burkhart SS: A new method for knotless fixation of an upper subscapularis tear. *Arthroscopy* 2011;27(6):861-866.

50. Mall NA, Chahal J, Heard WM, et al: Outcomes of arthroscopic and open surgical repair of isolated subscapularis tendon tears. *Arthroscopy* 2012;28(9):1306-1314.

51. Jeong JY, Pan HL, Song SY, Lee SM, Yoo JC: Arthroscopic subscapularis repair using single-row mattress suture technique: Clinical results and structural integrity. *J Shoulder Elbow Surg* 2018;27(4):711-719.

A level IV study of isolated or combined arthroscopic subscapularis repairs in 68 patients with short-term follow-up demonstrated a high healing rate (91%) using a single-row mattress technique. Constant and ASES scores improved significantly (50 and 47 preoperative versus 76 and 81 postoperative, respectively), but a small strength deficit (mean 0.7 kg in belly-press position, $P = 0.015$) persisted compared with the contralateral shoulder. Level of evidence: IV.

Chapter 19

Arthroscopic Management of Multidirectional Instability

Perry O. Hooper, DO • Brett McCoy, MD • Michael J. Griesser, MD • Anthony Miniaci, MD

ABSTRACT

Patients with multidirectional instability (MDI) can be a challenging entity to treat. Although commonly seen in young repetitive overhead athletes such as swimmers, MDI is not limited to this population. Bilateral involvement, frank instability events, and activities where pain occurs should all be gleaned during the initial evaluation of the patient. The physical examination portion should include a generalized ligamentous laxity evaluation and visualization of dynamic scapular movements along with a thorough shoulder examination. It is prudent to send MDI patients to dedicated formal physical therapy, typically 6 months, before entertaining a surgical procedure. However, certain patient populations may respond poorly to physical therapy and benefit from surgical intervention. Arthroscopic plication management and open capsular shift surgeries yield similar patient-reported outcomes and equivalent risks of postoperative instability events. Arthroscopic thermal shrinkage should not be included as a treatment measure in the MDI population. Surgical technique pearls include avoidance of overtightening leading to loss of motion and attention to the proximity of the axillary nerve to avoid injury.

Keywords: atraumatic; instability; multidirectional; shoulder

Dr. Griesser or an immediate family member serves as a board member, owner, officer, or committee member of the Society of Tennis Medicine and Science. Dr. Miniaci or an immediate family member has received royalties from Arthrosurface; is a member of a speakers' bureau or has made paid presentations on behalf of Arthrosurface; serves as a paid consultant to or is an employee of Arthrosurface and Trice; has stock or stock options held in Arthrosurface, DePuy, A Johnson & Johnson Company, Medtronic, Stryker, Trice, and Zimmer; has received research or institutional support from Arthrosurface; has received nonincome support (such as equipment or services), commercially derived honoraria, or other non–research-related funding (such as paid travel) from Arthrosurface and Stryker; and serves as a board member, owner, officer, or committee member of the American Orthopaedic Society for Sports Medicine, the American Shoulder and Elbow Surgeons, the Arthroscopy Association of North America, and the International Society of Arthroscopy, Knee Surgery, and Orthopaedic Sports Medicine. Neither of the following authors nor any immediate family member has received anything of value from or has stock or stock options held in a commercial company or institution related directly or indirectly to the subject of this chapter: Dr. Hooper and Dr. McCoy.

Introduction

Although the understanding of shoulder instability has improved through advances in preclinical, clinical research, and imaging, multidirectional instability (MDI) continues to be a difficult clinical diagnosis. This complex condition was first described in 1980 and has since been extensively studied.[1] MDI is defined as symptomatic, involuntary instability of the glenohumeral joint in two or more directions (inferior, anterior, and posterior).[2] The mnemonic AMBRI (*a*traumatic, *m*ultidirectional, *b*ilateral, *r*ehabilitation, *i*nferior capsular shift) has been used to describe MDI.[3] However, many inconsistencies in the characterization and the description of MDI have made it difficult to define its prevalence and compare research results.[4]

Despite published results indicating a good or an excellent outcome for more than 80% of patients after nonsurgical treatment including physical therapy,[5] not all patients improve with therapy alone. For these patients, open or arthroscopic surgical stabilization may be indicated.[6] The initial open surgical treatments focused on reducing laxity by decreasing joint volume with capsular retensioning, specifically in the inferior region.[7] Improved arthroscopic techniques and instrumentation and an improved understanding of pathoanatomy have led to the development of minimally invasive surgical methods for treating this complex condition.[8-10]

This chapter is adapted from McCpy B, Hussain WM, Griesser MJ, Miniaci A: Arthroscopic treatment of multidirectional instability, in Nicholson MD, ed: *Orthopaedic Knowledge Update: Shoulder and Elbow*, ed 4. Rosemont, IL, American Academy of Orthopaedic Surgeons, 2013, pp 297-305.

Pathoanatomy

The glenohumeral articulation allows excellent range of motion in the shoulder. Disruption of the delicate balance between stability and flexibility can predispose an individual to MDI. It is important to understand that laxity is not directly correlated with instability, and to some extent, both dynamic and static restraints may be able to compensate for structurally deficient elements. Laxity does play an important role, however, and it can become symptomatic when compensatory mechanisms fail.[11] In contrast to patients with traumatic instability, patients with laxity may have an isolated labrocapsular laxity without a definite labral tear. Nonetheless, patients with chronic instability from MDI can have secondary labral pathology, including tearing, despite the primarily atraumatic nature of the condition.[9,12]

The static stabilizing structures of the shoulder include both bony and ligamentous elements. The shallow concavity of the glenoid acts with the labrum to provide a minor but key contribution to shoulder stability; investigators have observed relatively flat cup surfaces in patients with MDI, compared with normal control patients.[11,13] A very small labrum can contribute to an overall decrease in effective glenoid depth. Glenoid version also can contribute to a propensity for instability.[11] The capsular ligaments, including the superior, middle, and inferior glenohumeral ligaments, have been well characterized; they serve to resist joint translation by reciprocally tightening or loosening, depending on extremity position. An absence or a deficiency of any of these structures can increase the predisposition to instability. Likewise, a defect in the rotator cuff interval has been proposed to increase the amount of inferior translation and may be present in MDI.[2,14] Conversely, a magnetic resonance arthrography evaluation found that the interval between the subscapularis and the supraspinatus (reflecting the size of the rotator cuff interval) was no greater in patients with MDI than in patients with other types of instability.[15] Dynamic stabilization occurs through musculotendinous elements that are most active in the midarc of the shoulder range of motion, where the capsuloligamentous structures are least effective.[2] The scapula provides a stable base for muscle activation creating precise concavity/compression ball and socket kinematics throughout arm motion.[16] Abnormalities or imbalances in the trapezius, rhomboid, and serratus anterior muscles can affect scapular rotation and ultimately shoulder stability. A study that confirmed the presence of abnormal scapular kinematics in patients with MDI emphasized the importance of incorporating directed stability exercises during rehabilitation.[17] The supraspinatus, infraspinatus, and teres minor vectors increase the contact force between the humeral head and the glenoid through concavity compression.[16] The muscle bellies of the rotator cuff serve as a direct reinforcement or block to prevent abnormal joint motion.[11] Active neuromuscular control and intact proprioceptive feedback mechanisms are necessary for functional dynamic stability of the glenohumeral joint. Differences in rotator cuff function were observed and the electromyography results of patients with MDI were compared with those of normal control patients during pulling, forward punching, elevation, and overhead throwing motions.[18] The irregularities in shoulders with MDI may diminish the ability of the rotator cuff to process and adjust its responses based on small variations in afferent proprioceptive input.

Variations in collagen and elastin may be present in patients with MDI compared with normal control patients. When collagen cross-links, collagen fibril diameter and density, and amino acid and elastin composition were compared, histochemical differences were found in tissue from shoulders with MDI or unidirectional instability compared with normal joints. Capsule from shoulders undergoing revision surgery for MDI differed from tissue harvested from shoulders undergoing primary surgical intervention for MDI. These analyses suggest an underlying connective tissue disorder in this cohort of patients with MDI.[19]

In addition to these factors, the presence of a large, redundant inferior capsule and the accompanying loss of negative intra-articular joint pressure may contribute to MDI. An increase in capsular volume is believed to contribute to a decrease in negative pressure that impairs stability. A cadaver study evaluated intra-articular pressure after capsular shift, before and after venting of the joint. Although the inferior capsular shift decreased joint volume and increased the responsiveness of intra-articular pressure to downward loading, the humeral head dislocated inferiorly in all specimens after venting, even after imbrication.[20] The labrum also is atypical in patients with MDI, and the capsulolabral complex does not have the bumper effect found in normal shoulders.

Clinical Evaluation

The diagnosis of MDI primarily is based on the clinical history and the physical examination. The patient's history may be characterized by nonspecific, activity-related shoulder pain that typically begins before the age of 30 years. The primary symptom can range from pain to instability. Decreases in athletic performance and strength may be present, with extremity numbness or paresthesias to a lesser extent.[11] Information as to the frequency, reproducibility, and severity of the symptoms as well as inciting or alleviating positions or activities can provide invaluable insight to the extent and the direction of instability. Connective tissue disorders, such as Ehlers-Danlos syndrome, with associated laxity and joint hypermobility are not uncommon in patients diagnosed with MDI, and both shoulders may be affected. Multidirectional laxity is most prevalent among repetitive overhead athletes, such as swimmers, volleyball players, and gymnasts.[11] Patients with relatively severe symptoms may have instability during more subtle activities, such as overhead lifting, holding objects at the side, or changing position while sleeping.[2,21]

Symptomatic MDI frequently is a result of repetitive microtrauma leading to capsular laxity.[7] Less commonly, a single inciting trauma or event may initiate symptoms. The clinician must maintain heightened awareness to ensure an appropriate diagnosis. MDI can appear as shoulder instability without anatomic injury, in contrast to anterior unilateral instability, which typically appears as anterior-inferior capsulolabral damage. MDI always should be considered in patients younger than 40 years who have persistent symptoms despite surgical stabilization.[11]

A patient who is able to voluntarily dislocate the shoulder can selectively control muscle contraction and relaxation to induce repetitive instability.[2] Voluntary dislocation often is associated with an emotional or a psychiatric disorder, and these patients typically have a poor outcome after surgical stabilization.[22] It is important to differentiate patients whose dislocation is related to secondary gain from those who are able to voluntarily induce shoulder dislocation but are careful to avoid provocative maneuvers or positions. These patients often self-protect or autoregulate positional instability, and typically they respond well to surgical stabilization.[11]

The physical examination begins with a visual inspection, with careful observation of any muscular atrophy, scapular asymmetry, or winging. Generalized laxity can be seen as metacarpal hyperextension, thumb-to-wrist opposition, knee and elbow recurvatum, patellar instability, or pes planus (**Figure 1**). The patient may exhibit a sulcus sign, characterized as a gap below the lateral border of the acromion when an inferiorly directed stress is applied to a relaxed adducted shoulder. A sulcus sign seen when the distal extremity is in external rotation (thereby increasing tension on the superior glenohumeral ligament) confirms greater laxity related to the superior glenohumeral ligament.

Although the diagnosis of MDI primarily is based on the history and the physical examination, radiographic images should be obtained. The primary purpose is to rule out an anatomic defect or assess for concomitant structural shoulder pathology, such as a Hill-Sachs or a reverse Hill-Sachs lesion or an avulsion of the glenohumeral ligaments. MRI can be obtained to assess the capsular anatomy, the labrum, the rotator cuff, and the biceps. CT is useful for assessing bone quality or defects.[7] In patients who have had unsuccessful earlier surgery for MDI, attention should be focused on the function and the strength of the individual rotator cuff muscles, particularly the subscapularis. Internal rotation strength may be decreased by as much as 30%, resulting in a loss of dynamic stabilization.[21,23]

Nonsurgical and Surgical Management Considerations

Determining the appropriate treatment of patients with a diagnosis of MDI requires careful interpretation of both subjective and objective findings. An algorithm to guide clinicians through this process is presented in **Figure 2**. It is important to note that patients whose pain is a key component of the clinical picture may have an etiology unrelated to hyperlaxity. Thus, the painful shoulder in a patient with MDI requires a broad differential diagnosis and a thorough workup. Any asymmetry discovered in the physical examination for instability requires an evaluation for mechanical derangement (eg, a labral or Bankart injury or a superior labrum anterior to posterior tear), in addition to MDI.

Nonsurgical Management

Nonsurgical management is considered the first-line treatment for most patients with MDI. Rehabilitation should treat scapulothoracic dyskinesia and include proprioceptive exercises and rotator cuff strengthening. A study of the nonsurgical management of MDI found that 35

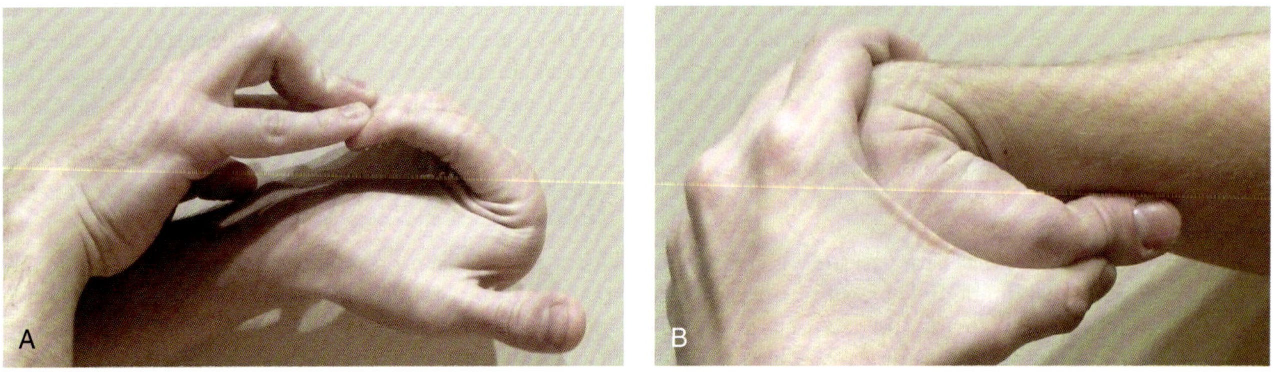

FIGURE 1 Photographs showing metacarpophalangeal hyperextension (**A**) and thumb-to-wrist opposition (**B**).

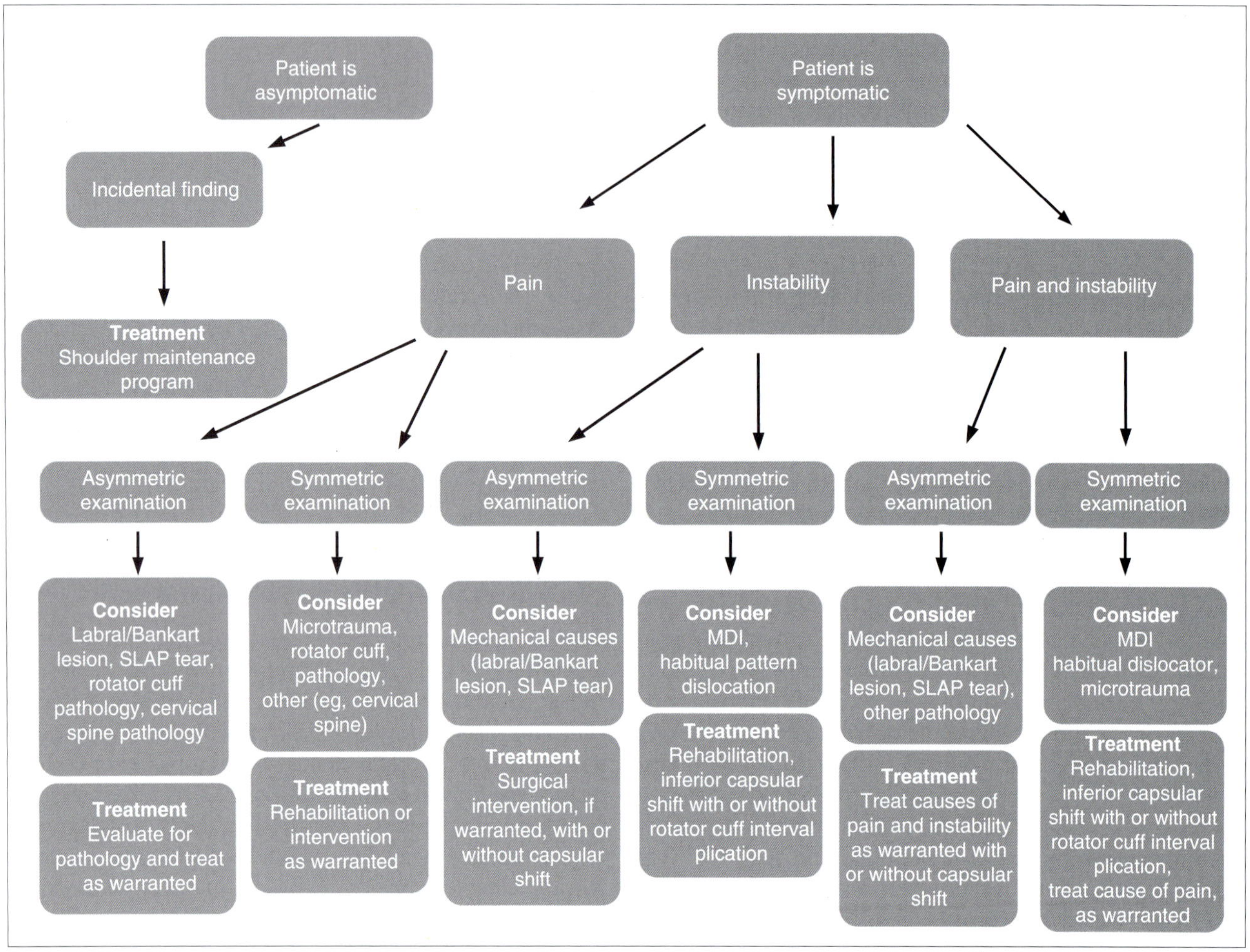

FIGURE 2 A flowchart for clinical use in deciding whether a patient has multidirectional instability (MDI) on the basis of the patient's primary symptoms and the clinician's examination findings, with treatment options based on the diagnosis.

of 39 patients had a good or an excellent result.[5] Subsequent research with long-term follow-up determined that young athletic patients have a relatively poor response to nonsurgical management; 49% of nonsurgically treated patients had a poor result, and 37% required surgery.[24] Shoulder kinematics were found not to return to normal with physical therapy alone, but a combination of therapy and capsular shift had adequately restored normal kinematics at 4-year follow-up.[25] Despite these findings, a minimum 6-month course of physical therapy was recommended before any surgical intervention.[25]

Surgical Manangement

Surgical intervention is reserved for patients with persistent disability despite rehabilitation. The goal of surgery is to treat the pathologic structures, and the focus is on decreasing the capsular volume using capsuloligamentous techniques. It is important to distinguish true MDI from traumatic instability in a patient with systemic hyperlaxity. In the original description of inferior capsular shift, more than half of the patients had an instability episode precipitated by significant trauma.[1] Although the presence of diffuse laxity in the setting of a Bankart repair was found to increase the failure rate, this is a different entity from true MDI.[26] The surgeon should carefully consider whether the patient's condition is a traumatic labral tear rather than true MDI. Relevant patient population data from the literature should be examined when making the diagnosis.

Arthroscopic Management Considerations

Historically, open procedures have been used to surgically treat MDI, but laboratory data have shown that open and arthroscopic surgery achieve a comparable amount of volume reduction.[27] In a cadaver model, 1-cm plication stitches decreased capsular volume by 10%, and five plication stitches achieved a volume reduction similar to that of an open shift.[28] A clinical study using the American Shoulder and Elbow Surgeons (ASES) Shoulder Index found a statistically favorable response to arthroscopic compared with open procedures. Patients with earlier surgery had a relatively low ASES score.[29] A 2012 systematic review of seven studies comparing open and arthroscopic treatment of MDI found no significant difference in recurrent instability, return to sports, loss of external rotation, or rate of complications. There was a slight trend toward improved return to sports after arthroscopic treatment.[30] This review appropriately excluded patients with a Bankart lesion but contained only level IV studies. This thought was further emphasized in a 2015 systematic review comparing open to arthroscopic surgical intervention in 861 shoulders, largely looking at postoperative instability events. The findings concluded equivalent risk for subsequent instability between the two surgical approaches with a dislocation rate of 7.5% and 7.8% in the open and arthroscopic treatments, respectively. The findings are difficult to interpret because of the inherent variation in disease processes and specific mechanisms of treatment. However, the literature suggests that in experienced hands, arthroscopic treatment can achieve the similar results as open surgery.[31] The arthroscopic treatment of MDI involves different techniques, the most common of which involve a capsular plication and/or rotator cuff interval closure. Thermal capsulorrhaphy has fallen out of favor because of reported high rates of failure, chondrolysis, and nerve injury.[31-33] Multiple laboratory studies have evaluated specific techniques for arthroscopic treatment. One study found that capsular plication alone decreased excess motion, but an additional rotator cuff interval closure was necessary to decrease glenohumeral translation.[34] A medial-lateral rotator cuff interval closure more effectively decreased posterior translation than a superior-inferior technique.[35] A comparison of three types of plication stitches found that the simple stitch was comparable to the figure-of-8 and mattress configurations.[35]

Limited clinical data are available on the outcomes of the arthroscopic treatment of MDI. Most of the studies extend only to midterm follow-up, and many of them include patients with a Bankart lesion. A retrospective study of 40 patients at 2- to 5-year follow-up after arthroscopic treatment of MDI found that 91% had satisfactory range of motion, 86% were able to return to sports with minimal or no limitation, and clinical outcome scores were good.[8] In a study of nine young overhead athletes with MDI who were treated with capsular plication and rotator cuff interval closure, seven had a good or an excellent result; seven returned to sports, but three returned at a lower level.[36]

Arthroscopic Technique

The examination under anesthesia is the first surgical step. All patients with MDI have inferior instability, but it is important to determine whether the primary direction is anterior or posterior. These findings should be compared with those of the contralateral shoulder. After the examination, the patient is positioned in the beach chair or the lateral position.

Establishing the posterior portal in a relatively lateral position is useful for subsequent capsular and labral work. One or two anterior portals should be established in the rotator cuff interval (**Figure 3**). A thorough diagnostic inspection of the shoulder should be conducted, with attention to the patulous nature of the rotator cuff interval and assessment for a Bankart-type labral injury (**Figure 4**). In MDI, the labrum may have some minor changes but should remain attached. Traction on the humerus will lead to a positive drive-through sign, which involves passing the scope from posterosuperior to anterior-inferior without obstruction from the glenohumeral joint (**Figure 5**).

Different treatment strategies exist for capsular plication and rotator cuff interval imbrication. Foremost, the surgeon should be aware of the axillary nerve that runs approximately 12.4 mm below the 6-o'clock position of

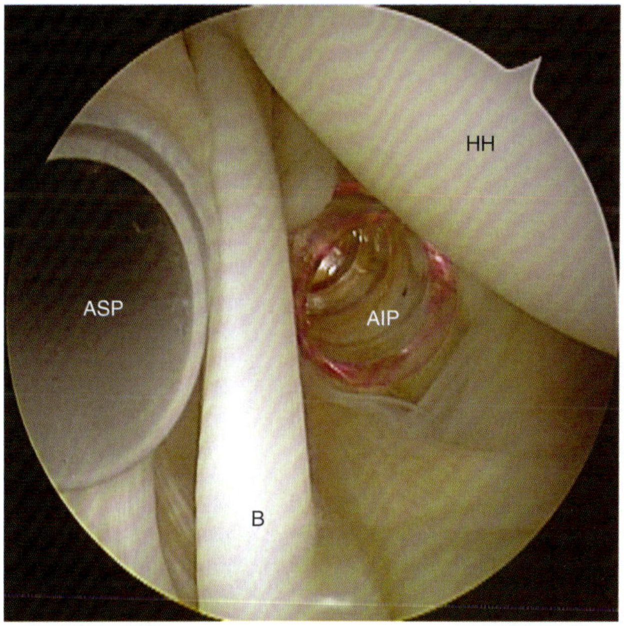

FIGURE 3 Arthroscopic image showing the anterosuperior portal (ASP) used for viewing and the anterior-inferior portal (AIP) used for instrumentation. B = biceps, HH = humeral head. (Reproduced from Ryu RKN: Multidirectional instability, in Galatz LM, ed: *Orthopaedic Knowledge Update: Shoulder and Elbow*, ed 3. Rosemont, IL, American Academy of Orthopaedic Surgeons, 2008, pp 303-312.)

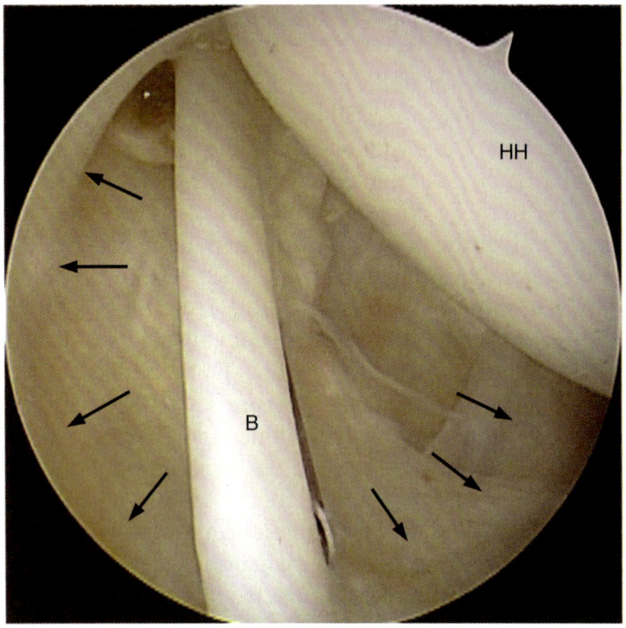

FIGURE 4 Arthroscopic image showing the patulous rotator cuff interval (arrows). B = biceps, HH = humeral head. (Reproduced from Ryu RKN: Multidirectional instability, in Galatz LM, ed: *Orthopaedic Knowledge Update: Shoulder and Elbow*, ed 3. Rosemont, IL, American Academy of Orthopaedic Surgeons, 2008, pp 303-312.)

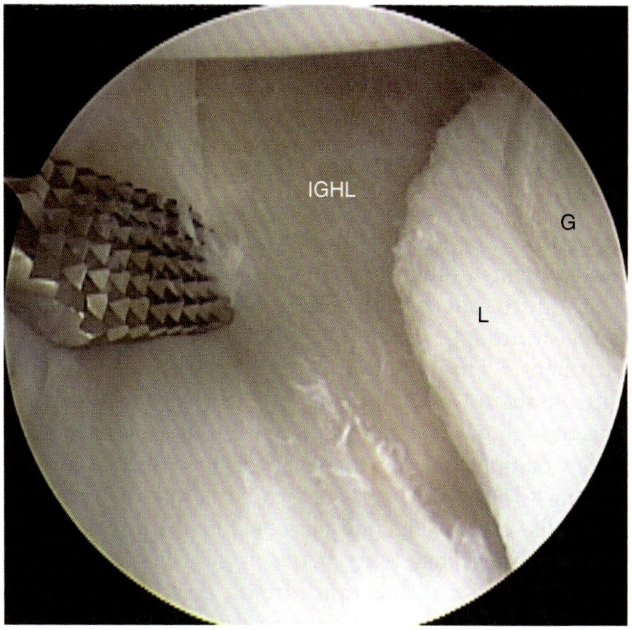

FIGURE 6 Arthroscopic image from the anterosuperior portal, showing careful rasping of the capsule to generate a healing response. G = glenoid, IGHL = inferior glenohumeral ligament, L = labrum. (Reproduced from Ryu RKN: Multidirectional instability, in Galatz LM, ed: *Orthopaedic Knowledge Update: Shoulder and Elbow*, ed 3. Rosemont, IL, American Academy of Orthopaedic Surgeons, 2008, pp 303-312.)

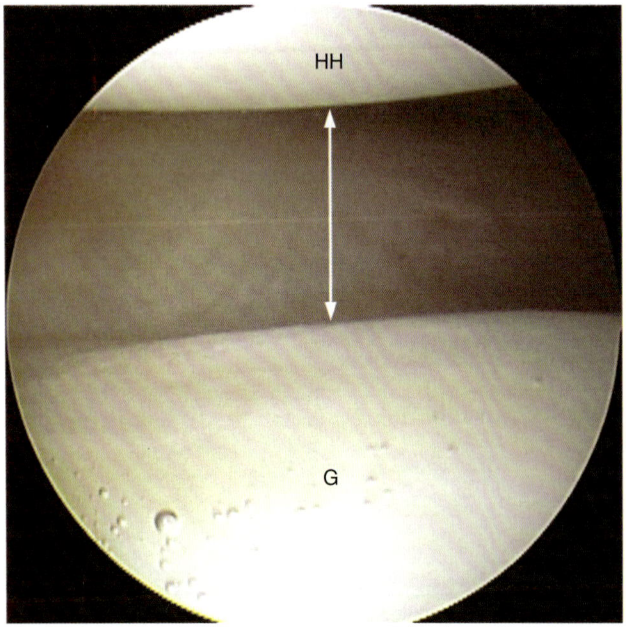

FIGURE 5 Arthroscopic image showing a positive drive-through sign (arrow). G = glenoid, HH = humeral head. (Reproduced from Ryu RKN: Multidirectional instability, in Galatz LM, ed: *Orthopaedic Knowledge Update: Shoulder and Elbow*, ed 3. Rosemont, IL, American Academy of Orthopaedic Surgeons, 2008, pp 303-312.)

the glenoid and can be protected by positioning the arm in abduction, external rotation, and slight traction.[37,38] Capsular abrasion is performed first and is followed by capsular plication in a sequential pattern that generally begins in the area of primary instability (anterior or posterior, **Figure 6**). It is important to progress from inferior to superior because each plication decreases the volume of the joint and thus inhibits visualization (**Figure 7**). Care must be taken to avoid shifting tissue in a medial to lateral direction because doing so can reduce the rotational motion of the shoulder. After treating the primary direction of instability, the tissue opposite the primary direction of instability is shifted to create a balanced shoulder (**Figure 8**). The centering of the humeral head on the glenoid is checked after sutures are in place, and the shoulder is taken through a range of motion. Sutures may rupture; they also can be removed and retensioned if there are limitations of motion. The sutures can be passed around the capsule and the labrum, or a glenoid suture anchor can be used. The optimal number of sutures, suture configuration, and suture material has not been determined. The senior author prefers three fiber wire suture anchors but will not hesitate to deploy more if the size and capsular laxity warrants it.

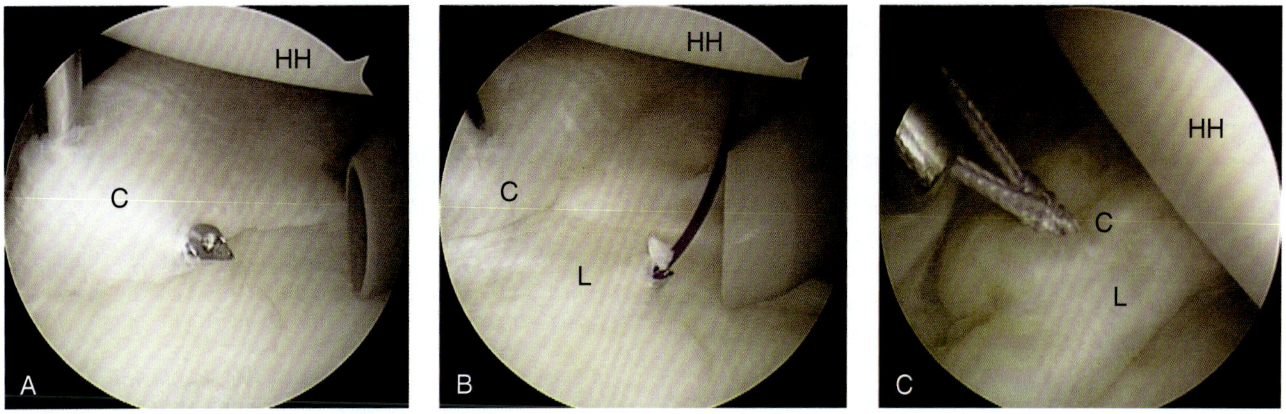

FIGURE 7 Arthroscopic images showing capsular tissue captured with first pass and shifted superiorly before the labrum is engaged (**A**); the suture hook passing through the labrum as the second step, with passage of absorbable suture (**B**); and knot tying on the capsular side of the tissue (**C**). C = capsular tissue, G = glenoid, HH = humeral head, L = labrum, PC = posterior cannula. (Reproduced from Ryu RKN: Multidirectional instability, in Galatz LM, ed: *Orthopaedic Knowledge Update: Shoulder and Elbow*, ed 3. Rosemont, IL, American Academy of Orthopaedic Surgeons, 2008, pp 303-312.)

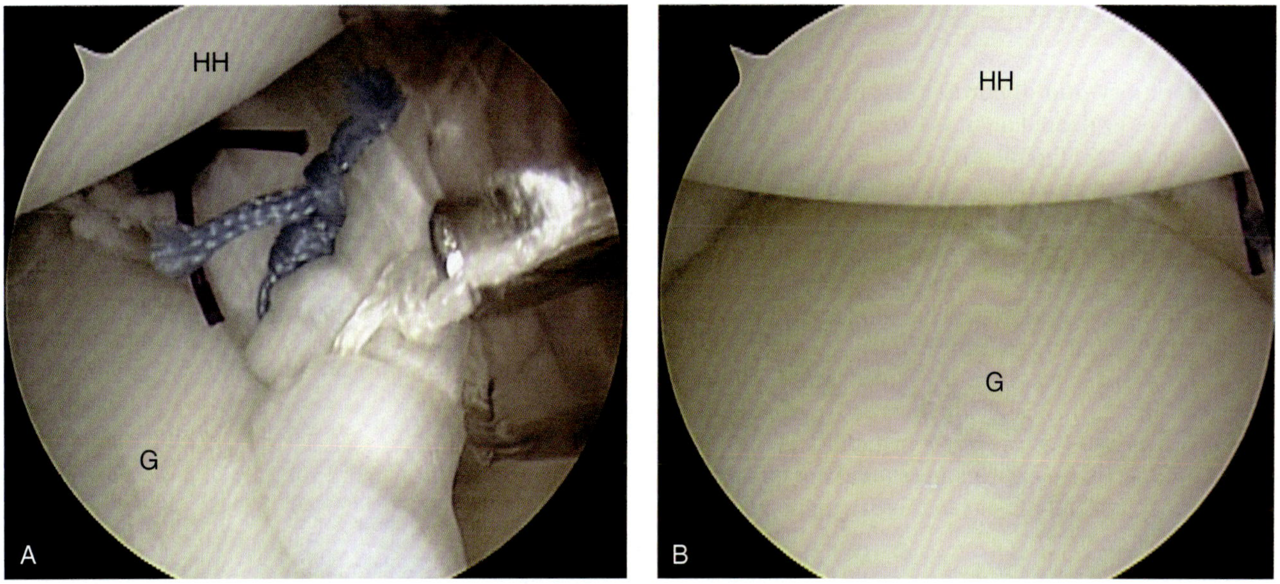

FIGURE 8 Arthroscopic images showing posterior capsular plication after the anterior-inferior component was treated (**A**), and the humeral head is balanced and well centered on the glenoid face after multiple plication sutures, as seen from the anterosuperior portal (**B**). G = glenoid, HH = humeral head. (Reproduced from Ryu RKN: Multidirectional instability, in Galatz LM, ed: *Orthopaedic Knowledge Update: Shoulder and Elbow*, ed 3. Rosemont, IL, American Academy of Orthopaedic Surgeons, 2008, pp 303-312.)

The role of rotator cuff interval closure is controversial. Most data supporting rotator interval closure are limited to cadaver studies, and there is minimal high-level clinical evidence. One study suggests no improvement in inferior instability but a decrease in motion.[15] It is important to avoid overtightening and a subsequent loss of external rotation; this can be prevented by positioning the arm in approximately 20° to 30° of external rotation during the repair. The techniques include both medial-lateral and superior-inferior closures.

Immobilization and Rehabilitation

Immobilization after surgery can be in a neutral position or in a position based on the direction of primary instability. For example, patients with posteroinferior instability can be immobilized in external rotation. Because postoperative stiffness is much less common than residual laxity after surgery for MDI, the recommendation is to proceed slowly with rehabilitation. Sling immobilization is maintained for 6 weeks (or a longer period if the joint remains supple). A gradual return of motion is obtained over a period as long as 6 months.

SUMMARY

MDI is a difficult clinical entity in terms of both diagnosis and management. It is important to appreciate that true MDI is atraumatic in nature. The first-line treatment is rehabilitation, but some data suggest that certain patients respond poorly to nonsurgical management. The current evidence for surgical intervention is not well defined with limitations in the heterogeneity of patients and treatment, but multiple studies suggest that arthroscopic treatment of MDI can achieve similar goals to open treatment. Continued higher level research in a prospective manner is warranted to define specific recommendations regarding surgical technique.

KEY STUDY POINTS

- Hyperlaxity and abnormal scapular movements should be evaluated on physical examination in the atraumatic MDI patient.
- Patients with atraumatic MDI should undergo formal physical therapy emphasizing periscapular exercises as a primary treatment before entertaining surgical intervention.
- Surgical intervention can be warranted after six months of conservative measures.
- Arthroscopic plication management and open capsular shift surgeries yield similar patient-reported outcomes and postoperative instability events. Arthroscopic thermal shrinkage should not be included as a treatment measure in this patient population.

Annotated References

1. Neer CS II, Foster CR: Inferior capsular shift for involuntary inferior and multidirectional instability of the shoulder: A preliminary report. *J Bone Joint Surg Am* 1980;62(6):897-908.

2. Bahu MJ, Trentacosta N, Vorys GC, Covey AS, Ahmad CS: Multidirectional instability: Evaluation and treatment options. *Clin Sports Med* 2008;27(4):671-689.

3. Thomas SC, Matsen FA III: An approach to the repair of avulsion of the glenohumeral ligaments in the management of traumatic anterior glenohumeral instability. *J Bone Joint Surg Am* 1989;71(4):506-513.

4. McFarland EG, Kim TK, Park HB, Neira CA, Gutierrez MI: The effect of variation in definition on the diagnosis of multidirectional instability of the shoulder. *J Bone Joint Surg Am* 2003;85(11):2138-2144.

5. Burkhead WZ Jr, Rockwood CA Jr: Treatment of instability of the shoulder with an exercise program. *J Bone Joint Surg Am* 1992;74(6):890-896.

6. Caprise PA Jr, Sekiya JK: Open and arthroscopic treatment of multidirectional instability of the shoulder. *Arthroscopy* 2006;22(10):1126-1131.

7. Cole B: *Surgical Techniques of the Shoulder, Elbow, and Knee in Sports Medicine*. Philadelphia, PA, WB Saunders, 2008.

8. Baker CL III, Mascarenhas R, Kline AJ, Chhabra A, Pombo MW, Bradley JP: Arthroscopic treatment of multidirectional shoulder instability in athletes: A retrospective analysis of 2- to 5-year clinical outcomes. *Am J Sports Med* 2009;37(9):1712-1720.

9. Alpert JM, Verma N, Wysocki R, Yanke AB, Romeo AA: Arthroscopic treatment of multidirectional shoulder instability with minimum 270 degrees labral repair: Minimum 2-year follow-up. *Arthroscopy* 2008;24(6): 704-711.

10. ElAttrache NS: *Surgical Techniques in Sports Medicine*. Philadelphia, PA, Lippincott, Williams & Wilkins, 2007.

11. Gaskill TR, Taylor DC, Millett PJ: Management of multidirectional instability of the shoulder. *J Am Acad Orthop Surg* 2011;19(12):758-767.

12. Werner AW, Lichtenberg S, Schmitz H, Nikolic A, Habermeyer P: Arthroscopic findings in atraumatic shoulder instability. *Arthroscopy* 2004;20(3): 268-272.

13. Kim SH, Noh KC, Park JS, Ryu BD, Oh I: Loss of chondrolabral containment of the glenohumeral joint in atraumatic posteroinferior multidirectional instability. *J Bone Joint Surg Am* 2005;87(1):92-98.

14. Schenk TJ, Brems JJ: Multidirectional instability of the shoulder: Pathophysiology, diagnosis, and management. *J Am Acad Orthop Surg* 1998;6(1):65-72.

15. Provencher MT, Dewing CB, Bell SJ, et al: An analysis of the rotator interval in patients with anterior, posterior, and multidirectional shoulder instability. *Arthroscopy* 2008;24(8):921-929.

16. Kibler WB, Thomas SJ, Sciascia AD: *The role of the scapula in the overhead athlete*, in *Mechanics, Pathomechanics and Injury in the Overhead Athlete*. Springer International Publishing, 2019, vol 11, pp 151-154.

17. Ogston JB, Ludewig PM: Differences in 3-dimensional shoulder kinematics between persons with multidirectional instability and asymptomatic controls. *Am J Sports Med* 2007;35(8):1361-1370.

18. Illyés A, Kiss RM: Electromyographic analysis in patients with multidirectional shoulder instability during pull, forward punch, elevation and overhead throw. *Knee Surg Sports Traumatol Arthrosc* 2007;15(5):624-631.

19. Rodeo SA, Suzuki K, Yamauchi M, Bhargava M, Warren RF: Analysis of collagen and elastic fibers in shoulder capsule in patients with shoulder instability. *Am J Sports Med* 1998;26(5):634-643.

20. Yamamoto N, Itoi E, Tuoheti Y, et al: The effect of the inferior capsular shift on shoulder intra-articular pressure: A cadaveric study. *Am J Sports Med* 2006;34(6):939-944.

21. Forsythe B, Ghodadra N, Romeo AA, Provencher MT: Management of the failed posterior/multidirectional instability patient. *Sports Med Arthrosc Rev* 2010;18(3):149-161.

22. Rowe CR, Pierce DS, Clark JG: Voluntary dislocation of the shoulder: A preliminary report on a clinical, electromyographic, and psychiatric study of twenty-six patients. *J Bone Joint Surg Am* 1973;55(3):445-460.

23. Warner JJ, Micheli LJ, Arslanian LE, Kennedy J, Kennedy R: Patterns of flexibility, laxity, and strength in normal shoulders and shoulders with instability and impingement. *Am J Sports Med* 1990;18(4):366-375.

24. Misamore GW, Sallay PI, Didelot W: A longitudinal study of patients with multidirectional instability of the shoulder with seven- to ten-year follow-up. *J Shoulder Elbow Surg* 2005;14(5):466-470.

25. Nyiri P, Illyés A, Kiss R, Kiss J: Intermediate biomechanical analysis of the effect of physiotherapy only compared with capsular shift and physiotherapy in multidirectional shoulder instability. *J Shoulder Elbow Surg* 2010;19(6):802-813.

26. Chechik O, Maman E, Dolkart O, Khashan M, Shabtai L, Mozes G: Arthroscopic rotator interval closure in shoulder instability repair: A retrospective study. *J Shoulder Elbow Surg* 2010;19(7):1056-1062.

27. Sekiya JK, Willobee JA, Miller MD, Hickman AJ, Willobee A: Arthroscopic multi-pleated capsular plication compared with open inferior capsular shift for reduction of shoulder volume in a cadaveric model. *Arthroscopy* 2007;23(11):1145-1151.

28. Ponce BA, Rosenzweig SD, Thompson KJ, Tokish J: Sequential volume reduction with capsular plications: Relationship between cumulative size of plications and volumetric reduction for multidirectional instability of the shoulder. *Am J Sports Med* 2011;39(3):526-531.

29. Yeargan SA III, Briggs KK, Horan MP, Black AK, Hawkins RJ: Determinants of patient satisfaction following surgery for multidirectional instability. *Orthopedics* 2008;31(7):647.

30. Jacobson ME, Riggenbach M, Wooldridge AN, Bishop JY: Open capsular shift and arthroscopic capsular plication for treatment of multidirectional instability. *Arthroscopy* 2012;28(7):1010-1017.

31. Longo UG, Rizzello G, Loppini M, et al: Multidirectional instability of the shoulder: A systematic review. *Arthroscopy* 2015:31(12):2431-2443.

    A systematic review of 24 articles evaluated postoperative instability in 861 shoulders treated surgically with either arthroscopic plication, arthroscopic thermal shrinkage, arthroscopic laser-assisted capsulorrhaphy, or open capsular shift. Findings found risk of subsequent instability event was equal between open capsular shift and arthroscopic plication with both approaches superior in this regard to arthroscopic thermal shrinkage and arthroscopic laser-assisted capsulorraphy. Level of evidence: IV.

32. D'Alessandro DF, Bradley JP, Fleischli JE, Connor PM: Prospective evaluation of thermal capsulorrhaphy for shoulder instability: Indications and results, two- to five-year follow-up. *Am J Sports Med* 2004;32(1): 21-33.

33. Hawkins RJ, Krishnan SG, Karas SG, Noonan TJ, Horan MP: Electrothermal arthroscopic shoulder capsulorrhaphy: A minimum 2-year follow-up. *Am J Sports Med* 2007;35(9):1484-1488.

34. Shafer BL, Mihata T, McGarry MH, Tibone JE, Lee TQ: Effects of capsular plication and rotator interval closure in simulated multidirectional shoulder instability. *J Bone Joint Surg Am* 2008;90(1):136-144.

35. Farber AJ, ElAttrache NS, Tibone JE, McGarry MH, Lee TQ: Biomechanical analysis comparing a traditional superior-inferior arthroscopic rotator interval closure with a novel medial-lateral technique in a cadaveric multidirectional instability model. *Am J Sports Med* 2009;37(6):1178-1185.

36. Voigt C, Schulz AP, Lill H: Arthroscopic treatment of multidirectional glenohumeral instability in young overhead athletes. *Open Orthop J* 2009;3:107-114.

37. Uno A, Bain GI, Mehta JA: Arthroscopic relationship of the axillary nerve to the shoulder joint capsule: An anatomic study. *J Shoulder Elbow Surg* 1999;8(3):226-230.

38. Price MR, Tillett ED, Acland RD, Nettleton GS: Determining the relationship of the axillary nerve to the shoulder joint capsule from an arthroscopic perspective. *J Bone Joint Surg Am* 2004;86(10):2135-2142.

Chapter 20

Superior Labrum Anterior to Posterior Lesions

James R. Andrews, MD • Meares Green, DO • Brett Shore, MD

ABSTRACT

In 1990, the term superior labrum anterior to posterior (SLAP) was applied to lesions of the superior labrum involving the long head of biceps, most notably in high-level overhead athletes. The proposed mechanisms for SLAP tear etiology are controversial and multiple theories have been hypothesized. In patients with symptomatic SLAP lesions, a thorough history and physical examination should be performed, including multiple tests to evaluate for labral pathology and shoulder instability. The management for SLAP lesions consists of nonsurgical and surgical options depending on multiple factors: age, activity level, symptoms, season versus off season, and tear type. Nonsurgical management can be attempted in low-demand and high-demand patients with an emphasis on rest from aggravating activities, NSAIDs, posterior capsular stretching, and rotator cuff strengthening. Surgical options can be considered after failed conservative treatment or acutely in a high-level athlete. The choice of surgical treatment is dependent on the type of lesion present and can include débridement, repair, débridement plus repair, or biceps tenodesis. Outcomes following SLAP repair have been variable in high-level athletes with difficulty in regaining preinjury health and performance but still this remains to be a good option.

Keywords: biceps; labral tear; overhead athlete; shoulder; SLAP

Dr. Andrews or an immediate family member has received royalties from Biomet Sports Medicine; serves as a paid consultant to or is an employee of Biomet Sports Medicine, Bauerfiend, Theralase, MiMedx, and Physiotherapy Associates; has stock or stock options held in Contessa Health, Patient Connection, and Connective Orthopaedics; has received research or institutional support from MiMedx; and serves as a board member, owner, officer, or committee member of the American Sports Medicine Institute, Board Member, the Andrews Research & Education Foundation Board Member, Contessa Health Advisory Board, FastHealth Advisor Board, MiMedx Advisory Board, Robins/Morton Board Member, Select Medical National Medical Director, and Theralase Advisory Board. Neither of the following authors nor any immediate family member has received anything of value from or has stock or stock options held in a commercial company or institution related directly or indirectly to the subject of this chapter: Dr. Green and Dr. Shore.

Introduction

Before the advent of shoulder arthroscopy, the etiology of shoulder dysfunction in the overhead athlete was believed to relate to external impingement of the undersurface of the acromion on the bursal side of the rotator cuff.[1] The primary treatment was open acromioplasty, which had poor results in overhead athletes; the failure rate was 50%, and only 22% returned to the preinjury level of play.[2] In 1985, lesions of the superior labrum associated with the long head of the biceps were first reported in high-level overhead athletes.[3] Fraying and detachment of the labrum were found, sometimes associated with tearing of the biceps tendon. These athletes also commonly had undersurface tearing of the rotator cuff. The proposed mechanism of this constellation of findings was attrition secondary to repetitive tension overloading on the rotator cuff and the biceps-labrum complex. In 1990, the term superior labrum anterior to posterior (SLAP) was applied to these lesions, and they were defined as starting posterior to the biceps anchor and extending anteriorly to involve the biceps anchor.[4] Four types of lesions were included in the initial Snyder classification, which later was expanded to include all identifiable pathology of the superior labrum. Several studies examined the pathogenesis, presentation, and treatment of SLAP lesions, thus improving understanding of these injuries and their management.

Classification

The original 4 types of SLAP lesions have been expanded to 10 types, although the original classification is still most widely used[4-6] (**Figure 1**). The interobserver reliability of this classification system has been inconsistent, although at least one study found good interobserver reliability among experienced surgeons.[7,8] A type I lesion is degenerative fraying of the inner margin of the superior labrum,

Section 4: Arthroscopy

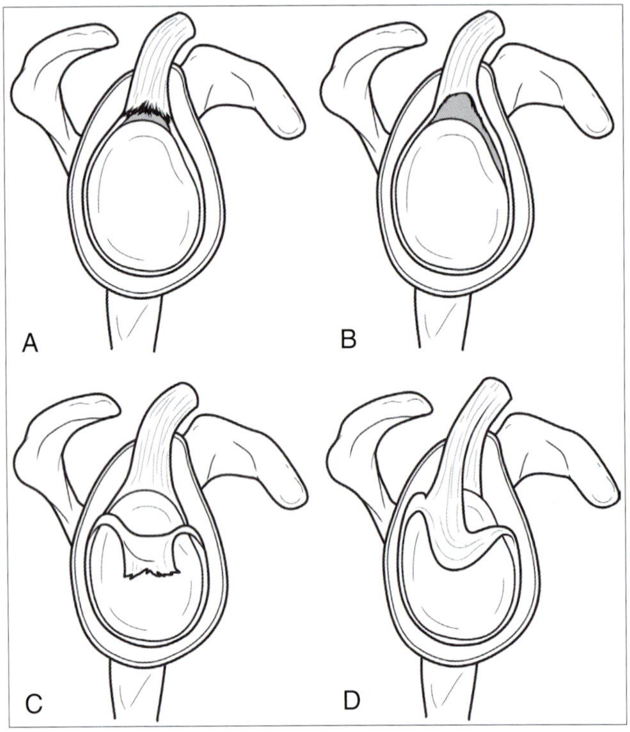

FIGURE 1 Schematic drawings showing the Snyder classification of superior labrum anterior to posterior (SLAP) lesions: types I (**A**), II (**B**), III (**C**), and IV (**D**).

without detachment of the labrum or the biceps anchor. Type I is the most common type of SLAP lesion; often it is asymptomatic and typically is found incidentally in middle-aged patients. A type II SLAP lesion is detachment of the superior labrum at the biceps insertion; this is the most common, clinically important type. Type II SLAP tears can be subcategorized as anterior, predominately posterior, or combined anterior and posterior (in relation to the biceps anchor) (**Figure 2**). Throwing athletes most commonly have posterior extension of the lesion. A type III SLAP lesion is characterized by a bucket-handle tear of the superior labrum, with displacement into the joint and an intact biceps anchor. A type IV SLAP lesion is a bucket-handle tear that extends into the biceps tendon, resulting in the appearance of a split tendon; part of the biceps anchor may still be attached to the superior glenoid. The additional Gartsman and Ryu types of SLAP lesions involve an associated instability lesion, such as a Bankart lesion, a posterior labral lesion, middle glenohumeral ligament involvement, or a 360° labral lesion (**Table 1**).

Anatomy and Biomechanics

The glenoid labrum is a fibrocartilaginous ring that surrounds and deepens the glenoid. The labrum also serves as the attachment point for the glenohumeral

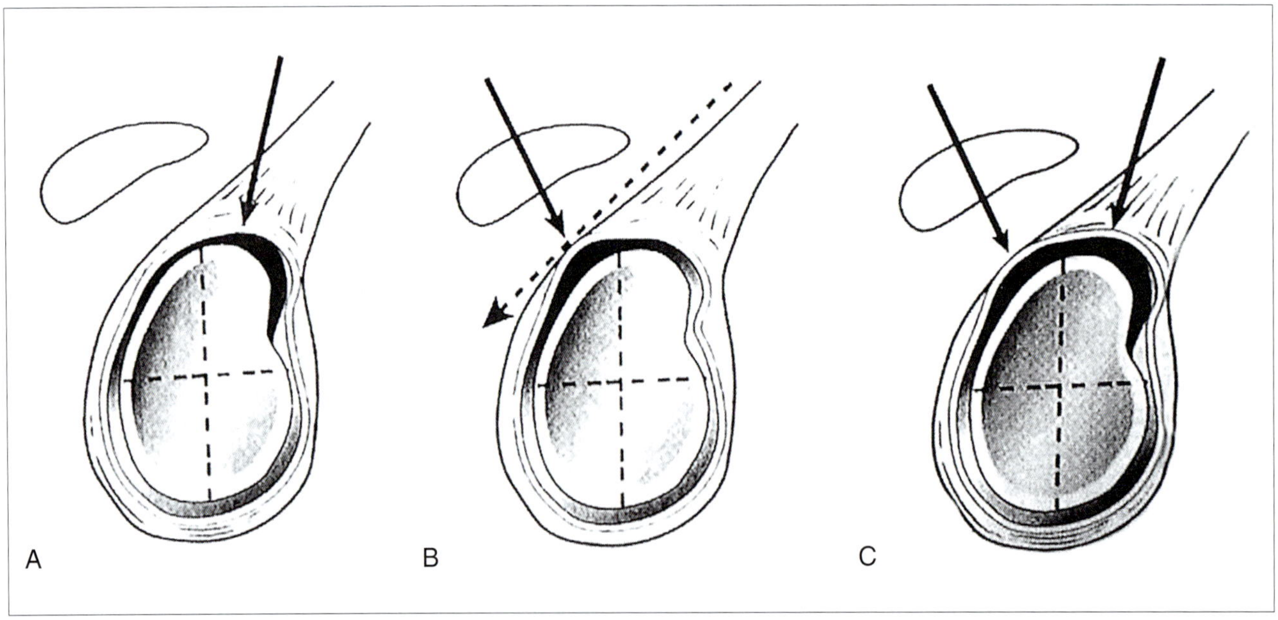

FIGURE 2 Schematic drawings showing the anterior (**A**), posterior (**B**), and combined anterior and posterior (**C**) subtypes of the Snyder type II superior labrum anterior to posterior (SLAP) lesion. Solid arrows = primary location of the tear (anterior, posterior, or combined anterior and posterior); dashed vertical and horizontal lines = glenoid quadrants; dashed arrow = orientation of the force producing a posterior SLAP tear (**B**). (Reproduced with permission from Morgan CD, Burkhart SS, Palmeri M, Gillespie M: Type II SLAP lesions: Three subtypes and their relationships to superior instability and rotator cuff tears. *Arthroscopy* 1998;14[6]:553-565.)

Table 1

The Classification of SLAP Lesions

Type	Description
I	Fraying of superior labrum
II	Detachment of biceps anchor and superior labrum
III	Bucket-handle tear of superior labrum with intact biceps anchor
IV	Bucket-handle tear of superior labrum extending into the biceps tendon
V	Extension of Bankart lesion to include detachment of the biceps anchor
VI	Anterior or posterior labral flap with type II biceps lesion
VII	Biceps anchor detachment extending into the middle glenohumeral ligament
VIII	Type II with posterior labral extension
IX	Type II with 360° labral detachment
X	Type II with posteroinferior labral detachment

SLAP = superior labrum anterior to posterior

ligaments and the biceps tendon. The superior labrum can be meniscoid in appearance and attached to the glenoid peripherally, or it can be firmly attached to the glenoid both centrally and peripherally. The long head of the biceps attaches to the posterosuperior labrum and the supraglenoid tubercle, which lies 5 mm medial to the superior glenoid rim. Approximately 40% to 60% of the biceps tendon fibers attach to the supraglenoid tubercle, with the remainder attaching directly to the labrum. The primary site of attachment of the biceps to the labrum varies; in most individuals, it attaches purely or primarily posterior, with some anterior component, but it also can be primarily anterior. The blood supply to the labrum comes through capsular and periosteal vessels that branch from the suprascapular, posterior humeral circumflex, and circumflex scapular arteries. The peripheral labrum has the greatest concentration of vessels, the central portion of the labrum is relatively avascular, and the superior labrum has the least robust blood supply.

The biceps tendon serves as a humeral head depressor and a secondary restraint to glenohumeral translation, particularly in abduction and external rotation.[9] A SLAP tear reduces resistance to external rotation force in the abducted and externally rotated position. Simulated SLAP lesions were found to increase anterior-inferior translation, increasing tension on the inferior glenohumeral ligament complex.[10] The biceps was found to have a greater stabilizing effect as glenohumeral stability decreased.[11]

The peel-back sign results from the effect of the throwing position on the superior labrum and the biceps anchor[12] (**Figure 3**). The throwing position of maximal abduction and external rotation forces the biceps tendon into a relatively posterior and vertically oriented position, twisting the posterosuperior labrum in the process. This motion is effectively resisted by the biceps anchor in an intact shoulder, but in the presence of a type II SLAP

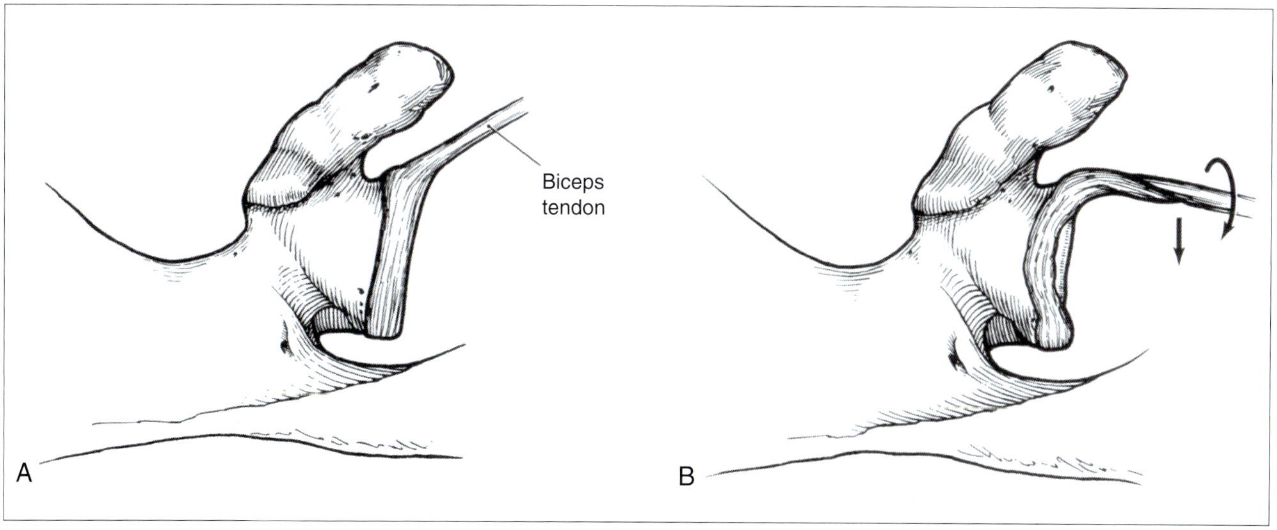

FIGURE 3 Schematic drawings showing a superior view of the resting position of the biceps anchor (**A**) and vertical force (arrows) transmitted to the posterosuperior labrum with abduction and external rotation (**B**). (Reproduced with permission from Burkhart SS, Morgan CD: The peel-back mechanism: Its role in producing and extending posterior type II SLAP lesions and its effect on SLAP repair rehabilitation. *Arthroscopy* 1998;14[6]:637-640.)

lesion, the labrum rotates medially over the glenoid and onto the posterior scapular neck. Repair of a type II SLAP lesion restores stability to the superior labrum and eliminates the peel-back sign.

Pathogenesis

The proposed mechanisms for the etiology of the SLAP lesion include repetitive overhead activity, traction, and compression, all of which have been evaluated in cadaver models. A single traumatic event is responsible for a SLAP lesion in patients who have not had an extended period of symptoms, and repetitive overhead activity is the cause specifically in throwing athletes. In a cadaver study, direct compression or impaction resulted in a SLAP lesion, particularly when the arm was flexed forward.[13] Another study found that traction with inferior subluxation consistently produced a SLAP lesion.[14]

The cause of type II SLAP lesions in overhead athletes is complex and controversial. In one proposal, glenohumeral internal rotation deficit (GIRD) accompanied by posterior capsular contracture leads to posterosuperior migration of the humeral head with abduction and external rotation and subsequently to increased shear and torsional forces at the biceps anchor.[12,15] Although evidence of this peel-back mechanism was observed during arthroscopic examination of the shoulder, there is little direct evidence that symptomatic GIRD with an associated posterior capsular contracture is a prerequisite for the development of a SLAP lesion. The peel-back mechanism may be the norm in overhead athletes who have increased external rotation, commonly with decreased internal rotation, in the throwing shoulder (**Figure 4**). It may be this hyperexternal rotation that puts abnormal stresses on the biceps anchor, independent of posterior capsular contracture. Internal impingement occurs when the posterosuperior rotator cuff is pinched between the greater tuberosity and the posterosuperior glenoid labrum at 90° abduction and 90° external rotation.[16] This impingement is repeated thousands of times in the late cocking phase of throwing, and it may cause a SLAP lesion.

Although each of these etiologies is plausible for type II SLAP lesions in overhead athletes, the so-called weed-pulling hypothesis probably provides an adequate explanation for a SLAP lesion in most patients.[17] The weed-pulling hypothesis suggests that SLAP tears are created by repetitively alternating forces during late cocking, which creates a posterior force on the biceps-labral complex, and deceleration-follow-through, which creates an anterior force. The result is the characteristic SLAP lesion in throwing athletes.

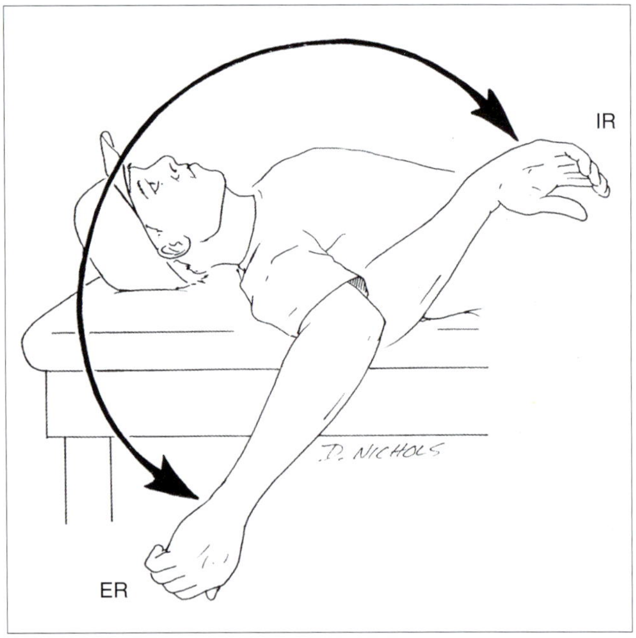

FIGURE 4 Schematic drawing showing the total arc of motion concept, in which external rotation (ER) + internal rotation (IR) = total motion. (Reproduced with permission from Wilk KE, Meister K, Andrews JR: Current concepts in the rehabilitation of the overhead throwing athlete. *Am J Sports Med* 2002;30[1]:136-151.)

Clinical Evaluation

Patients with a symptomatic SLAP lesion broadly fall into two groups: overhead athletes, most of whom are baseball pitchers (although some are baseball position players, swimmers, tennis players, javelin throwers, or volleyball players), and people who have undergone an acute traumatic event causing traction or compression. SLAP lesions also develop in military personnel because of the rigorous and repetitive nature of their training. Military personnel who underwent shoulder arthroscopy were found to have a 22% incidence of SLAP lesions, 69% of which were type II.[18]

An accurate and thorough history of symptoms is critical to patient evaluation for a SLAP lesion. An overhead athlete may describe a vague onset of symptoms of somewhat unclear duration, without a clear inciting event. It is important to elicit the nature of the overhead activity, including changes in velocity, mechanics, stamina, and pain. The symptoms of internal impingement often are similar to those of a SLAP lesion, including vague pain and so-called dead arm syndrome with hard throwing. Dead arm syndrome was redefined in 2000 as an inability to throw with preinjury velocity and control because of pain and unease in the throwing shoulder.[19] Mechanical symptoms such as locking, catching, or popping may be present, especially with rotational shoulder motions.

Several tests should be used in combination with a thorough history, although their overall reliability is highly variable. Positive test results are suggestive rather than diagnostic of a SLAP lesion.

The physical examination for a suspected SLAP lesion should include evaluation for scapular dysfunction or pathologic shoulder motion (such as GIRD or crepitus) as well as provocative tests for shoulder pathology. Muscular atrophy should be evaluated; atrophy of the infraspinatus suggests a spinoglenoid notch ganglion cyst, which has been associated with SLAP lesions. In the absence of other pathology, a patient with a SLAP lesion should have normal rotator cuff strength and active shoulder motion (in a throwing athlete, defined as a less-than-25° difference between the dominant and nondominant arms). The examination for shoulder instability is critical for detecting associated labral pathology; the anterior apprehension-relocation and posterior load-and-shift tests should be included. The O'Brien active compression, biceps load II, forced shoulder abduction and elbow flexion, dynamic labral shear, Crank, and resisted supination external rotation tests also have been described for detecting a SLAP lesion[20-25] (**Figure 5**).

An evaluation of several well-described and new tests found that the dynamic labral shear test was the most accurate single test, and the dynamic labral shear and O'Brien tests were the most useful combination for detecting a SLAP lesion.[26] A 2009 meta-analysis of studies that evaluated the clinical usefulness of provocative tests for SLAP lesions found that the active compression, Crank, and Speed tests were the most sensitive and specific, and the anterior slide test was significantly less accurate.[27] A case-control study found that the biceps load II test was the most accurate in identifying a SLAP-only lesion, and the O'Brien, dynamic labral shear, Speed, and labral tension tests did not accurately identify SLAP lesions.[28] However, there was objection that the dynamic labral shear test was incorrectly performed in this study. The test is correctly performed with the patient supine and the shoulder off the side of the table, with the scapula supported but the humerus free. The shoulder is brought into 90° abduction, and the elbow is flexed to 90°. The shoulder is externally rotated to its natural limit, the elbow is dropped back to its natural limit of horizontal abduction, and the shoulder is passively elevated while horizontal abduction and external rotation are maintained. A positive test reproduces the patient's pain when the shoulder is moved through the arc of motion (usually 90° to 120°); a painful click may be felt. The active compression test is performed with downward pressure on a patient's arm while the shoulder is flexed to 90°, the elbow is extended, the arm is slightly adducted (at 10° to 15°), and the hand is first in maximal pronation and then in supination. The test is positive if the pain from the test in pronation is reduced or eliminated in supination. The Speed test is performed with downward pressure on the arm while the shoulder is flexed to 60° and the elbow is extended. The test is positive if the pain is localized to the bicipital groove. The Crank test is performed with the

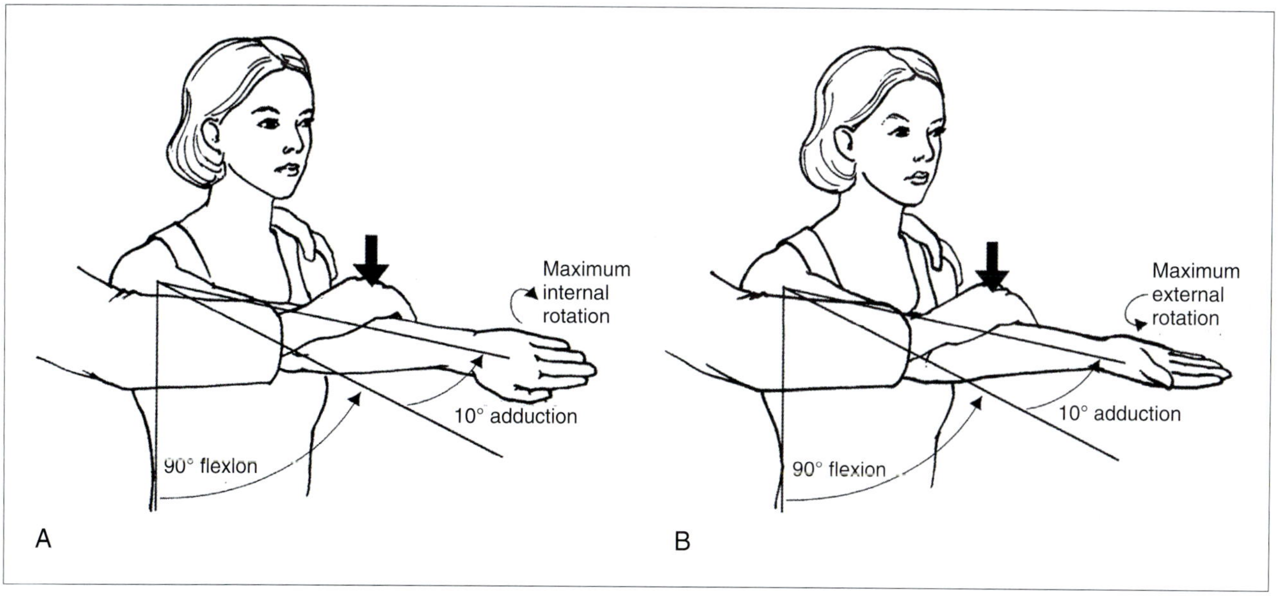

FIGURE 5 Schematic drawings showing the O'Brien active compression test. A downward force is resisted while the flexed and adducted shoulder is rotated internally (**A**) or externally (**B**). The reduction of symptoms in external rotation is a positive test. (Reproduced with permission from Parentis MA, Jobe CM, Pink MM, Jobe FW: An anatomic evaluation of the active compression test. *J Shoulder Elbow Surg* 2004;13[4]:410-416.)

shoulder elevated to 160° and an axial load applied while the humerus is internally and externally rotated. The test is positive with pain in external rotation, and clicking or catching also may occur. The biceps load II test is performed with the patient supine, the shoulder abducted to 120°, the elbow flexed to 90°, and the forearm supinated. The shoulder is maximally externally rotated, and the patient flexes the elbow against resistance. In a positive test, the patient's pain is reproduced.

Imaging

The initial imaging studies are plain radiographs (the AP, scapular AP, axillary, and outlet views), which are not specific for SLAP lesions but can help identify other shoulder pathology. MRI is the study of choice for identifying SLAP lesions as well as concomitant labral, chondral, and rotator cuff pathology. Although the benefit of magnetic resonance arthrography (MRA) for identifying labral pathology has been extensively debated, it is quite useful for identifying subtle lesions of the labrum when intra-articular contrast is added. The abduction and external rotation view accentuates both superior and anterior labral pathology and is useful because of the anatomic variability of the superior labrum.[29] External rotation of the shoulder was found to improve the sensitivity and specificity of MRA for identifying SLAP lesions.[30] MRA findings consistent with a SLAP lesion include increased signal in the superior labrum with T2-weighting and the appearance of contrast between the glenoid and the superior labrum on coronal MRA (**Figure 6**). Identification of an anterosuperior labral tear on axial MRI or MRA also suggests a SLAP lesion. MRI is useful for identifying suprascapular and spinoglenoid cysts that may be associated with a SLAP lesion.

MRI for identifying SLAP lesions has a reported sensitivity of 67% to 98% and a specificity of 63% to 100%.[31-35] A side-by-side comparison using a 3-T magnet found that MRA had greater sensitivity than conventional MRI (83% versus 98%).[36] CT arthrography was found to be accurate and have good interobserver reliability for identifying SLAP lesions, comparable that of MRA for labral pathology.[37]

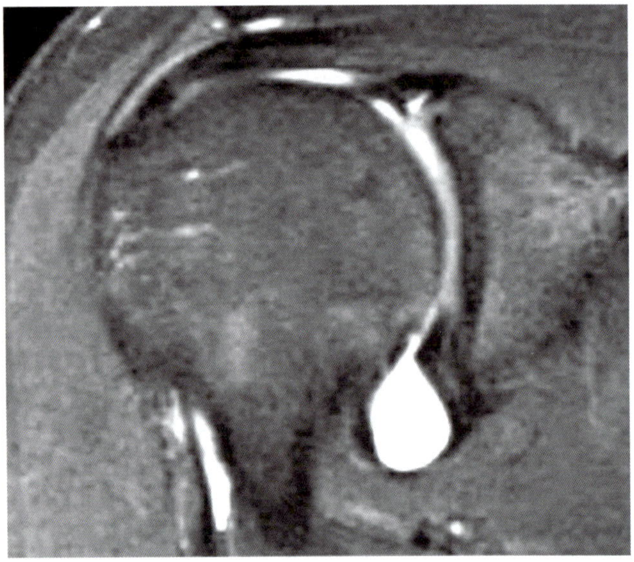

FIGURE 6 T2-weighted coronal magnetic resonance arthrogram showing dye tracking between the superior labrum and the glenoid. (Reproduced from Keener JD, Brophy RH: Superior labral tears of the shoulder: Pathogenesis, evaluation, and treatment. *J Am Acad Orthop Surg* 2009;17[10]:627-637.)

Management

Nonsurgical Management

The nonsurgical treatment of a SLAP lesion consists of rest from the inciting activity, anti-inflammatory drugs, posterior capsular stretching, and strengthening of the rotator cuff and scapular stabilizers. A four-phase protocol is used for rehabilitation in athletes with a shoulder condition such as a SLAP tear, rotator cuff pathology, tendinitis, GIRD, or internal impingement.[39] The goals in the acute phase are to reduce pain, decrease inflammation, restore normal motion (especially internal rotation and horizontal adduction), and restore muscle strength and proprioception. The intermediate phase focuses on progressively increasing strength, improving flexibility, and facilitating neuromuscular control. In the advanced strengthening phase, aggressive strengthening drills, functional drills, and plyometrics are used. The final phase is the return to throwing (or other overhead sport) phase; it includes an interval throwing program or another sport-specific progression until pain-free athletic participation is achieved. In one study, nonsurgical treatment was successful in 19 of 39 patients (49%), but the remaining patients required surgery after unsuccessful nonsurgical treatment.[40] Before surgical intervention is considered, the athlete should attempt to regain full motion nonsurgically, especially in internal rotation.

Surgical Management

Surgical management of a SLAP lesion generally is performed arthroscopically. Several techniques can be chosen, depending on the type of lesion, activity level of the patient, and associated pathology. The indications for surgical treatment generally include 3 months of unsuccessful nonsurgical treatment, although early surgical intervention can be considered for a high-level overhead athlete, particularly in the off-season. For an in-season athlete who can perform despite the pain associated with a SLAP lesion, surgical treatment can be delayed until the season ends. The management of SLAP lesions in patients who are not high-level athletes has been heavily debated, and questions remain as to which patients can benefit from surgery and which procedure should be used. Surgical management of a SLAP lesion is recommended if nonsurgical management has been unsuccessful, the patient's symptoms and examination findings are correlated with those of a SLAP lesion, and the biceps anchor is unstable on arthroscopy. Biceps tenodesis was traditionally favored in patients older than 40 years, but recent trends have favored tenodesis at a younger age.

The choice of surgical management depends on the type of SLAP lesion, as determined using the original four-type Snyder classification. Other classification types essentially consist of a SLAP lesion plus an instability lesion, which generally is surgically managed as it would be in the absence of extension into the superior labrum. The recommendation is to repair the SLAP lesion concomitant with the instability procedure. A type I SLAP lesion can be managed with gentle débridement back to a stable base but, in the absence of symptoms, may not require surgical management. A type II SLAP lesion by definition destabilizes the biceps anchor. Reattachment of the biceps-labrum complex to the superior glenoid generally is required, but primary biceps tenodesis can be used in revision surgery or for a patient who is older than 40 years or relatively inactive. A type III SLAP lesion can be treated with débridement of the bucket-handle labrum and repair of any unstable labral rim. In addition, the middle glenohumeral ligament should be repaired if it is attached to the bucket-handle labrum. The choice of surgical management of a type IV lesion depends on the severity of the injury to the biceps tendon. With minimal biceps involvement, débridement of the biceps plus labral repair is appropriate, but the management option for a severely injured biceps is open or arthroscopic primary biceps tenodesis.

Surgical Technique

Many techniques of SLAP repair have been described; the technique preferred by this chapter's authors is described here (**Figures** 7 and 8). Beach-chair or lateral decubitus positioning of the patient can be used for arthroscopy. The posterior portal should be established in standard fashion. It can be helpful to establish a very medial portal (near the glenoid) if a Bankart lesion is also present; a more lateral portal is helpful for a SLAP lesion with substantial posterior extension. An anterior portal is established in the rotator cuff interval, and diagnostic arthroscopy is performed to identify any concomitant pathology. Additional portals are used for anchor placement, depending on the nature of the SLAP lesion, including an accessory lateral portal (approximately 1 cm from the anterolateral corner of the acromion), the portal of Wilmington (approximately 1 cm anterolateral to the posterolateral corner of the acromion), and the Neviaser portal, which can be used for suture passage. It is rarely necessary to establish all of these portals. A cannula should be used only in the anterior portal, not through the rotator cuff.[41] Any portal through the rotator cuff should be made with a No. 11 blade oriented in line with the fibers of the rotator cuff to minimize iatrogenic pathology.

The SLAP lesion should be probed and classified to determine the appropriate surgical management option. Determining the stability of the biceps anchor is critical. The labrum should be freed from the glenoid, essentially

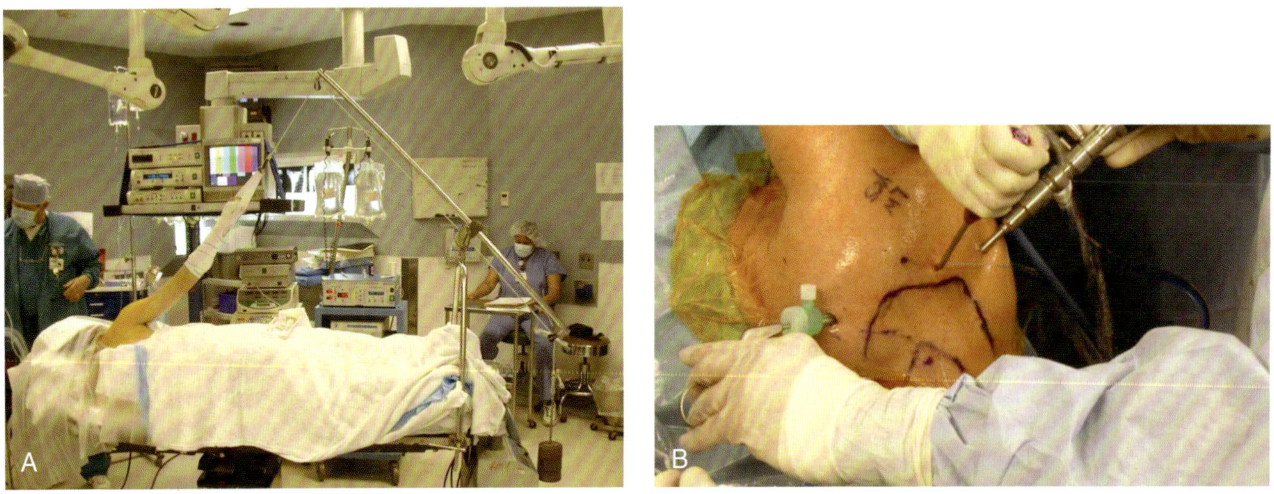

FIGURE 7 Photographs showing repair of a superior labrum anterior to posterior (SLAP) lesion. **A**, The lateral decubitus patient position is preferred for an all-arthroscopic procedure, but the beach-chair position also can be used. **B**, The position of the anterior portal (green cannula), the posterior viewing portal, and an accessory portal for anchor placement (not always necessary) are shown.

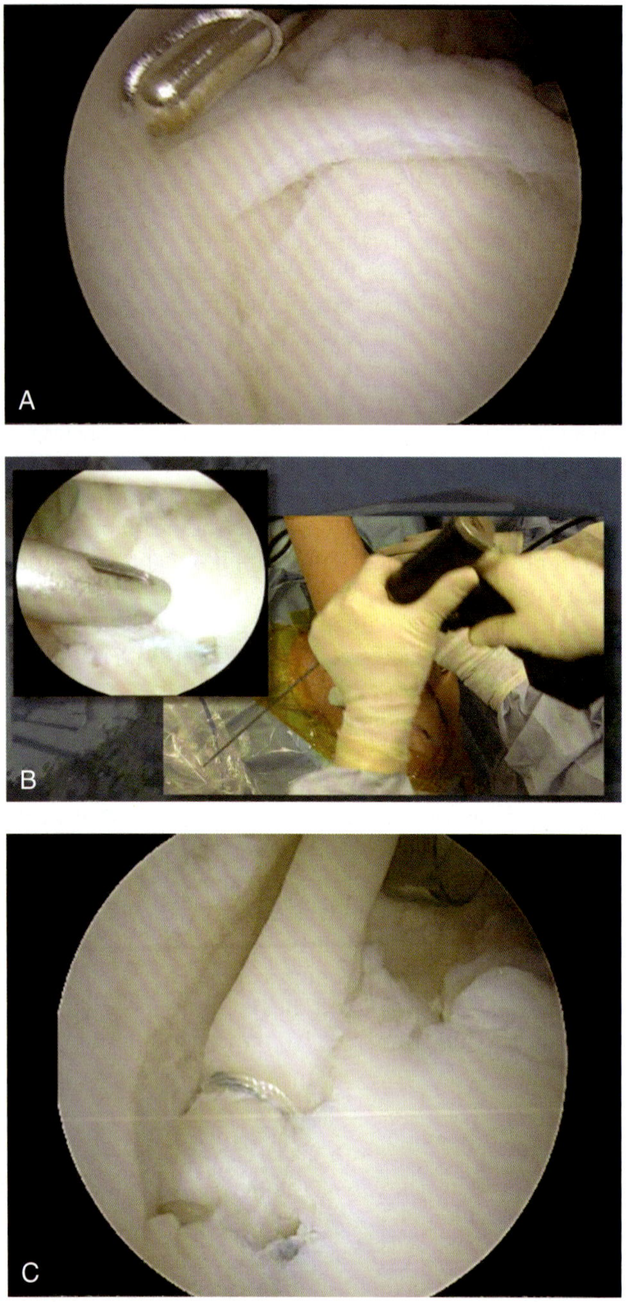

FIGURE 8 Photograph and arthroscopic images showing repair of a superior labrum anterior to posterior (SLAP) lesion. **A**, Biceps anchor involvement in the lesion. The labrum is elevated from the glenoid, and a shaver is used to prepare the superior glenoid rim by removing soft tissue and leaving a bleeding bony bed. **B**, Anchors are placed at the superior glenoid margin, most commonly just anterior and posterior to the biceps tendon, through the standard portals or an accessory posterior portal. **C**, The completed SLAP repair with knotless biocomposite anchors.

completing the tear. The next step is the preparation of a bleeding bony bed for healing, as in any labral repair. This step typically is done from the anterior portal. Good control of the shaver, commonly used on the reverse setting, is important to avoid the tendency to skive during preparation on the glenoid face. The next step is anchor placement at the articular margin; the use of suture tacks has largely been abandoned because of reports of synovitis and articular damage.[42,43] The choice of anchors has evolved over the years and trends are now supporting knotless anchors to avoid impingement. A retrospective case series reviewed 11 patients with knot-induced pain and mechanical symptoms after arthroscopic fixation of unstable type II SLAP lesions, which required a secondary procedure for knot removal. The patients had significant improvement in objective scores, subjective scores, and pain relief.[69] Standard biocomposite knotless suture anchors are preferred. One anchor should be placed anterior to the biceps anchor, using a spinal needle to identify the appropriate angle of approach from the accessory lateral portal (45° from the center of the glenoid). This portal usually can be used to place one anchor posterior to the biceps, but the portal of Wilmington should be used if the SLAP lesion has substantial posterior extension. It is important to avoid compromising the anchor placement or the orientation to save a portal. Suture passage can be accomplished using a suture retrieval device that passes through a spinal needle, a rigid retrograde suture-passing device, a curved suture loop, or a suture-retrieving instrument. The suture configuration can be a simple loop, in which only one suture limb is passed around the superior labrum, or a mattress stitch, in which both limbs are passed. Biomechanical data suggest that one mattress suture has a higher load to failure than one simple suture, one double-loaded anchor provides a load to failure equivalent to that of two single-loaded anchors, and two posterior anchors are equivalent to one anterior and one posterior anchor (on a posteriorly directed vector simulating the peel-back mechanism).[45-47] Surgical management of any paralabral cyst can be performed concomitantly and usually arthroscopically.[48] A paralabral cyst may resolve without direct decompression through repair of the SLAP lesion, but direct decompression is preferred if there is substantial muscle atrophy.[49]

Postoperative Care

The choice of a specific rehabilitation protocol after SLAP lesion repair depends on the nature of the repair (a slower progression is required for a relatively extensive tear) as well as any additional pathology identified during surgery.[50] The first 6 weeks of the postoperative period are focused on regaining range of motion and dynamic stability of the shoulder, and the next 6 weeks are devoted to strengthening and regaining proprioception.

Rehabilitation can be fairly aggressive after a simple débridement procedure, but repair of a type II SLAP lesion requires a more gradual, structured protocol. For the first 4 weeks, the allowable range of motion is below 90° of elevation; internal rotation is allowed to a greater extent than external rotation. Full motion is to be obtained by 8 weeks after surgery, with throwing motion by 12 weeks. Isometric strengthening is initiated immediately after surgery to promote dynamic stabilization, but weight-bearing exercises are avoided until 7 weeks have passed, and biceps strengthening is initiated after 12 weeks.

Rehabilitation after a type IV lesion repair is similar to that for a type II lesion, with additional emphasis on management of the biceps tendon. If the biceps was released, active biceps exercises begin at 6 weeks. If a tenodesis was performed, it is advisable to begin active biceps exercises after 12 weeks.

Outcomes

Most reports of SLAP lesion outcomes have focused on type II lesions. At 1-year follow-up, 78% of the patients who underwent simple débridement of a SLAP lesion had an excellent result, but at 2-year follow-up, only 63% had an excellent result, and only 44% had returned to sports.[51]

Studies have focused on outcomes of baseball players following arthroscopic SLAP repair. A study of 216 baseball players who had isolated SLAP repair or SLAP repair with débridement of partial-thickness(<25%) rotator cuff repair had a minimal follow-up of 2 years. Of the 216 players, 133 players were contacted and had 62% successful return to play (59% for pitchers and 76% for nonpitchers).[70] A retrospective review of 24 Major League Baseball pitchers found 62.5% were able to return to play after SLAP repair. Of those who were able to return to play, 87.5% were able to return to prior performance.[71]

The results of a SLAP lesion repair depend on the method of fixation. The use of bioabsorbable tacks has led to relatively poor outcomes, particularly as related to night pain, the expected level of postoperative activity, and return to sports.[41,52] Arthroscopic repair of a SLAP lesion was found to eliminate the peel-back sign, with a 97% rate of good or excellent results.[53] At 1-year follow-up, 44 of 53 pitchers (87%) had returned to play. The results were worse in patients with an undersurface rotator cuff tear, all of whom had a substantial internal rotation deficit. A study of 23 elite overhead athletes found relatively poor return to play results in patients who had an undersurface rotator cuff tear.[54] At a mean 38-month follow-up, 22 patients (96%) had a good to excellent American Shoulder and Elbow Index score. However, only 12 patients (52%) had a good to excellent score on the Kerlan-Jobe Orthopaedic Clinic measure,[55] and 13 (57%) had returned to play. A 2009 prospective study of 47 patients found that 40 (87%) had a good to excellent result at an average 2.7-year follow-up, with better patient-reported outcomes and a higher return to play rate in patients with an acute traumatic event than in those with an atraumatic etiology.[56] At an average 3.5-year follow-up, overhead athletes had an overall satisfaction rate of 93%, a perceived rate of return to preinjury performance of 84%, and average American Shoulder and Elbow Surgeons and Kerlan-Jobe Orthopaedic Clinic scores of 87.9 and 73.6, respectively.[57]

An 87% overall rate of good to excellent results was found in a study of patients with an average age of 39.7 years.[58] Sixty-five percent of patients with a workers' compensation claim had good to excellent results versus 95% of patients with no claim, and there was a trend toward worse results that did not reach statistical significance in patients older than 40 years. Similarly, another study found no significant difference in outcomes after SLAP repair based on age younger or older than 40 years.[59] Good results were reported for concomitant SLAP and rotator cuff repairs in older patients (mean age, 57 years).[60] A study of patients aged 45 to 60 years found débridement of type II SLAP lesions to be superior to repair in combination with rotator cuff repair.[61] Data are limited on revision SLAP repair, but in one small study, revision repair had significantly worse results in 12 patients than primary repair in historical control patients, particularly in patients who were overhead athletes or had a workers' compensation claim.[62]

Primary biceps tenodesis has been proposed as a reasonable alternative for managing a SLAP lesion, particularly in patients who are older or not involved in overhead sports. A comparison of results in primary arthroscopic tenodesis and SLAP repair found significantly better Constant scores, satisfaction, and return to play after tenodesis. The patients treated with tenodesis were significantly older than those treated with repair (average age, 52 and 37 years, respectively), and extrapolation of the data to a younger patient population is problematic.[63] A systematic comparison review compared labral repair versus biceps tenodesis for isolated SLAP II tears, similar objective and subjective clinical outcomes, return to activity, and complications occurred.[72] A systematic review analyzed the surgical management of superior labral injuries in patients aged 40 years or older found increasing age and worker's compensation were independent risk factors for decreased patient satisfaction and increased complications, including postoperative stiffness and revision surgeries following SLAP repair. The evidence supported biceps tenodesis or tenotomy in the older population.[73]

Surgical trends for the surgical management of SLAP tears have shifted over the past decade. An epidemiology study from 2004 to 2009 evaluated 25,574 cases of arthroscopic SLAP repair. The incidence of repair increased from 17.0 per 10,000 patients in 2004 to 28.1

per 10,000 patients in 2009.[74] A study comparing the incidence of SLAP repair versus biceps tenodesis and tenotomy from 2002 to 2011 found the proportion of isolated SLAP repair decreased from 68.3% to 44.8%, whereas biceps tenodesis increased from 1.9% to 18.8%. In the patients who underwent rotator cuff repair, biceps tenotomy or tenodesis increased from 6.0% to 28.0% and SLAP repair decreased from 60.2% to 15.3%.[75] A retrospective study analyzed 46,650 SLAP tear diagnoses from 2007 to 2016 with 3,347 patients who underwent surgical treatment. There was a 69% decrease in isolated SLAP repair during this period and a 370% increase in biceps tenodesis; there was a 1,500% increase in biceps tenodesis performed in patients older than 40 years.[76]

Complications

The most common complication of SLAP repair is postoperative stiffness with decreased range of motion, which can be minimized with adequate postoperative physical therapy. Additional reported complications include night pain with penetration of the rotator cuff, synovitis, and chondral damage related to loose bodies and metallic anchors.[52,64-66] Isolated suprascapular nerve injury has been reported.[67,68]

SUMMARY

SLAP lesions are commonly found in two distinct populations: patients who have had a single traumatic event and those who participate in overhead sports. The classic type II SLAP lesion is found in the dominant arm of a male overhead athlete younger than 40 years. The pathogenesis of SLAP lesions in overhead athletes is controversial. The clinical evaluation for a SLAP lesion is somewhat unreliable; an accurate diagnosis is dependent on high-quality imaging (3-T MRA) and can be confirmed arthroscopically. Nonsurgical treatment sometimes is effective, but surgical repair is the standard for overhead athletes. Surgical repair of a SLAP lesion has good results with respect to pain and overall shoulder function, but return to high-level athletic activity is less predictable. The preferred surgical technique for SLAP repair is performed arthroscopically with anatomic reduction of the biceps anchor to the glenoid with the use of knotless anchors. Biceps tenodesis is an alternate surgical option with comparable results to labral repair and is the preferred treatment for patients older than 40 years. Major complications are uncommon with modern repair techniques. Structured rehabilitation based on the extent of the injury and the nature of the repair is important to a successful outcome.

KEY STUDY POINTS

- SLAP lesion is a relatively new pathology involving the superior labral biceps complex becoming detached from the glenoid rim.
- SLAP lesions are most commonly found in overhead athletes but can be found in the general population. Acute and traumatic events can be caused by direct compression or by traction with inferior subluxation. The pathogenesis of type II SLAP lesions in the overhead athletes is controversial with the proposed etiologies involving internal impingement or the peel-back mechanism.
- The clinical evaluation for SLAP lesions includes a thorough history and physical examination. Multiple special tests can be used including dynamic labral shear, O'Brien's active compression, biceps load II, Crank, Speed, and shoulder instability examination.
- Surgical management of SLAP lesions depends on age, activity level, and tear type. A trial of nonsurgical management should be considered as first-line therapy. Surgical treatment can be considered after failure of nonsurgical treatment or acutely in the elite athlete. The use of knotless suture anchor fixation is the preferred fixation method to avoid knot impingement.
- Outcomes following SLAP repair is variable with difficulty regaining preinjury status in high-demand throwers but this still remains a good option.

Annotated References

1. Neer CS II: Anterior acromioplasty for the chronic impingement syndrome in the shoulder: A preliminary report. *J Bone Joint Surg Am* 1972;54(1):41-50.

2. Tibone JE, Jobe FW, Kerlan RK, et al: Shoulder impingement syndrome in athletes treated by an anterior acromioplasty. *Clin Orthop Relat Res* 1985;(198):134-140.

3. Andrews JR, Carson WG Jr, McLeod WD: Glenoid labrum tears related to the long head of the biceps. *Am J Sports Med* 1985;13(5):337-341.

4. Snyder SJ, Karzel RP, Del Pizzo W, Ferkel RD, Friedman MJ: SLAP lesions of the shoulder. *Arthroscopy* 1990;6(4):274-279.

5. Maffet MW, Gartsman GM, Moseley B: Superior labrum-biceps tendon complex lesions of the shoulder. *Am J Sports Med* 1995;23(1):93-98.

6. Powell SE, Nord KD, Ryu RK: The diagnosis, classification and treatment of SLAP lesions. *Oper Tech Sports Med* 2004;12:99-110.

7. Gobezie R, Zurakowski D, Lavery K, Millett PJ, Cole BJ, Warner JJ: Analysis of interobserver and intraobserver variability in the diagnosis and treatment of SLAP tears using the Snyder classification. *Am J Sports Med* 2008;36(7):1373-1379.

8. Jia X, Yokota A, McCarty EC, et al: Reproducibility and reliability of the Snyder classification of superior labral anterior posterior lesions among shoulder surgeons. *Am J Sports Med* 2011;39(5):986-991.

9. Kumar VP, Satku K, Balasubramaniam P: The role of the long head of biceps brachii in the stabilization of the head of the humerus. *Clin Orthop Relat Res* 1989;(244):172-175.

10. Pagnani MJ, Deng XH, Warren RF, Torzilli PA, Altchek DW: Effect of lesions of the superior portion of the glenoid labrum on glenohumeral translation. *J Bone Joint Surg Am* 1995;77(7):1003-1010.

11. Warner JJ, McMahon PJ: The role of the long head of the biceps brachii in superior stability of the glenohumeral joint. *J Bone Joint Surg Am* 1995;77(3):366-372.

12. Burkhart SS, Morgan CD: The peel-back mechanism: Its role in producing and extending posterior type II SLAP lesions and its effect on SLAP repair rehabilitation. *Arthroscopy* 1998;14(6):637-640.

13. Clavert P, Bonnomet F, Kempf JF, Boutemy P, Braun M, Kahn JL: Contribution to the study of the pathogenesis of type II superior labrum anterior-posterior lesions: A cadaveric model of a fall on the outstretched hand. *J Shoulder Elbow Surg* 2004;13(1):45-50.

14. Bey MJ, Elders GJ, Huston LJ, Kuhn JE, Blasier RB, Soslowsky LJ: The mechanism of creation of superior labrum, anterior, and posterior lesions in a dynamic biomechanical model of the shoulder: The role of inferior subluxation. *J Shoulder Elbow Surg* 1998;7(4):397-401.

15. Burkhart SS, Morgan CD, Kibler WB: The disabled throwing shoulder: Spectrum of pathology. Part I: Pathoanatomy and biomechanics. *Arthroscopy* 2003;19(4):404-420.

16. Walch G, Boileau P, Noel E, Donell ST: Impingement of the deep surface of the supraspinatus tendon on the posterosuperior glenoid rim: An arthroscopic study. *J Shoulder Elbow Surg* 1992;1(5):238-245.

17. Jazrawi LM, McCluskey GM III, Andrews JR: Superior labral anterior and posterior lesions and internal impingement in the overhead athlete. *Instr Course Lect* 2003;52:43-63.

18. Kampa RJ, Clasper J: Incidence of SLAP lesions in a military population. *J R Army Med Corps* 2005;151(3):171-175.

19. Burkhart SS, Morgan CD, Kibler WB: Shoulder injuries in overhead athletes: The "dead arm" revisited. *Clin Sports Med* 2000;19(1):125-158.

20. O'Brien SJ, Pagnani MJ, Fealy S, McGlynn SR, Wilson JB: The active compression test: A new and effective test for diagnosing labral tears and acromioclavicular joint abnormality. *Am J Sports Med* 1998;26(5):610-613.

21. Kim SH, Ha KI, Ahn JH, Kim SH, Choi HJ: Biceps load test II: A clinical test for SLAP lesions of the shoulder. *Arthroscopy* 2001;17(2):160-164.

22. Nakagawa S, Yoneda M, Hayashida K, Obata M, Fukushima S, Miyazaki Y: Forced shoulder abduction and elbow flexion test: A new simple clinical test to detect superior labral injury in the throwing shoulder. *Arthroscopy* 2005;21(11):1290-1295.

23. Liu SH, Henry MH, Nuccion SL: A prospective evaluation of a new physical examination in predicting glenoid labral tears. *Am J Sports Med* 1996;24(6):721-725.

24. Myers TH, Zemanovic JR, Andrews JR: The resisted supination external rotation test: A new test for the diagnosis of superior labral anterior posterior lesions. *Am J Sports Med* 2005;33(9):1315-1320.

25. Cheung EV, O'Driscoll SW: *Abstract: The dynamic labral shear test for superior labral anterior posterior tears of the shoulder. 74th Annual Meeting Proceedings.* Rosemont, IL, American Academy of Orthopaedic Surgeons, 2007, p 574.

26. Ben Kibler W, Sciascia AD, Hester P, Dome D, Jacobs C: Clinical utility of traditional and new tests in the diagnosis of biceps tendon injuries and superior labrum anterior and posterior lesions in the shoulder. *Am J Sports Med* 2009;37(9):1840-1847.

27. Meserve BB, Cleland JA, Boucher TR: A meta-analysis examining clinical test utility for assessing superior labral anterior posterior lesions. *Am J Sports Med* 2009;37(11):2252-2258.

28. Cook C, Beaty S, Kissenberth MJ, Siffri P, Pill SG, Hawkins RJ: Diagnostic accuracy of five orthopedic clinical tests for diagnosis of superior labrum anterior posterior (SLAP) lesions. *J Shoulder Elbow Surg* 2012;21(1):13-22.

29. Borrero CG, Casagranda BU, Towers JD, Bradley JP: Magnetic resonance appearance of posterosuperior labral peel back during humeral abduction and external rotation. *Skeletal Radiol* 2010;39(1):19-26.

30. Jung JY, Ha DH, Lee SM, Blacksin MF, Kim KA, Kim JW: Displaceability of SLAP lesion on shoulder MR arthrography with external rotation position. *Skeletal Radiol* 2011;40(8):1047-1055.

31. Connell DA, Potter HG, Wickiewicz TL, Altchek DW, Warren RF: Noncontrast magnetic resonance imaging of superior labral lesions: 102 cases confirmed at arthroscopic surgery. *Am J Sports Med* 1999;27(2):208-213.

32. Bencardino JT, Beltran J, Rosenberg ZS, et al: Superior labrum anterior-posterior lesions: Diagnosis with MR arthrography of the shoulder. *Radiology* 2000;214(1):267-271.

33. Jee WH, McCauley TR, Katz LD, Matheny JM, Ruwe PA, Daigneault JP: Superior labral anterior posterior (SLAP) lesions of the glenoid labrum: Reliability and accuracy of MR arthrography for diagnosis. *Radiology* 2001;218(1):127-132.

34. Tung GA, Entzian D, Green A, Brody JM: High-field and low-field MR imaging of superior glenoid labral tears and associated tendon injuries. *AJR Am J Roentgenol* 2000;174(4):1107-1114.

35. Pandya NK, Colton A, Webner D, Sennett B, Huffman GR: Physical examination and magnetic resonance imaging in the diagnosis of superior labrum anterior-posterior lesions of the shoulder: A sensitivity analysis. *Arthroscopy* 2008;24(3):311-317.

36. Magee T: 3-T MRI of the shoulder: Is MR arthrography necessary? *AJR Am J Roentgenol* 2009;192(1):86-92.

37. Kim YJ, Choi JA, Oh JH, Hwang SI, Hong SH, Kang HS: Superior labral anteroposterior tears: Accuracy and interobserver reliability of multidetector CT arthrography for diagnosis. *Radiology* 2011;260(1):207-215.

38. Oh JH, Kim JY, Choi JA, Kim WS: Effectiveness of multidetector computed tomography arthrography for the diagnosis of shoulder pathology: Comparison with magnetic resonance imaging with arthroscopic correlation. *J Shoulder Elbow Surg* 2010;19(1):14-20.

39. Wilk KE, Obma P, Simpson CD, Cain EL, Dugas JR, Andrews JR: Shoulder injuries in the overhead athlete. *J Orthop Sports Phys Ther* 2009;39(2):38-54.

40. Edwards SL, Lee JA, Bell JE, et al: Nonoperative treatment of superior labrum anterior posterior tears: Improvements in pain, function, and quality of life. *Am J Sports Med* 2010;38(7):1456-1461.

41. O'Brien SJ, Allen AA, Coleman SH, Drakos MC: The trans-rotator cuff approach to SLAP lesions: Technical aspects for repair and a clinical follow-up of 31 patients at a minimum of 2 years. *Arthroscopy* 2002;18(4):372-377.

42. Freehill MQ, Harms DJ, Huber SM, Atlihan D, Buss DD: Poly-L-lactic acid tack synovitis after arthroscopic stabilization of the shoulder. *Am J Sports Med* 2003;31(5):643-647.

43. Sassmannshausen G, Sukay M, Mair SD: Broken or dislodged poly-L-lactic acid bioabsorbable tacks in patients after SLAP lesion surgery. *Arthroscopy* 2006;22(6):615-619.

44. Oh JH, Lee HK, Kim JY, Kim SH, Gong HS: Clinical and radiologic outcomes of arthroscopic glenoid labrum repair with the BioKnotless suture anchor. *Am J Sports Med* 2009;37(12):2340-2348.

45. Domb BG, Ehteshami JR, Shindle MK, et al: Biomechanical comparison of 3 suture anchor configurations for repair of type II SLAP lesions. *Arthroscopy* 2007;23(2):135-140.

46. Baldini T, Snyder RL, Peacher G, Bach J, McCarty E: Strength of single- versus double-anchor repair of type II SLAP lesions: A cadaveric study. *Arthroscopy* 2009;25(11):1257-1260.

47. Morgan RJ, Kuremsky MA, Peindl RD, Fleischli JE: A biomechanical comparison of two suture anchor configurations for the repair of type II SLAP lesions subjected to a peel-back mechanism of failure. *Arthroscopy* 2008;24(4):383-388.

48. Westerheide KJ, Dopirak RM, Karzel RP, Snyder SJ: Suprascapular nerve palsy secondary to spinoglenoid cysts: Results of arthroscopic treatment. *Arthroscopy* 2006;22(7):721-727.

49. Youm T, Matthews PV, ElAttrache NS: Treatment of patients with spinoglenoid cysts associated with superior labral tears without cyst aspiration, debridement, or excision. *Arthroscopy* 2006;22(5):548-552.

50. Wilk KE, Reinold MM, Dugas JR, Arrigo CA, Moser MW, Andrews JR: Current concepts in the recognition and treatment of superior labral (SLAP) lesions. *J Orthop Sports Phys Ther* 2005;35(5):273-291.

51. Cordasco FA, Steinmann S, Flatow EL, Bigliani LU: Arthroscopic treatment of glenoid labral tears. *Am J Sports Med* 1993;21(3):425-430, discussion 430-431.

52. Cohen DB, Coleman S, Drakos MC, et al: Outcomes of isolated type II SLAP lesions treated with arthroscopic fixation using a bioabsorbable tack. *Arthroscopy* 2006;22(2):136-142.

53. Morgan CD, Burkhart SS, Palmeri M, Gillespie M: Type II SLAP lesions: Three subtypes and their relationships to superior instability and rotator cuff tears. *Arthroscopy* 1998;14(6):553-565.

54. Neri BR, ElAttrache NS, Owsley KC, Mohr K, Yocum LA: Outcome of type II superior labral anterior posterior repairs in elite overhead athletes: Effect of concomitant partial-thickness rotator cuff tears. *Am J Sports Med* 2011;39(1):114-120.

55. Alberta FG, ElAttrache NS, Bissell S, et al: The development and validation of a functional assessment tool for the upper extremity in the overhead athlete. *Am J Sports Med* 2010;38(5):903-911.

56. Brockmeier SF, Voos JE, Williams RJ III, Altchek DW, Cordasco FA, Allen AA: Hospital for special surgery sports medicine and shoulder service: Outcomes after arthroscopic repair of type-II SLAP lesions. *J Bone Joint Surg Am* 2009;91(7):1595-1603.

57. Neuman BJ, Boisvert CB, Reiter B, Lawson K, Ciccotti MG, Cohen SB: Results of arthroscopic repair of type II superior labral anterior posterior lesions in overhead athletes: Assessment of return to preinjury playing level and satisfaction. *Am J Sports Med* 2011;39(9): 1883-1888.

58. Denard PJ, Lädermann A, Burkhart SS: Long-term outcome after arthroscopic repair of type II SLAP lesions: Results according to age and workers' compensation status. *Arthroscopy* 2012;28(4):451-457.

59. Alpert JM, Wuerz TH, O'Donnell TF, Carroll KM, Brucker NN, Gill TJ: The effect of age on the outcomes of arthroscopic repair of type II superior labral anterior and posterior lesions. *Am J Sports Med* 2010;38(11):2299-2303.

60. Forsythe B, Guss D, Anthony SG, Martin SD: Concomitant arthroscopic SLAP and rotator cuff repair. *J Bone Joint Surg Am* 2010;92(6):1362-1369.

61. Abbot AE, Li X, Busconi BD: Arthroscopic treatment of concomitant superior labral anterior posterior (SLAP) lesions and rotator cuff tears in patients over the age of 45 years. *Am J Sports Med* 2009;37(7):1358-1362.

62. Park S, Glousman RE: Outcomes of revision arthroscopic type II superior labral anterior posterior repairs. *Am J Sports Med* 2011;39(6):1290-1294.

63. Boileau P, Parratte S, Chuinard C, Roussanne Y, Shia D, Bicknell R: Arthroscopic treatment of isolated type II SLAP lesions: Biceps tenodesis as an alternative to reinsertion. *Am J Sports Med* 2009;37(5):929-936.

64. Edwards DJ, Hoy G, Saies AD, Hayes MG: Adverse reactions to an absorbable shoulder fixation device. *J Shoulder Elbow Surg* 1994;3(4):230-233.

65. Burkart A, Imhoff AB, Roscher E: Foreign-body reaction to the bioabsorbable Suretac device. *Arthroscopy* 2000;16(1):91-95.

66. Kaar TK, Schenck RC Jr, Wirth MA, Rockwood CA Jr: Complications of metallic suture anchors in shoulder surgery: A report of 8 cases. *Arthroscopy* 2001;17(1): 31-37.

67. Yoo JC, Lee YS, Ahn JH, Park JH, Kang HJ, Koh KH: Isolated suprascapular nerve injury below the spinoglenoid notch after SLAP repair. *J Shoulder Elbow Surg* 2009;18(4):e27-e29.

68. Kim SH, Koh YG, Sung CH, Moon HK, Park YS: Iatrogenic suprascapular nerve injury after repair of type II SLAP lesion. *Arthroscopy* 2010;26(7):1005-1008.

69. Park JG, Cho NS, Kim JY, Song JH, Hong SJ, Rhee YG: Arthroscopic knot removal for failed superior labrum anterior-posterior repair secondary to knot-induced pain. *Am J Sports Med* 2017;45(11):2563-2568. doi:10.1177/0363546517713662.

    A case series of 11 patients with knot-induced pain after surgical fixation of unstable type II SLAP lesions. Sharp pain and clicking were the most common symptoms. At a mean of 3 weeks, the majority of patients had dramatic pain relief, and all patients had a negative compression-rotation test at 6 weeks. Level of evidence: IV.

70. Gilliam BD, Douglas L, Fleisig GS, et al: Return to play and outcomes in baseball players after superior labral anterior-posterior repairs. *Am J Sports Med* 2017;46(1):109-115. doi:10.1177/0363546517728256.

    This is a case series of 216 baseball players who underwent SLAP repair. One hundred thirty-three were reached by phone for follow-up interview. Overall 62% successfully returned to play. Return-to-play rates were 59% for pitchers and 76% for nonpitchers. The percentage of players who felt the same or better at follow-up compared with preinjury was higher among nonpitchers. Level of evidence: IV.

71. Smith R, Lombardo DJ, Petersen-Fitts GR, et al: Return to play and prior performance in Major League Baseball pitchers after repair of superior labral anterior-posterior tears. *Orthop J Sports Med* 2016;4(12):2325967116675822.

    This descriptive epidemiological study determined return to play rate of Major League Baseball pitchers who underwent SLAP repair between 2003 and 2010. 62.5% were able to return to play at the Major League Baseball level after SLAP repair surgery. Pitchers had a significant decrease in innings pitched following surgery. Level of evidence: IV.

72. de Sa D, Arakgi ME, Lian J, Crum RJ, Lin A, Lesniak BP: Labral repair versus biceps tenodesis for primary surgical management of type II superior labrum anterior to posterior tears: A systematic review. *Arthroscopy* 2019;35(6):1927-1938. doi:10.1016/j.arthro.2018.12.015.

    This systematic review of 23 studies compared SLAP repair versus biceps tenodesis (BT) for primary surgical management of type II SLAP lesions. SLAP repair was performed on 781 patients (mean age 35 years), and BT was performed on 100 patients (mean age 44 years). Similar scores were found in both the repair and BT groups. Level of evidence: III.

73. Erickson J, Lavery K, Monica J, Gatt C, Dhawan A: Surgical treatment of symptomatic superior labrum anterior-posterior tears in patients older than 40 years. *Am J Sports Med* 2014;43(5):1274-1282. doi:10.1177/0363546514536874.

    This systematic review analyzed published data on surgical management of SLAP tears in patients older than or of age 40 years. Multiple articles demonstrated higher failure rates and revision surgery rates in the older cohort with primary SLAP repair. Age older than 40 years and worker's compensation were found to be independent risk factors for increased surgical complications. Level of evidence: III.

74. Zhang AL, Kreulen C, Ngo SS, Hame SL, Wang JC, Gamradt SC: Demographic trends in arthroscopic SLAP repair in the United States. *Am J Sports Med* 2012;40(5):1144-1147. doi:10.1177/0363546512436944.

75. Mackinnon-Patterson B, Creighton RA, Spang JT, Kamath GV: Surgical trends in the treatment of superior labrum anterior and posterior (SLAP) lesions of the shoulder. Analysis of data from the American Board of Orthopaedic Surgery certification examination database. *Orthop J Sports Med* 2014;2(2 suppl):2325967114s00095. doi:10.1177/2325967114s00095.

    This is a level III cohort study analyzing surgical trends for SLAP lesions between 2002 and 2011. The proportion of SLAP repairs decreased from 69.3% to 44.8% and biceps tenodesis increased from 1.9% to 18.8%. Practice trends for orthopaedic board candidates indicate that the proportion of SLAP repairs has decreased over time, with an increase in biceps tenodesis and tenotomy. Level of evidence: IV.

76. Cvetanovich GL, Gowd AK, Agarwalla A, Forsythe B, Romeo AA, Verma NN: Trends in the management of isolated SLAP tears in the United States. *Orthop J Sports Med* 2019;7(3):232596711983399. doi:10.1177/2325967119833997.

    This is a descriptive epidemiology study of trends in the management of isolated SLAP tears in the United States. The management of isolated SLAP tears has shifted from 2007 to 2016 with an increase in the frequency of biceps tenodesis and a decline in the frequency of SLAP repair. Level of evidence: IV.

Chapter 21

Arthroscopic Management of the Arthritic Shoulder

Emilie V. Cheung, MD • Marc Safran, MD • John G. Costouros, MD

ABSTRACT

Glenohumeral osteoarthritis in young, active patients is challenging to manage because these patients have higher activity demands and longer life expectancy, which would limit the durability of the prosthetic replacement. When conservative modalities such as viscosupplementation, activity modification, and anti-inflammatory modalities have failed, arthroscopic treatment can be a reasonable treatment option. In this chapter, the arthroscopic management of glenohumeral osteoarthritis has been discussed.

Keywords: arthritis; arthroscopy; capsular release; debridement; shoulder

Introduction

The management of glenohumeral osteoarthritis (GHOA) in the young and active patient continues to pose a clinical challenge to the orthopaedic surgeon. The definition of young is based on chronological age as well as physiological age and must be made in the context of activity demands and patient expectations. In addition to GHOA, other pain generators, including the acromioclavicular joint, long head of the biceps, or rotator cuff complex, may play a much large role in shoulder pain and dysfunction. Although total shoulder arthroplasty (TSA) has been shown to reliably provide pain relief and functional improvement in patients with GHOA, the clinical results are less successful, less durable, and frequently less attractive to the younger active patient.[1-3] This patient population has greater expectations for postoperative pain relief and functional improvement; often desires to participate in higher impact activities, which can accelerate the risk of prosthetic loosening; is less inclined to agree to or comply with postoperative activity restrictions; and has increased longevity to allow for more problems to evolve over time.[4]

The authors of a 2004 study[2] reported on 78 arthritic shoulders in patients aged 50 years or younger treated with either hemiarthroplasty or TSA with a minimum 15-year follow-up. The estimated survival rate, defined as being free of revision, for hemiarthroplasty was 75% and for TSA was 84% at 20 years. There was marked long-term pain relief and improvement in motion with shoulder arthroplasty. However, with the Neer clinical rating system, nearly half of these patients were found to have an unsatisfactory result, mostly because of limitations in motion. The authors concluded that great care must be exercised, and alternative methods of treatment considered, before shoulder joint replacement arthroplasty is offered to patients aged 50 years or younger. Reasons for revision surgery after TSA include infection, glenoid loosening, and rotator cuff tearing. The authors of a 2010 study[1] reported on a similar experience and demonstrated inferior outcomes in patients younger than 50 years undergoing shoulder arthroplasty primarily because of a greater distribution of more complex pathologics including capsulorrhaphy arthropathy, inflammatory arthropathy, osteonecrosis, posttraumatic arthropathy, and postarthroscopic glenohumeral chondrolysis.[3,5] The authors of a 2013 study reported on 2,981 primary shoulder arthroplasties over a 5-year period and noted that patients younger than 60 years had a twofold higher rate of revision primarily because of dissatisfaction of hemiarthroplasty in younger patients.[3]

Dr. Cheung or an immediate family member serves as a paid consultant to or is an employee of Exactech, Inc. and serves as a board member, owner, officer, or committee member of the American Academy of Orthopaedic Surgeons. Dr. Safran or an immediate family member has received royalties from DJ Orthopaedics, Smith & Nephew, and Stryker; is a member of a speakers' bureau or has made paid presentations on behalf of Medacta and Smith & Nephew; serves as a paid consultant to or is an employee of Medacta; serves as an unpaid consultant to Biomimedica; has stock or stock options held in Biomimedica; has received research or institutional support from Smith & Nephew; and serves as a board member, owner, officer, or committee member of the International Society for Hip Arthroscopy and the International Society of Arthroscopy, Knee Surgery, and Orthopaedic Sports Medicine. Dr. Costouros or an immediate family member has received royalties from Shoulder Innovations and Wright Medical Technology, Inc.; is a member of a speakers' bureau or has made paid presentations on behalf of DJ Orthopaedics; serves as a paid consultant to or is an employee of DJ Orthopaedics, Shoulder in Motion, Tornier, and Wright Medical Technology, Inc.; and has received research or institutional support from Tornier.

Although nonsurgical treatment should always be the first step in treatment, it may not provide satisfactory pain relief, and patients may become frustrated by their functional decline with activities of daily living and recreational pursuits. The literature is inconsistent and the published studies in our peer-reviewed literature are underpowered with respect to steroid injection, viscosupplementation, and newer biologic agents including platelet-rich plasma and other stem-cell therapies.[6-8] Similarly, manual physical therapy has not been shown to provide significant improvement in pain or function in patients with GHOA.[9] However, one prospective randomized study demonstrated superior shoulder scores at short-term follow-up with hyaluronic acid injection when compared with a control group in patients with GHOA.[10]

Arthroscopic treatment is a reasonable option for this challenging subset of patients. This includes arthroscopic débridement, removal of loose bodies, chondroplasty, capsular release, and treatment of other associated pathologies that contribute to pain. The largest published experience is derived from Millett who has popularized the term CAM for comprehensive arthroscopic management and has reported favorable results in select patients with 85% survivorship at 2 years, noting that patients with >2 mm of glenohumeral joint space achieved better clinical results.[11] The benefits of arthroscopy are well-described and include smaller incisions, shorter surgical time, less bleeding and postoperative pain, lower rates of infection, outpatient surgery, a faster overall recovery relative to prosthetic replacement, and lack of long-term restrictions.

The Outerbridge[12] classification, although originally used to describe chondral and osteochondral lesions of the patella, has been used clinically to describe chondral and osteochondral lesions in other joints, including the shoulder. Outerbridge grade I lesions are characterized by softening of the articular surface, grade II is characterized by fissuring of the hyaline articular cartilage, grade III is characterized by fibrillation of cartilage, and grade IV is exposed subchondral bone. Chondromalacia is addressed at the time of shoulder arthroscopy with débridement of the articular surface with grade III or IV lesions to create a smoother bearing surface and to remove loose chondral flaps, which may be causing mechanical pain.

Imaging Studies

Radiographic studies should include a true AP view, or Grashey view, of the shoulder, performed perpendicular to the scapular plane, rather than to the plane of the body. The x-ray beam is angled approximately 40° laterally to obtain proper view of the glenohumeral joint space. In addition, an axillary view of the shoulder is performed to evaluate for eccentric glenoid wear and the presence of glenohumeral subluxation (**Figure 1**). Radiographic changes of osteoarthritis include joint space narrowing, inferior humeral osteophyte formation, subchondral cyst formation, and subchondral sclerosis (**Figure 2**).

The Samilson and Prieto[13] radiologic classification system has been used to describe the degree of shoulder arthropathy. Mild arthrosis, by definition, includes inferior humeral head and/or glenoid exostosis <3 mm in height. Moderate arthrosis includes inferior humeral head and/or glenoid exostosis measuring 3 to 7 mm in size with slight glenohumeral irregularity. Severe arthrosis includes inferior humeral head and/or glenoid exostosis measuring >7 mm and glenohumeral joint space narrowing and sclerosis.

MRI is useful to identify concomitant pathologies such as rotator cuff tearing, labral or biceps pathology, and focal chondral lesions. Preoperative diagnosis is useful for managing expectations during the preoperative discussion. These lesions can be addressed at the time of surgery.

Clinical Examination

Frequently, arthritis does not occur in isolation. Coexistent shoulder pathology may include subacromial impingement, rotator cuff tears, acromioclavicular joint arthritis, long head biceps tendinopathy, capsular

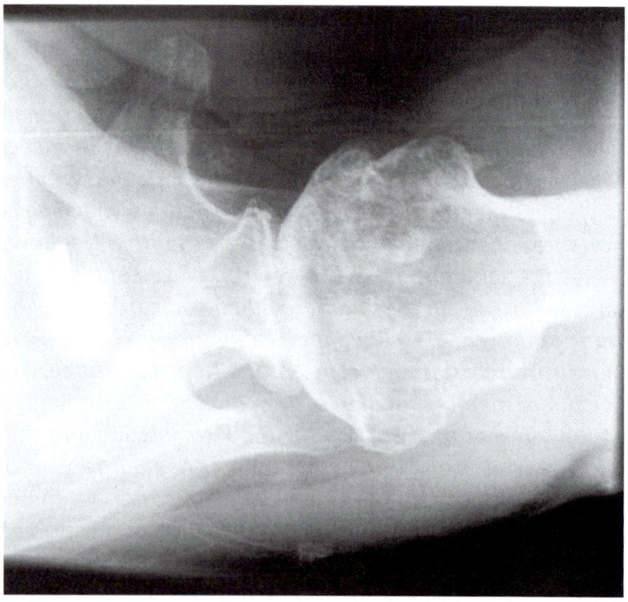

FIGURE 1 Axillary radiograph of a patient with a humeral head that is out of round (flattening) and an asymmetric glenoid wear resulting in a biconcave glenoid, an apex at the center of the glenoid, because of posterior glenoid wear.

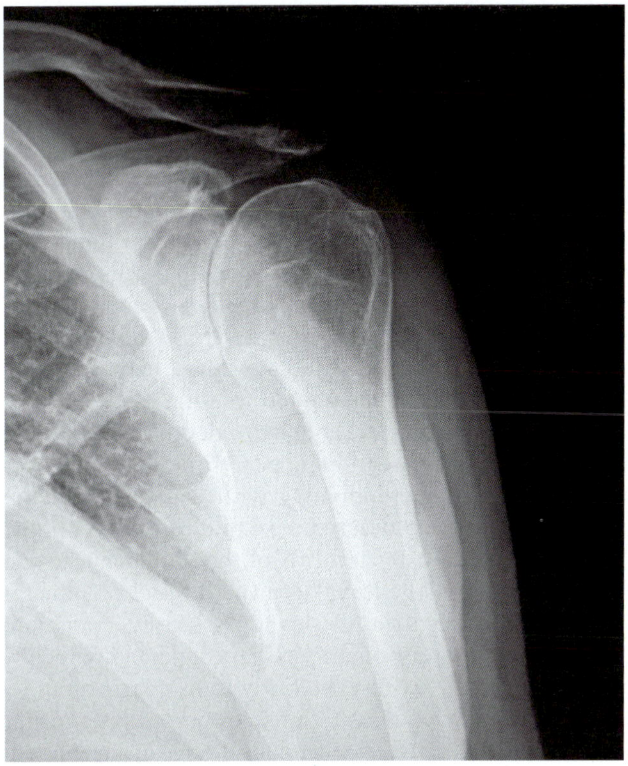

FIGURE 2 Shoulder AP radiograph demonstrates changes of osteoarthritis include joint space narrowing, inferior humeral osteophyte formation, subchondral cyst formation, and subchondral sclerosis.

contracture, labral tears, and suprascapular neuropathy. Referred pain to the shoulder, for instance cervical spine pathology, must always be evaluated as a potential cause of pain and loss of function. A detailed and comprehensive physical examination can help to guide the surgeon in identifying other potential pain generators in the shoulder in addition to advanced osteoarthritis. These other causes of shoulder pain may be addressed at the time of surgery.

Contraindications for Surgery

Contraindications for surgery include those parameters similar to any surgical procedure, including patients with medical comorbidities, which preclude general anesthesia or active infection. A relative contraindication is the patient who is medically unfit to undergo general anesthesia because shoulder arthroscopic débridement may be achieved using regional anesthesia (interscalene block), provided the anesthesiologist is comfortable with this technique.

Indications for Surgery

Indications for surgery include patients in whom nonsurgical treatment has failed for at least 3 months. Nonsurgical treatment includes a trial of physical therapy for maintenance of range of motion and oral nonsteroidal anti-inflammatory medications. Intra-articular injection of corticosteroid or another agent described earlier (viscosupplementation, platelet-rich plasma, etc) may be considered but is not a routine part of the treatment algorithm for the current authors.

Many consider arthroscopic débridement in the treatment algorithm of shoulder arthritis for young, active patients and for elderly patients with medical comorbidities that would preclude prosthetic replacement. Physiologically young patients (age less than 60 years) with the diagnosis of mild to moderate osteoarthritis, mild loss in range of motion, and concentric wear of the glenohumeral joint may be the best candidates for surgery. In patients whose occupation requires heavy manual labor or lifting or who participate in contact sports, TSA is often not recommended because of concern for glenoid component loosening. These patients may be best served with a less invasive procedure such as arthroscopic débridement. Shoulder arthroscopy has been shown to be a safe procedure with a low complication rate.[14,15] However, it is generally accepted that arthroscopic treatment of shoulder arthritis is a temporizing procedure, and not definitive. Those who undergo arthroscopic débridement still often need a prosthetic replacement some years after the arthroscopic procedure.

Surgical Technique

The surgical technique includes a complete diagnostic arthroscopy of the glenohumeral joint and subacromial space (**Figures 3** and **4**). Regional anesthesia, specifically interscalene blockade, is effective not only for postoperative pain control but also to facilitate working in a contracted joint. A technical consideration in advanced osteoarthritis is that the glenohumeral joint space is extremely narrowed because of the disease itself and the presence of capsular contracture. In a tight shoulder, traction may be applied to the humeral head while introducing the arthroscope into the glenohumeral joint to avoid inadvertent chondral injury by the trocar. Another helpful technique is to introduce the trochar more superiorly than normal when entering the joint, near the superior aspect of the humeral head at the joint line. Another way to address this potential problem is to use a disposable plastic cannula to enter the joint initially followed by replacement of the metallic cannula over a switching stick.

A standard anterior working portal located within the rotator interval is created by an outside-in technique. Coexistent lesions that may be potential sources of shoulder pain may also need to be addressed at the time of surgery. Loose osteochondral fragments are removed. A motorized shaver is used to débride osteochondral lesions, and

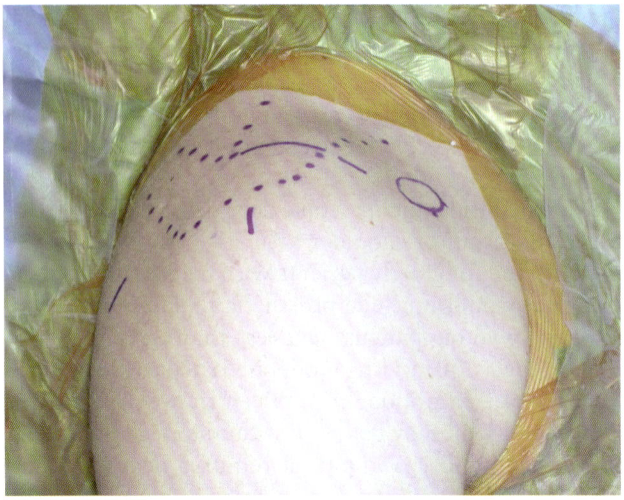

FIGURE 3 Clinical photograph showing standard shoulder arthroscopy setup for beach-chair position of a right shoulder. Bony landmarks are marked. The scapular spine and clavicle are marked by the dotted lines. The acromioclavicular joint is marked by the long solid line. The coracoid is marked by the circle. The standard locations of the posterior, lateral, and anterior portals are marked.

unstable flaps are débrided to a stable base with a shaver, curet, and/or rongeur. Outerbridge grade III articular cartilage is débrided to smooth tapering margins.

Large inferior humeral head osteophytes may cause mechanical symptoms such as locking and crepitus. If

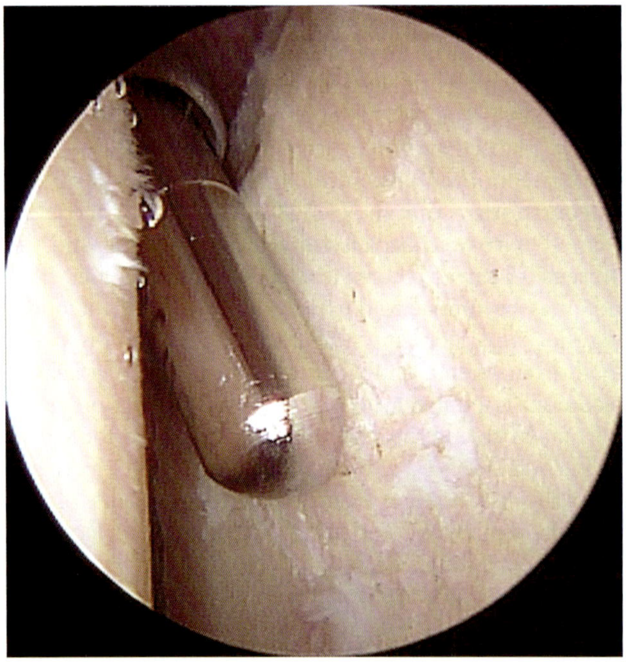

FIGURE 4 Arthroscopic view of the glenohumeral joint through the standard posterior viewing portal of a left shoulder. There is severe degenerative joint disease affecting the humeral head and glenoid articular surfaces.

the surgeon feels comfortable with this technique, large inferior osteophytes from the humeral head may be shaved down by a motorized burr. The risk to injury to the axillary nerve must be noted during débridement of osteophytes near the axillary pouch.[16]

Microfracture technique or drilling of intact subchondral bone may be performed for focal lesions. The intention is that the bleeding bed of subchondral bone may lead to influx of pluripotent mesenchymal cells, leading to fibrocartilage deposition, filling the articular defect. After the cartilage defect is prepared to a stable rim, the zone of calcified cartilage is removed at the base of the lesion with a curet. Then a microfracture awl is used to penetrate the subchondral bone to a depth of 2 mm with a 2 mm spacing between bony penetrations[17] (**Figure 5**).

Arthroscopic glenoidplasty with osteocapsular arthroplasty has been described as an effective technique for patients with osteoarthritis of the shoulder who are unsuitable for prosthetic replacement. If the glenohumeral joint is not concentric, this is addressed by correcting the articular contour of the misshapen glenoid, which is characteristically worn posteriorly in osteoarthritis. An arthroscopic burr and rasp is used to contour the anterior glenoid, or smooth the osteochondral ridge in a biconcave glenoid, converting it into a concentric concave shape. As a result pain and motion are improved on. Multiple portals may need to be created to gain access to large osteophytes around the humeral head. Arthroscopic synovectomy and capsular release are performed, if indicated. This may restore the position of the humeral head and may theoretically increase the joint contact surface area, but it is a technically challenging procedure and should be reserved for the experienced shoulder arthroscopist.

Arthroscopic débridement alone will not restore motion in patients who have capsular contractures. Capsular contractures exist in about 30% of patients undergoing arthroscopic débridement of shoulder osteoarthritis.[18,19] Therefore, capsular release is recommended when the patient has lost significant motion and may help reestablish a concentric joint. However, preoperative evaluation should include careful inspection of the radiographs to be sure the humeral head is still round and the joint concentric, as a flat humeral head will not rotate, even after capsular release. Some surgeons think that capsular releases also reduce the contact pressures, which may then reduce pain.

The capsular release may be performed using a radiofrequency device or a handheld biting instrument. A standard anterior working portal is created by an outside-in technique through the rotator interval. The rotator interval capsule and coracohumeral ligament is incised 1 cm lateral to the glenoid rim with the radiofrequency device. The thick capsular tissue within the rotator interval is completely

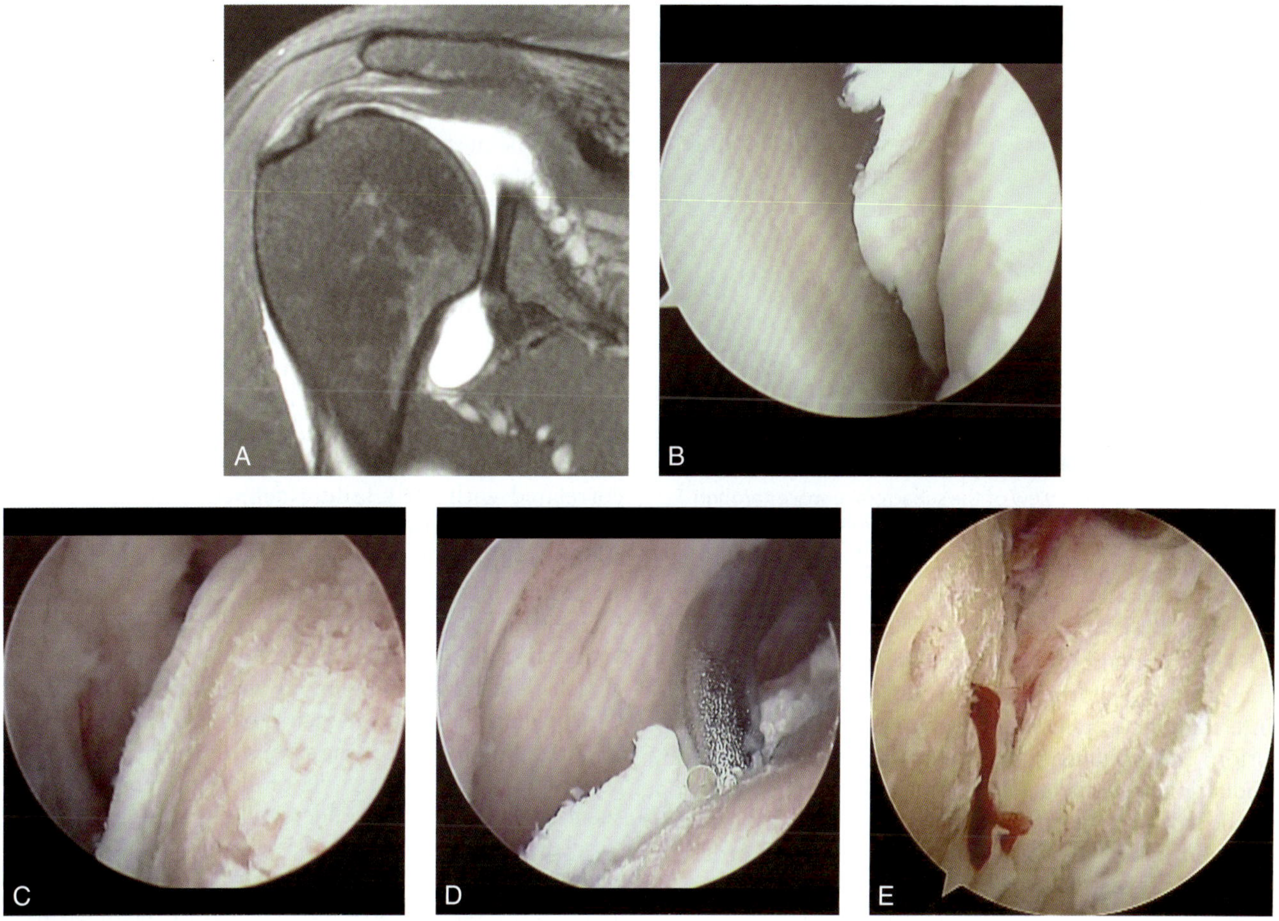

FIGURE 5 An isolated full-thickness chondral lesion of the humeral head. **A,** Magnetic resonance image revealing the lesion preoperatively. **B,** Intraoperative arthroscopic photograph showing the lesion with a flap of articular cartilage at the edge of the lesion. **C,** Intraoperative arthroscopic photograph showing the lesion after débridement with a curet. **D,** Intraoperative arthroscopic photograph of the microfracture awl penetrating the subchondral bone. **E,** Intraoperative arthroscopic photograph from another patient who underwent microfracture of the humeral head demonstrating blood leaking out of a hole in the bone made by the awl.

released, followed by release of the middle glenohumeral ligament. The exposure of rotator interval tissue may be facilitated by external rotation of the arm in adduction. Care should be taken to preserve the subscapularis tendon, as well as the medial aspect of the biceps sling to prevent destabilizing the biceps tendon. The thick capsule covering the subscapularis should be released to the anterior-inferior capsular pouch. One can differentiate between the subscapularis and the capsule by the appearance of the subscapularis tendon fibers, which are oriented transversely, whereas the capsule has an amorphous appearance.

The posterior capsular release may be performed by viewing through the anterior portal and instrumentation placed through the posterior portal. The posterior capsule and associated glenohumeral ligament is generally less robust than the anterior capsular structures. Internal rotation during the release may assist in visualization of the posterior capsule.

Release of the inferior capsule should be performed with the arm in adduction to minimize risk of injury to the axillary nerve, which is often in close proximity to the inferior glenoid. Rather than risk injury to the axillary nerve with radiofrequency or direct mechanical injury, some surgeons prefer to complete the inferior release with manual manipulation by placing the arm in maximal forward elevation while stabilizing the scapula.

The subacromial space is then entered to perform a subacromial decompression (**Figure 6**), and a distal clavicle excision may also be performed if indicated. It is considered that the subacromial bursectomy is critical to the success of arthroscopic débridement of the shoulder for glenohumeral arthritis. A radiofrequency device is used for ablation of the subacromial bursa. Care is taken to preserve the coracoacromial ligament, especially in the context of a massive rotator cuff tear to help reduce the risk of humeral head anterosuperior escape.

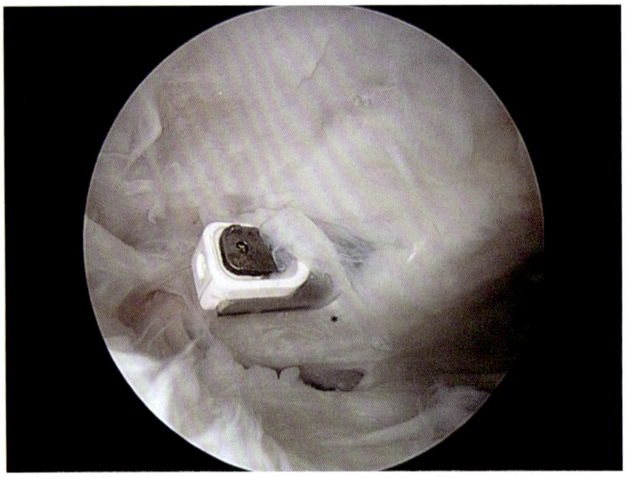

FIGURE 6 Arthroscopic view of the subacromial space through the posterior portal of a right shoulder. Bursectomy has been performed with a radiofrequency probe and arthroscopic shaver. The coracoclavicular ligament has been left intact (shiny structure). The rotator cuff is intact, in the lower part of the arthroscopic field.

A manipulation of the shoulder under anesthesia is then gently performed. This leads to disruption of the inferior capsular fibers that remain at the 6-o'clock position. Manipulation is performed in forward flexion, abduction, external rotation at the side, internal rotation at the side, external rotation in abduction, and internal rotation in abduction. Motion achieved is recorded in the surgical report.

Postoperative Rehabilitation

After surgery, a sling is used for comfort only and the patient is encouraged to move the arm actively, and passively. The patient is referred to physical therapy immediately after surgery for aggressive passive and active range of motion exercises to maintain the motion achieved during surgery and prevent the development of adhesions. The patient should be educated in obtaining forward elevation in the scapular plane, external rotation at the side, external rotation in abduction, and internal rotation. Exercises performed in the supine position limit scapulothoracic motion and help isolate the glenohumeral joint. In addition to supervised physical therapy, these exercises should be performed several times daily on a home program. Cryotherapy is routinely useful for control of postoperative swelling and pain control. Use of anti-inflammatory medications may also be helpful in the postoperative period. Strengthening exercises are generally incorporated as postoperative range of motion improves and pain subsides.

Results

Arthroscopic management of early shoulder arthritis has been shown to be an effective treatment option in most studies with relatively short-term follow-up.[20] Patients with early osteoarthritis can benefit from arthroscopic treatment for coexistent pathology such as arthroscopic bursectomy, labral débridement, or débridement of partial-thickness rotator cuff tears.[19,21]

The authors of 2017 study[22] reported on 107 shoulders in 98 patients with minimum 2-year follow-up who underwent comprehensive arthroscopic management (CAM). The procedure includes glenohumeral chondroplasty, capsular release, synovectomy, humeral osteoplasty, axillary nerve neurolysis, subacromial decompression, loose body removal, microfracture, and biceps tenodesis. All shoulders met criteria for TSA, but the patients opted for joint preservation with arthroscopic management. There were a number of radiographic features that were correlated with early failure defined as progression to TSA during the study. Patients in whom the CAM procedure failed had significantly less preoperative joint space than in patients in whom the procedure succeeded. Higher grades of osteoarthritis and age older than 50 years were also associated with failure. Shoulders with Walch type B2 and C glenoid were significantly more likely to fail than were Walch types A1, A2, and B1.[22]

In a follow-up study, the same group reported on outcomes with a minimum 5-year follow-up. Forty-six consecutive patients (49 shoulders) who underwent a CAM procedure at a minimum of 5 years from surgery were included. Survivorship was 95.6% at 1 year, 86.7% at 3 years, and 76.9% at 5 years. This study demonstrated, in a very selective group of patients, significant improvements in midterm clinical outcomes and high patient satisfaction after the arthroscopic CAM procedure for GHOA. The authors concluded that the CAM procedure can provide reasonable outcomes and should be considered an effective procedure in appropriately selected patients. Further studies are warranted to evaluate longer term outcomes after this procedure.[23]

The authors of 2002 study[18] evaluated the effectiveness of arthroscopy on focal chondral defects and found that arthroscopic management of patients with isolated, focal grade IV chondral lesions of the glenohumeral joint (no radiographic evidence of arthritis) was effective. Significant pain relief was documented in 88% of patients, and continued for 28 months or greater. The addition of concomitant procedures, such as acromioplasty, distal clavicle resection, labral débridement, or labral repair, did not have a negative impact on the functional results. The authors recommended arthroscopic capsular release in patients with a loss of passive shoulder motion. Osteochondral lesions greater than 2 cm^2 were associated with return of pain and failure of this procedure.

The authors of a 2008 study[24] reported on the outcomes of arthroscopic management of 20 shoulders in 19 patients younger than 55 years with grade II-IV

Outerbridge change. In addition to arthroscopic débridement, 9 patients had concomitant subacromial decompressions and 4 additional patients had subacromial bursectomy without acromioplasty (13 of 19 patients had subacromial bursectomies). At a minimum 12-month follow-up (average, 20 months, 12 to 33 months), three had progressed to shoulder arthroplasty, with a survivorship of 85%. It was found that the outcome scores were similar for those with chondral injury grade II to III and those with grade IV change. The investigators did find that those with unipolar lesions (glenoid or humeral head) did better when compared with those individuals with chondral loss on both sides of the joint. They also found that nine patients rated their shoulder greater than 80% (five had grade IV). Overall, the ASES score was 75 in these patients post arthroscopy.

A 2007 study reported on the treatment of GHOA with débridement and capsular release in eight patients with short-term follow-up, noting improvement in pain and functional outcome scores.[25] The concept of capsular release to gain motion in the presence of arthritis is most beneficial in those with concentric wear. In patients with posterior wear, a biconcave glenoid and flat humeral head with osteophytes will unlikely gain motion with a capsular release and may increase pain. Although osteophyte excision has not been studied extensively, early reports suggest that this may improve the outcomes of arthroscopic débridement.[17]

The authors of a 2010 study[26] reported favorable results on pain relief and recovery of shoulder function in 55 out of 71 selected patients at an average follow-up of just over 2 years. These authors studied these 71 patients who underwent surgery by one of four surgeons. These patients were a mixed group, with 20 subjects having had prior operations. Radiographically, the patients rated between 0 and 4 on the Samilson-Prieto scale, and all had Outerbridge grade II-IV lesions. These patients were self-selected in that they chose the arthroscopic option themselves, because they were not considered to be candidates for arthroplasty based on the degree of disease on radiography, the patient's age or activity level, and/or the patient's desire to avoid arthroplasty. These patients underwent a variety of concomitant procedures: 44 capsular release, 14 biceps tenodesis/tenotomy, 11 microfracture, 12 loose body/osteophyte removal, and 28 subacromial decompression. The data were not studied with respect to these additional procedures, so the effect of any additional procedure is not clear. Sixteen patients (22%) were converted to a total shoulder replacement (TSR) at an average 10 months post arthroscopy. The other 55 patients did not require a TSR at 27-month follow-up (12 to 90 months). Of those who were converted to a TSR, indicating that this procedure offers limited benefit in patients with more advanced OA. Conversely, those not converted to a TSR had a mean joint space width of 2.6 mm and a mean OA grade of 1.9.

Microfracture of the shoulder has been used for the treatment of focal chondral lesions of the humerus and glenoid and is largely based on techniques derived from the knee. The authors of a 2009 study reported on the use of microfracture for the treatment of full-thickness lesions of the shoulder in 30 patients with a mean age of 43 years at minimum 2-year follow-up.[17] Although 19% of patients were clinical failures and required another shoulder surgery at a mean follow-up of 47 months, the remaining patients reported improvements in pain relief and functional scores. The procedure was most effective in unipolar lesions affecting the humerus only and smaller lesions.

SUMMARY

In conclusion, arthroscopic débridement and capsular release for management of the osteoarthritic shoulder is an effective treatment option in the young, active patient. Concomitant shoulder pathologies, such as rotator cuff disease, impingement syndrome, biceps and labral pathology, and acromioclavicular arthritis should be addressed at the time of surgery. Early reported results have been encouraging with regard to pain relief and restoration of function in short-term follow-up, even in patients with severe glenohumeral arthritis. The benefits of capsular release, osteophyte excision, and microfracture are still under investigation. Arthroscopic débridement provides a treatment alternative for selected patients and may delay the need for prosthetic replacement.

KEY STUDY POINTS

- Arthroscopic management of glenohumeral osteoarthritis (GHOA) provides a treatment alternative for selected patients and may delay the need for prosthetic replacement.
- It is important to inform patients about the limitations of the procedure.
- Patients with less joint space and pathologic posterior glenoid shape are more likely to progress to early failure.

Annotated References

1. Saltzman MD, Mercer DM, Warme WJ, Bertelsen AL, Matsen FA: Comparison of patients undergoing primary shoulder arthroplasty before and after the age of fifty. *J Bone Joint Surg Am* 2010;92(1):42-47. doi:10.2106/JBJS.I.00071.

2. Sperling JW, Cofield RH, Rowland CM: Minimum fifteen-year follow-up of Neer hemiarthroplasty and total shoulder arthroplasty in patients aged fifty years or younger. *J Shoulder Elbow Surg* 2004;13(6):604-613. doi:10.1016/S1058274604001296.

3. Dillon MT, Inacio MCS, Burke MF, Navarro RA, Yian EH: Shoulder arthroplasty in patients 59 years of age and younger. *J Shoulder Elbow Surg* 2013;22(10):1338-1344. doi:10.1016/j.jse.2013.01.029.

   This was a retrospective cohort study of 2981 primary arthroplasties. Younger patients (<60 years) had a two times higher risk of revision than older patients. Level of evidence: III.

4. Johnson MH, Paxton ES, Green A: Shoulder arthroplasty options in young (<50 years old) patients: Review of current concepts. *J Shoulder Elbow Surg* 2015;24(2):317-325. doi:10.1016/j.jse.2014.09.029.

   Current concepts review on shoulder arthroplasty in young patients, with concerns of survivorship because of implant failure and functional deterioration.

5. Rao AJ, Johnston TR, Harris AHS, Smith RL, Costouros JG: Inhibition of chondrocyte and synovial cell death after exposure to commonly used anesthetics: Chondrocyte apoptosis after anesthetics. *Am J Sports Med* 2014;42(1):50-58. doi:10.1177/0363546513507426.

   This is an analysis of chondrocyte apoptosis after exposure to local anesthetics. Apoptosis occurred in a time-dependent fashion. 0.5% bupivacaine and 1:1000 epinephrine demonstrated more than 60% cell death.

6. Takamura KM, Chen JB, Petrigliano FA: Nonarthroplasty options for the athlete or active individual with shoulder osteoarthritis. *Clin Sports Med* 2018;37(4):517-526. doi:10.1016/j.csm.2018.05.003.

   After nonsurgical management fails, arthroscopic débridement with concomitant procedures to address potential pain generators may be an option in small, contained, unipolar lesions.

7. Di Giacomo G, De Gasperis N: The role of hyaluronic acid in patients affected by glenohumeral osteoarthritis. *J Biol Regul Homeost Agents* 2015;29(4):945-951.

   Patients with shoulder OA were divided into two groups. Group 1 received five intra-articular injections of Hyalgan and physiotherapy. Group 2 received only physiotherapy. There was a significant difference between the groups, with the Hyalgan group demonstrating greater and long-lasting efficacy of Hyalgan injections at 5 months. Level of evidence: II.

8. Kothari SY, Srikumar V, Singh N: Comparative efficacy of platelet rich plasma injection, corticosteroid injection and ultrasonic therapy in the treatment of periarthritis shoulder. *J Clin Diagn Res* 2017;11(5):RC15-RC18. doi:10.7860/JCDR/2017/17060.9895.

   In this randomized trial, patients with shoulder OA who received PRP injection, corticosteroid, or ultrasound therapy were compared. PRP treatment resulted in significant improvements over corticosteroid and ultrasound therapy, in motion, VAS score, and QuickDASH score at 12 weeks. Level of evidence: II.

9. Crowell MS, Tragord BS: Orthopaedic manual physical therapy for shoulder pain and impaired movement in a patient with glenohumeral joint osteoarthritis: A case report. *J Orthop Sports Phys Ther* 2015;45(6):453-461, A1-3. doi:10.2519/jospt.2015.5887.

   Treatment consisted of five sessions of physiotherapy over 4 weeks. Short-term improvements in self-reported function and pain were maintained at 1 year. Level of evidence: IV.

10. Di Giacomo G, de Gasperis N: Hyaluronic acid intra-articular injections in patients affected by moderate to severe glenohumeral osteoarthritis: A prospective randomized study. *Joints* 2017;5(3):138-142. doi:10.1055/s-0037-1605389.

    In this randomized trial, patients with shoulder OA who received intra-articular HA injection and physiotherapy, and physiotherapy only were compared. The combination of injection and physiotherapy was more effective than physiotherapy alone in reducing pain and improving shoulder scores. Level of evidence: II.

11. Millett PJ, Horan MP, Pennock AT, Rios D: Comprehensive Arthroscopic Management (CAM) procedure: Clinical results of a joint-preserving arthroscopic treatment for young, active patients with advanced shoulder osteoarthritis. *Arthroscopy* 2013;29(3):440-448. doi:10.1016/j.arthro.2012.10.028.

    The CAM procedure reduced pain, improved function, and provided short-term durability in 30 patients with advanced shoulder OA, as an alternative to arthroplasty. Survivorship was 85% at 2 years. Level of evidence: IV.

12. Outerbridge RE, Dunlop JA: The problem of chondromalacia patellae. *Clin Orthop Relat Res* 1975;(110):177-196. doi:10.1097/00003086-197507000-00024.

13. Samilson RL, Prieto V: Dislocation arthropathy of the shoulder. *J Bone Joint Surg Am* 1983;65(4):456-460.

14. Bigliani LU, Flatow EL, Deliz ED: Complications of shoulder arthroscopy. *Orthop Rev* 1991;20(9):743-751.

15. Small NC: Complications in arthroscopic surgery of the knee and shoulder. *Orthopedics* 1993;16(9):985-988.

16. Millett PJ, Gaskill TR: Arthroscopic management of glenohumeral arthrosis: Humeral osteoplasty, capsular release, and arthroscopic axillary nerve release as a joint-preserving approach. *Arthroscopy* 2011;27(9):1296-1303. doi:10.1016/j.arthro.2011.03.089.

17. Millett PJ, Huffard BH, Horan MP, Hawkins RJ, Steadman JR: Outcomes of full-thickness articular cartilage injuries of the shoulder treated with microfracture. *Arthroscopy* 2009;25(8):856-863. doi:10.1016/j.arthro.2009.02.009.

18. Cameron BD, Galatz LM, Ramsey ML, Williams GR, Iannotti JP: Non-prosthetic management of grade IV osteochondral lesions of the glenohumeral joint. *J Shoulder Elbow Surg* 2002;11(1):25-32. doi:10.1067/mse.2002.120143.

19. Ogilvie-Harris DJ, Wiley AM: Arthroscopic surgery of the shoulder. A general appraisal. *J Bone Joint Surg Br* 1986;68(2):201-207.

20. Elser F, Braun S, Dewing CB, Millett PJ: Glenohumeral joint preservation: Current options for managing articular cartilage lesions in young, active patients. *Arthroscopy* 2010;26(5):685-696. doi:10.1016/j.arthro.2009.10.017.

21. Weinstein DM, Bucchieri JS, Pollock RG, Flatow EL, Bigliani LU: Arthroscopic debridement of the shoulder for osteoarthritis. *Arthroscopy* 2000;16(5):471-476. doi:10.1053/jars.2000.5042.

22. Mitchell JJ, Warner BT, Horan MP, et al: Comprehensive arthroscopic management of glenohumeral osteoarthritis: Preoperative factors predictive of treatment failure. *Am J Sports Med* 2017;45(4):794-802. doi:10.1177/0363546516668823.

    The CAM procedure was performed in 107 shoulders. 16% progressed to TSA at a mean of 2 years. Radiographic features that were correlated with early failure included those with less joint space, grade of OA, and Walch type B2 and C glenoids. Level of evidence: III.

23. Mitchell JJ, Horan MP, Greenspoon JA, Menge TJ, Tahal DS, Millett PJ: Survivorship and patient-reported outcomes after comprehensive arthroscopic management of glenohumeral osteoarthritis: Minimum 5-year follow-up. *Am J Sports Med* 2016;44(12):3206-3213. doi:10.1177/0363546516656372.

    The CAM procedure was performed in 49 shoulders. This study demonstrates significant improvements in midterm clinical outcomes and high patient satisfaction after the arthroscopic CAM procedure for GHOA, with a 76.9% survivorship rate at a minimum of 5 years postoperatively. Level of evidence: IV.

24. Kerr BJ, McCarty EC: Outcome of arthroscopic débridement is worse for patients with glenohumeral arthritis of both sides of the joint. *Clin Orthop Relat Res* 2008;466(3):634-638. doi:10.1007/s11999-007-0088-0.

25. Richards DP, Burkhart SS: Arthroscopic debridement and capsular release for glenohumeral osteoarthritis. *Arthroscopy* 2007;23(9):1019-1022. doi:10.1016/j.arthro.2006.11.016.

26. Van Thiel GS, Sheehan S, Frank RM, et al: Retrospective analysis of arthroscopic management of glenohumeral degenerative disease. *Arthroscopy* 2010;26(11):1451-1455. doi:10.1016/j.arthro.2010.02.026.

Section 5

Principles of Clinical Information

SECTION EDITORS:

T. BRADLEY EDWARDS, MD
BRENT J. MORRIS, MD

Chapter 22

Proximal Humeral Anatomy and Prosthetic Reconstruction

Christopher R. Chuinard, MD, MPH, FAOA, FAAOS

ABSTRACT

Anatomic shoulder arthroplasty is used for the management of glenohumeral arthritis. Its origins go back over 100 years, but successful arthroplasty was not achieved until the middle of the 20th century. As clinical and biomechanical research has improved, the designs, the fixation methods, implant sizes and shapes, and surface materials have evolved anatomic shoulder arthroplasty to a reliable, durable treatment option. Soft-tissue considerations and surgical technique continue to be variables that influence the outcome.

Keywords: anatomic; arthroplasty; humeral; prosthetic; replacement; shoulder

Introduction

The history of proximal humeral arthroplasty dates from 1893, when French surgeon Jules Émile Péan performed a two-stage procedure (resection followed by staged implantation) on a patient with extensive tuberculosis osteomyelitis.[1] The implant was crafted by a dentist, had a platinum shaft, and was more similar to a modern reverse prosthesis than a nonconstrained design. The prosthesis performed admirably for a short time but eventually failed because of recurrent infection. Péan had been inspired by Themistocles Gluck, a German surgeon who designed several proximal humeral replacements, including one with modular ivory heads.[1] Both surgeons were prescient in their approaches but not in their execution. Modern arthroplasty has little use for noble metals and ivory resurfacing, but it has benefited from more than a century of development. Prostheses have evolved into approximations of native humeral anatomy as well as designs that do not resemble anything in nature.

Dr. Chuinard or an immediate family member has received royalties from Shoulder Innovations and Wright Medical Technology, Inc.; is a member of a speakers' bureau or has made paid presentations on behalf of DJ Orthopaedics; serves as a paid consultant to or is an employee of DJ Orthopaedics, Shoulder in Motion, Tornier, and Wright Medical Technology, Inc.; and has received research or institutional support from Tornier.

Humeral Anatomy

The goal of an unconstrained primary arthroplasty is to re-create normal, patient-specific humeral anatomy. To reproducibly and reliably accomplish this goal, the surgeon must understand normal humeral anatomy, glenoid anatomy, and glenohumeral kinematics. The primary consideration for glenohumeral arthroplasty is the humerus itself. It is important to understand the relationship between the articular surface and the axis of motion. Because the normative shape of the humeral head may be lost during arthroplasty, the surgeon must understand relationships between humeral size, shape, and radius of curvature for accurate reproduction of the anatomy.

Humeral Head Size and Shape

Although multiple cadaver studies have provided some average values for humeral head size and shape, the reported norms vary. The articular surface of the humeral head approximates one-third of a sphere, but it becomes slightly ellipsoid at the periphery, averaging 2 mm less in the axial plane than in the coronal plane.[2-6] Because of this relationship, there is a fairly constant ratio between humeral head diameter and thickness; this implies that there is a single head height for each radius.[2-8] The average thickness of the humeral head radius of curvature is 24 mm in men and 19 mm in women. The average humeral head diameter is 2 mm greater in both dimensions in men than in women.[4,8,9] Studies reported an average humeral head diameter of 43.4 mm or 44.5 mm at the anatomic neck.[2-4] Across studies, there is a fairly consistent 70% to 80% ratio of humeral head radius to humeral head height. The between-study variations may have to do with differing methodologies[4-11] (**Figure 1**).

Mathematical models demonstrate that oval heads fit the native articular geometry with three times less error than spherical models; studies demonstrated a 12% difference in the radii between the frontal and sagittal planes, and, as a result, using the superior-inferior dimension to select a spherical prosthetic head may result in a head that is too large.[5,12,13] By contrast, using the anterior-posterior dimension may result in selecting a head that is too small.[12,13] In a 2016 study, 79 human cadaver humeri were mathematically modeled, the results

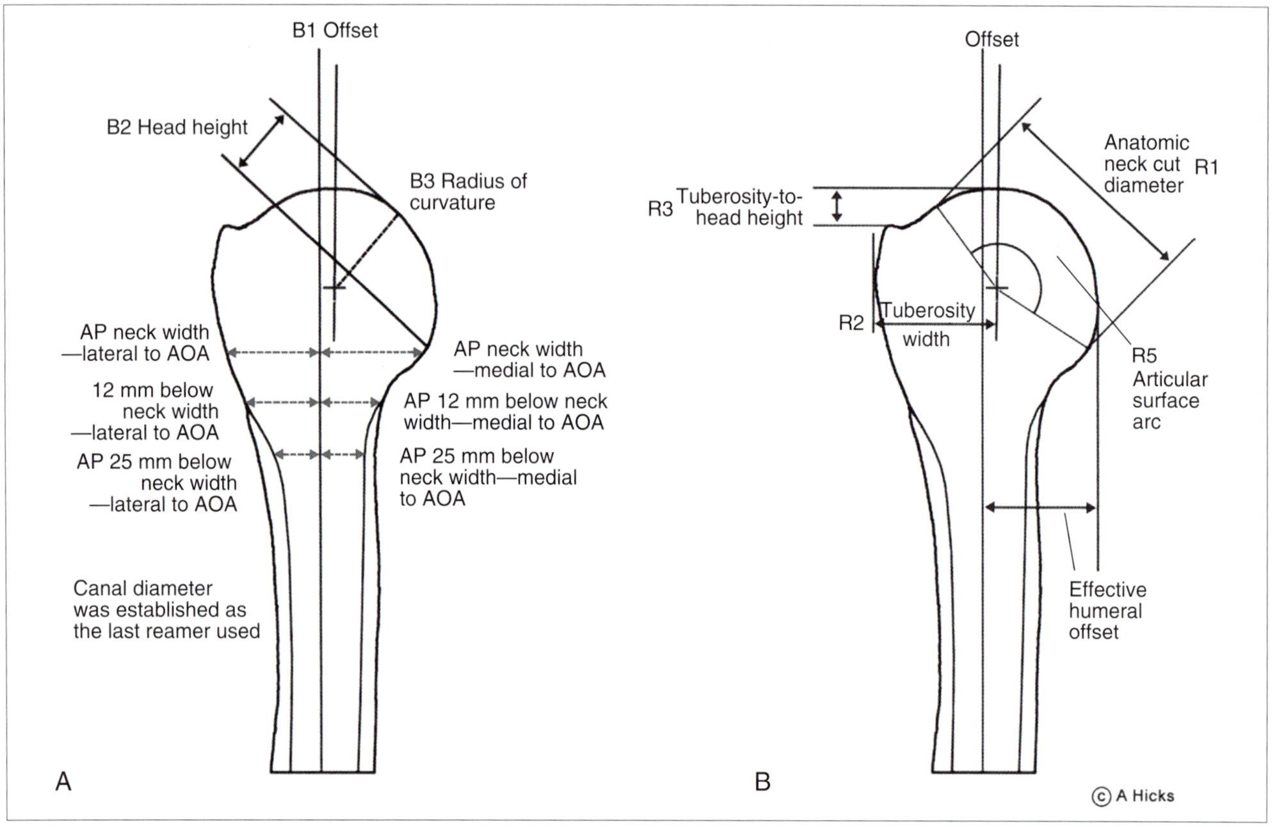

FIGURE 1 **A** and **B**, Illustrations of the key anatomic relationships in humeral arthroplasty. AOA = anatomic orthopaedic axis, B = biomechanics parameter, I = intraosseous parameter, R = redundant parameter. (Reprinted from J Shoulder Elbow Surg 16[suppl 3]. Wirth MA, Ondrla J, Southworth C, Kaar K, Anderson BC, Rockwood CA III: Replicating proximal humeral articular geometry with a third-generation implant: A radiographic study in cadaveric shoulders, S111-S116. Copyright © 2007 Journal of Shoulder and Elbow Surgery Board of Trustees. doi:10.1016/j.jse.2006.09.008.)

of which showed that the humeral heads became more oval as they increased in size.[14] Furthermore, a 2013 study demonstrated superior range of motion, translation, and glenohumeral kinematics when comparing spherical to nonspherical prosthetic humeral heads in their model.[12] In a follow-up study, nonspherical heads provided more glenohumeral translation, regardless of glenoid conformity.[13] The clinical relevance of these studies remains unknown; however, as the goal is more anatomic designs, ovoid heads paired with conforming glenoids may be an important area of research.

The use of a large prosthetic head was found to constrain the first and last 20° of abduction, leading to proximal humeral migration, loss of external rotation, and more posterior translation. Using a smaller head led to an inferior migration.[10] An increase in humeral head height to 5 mm above normal will significantly reduce motion, and a reduction of an equal amount can decrease joint excursion by 24°.[7] A displacement of 5 mm, corresponding to 20% of the radius of the humeral head, altered the lever arm of the rotator cuff by 20%.[15]

Humeral Neck-Shaft Angle

The angle between the center line of the humeral head and the axis of the humeral canal is the neck-shaft angle (**Figure 2**). Reported values range from 129.6° to 137.0°, with a weighted average of 134.4°.[2-5,16] A study of 2,058 cadaver humeri found that 78% of the humeri fell between 130° and 140°, with 135° being the most common measurement and a mean of 134.7° (range, 115° to 148°).[17] The clinical relevance is that an extreme varus or valgus angle can make prosthetic reconstruction challenging unless an adaptable prosthesis is used. However, variations in cutting technique allowed appropriate reconstruction of the articular surface with a fixed-angle prosthesis. For a varus neck-shaft angle, the humeral osteotomy should begin at the superolateral point; for a valgus neck-shaft angle, the osteotomy should begin from the inferomedial point[14] (**Figure 3**). Because alterations of the neck-shaft angle during prosthetic reconstruction could lead to a change in the length of the abductor muscles, thereby shifting the center of rotation and leading to impingement or rotator cuff dysfunction, the surgeon must mate the prosthesis with the line of the humeral head

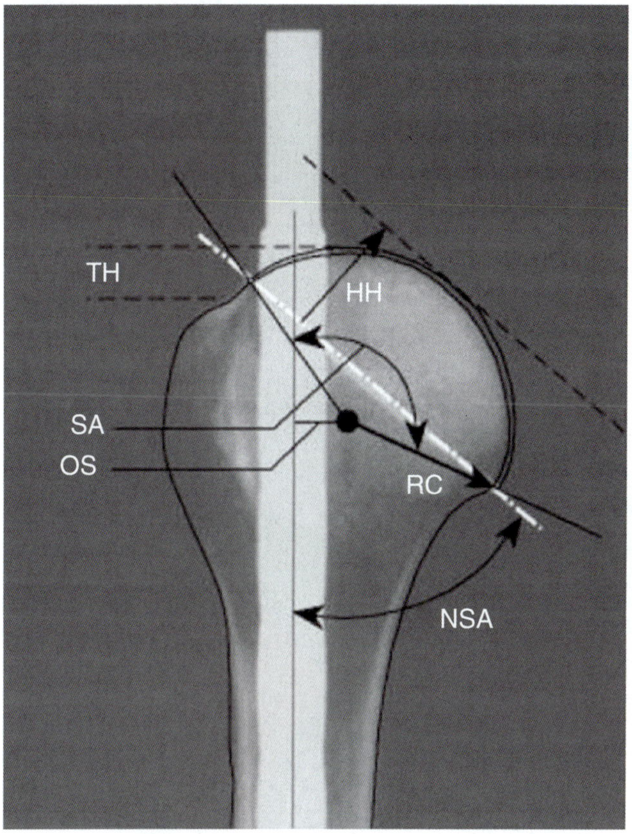

FIGURE 2 True AP radiograph showing the coronal anatomic parameters of the proximal humerus. Black dot = center of rotation, dashed white line = base of articular surface, HH = humeral head height, NSA = neck-shaft angle, OS = medial offset, RC = radius of curvature, TH = tuberosity-to-head height, vertical black line = center line of reamed canal. (Adapted from J Shoulder Elbow Surg 14[Suppl 1]. Pearl ML: Proximal humeral anatomy in shoulder arthroplasty: Implications for prosthetic design and surgical technique, S99-S104. Copyright © 2005 Journal of Shoulder and Elbow Surgery Board of Trustees. doi:10.1016/j.jse.2004.09.025.)

resection and restore the appropriate articular surface arc to the humerus.[17-19]

Humeral Head Offset

It is important to consider the offset of the center of rotation of the humeral head from the axis of the humeral shaft in both the transverse and the coronal planes. Because the center of rotation of the humeral head is not coincident with the axis of the humeral shaft (the so-called orthopaedic axis), small variations in position can lead to large alterations in glenohumeral kinematics. The orthopaedic axis represents the central reaming axis of the humerus; the actual center of rotation of the humeral head lies an average 2.1 mm posterior (ranges 2 to 4 mm in the axial plane) and 6.6 mm medial (ranges 6 to 9 mm in the coronal plane) to the humeral axis, thus creating a combined center of rotation that is posteromedial to the longitudinal axis of the humeral canal[2,5,8,16,19-22] (**Figure 4**).

Humeral Head Retroversion

Humeral head retroversion or retrotorsion is the angle between the epicondylar axis of the distal humerus and the central axis of the humeral head. Reported humeral retroversion values range from 17.9° (± 13.7°) to 21.4° (± 3.3°). Humeral head retroversion may be more affected than other parameters by patient age, sex, and ethnicity, and it can vary between sides in the same individual.[2,23-26] A correlation may exist between the position of the bicipital groove and the equator of the humeral head; the bicipital groove lies an average of 8 to 9 mm from the equator, allowing it to be used as an additional landmark for humeral retroversion.[5,23-25] When CT was used to determine retroversion in 120 cadavers, an average of 17.6° of retroversion was measured from the transepicondylar axis, and an average of 28.8° was measured from the forearm axis.[27] A three-dimensional laser analysis of the articular surface yielded an average retroversion of 18.6°, with articular geometry approximating a centroid.[23] Another study found that retroversion could be reliably measured based on the lateral margin of the lesser tuberosity and arrived at an average of 48°.[28] The researchers measured 185 dry bone specimens with a special jig to determine that the lesser tuberosity was a more reliable reference point than the bicipital groove or the transepicondylar line. Many humeral systems for arthroplasty reconstruction reference retroversion based on the axis of the forearm. When relying on a humeral cutting guide that uses the forearm for reference, the surgeon should account for natural variation by considering the 10° to 15° carrying angle and visualizing the insertion of the rotator cuff before performing the humeral osteotomy[20] (**Figure 5**).

Humeral Shaft Morphology

In the past 10 years, increasing attention has been given to the proximal humeral shaft and metaphyseal morphology. Three morphotypes of the proximal humerus were identified: low offset, standard, and high offset[5] (**Figure 6**). These terms refer to the relative amount of offset of the head to the humeral shaft in the metaphyseal segment. Decreasing the offset may make the insertion of a straight stem more difficult. Curved stems, so-called finless stems, and reduced-geometry stems were developed based on improved understanding of this anatomy. As more attention was directed to creating adaptable prostheses, the limitations of some press-fit designs became apparent. Some press-fit stems displaced the center of rotation superiorly and laterally by 12 and 8 mm, respectively, leading to rotator cuff dysfunction.[29,30] Elevation of the prosthetic humeral head by as little as 5 mm can decrease the moment arms of the rotator cuff musculature and can even change their vectors when the arm is adducted.[31-33] The greater-tuberosity-to -humeral-head height averages 6 mm; if the humerus is too

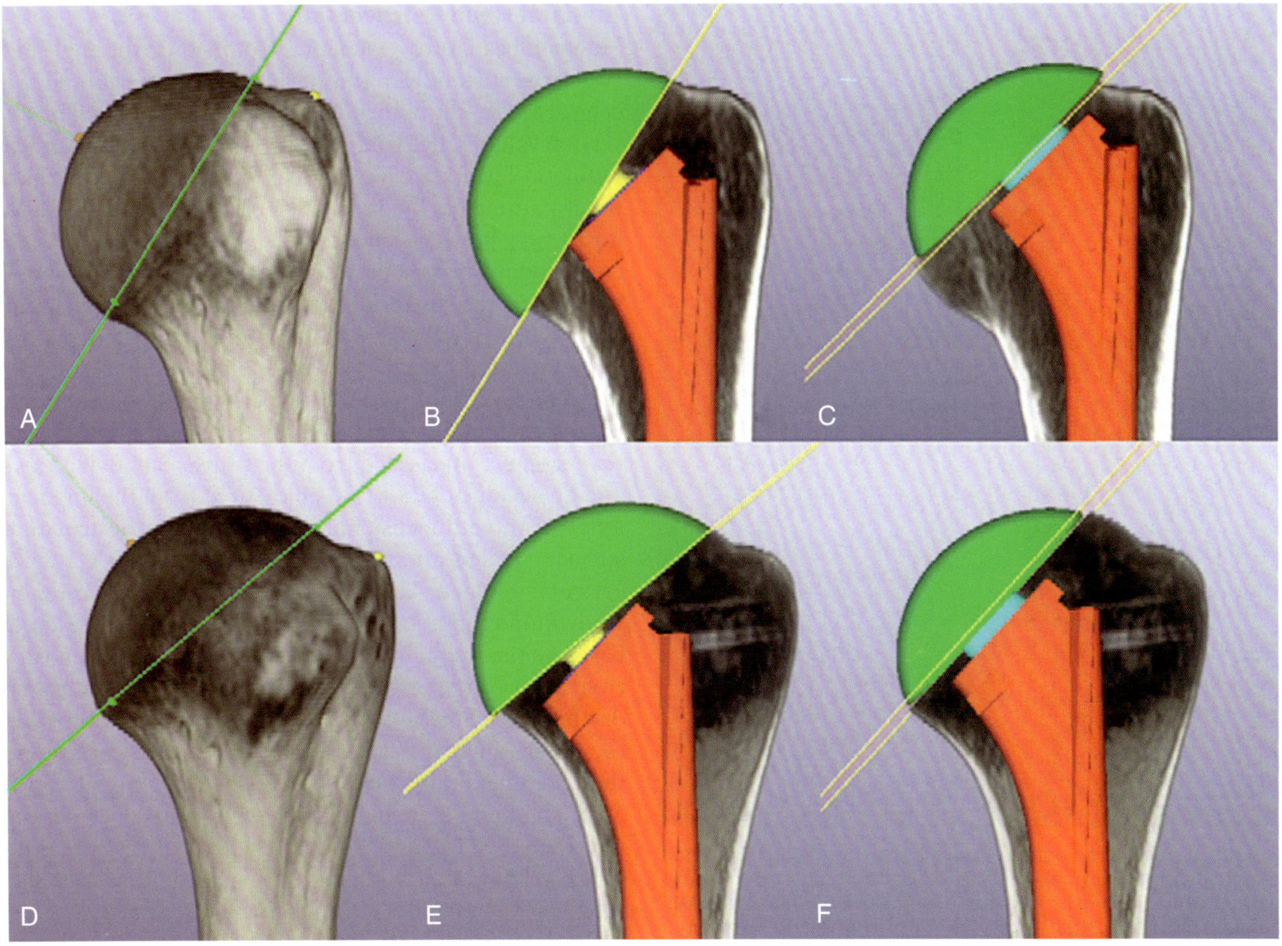

FIGURE 3 Schematic drawings showing neck-shaft angle reconstructions using adjustable-angle and fixed-angle devices. A humerus with a varus neck-shaft angle (**A**) can be treated with an adjustable-angle device and a humeral osteotomy at the anatomic neck (**B**) or a fixed-angle prosthesis and a 135° osteotomy with a modified cut from the superolateral point of the neck plane (**C**). A humerus with a valgus neck-shaft angle (**D**) can be treated with an adjustable-angle device and a humeral osteotomy at the anatomic neck (**E**) or a fixed-angle prosthesis and a 135° osteotomy with a modified cut from the superolateral point of the neck plane (**F**). Green line = anatomic neck (defining the native neck-shaft angle), yellow line = prosthetic neck and neck-shaft angle. Blue area = fixed-angle prosthetic neck, green area = prosthetic humeral head, red area = prosthetic body, yellow area = variable-angle prosthetic neck. (Reproduced with permission from Jeong J, Bryan J, Iannotti JP: Effect of a variable prosthetic neck-shaft angle and the surgical technique on replication of normal humeral anatomy. *J Bone Joint Surg Am* 2009;91[8]:1932-1941. doi:10.2106/JBJS.H.00729.)

high, the inferior capsule will be overly tight with the arm in abduction, and the rotator cuff will be under excessive tension with the arm in adduction[4,34] (**Figure 1**).

Prosthesis Design Considerations

First-Generation, Second-Generation, and Third-Generation Humeral Implants

Modern shoulder arthroplasty began with Charles Neer's monoblock design in 1951.[35] This system offered five stem diameters and one humeral head size. The stem resembled a modern fracture stem, with fenestrations to allow bony growth. Neer's early success with this implant led to the 1974 introduction of an implant that borrowed from successful hip arthroplasty, with a cemented stem, two humeral head options, and a polyethylene glenoid component. The second generation of shoulder arthroplasty was launched by the introduction of modularity between the humeral head and shaft to allow a more anatomic reconstruction. This system facilitated more anatomic placement of the humeral head relative to the tuberosities and the rotator cuff, allowing easier soft-tissue tensioning by providing different head heights and variable offset between the shaft and the head.[36] However, many second-generation stems had a gap between the head and the collar of the stem: a smaller head size and a corresponding loss of articular surface arc led to premature contact between the nonarticular portions of the humerus and glenoid.[29,30] The step-off between the collar of the stem and the humeral head with a second-generation

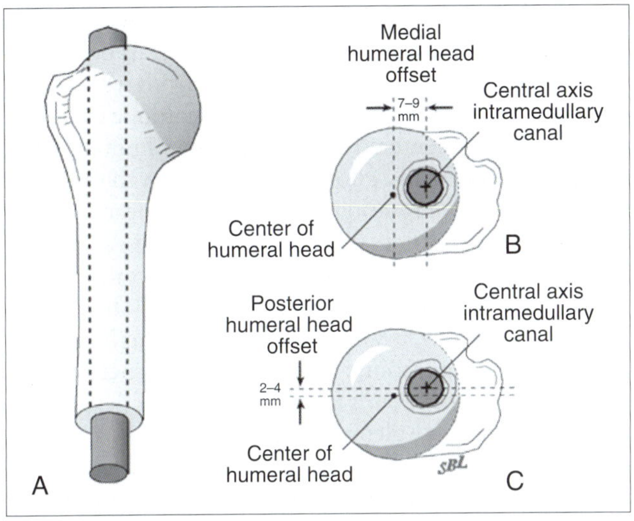

FIGURE 4 Schematic drawings showing the humeral head offset. **A**, The central axis of the intramedullary canal. **B**, The humeral head offset in the coronal plane (approximately 7 to 9 mm medial to the central axis of the intramedullary canal). **C**, The humeral head offset in the axial plane (2 to 4 mm posterior to the central axis of the intramedullary canal). (Reproduced with permission from Iannotti JP, Lippitt SB, Williams GR Jr: Variation in neck-shaft angle: Influence in prosthetic design. *Am J Orthop (Belle Mead NJ)* 2007;36[12 suppl 1]:9-14.)

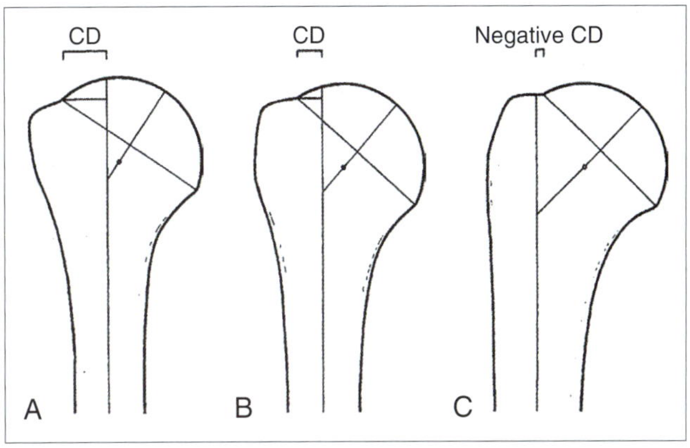

FIGURE 6 Schematic drawings showing proximal humeral morphology and the types of offset of the articular surface relative to the proximal metaphysis: high offset (**A**), standard (**B**), and low offset (**C**). CD = critical distance or greater tuberosity offset, defined as the distance between the medial insertion of the supraspinatus and the longitudinal axis of the humeral shaft; as the CD decreases, insertion of a straight-stemmed prosthesis becomes more difficult. Angled lines = humeral head inclination angle relative to the shaft, dot = geometric center of rotation, vertical line = longitudinal axis of the humeral shaft. (Reprinted from J Shoulder Elbow Surg 11[4]. Hertel R, Knothe U, Ballmer FT: Geometry of the proximal humerus and implications for prosthetic design, 331-338. Copyright © 2002 Journal of Shoulder and Elbow Surgery Board of Trustees. doi:10.1067/mse.2002.124429.)

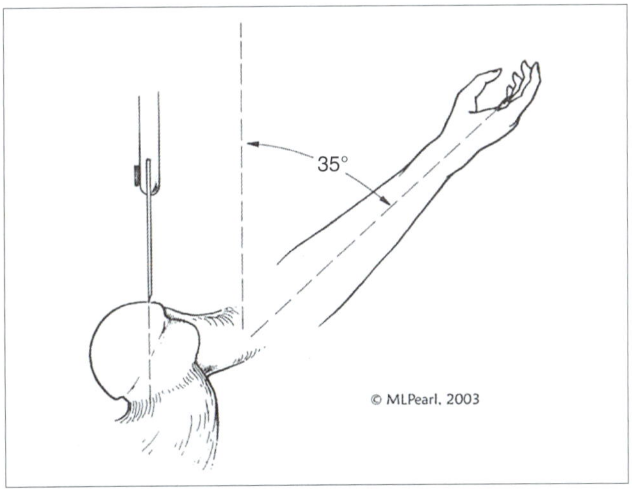

FIGURE 5 Schematic drawing showing a humeral osteotomy made in excessive retroversion. With a standard osteotomy at 35° of retroversion, anatomic reconstruction is difficult, and there is a risk of violating the rotator cuff. (Reprinted from J Shoulder Elbow Surg 14[1 suppl 1]. Pearl ML: Proximal humeral anatomy in shoulder arthroplasty: Implications for prosthetic design and surgical technique, S99-S104. Copyright © 2005 Journal of Shoulder and Elbow Surgery Board of Trustees. doi:10.1016/j.jse.2004.09.025.)

implant made it easy to overstuff the joint or position the humeral head in an overly superior position relative to the greater tuberosity.[19] Usually, soft-tissue tensioning is easiest to judge when the humeral head rests on the cut surface, but implants with a step-off between the stem and the head made this step challenging. Most second-generation implants have a preset neck-shaft angle that necessitates a cut using a specific osteotomy guide. Cementing these implants may improve the ability to accurately reproduce the anatomy, but they can be unforgiving when press fit.

The modern adaptable shoulder prosthesis is based on anatomic norms.[2,3] These third-generation stems have multiple areas of adjustment to account for variation in neck-shaft angle as well as more anatomic head sizes and variable offset. Compared with a second-generation implant, the anatomic implant more accurately restored glenohumeral motion and minimize eccentric loading of the glenoid. Furthermore, the second-generation implant produced eight times the joint reactive force at the superior aspect of the glenoid.[37] Further evolution of implant adaptability has allowed near-normalization of the center of rotation in prosthetic reconstruction of the proximal humerus.[38] With a third-generation implant, the surgeon can perform an anatomic osteotomy of the humeral head and be confident that the prosthesis will reproduce the anatomy. The prosthesis can be adapted to the patient, rather than the patient adapted to the prosthesis. Cementation of the stem can provide an additional degree of freedom in third-generation as well as second-generation implants.

Long-Stem, Short-Stem, and No-Stem Humeral Implants and Humeral Resurfacing

Over the past years, increasing attention has been directed to the shaft portion of the humeral implant. The concepts of hip arthroplasty have been extended to shoulder arthroplasty. Many of the original concepts of humeral implants were based on those of femoral implants. Resurfacing shoulder arthroplasty also was adapted from the hip precedent and has been used for several years. The resurfacing should remove only the remaining cartilage and underlying subchondral bone, with the intent of easily reproducing the offset, the radius of curvature, the diameter, and the head height of the proximal humerus while preserving proximal humeral bone stock and avoiding stem-associated complications.[39-41]

Advocates of resurfacing believe that this bone-preserving operation may be preferable to total or stemmed hemiarthroplasty in young, active patients.[39-45] Conversion to a stemmed implant or an arthrodesis is thought to be easy. In a study of 36 patients younger than 55 years who underwent a resurfacing hemiarthroplasty, there was no short-term implant loosening or glenoid wear, and 35 patients reported high satisfaction.[41] If a stem is not used, re-creating the instant center of rotation may be easier because the position of the articular surface is not dictated by the humeral canal. In total shoulder arthroplasty, however, the approach to the glenoid is challenging if the humerus is not resected (**Figure 7, A**). Caution should be exercised if there is insufficient bone stock, osteopenic bone, significant osteonecrosis, or proximal humeral deformity. In some patients with a focal cartilaginous defect or osteonecrosis, it may be necessary to resurface the isolated pathologic area[45] (**Figure 7, B**).

Current stem designs focus on metaphyseal fixation of the humeral stem. These designs derive their press fit from the proximal metaphyseal bone rather than more distal cortical bone, that is, the DePuy Global. Studies from Europe showed promise with stemless or canal-sparing implants that have purchase in the metaphysis below the resection plane. Stemless designs differ from resurfacing implants in that the surgeon makes an anatomic head cut, and the device is centered on the cut, thus eliminating the concerns of offset and allowing the surgeon to re-create the native center of rotation independent of the axis of the humeral shaft. With fixation in the metaphyseal region, there is no stem to force the device into varus or incorrect version. Early studies have reported good short-term clinical success, even with distorted proximal humeral anatomy, after anatomic humeral reconstruction and glenoid replacement with a bone-conserving device that allowed traditional glenoid exposure.[47-49] The use of a stemless implant may not be preferable in patients with osteoporotic bone, many of whom are older women.[49,50]

The advantages of a design with a relatively long stem are the larger bone-implant interface to distribute the forces and the larger surface area to resist rotational or torsional loads, which lead to good long-term stability. The disadvantages include stem-related complications, such as intraoperative or postoperative periprosthetic fracture, alterations in kinematics, and difficult revision. The advantages of a stemless device include the preservation of proximal bone, which may be an advantage for later revision or repair of a rotator cuff tear. Because the humeral head is resected in the same fashion as in a primary arthroplasty, access to the glenoid is facilitated. Stemless implants have less metal and therefore may be less stiff, share more load across the bone, and may have better long-term survivability.[47]

Humeral resurfacing may be necessary if hemiarthroplasty is indicated. A relatively young patient, a patient with distorted proximal humeral anatomy (as with fracture sequelae), or a patient with a pristine concentric glenoid may be an ideal candidate for resurfacing rather than stemmed hemiarthroplasty or traditional total

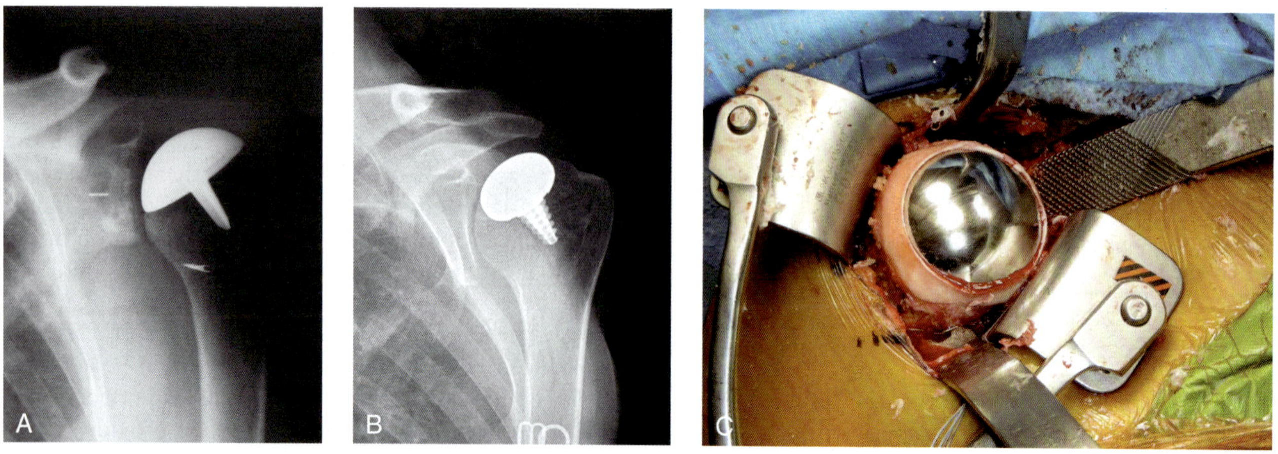

FIGURE 7 **A**, Grashey radiograph showing a resurfacing total shoulder arthroplasty. Grashey radiograph (**B**) and intraoperative photograph of the same patient (**C**) showing a focal resurfacing to treat osteonecrosis.

shoulder arthroplasty.[41] Because the proximal humerus is reamed or milled to accommodate a metallic shell that restores a smooth, spherical articular surface, advocates claim that the resurfacing procedure can easily re-create the anatomic instant center of rotation of the humerus. However, the joint can be easily overstuffed, and care must be taken to ensure that the guide pin is perpendicular to the plane of the anatomic neck before humeral preparation.[42,43,46] The same soft-tissue releases as in a total shoulder arthroplasty should be performed to ensure adequate exposure of the humerus during preparation, but good long-term satisfaction and survivorship are possible.[44,45,51]

The short-stemmed implant represents a compromise between conventional and stemless or resurfacing stem designs (**Figure 8**). A shorter stem can provide the rotational control and excellent stability of a traditional stemmed design but obtains its press-fit biologic fixation in the metaphysis of the proximal humerus, and newer implants take an anthropomorphic design that increases in canal filling dimensions as the implant increases in size. Long-term follow-up may reveal that the short stem provides less stress shielding, with accompanying proximal humeral osteolysis or resorption because the forces are concentrated adjacent to the humeral head rather than distally to the humeral shaft. Although the short-stemmed implant may be subject to the same long-term issues as a longer stemmed device, near-term data are promising. Furthermore, the shorter-stemmed implant holds promise for bone-conserving arthroplasty, which may be important in revision surgery or the treatment of future pathology such as rotator cuff disease. Therefore, modern stem design has focused on metaphyseal fixation for the humerus, abandoning distal fixation that was an evolution of hip stem design. These designs derive their press fit from the proximal metaphyseal bone, rather than more distal cortical bone. Now almost every domestically available manufacturer offers shorter stemmed options that derive their stability from the metaphyseal cancellous bone; furthermore, most stems offer convertibility to a reverse. With the migration toward shorter, more metaphyseal filling stems, longer stems are being reserved for revision or fracture applications.

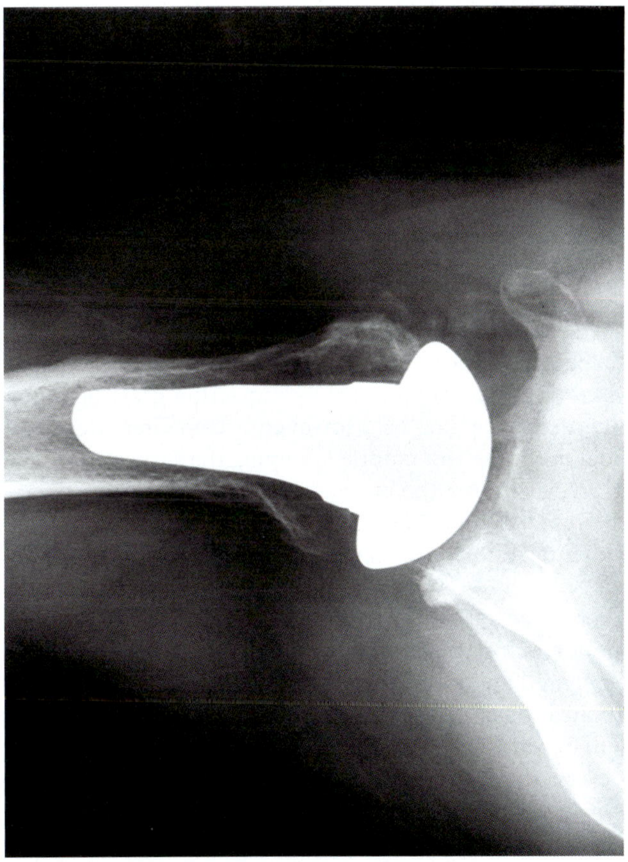

FIGURE 8 Axillary radiograph showing a fibrous union after a lesser tuberosity osteotomy. The patient had no deficit.

Bony (Anatomic) and Soft-Tissue Balancing

For proper postarthroplasty functioning, the reconstruction must restore the anatomy, and the muscle forces must be appropriately balanced. Most often, soft-tissue balancing involves releasing excessively tight tissues from the anterior aspect of the joint to allow appropriate alignment, stability, and range of motion. Less commonly, it may be necessary to plicate redundant soft tissues in the posterior aspect of the joint. Humeral head size fell within eight fixed combinations in 85% of the population; therefore, the implant size can be selected to provide the ideal amounts of range of motion, stability, and translation. Implant head height or thickness can be varied to alter the relative soft-tissue tension.[4,21,52]

The concept of bony balancing implies that the humeral anatomy will be reconstructed to essentially the native dimensions, or, at a minimum, those determined by the humeral head resection.[3] Under the assumption that humeral head thickness is related to the diameter of the anatomic neck or the resection plane, the resection will predetermine the humeral head thickness.[2] Therefore, when the osteophytes are removed, the anatomic neck identified, and the resection is performed, the critical steps have been completed and what remains is primarily a matter of covering the resection.

The subsequent restoration of the bony anatomy should restore normal glenohumeral kinematics. Overstuffing can occur with a proper cut if the stem is placed in a varus position or if the stem is placed correctly but the head cut is inadequate.[19,31-33] In either case, the head should be centered on the metaphysis; this task is made easier by using a modern adaptable implant, which can minimize the difference between bone and soft-tissue balancing. The superior aspect of the head should sit 5 to 10 mm above the summit of the greater tuberosity.[4,7,8,34] The offset of the humeral shaft necessitates the use of an offset head more often than a centered head.[2,3,5] If the particular system lacks a centered option, the surgeon must choose the appropriate direction for overhang; with a lesser tuberosity osteotomy, an anterior overhang may mate well with the area reconstituted by the osteotomy. Alternatively, a cemented stem can be used, as is more commonly done in Europe than in the United States. A cemented stem allows the surgeon to float the humeral implant into the ideal location for reconstructing the articular geometry.

If the soft tissues appear symmetrically tight, the humeral head may be too large or the resection may be inadequate.[52] Attention should be directed to the capsule, ensuring that the soft-tissue releases have been adequate. To correct excessive posterior translation, the humeral head size can be increased at the expense of range of motion (external rotation); more posterior offset can be placed; or posterior plication sutures can be placed in the capsule or through the humerus (as in repair of a posterior humeral avulsion of the glenohumeral ligament).[51,52] After soft-tissue reconstruction, the arm should allow 40° of external rotation in the adducted position; the head should translate 50% of the width of the glenoid with a posteriorly directed force; and there should be 60° of internal rotation with the arm in the abducted position.[53] (This is the so-called 40-50-60 rule.)

Cemented and Noncemented Fixation

Fixation is a relative term because bone is a dynamic, living structure. Immediately after surgery, the bone-implant interface is different from the interface at 2-year follow-up. As the surgical trauma is replaced by a zone of healing, the thinner the transition zone is, the better the force is distributed to the surrounding bone. The surgeon must create an environment that supports appropriate force transmission between the implant and the bone so that the component does not loosen over time, leading to pain or prosthetic failure. Until material science creates an implant that replicates the stiffness of the native tissues, there will be a relative mismatch between the implant and the bone. This mismatch in stiffness leads to micromotion and eventual loosening of the implant.[54] The prosthetic design and interface should be loaded in compression to distribute the forces as evenly as possible in an attempt to keep micromotion to less than 70 μm. Minimizing the load across the interface for the first 6 to 12 weeks may encourage maturation of the healing zone but is not practical. Therefore, it is important to distribute the forces as evenly as possible to minimize shear and maximize compression. To achieve even force distribution, the implant must register appropriately with the native glenoid or the glenoid component, articulating with as much rotational kinematics as possible and minimizing rolling or gliding.[55]

A noncemented prosthesis is designed to achieve initial fixation through a macroscopic interlock between the surface of the prosthesis and the bone. It is essential to minimize the shear forces that occur if the implant pistons within the canal or convert them to compressive force at the bone-implant interface. Impaction bone grafting may enhance the metaphyseal fit and prevent the stem from moving into varus.[56] Ideally, the forces should be transmitted through the implant to the bone, resulting in minimal shear stresses at the bone-prosthesis interface and transmitting the load to the bone in series rather than in parallel or by load sharing.[57] The next phase allows bone ingrowth or ongrowth at the interstices of the prosthesis to lock it in place. This is a dynamic process because bone is constantly turning over.[54] Some prosthetic designs have fared better than others, and recent radiographic concerns have been raised that a collared or distally press-fit implant may stress shield proximally, leading to bone resorption along the medial calcar.[58] Proximal humeral bone loss results in more micromotion and ultimately to prosthetic loosening.[59] Metaphyseal press fit was more efficacious than distal stem press fit, and this design trend has continued in the evolution of smaller tapered stems.[60]

The practical concerns and considerations related to press-fit designs have to do with the relative ease of implantation rather than the stability of the initial press fit. Large fins can force the stem into a varus position, may not always align with the cut, or may force the stem into poor inclination or version. Smaller cylindrical bodies have been replaced by those with a more proximal wedge shape to prevent settling within the bone; a tight metaphyseal fit can be augmented by impaction grafting along the medial calcar.[56,60] However, a cemented stem can float in the cement mantle, allowing the surgeon to place it precisely over the cut surface to accurately re-create the resected anatomy and center of rotation. Published loosening rates with unconstrained shoulder arthroplasty range from zero with a bony ingrowth model or 1.5% in a cemented application to 10.0% with a limited-ingrowth monoblock stem, and some studies suggest that certain cemented stem designs may outperform noncemented applications.[55,61-64] It is important to recognize that there will be variation based on the suitability of the stem for the specific application; for example, the results are poor if a stem designed for a cemented application is used as a press-fit stem or vice versa. A study of 1,584 primary arthroplasties identified risk factors for humeral component failure, including male sex, relatively young age, a metal-backed glenoid, and posttraumatic arthropathy.[61] Improved rotational micromotion was found with a proximal cemented stem compared with a press-fit stem, and there was no advantage to full cementation.[65] Therefore, in a patient without a fracture, it may be preferable to proximally apply cement only to the metaphyseal portion of the stem before implantation. A level I study that compared cemented and noncemented implantation of a specific stem found better outcomes in terms of range of motion, strength, and quality of life when the cemented application was used.[66]

Soft-Tissue Considerations

The subscapularis is critical for successful function after anatomic shoulder arthroplasty. A rotator cuff tear or subscapularis deficiency was identified in 72% of painful shoulder arthroplasties, and subscapularis deficiency was implicated in poor long-term outcomes.[67-69] Some studies regarding transosseous subscapularis repair in shoulder arthroplasty found a 25% rate of subscapularis deficiency.[70] Concern over the integrity of subscapularis repair has led to the development of alternative approaches to tenotomy.[71] The variations range from a periosteal sleeve elevation to several types of lesser tuberosity osteotomy, in which the tendon and the capsule usually are taken together to preserve blood supply (**Figure 9**). Biomechanically, a superior load to failure was found with a lesser tuberosity osteotomy and a double-row repair, although more recent studies found little difference in repair strength with osteotomy or tenotomy.[69,72-76] Of 45 patients, 41 had a negative lift-off test, and all 45 had a negative belly-press test result after routine tenotomy and repair.[77] Excellent bone-to-bone healing and excellent clinical results were reported after a lesser tuberosity osteotomy; nonetheless, 44% of the patients had fatty infiltration of the muscle belly.[68,69] Better function of the subscapularis was found in patients who underwent osteotomy compared with a historical cohort of patients who underwent tenotomy.[78] Ultimately, surgeon experience and preference may dictate the approach to the subscapularis and its repair.

A report of a subscapularis-sparing approach through the rotator cuff interval noted the advantage of immediate full activity without limitation. A subscapularis-sparing approach is technically demanding and requires specialized instruments and may not be suitable for patients with a stiff shoulder, a large inferior osteophyte, or a large deltoid.[79] In the 22 studied patients, the concerns were nonanatomic humeral head osteotomies in 6, residual inferior humeral neck osteophytes in 8, and the humeral head prosthesis undersized in 5.[79] In a similar manner, the authors of a 2015 study studied a cohort of 96 patients randomized to a traditional (n = 50) or a subscapularis-sparing approach (n = 46).[80] Seven patients (15%) in the subscapularis-sparing approach were removed from the study as they required a tenotomy to safely complete the procedure.[80] Radiographically, 29% of the subscapularis patients had residual inferior osteophytes, and 23% demonstrated humeral head diameters that were off by >4 mm compared with only 8% in the traditional approach.[80] The authors of a 2015 study have demonstrated excellent results with a subscapularis-sparing approach for humeral head hemiarthroplasty that maintains the upper tendinous portion while releasing the distal muscular portion.[81]

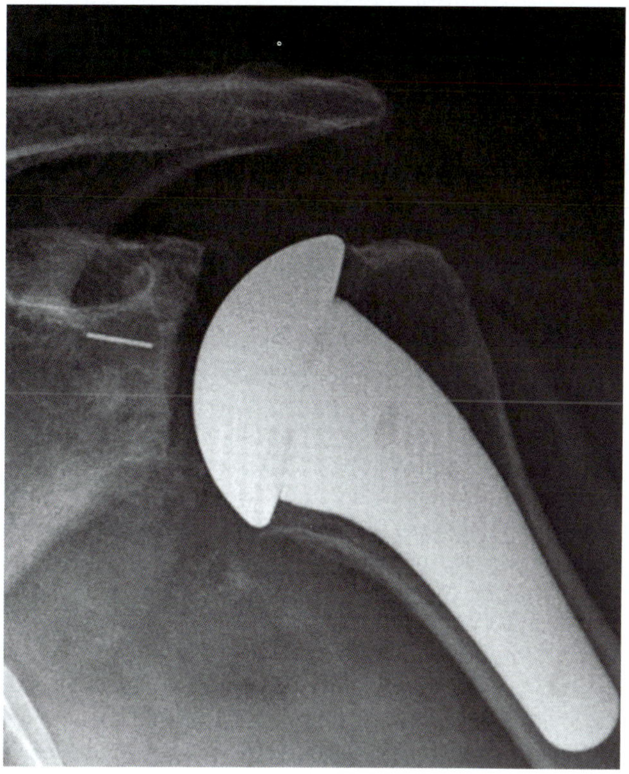

FIGURE 9 Grashey view of an early short-stem design.

Future Directions

Because concerns about glenoid wear or glenoid implant prosthetic loosening still remain, research continues regarding prosthetic reconstruction that provides as much pain relief as a total shoulder arthroplasty while requiring less surgical time, being less difficult, and being less expensive. The creation of a humeral implant that is less stiff and provides improved wear characteristics over current materials is desirable. No hard-on-hard bearings (both the head and the socket consist of a hard material, such as metal-on-metal or ceramic-on-ceramic) are commercially available for shoulder arthroplasty; research is being done for suitable applications, but the current state-of-the-art for an anatomic shoulder remains a hard humeral bearing surface such as metal or ceramic as opposed to a softer plastic bearing on the glenoid side.[82] Composite materials may be better suited to the humerus rather than ceramic or metal-on-metal applications. With a modulus of elasticity of 29.4 GPa, pyrolytic carbon may be a future option for shoulder arthroplasty because it is closer to the modulus of cortical bone (23 GPa) and may exhibit better wear characteristics against cartilage, making it ideal for consideration in a hemiarthroplasty.[83] Pyrolytic carbon has been used in mechanical heart valves since the 1960s and for small-joint arthroplasty since 1979; in Europe, several hundred pyrolytic carbon humeral arthroplasties have been performed[84] (**Figure 10**). The authors of a 2017 study documented the minimum 2-year results of 67 of the snooker ball pyrocarbon interposition shoulder arthroplasties; this was a young cohort with a mean age of 51 years at the time of implantation (**Figure 10, A** and **B**).[85] Seven patients (10%) underwent revision at a mean of 4 years and 2 were lost and 3 were excluded, leaving 55 patients whose Constant score improved from a mean of 34.1 to 66.1; radiographic evaluation showed glenoid erosion in 6 patients and tuberosity thinning in 3.[85] Overall, the authors reported results on par with hemiarthroplasty but inferior to total shoulder arthroplasty.[85] The material itself seems to be suited for the task, but the size of the implant was 4 mm smaller than that of the native humeral head, which may have led to the mediocre results.[85] In comparison, the authors studied 65 patients who underwent hemiarthroplasty with a modular stem and pyrolytic carbon humeral head; at 2 years, the survivability was 95.3% (two revisions for persistent glenoid pain and one for cuff failure).[86] The mean postoperative Constant score was 74.8 with no progressive glenoid erosion.[86] The authors concluded that pyrocarbon hemiarthroplasty was a good option for primary osteoarthritis or osteonecrosis or postcapsulorrhaphy arthritis; however, the results for fracture sequelae (posttraumatic osteoarthritis or osteonecrosis) were poor—in fact, better results were observed with the pyrocarbon interposition shoulder arthroplasty.[86] An investigational device exemption is currently under way in the United States for the pyrolytic carbon humeral hemiarthroplasty.

Although hemiarthroplasty remains an option, the benchmark for prosthetic shoulder replacement is total shoulder arthroplasty. Modern unconstrained shoulder arthroplasty attempts reconstruction of the native proximal humeral anatomy, thereby relieving pain and restoring normal glenohumeral kinematics. The evolution of prosthesis design has led to modular implants that adapt to patient anatomy while minimizing surgical trauma and improving long-term implant survivability. Therefore, stem design has evolved to smaller, cancellous secured implants that are convertible, so-called fourth-generation implants[87-91] (**Figure 11**). Reports of an early design showed some maladaptive bone remodeling that was likely the result of stress shielding in implants that lacked proximal porous coating or in implants that made distal cortical contact.[90,92] Other studies have shown that minimal canal filling with the porous-coated implant had very minimal bone changes.[93] A study comparing a traditional stemmed implant to the short-stemmed iteration demonstrated significantly less stress shielding with the short-stemmed version.[94] Furthermore, the authors of a 2016 study, by comparing traditional stems with both short stems and stemless options, demonstrated that reducing humeral stem length allows for normal stress distribution in the proximal humerus.[95]

The recent proliferation of stemless implants is the result of early European success. Biomet's TESS, Zimmer Biomet, Warsaw, IN (introduced in 2004) and Arthrex's Eclipse, Arthrex, Naples, FL (introduced in 2005) have excellent clinical history with 8- to 9-year outcomes and

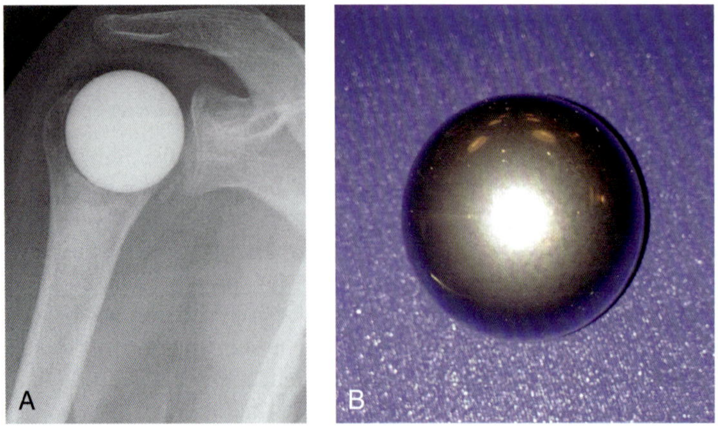

FIGURE 10 Three pyrolytic carbon implants are commercially available in Europe. Grashey radiograph (**A**) and photograph (**B**) showing the so-called snooker ball implant (Tornier). (Panel A, Courtesy of Gilles Walch, MD.)

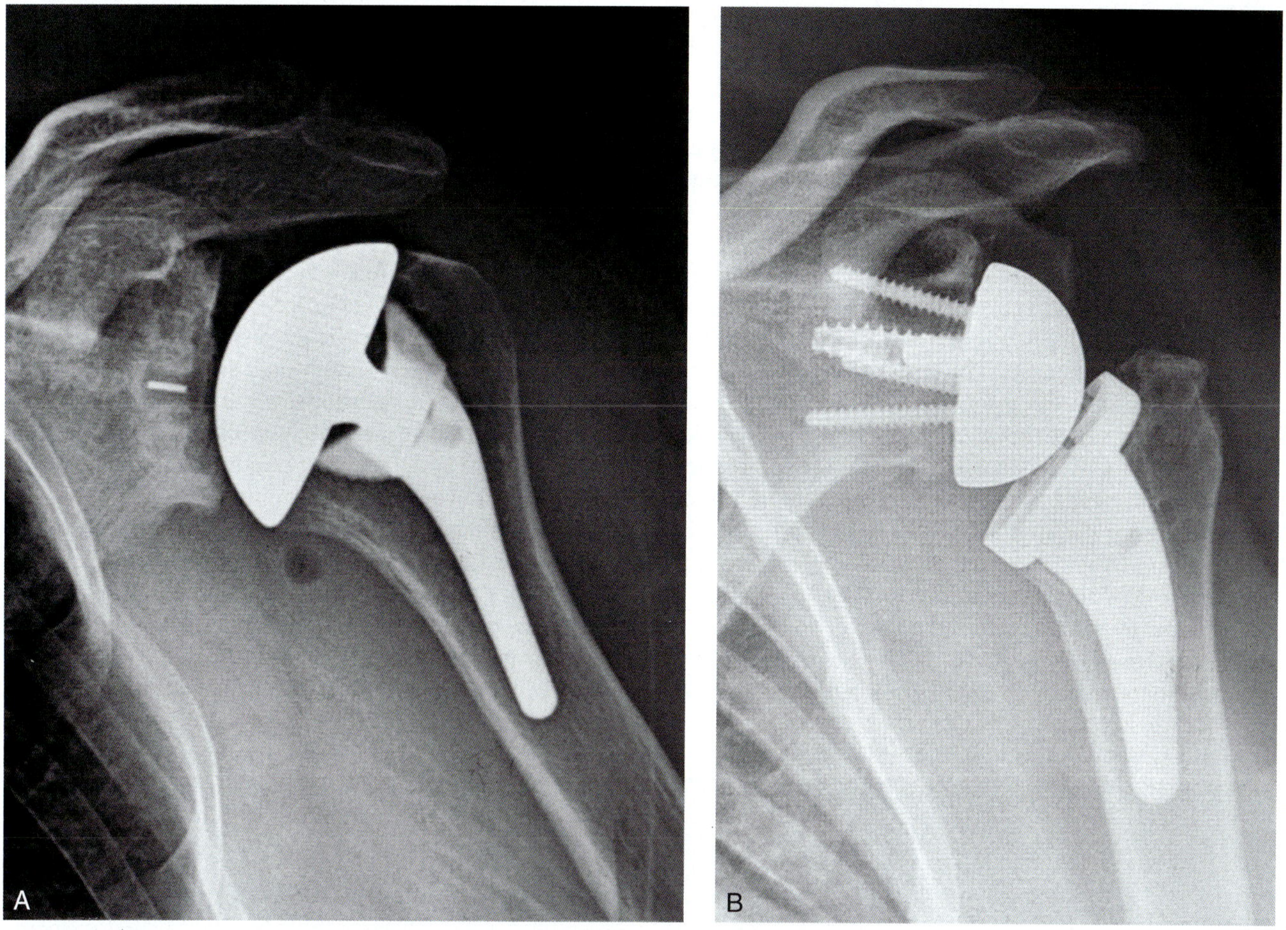

FIGURE 11 Grashey radiograph of a microstemmed convertible implant (**A**); Grashey radiograph of a short-stemmed anatomic that had been converted to a reverse shoulder after the patient suffered failure of the rotator cuff (**B**).

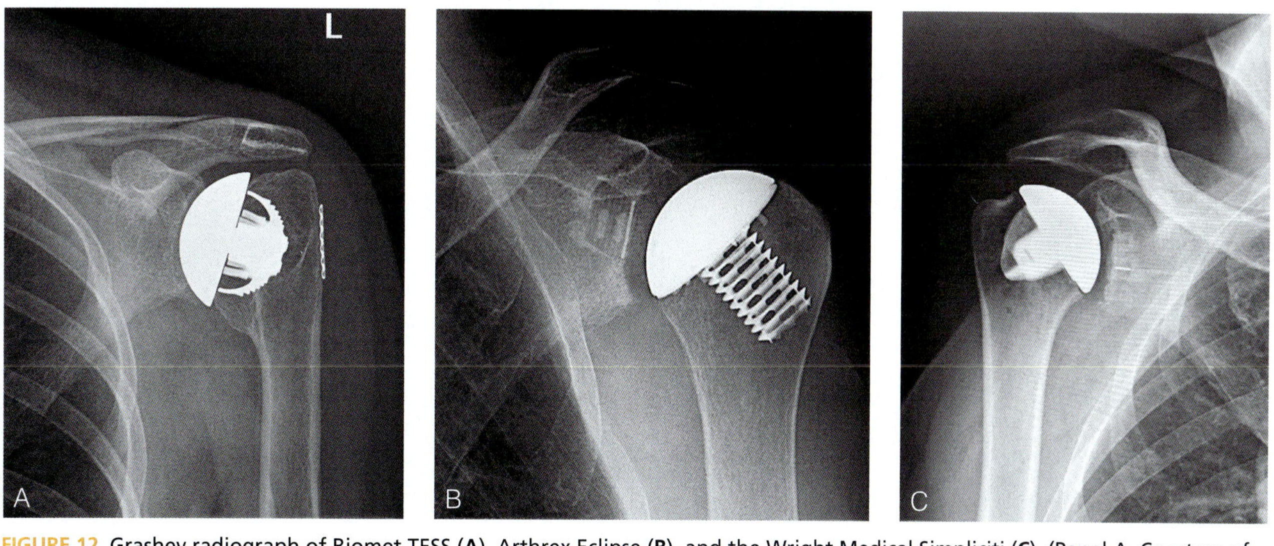

FIGURE 12 Grashey radiograph of Biomet TESS (**A**), Arthrex Eclipse (**B**), and the Wright Medical Simpliciti (**C**). (Panel A, Courtesy of George Athwal, MD. Panel B, Courtesy of Arthrex®, Naples, Florida 2020.)

survivability that rival traditional stemmed implants[96,97] (**Figure 12, A** and **B**).[96,97] Concerns about proximal humeral bone density may make these stemless implants less desirable in patients with osteoporotic bone, especially elderly females, but radiologic changes, likely due to stress shielding, have not been shown to have a negative effect on the outcome.[98,99] The Simpliciti device was the first stemless implant to be approved for use in the United States after an investigational device exemption; the data from this clinical trial and others that have followed show that this stemless implant functions comparably to traditional stemmed implants (**Figure 12, C**).[100,101] Currently, there are six stemless options available in the United States: Tornier Simpliciti (the first), Zimmer/Biomet Sidus and Nano, DePuy Icon, Exactech Equinoxe Stemless, and the Arthrex Eclipse. There are several more options in Europe both for anatomic and reverse applications.

A precision multiplanar cut humeral implant, indicated for both total arthroplasty and hemiarthroplasty, has recently come to market; rather than reconstructing the articular surface as a hemisphere, the designers have adopted an ovoid shape to better replicate the shape and kinematics of the glenohumeral joint[102,103] (**Figure 13**). Short-term data show promise, as the device may more accurately reproduce humeral anatomy than traditional designs.

SUMMARY

Humeral stems are reducing in size or disappearing completely. As designs become more anatomic, good clinical success has been reported even for cases of distorted proximal humeral anatomy. There are some data to suggest that stemless implants may produce less initial surgical pain, shorter surgical times, less blood loss, and fewer intraoperative humeral complications, while having the potential for longer clinical success because of better load sharing characteristics, and there may be advantages for easier revision.[95-100] However, malpositioning of the implant from an improper head cut or poor surgical technique can create just as many problems because improved prosthesis design is not a substitute for rigorous surgical technique. Soft-tissue considerations still are of paramount importance for providing long-term stability and functionality after reconstruction. Short-term to medium-term data

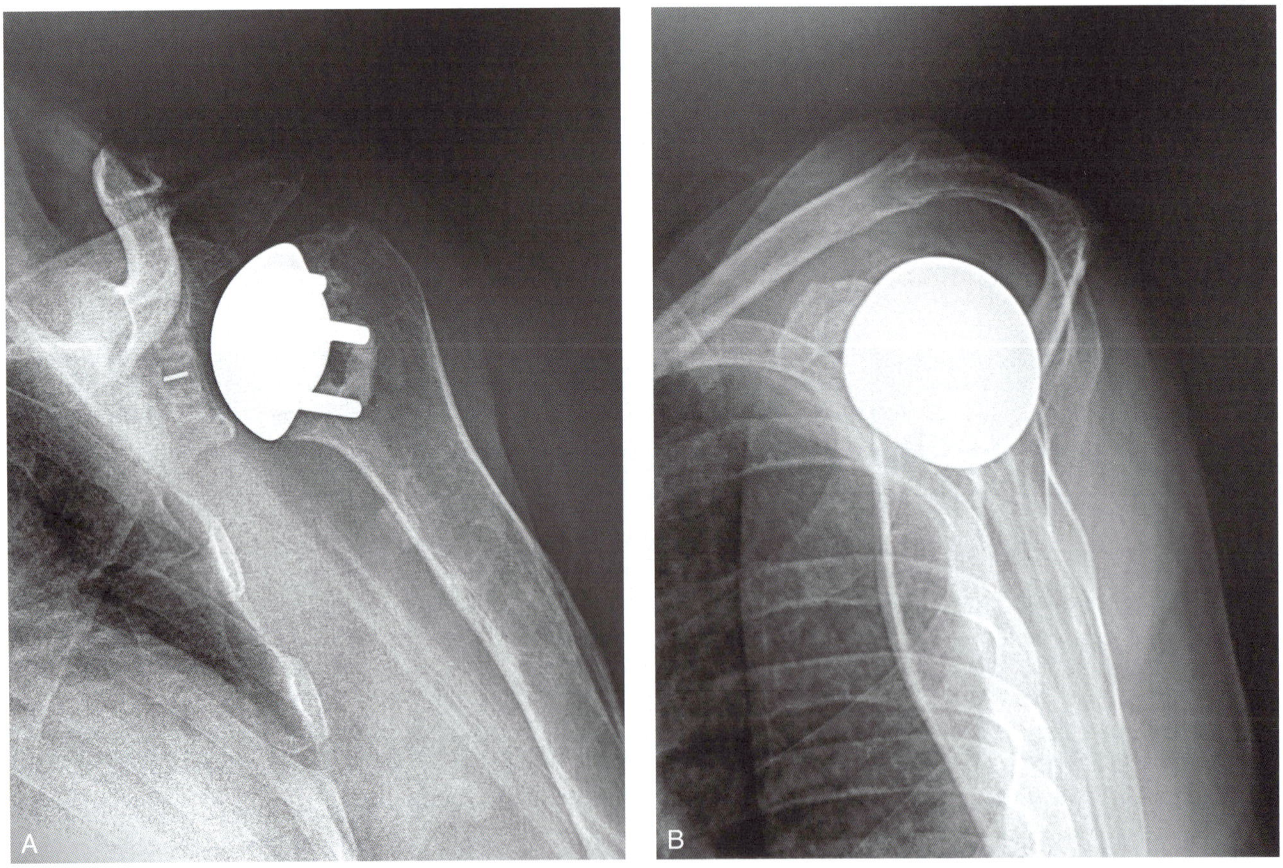

FIGURE 13 Grashey (**A**) and outlet (**B**) radiographs of an ovoid anatomic humeral implant used in a case of proximal humeral deformity.

demonstrate that stemless implants perform as well as traditional stemmed implants; it will take much longer follow-up studies to determine if stem designs confer any true advantage (other than ease of removal) over stemmed implants. Material science may provide compounds with biomechanical properties similar to those of the host bone and thereby increase device longevity.

KEY STUDY POINTS

- The humeral side of anatomic shoulder arthroplasty has become more anatomic as research has better defined key anatomic parameters of the humerus.
- Proximal humeral geometry has both offset and version that should be mimicked for better long-term outcomes with shoulder arthroplasty.
- Shorter stem designs that allow for more normal force transmission will predominate primary shoulder arthroplasty, relegating longer stem designs to revision applications.
- The search continues for more biologically compatible implants.

Annotated References

1. Bankes MJ, Emery RJ: Pioneers of shoulder replacement: Themistocles Gluck and Jules Emile Péan. *J Shoulder Elbow Surg* 1995;4(4):259-262.

2. Boileau P, Walch G: The three-dimensional geometry of the proximal humerus: Implications for surgical technique and prosthetic design. *J Bone Joint Surg Br* 1997;79(5):857-865.

3. Walch G, Boileau P: Prosthetic adaptability: A new concept for shoulder arthroplasty. *J Shoulder Elbow Surg* 1999;8(5):443-451.

4. Iannotti JP, Gabriel JP, Schneck SL, Evans BG, Misra S: The normal glenohumeral relationships: An anatomical study of one hundred and forty shoulders. *J Bone Joint Surg Am* 1992;74(4):491-500.

5. Hertel R, Knothe U, Ballmer FT: Geometry of the proximal humerus and implications for prosthetic design. *J Shoulder Elbow Surg* 2002;11(4):331-338.

6. Pearl ML: Proximal humeral anatomy in shoulder arthroplasty: Implications for prosthetic design and surgical technique. *J Shoulder Elbow Surg* 2005;14(1 suppl S):S99-S104.

7. Pearl ML, Volk AG: Coronal plane geometry of the proximal humerus relevant to prosthetic arthroplasty. *J Shoulder Elbow Surg* 1996;5(4):320-326.

8. Robertson DD, Yuan J, Bigliani LU, Flatow EL, Yamaguchi K: Three-dimensional analysis of the proximal part of the humerus: Relevance to arthroplasty. *J Bone Joint Surg Am* 2000;82(11):1594-1602.

9. Wataru S, Kazuomi S, Yoshikazu N, Hiroaki I, Takaharu Y, Hideki Y: Three-dimensional morphological analysis of humeral heads: A study in cadavers. *Acta Orthop* 2005;76(3):392-396.

10. Vaesel MT, Olsen BS, Søjbjerg JO, Helmig P, Sneppen O: Humeral head size in shoulder arthroplasty: A kinematic study. *J Shoulder Elbow Surg* 1997;6(6):549-555.

11. Wirth MA, Ondrla J, Southworth C, Kaar K, Anderson BC, Rockwood CA III: Replicating proximal humeral articular geometry with a third-generation implant: A radiographic study in cadaveric shoulders. *J Shoulder Elbow Surg* 2007;16(suppl 3):S111-S116.

12. Jun BJ, Iannotti JP, McGarry MH, Yoo JC, Quigley RJ, Lee TQ: The effects of prosthetic humeral head shape on glenohumeral joint kinematics: A comparison of non-spherical and spherical prosthetic heads to the native humeral head. *J Shoulder Elbow Surg* 2013;22:1423-1432.

    In this model, ovoid heads, which better approximate native anatomy, demonstrate improved glenohumeral kinematics compared with heads derived from spheroid geometry. In fact, at all positions tested, the nonspherical heads did not differ from the native heads; however, the spherical heads exhibited decreased motion and decreased translation of the humeral head.

13. Jun BJ, Lee TQ, McGarry MH, Quigley RJ, Shin SJ, Iannotti JP: The effects of prosthetic humeral head shape on glenohumeral joint kinematics during humeral axial rotation in total shoulder arthroplasty. *J Shoulder Elbow Surg* 2016;25:1084-1093.

    The results showed that ovoid heads replicated native glenohumeral translation during axial rotation regardless of glenoid conformity, whereas spheroid heads exhibited almost no glenohumeral translation with increasing levels of mismatch.

14. Humphrey CS, Sears BW, Curtin MJ: An anthropometric analysis to derive formulae for calculating the dimensions of anatomically shaped humeral heads. *J Shoulder Elbow Surg* 2016;25:1532-1541.

    The authors created a formula derived from measurements of cadaver humeri that can predict the size and shape of an ovoid anatomic humeral head for an arthroplasty, showing that the elliptical shape at the base of the head increases as the head size increases.

15. Fischer LP, Carret JP, Gonon GP, Dimnet J: Etude cinématique des mouvements de l'articulation scapulohumérale (articulatio humeri). *Rev Chir Orthop Reparatrice Appar Mot* 1977;63(suppl 2):108-115.

16. Roche C, Angibaud L, Flurin PH, Wright T, Fulkerson E, Zuckerman J: Anatomic validation of an "anatomic" shoulder system. *Bull Hosp Jt Dis* 2006;63(3-4):93-97.

17. Jeong J, Bryan J, Iannotti JP: Effect of a variable prosthetic neck-shaft angle and the surgical technique on replication of normal humeral anatomy. *J Bone Joint Surg Am* 2009;91(8):1932-1941.

18. Takase K, Yamamoto K, Imakiire A, Burkhead WZ Jr: The radiographic study in the relationship of the glenohumeral joint. *J Orthop Res* 2004;22(2):298-305.

19. Iannotti JP, Spencer EE, Winter U, Deffenbaugh D, Williams G: Prosthetic positioning in total shoulder arthroplasty. *J Shoulder Elbow Surg* 2005;14(1 suppl S):111S-121S.

20. Pearl ML, Volk AG: Retroversion of the proximal humerus in relationship to prosthetic replacement arthroplasty. *J Shoulder Elbow Surg* 1995;4(4):286-289.

21. Pearl ML, Kurutz S, Postacchini R: Geometric variables in anatomic replacement of the proximal humerus: How much prosthetic geometry is necessary? *J Shoulder Elbow Surg* 2009;18(3):366-370.

22. Iannotti JP, Lippitt SB, Williams GR Jr: Variation in neck-shaft angle: Influence in prosthetic design. *Am J Orthop (Belle Mead NJ)* 2007;36(12 suppl 1):9-14.

23. Harrold F, Wigderowitz C: A three-dimensional analysis of humeral head retroversion. *J Shoulder Elbow Surg* 2012;21(5):612-617.

24. Tillett E, Smith M, Fulcher M, Shanklin J: Anatomic determination of humeral head retroversion: The relationship of the central axis of the humeral head to the bicipital groove. *J Shoulder Elbow Surg* 1993;2(5):255-256.

25. Doyle AJ, Burks RT: Comparison of humeral head retroversion with the humeral axis/biceps groove relationship: A study in live subjects and cadavers. *J Shoulder Elbow Surg* 1998;7(5):453-457.

26. Edelson G: Variations in the retroversion of the humeral head. *J Shoulder Elbow Surg* 1999;8(2):142-145.

27. Hernigou P, Duparc F, Hernigou A: Determining humeral retroversion with computed tomography. *J Bone Joint Surg Am* 2002;84(10):1753-1762.

28. Hromádka R, Kubena AA, Pokorný D, Popelka S, Jahoda D, Sosna A: Lesser tuberosity is more reliable than bicipital groove when determining orientation of humeral head in primary shoulder arthroplasty. *Surg Radiol Anat* 2010;32(1):31-37.

29. Pearl ML, Kurutz S: Geometric analysis of commonly used prosthetic systems for proximal humeral replacement. *J Bone Joint Surg Am* 1999;81(5):660-671.

30. Pearl ML, Kurutz S, Robertson DD, Yamaguchi K: Geometric analysis of selected press fit prosthetic systems for proximal humeral replacement. *J Orthop Res* 2002;20(2):192-197.

31. Nyffeler RW, Sheikh R, Jacob HA, Gerber C: Influence of humeral prosthesis height on biomechanics of glenohumeral abduction: An in vitro study. *J Bone Joint Surg Am* 2004;86(3):575-580.

32. Favre P, Moor B, Snedeker JG, Gerber C: Influence of component positioning on impingement in conventional total shoulder arthroplasty. *Clin Biomech (Bristol, Avon)* 2008;23(2):175-183.

33. Williams GR Jr, Wong KL, Pepe MD, et al: The effect of articular malposition after total shoulder arthroplasty on glenohumeral translations, range of motion, and subacromial impingement. *J Shoulder Elbow Surg* 2001;10(5):399-409.

34. Takase K, Imakiire A, Burkhead WZ Jr: Radiographic study of the anatomic relationships of the greater tuberosity. *J Shoulder Elbow Surg* 2002;11(6):557-561.

35. Neer CS II: Articular replacement for the humeral head. *J Bone Joint Surg Am* 1955;37-A(2):215-228.

36. Fenlin JM Jr, Vaccaro A, Andreychik D, Lin S: Modular total shoulder: Early experience and impressions. *Semin Arthroplasty* 1990;1(2):102-111.

37. Büchler P, Farron A: Benefits of an anatomical reconstruction of the humeral head during shoulder arthroplasty: A finite element analysis. *Clin Biomech (Bristol, Avon)* 2004;19(1):16-23.

38. Irlenbusch U, End S, Kilic M: Differences in reconstruction of the anatomy with modern adjustable compared to second-generation shoulder prosthesis. *Int Orthop* 2011;35(5):705-711.

39. Hammond G, Tibone JE, McGarry MH, Jun BJ, Lee TQ: Biomechanical comparison of anatomic humeral head resurfacing and hemiarthroplasty in functional glenohumeral positions. *J Bone Joint Surg Am* 2012;94(1):68-76.

40. Jensen KL: Humeral resurfacing arthroplasty: Rationale, indications, technique, and results. *Am J Orthop (Belle Mead NJ)* 2007;36(12 suppl 1):4-8.

41. Bailie DS, Llinas PJ, Ellenbecker TS: Cementless humeral resurfacing arthroplasty in active patients less than fifty-five years of age. *J Bone Joint Surg Am* 2008;90(1):110-117.

42. Thomas SR, Sforza G, Levy O, Copeland SA: Geometrical analysis of Copeland surface replacement shoulder arthroplasty in relation to normal anatomy. *J Shoulder Elbow Surg* 2005;14(2):186-192.

43. Thomas SR, Wilson AJ, Chambler A, Harding I, Thomas M: Outcome of Copeland surface replacement shoulder arthroplasty. *J Shoulder Elbow Surg* 2005;14(5):485-491.

44. Pritchett JW: Long-term results and patient satisfaction after shoulder resurfacing. *J Shoulder Elbow Surg* 2011;20(5):771-777.

45. Burgess DL, McGrath MS, Bonutti PM, Marker DR, Delanois RE, Mont MA: Shoulder resurfacing. *J Bone Joint Surg Am* 2009;91(5):1228-1238.

46. Scalise J, Miniaci A, Iannotti J: Resurfacing arthroplasty of the humerus: Indications, surgical technique, and clinical results. *Tech Shoulder Elbow Surg* 2007;8:152-160.

47. Huguet D, DeClercq G, Rio B, Teissier J, Zipoli B, TESS Group: Results of a new stemless shoulder prosthesis: Radiologic proof of maintained fixation and stability after a minimum of three years' follow-up. *J Shoulder Elbow Surg* 2010;19(6):847-852.

48. Collin P, McGourbey G, Boileau P, Walch G: Complications of the Simpliciti stemless prosthesis, in Walch G, Boileau P, Molé D, Favard L, Lévigne C, Sirveaux F, eds: *Shoulder Concepts 2012: Complications in Shoulder Arthroplasty.* Montpellier, France, Sauramps Medical, 2012, pp 57-61.

49. Tauber M, Habermeyer P, Magosch P: Is a stemless prosthesis better?, in Walch G, Boileau P, Molé D, Favard L, Lévigne C, Sirveaux F, eds: *Shoulder Concepts 2012: Complications in Shoulder Arthroplasty.* Montpellier, France, Sauramps Medical, 2012, pp 49-56.

50. Barvencik F, Gebauer M, Beil FT, et al: Age- and sex-related changes of humeral head microarchitecture: Histomorphometric analysis of 60 human specimens. *J Orthop Res* 2010;28(1):18-26.

51. Williams G, Iannotti J: Unconstrained prosthetic arthroplasty for glenohumeral arthritis with an intact or repairable rotator cuff: Indications, techniques, and results, in Iannotti J, Williams G, eds: *Disorders of the Shoulder*, ed 2. Philadelphia, PA, Lippincott Williams & Wilkins, 2007, pp 713-715.

52. Harryman DT, Sidles JA, Harris SL, Lippitt SB, Matsen FA III: The effect of articular conformity and the size of the humeral head component on laxity and motion after glenohumeral arthroplasty: A study in cadavera. *J Bone Joint Surg Am* 1995;77(4):555-563.

53. Matsen F, Clinton J, Rockwood C, Wirth M, Lippitt S: *The Shoulder*, ed 4. Philadelphia, PA, Saunders, 2009, pp 1093-1096.

54. Jobe CM, Phipatanakul WP, Bowsher JG: *Revision and Complex Shoulder Arthroplasty.* Philadelphia, PA, Wolters Kluwer/Lippincott Williams & Wilkins, 2010, pp 83-94.

55. Cofield R: Loosening of cemented and uncemented humeral stems, in Walch G, Boileau P, Molé D, Favard L, Lévigne C, Sirveaux F, eds: *Shoulder Concepts 2012: Complications in Shoulder Arthroplasty.* Montpellier, France, Sauramps Medical, 2012, pp 23-27.

56. Boorman RS, Hacker S, Lippitt SB, Matsen FA: A conservative broaching and impaction grafting technique for humeral component Placement and fixation in shoulder arthroplasty: The Procrustean method. *Tech Shoulder Elbow Surg* 2001;2:172-173.

57. Orr TE, Carter DR: Stress analyses of joint arthroplasty in the proximal humerus. *J Orthop Res* 1985;3(3):360-371.

58. Edwards B: Can a short-stem avoid the potential complications of the longer stems? The Aequalis Ascend experience, in Walch G, Boileau P, Molé D, Favard L, Lévigne C, Sirveaux F, eds: *Shoulder Concepts 2012: Complications in Shoulder Arthroplasty.* Montpellier, France, Sauramps Medical, 2012, pp 147-149.

59. Cuff D, Levy JC, Gutiérrez S, Frankle MA: Torsional stability of modular and non-modular reverse shoulder humeral components in a proximal humeral bone loss model. *J Shoulder Elbow Surg* 2011;20(4):646-651.

60. Matsen FA III, Iannotti JP, Rockwood CA Jr: Humeral fixation by press-fitting of a tapered metaphyseal stem: A prospective radiographic study. *J Bone Joint Surg Am* 2003;85(2):304-308.

61. Cil A, Veillette CJ, Sanchez-Sotelo J, Sperling JW, Schleck CD, Cofield RH: Survivorship of the humeral component in shoulder arthroplasty. *J Shoulder Elbow Surg* 2010;19(1):143-150.

62. Gonzalez JF, Alami GB, Baque F, Walch G, Boileau P: Complications of unconstrained shoulder prostheses. *J Shoulder Elbow Surg* 2011;20(4):666-682.

63. Sperling JW, Cofield RH, O'Driscoll SW, Torchia ME, Rowland CM: Radiographic assessment of ingrowth total shoulder arthroplasty. *J Shoulder Elbow Surg* 2000;9(6):507-513.

64. Throckmorton TW, Zarkadas PC, Sperling JW, Cofield RH: Radiographic stability of ingrowth humeral stems in total shoulder arthroplasty. *Clin Orthop Relat Res* 2010;468(8):2122-2128.

65. Harris TE, Jobe CM, Dai QG: Fixation of proximal humeral prostheses and rotational micromotion. *J Shoulder Elbow Surg* 2000;9(3):205-210.

66. Litchfield RB, McKee MD, Balyk R, et al: Cemented versus uncemented fixation of humeral components in total shoulder arthroplasty for osteoarthritis of the shoulder: A prospective, randomized, double-blind clinical trial – A JOINTs Canada Project. *J Shoulder Elbow Surg* 2011;20(4):529-536.

67. Sperling JW, Potter HG, Craig EV, Flatow E, Warren RF: Magnetic resonance imaging of painful shoulder arthroplasty. *J Shoulder Elbow Surg* 2002;11(4):315-321.

68. Gerber C, Yian EH, Pfirrmann CA, Zumstein MA, Werner CM: Subscapularis muscle function and structure after total shoulder replacement with lesser tuberosity osteotomy and repair. *J Bone Joint Surg Am* 2005;87(8):1739-1745.

69. Gerber C, Pennington SD, Yian EH, Pfirrmann CA, Werner CM, Zumstein MA: Lesser tuberosity osteotomy for total shoulder arthroplasty: Surgical technique. *J Bone Joint Surg Am* 2006;88(suppl 1, pt 2):170-177.

70. Liem D, Kleeschulte K, Dedy N, Schulte TL, Steinbeck J, Marquardt B: Subscapularis function after transosseous repair in shoulder arthroplasty: Transosseous subscapularis repair in shoulder arthroplasty. *J Shoulder Elbow Surg* 2012;21(10):1322-1327.

71. Armstrong A, Lashgari C, Teefey S, Menendez J, Yamaguchi K, Galatz LM: Ultrasound evaluation and clinical correlation of subscapularis repair after total shoulder arthroplasty. *J Shoulder Elbow Surg* 2006;15(5):541-548.

72. Krishnan SG, Stewart DG, Reineck JR, Lin KC, Buzzell JE, Burkhead WZ: Subscapularis repair after shoulder arthroplasty: Biomechanical and clinical validation of a novel technique. *J Shoulder Elbow Surg* 2009;18(2):184-192, discussion 197-198.

73. Van Thiel GS, Wang VM, Wang F-C, et al: Biomechanical similarities among subscapularis repairs after shoulder arthroplasty. *J Shoulder Elbow Surg* 2010;19(5):657-663.

74. Van den Berghe GR, Nguyen B, Patil S, et al: A biomechanical evaluation of three surgical techniques for subscapularis repair. *J Shoulder Elbow Surg* 2008;17(1):156-161.

75. Giuseffi SA, Wongtriratanachai P, Omae H, et al: Biomechanical comparison of lesser tuberosity osteotomy versus subscapularis tenotomy in total shoulder arthroplasty. *J Shoulder Elbow Surg* 2012;21(8):1087-1095.

76. Ahmad CS, Wing D, Gardner TR, Levine WN, Bigliani LU: Biomechanical evaluation of subscapularis repair used during shoulder arthroplasty. *J Shoulder Elbow Surg* 2007;16(suppl 3):S59-S64.

77. Caplan JL, Whitfield B, Neviaser RJ: Subscapularis function after primary tendon to tendon repair in patients after replacement arthroplasty of the shoulder. *J Shoulder Elbow Surg* 2009;18(2):193-196, discussion 197-198.

78. Qureshi S, Hsiao A, Klug RA, Lee E, Braman J, Flatow EL: Subscapularis function after total shoulder replacement: Results with lesser tuberosity osteotomy. *J Shoulder Elbow Surg* 2008;17(1):68-72.

79. Lafosse L, Schnaser E, Haag M, Gobezie R: Primary total shoulder arthroplasty performed entirely thru the rotator interval: Technique and minimum two-year outcomes. *J Shoulder Elbow Surg* 2009;18(6):864-873.

80. Ding DY, Mahure SA, Akuoko JA, Zuckerman JD, Kwon YW: Total shoulder arthroplasty using a subscapularis-sparing approach: A radiographic analysis. *J Shoulder Elbow Surg* 2015;24:831-837.

The authors demonstrated that although their approach results in a successful reconstruction, humeral head size mismatch and retained osteophytes are a concern that could lead to potential problems for the long-term success.

81. Savoie FH, Charles R, Casselton J, O'Brien MJ, Hurt JA: The subscapularis-sparing approach in humeral head replacement. *J Shoulder Elbow Surg* 2015;24(4):606-612.

The authors credit this approach with the ability to effectively perform humeral head replacement with a decreased rate of subscapularis failure by leaving the upper tendinous portion of the subscapularis intact. Level of evidence: IV.

82. Williams GR Jr, Iannotti JP: Alternative bearing surfaces – Do we need them? *Am J Orthop (Belle Mead NJ)* 2007;36(12 suppl 1):15-17.

83. Cook SD, Thomas KA, Kester MA: Wear characteristics of the canine acetabulum against different femoral prostheses. *J Bone Joint Surg Br* 1989;71(2):189-197.

84. Stanley J, Klawitter J, More R: Joint replacement technology, in Revell P, ed: *Joint Replacement Technologies*. Boca Raton, FL, CRC Press, 2008, pp 631-656.

85. Garret J, Godeneche A, Boileau P, et al: Pyrocarbon interposition shoulder arthroplasty: Preliminary results from a prospective multicenter study at 2 years of follow-up. *J Shoulder Elbow Surg* 2017;26(7):1143-1151.

Pyrolytic carbon interposition arthroplasty offers results that are equivalent to traditional hemiarthroplasty but inferior to those of total shoulder arthroplasty.

86. Garret J, Harly E, Le Huec JC, Brunner U, Rotini R, Godenèche A: Pyrolytic carbon humeral head in hemi-shoulder arthroplasty: Preliminary results at 2-year follow-up. *JSES Open Access* 2019;3(1):37-42.

The authors show that pyrolytic carbon hemiarthroplasty provides good outcomes for most indications but not for posttraumatic fracture sequel.

87. Jost PW, Dines JS, Griffith MH, Angel M, Altchek DW, Dines DM: Total shoulder arthroplasty utilizing mini-stem humeral components: Technique and short-term results. *HSS J* 2011;7(3):213-217.

88. Guiseffi SA, Streubel P, Sperling J, Sanchez-Sotelo J: Short-stem uncemented primary reverse shoulder arthroplasty: Clinical and radiological outcomes. *Bone Joint J* 2014;96-B(4):526-529.

    Reverse shoulder arthroplasty with a short stem can provide safe, reliable outcomes.

89. Harmer L, Throckmorton T, Sperling JW: Total shoulder arthroplasty: Are the humeral components getting shorter? *Curr Rev Musculoskelet Med* 2016;9(1):17-22.

    The authors describe theoretical advantages of preserved bone stock, less stress shielding, eliminating the diaphyseal stress riser, ease of stem removal at revision, and humeral head placement independent from the humeral shaft axis with implants that have shorter and shorter stems.

90. Szerlip BW, Morris BJ, Laughlin MS, Kilian CM, Edwards TB: Clinical and radiographic outcomes after total shoulder arthroplasty with an anatomic press-fit short stem. *J Shoulder Elbow Surg* 2018;27(1):10-16.

    Short-stem components provide equivalent outcomes to longer stem components; however, the authors did report higher loosening rates with a short stem that lacked proximal porous coating. Level of evidence: II.

91. Romeo AA, Thorsness RJ, Sumner SA, Gobezie R, Lederman ES, Denard PJ: Short-term clinical outcome of an anatomic short-stem humeral component in total shoulder arthroplasty. *J Shoulder Elbow Surg* 2018;27(1): 70-74.

    This clinical outcome study demonstrates good short-term results with an anatomic short-stem arthroplasty. Level of evidence: IV.

92. Casagrande DJ, Parks DL, Torngren T, et al: Radiographic evaluation of short-stem press-fit total shoulder arthroplasty: Short-term follow-up. *J Shoulder Elbow Surg* 2016;25(7):1163-1169.

    This study demonstrated higher loosening rates with one particular implant at short-term follow-up. Level of evidence: IV.

93. Raiss P, Schnetzke M, Wittmann T, et al: Postoperative radiographic findings of an uncemented convertible short stem for anatomic and reverse shoulder arthroplasty. *J Shoulder Elbow Surg* 2019;28(4):715-723.

    This study demonstrated good results with a short-stemmed component; however, the authors noted that radiographic changes were associated with a higher percentage of canal fill or cortical contact. Level of evidence: IV.

94. Denard PJ, Noyes MP, Walker JB, et al: Proximal stress shielding is decreased with a short stem compared with a traditional-length stem in total shoulder arthroplasty. *J Shoulder Elbow Surg* 2018;27(1):53-58.

    Short-stem arthroplasties demonstrated equal clinical results to the long stem cohort but had lower rates of radiographic stress shielding. Level of evidence: III.

95. Razfar N, Reeves JM, Langohr DG, Willing R, Athwal GS, Johnson JA: Comparison of proximal humeral bone stresses between stemless, short stem, and standard stem length: A finite element analysis. *J Shoulder Elbow Surg* 2016;25(7):1076-1083.

    Short-stem designs transfer stresses closer to the normal humerus.

96. Hawi N, Magosch P, Tauber M, Lichtenberg S, Habermeyer P: Nine-year outcome after anatomic stemless shoulder prosthesis: Clinical and radiologic results. *J Shoulder Elbow Surg* 2017;26(9):1609-1615.

    Midterm to longer term follow-up of this stemless design is equivalent to that of longer stem designs. Level of evidence: IV.

97. Beck S, Beck V, Wegner A, Dudda M, Patsalis T, Jäger M: Long-term survivorship of stemless anatomical shoulder replacement. *Int Orthop* 2018;42(6):1327-1330.

    This stemless design demonstrated excellent clinical results at 8 years with a 93.5% survivorship.

98. Santos B, Quental C, Folgado J, Sarmento M, Monteiro J: Bone remodelling of the humerus after a resurfacing and a stemless shoulder arthroplasty. *Clin Biomech (Bristol, Avon)* 2018;59:78-84.

    Stemless designs provide better bone loading than resurfacing, but both may not be well suited for patients with proximal humeral bone density issues.

99. Heuberer PR, Brandl G, Pauzenberger L, Laky B, Kriegleder B, Anderl W: Radiological changes do not influence clinical mid-term outcome in stemless humeral head replacements with hollow screw fixation: A prospective radiological and clinical evaluation. *BMC Musculoskelet Disord* 2018;19(1):1-9.

    Radiologic changes, likely resulting from stress shielding, affected 37% of the stemless implants in this cohort; however, the radiographic findings had no bearing on the results.

100. Churchill RS, Chuinard C, Wiater JM, et al: Clinical and radiographic outcomes of the Simpliciti canal-sparing shoulder arthroplasty system: A prospective two-year multicenter study. *J Bone Joint Surg Am* 2016;98(7):552-560.

     The authors demonstrated excellent clinical and radiologic outcomes with a stemless design that were equivalent to those of a stemmed design. Level of evidence: IV.

101. Pinto MC, Archie AT, Mosher ZA, et al: Radiographic restoration of native anatomy: A comparison between stemmed and stemless shoulder arthroplasty. *J Shoulder Elbow Surg* 2019;28(8):1595-1600.

Radiographic parameters were compared to evaluate the ability of stemmed versus stemless implants to reconstruct humeral anatomy; both designs resulted in nearly equivalent reconstruction, with stemless designs favoring restoration of the neck shaft angle. Level of evidence: III.

102. Goldberg SS, Baranek ES: Total shoulder arthroplasty using a bone-sparing, precision multiplanar humeral prosthesis. *Am J Orthop (Belle Mead NJ)* 2018;47:1-10.

The authors demonstrate excellent anatomic reconstruction with a novel humeral implant.

103. Baranek ES, Trofa DP, Levine WN, Goldberg SS: Accuracy of humeral implant positioning using a canal-sparing total shoulder arthroplasty system. *J Shoulder Elbow Arthroplast* 2019;3:1-8.

The authors provide evidence that a multiplanar implant can provide better anatomic reconstruction than traditional stemmed designs.

Chapter 23

Glenoid Anatomy and Prosthetic Reconstruction

Patric Raiss, MD • T. Bradley Edwards, MD • Gilles Walch, MD

ABSTRACT

Treatment of the osteoarthritic glenoid is the unsolved problem in anatomic total shoulder arthroplasty, especially in the long term. Multiple implant concepts, fixation methods, and surgical techniques have been introduced in the past with varying results. New technologies like three-dimensional preoperative planning tools and patient-specific instruments were developed helping surgeons to better understand the pathology and erosion patterns and positioning of the implants. This chapter gives an overview of the possible treatment options of the osteoarthritic glenoid and the outcomes of the different procedures.

Keywords: anatomic shoulder replacement; glenoid component; glenoid loosening; shoulder arthroplasty; shoulder joint

Dr. Raiss or an immediate family member is a member of a speakers' bureau or has made paid presentations on behalf of Wright Medical Technology, Inc.; serves as a paid consultant to or is an employee of Wright Medical Technology, Inc.; and serves as a board member, owner, officer, or committee member of DVSE. Dr. Edwards has received royalties from DJ Orthopaedics, Orthohelix, Shoulder Options, Tornier, and Wright Medical Technology, Inc.; is a member of a speakers' bureau or has made paid presentations on behalf of DJ Orthopaedics, Tornier, and Wright Medical Technology, Inc.; serves as a paid consultant to or is an employee of DJ Orthopaedics, Enhatch, Shoulders In Motion, Smith & Nephew, United Orthopedic Company, and Wright Medical Technology, Inc.; has received research or institutional support from Tornier and Wright Medical Technology, Inc.; has received nonincome support (such as equipment or services), commercially derived honoraria, or other non–research-related funding (such as paid travel) from Tornier and Wright Medical Technology, Inc.; and serves as a board member, owner, officer, or committee member of the American Shoulder and Elbow Surgeons. Dr. Walch or an immediate family member has received royalties from Wright Medical Technology, Inc.; serves as a paid consultant to or is an employee of Wright Medical Technology, Inc.; has received nonincome support (such as equipment or services), commercially derived honoraria, or other non–research-related funding (such as paid travel) from Wright Medical Technology, Inc.; and serves as a board member, owner, officer, or committee member of the French Orthopaedic Society (SOFCOT) Board.

Introduction

Hemiarthroplasty of the proximal humerus is a standard procedure for treating degenerative pathologies of the glenohumeral joint, and it can lead to good results. However, resurfacing of the glenoid bone has many advantages. Total shoulder arthroplasty has been described as superior for pain relief, functional outcome, and patient satisfaction compared with hemiarthroplasty.[1] The major concern in total shoulder arthroplasty is loosening of the glenoid component, which has been frequently observed at mid- and long-term follow-up.[2-6] Therefore, some surgeons avoid implanting a glenoid component, especially in relatively young patients with a high level of activity and a long life expectancy.[7,8] The outcomes have varied with the use of different fixation concepts (cemented or noncemented) and glenoid component designs (keeled or pegged, flat-back or convex-back) and with or without posterior augmentation. Native glenoid morphology may have an influence on survival rates of glenoid components.[9] During prior decades, glenoid morphology was classified by using two-dimensional CT scans; however, large variations in measuring version and inclination have been described.[10] The introduction of three-dimensional (3D) planning software has allowed standardized analysis of glenoid morphology and virtual implantation of components.

Glenoid Anatomy

Knowledge of the anatomy of the glenoid is crucial for every shoulder surgeon, especially when total shoulder arthroplasty is being considered. The surgeon needs to know the version, inclination, height, width, and shape of the patient's glenoid.[11] A surgical plan can be formulated using this information.

The glenoid cavity is covered with cartilage, with the thinnest part in the center. The thickness of the cartilage increases from the center to the periphery. The cartilage terminates at the glenoid labrum, which consists of strong fibrocartilage. The morphology of the glenoid surface can be described as the shape of a pear or an inverted comma. The supraglenoid tubercle with its insertion of the long head of the biceps tendon is the superior point of the glenoid, and the infraglenoid tubercle with its insertion of the long head of the triceps tendon is the inferior point. Multiple studies have analyzed the average dimensions of the glenoid surface in nonarthritic shoulders, with slightly differing results.[12-15] Mean glenoid height measured from superior to inferior was found to range from 35 to 39 mm, and mean glenoid width to range from 23 to 29 mm.[12-15] In arthritic shoulders, a mean glenoid height of 40.2 mm (SD 4.9 mm), a mean width of 29 mm (SD 4.3 mm), and a mean radius of curvature of 35.4 mm (SD 7.8 mm) were described. An analysis of the articulating surface area and the volume of the glenoid vault found a mean surface area of 8.7 cm^2 and a volume of 11.9 cm^3.[14] These findings illustrate that glenoid anatomy in the osteoarthritic shoulder is different compared with nonarthritic joints. This may have influence on glenoid prosthetic reconstruction and on glenoid component fixation and design.[16,17]

The morphology of the osteoarthritic glenoid has been described by the authors of a 1999 study.[18] Three different types of glenoid morphology were defined by using axial CT scans. Concentric glenoids (type A glenoids) were subdivided into type A1 (no erosion) and A2 (with central erosion). Glenoids with posterior subluxation of the humeral head were defined as type B glenoids and subdivided into B1 (narrowing of the posterior joint space with subchondral sclerosis and osteophytes) and B2 (biconcavity with excessive retroversion). Glenoids with a dysplastic origin and a retroversion of >25° and a centered or slightly posteriorly subluxated humeral head were defined as type C. This original classification was modified by the authors of a 2016 study, and the glenoid morphologies B3 and D were added.[19] A B3 glenoid was defined as monoconcave and posteriorly worn with at least 15° of retroversion or at least 70% of posterior humeral head subluxation or both. Glenoids with anteversion >4° with or without anterior subluxation of the humeral head were defined as type D.

Preoperative Planning and Patient-Specific Instrumentation

Recently, 3D planning software has been developed for planning the prosthetic reconstruction of the joint prior to surgery. Standardized segmentations and reconstructions of the affected shoulders can be determined based on a CT scan. In addition to qualitative bony erosion, glenoid version and inclination and humeral head subluxation can be measured in a standardized fashion (**Figure 1**). Moreover, range of motion can be tested virtually and potential mechanical impingement can be detected and addressed. The authors of a 2018 study have described that fully automated 3D planning tools may improve preoperative planning, improve surgeon efficiency, and eliminate inter- and intraobserver discrepancies.[20] Moreover,

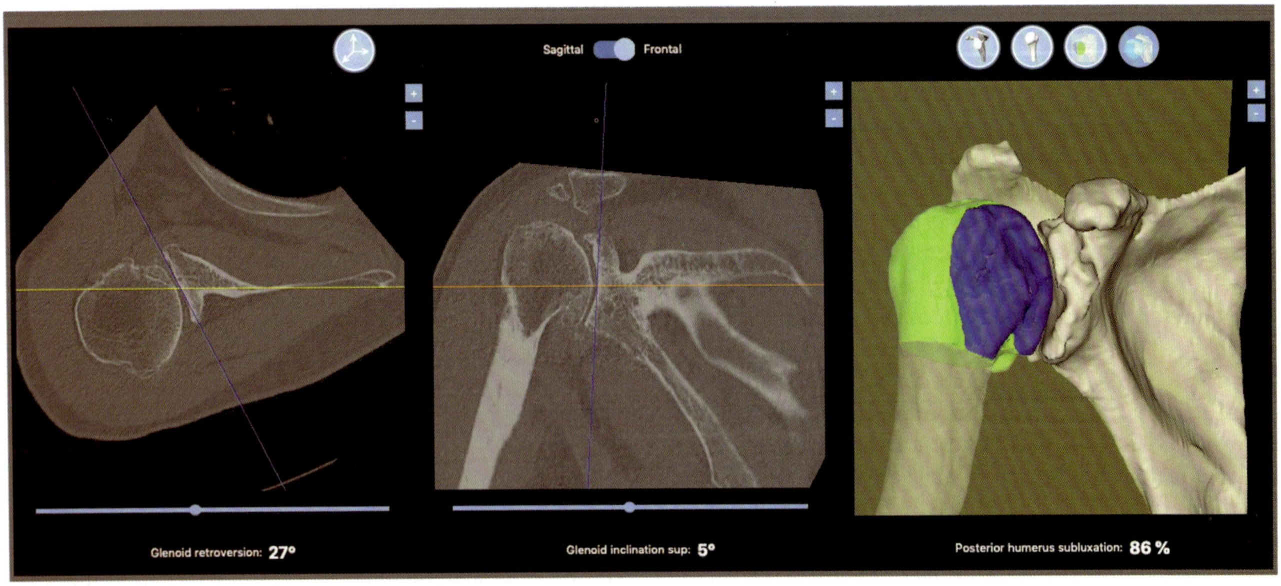

FIGURE 1 Overview of a three-dimensional planning tool showing the glenohumeral joint based on a CT data set after segmentation and reconstruction. Glenoid version and inclination are measured in a standardized fashion.

measurement of glenoid inclination and version seem to be more precise when performed utilizing automated 3D tools compared with conventional two-dimensional planning. It has also been described that the decision-making process and implant choice can be influenced when 3D planning is performed.[21] The authors of a 2018 study have shown that there can be a substantial difference between planning tools in glenoid version and inclination measurements.[22] In their study, two different planning tools were compared in 63 cases. A difference of >10° of glenoid version and inclination was found in 11% and 19% of the cases, respectively. These findings illustrate the need to evaluate differences between measurement systems.

3D planning software also provides data to create patient-specific instrumentation (PSI) for accurate placement of the central glenoid guide pin during surgery. Sterile 3D models of the glenoid can be developed helping the surgeon to better understand the patient's anatomy and assist in placement of the central guide pin. There are several studies published on the results of PSI in cadaveric and clinical trials. The authors of a 2018 study published a review article on the results of PSI compared with standard instrumentation techniques and concluded that PSI may improve guide pin positioning within a few millimeters.[23] Additionally, the number of outliers can be minimized using this technique. The authors of a 2019 study reported the results of a prospective study on 173 cases treated with total shoulder arthroplasty.[24] Patients were divided into three groups: (1) standard instrumentation group, (2) single-use PSI group, and (3) reusable PSI group. Overall, no differences were found between groups regarding placement of the central guide pins. Long-term results are necessary to clarify the hypothetical benefit of PSI.

Prosthetic Considerations

Glenoid components can be fixed with or without the use of bone cement or in a hybrid fashion. Several implant designs and fixation concepts are available.

Noncemented Glenoid Components

Higher rates of revision surgery and complications have been reported with the use of noncemented metal-backed glenoid components than with cemented components. A prospective, double-blinded randomized study compared the results of using a noncemented metal-backed bone ingrowth glenoid component with the results of using a cemented keeled flat-back component (each in 20 shoulders).[2] The rate of radiolucent lines around the components was significantly higher in the shoulders with a cemented component (85% versus 25%, $P < 0.01$), but loosening was found in four shoulders with a noncemented metal-backed component (20%) and three implant revisions were required

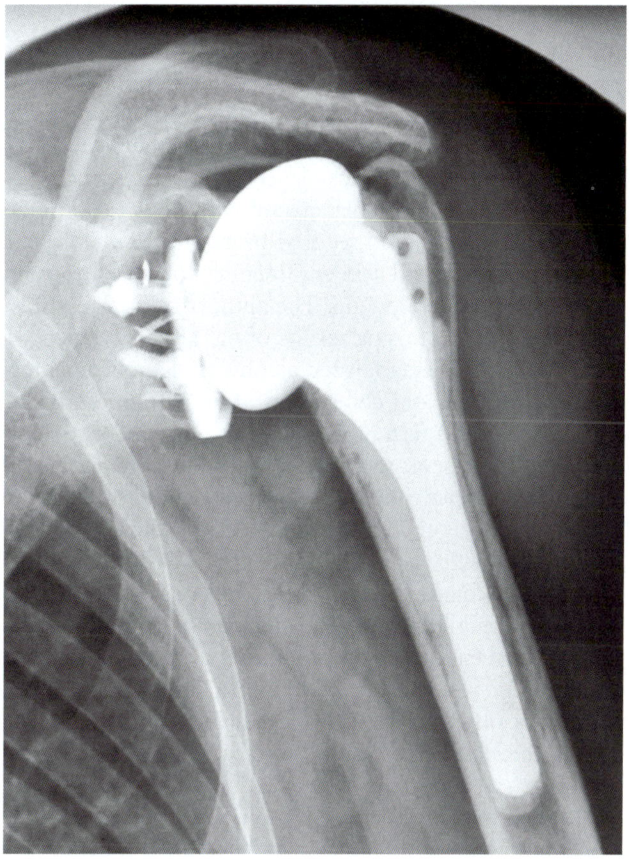

FIGURE 2 AP radiograph showing a total shoulder replacement 14 years after implantation of a cemented stem with a noncemented metal-back glenoid component. Proximal migration of the humerus and gross loosening of the glenoid component with breakage of one screw and wear of the polyethylene inlay can be seen.

(Figure 2). No loosening was detected in the shoulders with a cemented component. The same group published their results of this implant in the long term in 2015.[25] Survival without revision surgery for the noncemented metal-backed glenoid was only 46% at 12 years. At a mean of 8.5 years, 37% of the metal-backed glenoid cohort underwent revision surgery and 80% of patients had evidence of polyethylene liner wear. In 2005, the results of 147 consecutive shoulder arthroplasties were reported at a mean 7.5-year follow-up.[26] In 11% of shoulders, the metal-backed glenoid component had been removed because of clinical failure, and an additional 8% of shoulders had asymptomatic broken hardware evident on radiographs. Multiple investigations have confirmed the high complication rates with the use of different metal-backed designs.[27-29] The most common complication is loosening of the component, followed by severe polyethylene wear or dissociation of the polyethylene from the metal portion of the implant. A 14% failure rate has been described for a noncemented glenoid component with a soft metal-backside and polyethelene liner.[27] All other components included in this study showed good osteointegration and fixation. Excellent mid- and long-term results for noncemented metal-backed glenoid components were described by the authors of a 2010 study.[30] In this study, 35 arthroplasties in 35 patients were performed between 1996 and 2005 using a metal-backed glenoid component consisting of a titanium alloy shell coated with porous titanium and hydroxyapatite and secured by two 6.5-mm screws. The researchers found neither loosening nor complications at a mean 6-year follow-up. The authors of a 2013 study also published promising results of metal-backed glenoid components.[31] They analyzed a convertible noncemented metal-backed glenoid component after 38 months in 37 cases. In the short term, the authors did not find any signs of radiolucency or loosening. Other studies have published results of a noncemented metal-backed glenoid component for osteoarthritis and rheumatoid arthritis. Survival of the component at 10 years was 93% for osteoarthritis and 89% for rheumatoid arthritis.[32,33] The authors of a 2013 study used an all polyethylene anchor pegged component in an noncemented fashion in 34 patients and analyzed the radiographic results after 28 months.[34] No signs of loosening were observed in 88% of cases. However, long-term data is needed for most of the noncemented glenoid components. Metal-backed components on the glenoid side have fallen into disfavor owing to poorer outcomes with longer follow-up, and the fact that the failure characteristics are more dire when compared with failed all-polyethylene components.

Cemented Glenoid Components

The results of using cemented all-polyethylene glenoid components have been well documented. The phenomenon of radiolucent lines around cemented glenoid implants is common, with reported rates of zero to 96%.[35] Although the radiolucent lines often are visible on immediate postoperative radiographs, their presence is not always predictive of component loosening or clinical symptoms.

The two predominant types of cemented glenoid components are keeled and pegged (**Figure 3**). An analysis of immediate postoperative radiographs of 328 total shoulder arthroplasties found significantly higher rates of radiolucent lines when a keeled component was used.[35] These data were supported by two prospective randomized studies that found significantly more radiolucent lines around keeled components than around pegged components at 2-year follow-up.[36,37] A biomechanical study found that the maximal tensile edge displacement was significantly less in pegged than in keeled components.[38] However, another study found no difference in the occurrence of radiolucent lines at a mean 4-year follow-up of 50 patients with a keeled component and 50 with a pegged component.[39]

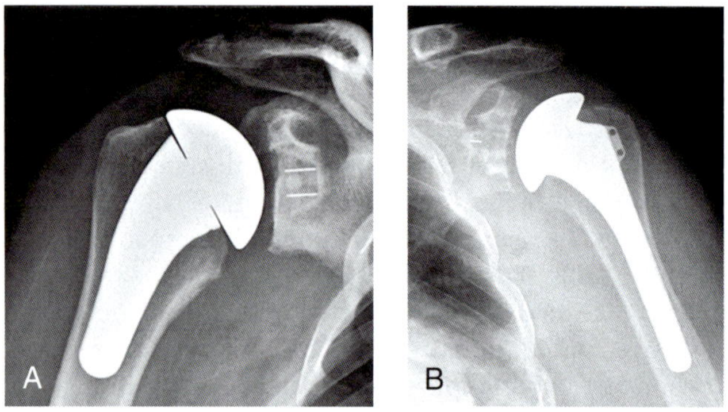

FIGURE 3 Immediate postoperative AP radiographs of a total shoulder replacement in which a noncemented stem is combined with a cemented keeled glenoid component (**A**) or a cemented pegged glenoid component (**B**).

The long-term results of using cemented keeled glenoid components have been well documented. Implant survival was reported on a series of 972 all-polyethylene cemented glenoid components, with revision as the end point.[6] The overall survival rate was 95% at 10 years and 92% at 15 years; at 15 years, the survival rate for the Cofield 1 prosthesis (Smith & Nephew) was 87%, and the rate for the Neer 2 prosthesis (Smith & Nephew) was 94%. The Cofield 2 prosthesis (Smith & Nephew) also had good survival, at 99% after 5 years and 94% after 10 years. Two multicenter studies of implant survival with a flat-back or a convex-back glenoid component had comparable results.[3,4] In patients with osteoarthritis but without a rotator cuff tear or preoperative instability, 263 total shoulder replacements with a cemented flat-back keeled glenoid were evaluated clinically and radiographically at a mean 10-year follow-up (range, 5 to 20 years).[3] Rates of implant survival with glenoid component revision as the end point were 94.5% at 10 years and 79.4% at 15 years. The results were less promising when radiographic loosening was defined as the end point; the survival rates were 80.3% at 10 years and only 33.6% at 15 years. The same investigators analyzed 333 total shoulder arthroplasties with a convex-back cemented glenoid component and reported survival rates of 99.7% at 5 years and 98.3% at 10 years, with revision of the glenoid component as the end point.[4] With radiologic loosening of the glenoid component as the end point, implant survival was 99.7% at 5 years but only 51.5% at 10 years. In both studies, significant associations were found between radiographic loosening and clinical deterioration in pain level, activity level, and shoulder motion.

A study of 518 cemented total shoulder arthroplasties with a convex-back or flat-back keeled glenoid component analyzed patterns of loosening of the glenoid component at a mean 8.6-year follow-up (range, 5 to 18 years).[40]

The three predominant mechanisms of failure were medial subsidence (in 7.9%), superior tilting (in 10%), and posterior tilting (in 6.4%). Medial subsidence of the glenoid component was associated with excessive reaming during glenoid preparation and complete removal of the subchondral bone ($P < 0.001$). The risk factors for superior tilting were an inferior position of the glenoid component, a superiorly oriented position of the glenoid component on the immediate postoperative radiographs, and superior migration of the humeral head ($P < 0.05$). The risk factors for posterior tilting were preoperative posterior subluxation of the humeral head and excessive reaming during glenoid preparation, with complete removal of the subchondral bone ($P < 0.01$). The overall rate of radiographic loosening was 32%, and the authors concluded that protection of the subchondral bone is important for long-term survival of the glenoid component.

Despite the promise shown by pegged glenoid components in comparative studies, few mid- to long-term data exist on these implants. One study with a follow-up period of 5 years reported that the pegged all-polyethylene Cofield 2 implant had a survival rate similar to that of keeled implants, with revision as the end point.[6] The pegged all-polyethylene Cofield 2 implant prosthesis differs from most current pegged implants in that it has three in-line pegs, rather than four or five pegs in a nonlinear configuration. Longer follow-up is needed to better elucidate any advantages of a pegged implant design over a keeled design. The results of a long-term study of this component showed a revision-free survival rate of 99% at 5 years and 83% at 10 years.[41] For radiographic component loosening, survival was 92% at 10 years and only 43% at 10 years. The authors of a 2017 study have shown in a prospective randomized study that no differences exist between cemented polyethylene keeled or pegged components for radiographic lucency, clinical outcomes or need for revision surgery at a follow-up of 8 years.[42] Moreover, the same group showed in a prospective randomized study that no difference was found between fully cemented conventional pegged polyethylene glenoid components and partially cemented finned central pegged polyethylene components with regard to radiolucency or loosening in the short-term after 35 months of follow-up.[43]

Flat-Back Versus Convex-Back Components

The backside of the glenoid can be flat or curved. Convex-back implants attempt to match the shape of the back of the implant to the concave surface of the patient's glenoid. Hemispherical reamers usually are available for glenoid preparation in a convex-back system. A flat reamer is used in bone preparation for a flat-back component. One disadvantage of flat-back components, in comparison with convex-back components, is that in general flat-back components require more extensive bone removal during reaming, because the convexity of the native glenoid must be reamed to a flat surface to match the shape of the back of the implant. Biomechanically, convex-back components were found to resist micromotion better than flat-back components.[38] However, clinical investigations have not shown either component to be superior.

The use of a keeled flat-back component has been shown to lead to more radiolucent lines in the short term, but this difference is mitigated at longer term follow-up.[44] A prospective study of 66 arthroplasties found a significant difference at 2-year follow-up between the mean Molé radiolucent line scores of the flat-back components (4.2 points) and the convex-back components (3.2 points).[45,46] At 10-year follow-up of the same patients, 56 arthroplasties had survived, but the mean radiolucent line score had increased to 9.8 points for the flat-back components and 8.3 points for the convex-back components.[44] This 10-year difference was not statistically significant, but the authors found that at 10-year follow-up patients younger than 60 years at the time of arthroplasty had a significantly higher radiolucent line score ($P < 0.03$), more radiolucent lines developed if the shoulder was dominant ($P < 0.017$), and the presence of radiolucent lines on immediate postoperative radiographs significantly predicted the progression of radiolucent lines ($P < 0.018$). This is the only study we are aware of comparing the clinical results of flat-back and convex-back glenoid components.

Backside Radius of Curvature of Glenoid Components

As mentioned earlier, it is crucial to protect the subchondral bone layer during preparation of the glenoid,[40] and it has been shown that the backside radius of curvature varies in osteoarthritic glenoids.[47] However, most anatomic glenoid components have only one backside radius of curvature regardless of the size of the implant. This can lead to over- or underreaming of the native glenoid resulting in inadequate implant seating. The number of implants available with different backside radiuses of curvatures on the market is limited. Short-term results have been published for keeled components[48] (Aequalis Perform, Wright Medical Inc, MN), pegged components,[49] and pegged design with an noncemented fluted central peg.[50] All radiographic results were satisfactory with a low rate of radiolucent lines and no loosening. However, long-term data are necessary to determine if these components do have a benefit compared with older designs.

Partially Cemented All-Polyethylene Components

Implant design has evolved during the past decade to include variations in component morphology, the number and location of fixation pegs, and the fixation method. The anchor-pegged glenoid implant (Anchor Peg Glenoid, DePuy; Cortiloc, Tornier) is a minimally cemented all-polyethylene design in which the finned central peg is impacted into the center drill hole without cement and the small peripheral pegs are conventionally cemented. Although the mechanism by which cancellous bone grows into the central peg is not understood, good results have been reported.[51-53] Several studies have been published showing comparable results to those of fully cemented pegged or keeled components. One different finding with this type of implant is the so-called ballooning around the central noncemented PE peg that represents osteolysis around the implant. At a mean 43-month follow-up, a CT-based study of 35 patients treated with this implant found bone ingrowth around the central noncemented peg in a mean 4.5 of the 6 fins in 32 implants (91%) and no bone ingrowth in 3 implants (9%).[52] Another study used radiographs under fluoroscopic control and detected bone formation around the fins of the anchor peg in 15 of 20 patients at a minimum 5-year follow-up.[51] Radiolucency or osteolysis (ballooning) was detected around the central peg in the remaining five patients. Another study of this type of implant radiographically followed 44 shoulders for a mean of 3 years.[53] When the classification system devised by the authors of a 2002 study was used to analyze cementing and seating of the glenoid components, 86% were scored as better cementing and better seating.[35] Osteolysis around the central peg was found in 7%, and 68% had adequate bone growth around the fins of the central peg. Gross loosening was detected in one implant. Comparable midterm results were published by several authors.[54,55] The authors of a 2012 study showed in a radiostereometric analysis that early migration of partially cemented components is associated with osteolysis around the central peg evident in three out of 11 cases in their study.[56] The authors of a 2016 study demonstrated in a biomechanical study that full cementation of all pegs outperforms partially cemented and noncemented PE components in component distraction and motion.[57]

Inset Glenoid Components

The authors of a 2011 study biomechanically compared fixation strength and stress distribution of a cemented polyethylene inset glenoid component with a conventional cemented polyethylene onlay peg component (Biomet, Warsaw, IN).[58] After 100,000 cycles, none of the implants loosened but inlay components showed less glenoid rim distractions. Finite element examination showed that inlay components had 87% reduction in displacement compared with onlay prostheses. The same group published a series of 21 cases with severe glenoid erosion and a glenoid vault depth of less than 15 mm at a mean follow-up of 8.7 years treated with the same inlay component.[59] At final follow-up, no loosening was observed and none of the components was revised. Although mechanical testing and finite element analysis showed that the inset implant had favorable results when compared with a conventional implant, it must be recognized that reaming through the cortex of the native glenoid prevents preservation of the subchondral bone, which is critical to the longevity of cemented keeled glenoid components.

Hybrid Glenoid Components

Hybrid glenoid components are usually made of polyethylene with one or more pegs that consists of titanium for bone ingrowth. The authors of a 2018 study analyzed 45 shoulders after a minimum follow-up of 5 years and found overall promising clinical results.[60] Radiographically, 42% of components had some lucency but were not judged to be at risk for loosening. One implant was loose. The authors of a 2019 study analyzed a large cohort of 316 cases treated with a hybrid cage glenoid component (Equinoxe, Exactech, Gainesville, FL) and compared the radiographic results with those of 316 matched cases with a fully cemented pegged polyethylene glenoid component.[61] The hybrid component showed significantly less radiolucent lines (9% versus 38%) and lower loosening/failure rates (2.6% versus 3.8%) and lower revision rates (2.5% versus 6.9%) after 50 months of follow-up.

Posterior Augmented Glenoid Components

Posterior augmented glenoid components are an option to address posterior glenoid wear. Commercially available implants are made out of polyethylene or a hybrid cage construct. Three different designs are currently on the market: full-wedge designs, half-wedge designs, and stepped designs. Full-wedge components (Equinoxe, Exactech, Gainesville, FL) are available with 8°, 12°, or 16° posterior augmentation. Half-wedge components (Aequalis Perform+; Wright Medical Group, Memphis, TN) with 15°, 25°, and 35° are available that correct 7°, 12°, and 17° of posterior wear, respectively. Stepped implants (Global StepTech anchor peg glenoid, DePuy Synthes, Warsaw, IN) have a central step in three different sizes (+3, +5, and +7 mm) and additional pegs for fixation. A correction of 10°, 15°, or 20° is possible with this implant. Biomechanical as well as 3D planning studies have demonstrated that bone removal of the native glenoid is less for full-wedge and half-wedge components compared with stepped components.[62,63] However, all designs have been described as viable options to address posterior glenoid wear in biomechanical testing.

Clinical studies are available for stepped and full-wedge designs currently. The authors of a 2015 study compared 24 cases treated with a full-wedge cemented polyethylene component for correction of posterior glenoid erosion with 24 cemented standard polyethylene components that underwent partial correction of the version by reaming.[64] After 30 months of follow-up, radiolucency was present in 60% of augmented components and 33% in cases with standard components. Moreover, one case in the augmented group had radiographic failure. The authors of a 2019 study compared 37 cases of augmented components with 37 cases of standard implants.[65] After a mean follow-up of 3.2 years, clinical outcomes and rates of radiolucency and revision surgeries were similar between groups. However, high failure rates were seen with the 16° augmented component, and the authors discontinued the use of this implant. The authors of a 2016 study reported on the short-term results (mean 35 months follow-up) of 21 cases treated with a stepped glenoid. There were no complications or revisions. Radiolucent lines around the components were detected in 24% of cases and bone ingrowth around the central peg was found in 95%.[66] The authors of a 2016 study also examined a small cohort at a mean of 36 months postoperatively.[67] They found osteointegration of the central peg in 63% of cases and osteolysis in one. The authors of a 2018 study analyzed 71 shoulders after a mean follow-up of 2.4 years with a stepped component.[68] No loosening of the components occurred, and no revisions were required. They stated that posterior erosion of the native glenoid and posterior humeral head subluxation can successfully be addressed by using this type of implant. As in all studies mentioned earlier, clinical parameters improved.

Posterior Augmentation of the Eccentric Glenoid With Bone Graft

Another possibility to address posterior glenoid erosion is to bone graft the defect with an augment from the humeral head or the iliac crest. The authors of a 2001 study reported on the long-term results of this procedure in 21 cases.[69] Correction of glenoid version was overall successful; however, five components failed leading to revision surgery. Of the seven patients available for follow-up, three rated their result as excellent, six satisfactory, and eight unsatisfactory. The authors of a 2013 study reported on a cohort of 13 cases that were treated with posterior bone augmentation.[70] Twelve patients were available for follow-up (mean 53 months), and in two cases glenoid component failure occurred (one after trauma and one after infection). Promising results were published by the authors of a 2017 study who followed 34 patients with a mean follow-up of 4 years after posterior glenoid bone grafting.[71] Normal glenoid retroversion was successfully restored and a decrease of humeral head subluxation resulted. All bone grafts incorporated completely, and no loosening occurred. In three cases broken or displaced screws were detected, and in another three cases the central metal marker of the keel was broken. However, no revision surgery for glenoid component loosening was necessary.

(Partial) Correction of Glenoid Version by Reaming

Posterior glenoid erosion can alternatively be corrected or partially corrected by reaming. The goal of this technique is to reduce the pathologic version of the arthritic glenoid allowing placement of a standard component without additional augmentation. Drawbacks of this procedure include the important anterior subchondral bone layer may be sacrificed, and the joint line will be medialized leading to a potential loss of tension of the rotator cuff muscles. Moreover, by reducing the bone stock, implant fixation may be compromised as the keel or pegs may penetrate the glenoid vault. The authors of a 2018 study have reported promising results in 59 patients that underwent this technique.[72] After a follow-up of 50 months, no revision for glenoid component failure was necessary, and no difference was found in the rate of progression of radiolucent lines for glenoids <20° of retroversion and >20° of retroversion.

Prosthetic Mismatch

The term prosthetic mismatch describes the difference in the radius of curvature between the glenoid and humeral components. The osseous radial glenohumeral mismatch can range from 8 to 9 mm, whereas the cartilaginous radial glenohumeral mismatch can be as small as 0.1 mm.[73] In total shoulder replacement, the range of prosthetic mismatch depends on the implant and ultimately is selected by the surgeon. A complete conformity between the humeral and glenoid components increases the contact area of the components and therefore decreases the contact pressure.[74] A conforming system, however, does not allow for the obligate translation that occurs as the humeral head translates on the glenoid. Consequently, increased forces are transmitted to the rim of the glenoid component.[75] This rim loading may increase the risk of glenoid component loosening.[76] Conversely, increasing glenohumeral mismatch reduces the contact area between the head and the glenoid components, resulting in increased contact pressure that can accelerate polyethylene wear and increase glenohumeral instability.[73-75] Most investigators recommend some mismatch of the components to avoid excessive loading of the glenoid rim.[73,74] Only one clinical study has analyzed the influence of the mismatch on the formation of radiolucent lines around cemented glenoid components.[73] In 319 shoulders treated with the Aequalis total shoulder arthroplasty system (Tornier), all patients had the same diagnosis of primary glenohumeral osteoarthritis, and a cemented keeled glenoid component was used. The patients were assigned to one of four glenohumeral radial mismatch groups: group 1, 0 to 4 mm; group 2, 4.5 to 5.5 mm; group 3, 6 to 7 mm; and group 4, more than 7 mm. At a mean 4.5-year follow-up, lower mean Molé radiolucent line scores were found in groups 3 and 4 (3.8 and 3.7 points, respectively) than in groups 1 and 2 (6.4 and 5.8 points, respectively). The authors concluded that a glenohumeral radial mismatch between 6 and 10 mm most favorably influences the development of radiolucent lines.

Polyethylene

Standard polyethylene glenoid components are made out of ultra-high–molecular-weight polyethylene. Newer materials have a cross-linked structure to reduce wear particles and to decrease osteolysis.[77] However, during cross-linking, free radicals are formed leading to oxidative degeneration of the ultra-high–molecular-weight polyethylene. Vitamin E can be incorporated into the ultra-high–molecular-weight polyethylene to reduce this process. Promising results with low wear rates have been published with potential clinical benefits in biomechanical shoulder studies as well as in clinical trials with short-term follow-up in hip and knee arthroplasty.[78,79]

Technical Considerations

Glenoid Preparation Technique

Adequate exposure of the glenoid surface is critical for preparation of the native glenoid during component implantation. Many techniques for glenoid exposure and preparation have been described. The preferred technique of the senior author is described here.

A humeral head retractor is inserted into the joint after tenotomy of the subscapularis tendon. After a release of the middle and inferior glenohumeral ligaments, the humeral head is retracted posteriorly to expose the anterior glenoid rim. The subscapularis tendon is placed into the subscapularis recess on the anterior scapula and held with an anterior glenoid rim retractor. The long head of the biceps tendon is released from its insertion on the supraglenoid tubercle and tenodesed at the upper border of the pectoralis major tendon using nonabsorbable suture. The glenoid labrum and capsule are released starting just anterior-inferior to the coracoid and terminating at the 5-o'clock or 7-o'clock position (in a right or left shoulder, respectively). The inferior capsule and lateral extent of the triceps tendon is released around to the 8-o'clock or 4-o'clock position (in a right or left shoulder, respectively). This inferior release is the key step for adequate glenoid exposure and implant insertion (**Figure 4**). The humeral head is dislocated anteriorly and resected. When the preparation of the humerus is complete, the proximal humerus is retracted posteriorly to expose the glenoid. Any residual cartilage can be removed from the glenoid using a curet. If a patient-specific instrument is used, all osteophytes must be preserved to place the instrument and guide pin correctly. If a patient-specific instrument is not used, glenoid osteophytes can be removed. The center of the glenoid surface is marked using an electrocautery. If a cannulated system is being used, the central guidewire can be inserted; a center hole can be drilled if a noncannulated system has been selected. A motorized reamer is used to prepare the surface of the glenoid. To protect the subchondral bone, which is important for implant longevity, minimal reaming is performed. If a posterior augmented component is used, additional reamers may be required. If a pegged component is being used, the remaining peg holes can be drilled. If a keeled component

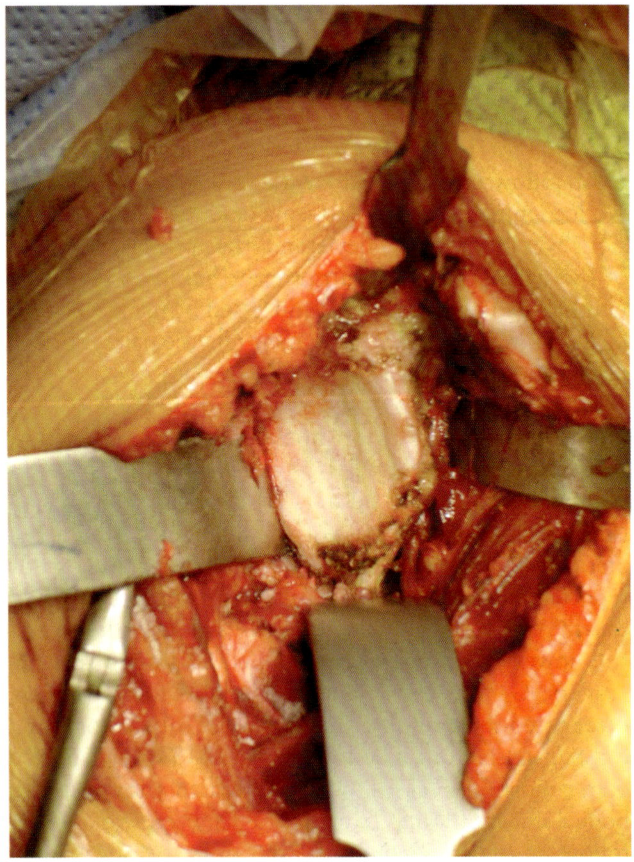

FIGURE 4 Photograph showing the exposure of a right glenoid after a deltopectoral approach was used. A Lambotte retractor is placed in the posterior part of the glenoid, and a Link retractor is placed in the anterior part. One Hohmann retractor is placed superoinferiorly at the glenoid.

is being used, the impaction technique is recommended. This technique involves minimal bone removal and uses a keel punch to impact the bone. It has been shown that this technique leads to significantly better radiolucent line scores around keeled glenoid components compared with a traditional curettage technique.[31] The implant can be fixed as recommended by the prosthesis manufacturer.

Cementing Technique

After glenoid preparation, the keel slot or the peg holes are irrigated by pulsatile lavage to remove blood and debris from the cancellous bone. The benefits of pulsatile lavage irrigation are well established in hip arthroplasty, although similar efficacy has not been proven in shoulder arthroplasty. The glenoid bone should be dried after irrigation. A comparison of three methods of drying the glenoid before keeled implant cementation (the use of thrombin-soaked gel foam, compressed gas lavage, or saline-solution lavage followed by simple sponge use) on immediate postoperative radiographs did not find a statistically significant difference in radiolucent lines around the glenoid component, based on the drying method.[80] In the weep-hole technique for drying the glenoid vault, a hole is drilled into the coracoid process to connect it to the glenoid vault, and continuous suction is performed over this hole during implant cementation.[81] A clinical study found significantly improved cement mantles and fewer radiolucent lines around keeled and pegged glenoid components when the weep-hole technique was used.[81] A CT-based in vitro study found significantly deeper cement penetration into the glenoid vault when the weep-hole technique was used compared with a standard technique.[82] A potential problem with this technique is that the drill hole might weaken the coracoid process leading to fracture.

Many types of cement are available, including slow- and fast-curing low-, medium-, or high-viscosity cements that may contain an antibiotic. The cement can be manually mixed in a bowl or can be mixed using a vacuum centrifuge to reduce porosity. No data are available comparing the outcomes of using different types of cement for glenoid component implantation.

Multiple techniques have been described for inserting the cement into the glenoid vault directly or with a syringe. In vitro syringe application was found to result in better cement penetration than manual application, and cement penetration was deeper in one patient with osteoporosis.[83] This finding was confirmed in a study that found a strong negative correlation between local bone mineral density in the glenoid vault and cement penetration.[84] Pressurization is a well-established method for improving cement penetration in hip and knee arthroplasty. A few studies have been published on this technique in total shoulder arthroplasty. The occurrence of radiolucent lines around all-polyethylene glenoid components was compared based on whether a free-hand packing technique or a new instrumented pressurization technique was used.[85] The incidence and thickness of radiolucent lines around the glenoid component were significantly greater on immediate postoperative radiographs after treatment with the free-hand technique ($P < 0.05$). Pegged glenoid components had significantly fewer radiolucent lines than keeled components ($P < 0.05$). When a 60-mL syringe was used in combination with a pressurizer sponge for cement application into the peg holes, 90% of the 69 shoulders had no radiolucent lines on immediate postoperative radiographs.[86] A size-matched pegged component used in combination with cement pressurization and the study authors' surgical technique was found to lead to a low incidence of radiolucent lines. Longer term follow-up data are not yet available. In 2012, a silicone pressurization device with a slot for a keeled component or a hole for a pegged component was introduced.[87] This device can easily be attached to a cement gun. In an in vitro study, the use of this device led to more homogenous and deeper cement penetration into the glenoid bone, in comparison with a conventional cementing technique. After pressurization of cement, the authors recommend holding the component in place until the cement polymerizes and removing any cement extrusion to avoid foreign bodies in the joint, which could induce third-body polyethylene wear. Holding the component during polymerization may not be necessary with anchor peg designs.

Future Directions

Glenoid loosening is the weak link in total shoulder arthroplasty. Glenoid loosening is especially problematic for relatively young patients who have a longer life expectancy and a higher activity level than most older patients.[7,8,88,89] Alternative bearing surfaces have been introduced for the purpose of avoiding conventional glenoid component implantation.

Biologic Resurfacing

One possibility for resurfacing the glenoid without implanting a conventional component is to use a soft-tissue graft. The principle is to create a smooth biologic glenoid surface and thereby reduce mechanical friction between the prosthetic humeral component and the glenoid.[90] Graft materials including meniscal allograft, joint capsule, fascia lata autograft, Achilles tendon allograft, and extracellular matrix products have been described.[90-92] In one study, 36 shoulders in patients with multiple diagnoses were treated with biologic glenoid resurfacing combined with humeral head replacement.[91] The anterior capsule was used in seven shoulders, autogenous fascia lata in 11 shoulders, and Achilles tendon allograft in 18 shoulders. At 2- to 15-year follow-up, the mean overall score on the American Shoulder and Elbow Surgeons Pain and Disability Index had improved to 91 points from 39 points before surgery. According to the Neer criteria, 50% of the patients were very satisfied with the result of surgery, 36% were satisfied, and 14% were not satisfied. All shoulders had a postoperative decrease in joint space, but there was no progression at 5 years. The patients in whom allograft was used had better results for glenohumeral mobility and radiographic glenoid erosion than those in whom autograft was used. Four additional procedures were performed; one was a débridement related to wound infection, and three were conversions to total shoulder arthroplasty. In all patients who underwent conversion to total shoulder arthroplasty, the anterior capsule had been initially used for glenoid resurfacing. An Achilles tendon allograft for biologic resurfacing of the glenoid was recommended.

In another study, contrary results were reported when hemiarthroplasty was combined with biologic resurfacing of the glenoid.[93] Thirteen patients (mean age, 34 years) underwent glenoid resurfacing with an Achilles tendon allograft in 11 patients, fascia lata autograft in one patient, or anterior capsule autograft in one patient. Only one patient was satisfied 3 years after the procedure. The remaining 12 patients underwent revision surgery. A total shoulder replacement was required in 10 patients because of severe shoulder pain and joint space narrowing. In two patients, an infection was treated with débridement and a resection arthroplasty. It was concluded that the graft material used in these patients was not durable and that biologic resurfacing of the glenoid should be pursued with caution.

In yet another study, 30 shoulders were treated using a metallic humeral head replacement and a meniscal allograft for resurfacing the glenoid.[92] Although there were significant improvements in all clinical outcome measures, 17% of the shoulders required revision surgery at 1-year follow-up. Two patients underwent conversion to a total shoulder replacement, and a third patient underwent graft removal with retention of the hemiarthroplasty. An infection requiring removal of all implants developed in one patient, and another patient underwent an arthroscopic débridement procedure.

Arthroscopic resurfacing of the glenoid using a patch without replacement of the humeral head led to a satisfactory result in 75% of patients at 3- to 6-year follow-up.[94] All scores on the Constant and American Shoulder and Elbow Surgeons measures were greatly improved. However, 25% of the patients underwent revision to a hemiarthroplasty. These inconsistent results led to the conclusion that biologic resurfacing may be a viable option for degenerative pathology of the shoulder joint in a young adult, but it should be used with caution. Prospective studies are needed to compare the results of techniques including biologic resurfacing, hemiarthroplasty, and total shoulder replacement.

The Ream-and-Run Procedure

Although hemiarthroplasty leads to inferior functional outcomes and less pain relief than total shoulder arthroplasty, it is a viable option for treating degenerative pathologies of the shoulder joint.[1] Specifically, in a relatively young patient glenoid component loosening is a concern. In shoulders with eccentric glenoid wear, the outcomes of hemiarthroplasty have been inferior compared with shoulders in which the humeral head is centered in the glenoid.[95] The so-called ream-and-run procedure was introduced as a means of correcting the biconcavity of eccentric glenoid wear without the use of a glenoid component.[96] During this procedure, the glenoid is prepared with a large-diameter reamer, and a humeral head 2 mm smaller than the diameter of curvature of the glenoid reamer is chosen.[75] It has been shown that the intrinsic stability of the reamed glenoid can be restored and that a fibrocartilaginous surface is created on the reamed surface, and more and more data are available as to the clinical and radiologic outcome of this type of procedure.[96-102] Ten-year results of this procedure have been described with overall satisfactory clinical findings and a revision rate of 16%.[98] Return to sport rates were described by the authors of a 2019 study and >90% of patients were able to play sports again after the procedure.[102] The results were comparable to those of patients who underwent total shoulder arthroplasty. Less promising results were found by the authors of a 2017 study who reported a revision rate of 25% in their cases after a follow-up of less than 3 years.[101]

Alternative Bearing Surfaces

Alternative bearing surfaces are mainly on the humeral side. Usually the humeral head is comprised of cobalt chrome. Some manufactures are using ceramic heads to reduce wear of the polyethylene on the glenoid side. Another potential advantage of a metal-free head is the hypoallergenic nature. Potential wear benefits were found by the authors of a 2017 study in a biomechanical study.[103] The overall results of total shoulder arthroplasty implanted with ceramic heads are promising;[104,105] however, long-term comparisons to standard bearings are missing.

Pyrocarbon is an alternative bearing surface on the humeral side that can be used either with a short stem or as a stemless prosthesis. However, this material has been used for hemiarthroplasty only and not yet in combination with glenoid components.[106-108]

SUMMARY

Significant improvement in function and pain relief can be expected after total shoulder replacement. However, the glenoid component continues to be the weak link in total shoulder arthroplasty. High rates of loosening have been described with cemented components. Noncemented metal-backed glenoid components have had high rates of failure in the past, and many have had to be abandoned. Newer noncemented designs have shown encouraging results; however, no long-term data are currently available. Other implant concepts or surgical techniques with posterior augmentation, inlay design, or varying backside radius of curvature have to be followed in the future. Preoperative 3D planning and the use of PSI may help improving the results in the long-term. However, further investigation is necessary to analyze the long-term results of using the newer glenoid implant concepts and designs and to identify the ideal treatment for the glenoid side of the shoulder.

KEY STUDY POINTS

- The glenoid component continues to be the weak link in total shoulder arthroplasty.
- 3D CT-based preoperative planning is an important tool to better understand the underlying pathology of the arthritic glenoid (eg, posterior erosion and inclination).
- Newer noncemented metal-backed glenoid components are oftentimes convertible to a reverse arthroplasty; however, long-term data are lacking.
- Results of cemented glenoid components are well documented even in the long term; however, high radiographic loosening rates have been reported.

Annotated References

1. Radnay CS, Setter KJ, Chambers L, Levine WN, Bigliani LU, Ahmad CS: Total shoulder replacement compared with humeral head replacement for the treatment of primary glenohumeral osteoarthritis: A systematic review. *J Shoulder Elbow Surg* 2007;16(4):396-402.

2. Boileau P, Avidor C, Krishnan SG, Walch G, Kempf JF, Molé D: Cemented polyethylene versus uncemented metal-backed glenoid components in total shoulder arthroplasty: A prospective, double-blind, randomized study. *J Shoulder Elbow Surg* 2002;11:351-359.

3. Young A, Walch G, Boileau P, et al: A multicentre study of the long-term results of using a flat-back polyethylene glenoid component in shoulder replacement for primary osteoarthritis. *J Bone Joint Surg Br* 2011;93:210-216.

4. Walch G, Young AA, Melis B, Gazielly D, Loew M, Boileau P: Results of a convex-back cemented keeled glenoid component in primary osteoarthritis: Multicenter study with a follow-up greater than 5 years. *J Shoulder Elbow Surg* 2010;20(3):385-394.

5. Raiss P, Bruckner T, Rickert M, Walch G: Longitudinal observational study of total shoulder replacements with cement: Fifteen to twenty-year follow-up. *J Bone Joint Surg Am* 2014;96:198-205. doi:10.2106/JBJS.M.00079.

   This is a retrospective study showing the 15- to 20-year results after cemented total shoulder arthroplasty in a longitudinal fashion. Level of evidence: IV.

6. Fox TJ, Cil A, Sperling JW, Sanchez-Sotelo J, Schleck CD, Cofield RH: Survival of the glenoid component in shoulder arthroplasty. *J Shoulder Elbow Surg* 2009;18:859-863.

7. Neyton L, Kirsch JM, Collotte P, et al: Mid- to long-term follow-up of shoulder arthroplasty for primary glenohumeral osteoarthritis in patients aged 60 or under. *J Shoulder Elbow Surg* 2019;28(9):1666-1673. doi:10.1016/j.jse.2019.03.006.

   This is a retrospective study showing the clinical and radiographic findings in a relatively young patient cohort after shoulder replacement. Level of evidence: III.

8. Sowa B, Bochenek M, Bülhoff M, et al: The medium- and long-term outcome of total shoulder arthroplasty for primary glenohumeral osteoarthritis in middle-aged patients. *Bone Joint J* 2017;99-B:939-943. doi:10.1302/0301-620X.99B7.BJJ-2016-1365.R1.

   This is an updated follow-up of a previous published study showing the the complications of total shoulder arthroplasty are increasing with longer follow-up. Level of evidence: IV.

9. Walch G, Moraga C, Young A, Castellanos-Rosas J: Results of anatomic nonconstrained prosthesis in primary osteoarthritis with biconcave glenoid. *J Shoulder Elbow Surg* 2012;21:1526-1533. doi:10.1016/j.jse.2011.11.030.

10. Bokor DJ, O'Sullivan MD, Hazan GJ: Variability of measurement of glenoid version on computed tomography scan. *J Shoulder Elbow Surg* 1999;8:595-598.

11. Schrumpf M, Maak T, Hammoud S, Craig EV: The glenoid in total shoulder arthroplasty. *Curr Rev Musculoskelet Med* 2011;4:191-199.

12. Churchill RS, Brems JJ, Kotschi H: Glenoid size, inclination, and version: An anatomic study. *J Shoulder Elbow Surg* 2001;10:327-332.

13. Mallon WJ, Brown HR, Vogler JB III, Martinez S: Radiographic and geometric anatomy of the scapula. *Clin Orthop Relat Res* 1992;(277):142-154.

14. Kwon YW, Powell KA, Yum JK, Brems JJ, Iannotti JP: Use of three-dimensional computed tomography for the analysis of the glenoid anatomy. *J Shoulder Elbow Surg* 2005;14:85-90.

15. Iannotti JP, Gabriel JP, Schneck SL, Evans BG, Misra S: The normal glenohumeral relationships. An anatomical study of one hundred and forty shoulders. *J Bone Joint Surg Am* 1992;74:491-500.

16. Rouleau DM, Lavoie F, Ogassawara R, et al: Glenoid version: How to measure it? Validity of different methods in two-dimensional computed tomography scans. *J Shoulder Elbow Surg* 2010;19:1230-1237.

17. Saha AK: The classic. Mechanism of shoulder movements and a plea for the recognition of "zero position" of glenohumeral joint. *Clin Orthop Relat Res* 1983;(173):3-10.

18. Walch G, Badet R, Boulahia A, Khoury A: Morphologic study of the glenoid in primary glenohumeral osteoarthritis. *J Arthroplasty* 1999;14:756-760.

19. Bercik MJ, Kruse K II, Yalizis M, Gauci MO, Chaoui J, Walch G: A modification to the Walch classification of the glenoid in primary glenohumeral osteoarthritis using three-dimensional imaging. *J Shoulder Elbow Surg* 2016;25:1601-1606. doi:10.1016/j.jse.2016.03.010.

    This is a radiographic analysis of osteoarthritic shoulders updating the initial Walch classification of the osteoarthritic glenoid morphology.

20. Boileau P, Cheval D, Gauci MO, Holzer N, Chaoui J, Walch G: Automated three-dimensional measurement of glenoid version and inclination in arthritic shoulders. *J Bone Joint Surg Am* 2018;100:57-65. doi:10.2106/JBJS.16.01122.

    This is a study on a fully automated 3D planning tool for shoulder replacement surgery. Compared with historical methods, measurement of glenoid inclination and retroversion and humeral head subluxation seems to be viable.

21. Werner BS, Hudek R, Burkhart KJ, Gohlke F: The influence of three-dimensional planning on decision-making in total shoulder arthroplasty. *J Shoulder Elbow Surg* 2017;26:1477-1483. doi:10.1016/j.jse.2017.01.006.

    This is a study on a 3D planning tool for shoulder replacement surgery showing that decision of treatment can be influenced by this tool. Level of evidence: III.

22. Denard PJ, Provencher MT, Lädermann A, Romeo AA, Parsons BO, Dines JS: Version and inclination obtained with 3-dimensional planning in total shoulder arthroplasty: Do different programs produce the same results? *JSES Open Access* 2018;2:200-204. doi:10.1016/j.jses.2018.06.003.

    This study compares two different 3D planning tools showing that differences in measuring of glenoid inclination and retroversion are possible between systems.

23. Villatte G, Muller AS, Pereira B, Mulliez A, Reilly P, Emery R: Use of Patient-Specific Instrumentation (PSI) for glenoid component positioning in shoulder arthroplasty. A systematic review and meta-analysis. *PLoS One* 2018;13:e0201759. doi:10.1371/journal.pone.0201759.

    This study shows that the use of PSI can be helpful in case of shoulder replacement surgery.

24. Iannotti JP, Walker K, Rodriguez E, Patterson TE, Jun BJ, Ricchetti ET: Accuracy of 3-dimensional planning, implant templating, and patient-specific instrumentation in anatomic total shoulder arthroplasty. *J Bone Joint Surg Am* 2019;101:446-457. doi:10.2106/JBJS.17.01614.

    This study shows that the use of PSI can be helpful in case of shoulder replacement surgery. Level of evidence: II.

25. Boileau P, Moineau G, Morin-Salvo N, et al: Metal-backed glenoid implant with polyethylene insert is not a viable long-term therapeutic option. *J Shoulder Elbow Surg* 2015;24:1534-1543. doi:10.1016/j.jse.2015.02.012.

    This is a study on long-term follow-up of uncemented glenoid components with high radiographic loosening rates. Level of evidence: IV.

26. Martin SD, Zurakowski D, Thornhill TS: Uncemented glenoid component in total shoulder arthroplasty. Survivorship and outcomes. *J Bone Joint Surg Am* 2005;87:1284-1292.

27. Fucentese SF, Costouros JG, Kuhnel SP, Gerber C: Total shoulder arthroplasty with an uncemented soft-metal-backed glenoid component. *J Shoulder Elbow Surg* 2010;19:624-631.

28. Groh GI: Survival and radiographic analysis of a cementless fluted pegged glenoid component. *J Shoulder Elbow Surg* 2010;19(8):1265-1268.

29. Taunton MJ, McIntosh AL, Sperling JW, Cofield RH: Total shoulder arthroplasty with a metal-backed, bone-ingrowth glenoid component. Medium to long-term results. *J Bone Joint Surg Am* 2008;90:2180-2188.

30. Castagna A, Randelli M, Garofalo R, Maradei L, Giardella A, Borroni M: Mid-term results of a metal-backed glenoid component in total shoulder replacement. *J Bone Joint Surg Br* 2010;92:1410-1415.

31. Katz D, Kany J, Valenti P, Gleyze P, El Kholti K: New design of a cementless glenoid component in unconstrained shoulder arthroplasty: A prospective medium-term analysis of 143 cases. *Eur J Orthop Surg Traumatol* 2013;23:27-34. doi:10.1007/s00590-012-1109-6.

    This is a retrospective study of uncemented glenoid components with promising short-term results.

32. Clement ND, Mathur K, Colling R, Stirrat AN: The metal-backed glenoid component in rheumatoid disease: Eight- to fourteen-year follow-up. *J Shoulder Elbow Surg* 2010;19:749-756. doi:10.1016/j.jse.2009.11.005.

33. Clement ND, Duckworth AD, Colling RC, Stirrat AN: An uncemented metal-backed glenoid component in total shoulder arthroplasty for osteoarthritis: Factors affecting survival and outcome. *J Orthop Sci* 2013;18:22-28. doi:10.1007/s00776-012-0308-7.

This is a study of mid-term follow-up of uncemented glenoid components with moderate failure rates. Level of evidence: IV.

34. De Wilde L, Dayerizadeh N, De Neve F, Basamania C, Van Tongel A: Fully uncemented glenoid component in total shoulder arthroplasty. *J Shoulder Elbow Surg* 2013;22:e1-e7. doi:10.1016/j.jse.2013.01.036.

This study includes short-term results of polyethylene glenoid components that were inserted in an uncemented fashion. Level of evidence: IV.

35. Lazarus MD, Jensen KL, Southworth C, Matsen FA III: The radiographic evaluation of keeled and pegged glenoid component insertion. *J Bone Joint Surg Am* 2002;84:1174-1182.

36. Gartsman GM, Elkousy HA, Warnock KM, Edwards TB, O'Connor DP: Radiographic comparison of pegged and keeled glenoid components. *J Shoulder Elbow Surg* 2005;14:252-257.

37. Edwards TB, Labriola JE, Stanley RJ, O'Connor DP, Elkousy HA, Gartsman GM: Radiographic comparison of pegged and keeled glenoid components using modern cementing techniques: A prospective randomized study. *J Shoulder Elbow Surg* 2010;19:251-257.

38. Anglin C, Wyss UP, Pichora DR: Mechanical testing of shoulder prostheses and recommendations for glenoid design. *J Shoulder Elbow Surg* 2000;9:323-331.

39. Throckmorton TW, Zarkadas PC, Sperling JW, Cofield RH: Pegged versus keeled glenoid components in total shoulder arthroplasty. *J Shoulder Elbow Surg* 2010;19:726-733.

40. Walch G, Young AA, Boileau P, Loew M, Gazielly D, Molé D: Patterns of loosening of polyethylene keeled glenoid components after shoulder arthroplasty for primary osteoarthritis: Results of a multicenter study with more than five years of follow-up. *J Bone Joint Surg Am* 2012;94:145-150.

41. McLendon PB, Schoch BS, Sperling JW, Sánchez-Sotelo J, Schleck CD, Cofield RH: Survival of the pegged glenoid component in shoulder arthroplasty: Part II. *J Shoulder Elbow Surg* 2017;26(8):1469-1476. doi:10.1016/j.jse.2016.12.068.

This is a retrospective study of cemented pegged glenoid components with high loosening rates in the long run. Level of evidence: IV.

42. Kilian CM, Press CM, Smith KM, et al: Radiographic and clinical comparison of pegged and keeled glenoid components using modern cementing techniques: Midterm results of a prospective randomized study. *J Shoulder Elbow Surg* 2017;26(12):2078-2085. doi:10.1016/j.jse.2017.07.016.

This prospective study shows no differences of radiolucent lines between keeled and pegged glenoid components in the midrun. Level of evidence: II.

43. Kilian CM, Morris BJ, Sochacki KR, et al: Radiographic comparison of finned, cementless central pegged glenoid component and conventional cemented pegged glenoid component in total shoulder arthroplasty: A prospective randomized study. *J Shoulder Elbow Surg* 2018;27:S10-S16. doi:10.1016/j.jse.2017.09.014.

This prospective randomized study shows good short-term results of two different pegged glenoid components. Level of evidence: II.

44. Collin P, Tay AK, Melis B, Boileau P, Walch G: A ten-year radiologic comparison of two-all polyethylene glenoid component designs: A prospective trial. *J Shoulder Elbow Surg* 2011;20:1217-1223.

45. Molé D, Roche O, Riand N, Levigne C, Walch G: Cemented glenoid components: Results in osteoarthritis and rheumatoid arthritis, in Walch G, Boileau P, eds: *Shoulder Arthroplasty*. Berlin/Heidelberg, Germany, Springer, 1999, pp 163-171.

46. Szabo I, Buscayret F, Edwards TB, Nemoz C, Boileau P, Walch G: Radiographic comparison of flat-back and convex-back glenoid components in total shoulder arthroplasty. *J Shoulder Elbow Surg* 2005;14:636-642.

47. Walch G, Mesiha M, Boileau P, et al: Three-dimensional assessment of the dimensions of the osteoarthritic glenoid. *Bone Joint J* 2013;95-B:1377-1382. doi:10.1302/0301-620X.95B10.32012.

This is a 3D CT study on the dimensions and shapes of osteoarthrtic glenoids.

48. Raiss P, Godenèche A, Wittmann T, et al: Short-term radiographic results of a cemented polyethylene keeled glenoid component with varying backside radiuses of curvature. *J Shoulder Elbow Surg* 2018;27:839-845. doi:10.1016/j.jse.2017.10.026.

This is a retrospective study on cemented keeled glenoid components with varying backside radiuses of curvature. Level of evidence: IV.

49. Dauzere F, Arboucalot M, Lebon J, Elia F, Bonnevialle N, Mansat P: Evaluation of thirty eight cemented pegged glenoid components with variable backside curvature: Two-year minimum follow-up. *Int Orthop* 2017;41:2353-2360. doi:10.1007/s00264-017-3635-7.

This is a retrospective study on cemented pegged glenoid components with varying backside radiuses of curvature. Level of evidence: IV.

50. Merolla G, Ciaramella G, Fabbri E, Walch G, Paladini P, Porcellini G: Total shoulder replacement using a bone ingrowth central peg polyethylene glenoid component: A prospective clinical and computed tomography study with short- to mid-term follow-up. *Int Orthop* 2016;40:2355-2363. doi:10.1007/s00264-016-3255-7.

    This study shows promising short-term results of a polyethylene glenoid component with cementation of the peripheral pegs only. Level of evidence: IV.

51. Churchill RS, Zellmer C, Zimmers HJ, Ruggero R: Clinical and radiographic analysis of a partially cemented glenoid implant: Five-year minimum follow-up. *J Shoulder Elbow Surg* 2010;19:1091-1097.

52. Arnold RM, High RR, Grosshans KT, Walker CW, Fehringer EV: Bone presence between the central peg's radial fins of a partially cemented pegged all poly glenoid component suggest few radiolucencies. *J Shoulder Elbow Surg* 2011;20:315-321.

53. Wirth MA, Loredo R, Garcia G, RockwoodJr CA, Southworth C, Iannotti JP: Total shoulder arthroplasty with an all-polyethylene pegged bone-ingrowth glenoid component: A clinical and radiographic outcome study. *J Bone Joint Surg Am* 2012;94:260-267. doi:10.2106/JBJS.J.01400.

54. Parks DL, Casagrande DJ, Schrumpf MA, Harmsen SM, Norris TR, Kelly JD II: Radiographic and clinical outcomes of total shoulder arthroplasty with an all-polyethylene pegged bone ingrowth glenoid component: Prospective short- to medium-term follow-up. *J Shoulder Elbow Surg* 2016;25:246-255. doi:10.1016/j.jse.2015.07.008.

    This study shows promising short-term results of a polyethylene glenoid component with cementation of the peripheral pegs only. Level of evidence: IV.

55. Wijeratna M, Taylor DM, Lee S, Hoy G, Evans MC: Clinical and radiographic results of an all-polyethylene pegged bone-ingrowth glenoid component. *J Bone Joint Surg Am* 2016;98:1090-1096. doi:10.2106/JBJS.15.00475.

    This study shows promising short-term results of polyethylene glenoid components with cementation of the peripheral pegs only. Level of evidence: IV.

56. Nuttall D, Haines JF, Trail IA: The early migration of a partially cemented fluted pegged glenoid component using radiostereometric analysis. *J Shoulder Elbow Surg* 2012;21:1191-1196. doi:10.1016/j.jse.2011.07.028.

57. Wiater BP, Moravek JE Jr, Kurdziel MD, Baker KC, Wiater JM: Biomechanical evaluation of all-polyethylene pegged bony ingrowth glenoid fixation techniques on implant micromotion. *Am J Orthop (Belle Mead NJ)* 2016;45:E211-E216.

    This study analyses implant micromotion in a specific anatomic glenoid design.

58. Gunther SB, Lynch TL, O'Farrell D, Calyore C, Rodenhouse A: Finite element analysis and physiologic testing of a novel, inset glenoid fixation technique. *J Shoulder Elbow Surg* 2011;21(6):795-803.

59. Gunther SB, Tran SK: Long-term follow-up of total shoulder replacement surgery with inset glenoid implants for arthritis with deficient bone. *J Shoulder Elbow Surg* 2019;28(9):1728-1736. doi:10.1016/j.jse.2019.01.020.

    This study shows promising long-term results of a glenoid component that is embedded into the native glenoid. Level of evidence: IV.

60. Nelson CG, Brolin TJ, Ford MC, Smith RA, Azar FM, Throckmorton TW: Five-year minimum clinical and radiographic outcomes of total shoulder arthroplasty using a hybrid glenoid component with a central porous titanium post. *J Shoulder Elbow Surg* 2018;27:1462-1467. doi:10.1016/j.jse.2018.01.012.

    A low rate of mechanical failure and a moderate rate of radiolucency of this particular implant are shown. Level of evidence: IV.

61. Friedman RJ, Cheung E, Grey SG, et al: Clinical and radiographic comparison of a hybrid cage glenoid to a cemented polyethylene glenoid in anatomic total shoulder arthroplasty. *J Shoulder Elbow Surg* 2019;28(12):2308-2231. doi:10.1016/j.jse.2019.04.049.

    Promising midterm results have been shown for the hybrid cage glenoid component at 50 months of follow-up. Level of evidence: III.

62. Sabesan VJ, Lima DJL, Whaley JD, Pathak V, Zhang L: Biomechanical comparison of 2 augmented glenoid designs: An integrated kinematic finite element analysis. *J Shoulder Elbow Surg* 2019;28:1166-1174. doi:10.1016/j.jse.2018.11.055.

    An augmented wedge glenoid component provides better implant fixation and stress profiles with less micromotions compared with stepped components.

63. Knowles NK, Ferreira LM, Athwal GS: Augmented glenoid component designs for type B2 erosions: A computational comparison by volume of bone removal and quality of remaining bone. *J Shoulder Elbow Surg* 2015;24:1218-1226. doi:10.1016/j.jse.2014.12.018.

    Virtual implantation of wedged glenoid components lead to less bone removal compared with stepped components.

64. Wright TW, Grey SG, Roche CP, Wright L, Flurin PH, Zuckerman JD: Preliminary results of a posterior augmented glenoid compared to an all polyethylene standard glenoid in anatomic total shoulder arthroplasty. *Bull Hosp Jt Dis* 2015;73(suppl 1):S79-S85.

This study shows promising short-term results of a posterior augmented glenoid component. Level of evidence: IV.

65. Priddy M, Zarezadeh A, Farmer KW, et al: Early results of augmented anatomic glenoid components. *J Shoulder Elbow Surg* 2019;28:S138-S145. doi:10.1016/j.jse.2019.04.014.

In this study, 16° full wedge components had a high failure rate and were discontinued. Components with less augmentation had similar results compared with standard glenoid components. Level of evidence: III.

66. Stephens SP, Spencer EE, Wirth MA: Radiographic results of augmented all-polyethylene glenoids in the presence of posterior glenoid bone loss during total shoulder arthroplasty. *J Shoulder Elbow Surg* 2016;26(5):798-803. doi:10.1016/j.jse.2016.09.053.

Good clinical results without complications or failures have been shown for this type of implant in the short term. Level of evidence: IV.

67. Favorito PJ, Freed RJ, Passanise AM, Brown MJ: Total shoulder arthroplasty for glenohumeral arthritis associated with posterior glenoid bone loss: Results of an all-polyethylene, posteriorly augmented glenoid component. *J Shoulder Elbow Surg* 2016;25:1681-1689. doi:10.1016/j.jse.2016.02.020.

A stepped posterior augmented glenoid component showed encouraging results in the short term. Level of evidence: IV.

68. Ho JC, Amini MH, Entezari V, et al: Clinical and radiographic outcomes of a posteriorly augmented glenoid component in anatomic total shoulder arthroplasty for primary osteoarthritis with posterior glenoid bone loss. *J Bone Joint Surg Am* 2018;100:1934-1948. doi:10.2106/JBJS.17.01282.

Posteriorly stepped augmented glenoid components can improve pathologic retroversion and posterior subluxation of the humeral head in B2 and B3 glenoids in the short term. Level of evidence: IV.

69. Hill JM, Norris TR: Long-term results of total shoulder arthroplasty following bone-grafting of the glenoid. *J Bone Joint Surg Am* 2001;83:877-883.

70. Sabesan V, Callanan M, Ho J, Iannotti JP: Clinical and radiographic outcomes of total shoulder arthroplasty with bone graft for osteoarthritis with severe glenoid bone loss. *J Bone Joint Surg Am* 2013;95:1290-1296. doi:10.2106/JBJS.L.00097.

Mixed results are shown of bone grafting of the eroded glenoid in combination with cemented glenoid components. Level of evidence: IV.

71. Nicholson GP, Cvetanovich GL, Rao AJ, O'Donnell P: Posterior glenoid bone grafting in total shoulder arthroplasty for osteoarthritis with severe posterior glenoid wear. *J Shoulder Elbow Surg* 2017;26:1844-1853. doi:10.1016/j.jse.2017.03.016.

Excellent results are presented in cases with posterior glenoid erosion treated with bone grafting and cemented keeled glenoid components. Level of evidence: IV.

72. Orvets ND, Chamberlain AM, Patterson BM, et al: Total shoulder arthroplasty in patients with a B2 glenoid addressed with corrective reaming. *J Shoulder Elbow Surg* 2018;27:S58-S64. doi:10.1016/j.jse.2018.01.003.

Partial correction of glenoid retroversion by reaming of the osteoarthritic glenoid shows good midterm results in this study. Level of evidence: IV.

73. Walch G, Edwards TB, Boulahia A, Boileau P, Mole D, Adeleine P: The influence of glenohumeral prosthetic mismatch on glenoid radiolucent lines: Results of a multicenter study. *J Bone Joint Surg Am* 2002;84:2186-2191.

74. Terrier A, Buchler P, Farron A: Influence of glenohumeral conformity on glenoid stresses after total shoulder arthroplasty. *J Shoulder Elbow Surg* 2006;15:515-520.

75. Matsen FA III, Bicknell RT, Lippitt SB: Shoulder arthroplasty: The socket perspective. *J Shoulder Elbow Surg* 2007;16:S241-S247.

76. Collins D, Tencer A, Sidles J, Matsen F III: Edge displacement and deformation of glenoid components in response to eccentric loading. The effect of preparation of the glenoid bone. *J Bone Joint Surg Am* 1992;74:501-507.

77. Wirth MA, Klotz C, Deffenbaugh DL, McNulty D, Richards L, Tipper J: Cross-linked glenoid prosthesis: A wear comparison to conventional glenoid prosthesis with wear particulate analysis. *J Shoulder Elbow Surg* 2009;18:130-137. doi:10.1016/j.jse.2008.06.015.

78. Alexander JJ, Bell SN, Coghlan J, Lerf R, Dallmann F: The effect of vitamin E-enhanced cross-linked polyethylene on wear in shoulder arthroplasty—A wear simulator study. *J Shoulder Elbow Surg* 2019;28(9):1771-1778. doi:10.1016/j.jse.2019.01.014.

Addition of vitamin E seems to reduce wear of the polyethylene glenoid component.

79. Lambert B, Neut D, van der Veen HC, Bulstra SK: Effects of vitamin E incorporation in polyethylene on oxidative degradation, wear rates, immune response, and infections in total joint arthroplasty: A review of the current literature. *Int Orthop* 2019;43:1549-1557. doi:10.1007/s00264-018-4237-8.

Tribology aspects of polyethylene with vitamin E have been overall positive.

80. Edwards TB, Sabonghy EP, Elkousy H, et al: Glenoid component insertion in total shoulder arthroplasty: Comparison of three techniques for drying the glenoid before cementation. *J Shoulder Elbow Surg* 2007;16:S107-S110.

81. Gross RM, High R, Apker K, Haggstrom J, Fehringer JA, Stephan J: Vacuum assist glenoid fixation: Does this technique lead to a more durable glenoid component? *J Shoulder Elbow Surg* 2011;20:1050-1060.

82. Hasan SA, Cox WK, Syed M, Suva LJ: Microcomputed tomography assessment of glenoid component cementation techniques in total shoulder arthroplasty. *J Orthop Res* 2010;28:559-564.

83. Nyffeler RW, Meyer D, Sheikh R, Koller BJ, Gerber C: The effect of cementing technique on structural fixation of pegged glenoid components in total shoulder arthroplasty. *J Shoulder Elbow Surg* 2006;15:106-111.

84. Raiss P, Pape G, Kleinschmidt K, et al: Bone cement penetration pattern and primary stability testing in keeled and pegged glenoid components. *J Shoulder Elbow Surg* 2011;20:723-731. doi:10.1016/j.jse.2010.09.006.

85. Klepps S, Chiang AS, Miller S, Jiang CY, Hazrati Y, Flatow EL: Incidence of early radiolucent glenoid lines in patients having total shoulder replacements. *Clin Orthop Relat Res* 2005;(435):118-125.

86. Barwood S, Setter KJ, Blaine TA, Bigliani LU: The incidence of early radiolucencies about a pegged glenoid component using cement pressurization. *J Shoulder Elbow Surg* 2008;17:703-708.

87. Raiss P, Sowa B, Bruckner T, et al: Pressurisation leads to better cement penetration into the glenoid bone: A cadaveric study. *J Bone Joint Surg Br* 2012;94:671-677.

88. Denard PJ, Wirth MA, Orfaly RM: Management of glenohumeral arthritis in the young adult. *J Bone Joint Surg Am* 2011;93:885-892. doi:10.2106/JBJS.J.00960.

89. Denard PJ, Raiss P, Sowa B, Walch G: Mid- to long-term follow-up of total shoulder arthroplasty using a keeled glenoid in young adults with primary glenohumeral arthritis. *J Shoulder Elbow Surg* 2013;22:894-900. doi:10.1016/j.jse.2012.09.016.

This study shows clinical and radiographic results of young patients who underwent cemented total shoulder replacement. Level of evidence: IV.

90. Burkhead WZ Jr, Krishnan SG, Lin KC: Biologic resurfacing of the arthritic glenohumeral joint: Historical review and current applications. *J Shoulder Elbow Surg* 2007;16:S248-S253.

91. Krishnan SG, Nowinski RJ, Harrison D, Burkhead WZ: Humeral hemiarthroplasty with biologic resurfacing of the glenoid for glenohumeral arthritis. Two to fifteen-year outcomes. *J Bone Joint Surg Am* 2007;89:727-734.

92. Nicholson GP, Goldstein JL, Romeo AA, et al: Lateral meniscus allograft biologic glenoid arthroplasty in total shoulder arthroplasty for young shoulders with degenerative joint disease. *J Shoulder Elbow Surg* 2007;16:S261-S266.

93. Elhassan B, Ozbaydar M, Diller D, Higgins LD, Warner JJ: Soft-tissue resurfacing of the glenoid in the treatment of glenohumeral arthritis in active patients less than fifty years old. *J Bone Joint Surg Am* 2009;91:419-424.

94. Savoie FH III, Brislin KJ, Argo D: Arthroscopic glenoid resurfacing as a surgical treatment for glenohumeral arthritis in the young patient: Midterm results. *Arthroscopy* 2009;25:864-871.

95. Hettrich CM, Weldon E III, Boorman RS, Parsons IM, Matsen FA III: Preoperative factors associated with improvements in shoulder function after humeral hemiarthroplasty. *J Bone Joint Surg Am* 2004;86:1446-1451.

96. Lynch JR, Franta AK, Montgomery WH Jr, Lenters TR, Mounce D, Matsen FA III: Self-assessed outcome at two to four years after shoulder hemiarthroplasty with concentric glenoid reaming. *J Bone Joint Surg Am* 2007;89:1284-1292.

97. Weldon EJ III, Boorman RS, Smith KL, Matsen FA III: Optimizing the glenoid contribution to the stability of a humeral hemiarthroplasty without a prosthetic glenoid. *J Bone Joint Surg Am* 2004;86:2022-2029.

98. Somerson JS, Matsen FA III: Functional outcomes of the ream-and-run shoulder arthroplasty: A concise follow-up of a previous report. *J Bone Joint Surg Am* 2017;99:1999-2003. doi:10.2106/JBJS.17.00201.

Overall promising results of this particular technique for glenoid preparation are demonstrated. Level of evidence: IV.

99. Somerson JS, Neradilek MB, Service BC, Hsu JE, Russ SM, Matsen FA III: Clinical and radiographic outcomes of the ream-and-run procedure for primary glenohumeral arthritis. *J Bone Joint Surg Am* 2017;99:1291-1304. doi:10.2106/JBJS.16.01201.

Short-term results of the ream and run procedure are encouraging in this study. Level of evidence: IV.

100. Somerson JS, Wirth MA: Self-assessed and radiographic outcomes of humeral head replacement with nonprosthetic glenoid arthroplasty. *J Shoulder Elbow Surg* 2015;24:1041-1048. doi:10.1016/j.jse.2014.10.022.

Over time, stable results can be achieved with this procedure without a difference between centric and eccentric glenoid erosions. Level of evidence: IV.

101. Getz CL, Kearns KA, Padegimas EM, Johnston PS, Lazarus MD, Williams GR Jr: Survivorship of hemiarthroplasty with concentric glenoid reaming for glenohumeral arthritis in young, active patients with a biconcave glenoid. *J Am Acad Orthop Surg* 2017;25:715-723. doi:10.5435/JAAOS-D-16-00019.

A high revision rate of the ream and run procedure was found in young patients with osteoarthritic shoulders in the short term. Level of evidence: IV.

102. Garcia GH, Gowd AK, Liu JN, Malaret MR, Cabarcas BC, Romeo AA: Return to sport following hemiarthroplasty with concentric reaming versus total shoulder arthroplasty: A matched pair analysis. *Orthopedics* 2019;42(5):276-284. doi:10.3928/01477447-20190627-05.

Both treatment options can lead to a high rate of return of sports.

103. Mueller U, Braun S, Schroeder S, et al: Influence of humeral head material on wear performance in anatomic shoulder joint arthroplasty. *J Shoulder Elbow Surg* 2017;26:1756-1764. doi:10.1016/j.jse.2017.05.008.

Polyethylene wear of the glenoid component could potentially be reduced by using a ceramic head.

104. Greiner S, Berth A, Kaab M, Irlenbusch U: Glenoid morphology affects the incidence of radiolucent lines around cemented pegged polyethylene glenoid components. *Arch Orthop Trauma Surg* 2013;133:1331-1339. doi:10.1007/s00402-013-1813-7.

Good radiographic and clinical results have been found for a cemented 2-peg glenoid component. Level of evidence: IV.

105. Berth A, Pap G: Stemless shoulder prosthesis versus conventional anatomic shoulder prosthesis in patients with osteoarthritis: A comparison of the functional outcome after a minimum of two years follow-up. *J Orthop Traumatol* 2013;14:31-37. doi:10.1007/s10195-012-0216-9.

Stemless humeral components have no disadvantage in clinical outcome parameters compared with conventional implants in this study. Level of evidence: IV.

106. Garret J, Godeneche A, Boileau P, et al: Pyrocarbon interposition shoulder arthroplasty: Preliminary results from a prospective multicenter study at 2 years of follow-up. *J Shoulder Elbow Surg* 2017;26:1143-1151. doi:10.1016/j.jse.2017.01.002.

Short-term results of a pyrocarbon ball inserted into the humeral metaphysis as hemiarthroplasty are shown. Level of evidence:IV.

107. Garret J, Harly E, Le Huec JC, Brunner U, Rotini R, Godenèche A, et al: Pyrolytic carbon humeral head in hemi-shoulder arthroplasty: Preliminary results at 2-year follow-up. *JSES Open Access* 2019;3:7-42. doi:10.1016/j.jses.2018.09.002.

Short-term clinical and radiographic results of a pyrocarbon head with a short humeral stem are shown. Level of evidence: IV.

108. Hudek R, Werner B, Abdelkawi AF, Gohlke F: Pyrocarbon interposition shoulder arthroplasty in advanced collapse of the humeral head. *Orthopäde* 2017;46:1034-1044. doi:10.1007/s00132-017-3495-2.

Short-term results of a pyrocarbon ball inserted into the humeral metaphysis as hemiarthroplasty are shown in this case series. Level of evidence: IV.

Chapter 24

Hemiarthroplasty and Reverse Shoulder Arthroplasty for Acute Proximal Humeral Fractures

Pascal Boileau, MD • Daniel Grant Schwartz, MD • Tjarco D. Alta, MD, PhD • Devin Lemmex, MD, FRCSC

ABSTRACT

Proximal humerus fractures remain a difficult problem to treat. Poor bone stock and fracture comminution often preclude anatomic reconstruction of the proximal humerus in the elderly population. Hemiarthroplasty and reverse shoulder arthroplasty remain viable procedures to restore function and eliminate pain in these situations. Complex proximal humerus fractures should be treated as massive rotator cuff tears and not simply as bony injuries. The integrity of the tuberosities is critical to achieve a favorable functional outcome. Modern fracture-specific stem designs and robust suture techniques have contributed to improved patient-reported and functional outcomes. Reverse shoulder arthroplasty has seen a rapid rise in its use for treating these difficult fractures with success, but longer term results are needed.

Keywords: hemiarthroplasty; proximal humerus fracture; reverse shoulder arthroplasty

Introduction

Proximal humeral fractures account for an estimated 5% of all fractures. In patients older than approximately 70 years, however, proximal humeral fractures are the third most common fracture (exceeded in incidence only by hip and distal radius fractures).[1] Only three- and four-part displaced proximal humeral fractures are typically treated with arthroplasty. The infrequent use of arthroplasty, combined with low interobserver and intraobserver agreement regarding surgeon treatment algorithms, contribute to the difficulty of managing proximal humeral fractures for even the most experienced surgeon.[2] Success requires a clear understanding of the indications, treatment options, prosthetic design rationales, and technical considerations related to tuberosity repair and prosthesis placement.

The author of a 1953 study, first described hemiarthroplasty for proximal humeral fractures; his satisfactory but imperfect results included a 90% rate of patients with an excellent or satisfactory result when prosthetic replacement was used for displaced three- and four-part fractures.[3,4] No subsequent study was able to replicate his results.[5,6] During the intervening decades, an understanding of metallurgy, an ability to create anatomic shoulder prostheses, and technical comprehension of tuberosity repair and prosthetic placement have improved the ability to restore the native anatomy with arthroplasty.

Reverse shoulder arthroplasty has become increasingly popular for treating proximal humeral fractures in patients older than 70 years, but the concept is not new. Grammont performed 22 reverse shoulder arthroplasties between 1989 and 1993 in patients with proximal humeral fractures or fracture sequelae.[7] Multiple reports have shown that reverse shoulder arthroplasty is a crucial tool in the arsenal of the orthopaedic surgeon.

Fracture Classification

In 1934, proximal humeral fractures were classified based on whether the anatomic fragment included the greater tuberosity, the lesser tuberosity, the surgical neck, or the humeral head.[8] This concept was expanded further to suggest that an anatomic fragment must be displaced at least 1 cm or angulated 45° to be considered part of a so-called displaced fracture.[9] Therefore, a four-part fracture would involve the humeral head displaced and/or angulated from the diaphysis, with both the greater and lesser tuberosities displaced and/or angulated. The more parts to the fracture, the more likely it is to involve compromise to the vascular supply of the humeral head.

Dr. Boileau or an immediate family member has received royalties from Wright Medical Technology, Inc. and serves as a paid consultant to or is an employee of CONMED Linvatec, Smith & Nephew, and Wright Medical Technology, Inc. Dr. Schwartz or an immediate family member serves as a paid consultant to or is an employee of Mitek and has stock or stock options held in Johnson & Johnson. Dr. Alta or an immediate family member is a member of a speakers' bureau or has made paid presentations on behalf of DePuy, A Johnson & Johnson Company. Neither Dr. Lemmex nor any immediate family member has received anything of value from or has stock or stock options held in a commercial company or institution related directly or indirectly to the subject of this chapter.

The Association for Osteosynthesis-Association for the Study of Internal Fixation (AO-ASIF) fracture classification system is not commonly used in clinical practice but is based on both comminution and the potential for disruption of the blood supply to the humeral head.[10] A type A fracture is entirely extra-articular and has one fracture line. A type B fracture also is entirely extra-articular but has two fracture lines. A type C fracture is intra-articular and is subclassified, in order of increasing severity, as a C1 fracture, indicating slight displacement, to a C3 fracture-dislocation, which carries the greatest risk for humeral head ischemia. The Hertel binary-based classification and the so-called LEGO classification are described but not commonly used in clinical practice.[11]

Indications and Contraindications for Arthroplasty

Hemiarthroplasty classically has been indicated for severe fracture patterns, including fracture-dislocations, certain three- and four-part fractures, humeral head-splitting fractures, and fractures involving more than 40% of the articular surface.[7,12-14] A valgus-impacted four-part fracture is relatively unlikely to lead to osteonecrosis of the humeral head, and some surgeons may treat it less aggressively than fractures with other patterns.[15] A preserved medial soft-tissue hinge, a metaphyseal fragment longer than 8 mm, and periosteal integrity may explain the relatively low risk of osteonecrosis in a valgus-impacted four-part fracture.[11] Patient age is somewhat controversial as an indication for hemiarthroplasty; some surgeons restrict hemiarthroplasty to patients older than 70 years, but others perform hemiarthroplasty for patients who are as young as 55 years, or even younger in some situations.[2,14,16] A discerning surgeon closely examines the physiologic age of the patient, including any coexisting medical conditions, and discusses all risks and benefits with the patient before the treatment decision is made.

Reverse shoulder arthroplasty is an alternative to hemiarthroplasty in patients with poor bone quality, typically seen in those older than 70 years.[17] Poor tuberosity bone stock, as a result of a comminuted fracture or osteoporosis, might preclude union with the shaft and the prosthesis, and this concern favors the choice of reverse shoulder arthroplasty. Preexisting rotator cuff arthropathy and massive rotator cuff rupture are additional indications for reverse shoulder arthroplasty.

Hemiarthroplasty and reverse shoulder arthroplasty are contraindicated if a patient has an active infection or is too medically unstable to tolerate surgery. Although there is no absolute minimum age for hemiarthroplasty or reverse shoulder arthroplasty, open reduction and internal fixation should be attempted for a relatively young patient with a heavily comminuted fracture. The surgeon should not choose hemiarthroplasty unless a patient is able to participate in a structured rehabilitation program because physical therapy is fundamental to obtaining a good result. Reverse shoulder arthroplasty should not be performed in patients with an axillary nerve palsy or insufficient glenoid bone stock to support a baseplate.

The Role of the External Rotator Cuff Muscles

In general, the surgeon should consider a displaced three- or four-part fracture of the proximal humerus as a massive rotator cuff tear that requires repair. The fractured tuberosities are displaced by medial traction of the rotator cuff muscles and tendons; the greater tuberosity is pulled posteromedially by the supraspinatus, infraspinatus, and teres minor, while the lesser tuberosity is pulled anteromedially by the subscapularis. The tuberosities must heal to the humeral shaft and to each other to achieve proper rotator cuff function. Greater tuberosity migration, malunion, or nonunion was found to be the major cause of poor outcomes after hemiarthroplasty to treat fracture.[5] Greater tuberosity positioning and healing are the keys to success. Because the shoulder is unfavorably balanced toward muscles of internal rotation (the pectoralis major, subscapularis, latissimus dorsi, and teres major muscles), loss of the greater tuberosity with its attached external rotator muscles (infraspinatus and teres minor) leaves the shoulder with no true external rotators. The surgeon must focus great attention on securely fixing the greater tuberosity; otherwise, the natural predominance of internal rotation in the shoulder could become even stronger in the face of tuberosity malunion or nonunion.

Greater tuberosity fixation and healing are important in reverse shoulder. Although reverse shoulder arthroplasty may allow restoration of active forward elevation in a rotator cuff-deficient shoulder, the absence of external rotator cuff muscles because of displacement or an improperly healed greater tuberosity leads to the absence of active external rotation. Active external rotation is of paramount importance for the patient's ability to control the position of the arm in space and perform activities of daily living (such as shaving, brushing teeth, combing hair, shaking a hand, opening a door, and using a spoon).[18,19] In the absence of external rotator muscles in greater tuberosity malunion or nonunion, there is no muscle to counteract the weight of the forearm during elevation or abduction, and the upper limb swings toward the trunk when attempting to elevate or abduct.

Repair of the tuberosities is often overlooked during reverse shoulder arthroplasty after trauma, but this omission predictably leads to a loss of external rotation and worse outcomes. Studies assessing the results of reverse shoulder arthroplasty and tuberosity healing found better functional outcome scores, abduction, forward flexion, and external rotation[19-26] (**Table 1**). To maximize the

Table 1

Results of Reverse Shoulder Arthroplasty for Proximal Humerus Fracture Based on Tuberosity Healing

Study (Year)	Number of Patients	Mean Patient Age, in Years	Mean Follow-Up, in Months (Range)	Mean Active External Rotation, in Degrees (±)	Mean Active Forward Elevation, in Degrees (±)	Mean Constant Score, Points (±)	Tuberosity Healing (%)
Boileau et al[21] (2019)	38	80	36 (28-44)	Union: 27 (12) Non- or malunion: 11 (12)	Union: 141 (25) Non- or malunion: 115 (26)	Union: 64 (15) Non- or malunion: 51 (12)	84
Chun et al[22] (2017)	38	80	36 (28-46)	Union: 29 (8) Non- or malunion: 10 (9)	Union: 125 (18) Non- or malunion: 127 (14)	Union: 67.9 (11.6) Non- or malunion: 63.9 (8.2)	37
Formaini et al[23] (2015)[a]	25	77	17 (NR)	29 (18)	117 (23)	NR	88
Gallinet et al[24] (2019)	119	79	>60 (NR)	Excision: 6 (8) Repair: 21 (18)	Excision: 100 (38) Repair: 126 (31)	Excision: 50 (18) Repair: 60 (14)	71
Reuther et al[25] (2019)	81	Healed: 78 Partial: 79 Unhealed: 77	Healed: 28 Partial: 28 Unhealed: 28	Healed: 19 (16) Partial: 14 (13) Unhealed: 11 (16)	Healed: 127 (28) Partial: 129 (35) Unhealed: 134 (27)	Healed: 60.3 (12.3) Partial: 61.5 (13.5) Unhealed: 62.3 (11.7)	45
Simovitch et al[19] (2019)	55	77	33.7 (24-62)	Union: 40 (18) Nonunion/excision: 28 (21)	Union: 131 (32) Nonunion/excision: 126 (32)	Union: 64.6 (12.5) Nonunion/ excision: 63.2	83
Torrens et al[26] (2018)	41	77	29 (24-37)	NR	NR	Healed: 61 Not healed: 61	68

NR = not reported.

[a]Did not distinguish results based on tuberosity healing.

ability to perform activities of daily living involving external rotation, tuberosity repair should be attempted for every patient. The surgeon must understand that, from a functional standpoint, positioning and healing of the greater tuberosity is crucial regardless of whether hemiarthroplasty or reverse shoulder arthroplasty is used.

Prosthesis Design Considerations

Advances in third-generation anatomic shoulder prostheses help to re-create the normal anatomy of the proximal humerus in patients with osteoarthritis.[6] However, conventional anatomic humeral prostheses can be too bulky to allow anatomic reduction of the tuberosities, and they allow only minimal contact between the tuberosities and the diaphysis. Because of the volume of metal around the neck, the probability of bony union is low, and the risk of tuberosity migration and malunion is high (**Figure 1**).

Accurate surgical placement of the tuberosities and their ability to heal have been correlated with improved clinical results.[5,27,28] Prosthetic stems that can aid in tuberosity placement and healing have been recently developed. A low-profile prosthesis with relatively little metal allows tuberosities to be reduced anatomically, with more space available for bone grafting to further promote healing (**Figure 2**). One low-profile stem incorporates a window into the metaphysis to allow placement of additional bone graft, which could facilitate union between the tuberosity fragments.[16] The metal around the metaphysis is roughened in some prostheses to increase bony stability by ingrowth into a rough hydroxyapatite-coated surface or a porous tantalum microsurface. However, caution must be taken when using a roughened metal surface if cerclage sutures placed around the neck of the prosthesis come into contact with a roughened surface. The roughened metal surface may abrade the cerclage sutures and impact tuberosity fixation. The use of a smooth medial prosthetic neck can avoid this problem.[6] With a lower profile fracture-dedicated implant, tuberosity migration and nonunion were reduced by 50%.[28]

Fracture-specific reverse shoulder arthroplasty stems have been developed. A hybrid implant with a smooth diaphysis allows cementation, and its roughened hydroxyapatite-coated proximal portion (with a window for bone grafting) promotes tuberosity consolidation[7] (**Figure 3**). The use of low-profile implants for both hemiarthroplasty and reverse shoulder arthroplasty is recommended to allow bone grafting and maximize the likelihood of tuberosity healing (**Figure 4**).

Fracture-Specific Stems

Hemiarthroplasty

In a study of 61 patients, postoperative Constant scores significantly improved if the greater tuberosity healed in an anatomic position ($P = 0.0004$) and the type of implant influenced both anatomic and functional outcomes. At a mean 45-month follow-up, the greater tuberosity was healed in an anatomic position in 26 of 30 patients (87%) with a fracture-specific stem and was healed at a mean 81-month follow-up in 14 of 31 patients (45%) with a conventional stem ($P < 0.0001$). Active forward elevation, active external rotation, and Constant scores were significantly better with a fracture-specific stem (136°, 34°, and 68°, respectively) than with a conventional stem (113°, 23°, and 58°, respectively; $P < 0.0001$). Regardless of the type of implant used, women and patients older than 75 years had significantly lower functional results and higher rates of tuberosity complication ($P < 0.0001$).[29]

Reverse Shoulder Arthroplasty

In a prospective multicenter cohort study, 75 consecutive patients (76 shoulders) with a displaced proximal humeral fracture were treated using a fracture-specific

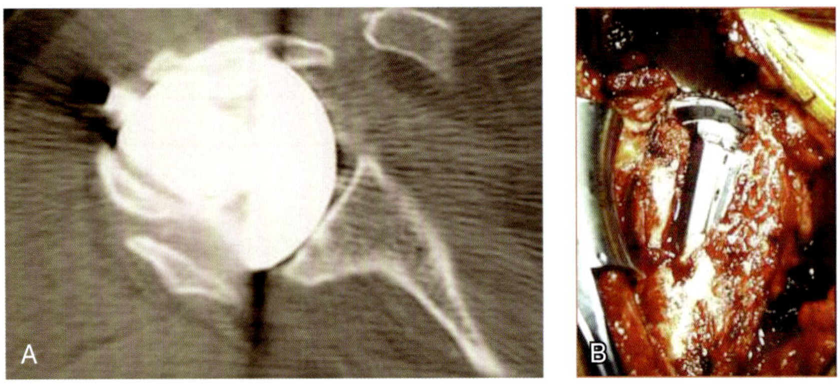

FIGURE 1 Axial CT (**A**) and a photograph from revision surgery (**B**) show that the design of a conventional anatomic hemiarthroplasty prosthesis is poorly adapted to the treatment of a proximal humeral fracture. The excess of metal at the neck level represents an obstacle to greater tuberosity positioning and acts as a barrier to healing. (Courtesy of Pascal Boileau, MD, Nice, France.)

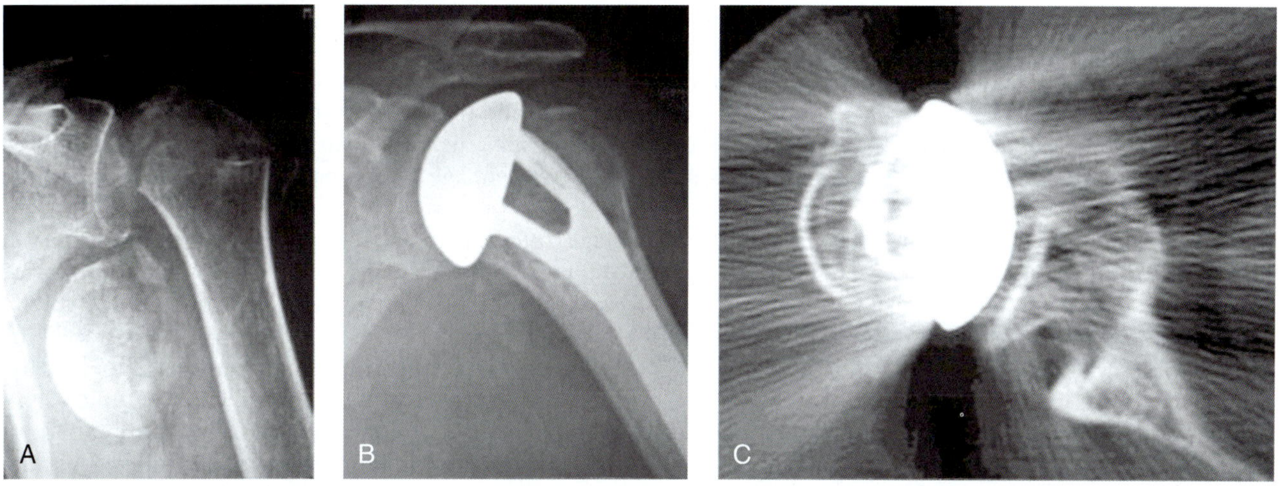

FIGURE 2 Proximal humeral reconstruction after a four-part fracture-dislocation, using a fracture-specific implant. **A**, Preoperative AP radiograph showing that the humeral head fragment is located in the axillary fold, disconnected from all capsular attachments, and devascularized. **B**, Postoperative AP radiograph showing anatomic tuberosity reconstruction around a fracture-specific stem. **C**, Axial CT showing accurate positioning of the tuberosities and cancellous bone harvested from the head fragment and used as a bone graft to promote tuberosity healing around the fracture stem. (Courtesy of Pascal Boileau, MD, Nice, France.)

reverse shoulder arthroplasty stem.[30] At a minimum 1-year follow-up of 49 patients (50 shoulders), the mean active mobility measurements were 131° (range, 40° to 170°) for anterior elevation, 24° (range, 0° to 50°) for external rotation, and five points (range, 0 to 10 points) for internal rotation. The mean score on a 10-point visual analog scale for pain was 1 (range, 0 to 5 points). The mean Constant score was 64 (range, 31 to 91 points) and 93% (range, 45% to 142%) when adjusted for age and gender. The mean subjective shoulder value was 70% (range, 50% to 90%). No complications were recorded, and no patient required further surgery. Forty-three shoulders (86%) had complete radiographic greater tuberosity healing. Five shoulders had early postoperative tuberosity migration, which healed in that position in two shoulders, led to nonunion and osteolysis in two shoulders, and led to osteolysis in one shoulder. Two

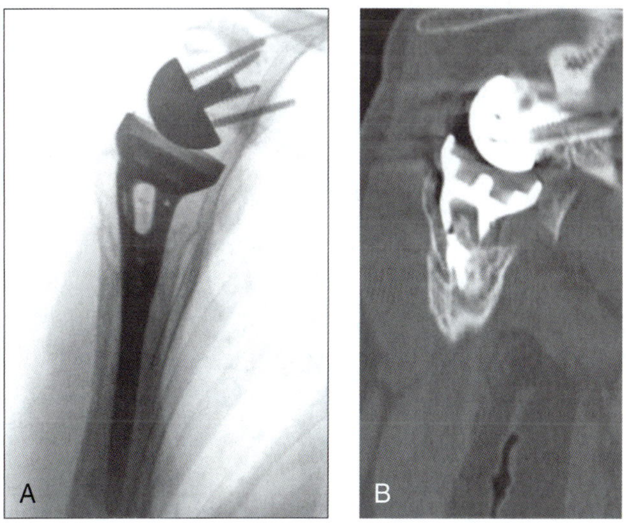

FIGURE 3 A fracture-specific implant 3 months after reverse shoulder arthroplasty. Tuberosity consolidation and union of the bone graft can be seen through the fracture stem window on an AP radiograph (**A**) and CT (**B**). (Courtesy of Pascal Boileau, MD, Nice, France.)

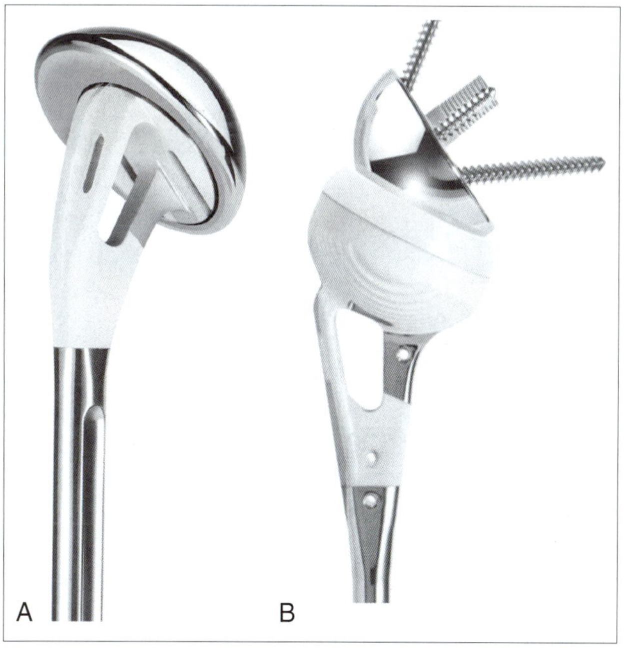

FIGURE 4 Photographs of the authors' preferred fracture-specific stem (Aequalis, Tornier) for hemiarthroplasty (**A**) and reverse shoulder arthroplasty (**B**). (Courtesy of Pascal Boileau, MD, Nice, France.)

shoulders had late tuberosity migration: one shoulder had a nonunion of the greater tuberosity with osteolysis, and the other had osteolysis alone. No glenoid or humeral loosening was observed.

Regardless of patient age, tuberosity healing can be achieved by reattachment and bone grafting around a fracture-specific reverse prosthesis. The use of a fracture-specific implant may encourage a reliable atmosphere for tuberosity healing.

Technical Considerations

Tuberosity Bone Grafting and Fixation

Because the healing of the tuberosities strongly affects clinical outcome, the technique for fixation should facilitate anatomic reduction and stable fixation.[5,27,28,31,32] The ideal construct uses six sutures—four horizontal cerclage sutures and two vertical tension band sutures—which securely fix the tuberosities to one another, to the prosthesis, and to the diaphysis to maximize interfragmentary stability[33] (**Figure 5**). Two sutures are placed in the tendon of teres minor, and two are placed in the tendon of infraspinatus. Two vertical sutures are placed in the humeral shaft, with one strand for the subscapularis and the supraspinatus and the other strand for the supraspinatus and the infraspinatus. The greater tuberosity is primarily fixed with two cerclage sutures passed medial to the prosthetic neck. The lesser tuberosity also is repaired with two cerclage sutures, with one strand each from the infraspinatus and teres minor cerclage sutures. The same technique is used for tuberosity repair with a reverse prosthesis.[17,33]

The Nice knot is a sliding knot that is self-stabilizing (nonslipping) and strong (because it uses a doubled suture) as well as easy to tie and tighten (**Figure 6**). This novel fixation technique has been successfully used for the past decade to fix fractured tuberosities around a hemiarthroplasty or a reverse shoulder arthroplasty.[34]

Prosthetic Positioning

Several methods have been proposed to restore humeral length after arthroplasty for fracture. The principle of restoring the native anatomy is a constant, regardless of

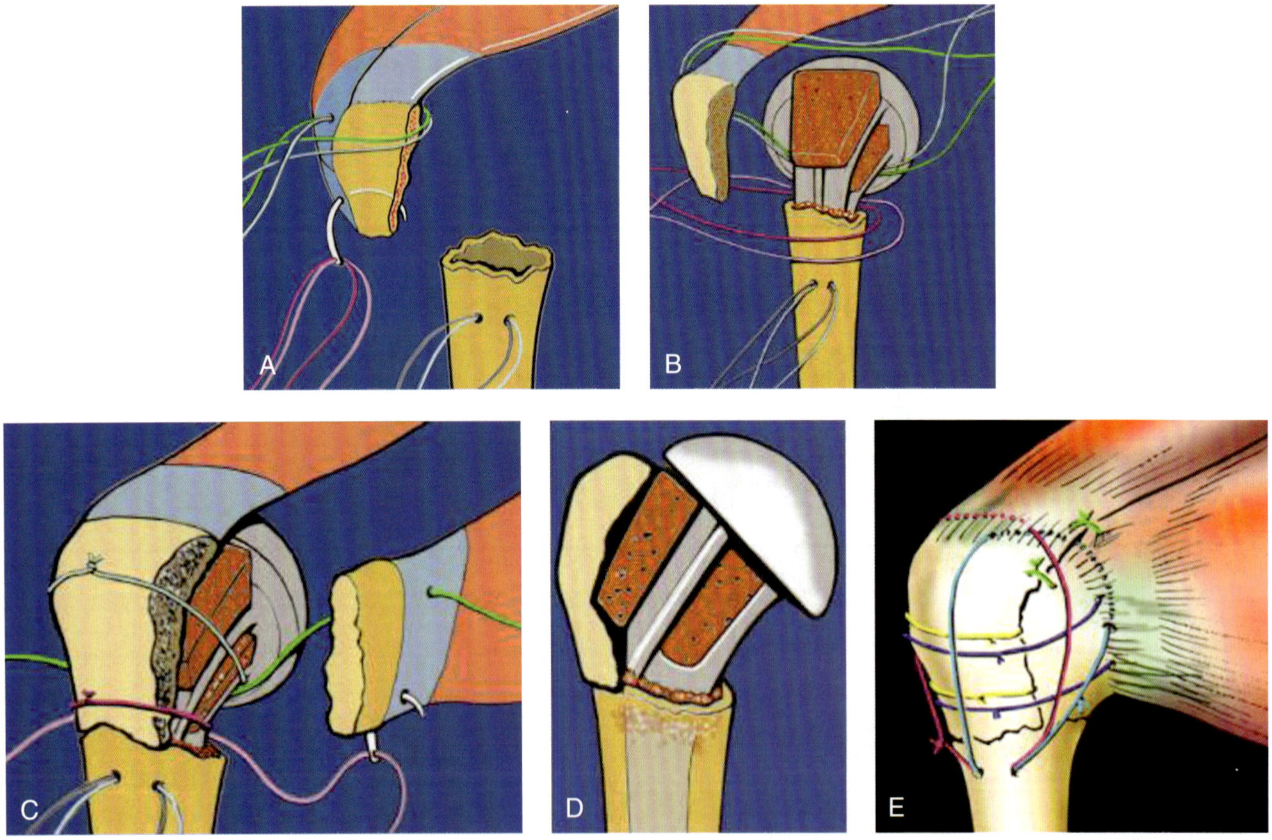

FIGURE 5 Schematic drawings showing a tuberosity repair. Six sutures are used, including four horizontal cerclages and two vertical tension band sutures. **A**, Two sutures are placed in the teres minor, two in the infraspinatus, and two in the humeral shaft. **B**, The four horizontal sutures are placed around the prosthetic neck. **C**, The greater tuberosity is primarily fixed with two horizontal cerclage sutures passed medial to the prosthetic neck. The lesser tuberosity is repaired with two additional horizontal cerclage sutures, and two vertical tension band sutures neutralize the construct. **D**, The fracture stem prosthesis with bone graft within the window. **E**, The final construct with the cerclage and tension band sutures tied. (Courtesy of Pascal Boileau, MD, Nice, France.)

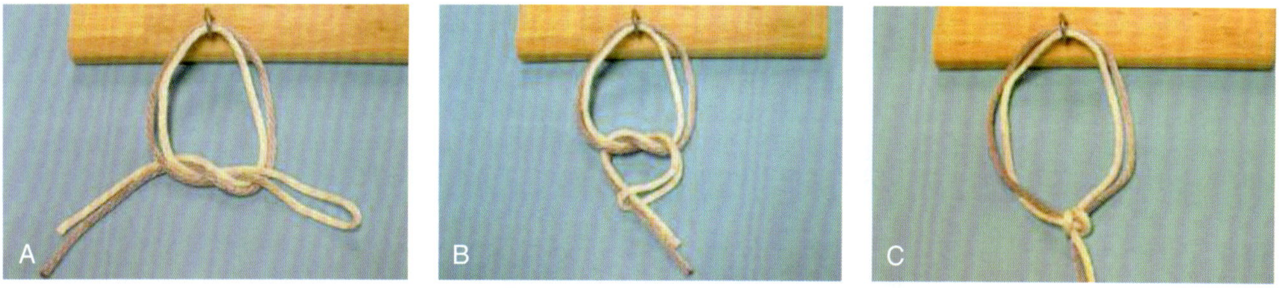

FIGURE 6 Photographs showing the double-suture Nice knot used for the fixation of the tuberosities around the prosthesis with cerclage sutures. A square knot is created (**A**), the two free strands are introduced into the loop (**B**), and the knot is created and tightened by pulling on both strands (**C**). Three half-hitch knots are added to definitively lock the knot. (Courtesy of Pascal Boileau, MD, Nice, France.)

whether the method is to restore the gothic arch between the lateral edge of the scapula and the medial humerus or to measure the distance from the superior edge of the pectoralis major to the superior aspect of the humeral head (mean, 5.5 cm).[35-37] Scaled radiographs of the injured and uninjured arms allow templating of the appropriate humeral height and humeral head size (**Figure 7**). With the help of a jig, it is easy to determine how much of the stem must remain out of the diaphysis to restore anatomic humeral length and, in turn, facilitate tuberosity repair (**Figure 8**). Implant-specific fracture-jigs can also help to restore retroversion, based on alignment with the forearm.

Results

Studies have confirmed a benefit to arthroplasty for traumatic fractures but still find the "satisfactory but imperfect" results noted decades ago.[4,9] A randomized controlled study of patients with a displaced four-part proximal humeral fracture found that patients treated with hemiarthroplasty had a significantly higher quality of life and lower pain scores than those treated nonsurgically.[38] This study underscores the importance of surgical treatment for some patients in preference to so-called "benign neglect." Decreased postoperative pain but imperfect range of motion are common findings in published reports.[39-45] The Norwegian Arthroplasty Register found an 8% revision rate for hemiarthroplasty within the first 10 years, and the rates for relatively young patients were even higher.[46] A nonrandomized study found similar functional results in patients with fracture after osteosynthesis or hemiarthroplasty, despite an older average age in the patients who underwent hemiarthroplasty.[47] Another study found poorer results after hemiarthroplasty than after open reduction and internal fixation.[32] These findings may

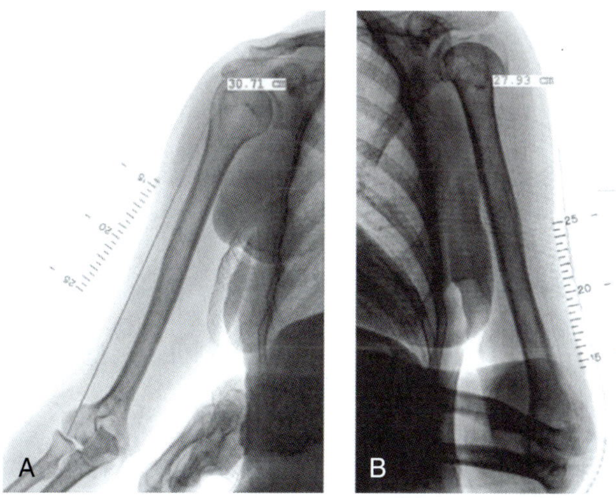

FIGURE 7 A scaled AP radiograph of a patient's uninjured arm (**A**) is used to create a template for the humeral height of the injured arm (**B**). (Courtesy of Pascal Boileau, MD, Nice, France.)

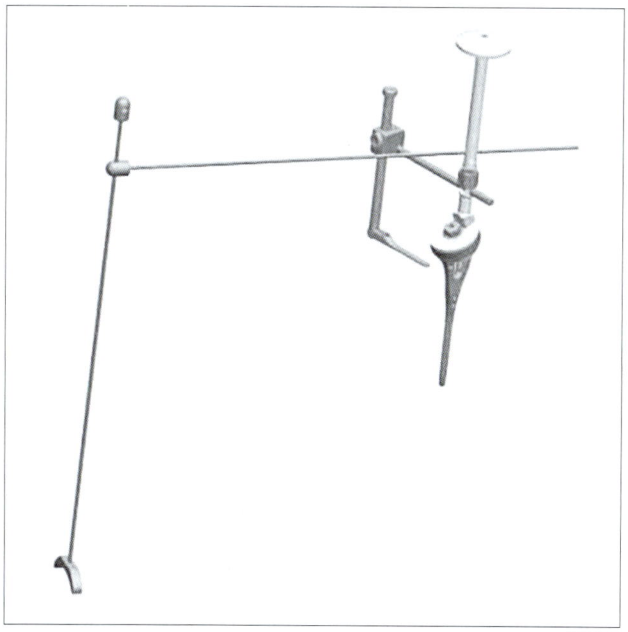

FIGURE 8 Photograph showing the fracture-jig (Tornier), which allows accurate control of the version and the height of the prosthesis during fracture reconstruction. (Courtesy of Pascal Boileau, MD, Nice, France.)

Table 2

Summary of Studies Comparing Reverse Shoulder Arthroplasty to Hemiarthroplasty for Proximal Humerus Fracture

Study (Year)	Number of Patients	Mean Patient Age, in Years	Mean Follow-Up, in Months (Range)	Mean Active External Rotation, in Degrees (±)	Mean Active Forward Elevation, in Degrees (±)	Mean Constant Score, Points (±)	Tuberosity Healing (%)
Baudi et al[48] (2014)	HA: 28 RSA: 25	HA: 71 RSA: 77	27.5 (NR)	HA: 23 (15) RSA: 15 (11)	HA: 89 (44) RSA: 131 (36)	HA: 42.3 (16.6) RSA: 56.2 (14.9)	HA: 37 RSA: 84
Bonnevialle et al[49] (2016)	HA: 57 RSA: 41	HA: 67 RSA: 78	HA: 39 (20-63) RSA: 39 (25-63)	HA: 28 (20) RSA: 23 (20)	HA: 112 (42) RSA: 130 (30)	HA: 54 (17) RSA: 57 (14)	HA: 72 RSA: 73
Sebastiá-Forcada et al[50] (2014)	HA: 31 RSA: 31	HA: 73 RSA: 74	HA: 27.7 (24-44) RSA: 29.4 (24-44)	HA: 3.3/10[a] RSA: 4.7/10[a]	HA: 79.8 RSA: 120.3	HA: 40 RSA: 56.1	HA: 56.7 RSA: 64.5

HA = hemiarthroplasty, RSA = reverse shoulder arthroplasty.
[a]Reported external rotation on a point system from 0 to 10, not degrees.

illustrate the importance of patient selection and surgeon experience in determining results. Despite the imperfect results, hemiarthroplasty has a definite place in the hands of an experienced orthopaedic surgeon.

Reverse shoulder arthroplasty is a newer technique than hemiarthroplasty, and evidence is emerging that supports its superiority to hemiarthroplasty in the context of elderly patients with complex proximal humerus fractures[48-50] (**Table 2**). This trend has also been corroborated in a recent meta-analysis where reverse shoulder arthroplasty outperformed hemiarthroplasty in all evaluated outcomes.[51] Glenoid notching after reverse shoulder arthroplasty for fracture has been a concern potentially lending to increased subjective pain, aseptic component loosening, and potentially revision surgery.[52] However, newer implant designs incorporating a lateralized glenosphere (either through the component itself or by bone grafting) have shown to decrease the incidence of scapular notching.[24] Additionally, the surgeon must be vigilant to implant the glenosphere baseplate at the inferior margin of the glenoid and avoid any superior tilt to the component. **Table 1** summarizes the results of reverse shoulder arthroplasty for the treatment of proximal humeral fractures.

KEY STUDY POINTS

- Arthroplasty options for proximal humerus fractures are favored when poor bone stock and fracture comminution preclude anatomic reconstruction with traditional open reduction and internal fixation techniques in the elderly population (older than70 years)
- Complex proximal humerus fractures should be treated as massive rotator cuff tears and not simply as bony injuries. Implant selection is important as bone grafting and tuberosity fixation options are critical to restoring the patient's ability to regain active external rotation.
- Complications after reverse shoulder arthroplasty for fracture include scapular notching, aseptic loosening, and instability. The rate of these complications can be minimized by a lateralized glenosphere, careful attention to humeral stem height, and anatomic tuberosity fixation.
- Reverse shoulder arthroplasty with preservation of the tuberosities is increasingly performed. Patient-reported outcomes and functional outcomes are beginning to favor reverse arthroplasty over hemiarthroplasty.

SUMMARY

Controversy remains regarding the optimal treatment of proximal humeral fractures. It can be difficult for the surgeon to determine whether a patient is best treated nonsurgically or with open reduction and internal fixation, hemiarthroplasty, or reverse shoulder arthroplasty. There is no consensus among surgeons as to appropriate management.[2] Ongoing investigations will be helpful for determining which fracture patterns may have a poor outcome, but clinical studies are beginning to show a trend that reverse shoulder arthroplasty may be superior to hemiarthroplasty. More importantly, however, is the importance of preservation and anatomic reduction of the greater tuberosity around the selected implant.

Annotated References

1. Baron JA, Barrett JA, Karagas MR: The epidemiology of peripheral fractures. *Bone* 1996;18(3 suppl):S209-S213.

2. Petit CJ, Millett PJ, Endres NK, Diller D, Harris MB, Warner JJ: Management of proximal humeral fractures: Surgeons don't agree. *J Shoulder Elbow Surg* 2010;19(3):446-451.

3. Neer CS, Brown TH Jr, McLaughlin HL: Fracture of the neck of the humerus with dislocation of the head fragment. *Am J Surg* 1953;85(3):252-258.

4. Neer CS II: Displaced proximal humeral fractures: II. Treatment of three-part and four-part displacement. *J Bone Joint Surg Am* 1970;52(6):1090-1103.

5. Boileau P, Krishnan SG, Tinsi L, Walch G, Coste JS, Molé D: Tuberosity malposition and migration: Reasons for poor outcomes after hemiarthroplasty for displaced fractures of the proximal humerus. *J Shoulder Elbow Surg* 2002;11(5):401-412.

6. Boileau P, Sinnerton RJ, Chuinard C, Walch G: Arthroplasty of the shoulder. *J Bone Joint Surg Br* 2006;88(5):562-575.

7. Sirveaux F, Roche O, Molé D: Shoulder arthroplasty for acute proximal humerus fracture. *Orthop Traumatol Surg Res* 2010;96(6):683-694.

8. Codman E: *The Shoulder: Rupture of the Supraspinatus Tendon and Other Lesions in or About the Subacromial Bursa*. Boston, MA, Thomas Todd, 1934.

9. Neer CS II: Displaced proximal humeral fractures: I. Classification and evaluation. *J Bone Joint Surg Am* 1970;52(6):1077-1089.

10. Müller ME: *Manual of Internal Fixation: Techniques Recommended by the AO-ASIF Group*, ed 3. Berlin, Germany, Springer, 1991, pp 118-125.

11. Hertel R, Hempfing A, Stiehler M, Leunig M: Predictors of humeral head ischemia after intracapsular fracture of the proximal humerus. *J Shoulder Elbow Surg* 2004;13(4):427-433.

12. Cadet ER, Ahmad CS: Hemiarthroplasty for three- and four-part proximal humerus fractures. *J Am Acad Orthop Surg* 2012;20(1):17-27.

13. Nho SJ, Brophy RH, Barker JU, Cornell CN, MacGillivray JD: Management of proximal humeral fractures based on current literature. *J Bone Joint Surg Am* 2007;89(suppl 3):44-58.

14. Voos JE, Dines JS, Dines DM: Arthroplasty for fractures of the proximal part of the humerus. *J Bone Joint Surg Am* 2010;92(6):1560-1567.

15. Iannotti JP, Ramsey ML, Williams GR Jr, Warner JJ: Nonprosthetic management of proximal humeral fractures. *Instr Course Lect* 2004;53:403-416.

16. Boileau P, Pennington SD, Alami G: Proximal humeral fractures in younger patients: Fixation techniques and arthroplasty. *J Shoulder Elbow Surg* 2011;20(2 suppl):S47-S60.

17. Sirveaux F, Navez G, Roche O, Mole D, Williams MD: Reverse prosthesis for proximal humerus fracture: Technique and results. *Tech Shoulder Elbow Surg* 2008;9:15-22.

18. Boileau P, Rumian AP, Zumstein MA: Reversed shoulder arthroplasty with modified L'Episcopo for combined loss of active elevation and external rotation. *J Shoulder Elbow Surg* 2010;19(2 suppl):20-30.

19. Simovitch RW, Roche CP, Jones RB, et al: Effect of tuberosity healing on clinical outcomes in elderly patients treated with a reverse shoulder arthroplasty for 3- and 4-part proximal humerus fractures. *J Orthop Trauma* 2019;33(2):e39-e45.

    This is a retrospective, multicenter database cohort study assessing clinical outcomes of greater tuberosity healing in those undergoing reverse shoulder arthroplasty for fracture. Patients with healed greater tuberosities had improved external rotation and ability to perform external rotation-type activities of daily living. Level of evidence: IV.

20. Gallinet D, Clappaz P, Garbuio P, Tropet Y, Obert L: Three or four parts complex proximal humerus fractures: Hemiarthroplasty versus reverse prosthesis. A comparative study of 40 cases. *Orthop Traumatol Surg Res* 2009;95(1):48-55.

21. Boileau P, Alta TJ, Decroocq L, et al: Reverse shoulder arthroplasty for acute fractures in the elderly: Is it worth reattaching the tuberosities? *J Shoulder Elbow Surg* 2019;28:437-444.

    Retrospective analysis of elderly patients who underwent reverse shoulder arthroplasty for three- and four-part proximal humerus fractures with a fracture-specific stem and standardized tuberosity suture fixation technique. A high rate of tuberosity healing was observed, which correlated with higher patient satisfaction and range of motion when compared with those who did not have functional tuberosities. Level of evidence: III.

22. Chun YM, Kim DS, Lee DH, Shin SJ: Reverse shoulder arthroplasty for four-part proximal humerus fracture in elderly patients: Can a healed tuberosity improve the functional outcomes? *J Shoulder Elbow Surg* 2017;26(7):1216-1221.

    This study is a comparison of patients who underwent reverse shoulder arthroplasty for proximal humerus fracture comparing those with healed tuberosities to those without. No difference in functional outcomes or range of motion was detected between the two groups. Level of evidence: III.

23. Formaini NT, Everding NG, Levy JC, Rosas S: Tuberosity healing after reverse shoulder arthroplasty for acute proximal humerus fractures: The "black and tan" technique. *J Shoulder Elbow Surg* 2015;24(11):e299-e306.

    This study reports on radiographic and clinical outcomes of those undergoing reverse shoulder arthroplasty for proximal humerus fracture using a hybrid cementation-impaction bone grafting technique. Patients showed a high tuberosity healing rate with restored external rotation. Level of evidence: IV.

24. Gallinet D, Cazeneuve JF, Boyer E, et al: Reverse shoulder arthroplasty for recent proximal humerus fractures: Outcomes in 422 cases. *Orthop Traumatol Surg Res* 2019;105(5):805-811.

    This is a retrospective, multicenter analysis of short- and long-term outcomes of reverse shoulder arthroplasty for proximal humerus fractures. Tuberosity fixation and healing was associated with improved patient-reported outcomes, range of motion, and fewer complications. Level of evidence: IV.

25. Reuther F, Petermann M, Stangl R: Reverse shoulder arthroplasty in acute fractures of the proximal humerus: Does tuberosity healing improve clinical outcomes? *J Orthop Trauma* 2019;33(2):e46-e51.

    This study reported functional outcomes of those patients who underwent reverse shoulder arthroplasty for proximal humerus fracture. Patients were separated into three groups based on tuberosity healing: healed, partially healed, and unhealed. No differences were detected between groups. Level of evidence: IV.

26. Torrens C, Alentorn-Geli E, Mingo F, Gamba C, Santana F: Reverse shoulder arthroplasty for the treatment of acute complex proximal humeral fractures: Influence of greater tuberosity healing on the functional outcomes. *J Orthop Surg (Hong Kong)* 2018;26(1):2309499018760132.

This study is an assessment of greater tuberosity healing on outcomes after reverse shoulder arthroplasty for proximal humerus fracture. No correlation between greater tuberosity healing and functional outcome was detected. Importantly, patient medical comorbidities were assessed with tuberosity healing and not age, or gender. Level of evidence: IV.

27. Kralinger F, Schwaiger R, Wambacher M, et al: Outcome after primary hemiarthroplasty for fracture of the head of the humerus: A retrospective multicentre study of 167 patients. *J Bone Joint Surg Br* 2004;86(2):217-219.

28. Loew M, Heitkemper S, Parsch D, Schneider S, Rickert M: Influence of the design of the prosthesis on the outcome after hemiarthroplasty of the shoulder in displaced fractures of the head of the humerus. *J Bone Joint Surg Br* 2006;88(3):345-350.

29. Boileau P, Winter M, Cikes A, et al: Can surgeons predict what makes a good hemiarthroplasty for fracture? in Boileau P, ed: *Shoulder Concepts 2012: Arthroscopy, Arthroplasty, and Fractures*. Paris, France, Sauramps Medical, 2012, pp 329-344.

30. Alta T, Decroocq L, Moineau G, et al: Paper No. OP16. *Reverse shoulder arthroplasty for the treatment of proximal humeral fractures in the elderly: Results with a minimum one-year follow-up. 24th Congress Scientific Program*. Saint Genis Laval, France. European Society for Surgery of the Shoulder and the Elbow, 2012, Available at: http://secec.com. Accessed September 10, 2012.

31. Mighell MA, Kolm GP, Collinge CA, Frankle MA: Outcomes of hemiarthroplasty for fractures of the proximal humerus. *J Shoulder Elbow Surg* 2003;12(6):569-577.

32. Solberg BD, Moon CN, Franco DP, Paiement GD: Surgical treatment of three and four-part proximal humeral fractures. *J Bone Joint Surg Am* 2009;91(7):1689-1697.

33. Boileau P, Walch G, Krishnan SG: Tuberosity osteosynthesis and hemiarthroplasty for four-part fractures of the proximal humerus. *Tech Shoulder Elbow Surg* 2000;1:96-109.

34. Boileau P, Rumian AP: A non-slipping and secure fixation of bone fragments and soft tissues useable in open and arthroscopic surgery, in Boileau P, ed: *Shoulder Concepts 2010: Arthroscopy and Arthroplasty*. Paris, France, Sauramps Medical, 2010, pp 245-251.

35. Krishnan SG, Bennion PW, Reineck JR, Burkhead WZ: Hemiarthroplasty for proximal humeral fracture: Restoration of the Gothic arch. *Orthop Clin North Am* 2008;39(4):441-450, vi.

36. Murachovsky J, Ikemoto RY, Nascimento LG, Fujiki EN, Milani C, Warner JJ: Pectoralis major tendon reference (PMT): A new method for accurate restoration of humeral length with hemiarthroplasty for fracture. *J Shoulder Elbow Surg* 2006;15(6):675-678.

37. Torrens C, Corrales M, Melendo E, Solano A, Rodríguez-Baeza A, Cáceres E: The pectoralis major tendon as a reference for restoring humeral length and retroversion with hemiarthroplasty for fracture. *J Shoulder Elbow Surg* 2008;17(6):947-950.

38. Olerud P, Ahrengart L, Ponzer S, Saving J, Tidermark J: Hemiarthroplasty versus nonoperative treatment of displaced 4-part proximal humeral fractures in elderly patients: A randomized controlled trial. *J Shoulder Elbow Surg* 2011;20(7):1025-1033.

39. Kontakis G, Koutras C, Tosounidis T, Giannoudis P: Early management of proximal humeral fractures with hemiarthroplasty: A systematic review. *J Bone Joint Surg Br* 2008;90(11):1407-1413.

40. Grönhagen CM, Abbaszadegan H, Révay SA, Adolphson PY: Medium-term results after primary hemiarthroplasty for comminute proximal humerus fractures: A study of 46 patients followed up for an average of 4.4 years. *J Shoulder Elbow Surg* 2007;16(6):766-773.

41. Antuña SA, Sperling JW, Cofield RH: Shoulder hemiarthroplasty for acute fractures of the proximal humerus: A minimum five-year follow-up. *J Shoulder Elbow Surg* 2008;17(2):202-209.

42. Fallatah S, Dervin GF, Brunet JA, Conway AF, Hrushowy H: Functional outcome after proximal humeral fractures treated with hemiarthroplasty. *Can J Surg* 2008;51(5):361-365.

43. Greiner SH, Kääb MJ, Kröning I, Scheibel M, Perka C: Reconstruction of humeral length and centering of the prosthetic head in hemiarthroplasty for proximal humeral fractures. *J Shoulder Elbow Surg* 2008;17(5):709-714.

44. Padua R, Bondì R, Ceccarelli E, Campi A, Padua L: Health-related quality of life and subjective outcome after shoulder replacement for proximal humeral fractures. *J Shoulder Elbow Surg* 2008;17(2):261-264.

45. Pavlopoulos DA, Badras LS, Georgiou CS, Skretas EF, Malizos KN: Hemiarthroplasty for three- and four-part displaced fractures of the proximal humerus in patients over 65 years of age. *Acta Orthop Belg* 2007;73(3):306-314.

46. Fevang BT, Lie SA, Havelin LI, Skredderstuen A, Furnes O: Risk factors for revision after shoulder arthroplasty: 1,825 shoulder arthroplasties from the Norwegian Arthroplasty Register. *Acta Orthop* 2009;80(1):83-91.

47. Bastian JD, Hertel R: Osteosynthesis and hemiarthroplasty of fractures of the proximal humerus: Outcomes in a consecutive case series. *J Shoulder Elbow Surg* 2009;18(2):216-219.

48. Baudi P, Campochiaro G, Serafini F, et al: Hemiarthroplasty versus reverse shoulder arthroplasty: Comparative study of functional and radiological outcomes in the treatment of acute proximal humerus fracture. *Musculoskelet Surg* 2014;98(suppl 1):19-25.

This study is a comparison of hemiarthroplasty against reverse shoulder arthroplasty for proximal humerus fracture with minimum 2-year follow-up. All patients underwent tuberosity fixation. Patients undergoing reverse shoulder arthroplasty showed improved functional outcomes and range of motion with an increased rate of tuberosity healing. Level of evidence: IV.

49. Bonnevialle N, Tournier C, Clavert P, et al: Hemiarthroplasty versus reverse shoulder arthroplasty in 4-part displaced fractures of the proximal humerus: Multicenter retrospective study. *Orthop Traumatol Surg Res* 2016;102(5):569-573.

    This study includes the short- and intermediate-term results comparing hemiarthroplasty to reverse shoulder arthroplasty for four-part proximal humerus fracture. The reverse shoulder arthroplasty group showed superior functional outcomes and fewer complications than the hemiarthroplasty group. A high rate of scapular notching was observed in the reverse shoulder arthroplasty group. Level of evidence: IV.

50. Sebastiá-Forcada E, Cebrian-Gomez R, Lizaur-Utrilla A, Gil-Guillen V: Reverse shoulder arthroplasty versus hemiarthroplasty for acute proximal humeral fractures. A blinded, randomized, controlled, prospective study. *J Shoulder Elbow Surg* 2014;23(10):1419-1426.

    This study is a randomized controlled trial comparing functional outcomes and range of motion of reverse shoulder arthroplasty versus hemiarthroplasty in the setting of proximal humerus fracture in those older than 70 years. Reverse shoulder arthroplasty showed superior functional outcomes and a lower revision rate. Patients with failed tuberosity healing had inferior outcomes irrespective of the prosthesis implanted. Level of evidence: I.

51. Austin DC, Torchia MT, Cozzolino NH, Jacobowitz LE, Bell JE: Decreased reoperations and improved outcomes with reverse total shoulder arthroplasty in comparison to hemiarthroplasty for geriatric proximal humerus fractures: A systematic review and meta-analysis. *J Orthop Trauma* 2019;33(1):49-57.

    This study is a meta-analysis of 15 studies comparing reverse shoulder arthroplasty to hemiarthroplasty for proximal humerus fractures. Reverse shoulder arthroplasty showed superior functional outcomes, range of motion, and revision surgery rate when compared with hemiarthroplasty. Level of evidence: III.

52. Cazeneuve JF, Cristofari DJ: Delta III reverse shoulder arthroplasty: Radiological outcome for acute complex fractures of the proximal humerus in elderly patients. *Orthop Traumatol Surg Res* 2009;95(5):325-329.

Chapter 25

Arthroplasty for Sequelae of Proximal Humeral Fractures

Armodios M. Hatzidakis, MD • Benjamin W. Sears, MD

ABSTRACT

Although most proximal humerus fractures can be successfully managed nonsurgically, a subset of patients will develop functional limitations and pain secondary to malunion, nonunion, osteonecrosis, instability, and secondary arthritis as a result of the fracture. Most of these patients can be successfully managed with prosthetic replacement. In general, the need for greater tuberosity osteotomy during subsequent arthroplasty intervention influences the most appropriate arthroplasty choice as patients who require arthroplasty with greater tuberosity osteotomy generally have worse functional outcomes than patients in whom a more normal greater tuberosity-humeral head relationship can be restored without osteotomy. Patients with humeral head impaction or necrosis (type I), or chronic dislocation (type II) typically do not require greater tuberosity osteotomy and can typically be successfully treated with an anatomic arthroplasty. Patients with proximal humeral nonunion (type III) can be treated with bone graft and internal fixation or reverse shoulder arthroplasty. Patients with severe anatomic distortion and tuberosity malunion (type IV) or irreparable rotator cuff deficiency are most reliably treated with reverse shoulder arthroplasty.

Keywords: arthroplasty; malunion; nonunion; proximal humerus fracture; sequelae

Dr. Hatzidakis or an immediate family member has received royalties from Wright Medical Technology, Inc; has made paid presentations on behalf of Wright Medical Technology, Inc; serves as a paid consultant to or is an employee of Medtronic and Wright Medical Technology, Inc; has stock or stock options held in Tornier; has received research or institutional support from Arthrex, Inc, Exactech, Inc, and Wright Medical Technology, Inc; and serves as a board member, owner, officer, or committee member of the American Shoulder and Elbow Surgeons. Dr. Sears or an immediate family member has received royalties from United Orthopedic Corporation; serves as a paid consultant to or is an employee of United Orthopedic Corporation; and has received research or institutional support from Arthrex, Inc and Tornier.

Introduction

Proximal humeral fractures are relatively common, accounting for approximately 185,000 emergency department visits annually in the United States.[1] Although most of these fractures are successfully treated nonsurgically, significant functional impairment can occur in the presence of osseous deformity, nonunion, or osteonecrosis and collapse resulting from the injury.[2-4] The delayed complications of proximal humeral fractures range from isolated tuberosity malunion or nonunion, which often can be managed with arthroscopic or open reduction and internal fixation, to a complex articular surface incongruency, which often leads to destruction of the articular surface and early-onset arthritis.[4,5] In patients with significant deformity of the proximal humeral anatomy or articular surface destruction, prosthetic arthroplasty may be the only reliable means of restoring a functional joint and providing pain relief.

Prosthetic arthroplasty for the management of the sequelae of proximal humeral fractures can be challenging because of injury complexity, rotator cuff insufficiency, bone loss, scarring, and distortion of the osseous anatomy. The decisions related to arthroplasty are even more challenging because patients with symptomatic proximal humeral fracture sequelae often are relatively young and active. Surgical treatment of such a patient can be difficult and has a less predictable outcome than for a patient with primary osteoarthritis.[3,6]

Fracture Sequelae Classification

The Boileau classification of proximal humeral fracture sequelae is based on a radiographic evaluation of 71 patients treated with nonconstrained (anatomic) arthroplasty.[2] The delayed fracture complications are classified into four types (**Figure 1**). Type I refers to a fracture sequela associated with impaction and humeral head collapse or necrosis, and type II refers to locked anterior or posterior proximal humeral dislocation or fracture-dislocation. Types I and II are categorized as intracapsular and have predictably good results after nonconstrained arthroplasty as long as glenoid bone stock is maintained. Fractures that proceed to surgical neck nonunion are type III, and those with a severe tuberosity malunion and gross proximal humeral deformity are type IV. Types III and IV are categorized as extracapsular and have less predictable outcomes after anatomic arthroplasty. An assessment of the need for greater tuberosity osteotomy or fixation during arthroplasty is a critical component of the classification system. Greater tuberosity nonunion or associated greater tuberosity osteotomy is consistently associated with poor results after nonconstrained shoulder arthroplasty, with the incidence of nonunited tuberosity osteotomy with anatomic shoulder arthroplasty at final follow-up reported at 36%.[2-4,7-9]

The Boileau classification is useful for surgical planning. Intracapsular sequelae (types I and II) are associated with minimal distortion of the proximal humeral anatomy and maintenance of the tuberosity-diaphysis continuity. Predictable, satisfactory results can generally be achieved with nonconstrained arthroplasty without tuberosity osteotomy (**Figure 2**). In these patients, a near-anatomic relationship of the greater tuberosity to the humeral head can be restored without the need for osteotomy. Using a modular and adaptable humeral prosthesis facilitates the restoration of this relationship. Using a convertible stem design may be advantageous for patients who may be a risk for possible conversion to a reverse arthroplasty in the future.

Extracapsular sequelae (types III and IV) are associated with severe distortion of proximal humeral anatomy and/or a disruption of the tuberosity-diaphysis continuity. In these patients, an unconstrained prosthesis has less predictable long-term results, primarily because of the difficulty or the impossibility of achieving greater tuberosity healing in a near-anatomic position with respect to the humeral prosthesis. Therefore, primary fixation with bone graft (for a type III nonunion) or a semiconstrained (reverse) prosthesis should be considered.

Indications and Contraindications to Arthroplasty

Prosthetic shoulder arthroplasty should be considered for a patient with symptomatic fracture sequelae, pain, and loss of function. The contraindications for arthroplasty include presence of an active infection, a severe neurologic injury, a comorbidity precluding a surgical procedure, or extremely poor bone quality or bony defects preventing adequate prosthetic fixation. The options include using an unconstrained shoulder prosthesis (hemiarthroplasty, humeral head resurfacing, and total shoulder arthroplasty) and the use of a semiconstrained prosthesis (reverse total shoulder arthroplasty).

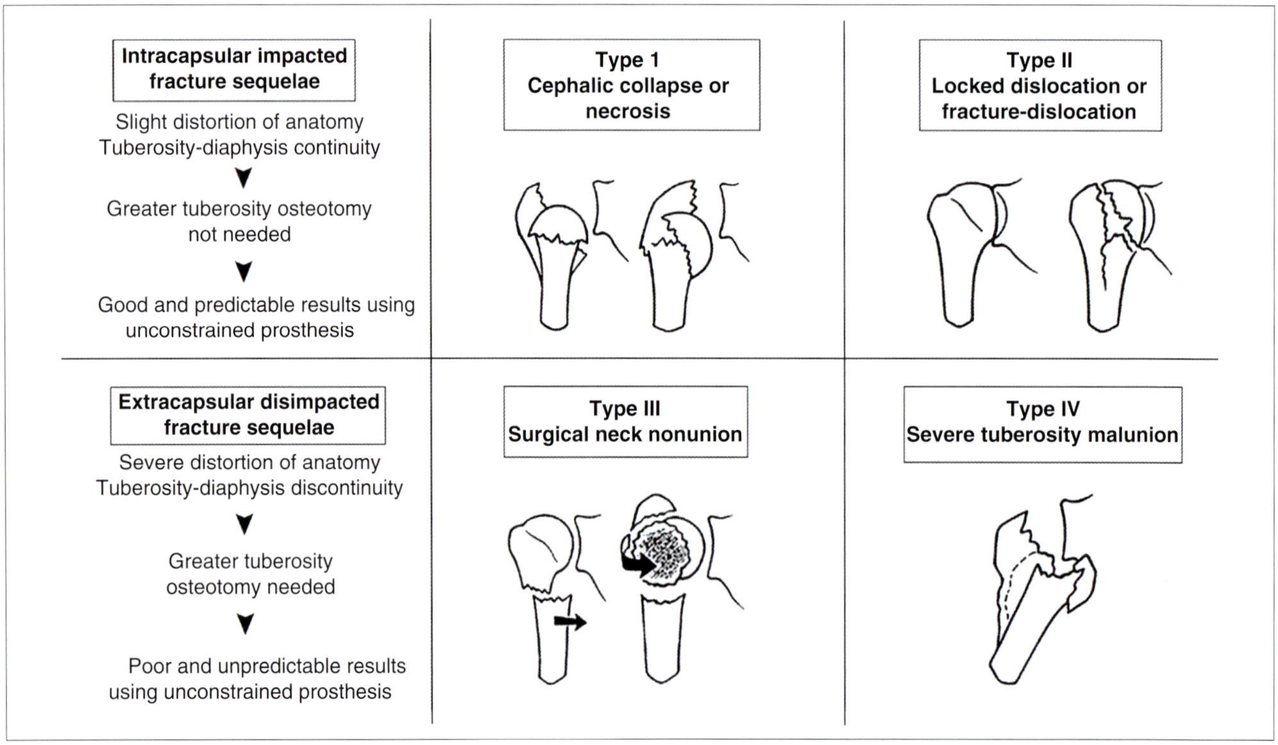

FIGURE 1 Illustration showing the Boileau classification of proximal humeral fracture sequelae. (Adapted with permission from Boileau P, Chuinard C, Le Huec JC, Walch G, Trojani C: Proximal humerus fracture sequelae: Impact of a new radiographic classification on arthroplasty. *Clin Orthop Relat Res* 2006;442:121-130. doi:10.1097/01.blo.0000195679.87258.6e.)

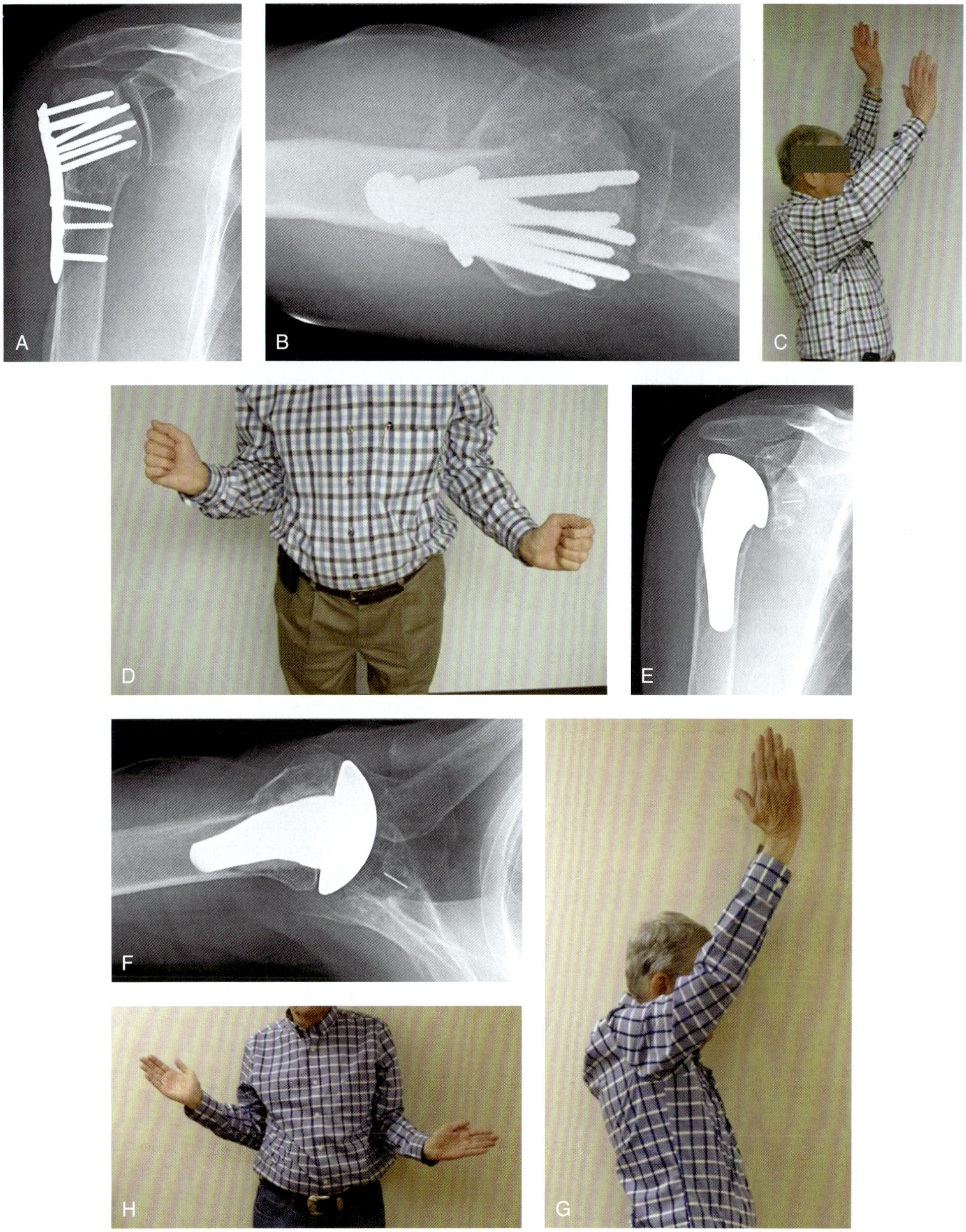

FIGURE 2 A 74-year-old male developed osteonecrosis and humeral head collapse (type I sequalae) 20 months after plate fixation of a proximal humeral fracture. Radiographs demonstrate osteonecrosis, humeral head collapse, and intra-articular screws penetration (**A** and **B**). Photographs demonstrating preoperative active forward flexion (**C**) and active external rotation (**D**). After revision to an anatomic total shoulder arthroplasty, the patient had excellent function at 5-year follow-up. AP (**E**) and axillary (**F**) radiographs as well as photographs demonstrating active forward flexion (**G**) and external rotation (**H**).

Hemiarthroplasty, Total Shoulder Arthroplasty, and Humeral Head Resurfacing

Hemiarthroplasty remains the treatment of choice if the fracture sequela involves minor tuberosity malunion or nonunion and the deformity of proximal humeral anatomy is minimal with no glenoid wear, as seen in type I or II fractures and some type III sequelae.[3,4] Advancements in prosthesis design (such as stemless, modularity, and head eccentricity with stemmed devices) have improved the ability of the implant to adapt to altered osseous anatomy. Total shoulder arthroplasty often is unnecessary because the patient has minimal arthritic changes to the glenoid, even if there are significant degenerative changes to the humeral head. However, degenerative changes in the glenoid are best seen at the time of surgery, and in these situations, resurfacing of the glenoid may result in the most predictable pain relief, return to function, and avoidance of revision.

Anatomic prostheses include those with a humeral stem, stemless implants, and resurfacing prostheses. Although stemmed implants have traditionally been preferred, their adaptability is limited by the intramedullary component. A stemless implant or resurfacing prosthesis is not constrained by the required connection to the humeral shaft, and this characteristic allows for increased adaptability in severe malunion, especially in relation to the neck-shaft angle. Good outcomes based on Constant shoulder scores were reported in 28 patients undergoing resurfacing arthroplasty for type I or II proximal humeral fracture sequelae, with only one reported complication.[10] Resurfacing arthroplasty was found to be a viable prosthetic option for patients with posttraumatic osteoarthritis, provided the patient had adequate bone stock and relative preservation of humeral head sphericity.[10] In patients with humeral head collapse or severely distorted anatomy, the use of stemless implants provides for more predicable implant osseous fixation than resurfacing arthroplasty.

Reverse Shoulder Arthroplasty

Reverse shoulder arthroplasty is most commonly used to treat fracture sequelae in lower demand patients with severe tuberosity malunion, nonunion, and/or rotator cuff deficiency.[11,12] Reverse shoulder arthroplasty greatly reduces the reliance on tuberosity positioning or rotator cuff function for glenohumeral motor power and stability, and it is the treatment of choice for patients who have low physical demands, severe tuberosity malunion, distortion of the proximal humeral anatomy (type IV sequelae), or sequelae with concurrent rotator cuff deficiency.[3,11,13] Reverse shoulder arthroplasty has resulted in good pain relief and postoperative elevation in patients older than 70 years who have intracapsular (type I or II) sequelae[4,13,14] (**Figure 3**). Reverse arthroplasty also can be used as a salvage procedure after failed hemiarthroplasty to treat fracture sequelae and should be considered as a primary treatment option in patients who have type I sequelae with a poor-quality or an irreparable rotator cuff. Patients with chronic anterior instability who undergo reverse arthroplasty have been shown to experience improved joint stability.[11] Additionally, several studies have reported good outcomes for use of reverse arthroplasty in patients with proximal humeral nonunion (type III sequela)[15-17] (**Figure 4**). The authors of a 2016 study[18] found the rate of osteoarthritis or rheumatoid arthritis is nearly doubled in patients with proximal humerus nonunion, with reverse arthroplasty being an obvious treatment for this condition. Relative contraindications for reverse arthroplasty include patient age and level of function and should be used cautiously for younger patients younger, regardless of the type of proximal humeral fracture sequelae; however, reverse arthroplasty may be the only treatment option for many patients with severe tuberosity nonunion, malunion, or a chronic locked dislocation and associated glenoid or humeral bone loss.[19]

Results

Several studies specifically examined the treatment of patients with chronic dislocation (type II sequela) using an anatomic prosthesis. A retrospective review of 11 patients with fixed anterior glenohumeral dislocation treated with a nonconstrained arthroplasty reported significant improvement in pain and function scores.[20] However, four patients (36%) had postoperative anterior instability, and definite radiographic loosening of the glenoid component developed in two of these four patients. Another study found that pain and function significantly improved in 12 patients with chronic posterior glenohumeral dislocation treated with nonconstrained shoulder arthroplasty; however, three patients (25%) required revision surgery for instability or component loosening.[21] Ultimately, anatomic shoulder arthroplasty for patients with a fixed shoulder dislocation reliably reduces pain and improves shoulder function but may be associated with residual instability and component loosening. The outcomes of anatomic arthroplasty for chronic posterior glenohumeral dislocation generally are better than the outcomes of arthroplasty for anterior dislocation.

In another study, 55 patients with proximal humeral sequelae underwent arthroplasty with an anatomic prosthesis for type I or II sequelae or reverse total shoulder arthroplasty for type III or IV sequelae.[15] The 36 patients with the anatomic prosthesis were followed for an average of 24 months, and the 19 patients with a reverse prosthesis were followed for an average of 19.3 months. Patients in both groups had significant postoperative

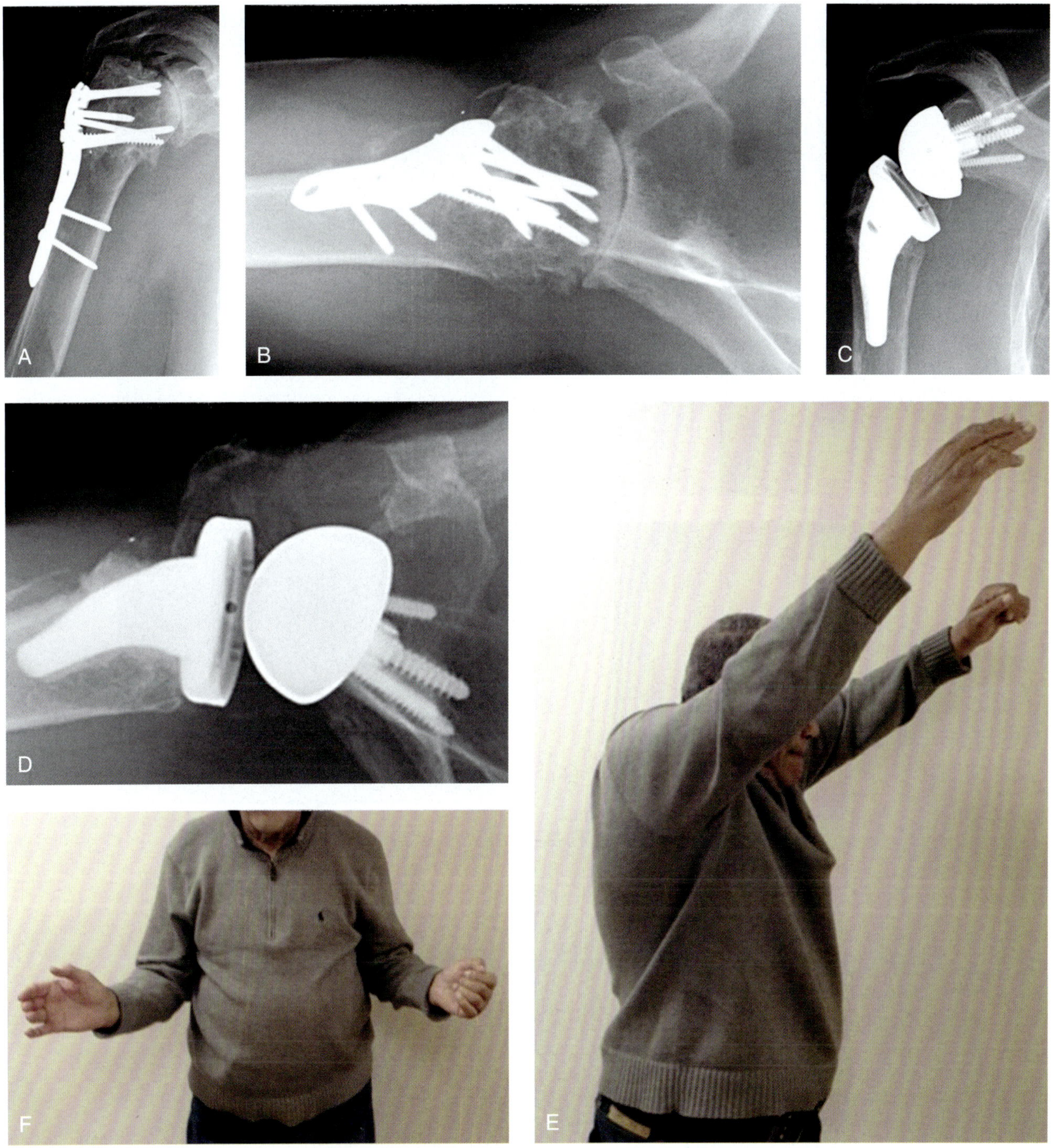

FIGURE 3 A 72-year-old underwent reverse total shoulder arthroplasty for severe glenohumeral osteoarthritis 4 years after plate fixation of a proximal humerus fracture (**A** and **B**). AP and axillary radiographs 1 year following reverse arthroplasty (**C** and **D**); photographs demonstrating active forward flexion and external rotation (**E** and **F**).

improvement in pain and function, although the extent of improvement relative to sequelae type was not reported. The mean Constant score increased from 19 to 68 points in patients with an anatomic prosthesis and from 9 to 47.5 points in patients with a reverse prosthesis.

The indications for reverse shoulder arthroplasty have broadened substantially. Although this procedure primarily is reserved for patients with low demands, its use as a salvage procedure in patients with fracture sequelae has allowed for the management of previously

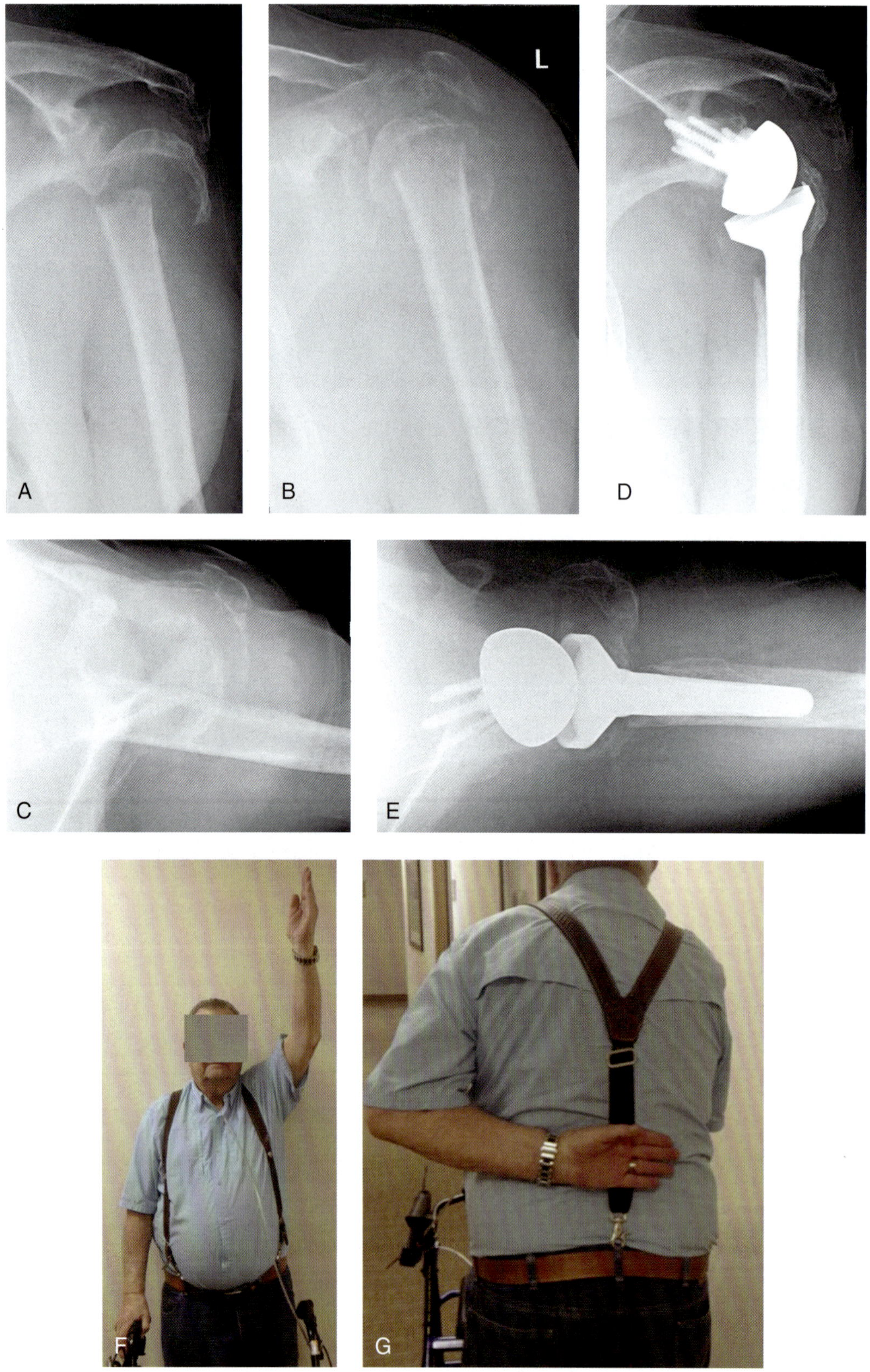

FIGURE 4 In a 77-year-old male with persistent nonunion of the tuberosities and surgical neck following an attempt (10 months) at conservative care for a proximal humerus fracture, radiographs demonstrate significant humeral head bone loss, as well as tuberosity and surgical neck nonunion with minimal to no glenoid bone loss (**A** through **C**). A reverse shoulder arthroplasty was performed. In the 1-year radiographs, the greater tuberosity was united to the reconstruction prosthesis (**D** and **E**). Photograph showing that the patient was able to achieve good active postoperative range of motion (1-year postoperative) (**F** and **G**).

untreatable glenohumeral disorders. Several studies have examined the role of reverse arthroplasty in proximal humeral fracture sequelae. The authors of a 2016 study reported on 32 patients with proximal humerus nonunion treated with reverse shoulder arthroplasty. They reported that reverse shoulder arthroplasty was an acceptable treatment for nonunion with significant improvements in Constant score and range of motion; however, 34% of patients had a postoperative dislocation that was associated with intraoperative resection of the tuberosities.[13] The authors of a 2012 study also reported significant improvement in motion, including rotation, as well as subjective shoulder scores in 18 patients with proximal humerus nonunion treated with reverse arthroplasty; however, five patients had postoperative complications, including prosthetic dislocation require revision in two patients. The researchers concluded that reverse arthroplasty improves function in patients with symptomatic proximal humeral nonunion that is not amenable to anatomic arthroplasty, albeit with a high complication rate.[16] In another study, 16 patients with proximal humeral malunion were treated with reverse shoulder arthroplasty for severe pain or functional limitations, without an osteotomy of the malunited tuberosities or remaining proximal humerus.[22] At 2-year follow-up, pain and function scores (including rotation) improved significantly on the American Shoulder and Elbow Surgeons score, the visual analog pain scale, and the Simple Shoulder Test, with no major complications. The researchers concluded that reverse arthroplasty for severe proximal humeral malunion yields satisfactory outcomes. The authors of the aforementioned 2016 study also reported significant improvement in Constant score and motion in 42 patients treated with reverse arthroplasty for type IV proximal humeral malunion with relatively low incidence of complications (9.5% complication rate) and a good or very good subjective rating postoperatively of 88%.[13]

Technical Considerations

Placement of Humeral Prosthesis Without Greater Tuberosity Osteotomy

If the proximal humerus is amenable to prosthesis placement without a tuberosity osteotomy (as in types I and II sequelae), the glenohumeral joint is exposed using a deltopectoral approach. Although it is important to maintain the healed position of the greater tuberosity if possible, a lesser tuberosity osteotomy can be performed to gain access to the joint and manage the subscapularis.[22] The subacromial, subdeltoid, and subcoracoid spaces should be cleared of scar tissue and mobilized to allow maximal exposure of the glenohumeral joint.

When access has been gained, the humeral head, rotator cuff, and glenoid surfaces are assessed. A humeral head cut should be planned with the goal of restoring natural glenohumeral anatomy (with the superior aspect of the implant resting 3 to 5 mm above the greater tuberosity), while preserving tuberosity integrity. In some patients with advanced necrosis (type I sequelae), the humeral head may be collapsed to the point that no cut is required. If a stemmed implant is selected, the stem should be thin and the implant should be impaction bone grafted or cemented to allow an increased offset when necessary. A stemless implant or resurfacing arthroplasty can be used to avoid humeral stem placement if a severe distortion of the neck-shaft angle is encountered.

Osteotomy of a Greater Tuberosity Malunion

Although arthroplasty of a greater tuberosity malunion has been shown to have significantly worse results with osteotomy than without osteotomy, the options for maintaining tuberosity integrity sometimes are limited because of tuberosity displacement, patient age, level of function, or the extent of degenerative changes.[3,4,7,8] The relative indications for tuberosity osteotomy include more than 1 cm of posterior displacement or an inability to adequately place the prosthesis because of altered anatomy.[23] Anatomic reconstruction with more relatively severe greater tuberosity malunion may result in less predictable return of shoulder function.

When a greater tuberosity osteotomy is required, the osteotomy should be made obliquely to allow as much contact area as possible for subsequent union. The insertion of the rotator cuff on the tuberosity should be protected, and the rotator cuff should be mobilized to optimize excursion. If possible, the distal periosteal connection to the tuberosity should be elevated but not severed, so the soft-tissue attachment and the blood supply to the osseous fragment are maintained. After prosthetic placement, bone graft from the humeral head should be placed along the proximal aspect of the implant and the tuberosity undersurface to augment healing. Finally, the tuberosities are secured around the implant using heavy, nonabsorbable cerclage sutures. Depending on the intraoperative range of motion, a limited program of passive shoulder range of motion can be initiated for the first 6 weeks after surgery to minimize stiffness and optimize healing of the greater tuberosity and subscapularis.

Arthroplasty for Proximal Humeral Nonunion

Open reduction and internal fixation, with or without bone grafting, is the first-line treatment of type III sequelae without advanced degenerative change. In patients with advanced arthritis or limited healing capability (poor bone quality or cavitation of the humeral head), humeral head replacement with an anatomic or a reverse prosthesis may provide the most optimal outcome[3,15,16] (**Figure 5**). Regardless of the type of prosthesis (anatomic or reverse), fixation and healing of the tuberosities to the humeral implant are critical for function, including active rotation after reverse arthroplasty.

A deltopectoral approach typically is used. The long head of the biceps tendon can be used as a guide to the rotator cuff interval. If possible, the lesser tuberosity should be left in continuity with the greater tuberosity, and the subscapularis is mobilized using a peel-down or a tenotomy to gain access to the joint. The humeral head cut should be made with great caution to preserve the viability of the greater tuberosity. After shaft preparation, the final humeral stem is skewered through the ring-shaped greater and lesser tuberosity fragment and cemented in the humeral diaphysis. The proximal fragment is grafted to the humeral shaft and the implant, and

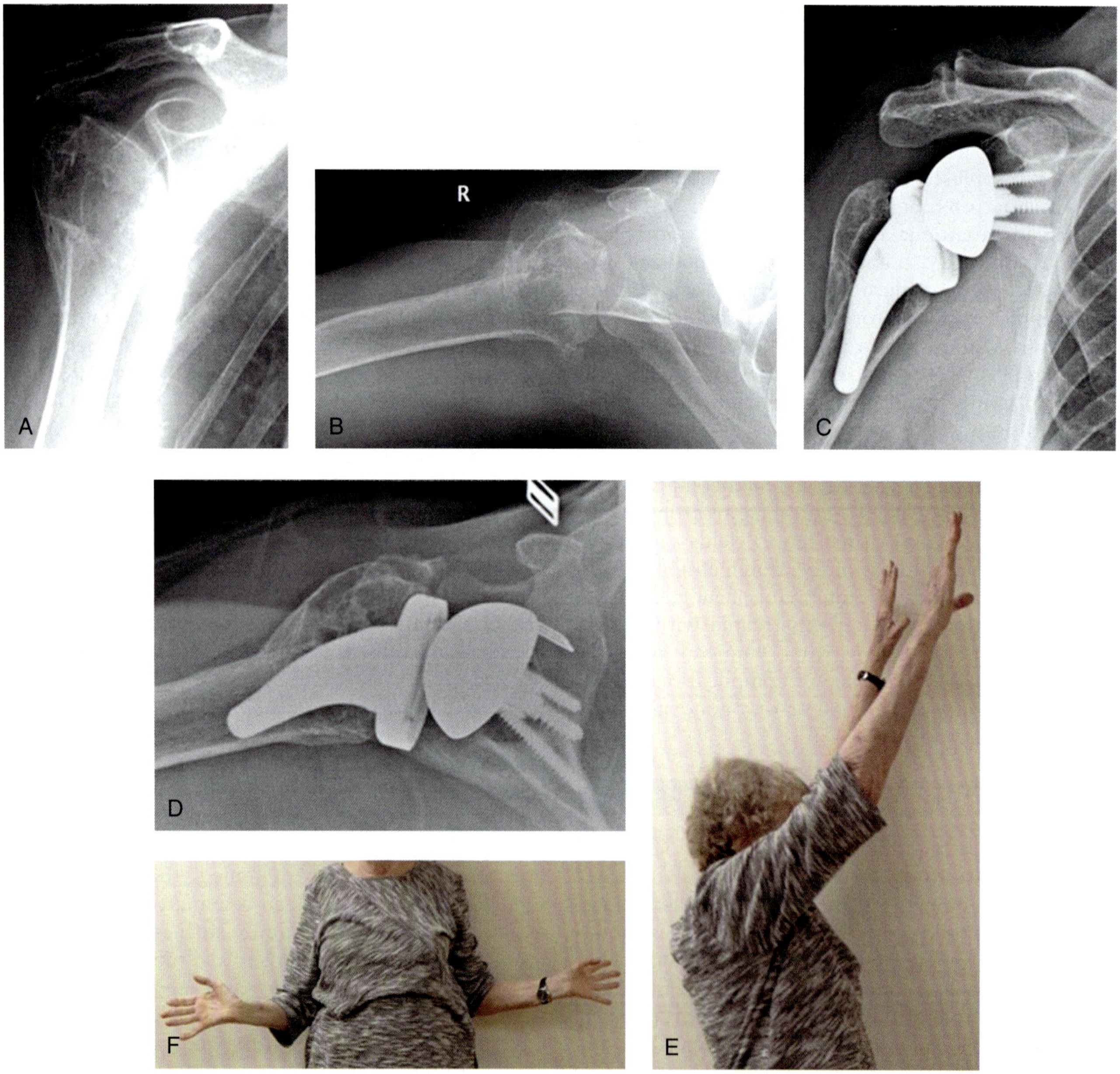

FIGURE 5 In a 77-year-old presented with greater tuberosity and surgical neck nonunion after 12 months of conservative management of a proximal humerus fracture, radiographs show nonunion and flattening of the humeral head (**A** and **B**). AP and axillary radiographs showing that she underwent a reverse arthroplasty (**C** and **D**). Photographs demonstrate that she has near full range of motion at 2 years postoperatively (**E** and **F**).

the subscapularis is repaired. Depending on the intraoperative range of motion, a limited program of passive shoulder range of motion can be initiated for the first 6 weeks after surgery.

Management of Chronic Locked Dislocations

Prosthetic replacement may be required for a patient who has a chronic glenohumeral dislocation (type II sequela) extending beyond 6 months after the index injury or involving a humeral defect of more than 40% of the articular surface.[22,24] For a posteriorly directed chronic dislocation with sufficient preserved glenoid bone, humeral arthroplasty is the treatment of choice. Posterior capsular plication can be considered if the posterior capsule is excessively patulous and stability is not achieved by restoring the architecture of the humeral head alone.

Patients with an anterior fracture-dislocation are at increased risk for instability compared with those with a posteriorly directed dislocation.[16] Bone graft may be necessary to augment a glenoid deficiency if the humerus is unstable or if the glenoid component is unsupported. The options for glenoid bone augmentation include using an osteotomized humeral head, an iliac crest autograft, coracoid transfer, or a distal tibial allograft. If there is concern for stability or if the rotator cuff is irreparable, reverse arthroplasty may be considered.

Future Directions

The indications and the techniques for treating proximal humeral fracture sequelae with anatomic or reverse shoulder arthroplasty continue to be advanced and refined. Healing of the greater tuberosity continues to be a critical factor in determining functional results after anatomic or reverse shoulder arthroplasty for treating an acute fracture or fracture sequelae. Evolving stemless designs allow for greater flexibility with implant insertion. Fracture stem designs for anatomic and reverse prostheses may improve the healing of the greater tuberosity with acute fractures and sequelae.[25]

Greater tuberosity osteotomy for proximal humeral malunion with reference to anatomic arthroplasty has been discussed in detail in the current literature.[9,10,15] Greater tuberosity osteotomy also may be required in reverse arthroplasty for proximal humeral malunion. The greater tuberosity often is displaced superiorly, laterally, and posteriorly in relation to the humeral shaft. Placement of a reverse humeral stem without greater tuberosity osteotomy sometimes leads to impingement of the malunited greater tuberosity with the acromion in abduction or with the acromion and/or the glenoid in external rotation. The impingement

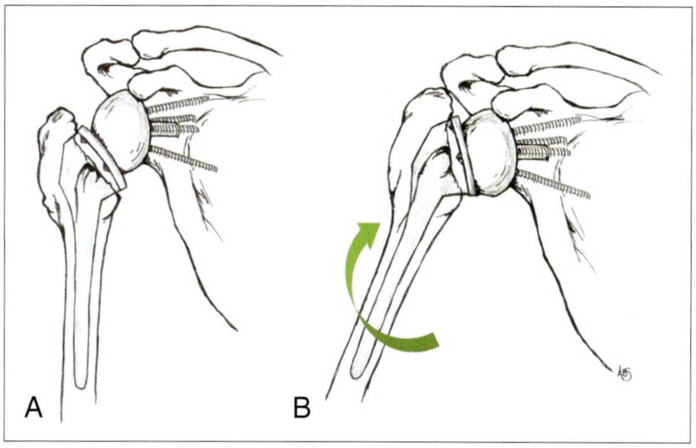

FIGURE 6 Schematic drawings showing reverse shoulder arthroplasty without greater tuberosity osteotomy in good position (**A**) and contact between the greater tuberosity and the acromion in elevation and external rotation (**B**). In patients with a severe greater tuberosity malunion, avoidance of a greater tuberosity osteotomy in reverse arthroplasty can complicate the surgical results secondary to acromial impingement. Greater tuberosity osteotomy may be indicated to avoid this impingement.

may result in decreased range of motion and instability (**Figure 6**). This factor may contribute to the less satisfactory outcomes of reverse shoulder arthroplasty for fracture sequelae when compared with the outcomes of reverse shoulder arthroplasty for rotator cuff tear arthropathy.

SUMMARY

Sequelae after proximal humeral fractures can cause significant pain and functional limitations, commonly leading to prosthetic replacement. Planning appropriate surgical management for these sequelae requires careful evaluation of the proximal humeral anatomy distortion and determination of the need for a greater tuberosity osteotomy. In general, patients who require arthroplasty with greater tuberosity osteotomy have worse functional outcomes than patients whose normal greater tuberosity-humeral head relationship can be restored without osteotomy. Patients with humeral head impaction or necrosis (type I), or chronic dislocation (type II) do not require greater tuberosity osteotomy and can be treated with an anatomic arthroplasty. Patients with proximal humeral nonunion (type III) often can be treated with bone graft and internal fixation, although recent studies have found good outcomes after reverse shoulder arthroplasty in some of these patients. Patients with severe anatomic distortion and tuberosity malunion (type IV) or irreparable rotator cuff deficiency are most reliably treated with reverse shoulder arthroplasty.

KEY STUDY POINTS

- Patients with humeral head impaction or necrosis (type I), or chronic dislocation (type II) do not require greater tuberosity osteotomy and can be treated with an anatomic arthroplasty.
- Patients with proximal humeral nonunion (type III) can be treated with bone graft and internal fixation or reverse shoulder arthroplasty.
- Patients with severe anatomic distortion and tuberosity malunion (type IV) or irreparable rotator cuff deficiency are most reliably treated with reverse shoulder arthroplasty.
- Reverse arthroplasty for proximal humeral nonunion (type III) has a high rate of complications including postoperative prosthetic dislocation.

Annotated References

1. Kim SH, Szabo RM, Marder RA: Epidemiology of humerus fractures in the United States: Nationwide Emergency Department Sample, 2008. *Arthritis Care Res (Hoboken)* 2012;64(3):407-414.

2. Boileau P, Trojani C, Walch G, Krishnan SG, Romeo A, Sinnerton R: Shoulder arthroplasty for the treatment of the sequelae of fractures of the proximal humerus. *J Shoulder Elbow Surg* 2001;10(4):299-308.

3. Boileau P, Chuinard C, Le Huec JC, Walch G, Trojani C: Proximal humerus fracture sequelae: Impact of a new radiographic classification on arthroplasty. *Clin Orthop Relat Res* 2006;442:121-130.

4. Cheung EV, Sperling JW: Management of proximal humeral nonunions and malunions. *Orthop Clin North Am* 2008;39(4):475-482, vii.

5. Martinez AA, Calvo A, Domingo J, Cuenca J, Herrera A: Arthroscopic treatment for malunions of the proximal humeral greater tuberosity. *Int Orthop* 2010;34(8):1207-1211.

6. Norris TR, Green A, McGuigan FX: Late prosthetic shoulder arthroplasty for displaced proximal humerus fractures. *J Shoulder Elbow Surg* 1995;4(4):271-280.

7. Antuña SA, Sperling JW, Sánchez-Sotelo J, Cofield RH: Shoulder arthroplasty for proximal humeral malunions: Long-term results. *J Shoulder Elbow Surg* 2002;11(2):122-129.

8. Mansat P, Guity MR, Bellumore Y, Mansat M: Shoulder arthroplasty for late sequelae of proximal humeral fractures. *J Shoulder Elbow Surg* 2004;13(3):305-312.

9. Jacobson JA, Duquin TR, Sanchez-Sotelo J, Schleck CD, Sperling JW, Cofield RH: Anatomic shoulder arthroplasty for treatment of proximal humerus malunions. *J Shoulder Elbow Surg* 2014;23(8):1232-1239.

   A retrospective review of 109 patients who underwent shoulder arthroplasty for proximal humerus malunions finding that most patients demonstrated improved pain and motion after surgery; however, postoperative instability was the most common complication leading to reoperation. Level of evidence: IV.

10. Pape G, Zeifang F, Bruckner T, Raiss P, Rickert M, Loew M: Humeral surface replacement for the sequelae of fractures of the proximal humerus. *J Bone Joint Surg Br* 2010;92(10):1403-1409.

11. Neyton L, Garaud P, Boileau P: Results of reverse shoulder arthroplasty in proximal humerus fracture sequelae, in Walch G, Boileau P, Mole D, Favard L, Levigne C, Sirveaux F, eds: *Reverse Shoulder Arthroplasty.* Montpellier, France, Sauramps Medical, 2006.

12. Stechel A, Fuhrmann U, Irlenbusch L, Rott O, Irlenbusch U: Reversed shoulder arthroplasty in cuff tear arthritis, fracture sequelae, and revision arthroplasty. *Acta Orthop* 2010;81(3):367-372.

13. Raiss P, Edwards TB, Collin P, et al: Reverse shoulder arthroplasty for malunions of the proximal part of the humerus (type-4 fracture sequelae). *J Bone Joint Surg Am* 2016;98(11):893-899.

    This is a retrospective, multicenter study of 42 patients with posttraumatic sequelae of the proximal humerus and malunions of the tuberosities who were treated with reverse shoulder arthroplasty between 2000 and 2010. Constant and motion score improved postoperatively with a 9.5% complication rate. The authors found reverse shoulder arthroplasty to be a viable treatment option for this diagnosis. Level of evidence: IV.

14. Martin TG, Iannotti JP: Reverse total shoulder arthroplasty for acute fractures and failed management after proximal humeral fractures. *Orthop Clin North Am* 2008;39(4):451-457, vi.

15. Kılıç M, Berth A, Blatter G, et al: Anatomic and reverse shoulder prostheses in fracture sequelae of the humeral head. *Acta Orthop Traumatol Turc* 2010;44(6):417-425.

16. Martinez AA, Bejarano C, Carbonel I, Iglesias D, Gil-Alvaroba J, Herrera A: The treatment of proximal humerus nonunions in older patients with the reverse shoulder arthroplasty. *Injury* 2012;43(supp 2):S3-S6.

17. Raiss P, Edwards TB, da Silva MR, Bruckner T, Loew M, Walch G: Reverse shoulder arthroplasty for the treatment of nonunions of the surgical neck of the proximal part of the humerus (type-3 fracture sequelae). *J Bone Joint Surg Am* 2014;96(24):2070-2076.

This is a retrospective review of 32 patients with proximal humeral nonunions managed with reverse shoulder arthroplasty. The authors found improvements in constant score and motion; however, 34% of patients were found to have postoperative instability. Preserving the tuberosities and rotator cuff improved stability. Level of evidence: IV.

18. Klement MR, Nickel BT, Bala A, Penrose CT, Zura RD, Garrigues GE: Glenohumeral arthritis as a risk factor for proximal humerus nonunion. *Injury* 2016;47(suppl 7):S36-S39.

    Meta-analysis of existing literature finding that nonunion rates after proximal humeral fracture in patients with preexisting osteo and rheumatoid arthritis were significantly higher than in those patients without preexisting glenohumeral arthritis. Level of evidence: III.

19. Raiss P, Edwards TB, Bruckner T, Loew M, Zeifang F, Walch G: Reverse arthroplasty for patients with chronic locked dislocation of the shoulder (type 2 fracture sequela). *J Shoulder Elbow Surg* 2017;26(2):279-287. doi:10.1016/j.jse.2016.05.028.

20. Matsoukis J, Tabib W, Guiffault P, et al: Primary unconstrained shoulder arthroplasty in patients with a fixed anterior glenohumeral dislocation. *J Bone Joint Surg Am* 2006;88(3):547-552.

21. Sperling JW, Pring M, Antuna SA, Cofield RH: Shoulder arthroplasty for locked posterior dislocation of the shoulder. *J Shoulder Elbow Surg* 2004;13(5):522-527.

22. Willis M, Min W, Brooks JP, et al: Proximal humeral malunion treated with reverse shoulder arthroplasty. *J Shoulder Elbow Surg* 2012;21(4):507-513.

23. Tauber M, Resch H: Prosthetic arthroplasty for delayed complications of proximal humerus fracture, in Cofield RH, Sperling JW, eds: *Revision and Complex Shoulder Arthroplasty*. Philadelphia, PA, Lippincott Williams & Wilkins, 2010.

24. Scalise JJ, Ciccone J, Iannotti JP: Clinical, radiographic, and ultrasonographic comparison of subscapularis tenotomy and lesser tuberosity osteotomy for total shoulder arthroplasty. *J Bone Joint Surg Am* 2010;92(7):1627-1634.

25. Krishnan SG, Reineck JR, Bennion PD, Feher L, Burkhead WZ Jr: Shoulder arthroplasty for fracture: Does a fracture-specific stem make a difference? *Clin Orthop Relat Res* 2011;469(12):3317-3323.

Chapter 26

Reverse Shoulder Arthroplasty for Chronic Shoulder Pathology

Randall J. Otto, MD • Phillip T. Nigro, MD • Mark A. Frankle, MD

ABSTRACT

Reverse shoulder arthroplasty is one of numerous advances in shoulder arthroplasty over the past half-century for the treatment of end-stage shoulder disease. Anatomic total shoulder arthroplasty has good results and is durable for the management of glenohumeral osteoarthritis with a balanced soft-tissue envelope. However, patients with arthritis and unbalanced soft tissues who are treated with total shoulder arthroplasty may have failure of the glenoid component caused by uneven forces. Reverse shoulder arthroplasty was developed to improve the outcomes of patients with a rotator cuff–deficient shoulder. The early failures of constrained devices led Grammont to develop a nonanatomic semiconstrained device. This device initially led to improved function and decreased pain. Over time, the design has been modified and has evolved into today's reverse shoulder prostheses. Because longer follow-up of these implants has shown durable results, the indications have expanded to include shoulder pathologies other than a rotator cuff–deficient shoulder, making it the fastest growing orthopaedic implant today.

Keywords: chronic shoulder pathologies; reverse shoulder arthroplasty; surgical indications

Dr. Otto or an immediate family member is a member of a speakers' bureau or has made paid presentations on behalf of DJ Orthopaedics and serves as a paid consultant to or is an employee of DJ Orthopaedics. Dr. Frankle or an immediate family member has received royalties from Cayenne Medical and DJO Surgical; is a member of a speakers' bureau or has made paid presentations on behalf of DJO Surgical; serves as a paid consultant to or is an employee of Cayenne Medical, DJO Surgical, and Synchrony Healthcare Communications; has received research or institutional support from DJO Surgical and Zimmer; and serves as a board member, owner, officer, or committee member of the American Academy of Orthopaedic Surgeons and the American Shoulder and Elbow Surgeons. Neither Dr. Nigro nor any immediate family member has received anything of value from or has stock or stock options held in a commercial company or institution related directly or indirectly to the subject of this chapter.

Introduction

The purpose of the reverse shoulder prosthesis is to provide a stable glenohumeral fulcrum to allow the deltoid to elevate the arm.[1] The reversed articulation blocks superior migration of the humerus, and the superiorly directed translational forces of the deltoid are converted into rotational moments. When a stable glenohumeral articulation is reestablished, the remaining rotator cuff muscles and periscapular musculature are able to restore humerus-trunk motion in conjunction with the deltoid.

Grammont designed the reverse prosthesis with a humeral component in extreme valgus (155°) and a hemispherical glenoid component directly centered on the fixation and the bony glenoid surface (**Figure 1**). This valgus humeral component was designed to tension the deltoid by lengthening the arm and to provide compression between the humeral socket and the glenosphere, thus stabilizing the articulation. In addition, medializing the center of rotation of the hemisphere could enhance the recruitment of deltoid muscle fibers, thereby allowing for a more efficient deltoid lever arm.[2] It was postulated that locating a humeral center of rotation as close as possible to the glenoid bone surface would decrease baseplate loosening.

Despite clinical improvements resulting from the use of the Grammont device, several mechanical problems emerged, including a substantial reduction in the impingement-free range of motion of the glenohumeral joint and a significant alteration in the proximal humeral lateral and inferior offset.[3,4] These deviations from the structural anatomic shoulder and the subsequent change in mechanics led to unforeseen complications including prosthetic abutment of bone and soft tissue (which leads to scapular notching) and loss of the appearance of the normal shoulder contour with the alteration in shoulder function. Numerous clinical and biomechanical studies have aimed at improving the prosthetic design and surgical technique of reverse shoulder arthroplasty (RSA).

Indications and Contraindications

Indications

The indications for RSA have continued to expand because it has become more widely used for treating patients

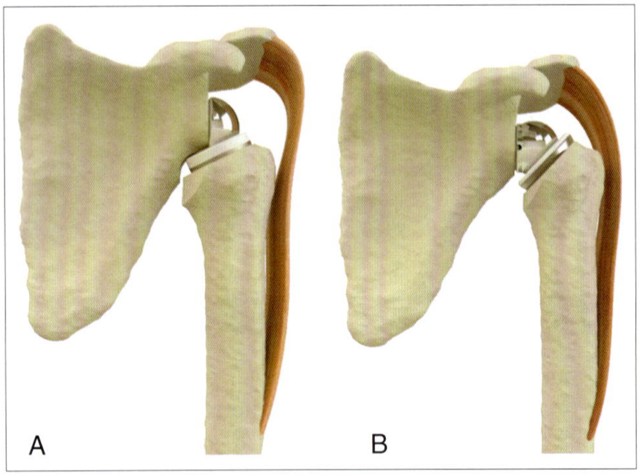

FIGURE 1 Computerized drawings showing a Grammont-style (**A**) and a lateral offset (**B**) reverse shoulder prosthesis.

with severe shoulder pathology. Originally, RSA was used for patients with glenohumeral arthritis in the setting of rotator cuff deficiency. More recently, the indications for RSA have expanded to many other shoulder pathologies. RSA has been successfully used for patients who have severe rotator cuff deficiency without glenohumeral arthritis; osteoarthritis with an intact rotator cuff; glenoid or humeral bone loss; chronic glenohumeral instability and postcapsulorrhaphy arthropathy; rheumatoid arthritis; a three-part or four-part proximal humeral fracture; proximal humerus fracture sequelae; or treatment of an infected shoulder arthroplasty, either in a single or a two-stage procedure. RSA is also successfully used for patients needing reconstruction after tumor resection and for patients who have failed a prior arthroplasty procedure including an unsuccessful hemiarthroplasty for fracture or rotator cuff tear arthropathy, total shoulder arthroplasty (TSA), or previous RSA.

RSA is considered if the patient reports pain not relieved by conservative measures and/or has significant impairment in shoulder function, which limits normal activities of daily living. Often patients have clinical evidence of pseudoparesis, or inability to raise the arm above 90° of flexion. Others can present with clinical or radiographic escape of the shoulder caused by lack of a stable fulcrum, most commonly in the anterosuperior direction. Although not required, residual posterior and anterior rotator cuff repair during surgery can aid in regaining rotational motion and strength after RSA. Future studies will continue to define and expand the indications for RSA.

Contraindications

Adequate deltoid muscle function is required for elevating the arm after RSA. Thus, historically RSA has been absolutely contraindicated if the patient has a nonfunctioning deltoid, probably as a result of neurologic injury, deltoid avulsion, extensive intramuscular scarring, or other neuromuscular injury. If the middle deltoid muscle belly is insufficient, it is unlikely the muscle will provide adequate function after RSA. There are recent reports of success with the use of RSA in a deltoid-deficient shoulder; however, caution should be used when considering RSA in this situation, and it should still be considered a relative contraindication.

Shoulder joint infection is a relative contraindication to performing RSA. However, RSA has been shown to be successful in the treatment of infectious processes with a single or two-stage procedure.[5,6] Success of a single-stage procedure is based on an appropriate débridement and removal of all previous implants, as well as long-term intravenous antibiotic therapy to eradicate the infection. However, in the setting of an active gross infection, an antibiotic spacer is the treatment of choice.

In the past, RSA had not been recommended for patients younger than 70 years because of concern about implant durability. However, there have been longer follow-up studies, including those with younger patients, with good clinical results.[7-14] The long-term clinical outcomes are similar to those in anatomic TSA. Although RSA should be used with caution in younger patients, it is no longer a relative contraindication for the procedure. The considerations in a younger patient include the severity of the clinical condition and pathology, pain, and reduction of shoulder function, as well as the patient's willingness to accept that the implant may not be sufficiently durable for their lifetime. In a patient who has relatively limited pathology (eg, a massive rotator cuff tear without arthritis), clinical severity plays an important role in predicting satisfaction. It is difficult to anticipate the extent of postoperative clinical improvement if the patient has a relatively good preoperative range of motion. Hence, integrating a patient's symptoms and pathology is critical for deciding on the appropriate treatment.

In the past, glenoid erosion was considered a strong contraindication to RSA. Recent studies have found that RSA can be successful in patients with glenoid deficiency.[15-20] RSA with glenoid bone grafting techniques has expanded its use in treating moderate or severe glenoid erosion.[15] In addition, implant design modifications have allowed for metallic augmentation on the glenoid baseplate to address bone deficiency and allow for adequate fixation. However, severe glenoid deficiency that precludes adequate implant fixation remains a contraindication to RSA.

The general contraindications to joint arthroplasty apply to patients being considered for RSA. These contraindications include severe medical illness, inability to tolerate surgery, inability to follow postoperative restrictions, and the presence of a metal allergy, although alternative bearing surfaces are being introduced to solve this issue. In addition, the surgeon must be aware of the learning curve required for RSA in the treatment of advanced pathology. As with any new technology, the surgeon's level of experience affects outcomes and complication rates.[21]

Changing Prosthetic Designs

The clinical limitations of the Grammont reverse shoulder devices led to the development of devices that maintained the reversed articulation while minimizing the distortion of humeral offset and maximizing the impingement-free range of motion of the glenohumeral joint. The current designs were developed to reduce the incidence of notching, lack of functional rotation, instability, and glenoid-sided failure. The changes have included the use of lateralized glenospheres, eccentric glenospheres, and humeral components placed in less valgus than the original design. Current prosthetic designs offer spheres with a center of rotation offset from the glenoid surface. These spheres are more ovoid than the original design and have a center of rotation as much as 10 mm lateral or 4 mm inferior to the surface of the glenoid.[22,23] Many current designs also have a more anatomic neck-shaft angle; in several designs, the neck-shaft angle is 135°, while others range between 145° and 147.5°.

Scapular Notching

Maximizing the impingement-free range of motion is critical not only for patient function but also for implant survivability, implant stability, and relief of unexplained pain. One consequence of decreasing the impingement-free range of motion is abutment of the scapular neck with the inferior aspect of the humeral socket when physiologic adduction is attempted (**Figure 2**). The adduction deficit leads to the radiographic appearance of a notch. Polyethylene wear and glenoid loosening are of concern with scapular notching. The presence of a notch and its size have a negative effect on clinical outcome scores and can cause glenoid component loosening.[24,25] Reduction in impingement-free range of motion increases the likelihood of prosthetic abutment with soft tissue or bone, leading to pain or levering out of the implant.

With a Grammont-style implant, maximal restoration of glenohumeral motion is prevented by the limited ability to adequately balance the soft tissues and provide a sufficient range of impingement-free motion. The surgical technique can be altered to avoid the adduction deficit. When a virtual simulation computer model was used to evaluate factors contributing to scapular notching, an adduction deficit was found to be best avoided by a varus humeral neck-shaft angle (130°).[3,4] The most important factor for maximizing the impingement-free range of motion in all planes of motion was the use of a glenosphere with a center of rotation lateral to the glenoid surface. Clinical studies have confirmed this conclusion; the risk of scapular notching is almost eliminated in the short term if a glenosphere with lateral offset is used.[26-31] However, longer follow-up has shown that scapular notching can continue to occur and progress over time. One modification of the Grammont device uses an autogenous bone graft between the glenoid and the baseplate to increase the lateral offset, although scapular notching still occurs at a high rate in this scenario, likely because of the valgus humeral component.[23]

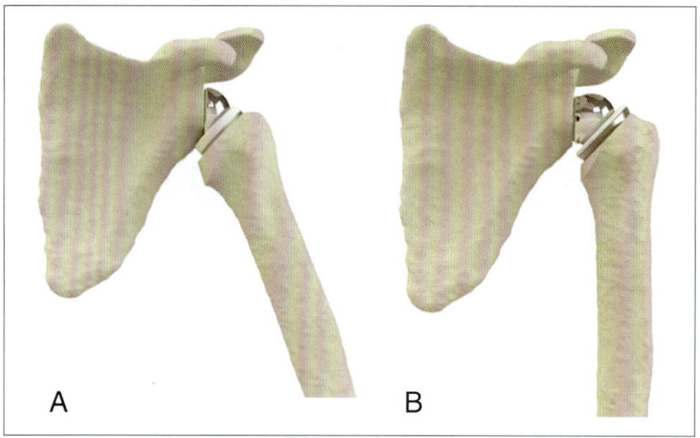

FIGURE 2 Computerized drawings showing a Grammont-style prosthesis (**A**) with an adduction deficit with abutment of inferior humerosocket with scapular neck and a lateral offset prosthesis (**B**) without abutment of inferior humerosocket with scapular neck.

Lack of External Rotation Improvement

The Grammont-style device repeatedly was found to improve function and provide pain relief, but the improvement in external rotation has been unreliable.[32-35] Grammont speculated that RSA could improve external rotation by allowing posterior deltoid recruitment, but few biomechanical data exist to support this theory.[36] Loss of external rotation strength might be explained by the altered anatomy seen in rotator cuff tear arthropathy, which can decrease the efficiency of contraction of the remaining rotator cuff. In addition, medializing the center of rotation causes slackening of the remaining rotator cuff muscles and prevents sufficient muscle contraction (**Figure 3**). Some evidence suggests that patients who do not have improvement in external rotation are less satisfied with their function.[33]

RSA implant designs with a lateral center of rotation allow more consistent external rotation improvement

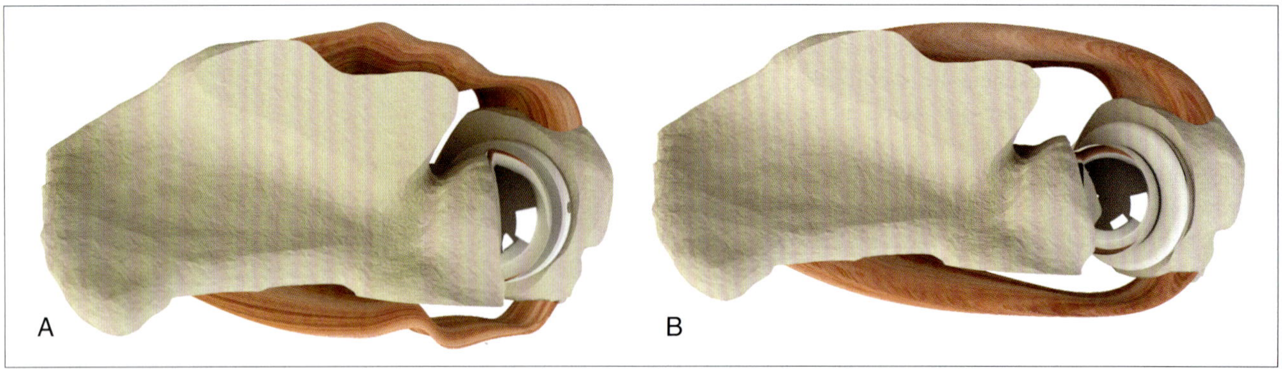

FIGURE 3 Computerized drawings showing slackening of the remaining rotator cuff external rotators with medial offset device (**A**) and tensioning of the remaining rotator cuff external rotators with lateral offset device (**B**).

than the Grammont prosthesis.[22] In patients with rotator cuff deficiency, the proximally migrated humerus may prevent the intact rotator cuff muscles from functioning properly. Positioning the humerus in a more anatomic position restores joint stability and tension to the remaining posterior rotator cuff muscles, leading to an improvement in external rotation. Several clinical studies confirmed that restoring the lateral offset of the humerus improves postoperative external rotation in patients with different pathologic conditions.[26-31] However, patients who have an absent or atrophic teres minor preoperatively will not have an improvement in external rotation postoperatively. These patients may require a latissimus dorsi/teres major transfer for improvement of external rotation.

Instability

Instability after RSA remains a concern. Rates of dislocation as high as 30% have been reported with the use of the Grammont design. The factors contributing to instability include glenosphere diameter, humeral socket constraint, soft-tissue tensioning, impingement, erroneous version of the prosthesis, and deltoid dysfunction.

Several researchers have suggested that the stability of the glenohumeral joint is improved by restoring muscle tension and thus increasing compression on the humerus.[26-31] The stability of the glenohumeral joint in a Grammont design is compromised with medialization of the humerus and subsequent slackening of the remaining rotator cuff muscles. Medialization of the humerus can turn the deltoid into a distracting force if there is glenoid bone loss and thereby can increase the possibility of dislocation.[36] An alternative method of improving stability with these implants is to lengthen the humerus and use a valgus humeral socket.[32] However, this method adds to the risk of acromial fracture, brachial plexopathy, deltoid overtensioning, and loss of motion. Increasing the glenoid-tuberosity distance by lateralizing the humerus is another method of improving stability by increasing the compressive forces across the glenohumeral joint. This can be performed with metallic or bony lateralization on the glenoid, or with an offset humeral socket shell on the humeral side.

Several prosthetic design factors including socket depth, glenosphere size, and compression forces were evaluated for their relation to instability.[37] The most important parameter for improving stability was increased compression forces across the joint, followed by increased humeral socket depth. The remaining rotator cuff muscle tension is restored by lateralizing the humerus, thus increasing the compression across the joint. Studies have found that lateralizing the humerus increases joint reactive forces.[37,38]

The initial management of a dislocation after RSA involves closed reduction followed by a period of sling immobilization. Open revision surgery is indicated if closed reduction is not possible or if instability recurs after closed reduction. It is important to identify the cause of dislocation to appropriately treat the patient surgically if this is required. Adequate inferior release of tissue around the implant should be performed to remove soft tissue that can impinge on the prosthesis and cause it to lever out. Soft-tissue tension should be assessed. A thicker polyethylene socket can be chosen to increase the lateral offset and tension. A more constrained socket or a larger glenosphere can be chosen to help improve stability. If these measures are not successful, the version and placement of the components should be considered as the cause of instability, as well as deltoid dysfunction.

Baseplate Failure

Failure of the attachment of the glenoid component to the bony glenoid has been reported by many authors.[22,31,39-44] All reverse components designed since 1985 are intended to allow bony ingrowth on the glenoid side. If ingrowth does not occur, the attachment is with fibrous tissue and is less durable. Factors that lead to failure to achieve ingrowth might include the design of the prosthesis, glenoid bone deficiency, and malpositioning of the component. Grammont's theory that centering the sphere over the fixation and the glenoid bone would eliminate the risk of glenoid failure has not been uniformly confirmed. As many as 50% of glenoid components failed in some early studies of patients who had rheumatoid arthritis or in whom scapular notching developed.[40,41] Other early devices also had high rates of mechanical failure rates.

In the original report of a device with an ovoid sphere and a center of rotation 10 mm from the glenoid surface, the glenoid component failure rate was almost 12%.[22] A 15° inferior tilt of the glenosphere has been shown to result in the most uniform compressive forces and the least micromotion at the bone-baseplate interface when a glenosphere with a lateral center of rotation was used.[45] This finding suggests a reduced risk of baseplate failure by tilting the glenoid component inferiorly. This was confirmed showing that a medialized glenosphere (the original Grammont design) has optimal force at a bone-baseplate interface with an inferior vertical tilt, compared with a baseplate perpendicular to the bony surface.[4] The most unstable components were superiorly tilted (**Figure 4**). This pattern was different if eccentric inferior glenospheres were selected, with inferior tilt providing the least stable mechanical environment.

A biomechanical analysis of baseplate constructs using locked 5.0-mm and unlocked 3.5-mm screw combinations found that baseplates fixed with 5.0-mm locked screws had better fixation and less micromotion.[46] A subsequent clinical study of a modified design using 5.0-mm locked screws and inferior tilt found that glenoid failure was reduced to 0.4% at a minimum 2-year follow-up.[30] There were no additional baseplate failures seen in this patient population as they were followed up for a minimum of 10 years.

When current implantation techniques are used, Grammont-style devices with locking-screw fixation have comparably low baseplate loosening rates, ranging from zero to 5% in patients who underwent primary RSA[25,32,35] and from zero to 8% in those who underwent RSA for rheumatoid arthritis or revision.[32,47,48] Modern techniques allow durable glenoid implant fixation with both Grammont-style and lateral offset devices. The glenoid fixation remains stable in the setting of decreased glenoid bone quality from patient disease or earlier arthroplasty.

Technical Considerations

Glenosphere Positioning

The incidence of scapular notching has been reduced through improved implant design. In addition, surgical technique has been altered to change the position of the glenosphere in an attempt to avoid inferior scapular neck impingement when the arm is at the side.[49] A biomechanical evaluation analyzed four different glenoid component positions to assess their influence on range of motion and mechanical impingement.[2] Placing the glenosphere beyond the inferior rim of the glenoid and tilting the component 15° were found to significantly reduce mechanical impingement. The importance of inferior glenosphere placement for avoiding impingement was subsequently validated clinically.[24]

Another biomechanical study used a computer simulation to determine the factors that can minimize the risk of an adduction deficit and subsequent impingement.[3] The second most important factor in avoiding inferior scapular impingement was found to be inferior placement of the glenosphere, and the most important factor was the use of a varus (130°) humeral neck-shaft angle.

Glenoid Bone Deficiency

In a normal shoulder, the glenoid center line is perpendicular to the glenoid surface and in approximately 10° of retroversion. The center line serves as a pillar of bone under which the humeral head rests, and this relationship is maintained throughout the range of motion with a coupling of glenohumeral and scapulothoracic motion. This relationship is disrupted by unbalanced forces in a rotator cuff–deficient shoulder, leading to mechanical alteration and pathologic glenoid wear patterns in as many as 36% of patients who undergo RSA.[50] Depending on the pathology, these wear patterns occur in a spectrum ranging from no wear to superior, anterior, posterior, and global wear. It is important to recognize the wear pattern for purposes of preoperative planning.

The glenoid component ideally is placed along the glenoid center line, where 2.5 to 3.5 cm of bone is accessible for fixation in a normally shaped glenoid. If the glenoid has substantial or eccentric wear, this placement is not always feasible. The use of an alternate glenoid center line has been proposed, in which the line is aimed at the dense bone where the scapular spine meets the scapular body.[50] This line is not always perpendicular to the remaining glenoid surface. The implantation of the glenoid component along this line allows the surgeon to achieve adequate bony fixation in the scapular body–scapular spine junction. Autogenous bone graft or allograft can be used to augment the deficient glenoid surface. Newer patient-specific planning software has provided advances to aid the surgeon in the surgical planning for these cases. In addition, several implant companies have designed metallic augmented glenoid baseplates to allow for correction of the glenoid bone deficiency while allowing for stable fixation and bony

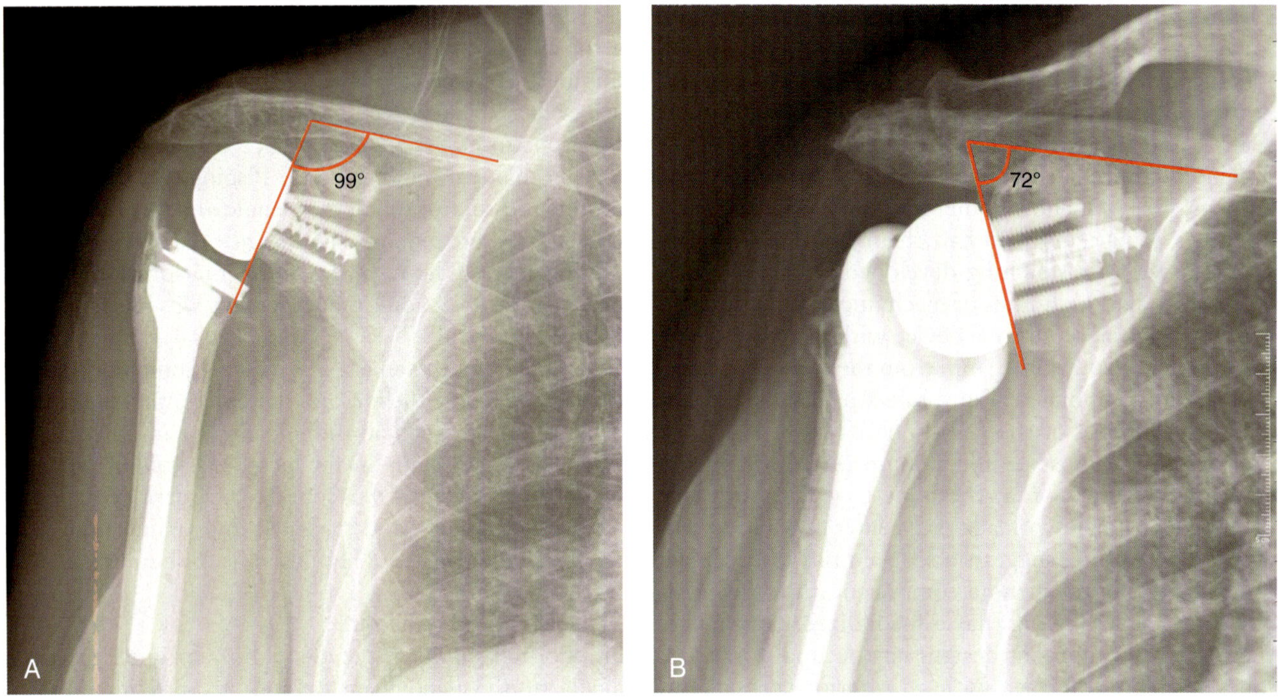

FIGURE 4 Grashey radiographs showing superior glenosphere tilt with baseplate failure (**A**) and inferior glenosphere tilt without baseplate failure (**B**).

ingrowth. Custom made implants are available, but no long-term data exist to support their use for this challenging problem.

Humeral Bone Loss

The use of RSA in the setting of proximal humeral bone loss was found to improve function and relieve pain.[27] However, proximal humeral bone deficiency resulted in high rates of instability, early prosthetic loosening, and rotational weakness.[27] The use of a proximal humeral allograft in conjunction with RSA improved results in patients with severe proximal humeral deficiency.[27,29] Longer follow-up of these patients has shown that survivorship in these cases is 88% at 5 years, 78% at 10 years, and 67% beyond 10 years.[51] The allograft also provides rotational stability for the humeral stem component. This factor is especially important with modular humeral components, which have a greater risk of mechanical failure than nonmodular humeral components when used in patients with proximal humeral bone loss.[52] The allograft also restores the natural contour of the proximal humerus and maintains the height of the prosthesis-bone construct and resists subsidence of the humeral implant, thereby helping to optimize deltoid tension. Finally, the allograft lateralizes the line of pull of the deltoid muscles to enhance the deltoid wrapping effect and increase the resultant force of the deltoid as a pulley.

Latissimus Dorsi Tendon Transfer

Patients who undergo RSA are less satisfied with their outcome if they do not have improvement in active external rotation, which is necessary for many activities of daily living.[33,53] Even with prosthetic design changes to lateralize the humerus for the purpose of restoring external rotation and strength, an absence or atrophy of the teres minor means that a patient will not have improvement in external rotation. The patient will have a hornblower's sign and an external rotation lag when the arm is at the side. The use of a modified latissimus dorsi–teres major tendon transfer has been proposed in conjunction with RSA in these patients to restore active elevation and external rotation, thereby improving patient function and satisfaction.[53-56]

Results

High complication rates were described in the initial reports of RSA used to treat patients with rotator cuff deficiency. Nonetheless, RSA has proved to be a durable treatment, even with the early generation implants. Refinements in implant technology and improved surgical techniques have led to findings of greater implant durability over time and lower complication rates. Specific results are outlined in **Tables 1** through **10**.

Table 1

Reverse Shoulder Arthroplasty Long-term Follow-up

Study (Year)	Number of Patients	Pathology (Number of Patients)	Average Follow-up	Preoperative/Postoperative Range of Motion: Forward Flexion	Abduction	External Rotation	Preoperative/ Postoperative Outcome Scores[a]	Complications
Devices With Medial Center of Rotation								
Guery et al[25] (2006)	57	Rotator cuff tear (48) Rheumatoid arthritis (6) Fracture (2) Revision (1)	69.6 mo	—	—	—	–/>30 (Constant) Survival: 88% at 72 mo, 58% at 120 mo	Infection (3), dislocation (3), glenoid loosening (3)
Favard et al[57] (2011)	148	Rotator cuff tear arthropathy	7.8 yr	69°/129°	—	5°/11°	24/62 (Constant)	22% complication rate
Melis et al[47] (2011)	68	Noncemented (34)	9.6 yr	–/123°	—	–/7°	–/53 (Constant)	Instability (4), humeral fracture (2), acromial fracture (1)
		Cemented (34)	9.6 yr	–/132°	—	–/11°	–/60 (Constant)	
Bacle et al[58] (2017)	87	Rotator cuff tear arthropathy (27) Failed arthroplasty (21) Rotator cuff tear (20) Posttraumatic arthritis (10) Primary arthritis (9)	150 mo	81°/131°	—	9°/9°	23/55 (Constant) 93% implant survival at 10 yr	10 delayed complications: humeral loosening (3), glenoid loosening (4), **unclear** (3)
Bassens et al[59] (2019)	74	Rotator cuff tear arthropathy (58) Fracture (3) Malunion (5) Osteonecrosis (3) Instability (3) Septic arthropathy (2)	113 mo	—	—	—	37.4/66.6 (Constant) 97% implant survival at 8 yr	—

(continued)

Table 1

Reverse Shoulder Arthroplasty Long-Term Follow-up (continued)

Study (Year)	Number of Patients	Pathology (Number of Patients)	Average Follow-up	Preoperative/Postoperative Range of Motion: Forward Flexion	Abduction	External Rotation	Preoperative/Postoperative Outcome Scores[a]	Complications
Gerber et al[60] (2018)	22	Rotator cuff tear	16 yr	53°/101°	55°/86°	20°/18°	23/58 (Constant) 73% survival at 10 yr 70% survival at 15 yr	Infection (6), mechanical block (1), dislocation (3), humeral loosening (2), glenoid loosening (2), scapular fracture (3), humeral fracture (1), polyethylene wear (1)
Devices With Lateral Center of Rotation								
Mulieri et al[26] (2010)	60	Rotator cuff tear without arthritis	52 mo	53°/134°	49°/125°	27°/51°	33/75 (ASES)	Proximal humerus fracture (1), failed baseplate (4), broken center screw (1), deep infection (1), hematoma (1), acromial fracture (2), scapular body fracture (1), dislocation (1)
Cuff et al[61] (2017)	42	Rotator cuff deficiency (19) Rotator cuff deficiency with arthroplasty (10) Failed rotator cuff surgery (13)	11 yr	70°/126°	65°/118°	18°/40°	35/74 (ASES) 90.7% implant survival at 10 yr	4 revisions: dislocation (3), humeral shaft fracture (1),

The numbers in parentheses are the total number (N) of patients with the complication.

[a]Measured using the Constant Shoulder Score or American Shoulder and Elbow Surgeons (ASES) Index.

Table 2

Reverse Shoulder Arthroplasty for Proximal Humeral Fracture

Study (Year)	Number of Patients	Average Follow-up	Preoperative/Postoperative Range of Motion: Forward Flexion	Abduction	External Rotation	Preoperative/ Postoperative Outcome Scores[a]	Complications
Bufquin et al[62] (2007)	43	22 mo	97°	86°	30°	44 (Constant)	Nerve injury (5), complex regional pain syndrome (3), dislocation (1), glenoid fracture (1), acromial fracture (1), deltoid anterior interval dehiscence (1)
Klein et al[63] (2008)	20	33 mo	122°	113°	25°	68 (ASES) 68 (Constant)	Recurrent dislocation (1), infection (2)
Gallinet et al[64] (2009)	16	12 mo	98°	—	9°	53 (Constant)	Deep infection (1), superficial infection (1), complex regional pain syndrome (1)
Cazeneuve and Cristofari[65] (2010)	36	6.6 yr	—	—	—	53 (Constant)	Complex regional pain syndrome (2), infection (1), dislocation (4), baseplate loosening (1)
Lenarz et al[66] (2011)	30	23 mo	139°	—	27°	78 (ASES)	Complex regional pain syndrome, deep vein thrombosis, and tuberosity resorption (1)
Ross et al[67] (2015)	29	54.9 mo	130°	113°	30°	89.3 (ASES) 70.9 (Constant) No revisions at final follow-up	Transient axillary nerve palsy (1)
Grubhofer et al[68] (2016)	52	35 mo	118°	111°	18°	64 (Constant)	Infection (2), periprosthetic fracture (1), hematoma (1)

(continued)

Table 2

Reverse Shoulder Arthroplasty for Proximal Humeral Fracture (continued)

Study (Year)	Number of Patients	Average Follow-up	Preoperative/Postoperative Range of Motion: Forward Flexion	Abduction	External Rotation	Preoperative/Postoperative Outcome Scores[a]	Complications
Shannon et al[69] (2016)	18 (acute)	36 mo	130°	—	42°	70.6 (ASES)	Infection (1)
	26 (failed ORIF)		133°	—	36°	64.6 (ASES)	Aseptic loosening (1), dislocation (1)
Chun et al[70] (2017)	14/38 united tuberosities	36.5 mo	125°	—	29°	74.3 (ASES) 67.9 (Constant)	Not listed
	24/38 nonunion tuberosities	37.3 mo	127°	—	10°	70.7 (ASES) 63.9 (Constant)	Not listed
Boileau et al[71] (2019)	38	36 mo	135° total group	—	24°	64 (Constant)	Pulmonary embolism (1), hematoma (1)
			141° healed tuberosities	—	27°	64 (Constant)	
			115° unhealed tuberosities	—	11°	51 (Constant)	

The numbers in parentheses are the total number (N) of patients with the complication.

ORIF = open reduction and internal fixation

[a]Measured using the Constant Shoulder Score or American Shoulder and Elbow Surgeons (ASES) Index.

Table 3

Reverse Shoulder Arthroplasty for Fracture Sequelae

Study (Year)	Number of Patients	Average Follow-up	Preoperative/Postoperative Range of Motion: Forward Flexion	Abduction	External Rotation	Preoperative/ Postoperative Outcome Scores[a]	Complications
Raiss et al[72] (2014)	32 proximal humerus nonunions	4 yr	42.9°/109.7°	—	0.5°/13.1°	14.2/46.6 (Constant)	Dislocation (11), infection (2)
Raiss et al[73] (2016)	42 proximal humerus malunions	4 yr	53.6°/120.5°	—	−5.4°/8.5°	19.7/54.9 (Constant)	Intraoperative humeral fracture (1), periprosthetic fracture (1), dislocation (1), aseptic loosening glenoid and humerus (1)
Dezfuli et al[74] (2016)	13 acute humeral fracture	34 mo	109°	103°	27°	82 (ASES) 70 (Constant)	Periprosthetic humeral fracture (1)
	13 malunion humerus	36 mo	109°	96°	22°	75 (ASES) 64 (Constant)	Infection (1)
	12 failed hemi	34 mo	103°	100°	3°	54 (ASES) 51 (Constant)	Infection (1)
	11 failed ORIF	24 mo	94°	94°	20°	59 (ASES) 59 (Constant)	Infection (1), periprosthetic humeral fracture (2)
Grubhofer et al[75] (2017)	54 failed ORIF	46 mo	59°/104°	54°/103°	13°/17°	26/55 (Constant)	Intraoperative humeral fracture (1), periprosthetic humeral fracture (1), infection (2), dislocation (1)

The numbers in parentheses are the total number (N) of patients with the complication.

ORIF = open reduction and internal fixation

[a]Measured using the Constant Shoulder Score or American Shoulder and Elbow Surgeons (ASES) Index.

Table 4

Reverse Shoulder Arthroplasty for Glenoid Bone Loss

Study (Year)	Number of Patients	Average Follow-up	Preoperative/Postoperative Range of Motion			Preoperative/ Postoperative Outcome Scores[a]	Graft Incorporation (%)	Complications
			Forward Flexion	Abduction	External Rotation			
Lorenzetti et al[16] (2017)	57 (glenoid allograft and autograft)	46 mo	70°/142°	65°/133°	29°/54°	37/75 (ASES)	98	Periprosthetic humerus fracture (1), aseptic loosening humerus (3), acromial fracture (5)
Jones et al[17] (2016)	44 (glenoid allograft and autograft)	41 mo	75°/116°	70°/102°	14°/26°	36/75 (ASES) 30/58 (Constant)	95	Graft failure (2), infection (2), dislocation (1), humeral loosening (1)
Lopiz et al[18] (2017)	20 (glenoid allograft and autograft)	26 mo	70°/113°	59°/104°	10°/13°	34/68 (ASES) 31/51 (Constant)	95	Baseplate loosening (1), acromial fracture (1), grade 3 notching (1), periprosthetic humeral fracture (1)
Ernstbrunner et al[19] (2017)	41 (glenoid allograft and autograft)	2.8 yr	—	59°/149°	—	–/77 (ASES)	78	Scapular spine fractures (2), broken humeral tray (1), posttraumatic fragmentation of the posterior aspect of the greater tuberosity (1), proximal humeral bone resorption (1), postoperative instability (1), heterotopic ossification leading to deltoid pain (1)
Tashjian et al[20] (2018)	14 (glenoid autograft)	2.6 yr	80°/130°	—	18°/29°	22/66 (ASES)	100	Baseplate loosening (1), dislocation (1), transient brachial plexus palsy (1)

The numbers in parentheses are the total number (N) of patients with the complication.
[a]Measured using the Constant Shoulder Score or American Shoulder and Elbow Surgeons (ASES) Index.

Table 5

Reverse Shoulder Arthroplasty With Humeral Bone Loss

Study (Year)	Number of Patients	Average Follow-up	Preoperative/Postoperative Range of Motion: Forward Flexion	Abduction	External Rotation	Preoperative/Postoperative Outcome Scores[a]	Graft Incorporation (%)	Complications
Sanchez-Sotelo et al[76] (2017)	26 with humeral allograft	4 yr	41°/98°	—	11°/31°	25 patients with no or mild pain 1 patient with moderate/severe pain	92	Infection (1), delayed wound healing (1), dislocation (1), allograft fracture (1), distal humeral fracture (1), delayed union (1)
Cox et al (2019)[51]	73 with humeral allograft	68 mo	49°/75°	45°/72°	15°/16°	34/51 (ASES)	100	Periprosthetic fractures (8), 4 dislocations (4), humeral loosening (3), glenosphere dissociations (2), infection (2)

The numbers in parentheses are the total number (N) of patients with the complication.

[a]Measured using the Constant Shoulder Score or American Shoulder and Elbow Surgeons (ASES) Index.

Table 6

Reverse Shoulder Arthroplasty for Instability

Study (Year)	Number of Patients	Average Follow-up	Preoperative/Postoperative Range of Motion: Forward Flexion	Abduction	External Rotation	Preoperative/Postoperative Outcome Scores[a]	Complications
Werner et al[77] (2014)	21 with chronic dislocation treated with glenoid bone graft	4.9 yr	35°/128°	25°/113°	2°/8°	6/57 (Constant)	Baseplate loosening (2)
Kurowicki et al[78] (2016)	24 with locked anterior dislocation	26 mo	60°/100°	45°/70°	–10°/30°	30/55 (ASES)	Acromial fracture (5), dislocation (2)
Cuff et al[79] (2018)	20 with postcapsulorrhaphy arthropathy	44 mo	130°/139°	—	22°/40°	38/79 (ASES)	Undefined complications (2)
Patel et al[80] (2019)	10 with prior anterior stabilization	4 yr	91°/138°	84°/128°	2°/31°	32/83 (ASES) 38/77 (Constant)	None
Hasler et al[81] (2019)	11 with instability	74 mo	80°/110°	60°/100°	25°/20°	25/53 (Constant)	Acromial fracture (1), persistent subjective instability (1)

The numbers in parentheses are the total number (N) of patients with the complication.

[a]Measured using the Constant Shoulder Score or American Shoulder and Elbow Surgeons (ASES) Index.

Table 7

Reverse Shoulder Arthroplasty (RSA) for Shoulder Arthritis With Intact Rotator Cuff

Study (Year)	Number of Patients	Average Follow-up	Preoperative/Postoperative Range of Motion: Forward Flexion	Abduction	External Rotation	Preoperative/ Postoperative Outcome Scores[a]	Complications
Mizuno et al[82] (2013)	27	54 mo	89°/152°	—	3°/27°	31/76 (Constant)	Glenoid loosening (1), transient nerve palsy (2), permanent nerve palsy (1)
Steen et al[83] (2015)	24	42 mo	38°/153°	60°/140°	5°/47°	43/80 (ASES)	Periprosthetic humeral fracture 18 mo after RSA (1)

The numbers in parentheses are the total number (N) of patients with the complication.
[a]Measured using the Constant Shoulder Score or American Shoulder and Elbow Surgeons (ASES) Index.

Table 8

Reverse Shoulder Arthroplasty for Rheumatoid Arthritis

Study (Year)	Number of Patients	Average Follow-up	Preoperative/Postoperative Range of Motion: Forward Flexion	Abduction	External Rotation	Preoperative/ Postoperative Outcome Scores[a]	Complications
Rittmiester et al[40] (2001)	7	54 mo	—	—	—	17/63 (Constant)	Revision (3), glenoid loosening (2), failed acromial open reduction and internal fixation (1)
Young et al[48] (2011)	18	3.8 yr	78°/139°	—	17°/46°	22/64.9 (Constant)	Acromial fracture (1), scapular spine fracture (1), coracoid fracture (1), greater tuberosity avulsion (2), transient axillary nerve palsy (1)
Holcomb et al[84] (2010)	21	36 mo	52°/126°	55°/116°	19°/33°	28/82 (ASES)	Periprosthetic glenoid fracture (1), infection (2), scapular spine fracture (1), intraoperative glenoid fracture (1), radiographic baseplate loosening (1)

The numbers in parentheses are the total number (N) of patients with the complication.
[a]Measured using the Constant Shoulder Score or American Shoulder and Elbow Surgeons (ASES) Index.

Section 5: Principles of Clinical Information

Table 9

Revision Reverse Shoulder Arthroplasty

Study (Year)	Number of Patients	Procedure And/or Pathology (Number of Patients)	Average Follow-up	Preoperative/Postoperative Range of Motion			Preoperative/ Postoperative Outcome Scores[a]	Complications
				Forward Flexion	Abduction	External Rotation		
Werner et al[35] (2005)	58	Primary rotator cuff tear arthroplasty (17) Revision arthroplasty (41)	38 mo	42°/100°	43°/90°	17°/12°	18/56 (Constant)	Overall (50%), revision surgery (33%) Hematoma (12), dislocation (5), infection (1), nerve lesion (1), glenoid loosening (3), humeral stem loosening (1), scapular fracture (4), polyethylene dissociation (1)
Boileau et al[32] (2006)	45	Primary rotator cuff tear arthroplasty (17) Revision after hemiarthroplasty (19) Revision for fracture sequelae (7)	40 mo	55°/121°	—	7°/11°	17/58 (Constant)	Dislocation (3), deep infection (3), aseptic humeral loosening (1), periprosthetic humeral fracture (2), intraoperative glenoid fracture (1), wound hematoma (1), acromial fracture (2), axillary nerve palsy (1)
Levy et al[27] (2007)	19	Revision of hemiarthroplasty	35 mo	49.7°/76.1°	42.2°/77.2°	—	29.1/61.2 (ASES)	Failed polyethylene (2), periprosthetic humeral fracture (1), humeral loosening (2), periprosthetic scapular fracture (2), baseplate loosening (2), infection (1), hematoma (1)

(continued)

Table 9

Revision Reverse Shoulder Arthroplasty (continued)

Study (Year)	Number of Patients	Procedure And/or Pathology (Number of Patients)	Average Follow-up	Preoperative/Postoperative Range of Motion			Preoperative/ Postoperative Outcome Scores[a]	Complications
				Forward Flexion	Abduction	External Rotation		
Levy et al[28] (2007)	29	Revision of hemiarthroplasty	35 mo	38.1°/72.7°	34.1°/70.4°	11.2°/17.6°	22.3/52.1 (ASES)	Periprosthetic fracture (1), polyethylene fracture (4), polyethylene dissociation (1), dislocation (4), infection (1), failed baseplate/broken screws (1), humeral stem loosening (1), radial nerve palsy (1)
Cuff et al[30] (2008)	96	Rotator cuff deficiency (70) Rotator cuff deficiency with arthroplasty (23) Proximal humeral nonunion (3)	27.5 mo	63.5°/118°	61°/109.5°	13.4°/28.2°	30/77.6 (ASES)	Dislocation (2), traumatic dislocation (2), traumatic acromial fracture (1), infection (2), hematoma (1), glenoid loosening (1)
Holcomb et al[85] (2009)	14	Reverse shoulder arthroplasty	33 mo	51°/118°	38°/112°	8°/22°	23/70 (ASES)	Glenoid failure (1), dislocation (1), hematoma (1)
Chacon et al[29] (2009)	25	Revision of hemiarthroplasty with allograft	30 mo	33°/82°	40°/82°	10°/18°	32/69 (ASES)	Recurrent instability (1), acromial fracture (1), allograft fracture (1), allograft and polyethylene fracture (1)
Walker et al[86] (2011)	22	Revision of failed total shoulder arthroplasty	40 mo	50°/130°	45°/100°	12.5°/49.5°	38.5/67.5 (ASES)	Scapula fracture (1), acromial fracture (1), dislocation (1), glenoid loosening (1), glenoid and humeral loosening (1)

Melis et al[87] (2011)	37	Conversion of total shoulder arthroplasty to reverse shoulder arthroplasty	47 mo	68°/121°	—	—	24/55 (Constant)	Glenoid loosening (3), instability (3), humeral subsidence (2), infection (2), hematoma (1)
Merolla et al[88] (2018)	157	Revision of failed hemiarthroplasty	49 mo	—	47°/108°	13°/27°	–/60 (ASES) Implant survivorship 93.3% at 5 yr	Glenoid component loosening (4), instability (3), humeral component disassembly (1), humeral stem loosening (1) and infection (2)
Stephens et al[89] (2016)	85	Revision of failed reverse	24 mo	74°/97°	71°/91°	22°/25°	46/53 (ASES)	Recurrent instability (2), recurrent infection (1)
Sheth et al[90] (2019)	110	Revision for failed total shoulder arthroplasty	57 mo	—	—	—	–/59 (ASES)	Scapular stress fracture (4), periprosthetic fracture (3), baseplate loosening (2), glenosphere dissociation (2), instability (2), infection (2), painful hardware (1), and greater tuberosity nonunion (1)
		Revision for failed hemiarthroplasty		—	—	—	–/66 (ASES)	

The numbers in parentheses are the total number (N) of patients with the complication.

[a]Measured using the Constant Shoulder Score or American Shoulder and Elbow Surgeons (ASES) Index.

Table 10

Reverse Shoulder Arthroplasty in Young Patients

Study (Year)	Number of Patients	Average Follow-up	Preoperative/Postoperative Range of Motion: Forward Flexion	Abduction	External Rotation	Preoperative/Postoperative Outcome Scores[a]	Complications
Muh et al[7] (2013)	67 patients younger than 60 yr	37 mo	55°/134°	—	10°/20°	40/72 (ASES)	Dislocation (5), infection (2), radial/ulnar nerve palsy (1), humeral stress fracture (1)
Ek et al[10] (2013)	46 patients younger than 65 yr	93 mo	72°/119°	67°/112°	27°/26°	34/74 (Constant)	Dislocation (7), infection (5), glenoid loosening (3), polyethylene wear (1), nerve palsy (2), soft-tissue impingement (1), nerve palsy (2), scapula fracture (3), periprosthetic humeral fracture (1)
Black et al[13] (2014)	32 patients younger than 65 yr with revision RSA	56 mo	–/115°	—	–/31°	–/70 (ASES)	Instability (1), glenoid loosening (2), nerve injury (1), hematoma (1), painful glenoid screw (1), scapular fracture (2), posterior rotator cuff deterioration (1)
	33 patients younger than 65 yr with primary RSA	55 mo	–/112°	—	–/35°	–/74 (ASES)	Instability (2), glenoid loosening (1), nerve injury (1), hematoma (1), deltoid rupture (1), scapular fracture (1)
Sameulsen et al[8] (2017)	67 patients younger than 65 yr	36 mo	—	58°/132°	20°/39°	Implant survival 91% at 5 yr	Instability (1), infection (1), hematoma (2), intraoperative glenoid fracture (1)
Ernstbrunner et al[9] (2017)	23 patients younger than 60 yr	11.7 yr	64°/117°	58°/111°	28°/26°	24/59 (Constant)	Dislocation (4), infection (2), glenoid component dissociation (1), stiffness (1), mechanical block (1)
Otto et al[11] (2017)	35 patients younger than 55 yr with revision RSA	62 mo	50°/86°	46°/79°	13°/16°	24/41 (ASES)	Humeral lucency (2), glenoid screw lucency (2), periprosthetic fractures (2), humeral dissociation (1), infection (1), recurrent instability (2)
	32 patients younger than 55 yr with primary RSA		65°/113°	52°/108°	11°/30°	28/59 (ASES)	Scapular fracture (1), symptomatic hardware (1), infection (4)
Leathers et al[14] (2018)	32 patients younger than 65 yr	3 yr	67°/133°	69°/127°	24°/40°	36/72 (ASES)	Radial nerve palsy (1), pneumothorax (1), heterotopic bone formation (1)
	50 patients older than 70 yr	3 yr	81°/117°	71°/110°	24°/27°	41/72 (ASES)	Nerve palsy (1), pneumothorax (1), heterotopic bone formation (1), hematoma (1), infection (2), acromial fracture (2), periprosthetic humeral fracture (2)

The numbers in parentheses are the total number (N) of patients with the complication.

[a]Measured using the Constant Shoulder Score or American Shoulder and Elbow Surgeons (ASES) Index.

SUMMARY

RSA has been historically used to treat rotator cuff deficiency arising from one of several etiologies. Multiple centers have reported on longer term follow-up using RSA implants for a variety of shoulder pathologies. The durability and outcomes seem to be similar to anatomic TSA in long-term studies. Because long-term results have shown successful outcomes, the indications have continued to expand, making RSA the fastest growing orthopaedic implant today. The refinement of implant design and surgical technique has led to the expansion of indications to include many different shoulder pathologies with predictable and reliable clinical outcomes. RSA is also being used in younger, more active patients, but longer follow-up on these patients is necessary to determine the ultimate implant durability in this population.

KEY STUDY POINTS

- RSA has been shown to be successful in a variety of shoulder pathologies in addition to rotator cuff arthropathy.
- Long-term results have shown that RSA is a durable and successful treatment option that has similar results to TSA in similar length follow-up.
- Complications after RSA have been reduced with improved implant design and surgical technique.
- The expanded indications and long-term success have led to RSA being the fastest growing orthopaedic implant today.

Annotated References

1. Grammont PM, Baulot E: Delta shoulder prosthesis for rotator cuff rupture. *Orthopedics* 1993;16(1):65-68.

2. Nyffeler RW, Werner CM, Gerber C: Biomechanical relevance of glenoid component positioning in the reverse Delta III total shoulder prosthesis. *J Shoulder Elbow Surg* 2005;14(5):524-528.

3. Gutiérrez S, Comiskey CA IV, Luo Z-P, Pupello DR, Frankle MA: Range of impingement-free abduction and adduction deficit after reverse shoulder arthroplasty: Hierarchy of surgical and implant-design-related factors. *J Bone Joint Surg Am* 2008;90(12):2606-2615.

4. Gutiérrez S, Levy JC, Lee WE III, Keller TS, Maitland ME: Center of rotation affects abduction range of motion of reverse shoulder arthroplasty. *Clin Orthop Relat Res* 2007;458:78-82.

5. Cuff DJ, Virani NA, Levy J, et al: The treatment of deep shoulder infection and glenohumeral instability with debridement, reverse shoulder arthroplasty and postoperative antibiotics. *J Bone Joint Surg Br* 2008;90(3):336-342.

6. Mercurio M, Castioni D, Ianno B, Gasparini G, Galasso O: Outcomes of revision surgery after periprosthetic shoulder infection: A systematic review. *J Shoulder Elbow Surg* 2019;28:1193-1203.

   A systematic review of 34 studies revealed 754 patients who underwent revision surgery after periprosthetic shoulder infections. *Cutibacterium acnes* was the most common microorganism seen. RSA had a lower prevalence of infection. Eradication rate was 96% with 1-stage, 93% with permanent spacers, 86% with 2-stage, 85% with resection arthroplasty, and 65% with irrigation and débridement alone. One-stage revision is recommended for periprosthetic shoulder infections with 2-stage procedures reserved for select cases in which the bacteria are unknown. Level of evidence: IV.

7. Muh SJ, Streit JJ, Wanner JP, et al: Early follow-up of reverse total shoulder arthroplasty in patients sixty years of age of younger. *J Bone Joint Surg* 2013;95:1877-1883.

   There were 67 RSA in patients younger than 60 years (mean 52.2 years) with a mean follow-up of 36.5 months. There were significant improvements in range of motion and functional outcomes. Patient satisfaction was determined by postoperative forward elevation greater than 100°. There was a 15% complication rate, including five dislocations, and a 43% scapular notching rate. seven reoperations (five revisions). Level of evidence: IV.

8. Samuelson BT, Wagner ER, Houdek MT, et al: Primary reverse shoulder arthroplasty in patients 65 years or younger. *J Shoulder Elbow Surg* 2017;26:e13-e17.

   There were 67 RSA in patients younger than 65 years (mean 60 years) with a mean follow-up of 3 years. The revision-free survival was 99% at 2 years and 91% at 5 years. The revision surgery–free survival was 97% and 90%, respectively. There was a 9% complication rate. Patients had improvements in pain, range of motion, and strength. Level of evidence: IV.

9. Ernstbrunner L, Suter A, Catanzaro S, Rahm S, Gerber C: Reverse total shoulder arthroplasty for massive, irreparable rotator cuff tears before the age of 60 years: Long-term results. *J Bone Joint Surg* 2017;99:1721-1729.

   There were 23 patients who underwent RSA at a mean age of 57 years (range, 47 to 59). The mean follow-up was 11.7 years (range, 8 to 19). There were significant improvements in functional outcomes and range of motion, which did not deteriorate beyond 10 years. Notching increased with time. The complication rate was 39% and the failure rate was 9%. Level of evidence: IV.

10. Ek ETH, Neukom L, Catanzaro S, Gerber C: Reverse total shoulder arthroplasty for massive irreparable rotator cuff tears in patients younger than 65 years old: Results after five to fifteen years. *J Shoulder Elbow Surg* 2013;22:1199-1208.

There were 46 RSA performed in patients with a mean age of 60 years (range, 46 to 64) with a mean follow-up of 93 months (range, 60 to 171). There were significant improvements in range of motion and functional outcomes. The complication rate was 37.5% and the failure rate was 15%. The revision surgery rate was 25%. Level of evidence: IV.

11. Otto RJ, Clark RE, Frankle MA: Reverse shoulder arthroplasty in patients younger than 55 years: 2- to 12-year follow-up. *J Shoulder Elbow Surg* 2017;26:792-797.

    There were 67 RSA in patients with a mean age of 47.9 years (range, 21 to 54) with an average follow-up of 62.3 months (range, 24 to 144). There were 32 primary RSA and 35 revision RSA for failed arthroplasty. There were similar degrees of improvements in range of motion and functional outcome between the groups. The complication rate was 22.4% and the revision surgery rate was 13.4%. The revision rate was 8.9% and the implant retention at 12 years was 91%. Level of evidence: IV.

12. Sershon RA, Van Thiel GS, Lin EC, et al: Clinical outcomes of reverse total shoulder arthroplasty in patients aged younger than 60 years. *J Shoulder Elbow Surg* 2014;23:395-400.

    There were 36 RSA in patients with a mean age of 54 years with a mean follow-up of 2.8 years. There were significant improvements in functional outcomes, range of motion, and pain. However, there was a 25% failure rate with an ASES score below 50. Level of evidence: IV.

13. Black EM, Roberts SM, Siegel E, Yannopoulos P, Higgins LD, Warner JJP: Reverse shoulder arthroplasty as salvage for failed prior arthroplasty in patients 65 years of age or younger. *J Shoulder Elbow Surg* 2014;23:1036-1042.

    There were 32 patients who underwent revision RSA for failed arthroplasty with an average of 55.3 months follow-up compared with 33 patients undergoing primary RSA with an average of 54.7 months follow-up. The average age of each group was 59.3 years. Subjective outcomes were worse in the revision group compared with the primary group but still had significant improvements from preoperative. There was a 28.1% complication rate in the revision group compared with 18.2% in the primary group. Level of evidence: III.

14. Leathers MP, Ialenti MN, Feeley BT, Zhang AL, Ma CB: Do younger patients have better results after reverse total shoulder arthroplasty? *J Shoulder Elbow Surg* 2018;27:S24-S28.

    Thirty-two patients younger than 65 years who underwent RSA were compared with 50 patients older than 70 years who underwent RSA. The mean follow-up was 3 years. There was no difference in ASES scores, but there was better range of motion in the younger patients compared with the older group. Complication rates were similar between groups. Level of evidence: III.

15. Klein SM, Dunning P, Mulieri P, Pupello D, Downes K, Frankle MA: Effects of acquired glenoid bone defects on surgical technique and clinical outcomes in reverse shoulder arthroplasty. *J Bone Joint Surg Am* 2010;92(5):1144-1154.

16. Lorenzetti A, Streit JJ, Cabezas AF, et al: Bone graft augmentation for severe glenoid bone loss in primary reverse total shoulder arthroplasty. *JB JS Open Access* 2017;2(3):e0015.

    There were 57 patients treated with RSA and glenoid bone grafting at a mean of 46 months follow-up. There were significant improvements in function, range of motion, and pain. There were four complications (7%) but no baseplate failures. Level of evidence: IV.

17. Jones RB, Wright TW, Zuckerman JD: Reverse total shoulder arthroplasty with structural bone grafting of large glenoid defects. *J Shoulder Elbow Surg* 2016;25:1425-1432.

    Forty-four patients underwent RSA with bulk structural graft for glenoid defects. There were 29 humeral head autografts, 1 iliac crest autograft, and 14 femoral head allografts. There were significant improvements in functional outcome scores. No difference was seen between autografts and allografts. Graft incorporation occurred in 81% of cases and there were six loose baseplates. The total complication rate was 13.6%. Level of evidence: IV.

18. Lopiz Y, Garcia-Fernandez C, Arriaza A, Rizo B, Marcelo H, Marco F: Midterm outcomes of bone grafting in glenoid defects treated with reverse shoulder arthroplasty. *J Shoulder Elbow Surg* 2017;26:1581-1588.

    There were 20 patients who underwent RSA with glenoid bone graft: 13 allografts and 7 autografts. There was a significant improvement in Constant scores at a mean of 26 months follow-up. Graft incorporation occurred in 95% of cases. There was a 20% complication rate with one case of glenoid loosening. Level of evidence: IV.

19. Ernstbrunner L, Werthel JD, Wagner E, Hatta T, Sperling JW, Cofield RH: Glenoid bone grafting in primary reverse total shoulder arthroplasty. *J Shoulder Elbow Surg* 2017;26:1441-1447.

    There were 41 patients who underwent RSA with glenoid bone graft (34 corticocancellous grafts and 7 structural grafts) at a mean of 2.8 years follow-up. There were significant improvements in clinical outcomes, range of motion, and pain. Glenoid incorporation occurred in 78% of patients and there was glenoid lucency present in 18%. None required revision surgery. Level of evidence: IV.

20. Tashjian RZ, Granger E, Chalmers PN: Structural glenoid grafting during primary reverse total shoulder arthroplasty using humeral head autograft. *J Shoulder Elbow Surg* 2018;27:e1-e8.

    There were 14 patients who underwent RSA with a large structural autograft for glenoid defect with a mean 2.6 years follow-up. There were three complications with one baseplate failure. There was 100% incorporation of the grafts. There were significant improvements in functional outcomes with an excellent patient satisfaction. Level of evidence: IV.

21. Kempton LB, Ankerson E, Wiater JM: A complication-based learning curve from 200 reverse shoulder arthroplasties. *Clin Orthop Relat Res* 2011;469(9):2496-2504.

22. Frankle M, Siegal S, Pupello D, Saleem A, Mighell M, Vasey M: The reverse shoulder prosthesis for glenohumeral arthritis associated with severe rotator cuff deficiency: A minimum two-year follow-up study of sixty patients. *J Bone Joint Surg Am* 2005;87(8):1697-1705.

23. Boileau P, Moineau G, Roussanne Y, O'Shea K: Bony increased-offset reversed shoulder arthroplasty: Minimizing scapular impingement while maximizing glenoid fixation. *Clin Orthop Relat Res* 2011;469(9):2558-2567.

24. Simovitch RW, Zumstein MA, Lohri E, Helmy N, Gerber C: Predictors of scapular notching in patients managed with the Delta III reverse total shoulder replacement. *J Bone Joint Surg Am* 2007;89(3):588-600.

25. Guery J, Favard L, Sirveaux F, Oudet D, Mole D, Walch G: Reverse total shoulder arthroplasty: Survivorship analysis of eighty replacements followed for five to ten years. *J Bone Joint Surg Am* 2006;88(8):1742-1747.

26. Mulieri P, Dunning P, Klein S, Pupello D, Frankle M: Reverse shoulder arthroplasty for the treatment of irreparable rotator cuff tear without glenohumeral arthritis. *J Bone Joint Surg Am* 2010;92(15):2544-2556.

27. Levy J, Frankle M, Mighell M, Pupello D: The use of the reverse shoulder prosthesis for the treatment of failed hemiarthroplasty for proximal humeral fracture. *J Bone Joint Surg Am* 2007;89(2):292-300.

28. Levy JC, Virani N, Pupello D, Frankle M: Use of the reverse shoulder prosthesis for the treatment of failed hemiarthroplasty in patients with glenohumeral arthritis and rotator cuff deficiency. *J Bone Joint Surg Br* 2007;89(2):189-195.

29. Chacon A, Virani N, Shannon R, Levy JC, Pupello D, Frankle M: Revision arthroplasty with use of a reverse shoulder prosthesis-allograft composite. *J Bone Joint Surg Am* 2009;91(1):119-127.

30. Cuff D, Pupello D, Virani N, Levy J, Frankle M: Reverse shoulder arthroplasty for the treatment of rotator cuff deficiency. *J Bone Joint Surg Am* 2008;90(6):1244-1251.

31. Valenti P, Sauzières P, Katz D, Kalouche I, Kilinc AS: Do less medialized reverse shoulder prostheses increase motion and reduce notching? *Clin Orthop Relat Res* 2011;469(9):2550-2557.

32. Boileau P, Watkinson D, Hatzidakis AM, Hovorka I: Neer Award 2005: The Grammont reverse shoulder prosthesis: Results in cuff tear arthritis, fracture sequelae, and revision arthroplasty. *J Shoulder Elbow Surg* 2006;15(5):527-540.

33. Simovitch RW, Helmy N, Zumstein MA, Gerber C: Impact of fatty infiltration of the teres minor muscle on the outcome of reverse total shoulder arthroplasty. *J Bone Joint Surg Am* 2007;89(5):934-939.

34. Wall B, Nové-Josserand L, O'Connor DP, Edwards TB, Walch G: Reverse total shoulder arthroplasty: A review of results according to etiology. *J Bone Joint Surg Am* 2007;89(7):1476-1485.

35. Werner CM, Steinmann PA, Gilbart M, Gerber C: Treatment of painful pseudoparesis due to irreparable rotator cuff dysfunction with the Delta III reverse-ball-and-socket total shoulder prosthesis. *J Bone Joint Surg Am* 2005;87(7):1476-1486.

36. Norris TR, Kelly JD, Humphrey CS: Management of glenoid bone defects in revision shoulder arthroplasty: A new application of the reverse total shoulder prosthesis. *Tech Shoulder Elbow Surg* 2007;8:37-46.

37. Gutiérrez S, Keller TS, Levy JC, Lee WE III, Luo Z-P: Hierarchy of stability factors in reverse shoulder arthroplasty. *Clin Orthop Relat Res* 2008;466(3):670-676.

38. Terrier A, Reist A, Merlini F, Farron A: Simulated joint and muscle forces in reversed and anatomic shoulder prostheses. *J Bone Joint Surg Br* 2008;90(6):751-756.

39. Boulahia A, Edwards TB, Walch G, Baratta RV: Early results of a reverse design prosthesis in the treatment of arthritis of the shoulder in elderly patients with a large rotator cuff tear. *Orthopedics* 2002;25(2):129-133.

40. Rittmeister M, Kerschbaumer F: Grammont reverse total shoulder arthroplasty in patients with rheumatoid arthritis and nonreconstructible rotator cuff lesions. *J Shoulder Elbow Surg* 2001;10(1):17-22.

41. Delloye C, Joris D, Colette A, Eudier A, Dubuc JE: Mechanical complications of total shoulder inverted prosthesis. *Rev Chir Orthop Reparatrice Appar Mot* 2002;88(4):410-414.

42. Frankle MA, Siegal S, Pupello DR, Gutierrez S, Griewe M, Mighell M: Coronal plane tilt angle affects risk of catastrophic failure in patients treated with a reverse shoulder prosthesis. *J Shoulder Elbow Surg* 2007;16:e46.

43. Seebauer L, Walter W, Keyl W: Reverse total shoulder arthroplasty for the treatment of defect arthropathy. *Oper Orthop Traumatol* 2005;17(1):1-24.

44. Sirveaux F, Favard L, Oudet D, Huquet D, Walch G, Molé D: Grammont inverted total shoulder arthroplasty in the treatment of glenohumeral osteoarthritis with massive rupture of the cuff: Results of a multicentre study of 80 shoulders. *J Bone Joint Surg Br* 2004;86(3):388-395.

45. Gutiérrez S, Walker M, Willis M, Pupello DR, Frankle MA: Effects of tilt and glenosphere eccentricity on baseplate/bone interface forces in a computational model, validated by a mechanical model, of reverse shoulder arthroplasty. *J Shoulder Elbow Surg* 2011;20(5):732-739.

46. Harman M, Frankle M, Vasey M, Banks S: Initial glenoid component fixation in "reverse" total shoulder arthroplasty: A biomechanical evaluation. *J Shoulder Elbow Surg* 2005;14(1 suppl):S162-S167.

47. Melis B, DeFranco M, Lädermann A, et al: An evaluation of the radiological changes around the Grammont reverse geometry shoulder arthroplasty after eight to 12 years. *J Bone Joint Surg Br* 2011;93(9):1240-1246.

48. Young AA, Smith MM, Bacle G, Moraga C, Walch G: Early results of reverse shoulder arthroplasty in patients with rheumatoid arthritis. *J Bone Joint Surg Am* 2011;93(20):1915-1923.

49. Lévigne C, Boileau P, Favard L, et al: Scapular notching in reverse shoulder arthroplasty. *J Shoulder Elbow Surg* 2008;17(6):925-935.

50. Frankle MA, Teramoto A, Luo Z-P, Levy JC, Pupello D: Glenoid morphology in reverse shoulder arthroplasty: Classification and surgical implications. *J Shoulder Elbow Surg* 2009;18(6):874-885.

51. Cox JL, McLendon PB, Christmas KN, Simon P, Mighell MA, Frankle MA: Clinical outcomes following reverse shoulder arthroplasty-allograft composite for revision of failed arthroplasty associated with proximal humeral bone deficiency: 2- to 15- year follow-up. *J Shoulder Elbow Surg* 2019;28:900-907.

There were 73 patients treated with RSA and proximal humeral allograft for proximal humeral bone loss with an average follow-up of 67.9 months. There were significant improvements in simple shoulder test and ASES scores. Total revision was required in 19% of patients (only two revisions for humeral loosening). The revision surgery–free survival rate of all reconstructions was 88% at 5 years, 78% at 10 years, and 67% beyond 10 years. Level of evidence: IV.

52. Cuff D, Levy JC, Gutiérrez S, Frankle MA: Torsional stability of modular and non-modular reverse shoulder humeral components in a proximal humeral bone loss model. *J Shoulder Elbow Surg* 2011;20(4):646-651.

53. Boileau P, Chuinard C, Roussanne Y, Bicknell RT, Rochet N, Trojani C: Reverse shoulder arthroplasty combined with a modified latissimus dorsi and teres major tendon transfer for shoulder pseudoparalysis associated with dropping arm. *Clin Orthop Relat Res* 2008;466(3):584-593.

54. Boileau P, Chuinard C, Roussanne Y, Neyton L, Trojani C: Modified latissimus dorsi and teres major transfer through a single delto-pectoral approach for external rotation deficit of the shoulder: As an isolated procedure or with a reverse arthroplasty. *J Shoulder Elbow Surg* 2007;16(6):671-682.

55. Boileau P, Rumian AP, Zumstein MA: Reversed shoulder arthroplasty with modified L'Episcopo for combined loss of active elevation and external rotation. *J Shoulder Elbow Surg* 2010;19(2 suppl):20-30.

56. Gerber C, Pennington SD, Lingenfelter EJ, Sukthankar A: Reverse Delta-III total shoulder replacement combined with latissimus dorsi transfer: A preliminary report. *J Bone Joint Surg Am* 2007;89(5):940-947.

57. Favard L, Levigne C, Nerot C, Gerber C, De Wilde L, Mole D: Reverse prostheses in arthropathies with cuff tear: Are survivorship and function maintained over time? *Clin Orthop Relat Res* 2011;469(9):2469-2475.

58. Bacle G, Nové-Josserand L, Garaud P, Walch G: Long-term outcomes of reverse total shoulder arthroplasty: A follow-up of a previous study. *J Bone Joint Surg Am* 2017;99:454-461.

There were 84 patients (87 RSA) evaluated for a minimum of 10 years follow-up. The mean follow-up was 150 months. There was a significant decrease in Constant scores at final follow-up compared with midterm results. There was a 29% complication rate and a 73% scapular notching rate. The 10-year overall survival rate with revision as the end point was 93%. Level of evidence: IV.

59. Bassens D, Decock T, Van Tongel A, De Wilde L: Long-term results of the Delta Xtend reverse shoulder prosthesis. *J Shoulder Elbow Surg* 2019;28:1091-1097.

There were 74 RSA with follow-up of at least 8 years with a mean follow-up of 113.1 months. There was a significant improvement in Constant scores at 5 years (91.1%), but this was significantly lower at the final follow-up (79.9%). This is represented by decreased range of motion and power. The overall survival rate was 97% at 8 years. Level of evidence: IV.

60. Gerber C, Canonica S, Catanzaro S, Ernstbrunner L: Longitudinal observational study of reverse total shoulder arthroplasty for irreparable rotator cuff dysfunction: Results after 15 years. *J Shoulder Elbow Surg* 2018;27:831-838.

There were 22 patients who underwent RSA with a minimum of 15-year follow-up. The mean follow-up was 16.1 years. The mean Constant score was significantly improved at final follow-up. There were also significant improvements in range of motion, pain, and subjective shoulder value, with no deterioration over 15 years. However, there was a substantial complication rate and failure rate in this population. The complication rate was 59%. There was a 55% reoperation rate and a 45% revision rate. Level of evidence: IV.

61. Cuff DJ, Pupello DR, Santoni BG, Clark RE, Frankle MA: Reverse shoulder arthroplasty for the treatment of rotator cuff deficiency: A concise follow-up, at a minimum of 10 years, of previous reports. *J Bone Joint Surg Am* 2017;99:1895-1899.

There were 42 RSA (40 patients) available for minimum 10-year follow-up. The average follow-up was 132 months. Patients had improvements in ASES and simple shoulder test scores for up to 5 years and these improvements were maintained at the latest follow-up of at least 10 years. The implant survivorship was 97% at 2 years, 94% at 5 years, and 90.7% at 10 years. Level of evidence: IV.

62. Bufquin T, Hersan A, Hubert L, Massin P: Reverse shoulder arthroplasty for the treatment of three- and four-part fractures of the proximal humerus in the elderly: A prospective review of 43 cases with a short-term follow-up. *J Bone Joint Surg Br* 2007;89(4):516-520.

63. Klein M, Juschka M, Hinkenjann B, Scherger B, Ostermann PA: Treatment of comminuted fractures of the proximal humerus in elderly patients with the Delta III reverse shoulder prosthesis. *J Orthop Trauma* 2008;22(10):698-704.

64. Gallinet D, Clappaz P, Garbuio P, Tropet Y, Obert L: Three or four parts complex proximal humerus fractures: Hemiarthroplasty versus reverse prosthesis. A comparative study of 40 cases. *Orthop Traumatol Surg Res* 2009;95(1):48-55.

65. Cazeneuve JF, Cristofari DJ: The reverse shoulder prosthesis in the treatment of fractures of the proximal humerus in the elderly. *J Bone Joint Surg Br* 2010;92(4):535-539.

66. Lenarz C, Shishani Y, McCrum C, Nowinski RJ, Edwards TB, Gobezie R: Is reverse shoulder arthroplasty appropriate for the treatment of fractures in the older patient? Early observations. *Clin Orthop Relat Res* 2011;469(12):3324-3331.

67. Ross M, Hope B, Stokes A, Peters SE, McLeod I, Duke PFR: Reverse shoulder arthroplasty for the treatment of three-part and four-part proximal humeral fractures in the elderly. *J Shoulder Elbow Surg* 2015;24:215-222.

    RSA was used for three-part and four-part proximal humerus fractures in 29 shoulders (28 patients) at an average follow-up of 54.9 months. Patients had good clinical and radiographic outcomes and there were no revisions. There was one axillary nerve palsy that resolved at 12 months. Level of evidence: IV.

68. Grubhofer F, Wieser K, Meyer DC, et al: Reverse total shoulder arthroplasty for acute head-splitting, 3- and 4-part fractures of the proximal humerus in the elderly. *J Shoulder Elbow Surg* 2016;25:1690-1698.

    RSA was used to treat 52 fractures (51 patients) at a mean age of 77 years with acute proximal humerus fractures. The mean follow-up was 35 months. There were four revisions. Patients had significant clinical improvements with Constant scores and subjective shoulder value. Patients with resected or secondarily displaced greater tuberosities had inferior clinical outcomes compared with healed tuberosities. Level of evidence: IV.

69. Shannon SF, Wagner ER, Houdek MT, Cross WW III, Sanchez-Sotelo J: Reverse shoulder arthroplasty for proximal humeral fractures: Outcomes comparing primary reverse arthroplasty for fracture versus reverse arthroplasty after failed osteosynthesis. *J Shoulder Elbow Surg* 2016;25:1655-1660.

    There were 18 patients who underwent RSA for acute fracture and 26 patients who underwent RSA after failed open reduction and internal fixation with a mean of 3 years follow-up. There was no difference in clinical outcomes with ASES scores or range of motion. Salvage RSA had a higher complication rate compared with primary RSA (8% versus 5%). Level of evidence: III.

70. Chun YM, Kim DS, Lee DH, Shin SJ: Reverse shoulder arthroplasty for four-part proximal humerus fracture in elderly patients: Can a healed tuberosity improve the functional outcomes? *J Shoulder Elbow Surg* 2017;26:1216-1221.

    Thirty-eight patients underwent RSA for four-part proximal humerus fractures. There were 14 patients with healed tuberosities and 24 patients with unhealed tuberosities. There was no difference in visual analog scale score, ASES score, Constant score, or forward elevation and internal rotation. However, there was a significant difference in external rotation, with healed tuberosities providing better postoperative external rotation. Level of evidence: III.

71. Boileau P, Alta TD, Decroocq L, et al: Reverse shoulder arthroplasty for acute fractures in the elderly: Is it worth reattaching the tuberosities? *J Shoulder Elbow Surg* 2019;28:437-444.

    Thirty-eight patients with an average age of 80 ± 4 years were treated with RSA for three-part and four-part proximal humerus fractures with an average follow-up of 36 ± 8 months. The tuberosity healing rate was 84%. Patients with healed tuberosities had improved forward elevation, external rotation, and patient satisfaction. Level of evidence: III.

72. Raiss P, Edwards TB, da Silva MR, Bruckner T, Loew M, Walch G: Reverse shoulder arthroplasty for the treatment of nonunions of the surgical neck of the proximal part of the humerus (type-3 fracture sequelae). *J Bone Joint Surg Am* 2014;96:2070-2076.

    There were 32 patients treated with RSA for proximal humerus nonunion with an average age of 68 years and a mean follow-up of 4 years. There was a significant improvement in Constant scores, flexion, and external rotation. There was a 41% complication rate leading to nine revisions (28%). The most common complication was dislocation (11 patients; 34%). Level of evidence: IV.

73. Raiss P, Edwards TB, Collin P, et al: Reverse shoulder arthroplasty for malunions of the proximal part of the humerus (type-4 fracture sequelae). *J Bone Joint Surg Am* 2016;98:893-899.

    There were 42 patients treated with RSA for proximal humerus malunions at an average age of 68 years and a mean follow-up of 4 years. There were significant improvements in Constant scores, active flexion, and external rotation. There was a 9.5% complication rate and a 98% satisfaction rate. Level of evidence: IV.

74. Dezfuli B, King JJ, Farmer KW, Struk AM, Wright TW: Outcomes of reverse total shoulder arthroplasty as primary versus revision procedure for proximal humerus fractures. *J Shoulder Elbow Surg* 2016;25:1133-1137.

    There were 49 patients who underwent RSA with proximal humerus fractures: 13 for acute fracture, 13 for malunion or nonunion, 12 for failed hemiarthroplasty, and 11 for failed open reduction and internal fixation. There were significant improvements in clinical outcomes and range of motion. The acute fracture group and fracture sequelae groups performed better than the failed hemiarthroplasty group. Level of evidence: III.

75. Grubhofer F, Wieser K, Meyer DC, Catanzaro S, Schürholz K, Gerber C: Reverse total shoulder arthroplasty for failed open reduction and internal fixation of fractures of the proximal humerus. *J Shoulder Elbow Surg* 2017;26:92-100.

    There were 54 fractures (53 patients) who underwent RSA for failed open reduction and internal fixation of a proximal humerus fracture. The mean follow-up was 46 months. There was a significant improvement in Constant scores, subjective shoulder value, and patient satisfaction. There was a 9% revision rate. Level of evidence: IV.

76. Sanchez-Sotelo J, Wagner ER, Sim FH, Houdek MT: Allograft-prosthetic composite reconstruction for massive proximal humeral bone loss in reverse shoulder arthroplasty. *J Bone Joint Surg Am* 2017;99:2069-2076.

    There were 26 patients who underwent RSA with allograft reconstruction for proximal humeral bone loss with an average follow-up of 4 years. There were improvements in pain, elevation, and external rotation. No difference was seen between primary and revision cases. There was one patient with delayed union at the graft site requiring bone grafting. The 2- and 5-year revision-free survival rate was 96%. Level of evidence: IV.

77. Werner BS, Böhm D, Abdelkawi A, Gohlke F: Glenoid bone grafting in reverse shoulder arthroplasty for long-standing anterior shoulder dislocation. *J Shoulder Elbow Surg* 2014;23:1655-1661.

    Twenty-one patients underwent RSA and anterior glenoid bone grafting for chronic anterior dislocation with a mean follow-up of 4.9 years. There were significant improvements in Constant scores. Two patients underwent revision because of baseplate loosening. Level of evidence: IV.

78. Kurowicki J, Triplet JJ, Momoh E, Moor MA, Levy JC: Reverse shoulder prosthesis in the treatment of locked anterior shoulders: A comparison with classic reverse shoulder indications. *J Shoulder Elbow Surg* 2016;25:1954-1960.

    Twenty-four patients underwent RSA for locked anterior dislocation compared to 48 controls with an average of 25.5 months follow-up. There were significant improvements in both groups in pain, function, and outcome scores. However, range of motion and functional outcomes were better in the control group compared with the locked anterior dislocation group. There were two patients in the anterior dislocation group who remained dislocated. Level of evidence: III.

79. Cuff DJ, Santoni BG: Anatomic total shoulder arthroplasty versus reverse total shoulder arthroplasty for post-capsulorrhaphy arthropathy. *Orthopedics* 2018;41(5):275-280.

    There were 19 TSA and 20 RSA used in patients with post-capsulorrhaphy arthropathy with a mean of 59.5 months and 43.8 months follow-up, respectively. There was no difference between the groups in functional outcomes. Forward elevation was better in the TSA group. However, the TSA group was less satisfied (84% versus 95%) and had a higher complication rate (21% versus 10%) and revision rate (16% versus zero) compared with the RSA group. Level of evidence: III.

80. Patel MK, Stone WZ, Struk AM, Farmer KW, Wright TW, King JJ: Shoulder arthroplasty after prior anterior stabilization procedures: Do reverses have better outcomes? *J Shoulder Elbow Surg* 2019;28:854-860.

    There were 15 TSA and 10 RSA after previous anterior stabilization procedures with an average follow-up of 3.3 and 4 years, respectively. RSA patients had greater improvements in range of motion, except internal rotation, and better ASES scores compared with TSA. TSA had a complication rate of 33% and a revision surgery rate of 20%. There were no complications or revision surgeries in the RSA group. Level of evidence: III.

81. Hasler A, Fornaciari P, Jungwirth-Weinberger A, Jentzsch T, Wieser K, Gerber C: Reverse shoulder arthroplasty in the treatment of glenohumeral instability. *J Shoulder Elbow Surg* 2019;28(8):1587-1594. doi:10.1016/j.jse.2019.02.001.

    There were 11 patients treated with RSA for instability matched to 22 patients treated with RSA for rotator cuff insufficiency. The median follow-up was 74 months. No significant difference was found between the groups in satisfaction, Constant scores, or complication rates. Range of motion was better in the control group but not statistically significant. Postoperative instability was not observed in either group. Level of evidence: III.

82. Mizuno N, Denard PJ, Raiss P, Walch G: Reverse total shoulder arthroplasty for primary glenohumeral osteoarthritis in patients with a biconcave glenoid. *J Bone Joint Surg Am* 2013;95:1297-1304.

    There were 27 RSA performed in patients with glenohumeral arthritis and a biconcave glenoid with a mean follow-up of 54 months. There was a significant improvement in Constant scores and range of motion. Complications occurred in 15% of patients with glenoid loosening in one patient. Scapular notching occurred in 37% of patients. There was no recurrence of posterior instability. Level of evidence: IV.

83. Steen BM, Cabezas AF, Santoni BG, et al: Outcome and value of reverse shoulder arthroplasty for treatment of glenohumeral osteoarthritis: A matched cohort. *J Shoulder Elbow Surg* 2015;24:1433-1441.

    Twenty-four patients who underwent RSA for glenohumeral osteoarthritis were compared with 96 patients who underwent TSA. Glenoid wear pattern, arthritis grade, and rotator cuff muscle quality were similar between groups. However, there was greater retroversion in the RSA group. Postoperative functional outcome scores were similar between groups. Five patients who underwent TSA had radiographic glenoid loosening. Patients were converted to RSA intraoperatively if there was improper glenoid component seating or persistent posterior subluxation. Level of evidence: III.

84. Holcomb JO, Hebert DJ, Mighell MA, et al: Reverse shoulder arthroplasty in patients with rheumatoid arthritis. *J Shoulder Elbow Surg* 2010;19(7):1076-1084.

85. Holcomb JO, Cuff D, Petersen SA, Pupello DR, Frankle MA: Revision reverse shoulder arthroplasty for glenoid baseplate failure after primary reverse shoulder arthroplasty. *J Shoulder Elbow Surg* 2009;18(5):717-723.

86. Walker M, Willis MP, Brooks JP, Pupello D, Mulieri PJ, Frankle MA: The use of the reverse shoulder arthroplasty for treatment of failed total shoulder arthroplasty. *J Shoulder Elbow Surg* 2012;21(4):514-522.

87. Melis B, Bonnevialle N, Neyton L, et al: Glenoid loosening and failure in anatomical total shoulder arthroplasty: Is revision with a reverse shoulder arthroplasty a reliable option? *J Shoulder Elbow Surg* 2012;21(3):342-349.

88. Merolla G, Wagner E, Sperling JW, Paladini P, Fabbri E, Porcellini G: Revision of failed shoulder hemiarthroplasty to reverse total arthroplasty: Analysis of 157 revision implants. *J Shoulder Elbow Surg* 2018;27:75-81.

There were 157 patients who underwent RSA for failed hemiarthroplasty with a mean of 49 months follow-up. Patients had significant improvements in functional outcome scores, pain, and range of motion. There were 11 revisions (7%) and the implant survivorship was 95.5% at 2 years and 93.3% at 5 years. Level of evidence: IV.

89. Stephens BC, Simon P, Clark RE, et al: Revision for a failed reverse: A 12-year review of a lateralized implant. *J Shoulder Elbow Surg* 2016;25:e115-e124.

There were 85 patients out of 1418 RSA who required return to the operating room for removal or exchange of components. The overall revision rate was 6%. The highest revision rate was for patients who had RSA for failed hemiarthroplasty (10%). Revision for baseplate failure was 2.5%. After a modification to the baseplate, this rate reduced to 0.3%. Range of motion and functional outcomes improved. Level of evidence: IV.

90. Sheth MM, Sholder D, Getz CL, Williams GR, Namdari S: Revision of failed hemiarthroplasty and anatomic total shoulder arthroplasty to reverse total shoulder arthroplasty. *J Shoulder Elbow Surg* 2019;28:1074-1081.

There were 110 patients who underwent revision RSA for failed shoulder arthroplasty with a mean follow-up of 57 months. Implant survival was 92% at 2 years and 74% at 5 years. There were modest improvements in pain, satisfaction, and functional outcomes. The complication rate was 20% and the reoperation rate was 11%. Level of evidence: IV.

Chapter 27

Complications of Reverse Shoulder Arthroplasty

Stephanie Muh, MD • Reuben Gobezie, MD

ABSTRACT

Understanding the complications associated with reverse total shoulder arthroplasty is critical with increasing utilization and expanding indications. Common intraoperative and postoperative complications, current treatment options, long-term outcomes, and future needs are discussed.

Keywords: complications; fracture; infection; reverse total shoulder; survivorship

Introduction

Long-term projections show that the demand for all types of shoulder arthroplasty will continue to increase.[1-4] As the indications for reverse shoulder arthroplasty (RSA) have expanded, the number of associated complications has grown. Overall complication rates of 11% to 50% have been reported after RSA.[5-11] Complication rates after primary RSA are higher than those for conventional primary total shoulder arthroplasty, and an even higher complication rate is reported after revision RSA, reaching of up to 69% in some cohorts.[7,9-13] The complications that are typically associated with RSA are related to the nonanatomic design of the prosthesis, its use in patients with abnormal morphology, and the surgeon's level of experience with RSA.[14,15] Higher complication and mortality rates were found to occur if the surgeon performs a relatively small number of shoulder arthroplasties.[11,12] Furthermore, severely obese patients, or those with a body mass index (BMI) greater than 35 kg/m^2, have also shown to have higher rates of complication after RSA.[10,11] The most common complications associated with RSA include joint infection, neurologic injury, instability, scapular notching, fracture, and baseplate failure.

Dr. Muh or an immediate family member serves as a paid consultant to or is an employee of DePuy, a Johnson & Johnson Company, Exactech, Inc., and FX Shoulder. Dr. Gobezie or an immediate family member has received royalties from Arthrex, Inc.; is a member of a speakers' bureau or has made paid presentations on behalf of Arthrex, Inc.; serves as a paid consultant to or is an employee of Arthrex, Inc.; has received research or institutional support from Arthrex, Inc.; serves as a board member, owner, officer, or committee member of Arthroscopy Association of North America, American Academy of Orthopaedic Surgeons, American Shoulder & Elbow Society and OREF.

Intraoperative Complications

Neurologic Injury

The reported incidence of neurologic injury after RSA ranges from 1% to 10%, but the injury often resolves spontaneously.[5,16-19] During RSA, moving the center of rotation more medially and distally lengthens the involved arm and tensions the brachial plexus.[20,21] The symptoms of neurologic injury vary from transitory pain to persistent dysesthesia and may include a catastrophic loss of shoulder function, particularly in a patient with a lesion of the axillary nerve.

A cadaver study found that nerve damage was related to the amount of strain of the brachial plexus.[20] The authors note that in rat models, an 8% lengthening of the sciatic nerve was critical for initiating blood flow arrest, and complete arrest of blood flow occurred at 15% of strain. It can be assumed that lengthening of other nerves can result in similar loss of vascularity. The cadaver study found that the brachial plexus sustained a large strain after RSA (as much as 19.3%). This finding suggests that lengthening caused by RSA may be a factor leading to brachial plexus injury in some patients.

A combination of intraoperative traction, limb manipulation, and lengthening of the arm necessitated by the nonanatomic design of the prosthesis contributes to the risk of neurologic injury. In a prospective study of 19 patients with primary RSA, 9 patients had subclinical electromyographic changes primarily involving the axillary nerve.[22] Compared with anatomic total shoulder arthroplasty, RSA led to an increased relative risk of 10.9 for postoperative nerve injury. The treated arm was lengthened a mean of 2.7 cm in RSA. However, eight of the nine nerve lesions spontaneously resolved within 6 months. A prospective study of intraoperative nerve injury in shoulder arthroplasty found a 56.7% incidence of nerve dysfunction or so-called nerve alerts during surgery.[23] Although none of the nerve alerts returned to baseline after retractor removal, most of these nerve alerts (76.7%) returned to baseline after the arm was repositioned into a neutral position from extreme external rotation, extension, abduction, or adduction for glenoid preparation. There was also a higher incidence of postoperative nerve dysfunction in patients with a history of previous open shoulder surgery and decreased motion (less than 10° passive external rotation with the elbow at the side). The researchers concluded that extreme arm positions should be minimized and patients with decreased motion and previous open surgery are at higher risk for neurologic injury.

Intraoperative Fracture

Intraoperative glenoid fracture is a rare but disastrous complication related to reaming and initial implant fixation. The common causes of glenoid fracture include a failure to start the reamer before making contact with the glenoid bone and during insertion of component if the baseplate is not inserted strictly in-line with prepared bone. Poor quality bone and severe glenoid erosion can contribute to glenoid fracture as well. Small fractures of the peripheral rim often can be ignored because they have no effect on stable fixation of the glenosphere. However, larger glenoid fractures that extend to the central portion are more problematic. Stable fixation of the glenoid, by augmented baseplate fixation or grafting, must be achieved before inserting the glenosphere. If a central screw baseplate design is used, the screw can be repositioned within the glenoid to achieve a similar outcome. If sufficient stability cannot be achieved, the RSA may need to be converted to a hemiarthroplasty.

Iatrogenic humeral fracture is the most common humeral complication. Patients often have osteopenia that places them at risk for fracture. The risk can be minimized by limiting the amount of torque placed on the humerus and maintaining awareness of humeral position during preparation, especially during instrumentation or reaming of the humeral canal when the arm is in an extended, adducted, and externally rotated position. A fracture at the humeral diaphysis should be reduced, and a long-stem humeral prosthesis can be placed. The radial nerve should be identified when a plate and cerclage wires are used for fracture reduction and fixation.

Postoperative Complications

Infection

Infection can be a devastating complication of RSA. A delay in diagnosis can lead to chronic pain, instability, poor functional motion, sepsis, or the need for extensive revision surgery. The reported rate of infection after conventional total shoulder arthroplasty is approximately 0.7%, but infection rates associated with RSA range from 1% to 15%.[6,8,17,24-27] Infection usually is related to a breach in sterile technique, postoperative hematoma formation, prolonged surgical time, or revision surgery. Not surprisingly, patients with a comorbidity, such as diabetes, inflammatory arthropathy, or another immunosuppressive disorder, are at an increased risk for infection. Patients undergoing revision surgery also are at increased risk for infection.

The diagnosis of infection in shoulder arthroplasty is challenging. The indolent nature of common shoulder pathogens leads to symptoms that usually are nonspecific in nature with pain being the primary report. *Cutibacterium acnes* (formerly known as *Propionibacterium acnes*), *Staphylococcus epidermidis*, and *Staphylococcus aureus* are common sources of infection related to shoulder surgery.[25] *C acnes* is the most common cause of infection after shoulder arthroplasty.[26,27] *C acnes* is a low virulent gram-positive, aerotolerant, non–spore-forming, anaerobic bacillus commonly found in normal flora of healthy skin and the sebaceous glands. There is an increased presence of *C acnes* around the shoulder and acromion higher than other regions of the body such as the hip or knee.[27] Successful diagnosis and treatment of *C acnes* infection remains challenging because of its low virulence. A patient with *C acnes* infection may report chronic nonspecific complaints, and laboratory values often are normal. Standard laboratory tests, such as C-reactive protein (CRP) level, erythrocyte sedimentation rate (ESR), and white blood cell counts, are routinely done but often are nondiagnostic for periprosthetic infection.[28,29]

In a retrospective review of 19 shoulder arthroplasties with confirmed periprosthetic infection, the optimized ESR cutoff (26 mm/hr) for detecting shoulder arthroplasty infection was found to have a sensitivity of 32% and specificity of 93%.[30] The optimized cutoff level for CRP (7 mg/L) had a sensitivity of 63% and specificity of 73%. The researchers concluded that ESR and CRP level had poor sensitivity for the diagnosis of shoulder implant infection.

Newer biochemical markers, including interleukin-6, tumor necrosis factor-α, and procalcitonin-C, have been investigated as diagnostic tools but have shown inconsistent results to aid in the diagnosis of infection. Alpha defensin testing of synovial fluid has been shown to have a sensitivity of 63% to 75% and specificity of 95% to 96% in predicting infection.[31,32] A sonication technique for the diagnosis of prosthetic shoulder infection was proposed as having better sensitivity and similar specificity compared with traditional intraoperative tissue culturing, but so far results are unreliable.[33] Adding to the difficulty of diagnosis is the relatively long incubation period needed to culture the organism; the average time for culture was reported to be 13.3 days (range, 4 to 21 days).[34] Next-generation sequencing has also been recently investigated as a way to improve diagnosis of periprosthetic joint infections.[35]

Perioperative infection prevention is critical. Perioperative antibiotics should be prophylactically administered within 1 hour of incision. A chlorhexidine scrub was found to be the most effective means of eliminating coagulase-negative *Staphylococcus* and *Cutibacterium* from the shoulder region.[36] Long surgical time also has been identified as a risk factor for infection.[37] The use of antibiotic-loaded bone cement was found to reduce the rate of deep infection in primary RSA compared with cement without antibiotics.[38] Some evidence suggests that hematoma formation in the dead space associated with RSA is a risk factor for infection.[39] Therefore, it is important to avoid postoperative hematoma formation by meticulous intraoperative hemostasis and consider the use postoperative placement of a drain.

The management of postoperative infection after RSA is similar to that after other total joint arthroplasty procedures. Several authors have noted that early administration of organism-specific antibiotics plays an important role in eradicating infection.[40] The current surgical treatment options include irrigation and débridement, antibiotic suppression, one-stage or two-stage revision surgery, resection arthroplasty, and arthrodesis.[41,42] Acute infection (of less than 6 weeks' duration) can be successfully managed with aggressive débridement, intravenous antibiotics, and polyethylene exchange, or with a single-stage reimplantation.[40,43,44] The best management of a chronic infection (of more than 3 months' duration) is controversial. The evidence is conflicting regarding the efficacy of one-stage and two-stage revision procedures for eradicating chronic infection.[40,42-45] Most experience has been with two-stage revision, in keeping with recommendations found in the lower extremity arthroplasty literature. The most reproducible results in terms of functional outcomes and infection eradication were found with a two-stage revision consisting of aggressive débridement, prosthesis removal, and the placement of a polymethyl methacrylate spacer, followed by 6 weeks of intravenous antibiotics and reimplantation.[41,45] Resection arthroplasty has been used for patients who are unable to undergo surgical reimplantation or have been unsuccessfully treated with every other option. Resection arthroplasty provides reasonable pain relief but limits postoperative function.

Scapular Notching

Scapular notching, first described in 1997, is a radiographic finding associated only with RSA (**Figure 1**). Scapular notching occurs when the medial edge of the humeral socket impinges on the inferior border of the glenoid. The incidence of scapular notching varies with the implant design. The incidence with the traditional Grammont-style RSA implant ranges from 19% to 96%.[6-8,17,19,46-48] Newer RSA implants with a lateral center of rotation and lateralized humerus appear to have a decreased incidence of scapular notching, with a range of zero to 16%.[24,46,49] Other factors, such as surgical approach, glenosphere positioning, native scapular anatomy (scapular neck length, glenoid erosion, and scapular neck angle), prosthesis neck angle, and patient activity level, also have been implicated in the development of scapular notching.[48,50,51] A biomechanical study of factors that cause impingement on the inferior scapular neck found that a relatively varus humeral component neck-shaft angle, inferior position of the glenosphere, and large glenosphere center-of-rotation offset were important in decreasing impingement.[51,52]

The diagnosis of scapular notching is made radiographically with a true AP (Grashey) view of the shoulder. Notching usually occurs 6 weeks to 14 months after surgery, but recent studies have shown continued progression with time. In the Sirveaux classification, a grade I notch is limited to the inferior scapular pillar, a grade II notch is in contact with the inferior screw of the baseplate, a grade III notch extends beyond the inferior screw, and a grade IV notch extends under the baseplate

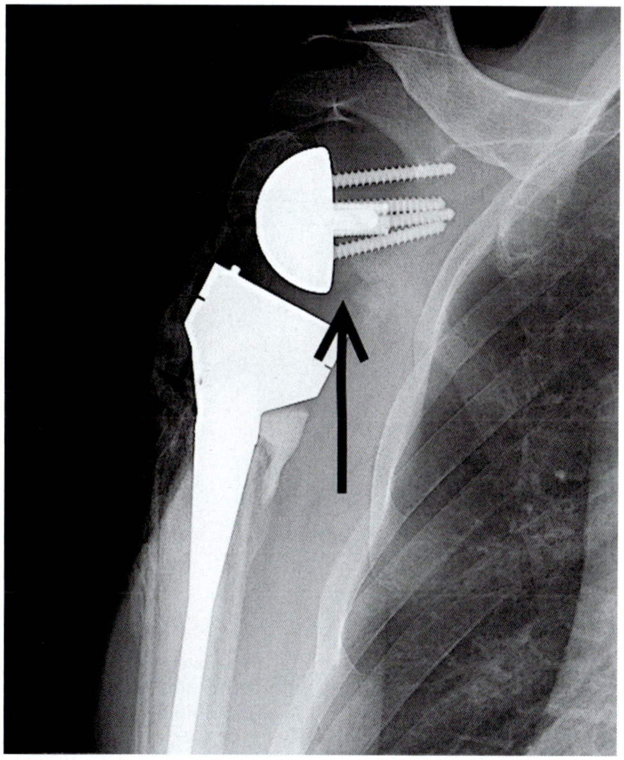

FIGURE 1 AP radiograph showing inferior scapular notching (arrow) after RSA.

and approaches the central peg[53] (**Figure 2**). Inferomedial scapular osteophytes commonly accompany scapular notching (**Figure 3**).

Controversy exists regarding the importance of scapular notching and whether it progresses over time. Scapular notching at a mean 4.5 months after surgery has been reported to stabilize at a mean 18 months after surgery,[51] whereas others report progression over time with a 48% incidence of notch progression at 1 year after surgery, 60% at 2 years, and 68% at 3 years, and the incidence of grade III and IV notching increased over time.[47] Long-term results have recently shown continued progression of scapular notching with 10-year follow-up.[54-57]

The implications of scapular notching have been debated. Several studies found that scapular notching was not correlated with scores on the Constant-Murley pain scale or with active forward flexion.[13,14,58-60] A negative correlation was found between scapular notching and the Constant-Murley score, the Subjective Shoulder Value, active forward flexion, and abduction.[5,47,51,53] Although the long-term implications of scapular notching are not well understood, most experts agree that surgical techniques should be undertaken to avoid notching, usually by placing the glenosphere as far inferior as possible. Designs incorporating a more lateralized center of rotation and designs such as the bony increased offset RSA have been introduced as a way to lateralize the glenoid component and avoid notching. In the bony increased offset RSA technique, lateralization is reproduced by placing bone graft (autogenous bone graft from humeral head, autogenous iliac crest, or allograft) on a baseplate designed with a relatively long central post to achieve host bone fixation. When the bone graft has healed, the center of rotation is maintained at the glenoid bone–prosthesis interface.[16]

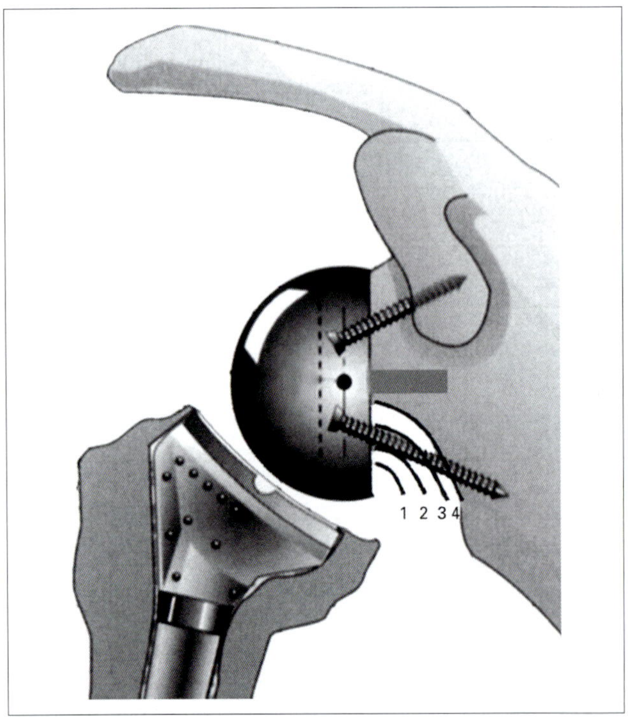

FIGURE 2 Schematic diagram of the Sirveaux classification of scapular notching. (Reproduced with permission from Sirveaux F, Favard L, Oudet D, Huquet D, Walch G, Molé D: Grammont inverted total shoulder arthroplasty in the treatment of glenohumeral osteoarthritis with massive rupture of the cuff: Results of a multicentre study of 80 shoulders. *J Bone Joint Surg Br* 2004;86[3]:388-395. doi:10.1302/0301-620X.86B3.14024.)

Instability

Dislocation remains one of the most common complications after RSA, with rates ranging from 1% to 31%.[7,8,11,12,17,19,21,25,61] Multiple factors contribute to instability, including body mass index, sex, soft-tissue tension, mechanical impingement, prosthesis version, proximal bone loss, prosthesis height, and axillary nerve dysfunction. One study showed strong association between a body mass index ≥ 30 kg/m^2, male gender, and previous RSA with atraumatic instability in the early postoperative period.[11] Patients undergoing RSA secondary to fracture sequelae have a higher rate of instability than those undergoing RSA for primary rotator cuff tear arthropathy, massive rotator cuff tear with pseudoparalysis, acute fracture, or instability arthropathy.[12] Adequate soft-tissue tension is critical for stability. If the patient lacks a functioning rotator cuff, appropriate lengthening of the deltoid is paramount and allows increased compression forces across the prosthesis to maintain stability. If the deltoid is not appropriately tensioned, the risk of dislocation is increased.[21] Surgical techniques such as minimizing humeral bone resection, positioning the glenosphere with an inferior tilt, and eccentric placement of the glenosphere allow the surgeon to gain stability by lowering the humerus relative to the glenoid and thus to increase deltoid tension. A prosthesis design with a more valgus head-neck angle, a larger glenosphere diameter, a lateral offset, or a thicker polyethylene insert also can be used to achieve appropriate soft-tissue tension. Mechanical impingement, in which the humeral component levers off the inferior aspect of the scapular neck, is a less common cause of instability that is often related to superior placement of the glenoid component. Another possible risk factor for instability is related to the status of the subscapularis tendon. There remains debate as to whether subscapularis repair improves stability.[12,62,63] The design of the implant likely plays an important role into the necessity for subscapularis repair as newer designs probably rely less on subscapularis repair for stability compared with older Grammont-style implants.

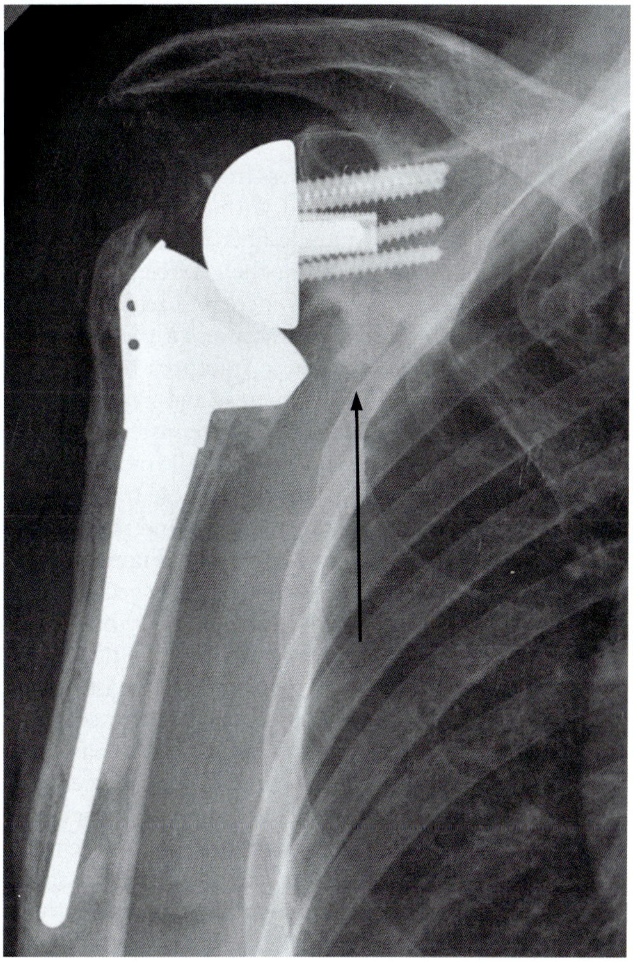

FIGURE 3 AP radiograph showing an inferior scapular osteophyte (arrow), which often occurs in conjunction with scapular notching.

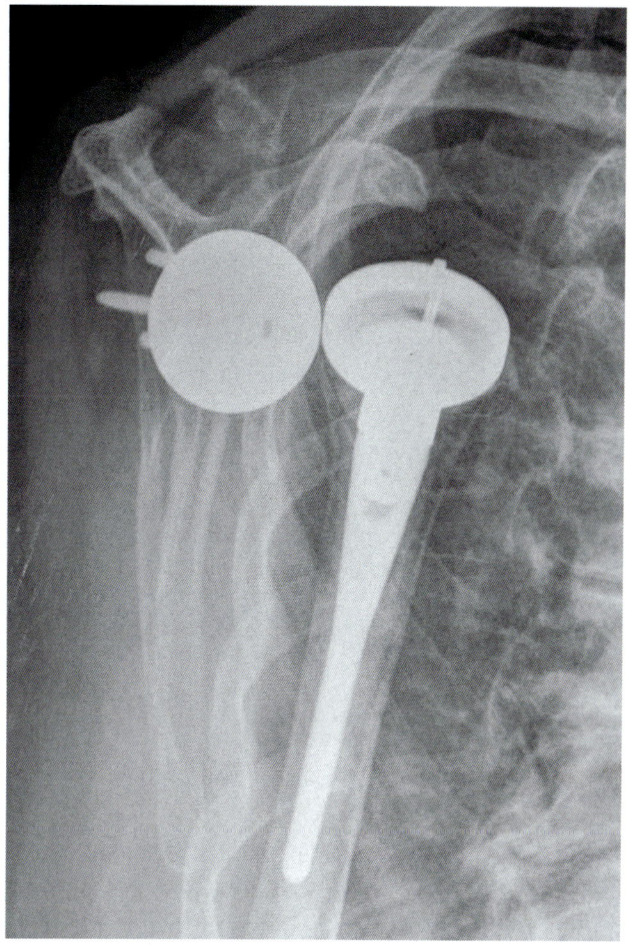

FIGURE 4 Scapular Y radiograph showing an anteriorly dislocated reverse shoulder prosthesis.

Most dislocations occur after a combination of extension, adduction, and internal rotation, as in a hand-behind-the-back position. The direction of dislocation is anterior (**Figures 4** and **5**). In most patients, the dislocated prosthesis can be treated with closed reduction. After the prosthesis is reduced, the shoulder should be examined under fluoroscopy to determine whether mechanical impingement is the cause of instability. If closed reduction of the prosthesis is not possible, the shoulder must be reduced with open measures or consideration of revision. An early atraumatic dislocation (within the first 3 months of surgery) may result from a technical error and may require revision, although an attempt at closed reduction is often tried before revision.[58] During revision surgery, the surgeon should evaluate for appropriate version, soft-tissue impingement, and appropriate tension of the deltoid. Any of these variables should be corrected to prevent recurrent instability. A late dislocation (more than 1 year after surgery) usually can be treated with closed reduction and a period of immobilization.[58]

Glenoid Baseplate Failure

Glenoid baseplate or component failure occurred after many of the early RSA designs (**Figures 6** and **7**).[24,64] In the early RSA designs, a glenosphere with a laterally offset center of rotation created excessive torque and shear forces at the junction of the baseplate and the glenoid bone. Innovations and implant design changes have decreased the rate of glenoid baseplate failure.[61,64] The Grammont reverse prosthesis medialized the center of rotation, which led to more concentric forces and reduced the torque at the prosthesis-bone junction. The Grammont design allowed stable fixation of the glenoid baseplate; implant survivorship was reported to be 84% at 10-year follow-up.[59]

The minimal implant pore size for achieving bony ingrowth is 150 μm.[60] Lack of bone ingrowth into the baseplate is associated with baseplate failure. Inferior tilt and the use of locking screws minimize forces at the baseplate-bone interface and thereby reduce the rate of failure, regardless of prosthesis design.[65] The addition of larger 5.0-mm peripheral locking screws helped to

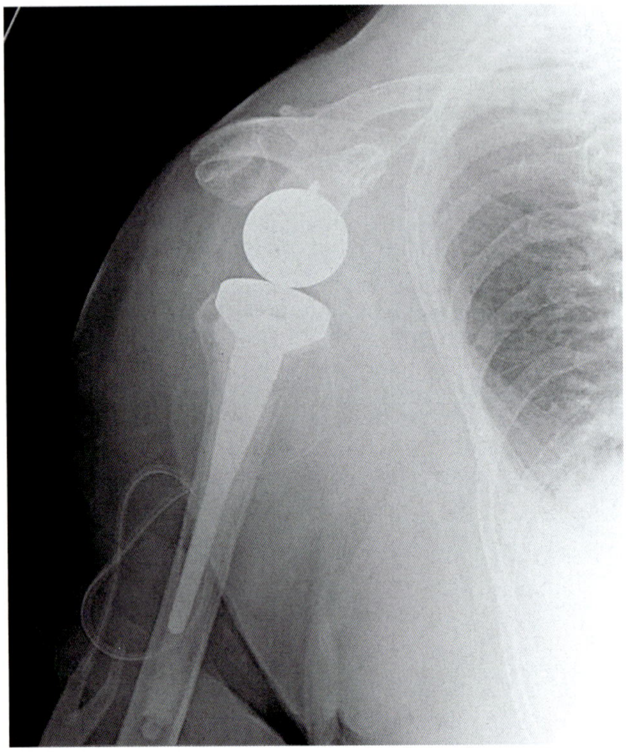

FIGURE 5 AP radiograph showing a reduced reverse shoulder prosthesis.

reduce the risk of mechanical baseplate failure in a device with a lateral eccentric center of rotation.[61] The reported rate of glenoid loosening is low with modern reverse prosthesis designs that incorporate locking technology in the baseplate. However, every effort should be made to optimally fix the glenosphere at the inferior border of the glenoid and into good bone stock.

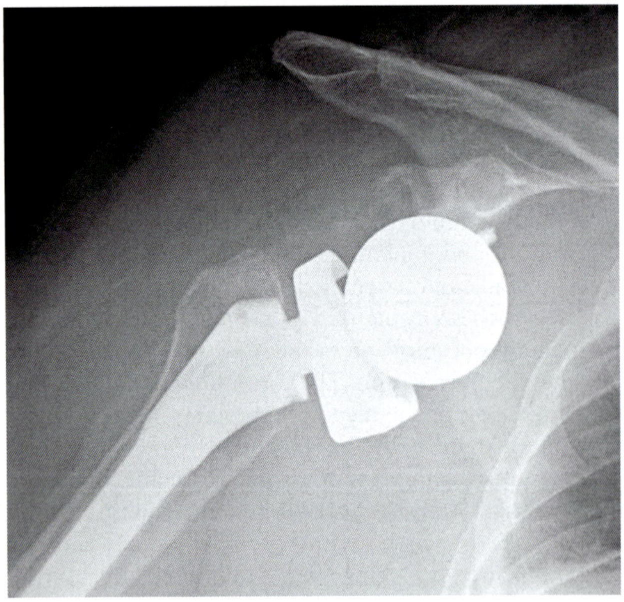

FIGURE 6 AP radiograph showing glenosphere failure with complete loss of fixation of the baseplate and rotational migration of the implant.

Scapular Fracture

Scapular spine and acromial stress fractures are also complications uniquely associated with RSA. The reverse total shoulder increases muscle fiber recruitment of the deltoid, which originates from the clavicle, acromion, and spine of the scapula. This increased tension on the deltoid is a possible cause of fractures of the acromion and spine of the scapula. These fractures received little attention historically, but interest and awareness on scapular fractures has increased. The reported incidence of scapular (scapular spine and acromial) fractures after RSA is 0.8% to 6.9%.[6,12,21,24,46,60,61,66] These fractures often appears within 1 year after surgery and may not be associated with a traumatic event[8,24,66,67] (**Figure 8**). The diagnosis of these fractures is a challenge because it is common for a patient to do well after surgery but have a sudden onset of pain or loss of function with no history of trauma. A deformity may not be obvious, but a key finding is point tenderness over the acromion or scapular spine. Radiographic imaging can also be difficult as many fractures can present without significant displacement. An axillary radiograph may be helpful to delineate between an acromial versus scapular spine fracture but are often unreliable with only a 78.8% accuracy. Often CT, single photon emission computed tomography, or MRI is necessary to identify the fracture.[68-70] A 4.4% rate of acromial stress fracture was reported in a retrospective review of 45 patients; the researchers thought that overtensioning of the deltoid might lead to acromial fracture in patients with severe osteoporosis or eroded acromial bone, as occurs with severe rotator cuff arthropathy.[64] A 0.8% rate was reported in a study of 457 patients.[66]

The treatment of scapular fractures is controversial. The outcome has been reported as satisfactory when minimally displaced fractures are treated nonsurgically with a period of immobilization.[22,24,61] In a study of 457 patients who underwent RSA, four patients had a postoperative acromial fracture. Three fractures were treated nonsurgically, and one was treated with an open reduction with tension band, which eventually failed and required hardware removal.[66] A persistent nonunion developed in two patients, and two patients healed with nonsurgical treatment, but had an inferior acromial tilt of at least 40°. The four patients with postoperative acromial fracture had a worse result in terms of Constant score, active elevation, and subjective satisfaction compared with other patients in the study. The optimal treatment could not be determined, but 6 weeks of nonsurgical treatment with an abduction splint was recommended to

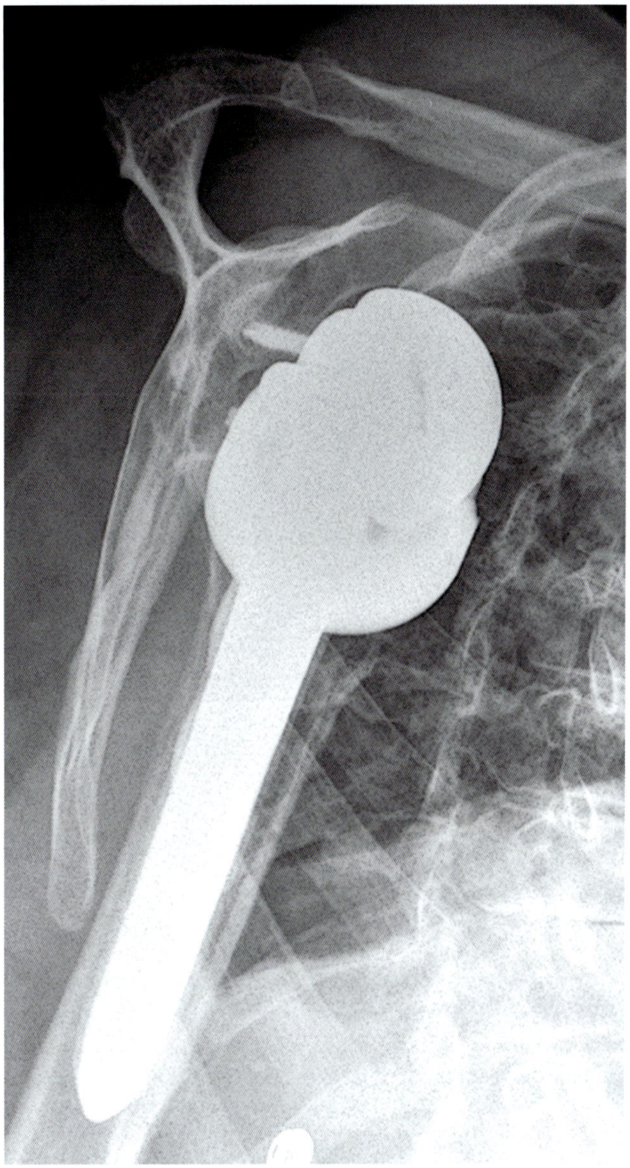

FIGURE 7 Scapular Y radiograph showing pullout and anterior migration and rotation of the entire glenosphere.

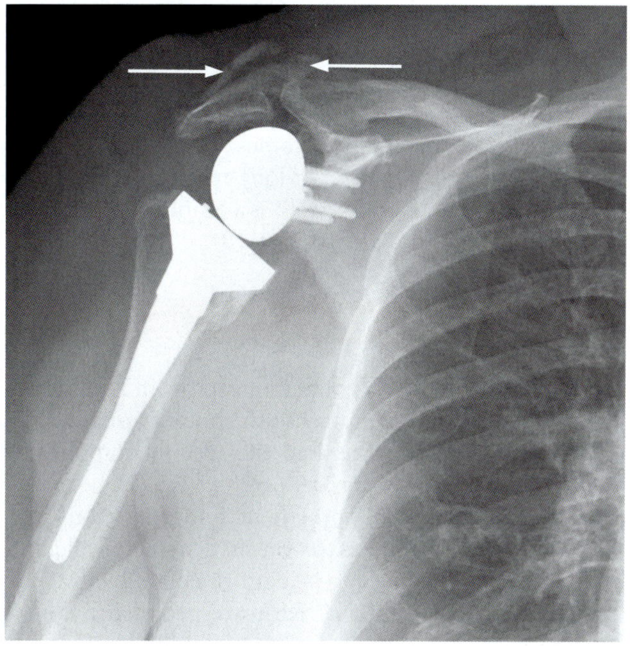

FIGURE 8 AP radiograph showing acromial fracture (arrows) with inferior tilting after reverse shoulder arthroplasty.

limit pain and acromial tilt. A high degree of suspicion was recommended whenever rehabilitation after RSA progresses slowly, is painful, or suddenly deteriorates within the first postoperative year.[66] Overall, functional results are often poor compared with patients without fracture.

Survivorship

Midterm results of RSA have been promising.[7,54,59,71] Overall, good results have been reported with up to 95% prosthetic survivorship at 8 years.[53] Despite the success with prosthetic survivorship, there is concern of functional decline after 6 to 8 years.[59,71] Although there have been multiple studies presenting data on midterm results, there are minimal data on long-term survivorship of RSA.[59,71] Longer term outcomes greater than 10 years have recently been reported. In a long-term follow-up study (150 months) of previously published midterm results (40 months), patients were found to have 93% overall prosthetic survival rate, but both absolute and relative Constant scores (55 and 86, respectively) significantly diminished compared with midterm results (63 and 90, respectively).[7,54] A systematic review of long-term outcomes with an average of 9.5 years follow-up found significant improvement with range of motion and functional outcomes compared with preoperative levels with no significant deterioration from 5 to 20 years.[55] Radiographic analysis demonstrated that scapular notching progressed with time with a rate up to 39%.[54-57] The clinical implications of this progressive scapular notching are still undetermined. Although the ultimate survivorship without failure is promising with reports of 84% to 87% survival at 15 years, there remains a concern for scapular notching, complications, and functional decline that should be considered.[54-57] The ultimate longevity of the RSA is not known, and there is a need for continued analysis in the future.

SUMMARY

Despite its higher complication rates in comparison with primary total shoulder arthroplasty, RSA has been shown to restore function and improve pain relief in appropriate patients. Complication rates will continue to decrease as surgeons become more experienced in the procedure. The long-term functional outcomes of RSA are still not clearly understood, and newer generation implants may have a significant effect on these outcomes. There is an obvious need for continued research of long-term functional and radiographic outcomes as well as complications of the reverse total shoulder arthroplasty.

KEY STUDY POINTS

- To minimize the risk of complications in RSA, the surgeon must be familiar with shoulder anatomy, the surgical exposure, and the specific complications related to this procedure.
- The diagnosis of periprosthetic joint infections in the shoulder continues to be a challenging problem, and newer tests need to be confirmed for accuracy.
- The midterm results of RSA are promising, and long-term outcomes support acceptable survivorship. However, more work is needed to decrease complication rates, better understand and prevent the progression of scapular notching, and to find for a future revision surgery solution after a failed RSA.

Annotated References

1. Jain NB, Yamaguchi K: The contribution of reverse shoulder arthroplasty to utilization of primary shoulder arthroplasty. *J Shoulder Elbow Surg* 2014;23(12):1905-1912.

   The overall trend of shoulder arthroplasty and the contribution of reverse total shoulder arthroplasty from 2009 to 2011 were evaluated. Reverse total shoulder arthroplasty indications have expanded and there is an increasing percentage of reverse total shoulder arthroplasty being performed as a primary shoulder replacement. Level of evidence: VI.

2. Day JS, Paxton ES, Lau E, Gordon VA, Abboud JA, Williams GR: Use of reverse total shoulder arthroplasty in the Medicare population. *J Shoulder Elbow Surg* 2015;24(5):766-772.

   Prevalence of reverse total shoulder arthroplasty in the medical population from 2011 was estimated. There is a similar amount of reverse total shoulder arthroplasties (37%) compared with that of total shoulder arthroplasty (42%). Lower volume surgeons perform reverse total shoulder arthroplasty more commonly than primary total shoulder arthroplasties. Level of evidence: VI.

3. Schairer WW, Nwachukwu BU, Lyman S, Craig EV, Gulotta LV: National utilization of reverse total shoulder arthroplasty in the United States. *J Shoulder Elbow Surg* 2015;24(1):91-97.

   The national utilization and indication of total shoulder arthroplasty, hemiarthroplasty, and reverse total shoulder arthroplasty in 2011 were compared. Reverse total shoulder arthroplasty was most commonly performed for rotator cuff arthropathy. Twenty-five percent of proximal humerus fractures were treated with reverse total shoulder arthroplasty. Level of evidence: VI.

4. Day JS, Lau E, Ong KL, Williams GR, Ramsey ML, Kurtz SM: Prevalence and projections of total shoulder and elbow arthroplasty in the United States to 2015. *J Shoulder Elbow Surg* 2010;19(8):1115-1120.

5. Cazeneuve JF, Cristofari DJ: The reverse shoulder prosthesis in the treatment of fractures of the proximal humerus in the elderly. *J Bone Joint Surg Br* 2010;92(4):535-539.

6. Naveed MA, Kitson J, Bunker TD: The Delta III reverse shoulder replacement for cuff tear arthropathy: A single-centre study of 50 consecutive procedures. *J Bone Joint Surg Br* 2011;93(1):57-61.

7. Wall B, Nové-Josserand L, O'Connor DP, Edwards TB, Walch G: Reverse total shoulder arthroplasty: A review of results according to etiology. *J Bone Joint Surg Am* 2007;89(7):1476-1485.

8. Werner CM, Steinmann PA, Gilbart M, Gerber C: Treatment of painful pseudoparesis due to irreparable rotator cuff dysfunction with the Delta III reverse-ball-and-socket total shoulder prosthesis. *J Bone Joint Surg Am* 2005;87(7):1476-1486.

9. Saltzman BM, Chalmers PN, Gupta AK, Romeo AA, Nicholson GP: Complication rates comparing primary with revision reverse total shoulder arthroplasty. *J Shoulder Elbow Surg* 2014;23(11):1647-1654.

   This retrospective review of 90-day postoperative complications compared primary versus revision reverse total shoulder arthroplasty. There was an increased complication rate in revision cases along with higher transfusion rate. Level of evidence: III.

10. Gupta AK, Chalmers PN, Rahman Z, et al: Reverse total shoulder arthroplasty in patients of varying body mass index. *J Shoulder Elbow Surg* 2014;23(1):35-42.

    This retrospective review compared different BMI and early postoperative complications in reverse total shoulder arthroplasty. Patients with BMI >35 kg/m2 had a higher complication rate and intraoperative blood loss; patients with BMI <25 kg/m2 also had higher complications rates. Level of evidence: III.

11. Chalmers N, Rahman Z, Romeo AA, Nicholson GP: Early dislocation after reverse total shoulder arthroplasty. *J Shoulder Elbow Surg* 2014;23(5):737-744.

    Overall incidence of 2.9% of early dislocations (<3 months) postoperatively after reverse shoulder arthroplasty was noted. Common associated factors included male sex, prior surgery, BMI >30 kg/m2, and no subscapularis repair at the time of surgery. Level of evidence: IV.

12. Trappey GJ IV, O'Connor DP, Edwards TB: What are the instability and infection rates after reverse shoulder arthroplasty? *Clin Orthop Relat Res* 2011;469(9):2505-2511.

13. Zumstein MA, Pinedo M, Old J, Boileau P: Problems, complications, reoperations, and revisions in reverse total shoulder arthroplasty: A systematic review. *J Shoulder Elbow Surg* 2011;20(1):146-157.

14. Walch G, Bacle G, Lädermann A, Nové-Josserand L, Smithers CJ: Do the indications, results, and complications of reverse shoulder arthroplasty change with surgeon's experience? *J Shoulder Elbow Surg* 2012;21(11):1470-1477.

15. Lyman S, Jones EC, Bach PB, Peterson MG, Marx RG: The association between hospital volume and total shoulder arthroplasty outcomes. *Clin Orthop Relat Res* 2005;432:132-137.

16. Boileau P, Moineau G, Roussanne Y, O'Shea K: Bony increased-offset reversed shoulder arthroplasty: Minimizing scapular impingement while maximizing glenoid fixation. *Clin Orthop Relat Res* 2011;469(9):2558-2567.

17. Boileau P, Watkinson D, Hatzidakis AM, Hovorka I: Neer Award 2005: The Grammont reverse shoulder prosthesis. Results in cuff tear arthritis, fracture sequelae, and revision arthroplasty. *J Shoulder Elbow Surg* 2006;15(5):527-540.

18. Wierks C, Skolasky RL, Ji JH, McFarland EG: Reverse total shoulder replacement: Intraoperative and early postoperative complications. *Clin Orthop Relat Res* 2009;467(1):225-234.

19. Valenti P, Sauzières P, Katz D, Kalouche I, Kilinc AS: Do less medialized reverse shoulder prostheses increase motion and reduce notching? *Clin Orthop Relat Res* 2011;469(9):2550-2557.

20. Van Hoof T, Gomes GT, Audenaert E, Verstraete K, Kerckaert I, D'Herde K: 3D computerized model for measuring strain and displacement of the brachial plexus following placement of reverse shoulder prosthesis. *Anat Rec (Hoboken)* 2008;291(9):1173-1185.

21. Lädermann A, Williams MD, Melis B, Hoffmeyer P, Walch G: Objective evaluation of lengthening in reverse shoulder arthroplasty. *J Shoulder Elbow Surg* 2009;18(4):588-595.

22. Lädermann A, Lübbeke A, Mélis B, et al: Prevalence of neurologic lesions after total shoulder arthroplasty. *J Bone Joint Surg Am* 2011;93(14):1288-1293.

23. Nagda SH, Rogers KJ, Sestokas AK, et al: Neer Award 2005: Peripheral nerve function during shoulder arthroplasty using intraoperative nerve monitoring. *J Shoulder Elbow Surg* 2007;16(3 suppl):S2-S8.

24. Frankle M, Siegal S, Pupello D, Saleem A, Mighell M, Vasey M: The reverse shoulder prosthesis for glenohumeral arthritis associated with severe rotator cuff deficiency: A minimum two-year follow-up study of sixty patients. *J Bone Joint Surg Am* 2005;87(8):1697-1705.

25. De Wilde L, Sys G, Julien Y, Van Ovost E, Poffyn B, Trouilloud P: The reversed Delta shoulder prosthesis in reconstruction of the proximal humerus after tumour resection. *Acta Orthop Belg* 2003;69(6):495-500.

26. Shields MV, Abdullah L, Namdri S: The challenge of Propionibacterium acnes and revision shoulder arthroplasty: A review of current diagnostic options. *J Shoulder Elbow Surg* 2016;25(6):1034-1040.

    A review of current literature regarding demographic, clinical, and radiographic predictors of *P acnes* infection. Alpha defensin showed the highest sensitivity (63%) in diagnosing *P acnes* infection. Level of evidence: V.

27. Patel A, Calfee RP, Plante M, Fischer SA, Green A: *Propionibacterium acnes* colonization of the human shoulder. *J Shoulder Elbow Surg* 2009;18(6):897-902.

28. Topolski MS, Chin PY, Sperling JW, Cofield RH: Revision shoulder arthroplasty with positive intraoperative cultures: The value of preoperative studies and intraoperative histology. *J Shoulder Elbow Surg* 2006;15(4):402-406.

29. Dodson CC, Craig EV, Cordasco FA, et al: Propionibacterium acnes infection after shoulder arthroplasty: A diagnostic challenge. *J Shoulder Elbow Surg* 2010;19(2):303-307.

30. Piper KE, Fernandez-Sampedro M, Steckelberg KE, et al: C-reactive protein, erythrocyte sedimentation rate and orthopedic implant infection. *PLoS One* 2010;5(2):e9358.

31. Ecker N, Kniker A, Gehrke T, et al: What is the diagnostic accuracy of alpha-defensin and leukocyte esterase test in periprosthetic shoulder infection? *Clin Orthop Relat Res* 2019;477(7):1712-1718.

    The accuracy of alpha defensin and leukocyte esterase for detecting periprosthetic shoulder infections was evaluated. Overall accuracy of alpha defensin was 91% with 75% sensitivity and 96% specificity. Overall accuracy of leukocyte esterase was 76% with 50% sensitivity and 85% specificity. Level of evidence: III.

32. Frangiamore SJ, Saleh A, Grosso MJ, et al: α-Defensin as a predictor of periprosthetic shoulder infection. *J Shoulder Elbow Surg* 2015;24(7):1021-1027.

    The diagnostic utility of alpha defensin in detecting periprosthetic infection was evaluated. Results show sensitivity of 63% and specificity of 95%. Level of evidence: III.

33. Piper KE, Jacobson MJ, Cofield RH, et al: Microbiologic diagnosis of prosthetic shoulder infection by use of implant sonication. *J Clin Microbiol* 2009;47(6):1878-1884.

34. Lutz MF, Berthelot P, Fresard A, et al: Arthroplastic and osteosynthetic infections due to Propionibacterium acnes: A retrospective study of 52 cases, 1995-2002. *Eur J Clin Microbiol Infect Dis* 2005;24(11):739-744.

35. Namdari S, Nicholson T, Abboud J, et al: Comparative study of cultures and next-generation sequencing in the diagnosis of shoulder prosthetic joint infections. *J Shoulder Elbow Surg* 2019;28(1):1-8.

    This study determined correlation between next-generation sequencing (NGS) and intraoperative cultures in revision shoulder arthroplasty. There was a fair concordance (0.333) between the diagnostic criteria for defining infection that included culture or NGS. Cultures resulted in monomicrobial results, whereas NGS suggested polymicrobial loads. Level of evidence: II.

36. Saltzman MD, Nuber GW, Gryzlo SM, Marecek GS, Koh JL: Efficacy of surgical preparation solutions in shoulder surgery. *J Bone Joint Surg Am* 2009;91(8):1949-1953.

37. Kanafani ZA, Sexton DJ, Pien BC, Varkey J, Basmania C, Kaye KS: Postoperative joint infections due to Propionibacterium species: A case-control study. *Clin Infect Dis* 2009;49(7):1083-1085.

38. Nowinski RJ, Gillespie RJ, Shishani Y, Cohen B, Walch G, Gobezie R: Antibiotic-loaded bone cement reduces deep infection rates for primary reverse total shoulder arthroplasty: A retrospective, cohort study of 501 shoulders. *J Shoulder Elbow Surg* 2012;21(3):324-328.

39. Cheung EV, Sperling JW, Cofield RH: Infection associated with hematoma formation after shoulder arthroplasty. *Clin Orthop Relat Res* 2008;466(6):1363-1367.

40. Weber P, Utzschneider S, Sadoghi P, Andress HJ, Jansson V, Müller PE: Management of the infected shoulder prosthesis: A retrospective analysis and review of the literature. *Int Orthop* 2011;35(3):365-373.

41. Sabesan VJ, Ho JC, Kovacevic D, Iannotti JP: Two-stage reimplantation for treating prosthetic shoulder infections. *Clin Orthop Relat Res* 2011;469(9):2538-2543.

42. Grosso MJ, Sabesan VJ, Ho JC, Ricchetti ET, Iannotti JP: Reinfection rates after 1-stage revision shoulder arthroplasty for patients with unexpected positive intraoperative cultures. *J Shoulder Elbow Surg* 2012;21(6):754-758.

43. Beekman PD, Katusic D, Berghs BM, Karelse A, De Wilde L: One-stage revision for patients with a chronically infected reverse total shoulder replacement. *J Bone Joint Surg Br* 2010;92(6):817-822.

44. Coste JS, Reig S, Trojani C, Berg M, Walch G, Boileau P: The management of infection in arthroplasty of the shoulder. *J Bone Joint Surg Br* 2004;86(1):65-69.

45. Sperling JW, Kozak TK, Hanssen AD, Cofield RH: Infection after shoulder arthroplasty. *Clin Orthop Relat Res* 2001;382:206-216.

46. Mulieri P, Dunning P, Klein S, Pupello D, Frankle M: Reverse shoulder arthroplasty for the treatment of irreparable rotator cuff tear without glenohumeral arthritis. *J Bone Joint Surg Am* 2010;92(15):2544-2556.

47. Lévigne C, Garret J, Boileau P, Alami G, Favard L, Walch G: Scapular notching in reverse shoulder arthroplasty: Is it important to avoid it and how? *Clin Orthop Relat Res* 2011;469(9):2512-2520.

48. Boileau P, Gonzalez JF, Chuinard C, Bicknell R, Walch G: Reverse total shoulder arthroplasty after failed rotator cuff surgery. *J Shoulder Elbow Surg* 2009;18(4):600-606.

49. Kempton LB, Balasubramaniam M, Ankerson E, Wiater JM: A radiographic analysis of the effects of prosthesis design on scapular notching following reverse total shoulder arthroplasty. *J Shoulder Elbow Surg* 2011;20(4):571-576.

50. Lévigne C, Boileau P, Favard L, et al: Scapular notching in reverse shoulder arthroplasty. *J Shoulder Elbow Surg* 2008;17(6):925-935.

51. Simovitch RW, Zumstein MA, Lohri E, Helmy N, Gerber C: Predictors of scapular notching in patients managed with the Delta III reverse total shoulder replacement. *J Bone Joint Surg Am* 2007;89(3):588-600.

52. Gutiérrez S, Levy JC, Frankle MA, et al: Evaluation of abduction range of motion and avoidance of inferior scapular impingement in a reverse shoulder model. *J Shoulder Elbow Surg* 2008;17(4):608-615.

53. Sirveaux F, Favard L, Oudet D, Huquet D, Walch G, Molé D: Grammont inverted total shoulder arthroplasty in the treatment of glenohumeral osteoarthritis with massive rupture of the cuff: Results of a multicentre study of 80 shoulders. *J Bone Joint Surg Br* 2004;86(3):388-395.

54. Bacle G, Nove-Josserand L, Garaud P, Walch G: Long-term outcomes of reverse total shoulder arthroplasty: A follow-up of a previous study. *J Bone Joint Surg Am* 2017;99(6):454-461.

    This is a follow-up study of previously reported midterm results. Overall prosthetic survival rate at 10 years was 93%. There was a significant decline in Constant scores from midterm to long-term results. There was a continued progression of scapular notching. Level of evidence: IV.

55. Ernstbrunner L, Andronic O, Grubhofer F, Camenzind RS, Wieser K, Gerber C: Long-term results of reverse total shoulder arthroplasty for rotator cuff dysfunction: A systematic review of longitudinal outcomes. *J Shoulder Elbow Surg* 2019;28(4):774-781.

This is a systematic review of midterm to long-term results for RSA with massive rotator cuff tears. There was no significant clinical decline in functional outcomes or range of motion. Progressive scapular notching was noted. Level of evidence: IV.

56. Gerber C, Canonica S, Catanzaro S, Ernstbrunner L: Longitudinal observational study of reverse total shoulder arthroplasty for irreparable rotator cuff dysfunction: Results after 15 years. *J Shoulder Elbow Surg* 2018;27(5):831-838.

    Long-term results of reverse total shoulder arthroplasty were reviewed. No significant decline in the Constant or the Subjective Shoulder Value score over time was observed. There was a significant decline with abduction over time. There was a 59% overall complication rate. Level of evidence: IV.

57. Ernstbrunner L, Suter A, Catanzaro S, Rahm S, Gerber C: Reverse total shoulder arthroplasty for massive, irreparable rotator cuff tears before the age of 60 years: Long-term results. *J Bone Joint Surg Am* 2017;99(20):1721-1729.

    Long-term results of RSA in patients younger than 60 years were reviewed. Postoperative significant subjective and functional improvement without evidence of deterioration with time was observed. Incidence of scapular notching increased with time. Level of evidence: IV.

58. Gerber C, Pennington SD, Nyffeler RW: Reverse total shoulder arthroplasty. *J Am Acad Orthop Surg* 2009;17(5):284-295.

59. Guery J, Favard L, Sirveaux F, Oudet D, Mole D, Walch G: Reverse total shoulder arthroplasty: Survivorship analysis of eighty replacements followed for five to ten years. *J Bone Joint Surg Am* 2006;88(8):1742-1747.

60. Jasty M, Bragdon C, Burke D, O'Connor D, Lowenstein J, Harris WH: In vivo skeletal responses to porous-surfaced implants subjected to small induced motions. *J Bone Joint Surg Am* 1997;79(5):707-714.

61. Cuff D, Pupello D, Virani N, Levy J, Frankle M: Reverse shoulder arthroplasty for the treatment of rotator cuff deficiency. *J Bone Joint Surg Am* 2008;90(6):1244-1251.

62. Edwards TB, Williams MD, Labriola JE, Elkousy HA, Gartsman GM, O'Connor DP: Subscapularis insufficiency and the risk of shoulder dislocation after reverse shoulder arthroplasty. *J Shoulder Elbow Surg* 2009;18(6):892-896.

63. Clark JC, Ritchie J, Song FS, et al: Complication rates, dislocation, pain, and postoperative range of motion after reverse shoulder arthroplasty in patients with and without repair of the subscapularis. *J Shoulder Elbow Surg* 2012;21(1):36-41.

64. Boileau P, Watkinson DJ, Hatzidakis AM, Balg F: Grammont reverse prosthesis: Design, rationale, and biomechanics. *J Shoulder Elbow Surg* 2005;14(1 suppl):S147-S161.

65. Gutiérrez S, Keller TS, Levy JC, Lee WE III, Luo ZP: Hierarchy of stability factors in reverse shoulder arthroplasty. *Clin Orthop Relat Res* 2008;466(3):670-676.

66. Walch G, Mottier F, Wall B, Boileau P, Molé D, Favard L: Acromial insufficiency in reverse shoulder arthroplasties. *J Shoulder Elbow Surg* 2009;18(3):495-502.

67. Neyton L, Erickson J, Ascione F, Bugelli G, Lunini E, Walch G: Grammont Award 2018. Scapular fractures in reverse shoulder arthroplasty (Grammont style): Prevalence, functional, and radiographic results with minimum 5-year follow-up. *J Shoulder Elbow Surg* 2019;28(2):260-267.

    Scapular spine fracture incidence of 1.3% with average final Constant score of 47 and flexion of 109° was observed. Overall, those with posteroperative scapular fracture had worse outcomes than those without fracture. Level of evidence: IV.

68. Mayne J, Bell S, Wright W, Coghlan J: Acromial and scapular spine fractures after reverse total shoulder arthroplasty. *Shoulder Elbow* 2016;8(2):90-100.

    The etiology, diagnosis, and treatment of acromial and scapular spine fractures were reviewed. Level of evidence: V.

69. Karthik K, Lau J, Sinha J, Tavakkolizadeh A: Scapular spine stress fractures: To fix or not to fix, our experience in a patient with bilateral fractures and review of the literature. *Int J Shoulder Surg* 2014;8(3):90-93.

    This study is a case report of bilateral scapular spine fractures with one side treated nonsurgically and the other with surgery. Both fractures healed with good functional outcomes. Level of evidence: V.

70. Otto RJ, Virani NA, Levy JC, Nigro PT, Cuff DJ, Frankle MA: Scapular fractures after reverse shoulder arthroplasty: Evaluation of risk factors and the reliability of a proposed classification. *J Shoulder Elbow Surg* 2013;22(11):1514-1521.

    Case-controlled comparison of scapular spine fractures after reverse shoulder arthroplasty with those of control patients found osteoporosis as a significant risk factor. Identifying decreased acromial-tuberosity distance and increased acromial tilt on radiographs aided in identification of fractures. Level of evidence: IV.

71. Favard L, Levigne C, Nerot C, Gerber C, De Wilde L, Mole D: Reverse prostheses in arthropathies with cuff tear: Are survivorship and function maintained over time? *Clin Orthop Relat Res* 2011;469(9):2469-2475.

Chapter 28

Indications and Outcomes for Revision Shoulder Arthroplasty

C. Scott Humphrey, MD • Andrew Green, MD

ABSTRACT

Revision shoulder arthroplasty presents a unique set of challenges for the orthopaedic surgeon. Identification of the cause of the failed shoulder arthroplasty and the associated pain can be difficult, and revision surgery can be technically complex with higher complication rates and inferior clinical results compared with primary arthroplasty. Nevertheless, revision shoulder arthroplasty often provides improvements in patient outcomes.

Keywords: arthroplasty; indications; outcomes; revision; shoulder

Introduction

Primary shoulder arthroplasty, anatomic and reverse, is generally successful. Recognition of favorable clinical outcomes and shifting patient demographics have led to increased popularity and utilization. From 2000 to 2010, the rate of shoulder arthroplasty performed for osteoarthritis in the United States increased 3.7-fold,1 and there was a fourfold increase in revision shoulder arthroplasty.[2] The demand for revision shoulder arthroplasty surgery is expected to continue to rise.

Revision surgery often improves patient outcomes, but it can be technically demanding and is associated with higher complication rates and inferior clinical results compared with primary arthroplasty. From the diagnostic ambiguity that is often associated with evaluation of the painful prosthetic shoulder to the mastery of the technical aspects of the surgery, revision shoulder arthroplasty presents a unique set of challenges for the orthopaedic surgeon.

Evaluation of the Failed Shoulder Arthroplasty

Causes of arthroplasty failure and the associated pain and dysfunction are often nebulous and multifactorial. The list of potential problems associated with failed shoulder arthroplasty is long and, at a minimum, includes component wear and loosening, instability, rotator cuff failure, periprosthetic fracture, implant malposition or improper sizing, glenoid bone erosion and arthrosis, periprosthetic infection, implant-related failure, heterotopic ossification, neurologic injury, complex regional pain syndrome, and inadequate postoperative rehabilitation.[3]

Pain and mechanical symptoms are common complaints from patients with failed shoulder arthroplasty. The diagnostic workup should include a comprehensive history and physical examination, imaging studies to include plain radiography and advanced imaging (CT, ultrasonography, and MRI), laboratory values, joint aspiration, nuclear scans, and electrodiagnostic studies, as appropriate.[3] A systematic approach to the patient workup is imperative. A history of an acute change in pain and function may suggest an anatomic or mechanical problem such as rotator cuff failure or component loosening.

Evaluation of serial plain radiographs may demonstrate changes that suggest humeral implant and/or glenoid component loosening. Grading systems have been described to classify the severity of loosening of the humeral component[4] (**Figure 1**), and for the glenoid components for anatomic[5] (**Figure 2**) and reverse[6] total shoulder arthroplasty (TSA). It should be kept in mind that the

Dr. Humphrey or an immediate family member has received royalties from Encore Medical; is a member of a speakers' bureau or has made paid presentations on behalf of DJO Surgical; serves as a paid consultant to or is an employee of DJO Surgical and United Orthopedic Corporation; and serves as a board member, owner, officer, or committee member of the American Shoulder and Elbow Surgeons and the Idaho Shoulder Education and Research Foundation. Dr. Green or an immediate family member has received royalties from Wright Medical Technology, Inc.; is a member of a speakers' bureau or has made paid presentations on behalf of DJ Orthopaedics; serves as a paid consultant to or is an employee of DJ Orthopaedics and Wright Medical Technology, Inc.; has stock or stock options held in IlluminOss Medical and Pfizer; has received research or institutional support from DJ Orthopaedics; has received nonincome support (such as equipment or services), commercially derived honoraria, or other non–research-related funding (such as paid travel) from Arthrex, Inc. and Smith & Nephew; and serves as a board member, owner, officer, or committee member of the American Academy of Orthopaedic Surgeons, the American Shoulder and Elbow Surgeons, and the American Shoulder and Elbow Surgeons.

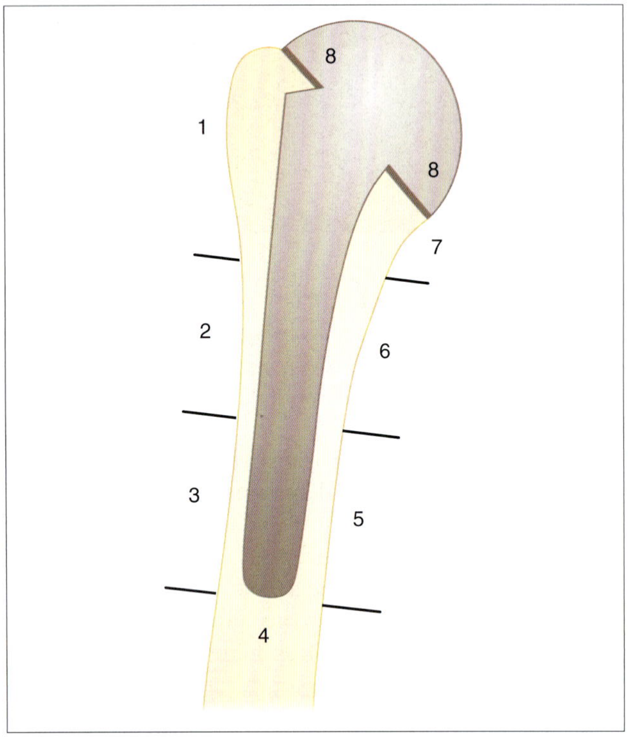

FIGURE 1 Illustration showing the Gruen zones adapted for the modern humeral stem: A humeral component is considered to be at risk when a lucent line 2 mm or greater in width was present in three or more of eight Gruen zones, or when at least two of three independent observers identified tilt or subsidence of the component.[4]

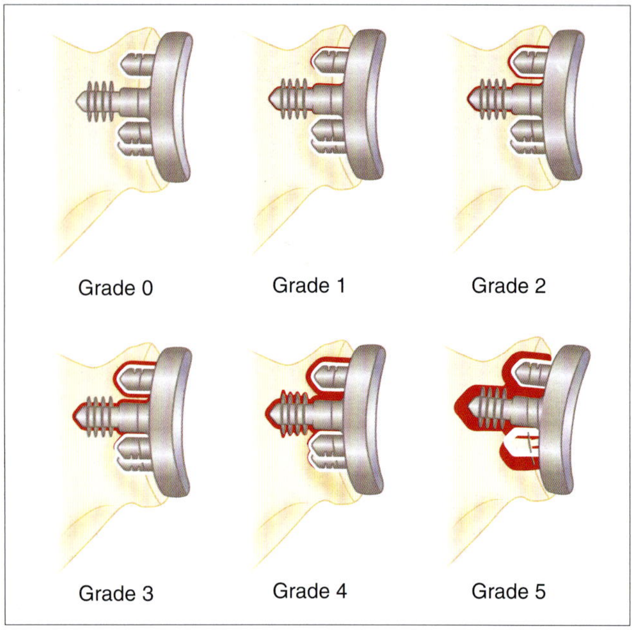

FIGURE 2 Illustration showing the grading system of the authors of a 2002 study,[5] which used to assess radiolucencies around a pegged glenoid. Grade 0, no lucencies; grade 1, incomplete lucencies around one or two pegs; grade 2, complete radiolucency (≤2 mm wide) around one peg only with or without other radiolucency around one other peg; grade 3, complete radiolucency (≤2 mm wide) around two or more pegs; grade 4, complete radiolucency (>2 mm wide) around two or more pegs; grade 5, gross loosening. (Redrawn with permission from Lazarus MD, Jensen KL, Southworth C, Matsen FA: The radiographic evaluation of keeled and pegged glenoid component insertion. *J Bone Joint Surg Am* 2002;84[7]:1174-1182.)

radiographic appearance of component loosening will vary depending on the implant design, and therefore these classification systems serve only as rough guidelines for the determination of component-related complications. In cases where plain radiograph findings are equivocal, a CT arthrogram and/or bone scintigraphy study may facilitate the diagnosis of loosening.

Rotator cuff failure is associated with weakness: internal rotation weakness with subscapularis injury, external rotation weakness with infraspinatus injury, and elevation weakness with supraspinatus injury. Plain radiographic findings can also suggest rotator cuff failure, acute or chronic. Elevation of the humeral head relative to the glenoid is consistent with supraspinatus and infraspinatus failure. Anterior subluxation is consistent with subscapularis failure.

Periprosthetic joint infection (PJI) should always be considered during the evaluation of a failed shoulder arthroplasty. A substantial proportion of revision shoulder arthroplasty cases have positive intraoperative cultures.[7] The standard preoperative evaluation for infection includes a peripheral white blood cell (WBC) count with differential, erythrocyte sedimentation rate (ESR), C-reactive protein (CRP), and joint aspiration for synovial fluid analysis and cultures. Unfortunately, preoperative tests are often negative even in cases that are later determined to have PJI.[8] Infection is confirmed in most cases with intraoperative tissue cultures. Indolent, late shoulder PJI is more commonly associated with male sex and implant loosening.

The Shoulder Group of the Second International Consensus Meeting on Periprosthetic Infections recently published guidelines for defining, preventing, evaluating, and managing periprosthetic shoulder infections.[9] Meeting any one of the following major criteria is diagnostic of definite periprosthetic shoulder infection: presence of a sinus tract from the skin surface to the prosthesis; gross intra-articular pus; and/or two positive tissue cultures with phenotypically identical virulent organisms. The weighted values for all minor criteria positive tests performed as part of the diagnostic evaluation of a failed shoulder arthroplasty are summed in **Tables 1** and **2**.

Indications for Revision Shoulder Arthroplasty

Regardless of the underlying pathology, persistent pain and dysfunction are the principal indications for revision TSA and are usually what drives the patient with failed shoulder arthroplasty to seek evaluation and treatment. A 2015 study found that the most common ICD-9 diagnosis codes at the time of revision surgery were unspecified

Table 1

Minor Criteria for Definition of Shoulder PJI

Minor Criteria	Weight
Unexpected wound drainage	4
Single positive tissue culture with virulent organism	3
Single positive tissue culture with low-virulence organism	1
Second positive tissue culture (identical low-virulence organism)	3
Humeral loosening	3
Positive frozen section (5 PMNs in ≤5 high-power fields)	3
Positive preoperative aspirate culture (low or high virulence)	3
Elevated synovial neutrophil percentage (>80%)[a]	2
Elevated synovial WBC count (>3,000 cells/mL)[a]	2
Elevated ESR (>30 mm/hr)[a]	2
Elevated CRP level (>10 mg/L)[a]	2
Elevated synovial α-defensin level	2
Cloudy fluid	2

CRP = C-reactive protein, ESR = erythrocyte sedimentation rate, PJI = periprosthetic joint infection, PMN = polymorphonuclear leukocyte, WBC = white blood cell
[a]Beyond 6 weeks from recent surgery.

Table 2

The Weighted Values for All Positive Tests Performed as Part of the Diagnostic Evaluation of a Failed Shoulder Arthroplasty Are Summed

- 6 or greater with identified organism indicates probable periprosthetic joint infection (PJI)
- 6 or greater without identified organism indicates possible PJI
- Fewer than 6:
  a. Single positive culture with virulent organism indicates possible PJI
  b. Two positive cultures with low-virulence organism indicates possible PJI
  c. Negative cultures or only single positive culture with low-virulence organism indicates PJI unlikely

Reprinted from *J Shoulder Elbow Surg* 2019;28[6S]. Garrigues GE, Zmistowski B, Cooper AM, Green A, ICM Shoulder Group. Proceedings from the 2018 International Consensus Meeting on Orthopedic Infections: the definition of periprosthetic shoulder infection, S8-S12, Copyright 2019, with permission from Elsevier.

mechanical complications of the implant (60%), shoulder pain (18%), dislocation of the prosthetic joint (12%), component loosening (10%), broken prosthesis (8%), cuff tear (7%), and infection (7%).[10] Common indications for revision surgery include glenoid arthrosis after hemiarthroplasty, glenohumeral instability, progressive bone loss, rotator cuff tear or dysfunction, component problems (wear, loosening, failure, malposition, or inadequate sizing), periprosthetic infection, and periprosthetic fracture. The last two indications warrant further discussion.

Periprosthetic Infection

Acute postoperative infection after primary shoulder arthroplasty is relatively uncommon and often presents with obvious signs and symptoms such as malaise, fever, wound erythema, and drainage. Acute PJI has been defined as any infection requiring irrigation and débridement within 6 weeks of the index arthroplasty or within 3 weeks of symptoms from a delayed-onset acute hematogenous infection.[11] If the infectious process is thought to be acute, it may be treated with irrigation and débridement (I&D) with or without implant removal, depending on the clinical situation. I&D along with chronic antibiotic suppression has been reported to allow component retention in 70% of shoulders presenting with an acute or delayed-onset acute hematogenous infection.[9,11] Alternatively, the implants can be removed and a temporary antibiotic-loaded cement spacer/prosthesis placed with the intention of staged revision after the infection has been adequately treated. Appropriate antibiotic treatment is coordinated with infectious disease consultants.

Patients with more than 3 weeks of symptoms are considered as having chronic infections.[11] Implants should be removed in cases of chronic infection with a virulent organism. A temporary antibiotic-loaded cement spacer/prosthesis is typically placed in such cases with the intention of staged revision after the infection has been adequately treated in coordination with an infectious disease specialist.

Chronic indolent infections associated with less virulent organisms such as coagulase-negative *Staphylococci* and *Cutibacterium acnes* (*C acnes*—formerly known as *Propionibacterium acnes*) are usually not obvious, more difficult to diagnosis, and require a high index of suspicion. Surgeons should have a high index of suspicion of infection in all revision shoulder arthroplasty cases and take appropriate diagnostic steps. Successful diagnosis and management of chronic periprosthetic infection are often hampered because clinical findings may be subtle, many of the traditional signs of infection are not present, and cultures may not be positive for as long as 2 weeks.[12]

Perioperative tests for chronic infection, including WBC, ESR, CRP, and bone scans (technetium, indium), have a high specificity and negative predictive value, but low sensitivity and positive predictive value.[13] None of these tests are adequate to predict whether intraoperative cultures will be positive.[8] Synovial fluid α-defensin can provide an additional data point to assist the clinician in determining whether PJI is present but is prone to false-positive results.[14] Polymerase chain reaction–restriction fragment length polymorphism testing is reported to be both sensitive and specific for identifying *C acnes* in tissue specimens within 24 hours, facilitating treatment decision making.[15]

At the time of revision surgery, the authors recommend obtaining intraoperative frozen section histology and cultures of multiple soft-tissue samples. *C acnes* is the most common bacterium isolated from specimens obtained during revision shoulder arthroplasty surgery.[7,8,16,17] *C acnes* has been found to be unevenly distributed within culture-positive shoulders[18]; therefore, sending multiple intraoperative tissue samples from varying locations within the shoulder joint is recommended when infection is suspected during revision arthroplasty to prevent missing the diagnosis. Factors associated with an increased likelihood of *C acnes* infection include male sex, humeral osteolysis and loosening, cloudy fluid, glenoid wear, and membrane formation.[16,19]

Humeral Periprosthetic Fracture

Periprosthetic fractures can occur after all types of shoulder arthroplasty and most commonly involve the humeral shaft, with greater tuberosity fractures being less common. Treatment is predicated on the location of the fracture (**Figure 3**), fixation of the humeral implant, status of the glenoid component, and individual patient factors.[20,21] Humeral stem length has an impact on the fracture location as well as the mode of surgical treatment. In a 2013 study of periprosthetic fracture management, the authors reported a complication rate of 39% and a revision surgery rate of 19%, and the prosthetic components were found to be loose in more than 50% of cases.[22]

Outcomes of Revision Shoulder Arthroplasty

Patients should be counseled that the clinical results of revision shoulder arthroplasty are typically inferior to the results of primary arthroplasty and that the risks of intraoperative and postoperative complication are higher. Data from two studies suggest that patients undergoing revisions because of component loosening or glenoid erosion can expect to have better outcomes than those whose revisions are performed for infection, instability, or other soft-tissue problems.[23,24]

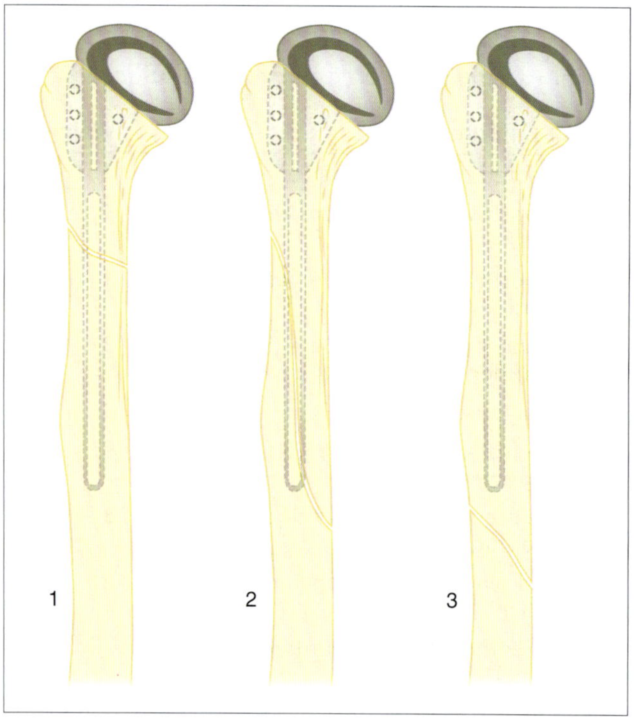

FIGURE 3 Illustration showing the fracture classification system of the authors of a 2008 study.[20] Type I fractures occur proximal to the tip of the prosthesis. Type II fractures occur proximal to the tip of the prosthesis and extend beyond the tip. Type III fractures originate below the tip of the prosthesis. (Reprinted from *J Shoulder Elbow Surg* 17[1]. Groh GI, Heckman MM, Wirth MA, Curtis RJ, Rockwood CA Jr: Treatment of fractures adjacent to humeral prostheses, 85-89. Copyright © 2008 Journal of Shoulder and Elbow Surgery Board of Trustees. doi:10.1016/j.jse.2007.05.007.)

Anatomic to Anatomic Prosthesis Revision

Patients undergoing revision to an anatomic TSA (aTSA) following painful hemiarthroplasty can achieve successful outcomes and implant survival rates.[25,26] Many authors report that although the clinical results of revision from a hemiarthroplasty to an aTSA can be excellent, there is a substantial risk of intraoperative complication, and the clinical outcomes are quite variable and, in many cases, unsatisfactory.[27-30] Patients with preoperative glenohumeral instability who develop glenoid component loosening after aTSA have limited if any improvement when revised to another anatomic arthroplasty.[31]

Similarly, patients with failed humeral hemiarthroplasty for fracture treatment do not predictably fare well when revised to aTSA. In a 2011 study,[30] only 12 of 34 patients (35%) who underwent revision to aTSA for painful glenoid arthrosis after hemiarthroplasty for fracture had a satisfactory result according to the modified Neer criteria rating.

In some cases, revision from failed aTSA due to glenoid failure can be addressed with revision to humeral head replacement. However, revision surgery gives predictably better clinical results when a total shoulder arthroplasty is performed rather than a hemiarthroplasty.[32] Although patients who have glenoid component revision experience a higher degree of satisfaction than those who undergo glenoid component removal, many patients with glenoid loosening have severe glenoid bone loss that precludes revision to another anatomic glenoid component.[31,33,34] Revision of aTSA to another aTSA is technically challenging, the results unreliable, and the need for further revision high.[35,36] Soft-tissue imbalance and glenohumeral instability are significantly associated with recurrent loosening. Some suggest that revision to reverse arthroplasty might be a more reliable option.

Anatomic to Reverse Prosthesis Revision

The original indication for reverse shoulder arthroplasty (RSA) was rotator cuff tear arthropathy (CTA). The indications for RSA have expanded with increased surgeon experience. There is a clear trend of increased use of reverse shoulder prostheses for revision shoulder arthroplasty surgery. In a recent article, the authors reported a much greater utilization of reverse prostheses (78%) for revision arthroplasty compared with aTSA prostheses (19%) or hemiarthroplasty (3%).[37] Revision to RSA has been shown to significantly improve patient-reported outcome scores compared with revision with hemiarthroplasty or aTSA.[38] Revision with RSA has been readily adapted to cases with scapular/glenoid bone loss that cannot be reconstructed with anatomic implants, as well as failed anatomic arthroplasty because of rotator cuff failure.

Although revision from aTSA to RSA often leads to better function and improved outcome scores compared with preoperative status, the patient-reported outcomes and satisfaction are inferior, and there are more complications compared with patients undergoing primary RSA for CTA.[39-44] On average, patients undergoing RSA for revision arthroplasty can expect improvements in function and shoulder scores to a mean of 50% of normal shoulders.[44]

Revision From Reverse to Reverse Shoulder Arthroplasty

There are a number of causes of failure that are specific to RSA, including instability, baseplate failure, scapular spine and acromial fractures, scapular notching, and humeral loosening. These cases can be extremely challenging, especially with regard to bone deficiency and joint stability. Although revision RSA to salvage a failed primary RSA can lead to better function and improved outcome scores compared with preoperative status, the results are less predictable and complication and revision rates are higher in patients undergoing revision surgery compared with those in patients with primary RSA for CTA.[40,45-49]

Several studies document that instability and infection are the most common problems that necessitate revision of RSA.[40,45,48,50,51] In patients with persistent instability or with risk factors for instability, the surgeon should consider using larger glenospheres and increasing lateral offset at the time of RSA.[52] Rates of infection are higher after revision than primary RSA.[53] Revision RSA for the management of glenoid baseplate mechanical failure can provide pain relief and restore function to the levels gained after the index RSA.[54] Age should not be used as an isolated reason to avoid revision surgery to RSA in patients older than 80 years.[55] Authors of a 2018 study reported that 51% of revision surgeries occur less than 6 months after the primary surgery and that male sex is associated with a significantly increased risk of revision.[56]

Technical Considerations

Humeral Stem Removal

Removal of the humeral stem is often required during revision surgery regardless of whether it is loose. Humeral stem removal may be required because of malposition. Stem removal may also be necessary for glenoid exposure. The stem must also be removed if an anatomic arthroplasty is being converted to a reverse and the original stem is not convertible.

Stem removal can be technically difficult. The most common complication is humeral fracture.[57] Intraoperative humeral fractures are reported to occur in 16% to 21% of shoulders undergoing revision surgery.[58,59] Fracture risk is reported to be greatest for female patients, patients with instability, and patients who have undergone previous hemiarthroplasties.[60] In a large registry study from 2017, it was found that females have over three times the risk of intraoperative fracture compared with males.[61]

A common belief is that press-fit components will be easier to remove in the revision setting than cemented components. However, this subject was examined in a 2018 study in which the authors found that the revision of humeral stems that had been placed with or without cement during the primary arthroplasty procedure demonstrated similar surgical time, need for intraoperative humeral osteotomy, and postoperative complication rates.[62] It has been shown that proximal cementation of the stem yields the same rotatory micromotion stability as full cementation while facilitating future explantation of the prosthesis.[63]

Two potential solutions to extract a well-fixed cemented or press-fit stem are a humeral window and a vertical humeral osteotomy (**Figure 4**). Humeral windows may facilitate controlled removal of well-fixed humeral components with a high rate of union, though a 20% humeral fracture rate has been noted.[64] In another study, a vertical humeral osteotomy was effective for the removal of the humeral prostheses with no perioperative

Section 5: Principles of Clinical Information

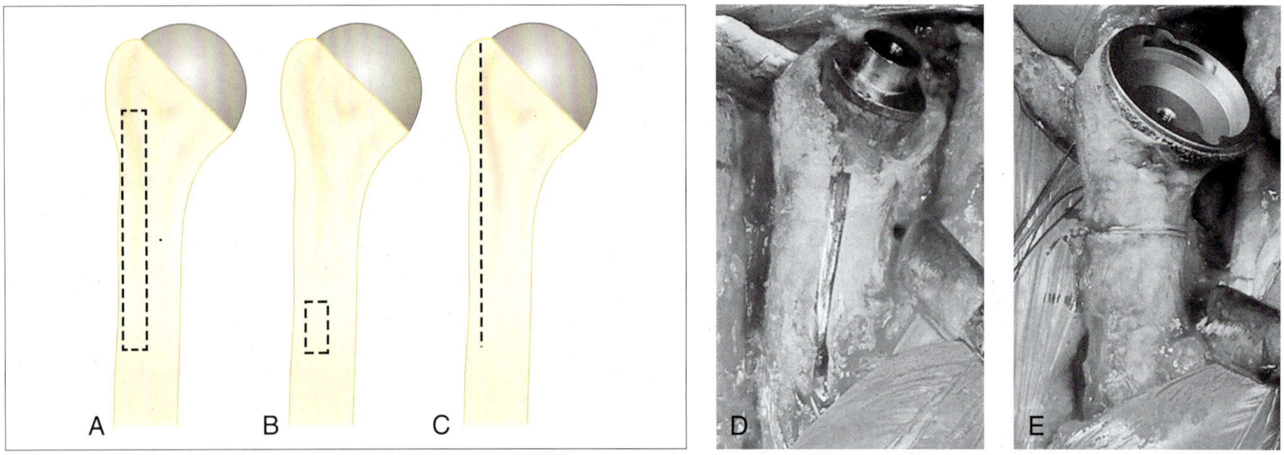

FIGURE 4 Illustration and photographs showing methods for removing a well-fixed humeral stem. **A**, An extensive humeral window. **B**, A limited, distal humeral window. **C**, A vertical humeral osteotomy. **D**, A vertical osteotomy allows access of thin cutting osteotomes to be inserted to break the prosthesis-bone coupling. This stem was removed without fracture complication. **E**, A reverse prosthesis was cemented into place after closure of the vertical osteotomy with suture. The pectoralis major tendon will be reattached using sutures that were placed through the bone before cementing.

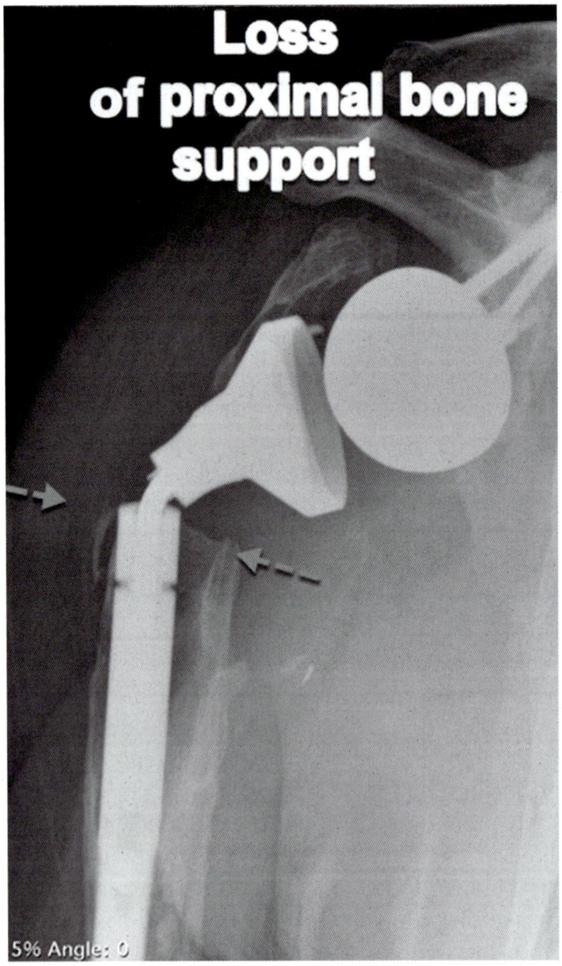

FIGURE 5 Radiograph showing that proximal humeral bone loss has compromised the necessary structural support for the stem, leading to mechanical failure of the implant. (Photo courtesy of Tom R. Norris, MD, San Francisco. Founding member and past-President, American Shoulder and Elbow Surgeons.)

or postoperative fractures.[65] Superiority of one technique over the other has not been substantiated to date[66] and should be left to surgeon preference and based on unique characteristics of each case.

The specific geometry and surface characteristics of a press-fit humeral stem can determine the difficulty of implant removal. Stems without fins and with smoother bone ingrowth/ongrowth surfaces are easier to remove. Various instruments including thin flexible osteotomes and high-speed burrs are useful for removal of press-fit stems. Most press-fit stems have only proximal surface treatment. Humeral prostheses that have a porous surface that runs the length of the stem are often extremely difficult to remove without significant bone destruction.

A question that often confronts the revision arthroplasty surgeon is whether to remove retained cement from the humeral canal after the humeral stem has been extracted. Rather than removing all of the cement, another option is to cement a smaller humeral stem within the retained, well-fixed cement mantle. Cement-within-cement fixation of the humeral component during revision RSA avoids removing retained cement with noted reasonable surgical times, good medium-term survival rates, and good pain relief and functional outcomes with low complications.[58]

Reconstruction for Bone Loss

Cases with associated proximal humeral bone loss have limited reconstruction options. A prosthesis that is not supported by surrounding proximal humeral bone is at increased risk for loosening and mechanical failure (**Figure 5**). Proximal humeral allograft may be used to restore proximal humeral bone stock, optimize deltoid tension, and maintain the correct height of the

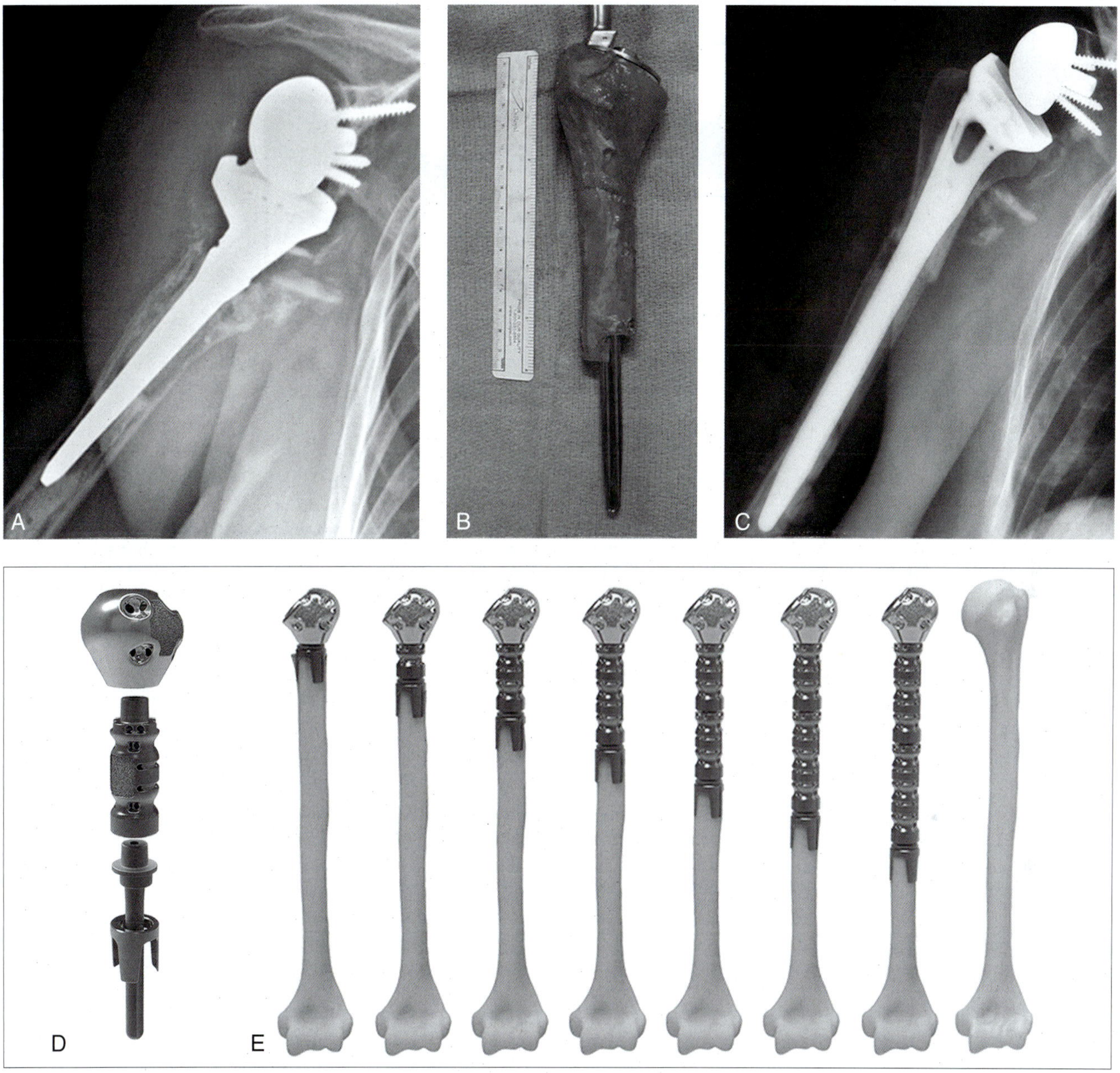

FIGURE 6 Proximal humeral bone loss presents a difficult challenge for reconstructive surgery. **A**, A preoperative radiograph demonstrating humeral component loosening with a severe proximal humerus bone defect. **B**, Photograph of a humeral allograft-prosthesis composite with step-cut. **C**, Postoperative radiograph. **D**, Photograph of a modular, reconstructive prosthesis (Equinoxe Humeral Reconstruction Prosthesis, Exactech, Inc), which is an alternative to the allograft-prothesis composite for managing proximal humeral bone loss. **E**, Photograph showing the modularity of the system, which allows the surgeon to replicate the proximal humeral anatomy for cases with varying amounts of proximal humeral bone loss. (**A** through **C**, Reproduced with permission from Boileau P: Complications and revision of reverse total shoulder arthroplasty. *Orthop Traumatol Surg Res* 2016;102[1 suppl]:S33-S43. Copyright © 2016 Elsevier Masson SAS. All rights reserved.)

prosthesis-bone construct. In a limited number of studies, the use of a reverse total shoulder allograft-prosthetic composite has been shown to provide pain relief and improved range of motion.[67,68] Alternatively, a reconstructive prosthesis can replicate the normal proximal humeral anatomy and obviate the need for allograft (**Figure 6**). It is unknown at this time whether one technique is superior to the other.

Reconstruction of sufficient glenoid bone stock is indispensable for reliable fixation of glenoid components.[69] Revision shoulder arthroplasty with glenoid bone grafting can produce good short-term outcomes.[70] Glenoid reconstruction surgery using bone-block autograft before[69] or during[71] revision arthroplasty may be considered in cases of extensive glenoid bone loss after primary shoulder arthroplasty. Tricortical iliac crest autograft can be used to

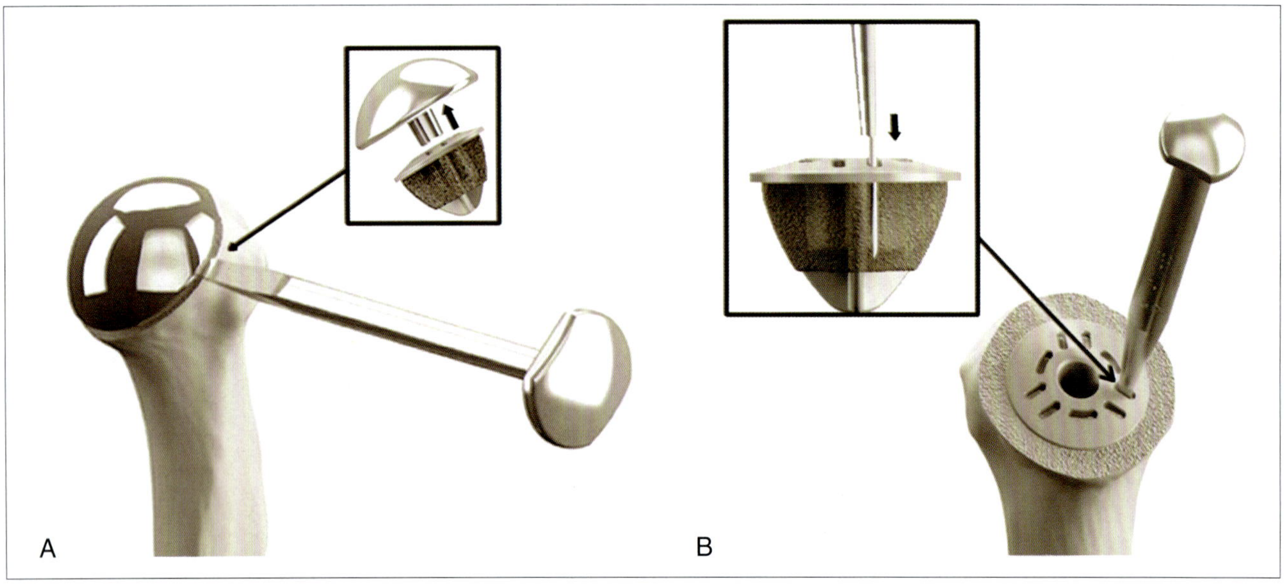

FIGURE 7 Photographs showing an example of an implant (Tornier Simpliciti, Wright Medical, Memphis, TN) that may be removed during revision cases with minimal humeral bone loss. The stemless prosthesis precludes the need for creation of a bone window or vertical osteotomy for implant removal. **A**, The humeral head is disengaged from the body of the implant. **B**, An osteotome is inserted through slots in the prosthesis body to sever bonding between the bone and the implant, allowing for uncomplicated removal of the implant with minimal bony destruction.

reconstruct a large glenoid defect, producing similar or better clinical outcomes compared with patients without bone loss.[71] Augmented glenoid components can also be used to reconstruct the glenoid in some bone-deficient cases.

Removable and Convertible Humeral Prostheses

Designers of newer prostheses have attempted to minimize the risk of intraoperative complications during revision surgery by incorporating prosthesis features that either facilitate implant removal with minimal bone loss (**Figure 7**), or permit the well-fixed components to be revised or converted without the need for removal from bone. When modular components are used for the index procedure (**Figures 8** and **9**), the complexity of the revision surgery can be minimized because removal of well-fixed components from the humeral and/or glenoid bone often becomes unnecessary.[26]

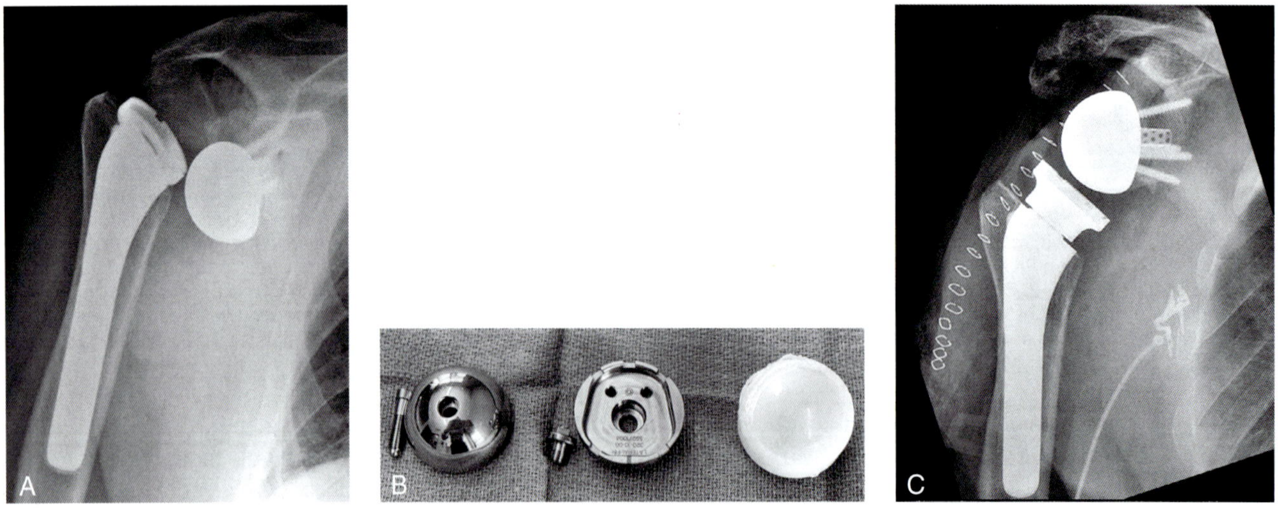

FIGURE 8 Radiographs and photograph showing a modular reverse prosthesis (Equinoxe, Exactech, Inc) was used for the index procedure. **A**, The patient presented with a history of recurrent posterosuperior dislocation. **B**, During the revision surgery, modular components including the glenosphere, humeral tray, and polyethylene cup were exchanged for larger ones. The stem and glenosphere baseplate were noted to be well fixed intraoperatively and were retained. **C**, A stable construct was achieved without intraoperative complication.

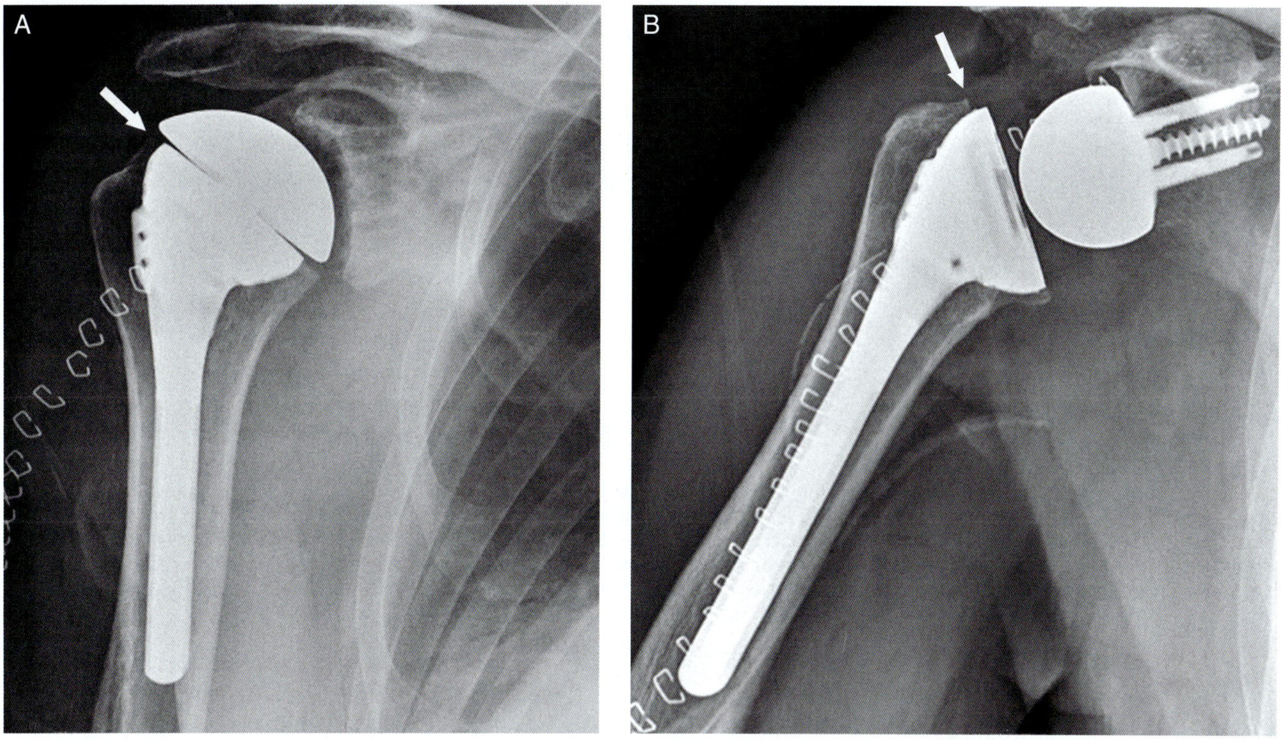

FIGURE 9 Radiographs showing an example of a convertible modular platform shoulder system (DJO AltiVate, DJO Global) in which the top of the shell of the inset humeral prosthesis is positioned flush with the anatomical neck bone cut (arrows). With convertible systems, stem removal is often unnecessary when revising from anatomic (**A**) to reverse (**B**) total shoulder arthroplasty (TSA). (Adapted with permission from Humphrey CS, Bravman JT: A method to facilitate improved positioning of a reverse prosthesis stem during arthroplasty surgery: The metaphyseal-centering technique. *Tech Shoulder Elb Surg* 2018;19[2]:67-74. doi:10.1097/BTE.0000000000000133.)

Several studies have documented the benefits of humeral stem retention versus extraction during revision surgery. The advantages of conversion arthroplasty with retention of the humeral stem include lower overall complications, blood loss, surgical time, and revision surgeries in comparison with stem exchange.[59,72-75] A 2018 pooled analysis that included 236 shoulders demonstrated significantly higher overall complications, fractures, surgical time, blood loss, and increased risk of revision surgery with humeral stem exchange.[72]

Although retention of the humeral stem appears to offer some advantages, conversion from anatomic to a reverse prosthesis cannot be achieved in about 25% of cases.[76] Reduction of the convertible reverse shoulder may not be possible because of a humeral component that was placed too high during the index procedure,[76] or because of severe soft-tissue contractures that do not allow the reverse shoulder prosthesis to be reduced with the original humeral stem in place despite appropriate soft-tissue releases.[73]

Convertible platform systems are believed to be generally beneficial, but there is a potential risk of excessive humeral lengthening[73] that comes with the use of a convertible onlay reverse stem (**Figure 10**). Neurologic complications[77] and scapular spine fractures[78] appear to correlate with arm lengthening. It was reported that use of an onlay reverse prosthesis resulted in a 4.3% incidence of scapular spine fracture, compared with a 1.3% rate with use of an inset Grammont-style reverse prosthesis.[78,79] Others, however, have reported that they could find no evidence of stress fractures of the acromion or scapular spine, neural injuries, or chronic regional pain syndrome at the postoperative follow-up despite a mean arm lengthening of 2.6 (0.9 to 4.7) cm.[73] Excessive arm lengthening during conversion from aTSA to a reverse prosthesis may potentially be avoided by use of an inset convertible platform system (**Figures 9** and **10**).[80] The overall cost of revision arthroplasty may be less when a platform system is used.[75] Additional studies are needed to elucidate the risks and benefits of using convertible platform arthroplasty systems.

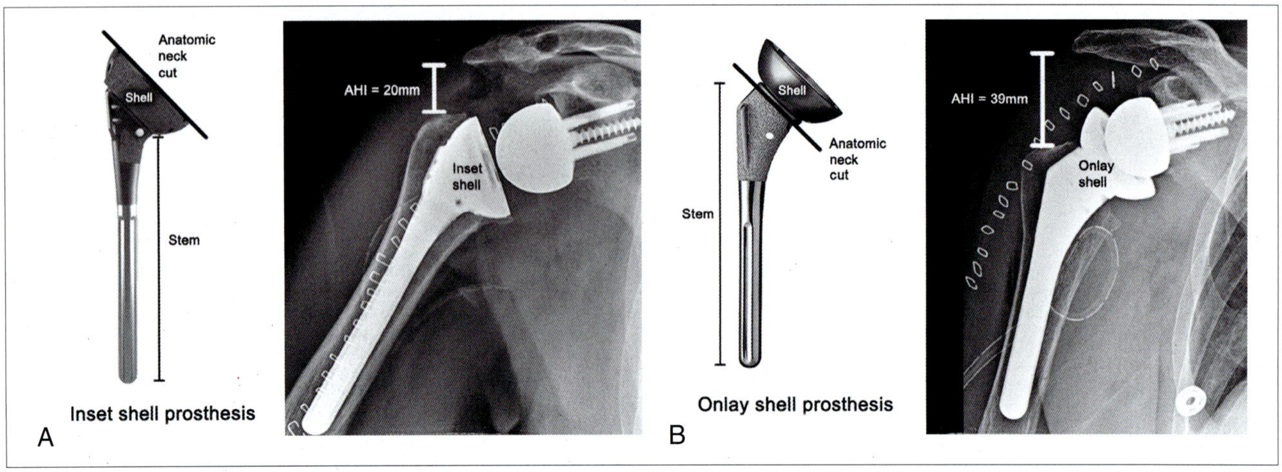

FIGURE 10 Photographs and radiographs showing reverse prostheses with an inset-shell design (**A**) versus an onlay-shell design (**B**). In this example, use of an onlay reverse prosthesis leads to increased humeral lengthening compared with that of the inset prosthesis, as can be seen by comparing the respective acromiohumeral interval (AHI) measurements. (Adapted with permission from Humphrey CS, Bravman JT: A method to facilitate improved positioning of a reverse prosthesis stem during arthroplasty surgery: The metaphyseal-centering technique. *Tech Shoulder Elb Surg* 2018;19[2]:67-74. doi:10.1097/BTE.0000000000000133.)

SUMMARY

Revision shoulder arthroplasty presents a unique set of challenges for the orthopaedic surgeon. Causes of arthroplasty failure and its associated pain are often nebulous and multifactorial. Revision surgery often leads to improvement in the patient's condition but can be technically difficult and is associated with higher complication rates and inferior clinical results compared with primary arthroplasty. Stemless, modular, and convertible platform arthroplasty systems may offer advantages over other prosthesis types in the revision setting.

KEY STUDY POINTS

- There are multiple causes of failed shoulder arthroplasty.
- Revision surgery is technically demanding and is associated with higher complication rates and inferior clinical results compared with primary arthroplasty.
- Evaluation with history, physical examination, imaging, and special testing is necessary before considering surgery.
- Periprosthetic infection should always be considered.
- Humeral osteotomy and humeral windows can be used to remove a well-fixed humeral component.
- Revision to reverse shoulder arthroplasty has advantages over revision to anatomic arthroplasty in many cases.
- Stemless, modular, and convertible platform arthroplasty systems may offer advantages over other prosthesis types in the revision setting.

Annotated References

1. Trofa D, Rajaee SS, Smith EL: Nationwide trends in total shoulder arthroplasty and hemiarthroplasty for osteoarthritis. *Am J Orthop (Belle Mead NJ)* 2014;43(4):166-172.

   From 2000 to 2010, the nationally adjusted population rate of shoulder arthroplasty performed for osteoarthritis increased 3.7-fold. Specifically, the population rate of TSA increased 5.0-fold and that of hemiarthroplasty increased 1.9-fold. In 2010, 80.3% of patients having shoulder arthroplasty for arthritis underwent TSA. Level of evidence: III.

2. Schwartz BE, Savin DD, Youderian AR, et al: National trends and perioperative outcomes in primary and revision total shoulder arthroplasty: Trends in total shoulder arthroplasty. *Int Orthop* 2015;39(2):271-276.

   This study demonstrates that the rate of TSA is rapidly increasing in the United States, with over a fourfold increase in revisions and fivefold increase in primaries over the 10 years studied. Level of evidence: III.

3. Wiater BP, Moravek JE Jr, Wiater JM: The evaluation of the failed shoulder arthroplasty. *J Shoulder Elbow Surg* 2014;23(5):745-758.

   This article provides a thorough and systematic approach to evaluation of the failed shoulder arthroplasty so that the most appropriate treatment pathway can be initiated. Level of evidence: V.

4. Sperling JW, Cofield RH, O'Driscoll SW, et al: Radiographic assessment of ingrowth total shoulder arthroplasty. *J Shoulder Elbow Surg* 2000;9(6):507-513.

5. Lazarus MD, Jensen KL, Southworth C, et al: The radiographic evaluation of keeled and pegged glenoid component insertion. *J Bone Joint Surg Am* 2002;84(7):1174-1182.

6. Sirveaux F, Favard L, Oudet D, et al: Grammont inverted total shoulder arthroplasty in the treatment of glenohumeral osteoarthritis with massive rupture of the cuff. Results of a multicentre study of 80 shoulders. *J Bone Joint Surg Br* 2004;86(3):388-395.

7. Kelly JD II, Hobgood ER: Positive culture rate in revision shoulder arthroplasty. *Clin Orthop Relat Res* 2009;467(9):2343-2348.

8. Topolski MS, Chin PY, Sperling JW, et al: Revision shoulder arthroplasty with positive intraoperative cultures: The value of preoperative studies and intraoperative histology. *J Shoulder Elbow Surg* 2006;15(4):402-406.

9. Garrigues GE, Zmistowski B, Cooper AM, et al: Proceedings from the 2018 International Consensus Meeting on Orthopedic Infections. *J Shoulder Elbow Surg* 2019;28(6S):S4-S99.

   The Shoulder Group of the Second International Consensus Meeting on Periprosthetic Infections recently published guidelines for defining, preventing, evaluating, and managing periprosthetic shoulder infections. Level of evidence: V.

10. Matsen FA III, Li N, Gao H, et al: Factors affecting length of stay, readmission, and revision after shoulder arthroplasty: A population-based study. *J Bone Joint Surg Am* 2015;97(15):1255-1263.

    Data were analyzed from the New York Statewide Planning and Research Cooperative System on 17,311 primary shoulder arthroplasties performed from 1998 to 2011 to identify factors associated with surgical revision. Revision was associated with younger patient age and osteoarthritis or traumatic arthritis. The most common diagnoses at the time of revision surgery were unspecified mechanical complications of the implant (60%), shoulder pain (18%), dislocation of the prosthetic joint (12%), component loosening (10%), a broken prosthesis (8%), a cuff tear (7%), and infection (7%). Level of evidence: III.

11. Dennison T, Alentorn-Geli E, Assenmacher AT, et al: Management of acute or late hematogenous infection after shoulder arthroplasty with irrigation, debridement, and component retention. *J Shoulder Elbow Surg* 2017;26:73-78.

    This study reports the outcomes and complications of I&D with component retention for acute and delayed-onset acute hematogenous periprosthetic shoulder infections. I&D allowed component retention in 70% of shoulders presenting with an acute or delayed-onset acute hematogenous infection. Most patients were prescribed chronic antibiotic suppression, and reasonable motion was maintained. Level of evidence: IV.

12. Dodson CC, Craig EV, Cordasco FA, et al: *Propionibacterium acnes* infection after shoulder arthroplasty: A diagnostic challenge. *J Shoulder Elbow Surg* 2010;19(2):303-307.

13. Ahmadi S, Lawrence TM, Sahota S, et al: Significance of perioperative tests to diagnose the infection in revision total shoulder arthroplasty. *Arch Bone Jt Surg* 2018;6(5):359-364.

    The purpose of this study was to evaluate the value of perioperative tests (periprosthetic tissue cultures, WBC count, ESR, CRP, bone scans, and intraoperative pathology readings). All of the perioperative tests had a high specificity and negative predictive value, but low sensitivity and positive predictive value. Level of evidence: III.

14. Kelly MP, Darrith B, Hannon CP, et al: Synovial fluid alpha-defensin is an adjunctive tool in the equivocal diagnosis of periprosthetic joint infection. *J Arthroplasty* 2018;33(11):3537-3540.

    In patients for whom the diagnosis of PJI is unclear because of recent antibiotic use, equivocal laboratory findings, or suspected false-negative or false-positive cultures, synovial fluid α-defensin can provide an additional data point to assist the clinician in determining whether PJI is present but is prone to false-positive results in this challenging population. Level of evidence: II.

15. Holmes S, Pena Diaz AM, Athwal GS, et al: Neer Award 2017: A rapid method for detecting *Propionibacterium acnes* in surgical biopsy specimens from the shoulder. *J Shoulder Elbow Surg* 2017;26(2):179-185.

    The authors developed a polymerase chain reaction–restriction fragment length polymorphism approach that is sensitive and specific for identification of *C acnes* in tissue specimens. Using this assay, a *C acnes*-positive tissue specimen can be confirmed within 24 hours of sampling, facilitating treatment decision making, targeted antibiotic therapy, and monitoring to minimize implant failure and revision surgery. Level of evidence: IV.

16. Pottinger P, Butler-Wu S, Neradilek MB, et al: Prognostic factors for bacterial cultures positive for *Propionibacterium acnes* and other organisms in a large series of revision shoulder arthroplasties performed for stiffness, pain, or loosening. *J Bone Joint Surg Am* 2012;94(22): 2075-2083.

17. Frangiamore SJ, Saleh A, Grosso MJ, et al: Early versus late culture growth of *Propionibacterium acnes* in revision shoulder arthroplasty. *J Bone Joint Surg Am* 2015;97(14):1149-1158.

    C acnes is the most commonly identified organism following revision shoulder arthroplasty. The proportion of positive cultures and the timing of culture growth may help to distinguish a true-positive from a false-positive culture result. Level of evidence: III.

18. Ahsan ZS, Somerson JS, Matsen FA III: Characterizing the *Propionibacterium* load in revision shoulder arthroplasty: A study of 137 culture-positive cases. *J Bone Joint Surg Am* 2017;99(2):150-154.

    The authors found that *C acnes* is unevenly distributed within culture-positive revised shoulders. A high percentage of specimens (mean, 43%; median, 50%) from the culture-positive shoulders showed no growth. As a result, the specimen number and source (explant, soft tissue, or fluid) have major influences on the culture results for a revised shoulder arthroplasty. Level of evidence: III.

19. Lucas RM, Hsu JE, Whitney IJ, et al: Loose glenoid components in revision shoulder arthroplasty: Is there an association with positive cultures? *J Shoulder Elbow Surg* 2016;25(8):1371-1375.

    Explanted glenoid components that were loose had a higher rate of culture positivity (56% [24/43]) in comparison to explanted glenoid components that were well fixed (13% [1/8]) ($P = 0.05$). Level of evidence: IV.

20. Groh GI, Heckman MM, Wirth MA, et al: Treatment of fractures adjacent to humeral prostheses. *J Shoulder Elbow Surg* 2008;17(1):85-89.

21. Kirchhoff C, Kirchhoff S, Biberthaler P: Classification of periprosthetic shoulder fractures. *Unfallchirurg* 2016;119(4):264-272.

    The authors present a new periprosthetic fracture classification system that encompasses the essential points of the existing classification systems while accounting for their deficiencies. Level of evidence: V.

22. Andersen JR, Williams CD, Cain R, et al: Surgically treated humeral shaft fractures following shoulder arthroplasty. *J Bone Joint Surg Am* 2013;95(1):9-18.

    The authors reviewed a consecutive series of patients with a humeral fracture around either an anatomic or a reverse shoulder prosthesis treated with either open reduction and internal fixation or revision shoulder arthroplasty. Fracture union occurred in 97% of patients. Complications occurred in 39%, and a revision surgery was required in 19% of the patients. More than half of the patients in this study were found to have a loose humeral component intraoperatively that required revision. Level of evidence: IV.

23. Sajadi KR, Kwon YW, Zuckerman JD: Revision shoulder arthroplasty: An analysis of indications and outcomes. *J Shoulder Elbow Surg* 2010;19(2):308-313.

24. Dines JS, Fealy S, Strauss EJ, et al: Outcomes analysis of revision total shoulder replacement. *J Bone Joint Surg Am* 2006;88(7):1494-1500.

25. Sheth MM, Sholder D, Abboud J, et al: Revision of failed hemiarthroplasty for painful glenoid arthrosis to anatomic total shoulder arthroplasty. *J Shoulder Elbow Surg* 2018;27(10):1884-1890.

    Anatomic TSA following hemiarthroplasty can achieve successful outcomes and implant survival rates. However, in their series, the complication rate was high (36%) and 21% of patients required revision surgery. Level of evidence: IV.

26. Groh GI, Wirth MA: Results of revision from hemiarthroplasty to total shoulder arthroplasty utilizing modular component systems. *J Shoulder Elbow Surg* 2011;20(5):778-782.

27. Sassoon AA, Rhee PC, Schleck CD, et al: Revision total shoulder arthroplasty for painful glenoid arthrosis after humeral head replacement: The nontraumatic shoulder. *J Shoulder Elbow Surg* 2012;21(11):1484-1491.

28. Hattrup SJ: Revision total shoulder arthroplasty for painful humeral head replacement with glenoid arthrosis. *J Shoulder Elbow Surg* 2009;18(2):220-224.

29. Rasmussen JV, Olsen BS, Al-Hamdani A, et al: Outcome of revision shoulder arthroplasty after resurfacing hemiarthroplasty in patients with glenohumeral osteoarthritis. *J Bone Joint Surg Am* 2016;98(19):1631-1637.

    In their series, the outcome of revision shoulder arthroplasty after failed resurfacing hemiarthroplasty was variable and, in many cases, disappointing. When resurfacing hemiarthroplasty is used in the management of osteoarthritis, revision cannot be counted on as a fallback. Level of evidence: II.

30. Rhee PC, Sassoon AA, Schleck CD, et al: Revision total shoulder arthroplasty for painful glenoid arthrosis after humeral head replacement: The posttraumatic shoulder. *J Shoulder Elbow Surg* 2011;20(8):1255-1264.

31. Deutsch A, Abboud JA, Kelly J, et al: Clinical results of revision shoulder arthroplasty for glenoid component loosening. *J Shoulder Elbow Surg* 2007;16(6):706-716.

32. Cil A, Veillette CJ, Sanchez-Sotelo J, et al: Revision of the humeral component for aseptic loosening in arthroplasty of the shoulder. *J Bone Joint Surg Br* 2009;91(1):75-81.

33. Antuna SA, Sperling JW, Cofield RH, et al: Glenoid revision surgery after total shoulder arthroplasty. *J Shoulder Elbow Surg* 2001;10(3):217-224.

34. Cheung EV, Sperling JW, Cofield RH: Revision shoulder arthroplasty for glenoid component loosening. *J Shoulder Elbow Surg* 2008;17(3):371-375.

35. Bonnevialle N, Melis B, Neyton L, et al: Aseptic glenoid loosening or failure in total shoulder arthroplasty: Revision with glenoid reimplantation. *J Shoulder Elbow Surg* 2013;22(6):745-751.

    In the authors' series, the overall rate of recurrent glenoid loosening (re-revision plus radiologic loosening) after reimplantation during revision surgery was 67%. This study suggests that revision of a TSA with reimplantation of an all-polyethylene cemented glenoid component does not solve the problem of glenoid loosening. Soft-tissue failure and prosthetic instability are underestimated preoperatively and may explain, in part, the high rate of recurrent glenoid loosening. Level of evidence: IV.

36. Sheth M, Sholder D, Padegimas EM, et al: Failure of anatomic total shoulder arthroplasty with revision to another anatomic total shoulder arthroplasty. *Arch Bone Jt Surg* 2019;7(1):19-23.

    Results of revision of aTSA to another aTSA were unpredictable and the revision rate was high. Reverse arthroplasty may be more reliable in this patient population. Level of evidence: IV.

37. Wagner ER, Chang MJ, Welp KM, et al: The impact of the reverse prosthesis on revision shoulder arthroplasty: Analysis of a high-volume shoulder practice. *J Shoulder Elbow Surg* 2019;28(2):e49-e56.

In a multicenter retrospective analysis, 274 revision shoulder arthroplasties were converted to an RSA (*n* = 182), aTSA (*n* = 68), or hemiarthroplasty (*n* = 24). Demographics, surgical indications, and types of prosthesis were analyzed. The number of revision arthroplasties increased over 12 years. From 2005 to 2010, TSA (33%) and hemiarthroplasty (16%) were used in similar rates as RSA (51%). From 2011 to 2016, there was a much higher incidence of revision arthroplasty with RSA (78%) compared with TSA (19%) or hemiarthroplasty (3%). The use of RSA for revision arthroplasty increased over time to become the majority by 2016. Level of evidence: III.

38. Kim K, Elbuluk A, Jia N, et al: Revision shoulder arthroplasty: Patient-reported outcomes vary according to the etiology of revision. *J Orthop* 2018;15(4):922-926.

Revision to RSA significantly improved patient-reported outcome scores compared with hemiarthroplasty or aTSA. Level of evidence: III.

39. Shields E, Wiater JM: Patient outcomes after revision of anatomic total shoulder arthroplasty to reverse shoulder arthroplasty for rotator cuff failure or component loosening: A matched cohort study. *J Am Acad Orthop Surg* 2019;27(4):e193-e198.

Revision of aTSA to RSA for component loosening or rotator cuff failure results in function comparable to primary RSA; however, more complications, worse subjective shoulder value scores, and lower patient satisfaction should be expected. Level of evidence: III.

40. Wall B, Nove-Josserand L, O'Connor DP, et al: Reverse total shoulder arthroplasty: A review of results according to etiology. *J Bone Joint Surg Am* 2007;89(7):1476-1485.

41. Stechel A, Fuhrmann U, Irlenbusch L, et al: Reversed shoulder arthroplasty in cuff tear arthritis, fracture sequelae, and revision arthroplasty. *Acta Orthop* 2010;81(3):367-372.

42. Valenti P, Kilinc AS, Sauzieres P, et al: Results of 30 reverse shoulder prostheses for revision of failed hemi- or total shoulder arthroplasty. *Eur J Orthop Surg Traumatol* 2014;24(8):1375-1382.

The purpose of this retrospective study was to evaluate the clinical and radiologic outcomes of a series of 30 reverse shoulder prostheses performed as revision of failed hemiarthroplasty or TSA. A total of 83% were satisfied (16 cases) or very satisfied (9 cases), and 17% were disappointed (5 patients). The mean Constant score increased from a mean of 25 to 52. The forward elevation changed from a mean of 55° (range 0 to 120) to 108° (range 40 to 160) ($P < 0.001$). There was no significant improvement of external rotation at 0° abduction (range 14° to 18°) or internal rotation (range 5 to 4.63). The complication rate was 26.6%. Level of evidence: IV.

43. Ortmaier R, Resch H, Matis N, et al: Reverse shoulder arthroplasty in revision of failed shoulder arthroplasty-outcome and follow-up. *Int Orthop* 2013;37(1): 67-75.

In revision shoulder arthroplasty, after failed primary shoulder arthroplasty, use of a reverse prostheis can improve the functional outcome, and patient satisfaction is usually high. Level of evidence: IV.

44. Austin L, Zmistowski B, Chang ES, et al: Is reverse shoulder arthroplasty a reasonable alternative for revision arthroplasty? *Clin Orthop Relat Res* 2011;469(9): 2531-2537.

45. Boileau P, Melis B, Duperron D, et al: Revision surgery of reverse shoulder arthroplasty. *J Shoulder Elbow Surg* 2013;22(10):1359-1370.

This study assesses the reasons for failure in RSA and evaluates the outcomes of revision RSA for 37 patients with RSA who had revision surgery between 1997 and 2009. Clinical and radiologic data were analyzed retrospectively with a minimum 2-year follow-up. The most common causes for RSA revision were prosthetic instability (48%); humeral loosening, derotation, or fracture (21%); and infection (19%). Only two patients (3%) had to be reoperated on for glenoid loosening. Underestimation of humeral shortening and excessive medialization were common causes of recurrent prosthetic instability. Proximal humeral bone loss was found to be a cause for humeral loosening or derotation. Previous surgery was found to be a potential cause of low-grade infection. The mean Constant score in patients who retained the RSA increased from 19 points before revision to 47 points at last follow-up ($P < 0.001$). The authors conclude that revision RSA often allows for a functional shoulder. Full-length scaled radiographs of both humeri are recommended to properly assess humeral shortening and excessive medialization before revision. Level of evidence: IV.

46. Boileau P, Watkinson D, Hatzidakis AM, et al: Neer Award 2005: The Grammont reverse shoulder prosthesis: Results in cuff tear arthritis, fracture sequelae, and revision arthroplasty. *J Shoulder Elbow Surg* 2006;15(5):527-540.

47. Saltzman BM, Chalmers PN, Gupta AK, et al: Complication rates comparing primary with revision reverse total shoulder arthroplasty. *J Shoulder Elbow Surg* 2014;23(11):1647-1654.

The purpose of this study was to describe the complication rates, types, timing, and risk factors after revision RSA, compared with primary RSA. Surgical complications were more frequent than medical complications in revision patients, occurring in 18% of primary cases and 62% of revisions. Multivariate logistic regression showed that revision status was the most significant predictor of overall ($P < 0.001$), minor ($P < 0.001$), surgical ($P < 0.001$), intraoperative ($P = 0.002$), and postoperative ($P < 0.001$) complication rates. Revision RSA has a significantly higher rate of complications than primary RSA. Level of evidence: III.

48. Wagner ER, Hevesi M, Houdek MT, et al: Can a reverse shoulder arthroplasty be used to revise a failed primary reverse shoulder arthroplasty?: Revision reverse shoulder arthroplasty for failed reverse prosthesis. *Bone Joint J* 2018;100-B(11):1493-1498.

The aim of this study was to determine the outcome of revision RSA when used as a salvage procedure for a failed primary RSA. A total of 27 revision RSAs were included in the study. The 5-year survival free of further revision was 85%. Smokers had a significantly increased risk of glenoid lucency ($P < 0.01$). Revision RSA, when used to salvage a failed primary RSA, can be a successful procedure. At intermediate follow-up, survival rates are reasonable, but dislocation and glenoid lucency remain a concern, particularly in smokers. Level of evidence: IV.

49. Black EM, Roberts SM, Siegel E, et al: Failure after reverse total shoulder arthroplasty: What is the success of component revision? *J Shoulder Elbow Surg* 2015;24(12):1908-1914.

This study examines the role of reimplantation and revision RSA after failed RSA, reporting outcomes and complications of this salvage technique. From 2004 to 2011, 16 patients underwent component revision and reimplantation after a prior failed RSA. Fourteen patients (88%) noted that they felt better postoperatively than before their original RSA and would go through the procedure again if given the option. Nine patients (56%) suffered major complications, and six of these (38% of cohort) ultimately underwent further procedures. The authors conclude that component revision and reimplantation can effectively relieve pain and improve function compared with baseline values, and patient satisfaction levels are moderately high despite significant complication and revision surgery rates. Level of evidence: IV.

50. Zumstein MA, Pinedo M, Old J, et al: Problems, complications, reoperations, and revisions in reverse total shoulder arthroplasty: A systematic review. *J Shoulder Elbow Surg* 2011;20(1):146-157.

51. Boileau P: Complications and revision of reverse total shoulder arthroplasty. *Orthop Traumatol Surg Res* 2016;102(1 suppl):S33-S43.

The functional results of revised RSA are inferior compared with those for primary prostheses and depend on the surgeon's experience and the number of RSAs performed, suggesting that patients should be referred to a tertiary center. Level of evidence: IV.

52. Hernandez NM, Chalmers BP, Wagner ER, et al: Revision to reverse total shoulder arthroplasty restores stability for patients with unstable shoulder prostheses. *Clin Orthop Relat Res* 2017;475(11):2716-2722.

Revision to RSA for prosthetic instability after aTSA is associated with reasonable implant survival and few complications. Approximately one in seven patients will have a recurrent dislocation. In patients with persistent instability or with risk factors for instability, consideration should be given for use of larger glenospheres and increasing the lateral offset at the time of RSA. Level of evidence: IV.

53. Trappey GJt, O'Connor DP, Edwards TB: What are the instability and infection rates after reverse shoulder arthroplasty? *Clin Orthop Relat Res* 2011;469(9):2505-2511.

54. Holcomb JO, Cuff D, Petersen SA, et al: Revision reverse shoulder arthroplasty for glenoid baseplate failure after primary reverse shoulder arthroplasty. *J Shoulder Elbow Surg* 2009;18(5):717-723.

55. Alentorn-Geli E, Clark NJ, Assenmacher AT, et al: What are the complications, survival, and outcomes after revision to reverse shoulder arthroplasty in patients older than 80 years? *Clin Orthop Relat Res* 2017;475(11):2744-2751.

Age should not be used as a reason to not consider revision surgery to RSA in patients older than 80 years. Level of evidence: IV.

56. Lehtimaki K, Rasmussen JV, Mokka J, et al: Risk and risk factors for revision after primary reverse shoulder arthroplasty for cuff tear arthropathy and osteoarthritis: A Nordic Arthroplasty Register Association study. *J Shoulder Elbow Surg* 2018;27(9):1596-1601.

The purpose of this study was to evaluate the survival of RSA and the risk factors for revision following RSA. RSA patients with CTA or osteoarthritis were identified from the Nordic Arthroplasty Register Association registry data (2004 to 2013). The study included 1904 patients. Revision was performed in 95 patients (5%), with a 10-year cumulative revision rate of 0.91. The most common reason for revision was infection ($n = 42$), followed by loosening ($n = 16$) and instability ($n = 12$). Most revisions occurred less than 6 months after the primary surgery. The overall midterm risk of revision after RSA for CTA was low (5%). Male sex was associated with a significantly increased risk of revision. Level of evidence: III.

57. Favard L: Revision of total shoulder arthroplasty. *Orthop Traumatol Surg Res* 2013;99(1 suppl):S12-S21.

During revision shoulder arthroplasty, the humeral stem must often be removed regardless of whether it is loose. However, its removal is very difficult and risky, and it often causes complications, with humerus fracture being the most common. Level of evidence: IV.

58. Wagner ER, Houdek MT, Hernandez NM, et al: Cement-within-cement technique in revision reverse shoulder arthroplasty. *J Shoulder Elbow Surg* 2017;26(8):1448-1453.

Cement-within-cement fixation of the humeral component in revision reverse shoulder arthroplasty is associated with a reasonable surgical time, good medium-term survival rates, and good pain relief and functional outcomes with low complications. This technique is an important consideration to preserve humeral bone stock and potentially humeral component and implant stability. Level of evidence: IV.

59. Dilisio MF, Miller LR, Siegel EJ, et al: Conversion to reverse shoulder arthroplasty: Humeral stem retention versus revision. *Orthopedics* 2015;38(9):e773-e779.

Patients who had retention of the humeral stem were compared with those who had stem revision. Humeral stem retention was associated with a significantly shorter surgical time (178.92 versus 237 minutes, $P = 0.02$). Minimal differences were observed for patient-reported outcomes. Of patients undergoing humeral stem removal, 21.4% had an intraoperative humeral shaft or tuberosity fracture compared with none in the stem retention group. The use of a platform shoulder arthroplasty system may benefit patients with failed shoulder arthroplasty undergoing conversion to RSA by avoiding humeral stem revision. Level of evidence: III.

60. Wagner ER, Houdek MT, Elhassan BT, et al: What are risk factors for intraoperative humerus fractures during revision reverse shoulder arthroplasty and do they influence outcomes? *Clin Orthop Relat Res* 2015;473(10):3228-3234.

Intraoperative humeral fractures occur in approximately 16% of shoulders undergoing revision surgery. Fractures during revision RSA are not uncommon secondary to the risks of component removal in revision surgery and poor remaining bone stock. The risk seems to be greatest for female patients, patients with instability, and patients who have undergone previous hemiarthroplasties. Level of evidence: IV.

61. Ingoe HM, Holland P, Cowling P, et al: Intraoperative complications during revision shoulder arthroplasty: A study using the National Joint Registry dataset. *Shoulder Elbow* 2017;9(2):92-99.

This is the largest registry study to date investigating the incidence and risk factors for intraoperative complications during revision shoulder arthroplasty (1,445 revision shoulder arthroplasties). Females have over three times the risk of intraoperative fractures compared with males. Periprosthetic fracture as an indication for revision carried the highest risk for any complication. Level of evidence: III.

62. Salesky MA, Grace TR, Feeley BT, et al: Effects of cemented versus press-fit primary humeral stem fixation in the setting of revision shoulder arthroplasty. *J Shoulder Elbow Surg* 2018;27(5):801-807.

Humeral stem fixation with or without cement during primary shoulder arthroplasty demonstrated similar surgical time, need for intraoperative humeral osteotomy, and postoperative complication rates in the setting of revision arthroplasty. Level of evidence: III.

63. Harris TE, Jobe CM, Dai QG: Fixation of proximal humeral prostheses and rotational micromotion. *J Shoulder Elbow Surg* 2000;9(3):205-210.

64. Sperling JW, Cofield RH: Humeral windows in revision shoulder arthroplasty. *J Shoulder Elbow Surg* 2005;14(3):258-263.

65. Van Thiel GS, Halloran JP, Twigg S, et al: The vertical humeral osteotomy for stem removal in revision shoulder arthroplasty: Results and technique. *J Shoulder Elbow Surg* 2011;20(8):1248-1254.

66. Sahota S, Sperling JW, Cofield RH: Humeral windows and longitudinal splits for component removal in revision shoulder arthroplasty. *J Shoulder Elbow Surg* 2014;23(10):1485-1491.

In both groups, there were no cases of malunion or clinical loosening. These data suggest that windows and longitudinal splits facilitate controlled removal of well-fixed components with high rate of union and low rate of intraoperative or postoperative sequelae. Level of evidence: IV.

67. Chacon A, Virani N, Shannon R, et al: Revision arthroplasty with use of a reverse shoulder prosthesis-allograft composite. *J Bone Joint Surg Am* 2009;91(1):119-127.

68. Cox JL, McLendon PB, Christmas KN, et al: Clinical outcomes following reverse shoulder arthroplasty-allograft composite for revision of failed arthroplasty associated with proximal humeral bone deficiency: 2- to 15-year follow-up. *J Shoulder Elbow Surg* 2019;28(5):900-907.

The purpose of this study was to report the results of a large cohort of patients treated with a reverse shoulder allograft-prosthetic composite.The revision surgery–free survival rate of all reconstructions was 88% (30 of 34) at 5 years, 78% (21 of 27) at 10 years, and 67% (8 of 12) beyond 10 years. The use of a reverse total shoulder allograft-prosthetic composite provides reliable pain relief and improved range of motion, with an acceptable rate of complications. Although ultimate function achieved is limited, patient satisfaction remains high. Level of evidence: IV.

69. Hoffelner T, Moroder P, Auffarth A, et al: Outcomes after shoulder arthroplasty revision with glenoid reconstruction and bone grafting. *Int Orthop* 2014;38(4):775-782.

Sufficient glenoid bone stock restoration is indispensable for reliable fixation of glenoid components and in turn a satisfactory clinical outcome. The authors describe a salvage procedure to be used in cases of extensive glenoid bone loss after primary shoulder arthroplasty. Results of glenoid reconstruction surgery using an iliac crest bone-block autograft before revision arthroplasty are reported. Level of evidence: IV.

70. Elhassan B, Ozbaydar M, Higgins LD, et al: Glenoid reconstruction in revision shoulder arthroplasty. *Clin Orthop Relat Res* 2008;466(3):599-607.

71. Kelly JD II, Zhao JX, Hobgood ER, et al: Clinical results of revision shoulder arthroplasty using the reverse prosthesis. *J Shoulder Elbow Surg* 2012;21(11):1516-1525.

72. Kirsch JM, Khan M, Thornley P, et al: Platform shoulder arthroplasty: A systematic review. *J Shoulder Elbow Surg* 2018;27(4):756-763.

Conversion arthroplasty with retention of the humeral stem is associated with lower overall complications, blood loss, surgical time, and revision surgeries in comparison with stem exchange. Level of evidence: IV.

73. Werner BS, Boehm D, Gohlke F: Revision to reverse shoulder arthroplasty with retention of the humeral component. *Acta Orthop* 2013;84(5):473-478.

    Modular systems allow retainment of a well-fixed humeral stem with good outcome. There is a risk of excessive humeral lengthening. Mean lengthening of the arm was 2.6 (0.9 to 4.7) cm without any neurologic complications. Level of evidence: IV.

74. Crosby LA, Wright TW, Yu S, et al: Conversion to reverse total shoulder arthroplasty with and without humeral stem retention: The role of a convertible-platform stem. *J Bone Joint Surg Am* 2017;99(9):736-742.

    Shoulder arthroplasty systems that use a convertible-platform humeral stem offer an advantage for revision TSA conversion in that a well-fixed, well-positioned humeral stem can be retained. There were significantly fewer complications as well as significantly decreased blood loss and surgical time when a convertible-platform stem was used ($P < 0.050$). Patients with component retention had slightly better postoperative range of motion. Level of evidence: III.

75. Crosby LA, Wright TW, Zuckerman JD: Revision total shoulder arthroplasty without humeral component removal. A preliminary report on the role of a platform humeral component. *Bull Hosp Jt Dis (2013)* 2015;73 suppl 1:S136-S139.

    There were significantly fewer complications as well as significantly decreased blood loss and surgical time when a convertible-platform stem was use ($P < 0.050$). Patients with stem retention had slightly better postoperative range of motion (active external rotation, 26° ± 23° versus 11° ± 23° [$P = 0.006$]; active forward elevation, 112° ± 37° versus 96° ± 33° [$P = 0.055$]). Level of evidence: III.

76. Kany J, Amouyel T, Flamand O, et al: A convertible shoulder system: Is it useful in total shoulder arthroplasty revisions? *Int Orthop* 2015;39(2):299-304.

    During revision surgery with a convertible prosthesis, the humeral stem was kept in three out of four cases. Most of the time, it was changed because of too high a position, making it impossible to reduce the RSA. A platform shoulder system allows much easier revisions. Level of evidence: IV.

77. Ladermann A, Lubbeke A, Melis B, et al: Prevalence of neurologic lesions after total shoulder arthroplasty. *J Bone Joint Surg Am* 2011;93(14):1288-1293.

78. Ascione F, Kilian CM, Laughlin MS, et al: Increased scapular spine fractures after reverse shoulder arthroplasty with a humeral onlay short stem: An analysis of 485 consecutive cases. *J Shoulder Elbow Surg* 2018;27(12):2183-2190.

    Scapular spine fractures have shown an increased prevalence after onlay-design reverse shoulder arthroplasty. The scapular spine fracture rate was 4.3% with use of an onlay reverse prosthesis. Functional results are limited in such cases, regardless of the fracture management. Level of evidence: IV.

79. Neyton L, Erickson J, Ascione F, et al: Grammont Award 2018: Scapular fractures in reverse shoulder arthroplasty (Grammont style): Prevalence, functional, and radiographic results with minimum 5-year follow-up. *J Shoulder Elbow Surg* 2019;28(2):260-267.

    Scapular fractures after Grammont-style (inset) RSAs are rare (1.3%). Final functional outcomes are poor regardless of acromial or spine fracture compared with primary RSA without fracture. Level of evidence: IV.

80. Humphrey CS, Bravman JT: A method to facilitate improved positioning of a reverse prosthesis stem during arthroplasty surgery: The metaphyseal-centering technique. *Tech Shoulder Elb Surg* 2018;19(2):67-74.

    The authors describe a surgical technique to allow an inset reverse humeral stem to be used for either anatomic or reverse shoulder arthroplasty. Excessive arm lengthening during conversion from aTSA to a reverse prosthesis may potentially be avoided by use of an inset convertible platform system. Level of evidence: IV.

Section 6

Trauma and Fractures

SECTION EDITOR:
ANAND M. MURTHI, MD

Chapter 29

Proximal Humerus Fractures

John-Erik Bell, MD, MS • Michael T. Torchia, MD, MS

ABSTRACT

Proximal humerus fractures are common injuries that follow a bimodal distribution, occurring in young patients after high-energy trauma and in elderly patients after low-energy falls. Fracture displacement follows a predictable pattern based on the muscular attachments around the proximal humerus. Most proximal humerus fractures are nondisplaced or minimally displaced and can be managed nonsurgically with good results. There are several options available for the surgical management of displaced proximal humerus fractures. Although new technology and recent outcome studies have refined the indications for the surgical management of proximal humerus fractures, this injury remains a challenge to surgeons from both a technical and decision-making standpoint.

Keywords: anatomy; evaluation; nonsurgical management; proximal humerus fractures; surgical management

Introduction

Proximal humeral fractures are the third most common extremity fragility fracture in individuals older than 65 years, behind hip and distal radius fractures.[1] Although these fractures most frequently occur in older adults as a consequence of low-energy trauma, as in a fall, they also occur in younger patients as a result of higher energy trauma. Most proximal humeral fractures are nondisplaced or minimally displaced, and usually they are managed nonsurgically. Nonsurgical management of a minimally displaced fracture leads to a predictably good outcome. The options for managing a displaced fracture include nonsurgical treatment, percutaneous pinning, open reduction and internal fixation (ORIF), and primary arthroplasty. The management of displaced fractures can be difficult, controversial, and fraught with complications. The aging of the US population and the widespread osteoporosis associated with aging means that rates of proximal humeral fracture will increase, as will those of other fragility fractures. Proximal humeral fractures are likely to impose a significant and increasing burden on the healthcare system.

Neither of the following authors nor any immediate family member has received anything of value from or has stock or stock options held in a commercial company or institution related directly or indirectly to the subject of this chapter: Dr. Bell and Dr. Torchia.

Anatomy and Classification

The epiphyseal lines of the proximal humerus was first described in 1934 and was divided into four anatomic fragments: the articular segment, the greater tuberosity, the lesser tuberosity, and the humeral shaft.[2] In a 2006 study a widely adopted classification system was built on parts defined as angulation of 45° or displacement of 1 cm of any of the four fragments.[3] Displacement of one of the parts is determined by its musculotendinous attachments. The supraspinatus and infraspinatus pull the greater tuberosity posteriorly and superiorly. The subscapularis pulls the lesser tuberosity anteriorly and medially. The pectoralis major and deltoid pull the humeral shaft proximally and medially, producing apex anterior angulation.

It is important to understand the vascularity of the proximal humerus because the risk of osteonecrosis is higher in some fracture patterns than in others, and this risk influences both the surgical indications and the prognosis. Originally the anterior circulation was considered to provide the dominant blood supply of the humeral head. The anterolateral branch of the anterior circumflex humeral artery enters bone at the junction of the intertubercular groove and the greater tuberosity proximally after ascending along the lateral aspect of the long head of the biceps, and it becomes the arcuate artery as it assumes an intraosseous course.[4] The importance of the posterior circulation has been emphasized later.[5,6] The posterior humeral circumflex artery was found to contribute 64% of the articular segment blood supply; this finding helps to explain why not all fractures with complete disruption of the anterior circulation go on to osteonecrosis.

The Neer system is straightforward and relatively easy to apply, but does not directly take into account the vascularity of the proximal humerus, and it has mediocre interobserver and intraobserver reliability.[7] The AO-ASIF

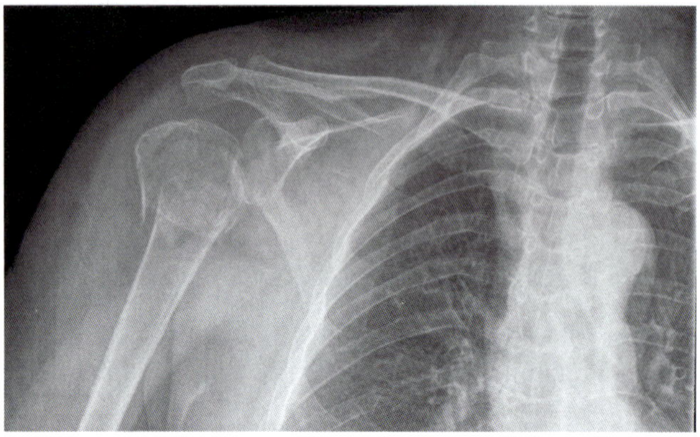

FIGURE 1 AP radiograph showing a valgus-impacted proximal humeral fracture.

classification system is based on both the fracture complexity and the extent of disruption of the humeral head blood supply. The three basic types are divided into a total of 27 groups and subgroups.[8] This classification system is comprehensive and correlated with outcomes and osteonecrosis, but it is very complex and has worse interobserver and intraobserver reliability than the Neer system.

The valgus-impacted fracture pattern was not part of the original Neer classification, but it was included in the updated 2002 Neer classification system.[9] In this three-part or four-part fracture pattern, the head position relative to the shaft is in valgus and impacted onto the shaft (**Figure 1**). The greater tuberosity is typically displaced superiorly relative to the head. It is important to recognize this pattern because the blood supply usually is preserved, in contrast to most displaced three-part and four-part fracture patterns. Rates of osteonecrosis are lower in valgus-impacted four-part fractures than in displaced four-part fractures and fracture dislocations presumably because of preservation of the medial hinge blood supply.[10,11]

The intimate anatomic relationship between nerves and fractured structures in the proximal humerus leads to a high rate of neurologic injury in these fractures. The rate of electromyography-documented axillary nerve abnormality is 58%, and the rate of suprascapular nerve abnormality is as high as 48%.[12] Injury of the axillary artery has been reported as a complication of proximal humeral fracture, most commonly with fracture dislocation.

Evaluation and Imaging

The patient history should include any preexisting shoulder symptoms that could indicate rotator cuff pathology, arthritis, or preinjury instability. The history also should include the mechanism of injury, any systemic comorbidities that might affect the safety of surgery or anesthesia, and the patient's social situation. The evaluation should include a thorough neurovascular examination, inspection of the skin, evaluation for associated injuries, and appropriate radiographs. The neurovascular examination should include the radial, median, ulnar, musculocutaneous (and lateral antebrachial cutaneous sensation), axillary, and suprascapular nerves. For the axillary nerve, deltoid muscle contraction and intact lateral shoulder sensation should be confirmed. The vascular examination always is important, even more so with dislocation of the glenohumeral joint. Doppler or angiogram imaging may be included if there is a question of vascular injury.

The standard shoulder trauma radiographs include the true AP, scapular Y, and axillary views. Additional radiographs to evaluate for specific pathology include internal-external rotation views for occult surgical neck or greater tuberosity fracture, the West Point axillary view for anterior glenoid rim fracture, and the Stryker notch view for a Hill-Sachs lesion. These specialized views have been largely supplanted by the ready availability of CT, which usually provides much more detailed information for surgical decision making and planning.

Decision Making and Nonsurgical Management

The characteristics of the patient as well as the fracture must be considered in determining the best treatment course. The patient's comorbidities, activity level, hand dominance, age, and ability to comply with postoperative restrictions and instructions are important considerations. Fracture characteristics including bone quality, fracture pattern and displacement, humeral head vascularity, and neurologic status also should factor into the decision-making process.

The risk of osteonecrosis of the humeral head increases with fracture complexity.[13] Predictors of vascular disruption include length of the metaphyseal head extension (less than 8 mm), fracture type, and integrity of the medial hinge.[14] The risk of osteonecrosis is increased in anatomic neck fractures, four-part displaced fractures, and all three-part fractures unless there is no fracture between the tuberosities. A longer metaphyseal extension is thought to be correlated with preservation of the posteromedial blood supply through the posterior humeral circumflex artery.

Nondisplaced and minimally displaced fractures should be managed nonsurgically. This treatment is not controversial and is widely accepted as the standard of care. Most patients, even those with a stable fracture, are treated with 2 to 4 weeks of sling immobilization. Early physical therapy is recommended and is associated with an improved outcome in stable fractures. Usually, gentle range-of-motion exercises are safe, beginning with pendulums and pulleys and progressing over the first few weeks to passive range of motion.[15] At 6 weeks, active-assisted and active range-of-motion exercises usually can begin, provided that radiographs show no further displacement and there is evidence of early healing. Patients typically have a good result. High radiographic union rates, good functional outcomes, low complication rates, and minimal differences between the injured and contralateral sides on validated outcome scales have been reported.[16,17]

Fracture dislocation can be managed in some patients with closed reduction and subsequent nonsurgical treatment. Prereduction radiographs should be scrutinized, however, because occult surgical neck fractures can become displaced during the reduction maneuver, potentially changing a nonsurgical fracture to a difficult surgical case (**Figure 2**). A dislocation with nondisplaced fracture lines may require general anesthesia with fluoroscopic imaging to minimize the amount of force required and avoid displacement.

The surgical indications are more controversial for displaced proximal humeral fractures. Generally speaking, young and/or very active patients with displaced fractures are treated more aggressively than elderly, low-demand patients, where the optimal treatment is more controversial. Most of the literature has focused on management of displaced fractures in the elderly. A recent prospective multicenter randomized clinical trial showed no difference in outcomes at both 2 and 5 years when comparing surgical versus nonsurgical management of displaced proximal humerus fractures.[18,19] ORIF with a locking plate was compared with nonsurgical management of displaced three-part fractures; no statistically significant difference in outcome was found, but 30% of the patients treated with ORIF required additional surgery.[20] Another prospective randomized controlled study compared hemiarthroplasty and nonsurgical management of displaced four-part fractures. The patients treated with hemiarthroplasty had significant improvement in pain and quality of life, but there was no between-group difference in range of motion.[21] A meta-analysis published in 2013 found no difference in clinical outcome scores between surgical and nonsurgical management of three-part and four-part proximal humerus fractures,[22] and a 2015 Cochrane review concluded that there is insufficient evidence to inform the decision on surgical versus nonsurgical management of displaced proximal humerus fractures.[23]

Because no definitive evidence supports a surgical or nonsurgical management strategy for displaced proximal humeral fractures, the treatment often is determined by the experience and preference of the surgeon. There are significant regional variations in the proportion of fractures managed surgically or nonsurgically.[24,25]

Surgical Management

Surgical management of proximal humeral fractures typically is done with the patient in the beach-chair or supine position. General or regional anesthesia or a combination is used. The fluoroscopy machine is parallel to the table to allow orthogonal views of the shoulder without the need to move the arm significantly. The standard deltopectoral approach and the deltoid-splitting (anterolateral) approach are most commonly used. The deltopectoral approach is extensile and utilitarian for both fracture fixation and arthroplasty, although reaching the lateral

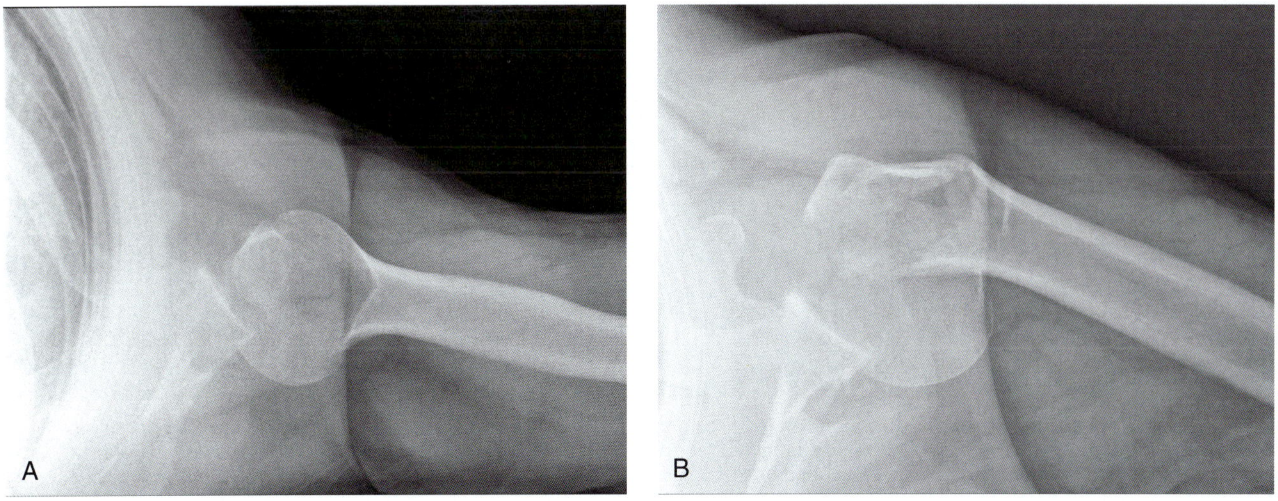

FIGURE 2 **A**, Axillary radiograph showing a posterior fracture dislocation with an engaging reverse Hill-Sachs lesion. A nondisplaced crack extends into the surgical neck. **B**, After an attempted closed reduction, the fracture has become displaced.

and posterior aspects of the proximal humerus can be difficult. The anterolateral deltoid-splitting approach provides excellent exposure of the lateral humerus and greater tuberosity for fracture fixation, but it places the axillary nerve at increased risk and is not extensile.[26]

Percutaneous pinning is becoming less popular in adults because techniques and implants for ORIF and arthroplasty are refined, but it remains an option for a surgical neck fracture or a valgus-impacted fracture with an intact medial hinge. Currently, its use is mostly confined to the pediatric population. Significant medial calcar communion is a relative contraindication to pinning. The advantages of percutaneous pinning include preservation of fracture hematoma and a minimal need for incision, soft-tissue stripping, and permanent hardware, as well as a relatively low risk of osteonecrosis. The disadvantages include technical difficulty, the need for hardware removal, and an inability to initiate early range-of-motion exercises because of less secure fixation and pin prominence. **Figure 3** illustrates the steps in percutaneous pinning. The results of percutaneous pinning generally are good.[27-30]

ORIF has become an established method of treatment since the introduction of locking-plate technology. The optimal fixation construct depends on both the fracture pattern and bone quality. Bone quality usually is poor, especially in the head. Frequently, the best fixation method for the tuberosities avoids the tuberosity bone entirely and consists of suture fixation in the rotator cuff tendon insertion. If significant metaphyseal comminution is present, a fixed-angle construct (a blade plate or locking plate) or intramedullary fixation is preferred to prevent failure into varus.

Locking plates initially were shown to be biomechanically superior to the existing fixation constructs including T plates and buttress plates. The key feature

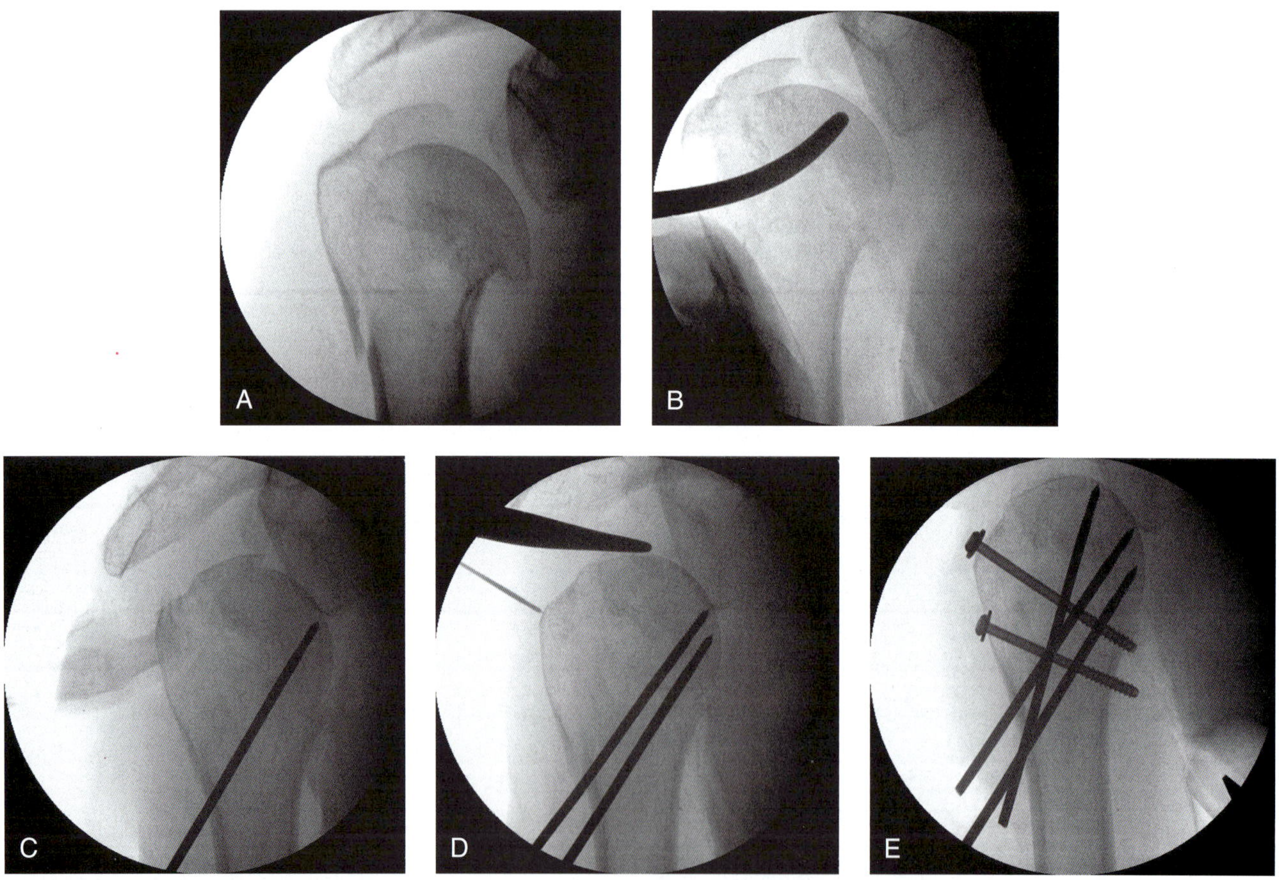

FIGURE 3 AP fluoroscopic images showing the technique for percutaneous pinning of a valgus-impacted three-part proximal humeral fracture. **A,** The humeral head is valgus impacted, and the greater tuberosity is elevated. **B,** A percutaneously placed hemostat is used to disimpact and elevate the head out of valgus. **C,** The head position is secured relative to the shaft using 2.8-mm terminally threaded pins. **D,** The percutaneous hemostat is used to reduce the greater tuberosity, which is provisionally fixed with guidewires for 4.0-mm cannulated screws. **E,** The cannulated screws with washers are advanced over guidewires to complete the construct.

of the proximal humeral locking plate is that the screws are directed toward the humeral head but are locked in different orientations, thereby increasing the pullout strength of the entire construct.[31-33] Locking-plate technology offers an option for ORIF in osteoporotic bone, for which arthroplasty or nonsurgical treatment had been the only other options. Locking-plate technology also offers a desirable option for young patients with relatively good bone stock who have a highly unstable high-energy fracture or a head-splitting fracture (**Figure 4**).

Although the use of locking plates has become popular and has allowed ORIF where it had not previously been possible, the associated rates of complications and revision surgery are high. Most of the reported complications are related to hardware and technique, and they underscore the difficulty of treating these fractures, even for experienced surgeons. Many studies have documented the high complication and revision surgery rates.[24,34-37] A large multicenter study of 187 patients reported a 34% complication rate when proximal humeral locking plates were used; 19% of the patients required a second, unplanned surgery within 12 months of the index procedure.[34] The complications include hardware penetration, varus collapse caused by loss of fixation, malunion, nonunion, infection, neurologic injury, adhesive capsulitis, and osteonecrosis, which often results in late hardware penetration as the humeral head collapses but the locked screws do not (**Figure 5**).

Attention to several specific points can minimize the risk of fixation-related complications. The most commonly reported early complication is screw penetration of the humeral head. This complication can best be avoided by measuring carefully, subtracting 5 mm from the measured length of each screw, and checking orthogonal images of all screws before leaving the operating room. Supplemental heavy suture fixation first through the rotator cuff bone–tendon junction and then through the plate can help prevent failure of tuberosity fixation or varus collapse. Most proximal humeral locking plates are designed to accommodate suture fixation through the proximal aspect. Salvage of failed proximal humeral ORIF is technically challenging. For some complications, such as osteonecrosis, chronic rotator cuff insufficiency, or tuberosity nonunion, conversion to arthroplasty may be the best option. For fixation failure caused by a technical factor, revision to blade plate fixation is a reasonable option because often there is sufficient residual bone stock in the head to allow a successful revision (**Figure 6**).

Augmentation of internal fixation constructs with intramedullary allograft has received attention since it was first described in 2008.[38] Biomechanical data have confirmed that intramedullary fibular strut augmentation of locking-plate fixation improves both maximal load to failure and initial construct stiffness.[39,40] This technique is most useful in fracture patterns with varus angulation and loss of medial support, and it has been shown to prevent varus collapse (**Figure 7**).

Primary shoulder arthroplasty is an option for three-part, four-part, and head-splitting fractures. The decision to perform arthroplasty rather than ORIF depends not only on the fracture pattern but also on patient characteristics including age, activity level, and expectations (**Figure 8**). The traditional standard has been hemiarthroplasty, but the reverse total shoulder prosthesis has become increasingly popular for managing these fractures, particularly in geriatric patients with relatively low physical demands.[41] The outcome of primary hemiarthroplasty is better than that of secondary arthroplasty after a proximal humeral fracture.[42] The most important factor in the outcome of hemiarthroplasty for fracture is the appropriate positioning and healing of the tuberosities.[43-45] Improper tuberosity position leads

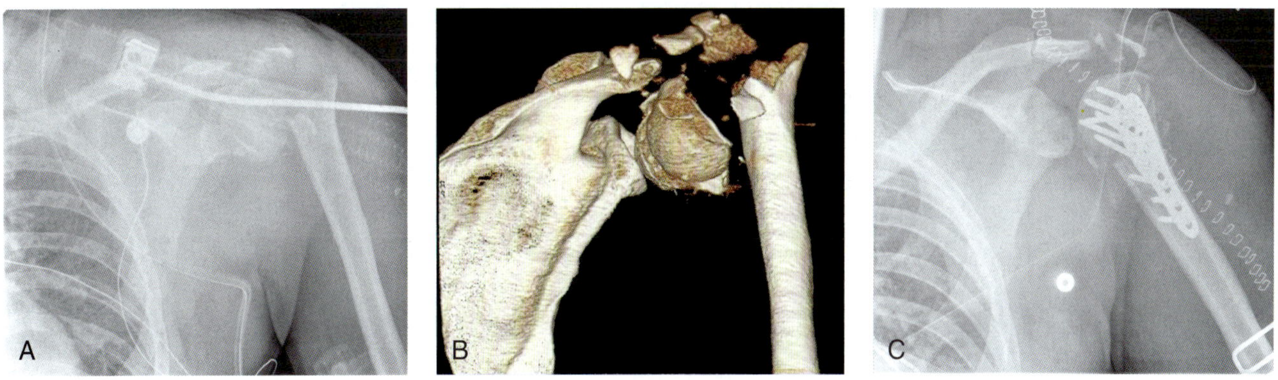

FIGURE 4 **A**, AP radiograph showing a high-energy comminuted four-part proximal humeral fracture in a 28-year-old man after a motor vehicle crash. **B**, Three-dimensional CT reconstruction showing intra-articular humeral head splitting. **C**, Postoperative AP radiograph showing open reduction and internal fixation with a locking proximal humerus plate.

Section 6: Trauma and Fractures

Section 6: Trauma and Fractures

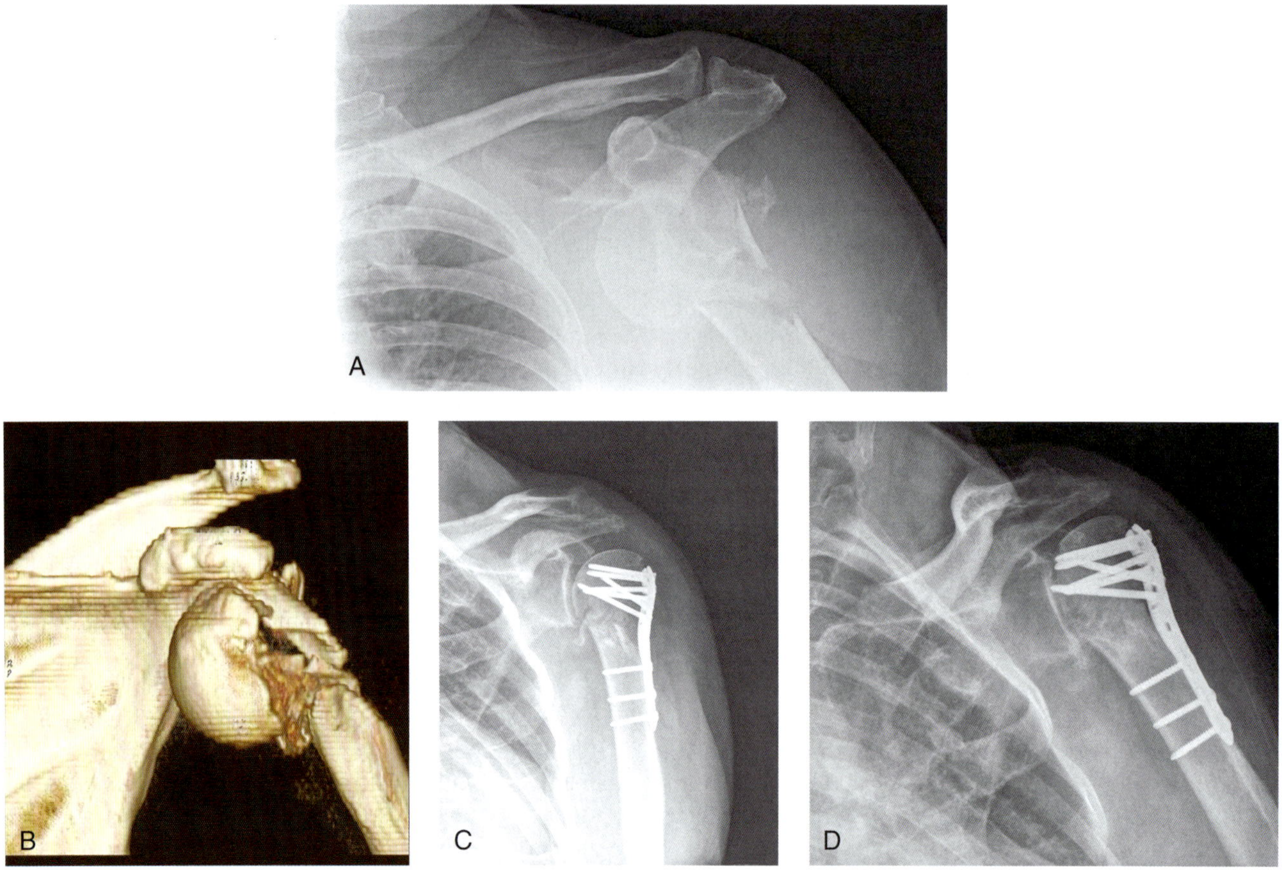

FIGURE 5 AP radiograph (**A**) and three-dimensional CT reconstruction (**B**) showing fracture dislocation of the proximal humerus in a 45-year-old man. **C**, Postoperative AP radiograph showing open reduction and internal fixation with a locking proximal humerus plate. **D**, AP radiograph 1 year after surgery showing osteonecrosis causing pain and crepitus. The humeral head has collapsed. Because the screws are locking, they did not back out as the head collapsed and remained fixed, eventually penetrating past the subchondral bone into the glenohumeral joint.

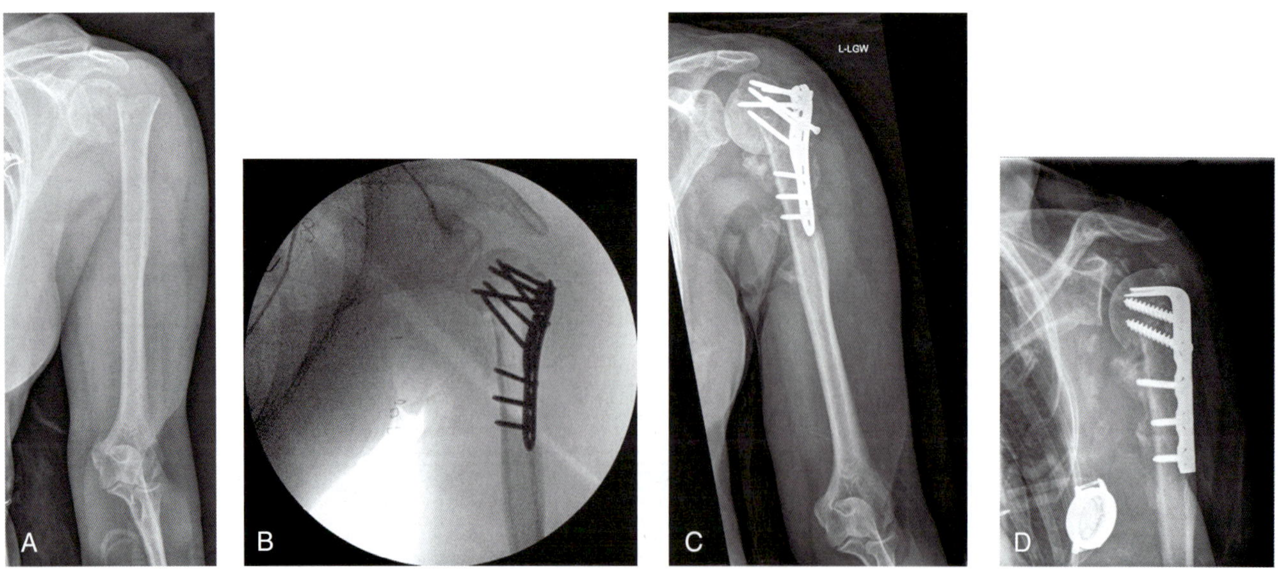

FIGURE 6 **A**, AP radiograph showing a displaced two-part proximal humeral fracture in a 60-year-old woman. **B**, AP fluoroscopic image showing initial treatment with a locking proximal humerus plate. **C**, AP radiograph showing varus collapse 6 weeks after surgery. **D**, AP radiograph showing revision to a 90° blade plate, which led to painless bony union.

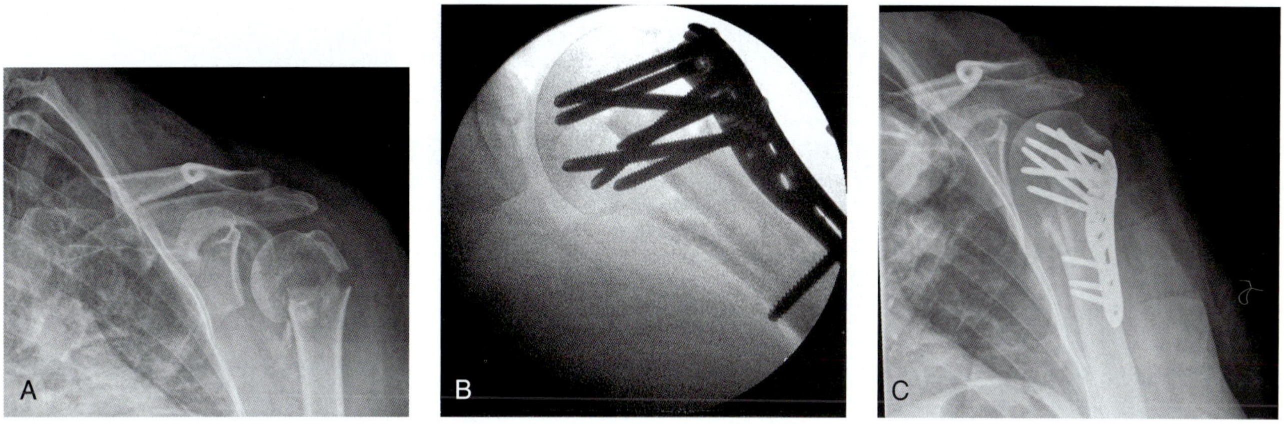

FIGURE 7 **A**, AP radiograph taken 4 weeks after a surgical neck two-part proximal humeral fracture in a 60-year-old patient with rheumatoid arthritis. The initial fracture treatment was nonsurgical, but the patient elected open reduction and internal fixation after progressive varus angulation and resorption at the fracture margins. AP fluoroscopic image (**B**) and AP radiograph (**C**) showing a standard proximal humeral locking plate applied with intramedullary fibular allograft strut for additional medial support against varus collapse.

to poor postoperative strength and range of motion.[45] The ideal construct for tuberosity repair should consist of both horizontally and vertically oriented heavy sutures placed directly through the bone-tendon junction of the rotator cuff and through the prosthesis, if possible. The medial circumferential cerclage suture is biomechanically important for the stability of the repair construct.[46]

Reverse total shoulder arthroplasty (RTSA) has become increasingly accepted as a reliable option for geriatric proximal humerus fractures and has been extensively studied over the past decade (**Figure 9**). The indications for reverse shoulder arthroplasty continue to be refined and outcome studies have shown promising results when used to treat proximal humeral fractures in geriatric patients with relatively low demands. Several studies have evaluated the outcome of reverse shoulder arthroplasty as the primary treatment of proximal humeral fracture. In the short term, the reverse arthroplasty predictably relieves pain and improves function.[47,48] In contrast to hemiarthroplasty, reverse shoulder arthroplasty can result in improved pain and function even if tuberosity healing does not occur. Nonetheless, tuberosity reconstruction is recommended with reverse arthroplasty for fracture to maximize external rotation function.[49] A

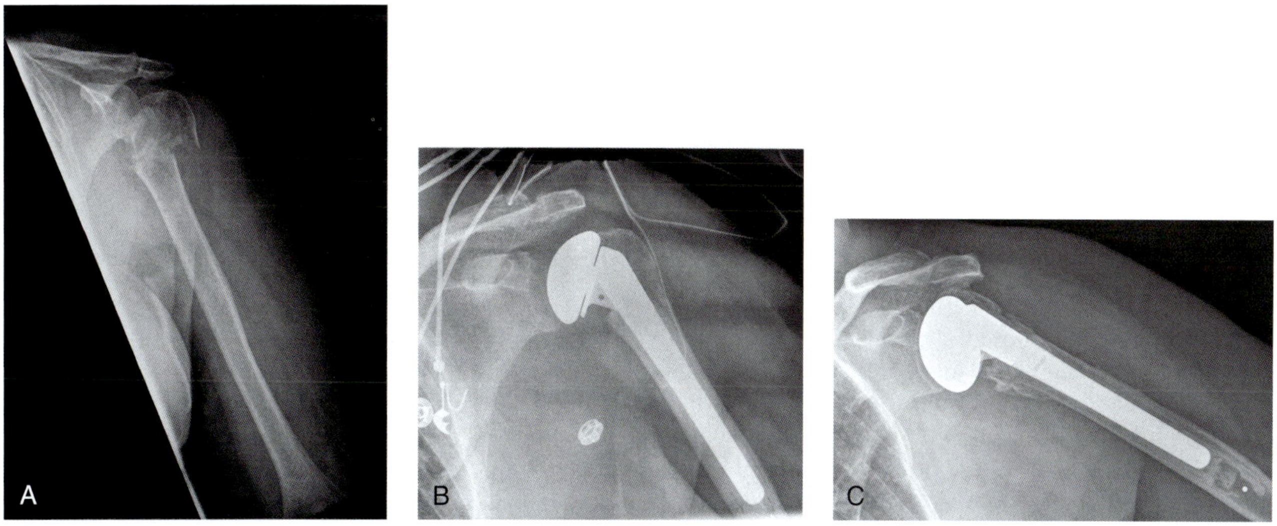

FIGURE 8 AP radiographs showing a displaced four-part proximal humeral fracture in an active 62-year-old woman before (**A**) and after (**B**) hemiarthroplasty. In (**B**), the tuberosity is in the appropriate position relative to the head. **C**, AP radiograph at 4-year follow-up, showing that the tuberosities are well healed. The patient had active forward elevation of 150° without pain.

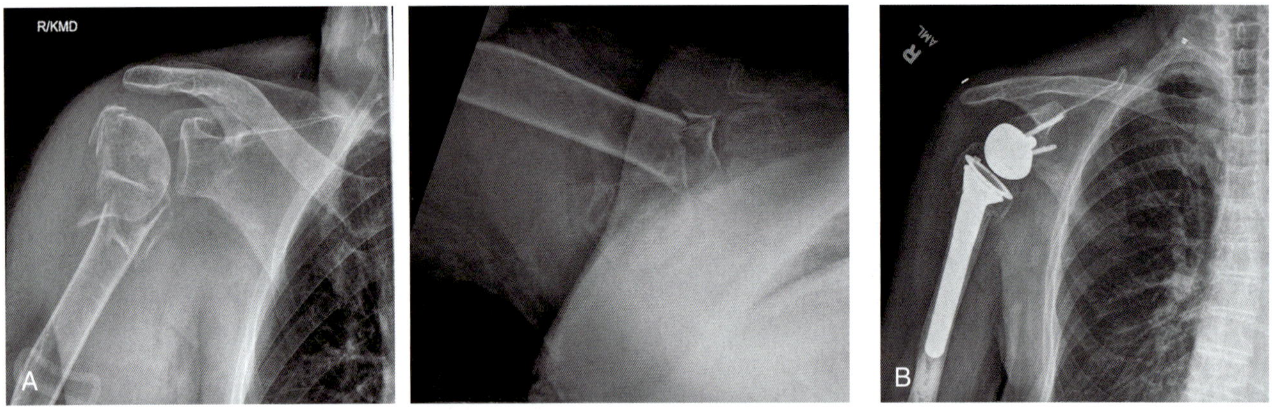

FIGURE 9 **A**, AP and axillary radiographs showing a comminuted four-part proximal humerus fracture in an 84-year-old woman. **B**, Post-surgical AP radiograph showing a cemented reverse total shoulder arthroplasty performed acutely in the same patient. At 6-month follow-up, the patient remains pain-free and is able to perform overhead activities.

recent meta-analysis demonstrated decreased reoperations, increased range of motion, and improved clinical outcome scores when comparing RTSA with hemiarthroplasty for the treatment of geriatric proximal humerus fractures.[50] There appears to be no difference in revision surgery rates, range of motion, and clinical outcome scores among patients with proximal humerus fractures treated acutely with RTSA compared with those who undergo RTSA in a delayed fashion.[51] Moreover, RTSA results in better outcomes among patients who develop proximal humerus fracture sequelae after nonsurgical treatment compared with those who develop sequelae after prior surgical intervention.[52] However, studies have documented mild deterioration in function and the development of lucent lines around the glenoid component at midterm follow-up.[53,54] Although early results have been promising, further studies are necessary to examine the long-term outcomes and timing of surgical intervention among patients treated with RTSA for proximal humerus fractures.

SUMMARY

Proximal humerus fractures are common, and incidence in the United States is likely to increase based on changing demographics. An understanding of the anatomy and vascularity of the proximal humerus is necessary to accurately classify these fractures and formulate an appropriate treatment plan. Each of the many treatment options has distinct indications and complications, some of which can be significant. There is consensus that nondisplaced and minimally displaced fractures should be managed nonsurgically, but no consensus exists on whether surgery improves outcomes significantly for displaced fractures or on the best surgical treatment for a given fracture pattern. More level I studies are needed to provide this evidence.

KEY STUDY POINTS

- Proximal humerus fractures are the third most common fracture in patients older than 65 years, and their incidence is expected to increase with the aging of the US population.
- Fracture displacement occurs in a predictable manner and is dictated by soft-tissue attachments around the proximal humerus.
- Most proximal humerus fractures are minimally displaced and can be managed nonsurgically.
- The advent of locked plating provides a biomechanically sound way to reconstruct the proximal humerus but can lead to a high rate of complications and revision surgeries, even among experienced surgeons.
- Reverse total shoulder arthroplasty (RTSA) is an increasingly popular option for nonreconstructable geriatric proximal humerus fractures and demonstrates better outcomes compared with hemiarthroplasty in the geriatric patient population.

Annotated References

1. Baron JA, Barrett JA, Karagas MR: The epidemiology of peripheral fractures. *Bone* 1996;18(3 suppl):S209-S213.

2. Codman E: *The Shoulder: Rupture of the Supraspinatus Tendon and Other Lesions in or About the Subacromial Bursa*. Brooklyn, NY, Miller, 1934.

3. Neer CS: The classic: Displaced proximal humeral fractures. Part I: Classification and evaluation. *Clin Orthop Relat Res* 2006;442:77-82.

4. Laing P: The arterial supply of the adult humerus. *J Bone Joint Surg Am* 1956;38-A(5):1105-1116.

5. Hettrich CM, Boraiah S, Dyke JP, Neviaser A, Helfet DL, Lorich DG: Quantitative assessment of the vascularity of the proximal part of the humerus. *J Bone Joint Surg Am* 2010;92(4):943-948.

6. Brooks C, Revell W, Heatley F: Vascularity of the humeral head after proximal humeral fractures. An anatomical cadaver study. *J Bone Joint Surg Br* 1993;75(1):132-136.

7. Siebenrock KA, Gerber C: The reproducibility of classification of fractures of the proximal end of the humerus. *J Bone Joint Surg Am* 1993;75(12):1751-1755.

8. Kellam JF, Meinberg EG, Agel J, Karam MD, Roberts CS: Introduction: Fracture and dislocation classification compendium – 2018 International comprehensive classification of fractures and dislocations committee. *J Orthop Trauma* 2018;32:S1-S170.

   This is the most recent orthopaedic trauma association (OTA) fracture classification scheme.

9. Neer CS: Four-segment classification of proximal humeral fractures: Purpose and reliable use. *J Shoulder Elbow Surg* 2002;11(4):389-400.

10. Jakob RP, Miniaci A, Anson PS, Jaberg H, Osterwalder A, Ganz R: Four-part valgus impacted fractures of the proximal humerus. *J Bone Joint Surg Br* 1991;73(2):295-298.

11. DeFranco MJ, Brems JJ, Williams GR Jr, Iannotti JP: Evaluation and management of valgus impacted four-part proximal humerus fractures. *Clin Orthop Relat Res* 2006;442:109-114.

12. Visser CP, Coene LNJ, Brand R, Tavy DL: Nerve lesions in proximal humeral fractures. *J Shoulder Elbow Surg* 2001;10(5):421-427.

13. Lee CK, Hansen HR: Post-traumatic avascular necrosis of the humeral head in displaced proximal humeral fractures. *J Trauma* 1981;21(9):788-791.

14. Hertel R, Hempfing A, Stiehler M, Leunig M: Predictors of humeral head ischemia after intracapsular fracture of the proximal humerus. *J Shoulder Elbow Surg* 2004;13(4):427-433.

15. Koval KJ, Gallagher MA, Marsicano JG, Cuomo F, McShinawy A, Zuckerman J: Functional outcome after minimally displaced fractures of the proximal part of the humerus. *J Bone Joint Surg Am* 1997;79(2):203-207.

16. Iyengar JJ, Devcic Z, Sproul RC, Feeley BT: Nonoperative treatment of proximal humerus fractures: A systematic review. *J Orthop Trauma* 2011;25(10):612-617.

17. Hanson B, Neidenbach P, de Boer P, Stengel D: Functional outcomes after nonoperative management of fractures of the proximal humerus. *J Shoulder Elbow Surg* 2009;18(4):612-621.

18. Rangan A, Handoll H, Brealey S, et al: Surgical vs nonsurgical treatment of adults with displaced fractures of the proximal humerus: The PROFHER randomized clinical trial. *J Am Med Assoc* 2015;313(10):1037-1047.

    This multicenter trial randomized 231 patients with displaced proximal humerus fractures to surgical or nonsurgical treatment. At 2 years, there was no difference in outcome scores, mortality, or complications between the two groups. Level of evidence: I.

19. Handoll H, Keding A, Corbacho B, Brealey S, Hewitt C, Rangan A: Five-year follow-up results of the PROFHER trial comparing operative and non-operative treatment of adults with a displaced fracture of the proximal humerus. *Bone Joint J* 2017;99-B(3):383-392.

    This article presented 5-year follow-up of the original PROFHER trial. Of the original 231 randomized patients, 176 were included in the 5-year follow-up. There was no significant difference in outcome scores between the surgical and nonsurgical treatment arms, confirming that the main findings of the PROFHER trial were unchanged at 5 years. Level of evidence: I.

20. Olerud P, Ahrengart L, Ponzer S, Saving J, Tidermark J: Internal fixation versus nonoperative treatment of displaced 3-part proximal humeral fractures in elderly patients: A randomized controlled trial. *J Shoulder Elbow Surg* 2011;20(5):747-755.

21. Olerud P, Ahrengart L, Ponzer S, Saving J, Tidermark J: Hemiarthroplasty versus nonoperative treatment of displaced 4-part proximal humeral fractures in elderly patients: A randomized controlled trial. *J Shoulder Elbow Surg* 2011;20(7):1025-1033.

22. Li Y, Zhao L, Zhu L, Li J, Chen A: Internal fixation versus nonoperative treatment for displaced 3-part or 4-part proximal humeral fractures in elderly patients: A meta-analysis of randomized controlled trials. *PLoS One* 2013;8(9):e75464.

    A meta-analysis of three randomized controlled trials with a total of 130 patients compared ORIF with nonsurgical management of displaced three-part and four-part proximal humeral fractures in elderly patients. Overall results demonstrated no functional difference between surgical and nonsurgical treatment among elderly patients with displaced three-part and four-part proximal humeral fractures. Level of evidence: II.

23. Handoll HH, Brorson S: Interventions for treating proximal humeral fractures in adults. *Cochrane Database Syst Rev* 2015;(11):CD000434.

    This Cochrane review article included 31 randomized controlled trials (1941 participants) pertinent to the management of proximal humerus fractures in adults. The authors concluded that there is high-quality or moderate-quality evidence that surgery does not result in a better outcome at 1 and 2 years after injury for patients with displaced proximal humerus fractures compared with nonsurgical management. Notably, the evidence did not cover the treatment of two-part tuberosity fractures, fractures in young patients, high-energy trauma, fracture-dislocations, or head-splitting fractures.

24. Bell JE, Leung BC, Spratt KF, et al: Trends and variation in incidence, surgical treatment, and repeat surgery of proximal humeral fractures in the elderly. *J Bone Joint Surg Am* 2011;93(2):121-131.

25. Sporer SM, Weinstein JN, Koval KJ: The geographic incidence and treatment variation of common fractures of elderly patients. *J Am Acad Orthop Surg* 2006;14(4):246-255.

26. Nicandri GT, Trumble TE, Warme WJ: Lessons learned from a case of proximal humeral locked plating gone awry. *J Orthop Trauma* 2009;23(8):607-611.

27. Herscovici D Jr, Saunders DT, Johnson MP, Sanders R, DiPasquale T: Percutaneous fixation of proximal humeral fractures. *Clin Orthop Relat Res* 2000;375:97-104.

28. Jaberg H, Warner J, Jakob R: Percutaneous stabilization of unstable fractures of the humerus. *J Bone Joint Surg Am* 1992;74(4):508-515.

29. Resch H, Povacz P, Fröhlich R, Wambacher M: Percutaneous fixation of three-and four-part fractures of the proximal humerus. *J Bone Joint Surg Br* 1997;79(2):295-300.

30. Magovern B, Ramsey ML: Percutaneous fixation of proximal humerus fractures. *Orthop Clin North Am* 2008;39(4):405-416.

31. Liew AS, Johnson JA, Patterson SD, King GJ, Chess DG: Effect of screw placement on fixation in the humeral head. *J Shoulder Elbow Surg* 2000;9(5):423-426.

32. Weinstein DM, Bratton DR, Ciccone WJ II, Elias JJ: Locking plates improve torsional resistance in the stabilization of three-part proximal humeral fractures. *J Shoulder Elbow Surg* 2006;15(2):239-243.

33. Hessmann MH, Sternstein W, Hansen M, Krummenauer F, Pol TF, Rommens M: Locked-plate fixation and intramedullary nailing for proximal humerus fractures: A biomechanical evaluation. *J Trauma* 2005;58(6):1194-1201.

34. Südkamp N, Bayer J, Hepp P, et al: Open reduction and internal fixation of proximal humeral fractures with use of the locking proximal humerus plate: Results of a prospective, multicenter, observational study. *J Bone Joint Surg Am* 2009;91(6):1320-1328.

35. Brunner F, Sommer C, Bahrs C, et al: Open reduction and internal fixation of proximal humerus fractures using a proximal humeral locked plate: A prospective multicenter analysis. *J Orthop Trauma* 2009;23(3):163-172.

36. Ricchetti ET, Warrender WJ, Abboud JA: Use of locking plates in the treatment of proximal humerus fractures. *J Shoulder Elbow Surg* 2010;19(2 suppl):66-75.

37. Röderer G, Erhardt J, Kuster M, et al: Second generation locked plating of proximal humerus fractures – A prospective multicentre observational study. *Int Orthop* 2011;35(3):425-432.

38. Gardner MJ, Boraiah S, Helfet DL, Lorich DG: Indirect medial reduction and strut support of proximal humerus fractures using an endosteal implant. *J Orthop Trauma* 2008;22(3):195-200.

39. Osterhoff G, Baumgartner D, Favre P, et al: Medial support by fibula bone graft in angular stable plate fixation of proximal humeral fractures: An in vitro study with synthetic bone. *J Shoulder Elbow Surg* 2011;20(5):740-746.

40. Bae JH, Oh JK, Chon CS, Oh CW, Hwang JH, Yoon YC: The biomechanical performance of locking plate fixation with intramedullary fibular strut graft augmentation in the treatment of unstable fractures of the proximal humerus. *J Bone Joint Surg Br* 2011;93(7):937-941.

41. Rosas S, Law TY, Kurowicki J, Formaini N, Kalandiak SP, Levy JC: Trends in surgical management of proximal humeral fractures in the Medicare population: A nationwide study of records from 2009 to 2012. *J Shoulder Elbow Surg* 2016;25(4):608-613.

    This retrospective review of Medicare patients between 2009 and 2012 evaluated trends in the treatment of 32,150 proximal humerus fractures. The authors found that the percentage of fractures managed surgically decreased from 16.2% to 13.9% over the time period examined. Moreover, the utilization rate of ORIF did not change, the utilization rate of hemiarthroplasty decreased, and the rate of reverse total shoulder arthroplasty increased. Level of evidence: IV.

42. Bosch U, Skutek M, Fremerey RW, Tscherne H: Outcome after primary and secondary hemiarthroplasty in elderly patients with fractures of the proximal humerus. *J Shoulder Elbow Surg* 1998;7(5):479-484.

43. Kralinger F, Schwaiger R, Wambacher M, et al: Outcome after primary hemiarthroplasty for fracture of the head of the humerus: A retrospective multicentre study of 167 patients. *J Bone Joint Surg Br* 2004;86(2):217-219.

44. Boileau P, Krishnan S, Tinsi L, Walch G, Coste J, Mole D: Tuberosity malposition and migration: Reasons for poor outcomes after hemiarthroplasty for displaced fractures of the proximal humerus. *J Shoulder Elbow Surg* 2002;11(5):401-412.

45. Frankle MA, Greenwald DP, Markee BA, Ondrovic LE, Lee WE III: Biomechanical effects of malposition of tuberosity fragments on the humeral prosthetic reconstruction for four-part proximal humerus fractures. *J Shoulder Elbow Surg* 2001;10(4):321-326.

46. Frankle MA, Ondrovic LE, Markee BA, Harris ML, Lee WE III: Stability of tuberosity reattachment in proximal humeral hemiarthroplasty. *J Shoulder Elbow Surg* 2002;11(5):413-420.

47. Lenarz C, Shishani Y, McCrum C, Nowinski RJ, Edwards TB, Gobezie R: Is reverse shoulder arthroplasty appropriate for the treatment of fractures in the older patient?: Early observations. *Clin Orthop Relat Res* 2011;469(12):3324-3331.

48. Bufquin T, Hersan A, Hubert L, Massin P: Reverse shoulder arthroplasty for the treatment of three-and four-part fractures of the proximal humerus in the elderly: A prospective review of 43 cases with a short-term follow-up. *J Bone Joint Surg Br* 2007;89(4):516-520.

49. Boileau P, Alta TD, Decroocq L, et al: Reverse shoulder arthroplasty for acute fractures in the elderly: Is it worth reattaching the tuberosities? *J Shoulder Elbow Surg* 2019;28(3):437-444.

This was a retrospective review of 38 displaced three-part or four-part proximal humerus fractures in the elderly patients treated with reattachement of the tuberosities around a reverse total shoulder arthroplasty. The 32 patients whose tuberosities healed had significantly higher range of motion and clinical outcome scores compared to the 6 patients whose tuberosities resorbed or resulted in a nonunion. Level of evidence: III.

50. Austin DC, Torchia MT, Cozzolino NH, Jacobowitz LE, Bell JE: Decreased reoperations and improved outcomes with reverse total shoulder arthroplasty in comparison to hemiarthroplasty for geriatric proximal humerus fractures: A systematic review and meta-analysis. *J Orthop Trauma* 2019;33(1):49-57.

This meta-analysis included 15 studies with 913 patients that directly compared hemiarthroplasty with reverse total shoulder arthroplasty in geriatric proximal humerus fractures. Reverse total shoulder arthroplasty had significantly better range of motion and clinical outcome scores as well as decreased revision surgery rates compared with hemiarthroplasty for the management of these fractures. Level of evidence: III.

51. Torchia MT, Austin DC, Cozzolino N, Jacobowitz L, Bell JE: Acute versus delayed reverse total shoulder arthroplasty for the treatment of proximal humeral fractures in the elderly population: A systematic review and meta-analysis. *J Shoulder Elbow Surg* 2019;28(4):765-773.

A meta-analysis compared reverse total shoulder arthroplasty performed in the acute setting with reverse total shoulder arthroplasty performed for the sequelae of proximal humerus fractures in the elderly. There was no difference in forward flexion, clinical outcome scores, or revision surgery rates between the two approaches, raising the possibility that a trial of nonsurgical treatment may be considered in this patient population. Level of evidence: IV.

52. Dezfuli B, King JJ, Farmer KW, Struk AM, Wright TW: Outcomes of reverse total shoulder arthroplasty as primary versus revision procedure for proximal humerus fractures. *J Shoulder Elbow Surg* 2016;25(7):1133-1137.

This retrospective review of 49 patients analyzed outcomes after RTSA performed for the following indications: acute proximal humerus fracture, nonunion or malunion of a proximal humerus fracture, failed hemiarthroplasty of a proximal humerus fracture, or failed ORIF of a proximal humerus fracture. The authors found that primary RTSA (for acute fractures or non/malunion) had better outcome scores compared with those performed as revision cases (for failed hemiarthroplasty or failed ORIF). Level of evidence: III.

53. Cazeneuve J, Cristofari DJ: The reverse shoulder prosthesis in the treatment of fractures of the proximal humerus in the elderly. *J Bone Joint Surg Br* 2010;92(4):535-539.

54. Cazeneuve JF, Cristofari DJ: Long term functional outcome following reverse shoulder arthroplasty in the elderly. *Orthop Traumatol Surg Res* 2011;97(6):583-589.

Chapter 30

Management of Severe Acute Proximal Humerus Fractures

Jennifer Tangtiphaiboontana, MD • Jonah Hébert-Davies, MD

ABSTRACT

Complex proximal humerus fractures are a challenging clinical entity, despite several advances in treatment over the past few decades. Although younger patients may benefit from open reduction and internal fixation, the risk for complications is unacceptably high in the older population. This has led many to suggest nonsurgical management be the mainstay of these fractures for this patient population. Unfortunately, for active patients this may lead to poor functional outcome, thus increasing the demand for a reliable solution to this problem. Although hemiarthroplasty was classically used to treat these fractures, the transition to reverse shoulder arthroplasty has given patients better outcomes, as long as complications are kept to a minimum. Although several questions remain unanswered, a fair amount of literature has been published on the topic of reverse shoulder arthroplasty for fractures and should be used to guide treatment using the best evidence available.

Keywords: proximal humerus fractures; reverse shoulder arthroplasty

Introduction

Proximal humerus fractures are the third most common fracture and are increasing in frequency with an aging population. Fragility fractures of the proximal humerus are often highly comminuted and displaced. The combination of poor bone quality and increased risk of osteonecrosis in comminuted fractures, with or without associated dislocations, presents several challenges in the elderly population and may preclude surgical treatment with plate osteosynthesis. This is particularly true of fractures with thin humeral head fragments and significant medial calcar comminution. Although the ideal management of proximal humerus fractures remains controversial, nonsurgical management of severe proximal humerus fracture may not be an acceptable treatment option, especially in high functioning, independent patients who wish to return to their prior level of activity. Classically, hemiarthroplasty was used as a treatment method for these complex fractures; however, unpredictable outcomes largely dependent on adequate healing of the tuberosities explain why many surgeons have stopped using this technique. General usage of the reverse shoulder arthroplasty (RSA) has increased dramatically since it was reintroduced over 15 years ago. Our understanding of biomechanics and design advancements with RSA has expanded its use for management of proximal humerus fractures, especially in the elderly population.[1,2] Other options have looked at supporting medial comminution and humeral head fragments with novel means (fibular strut, nitinol cage) to help avoid collapse and failure, however results are. This chapter will focus on the management of complex proximal humerus fractures using RSA and what specific issues have been reported in the evolving literature (**Figure 1**).

Nonsurgical Management Versus RSA

Although most undisplaced or minimally displaced fractures can adequately be managed without surgery, nonsurgical management of complex proximal humerus fracture is often reserved for low-demand, elderly patients or those with serious medical comorbidities who would not tolerate the stress of surgery and anesthesia. Specific fracture patterns with posteromedial impaction or displaced greater and lesser tuberosities have been shown to have inferior outcomes if allowed to heal in a nonanatomic position.[3] Although several studies have suggested that nonsurgical management of proximal humerus fractures have similar outcomes to surgical management, these studies compared nonsurgical management to hemiarthroplasty or fixation.[4-8]

Dr. Hébert-Davies or an immediate family member serves as a paid consultant to or is an employee of Globus Medical and Synthes. Neither Dr. Tangtiphaiboontana nor any immediate family member has received anything of value from or has stock or stock options held in a commercial company or institution related directly or indirectly to the subject of this chapter.

This chapter is adapted from Jo MJ, Gardner MJ: Treatment of severe acute proximal humeral fractures, in Nicholson GP, ed: *Orthopaedic Knowledge Update: Shoulder and Elbow*, ed 4. Rosemont, IL, American Academy of Orthopaedic Surgeons, 2013, pp 419-430.

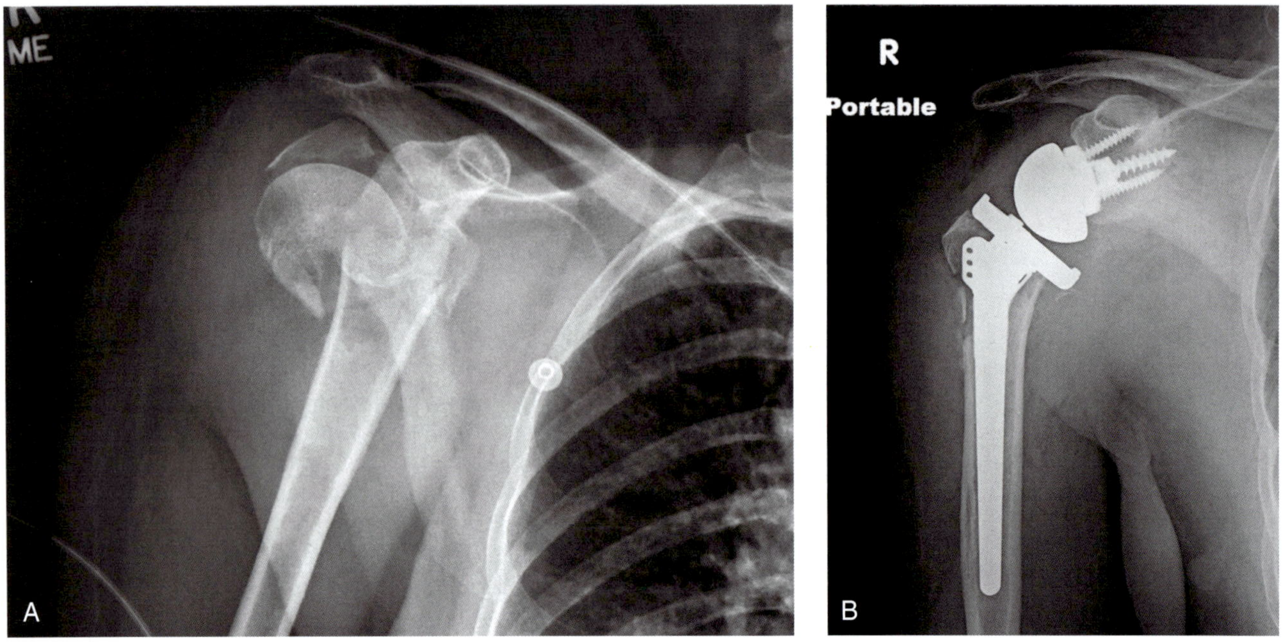

FIGURE 1 AP shoulder radiographs showing a displaced four-part proximal humerus in a 74-year-old woman before (**A**) and after (**B**) noncemented reverse shoulder arthroplasty. In (**B**), the tuberosity is reduced to the appropriate position.

There are a limited number of studies directly comparing the outcomes of nonsurgical management with those of RSA for severe proximal humerus fractures. A 2017 study[9] found no difference between shoulder motion and outcomes between nonsurgical management and RSA in patients with three-part and four-part proximal humerus fractures. In contrast, the authors of a 2019 study found that those who underwent primary RSA for three-part and four-part proximal humerus fractures had higher Constant-Murley scores, better shoulder motion, and higher satisfaction than patients who were treated nonsurgically.[10] In patients aged ≥70 years with a high level of independence, primary RSA for complex proximal humerus fractures results in good early function, reliable pain control, and return to prior level of independent living at a mean follow-up of 1 year.[11] RSA has also been shown to be a more cost-effective treatment option when compared with hemiarthroplasty or surgical fixation, as long as the rate of complications can be maintained in an expected range.[12,13]

Specific Considerations of Reverse Shoulder Arthroplasty

The use of RSA for treatment of proximal humerus fractures in the elderly population is growing. Results of recent studies evaluating the outcomes of RSA for proximal humerus fractures are outlined in **Table 1**. The relative indications for RSA include fractures at high risk for failure or inferior functional results from plate osteosynthesis or hemiarthroplasty such as irreparable fracture, humeral head osteonecrosis, poor tuberosity bone quality with osteoporosis and/or comminution, and preexisting chronic rotator cuff tear or arthritis. Absolute contraindications for RSA include permanent axillary nerve dysfunction or global deltoid muscle dysfunction. Relative contraindications include associated acromion or scapular spine fracture that may displace with deltoid tensioning, or glenoid fractures or deficiency that precludes stable baseplate implantation.

Approach

The deltopectoral approach with the patient in the beach-chair position is the most commonly used approach and allows for adequate exposure of the proximal humerus and access to the fracture fragments for suture fixation, avoids violating the deltoid muscle, and reduces the risk to the axillary nerve. The anterosuperior is another described approach that splits the deltoid between the anterior and middle thirds, provides easier glenoid access, and avoids disrupting the anterior shoulder soft tissues. A study comparing the deltopectoral and the anterosuperior approach for RSA found a decreased rate of dislocation, scapular notching, and acromial fracture with the anterosuperior approach at 2-year follow-up but no difference in Constant-Murley scores or active motion.[28] Despite these findings, the anterosuperior approach is not recommended for fractures because of the limited access to the humeral shaft, lesser tuberosity, and requirement for deltoid reattachment. Furthermore, the removal of the proximal humerus head in fracture cases renders glenoid access much easier and obviates the need for the anterosuperior approach.

Table 1

Recent Studies of Reverse Shoulder Arthroplasty for Three-Part and Four-Part Proximal Humerus Fractures

Study (Year)	Stem Fixation	Prosthesis	Patients (*N*)	Mean Follow-Up (Months)	Mean Patient Age (Years)	Outcome Measures (Mean Score)	Forward Elevation (Mean Degrees)	External Rotation (Mean Degrees)	Tuberosity Union (%)
Gallinet et al[14] (2013)	Cemented	Delta III DePuy Zimmer Reverse Anatomic Shoulder Aequialis Reverse Fracture	53	24	76.9	DASH: 35.7 CMS: 55.9	106	7	66
Sebastia-Forcada et al[15] (2014)	Noncemented	SMR Modular Shoulder System	31	29.4	74.7	DASH: 17.5 UCLA: 29.1 CMS: 56.1	120	5	64.5
Cazeneuve[16] (2014)	Cemented	Delta III DePuy	23	86	75.5	CMS: 60	>120	1.1*	NR
Garofalo et al[17] (2015)	Cemented	Aequialis Reverse Fracture	87	27	76.2	NR	138	29	75
Ross et al[18] (2015)	Both	SMR Modular Shoulder System Delta III DePuy	21	54.8	79	VAS: 2.2 ASES: 89 CMS: 88	130	30	NR
Formaini et al[19] (2015)	Cemented	DJO Reverse Shoulder Prosthesis	25	17	77	VAS: 2 ASES: 71 SST: 7	117	29	88
Youn et al[20] (2016)	Noncemented	SMR Modular Shoulder System	33	36	76.5	VAS: 2 ASES: 75.9 CMS: 54.1	114		90
Grubhofer et al[21] (2016)	Both	Zimmer Reverse Anatomic Shoulder	51	35	77	SSV: 83 CMS: 62	118	18	86
Chun et al[22] (2017)	Cemented	Aequialis Reverse Fracture	38	36.9	80.4	VAS: 1.5 ASES: 72.5 CMS: 65.9	126	20	37

(continued)

Table 1

Recent Studies of Reverse Shoulder Arthroplasty for Three-Part and Four-Part Proximal Humerus Fractures (continued)

Study (Year)	Stem Fixation	Prosthesis	Patients (*N*)	Mean Follow-Up (Months)	Mean Patient Age (Years)	Outcome Measures (Mean Score)	Forward Elevation (Mean Degrees)	External Rotation (Mean Degrees)	Tuberosity Union (%)
Ohl et al[23] (2018)	Both	Six implants used	420	28	77.7	SSV: 70 CMS: 57	115	17	40.2
Simovitch et al[24] (2019)	Both	Equinoxe Exactech	55	33.7	77	ASES: 78.3 UCLA: 28.2 SST: 8.8 CMS: 64.1	130	36	83
Reuther et al[25] (2019)	Cemented	Affinis Fracture Inverse	81	24.8	78.5	ASES: 76.1 CMS: 61.1	129	16	45.6
Wright et al[26] (2019)	Noncemented	Zimmer Trabecular Metal stem Zimmer Trabecular Metal or DJO Reverse Shoulder Prosthesis baseplate	21	56	71	ASES: 82 SSV: 69.4	130	32	70
Boileau et al[27] (2019)	Cemented	Aequialis Reverse Fracture	38	36	80	CMS: 64	135	24	84

ASES = American Shoulder and Elbow Surgeons score, CMS = Constant-Murley score, DASH = Disabilities of the Arm, Shoulder and Hand score, NR = not reported, SST = simple shoulder test, SSV = subjective shoulder value, UCLA = University of California, Los Angeles score, VAS = visual analog scale.
*Indicates range of motion based on points system as part of the Constant-Murley score.

Humeral Height and Stem Fixation

Humeral stem height plays a critical role in stability, and the proper height can be challenging to determine especially in comminuted fractures. If the medial calcar of the proximal humerus is still present, this may also be used to determine the height of the prosthesis by positioning the medial aspect of the stem along the calcar. Contralateral shoulder radiographs can also be used to help with proper stem height.[17,29]

The humeral stem may be cemented or press-fit with impaction bone grafting. Impaction grafting is done by placing the cancellous graft harvested from the fracture humeral head along the peripheral aspects of the humeral canal and using a broach to impact the bone in place. Special care must be taken to identify any fracture lines that may extend into the shaft and could compromise stem fixation. If there are concerns regarding the stability of the humeral stem, particularly in osteoporotic bone or patients with a capacious humeral canal, additional stability with cement fixation may be needed.

Noncemented humeral stems offer several theoretical advantages including reduced operating time, avoiding morbidity associated with using cement, and allowing for adjustment of the humeral component after implantation in the case of persistent instability despite modularity adjustments. There have been few studies evaluating the outcomes of noncemented stems for fractures and most have demonstrated good results.[15,20,26] The authors of a 2016 study[20] reported that only 10% of patients treated with noncemented RSA for proximal humerus fractures had radiographic findings that were at risk for loosening at 3-year follow-up, but there were no signs of stem subsidence. No patients required revision surgery and all had good clinical outcomes. The authors of a 2019 study reported similar findings with noncemented stems and found that 97% of their patients had stable humeral fixation and good clinical outcomes.[26] A comparative study evaluating the outcomes of cemented versus noncemented RSA for proximal humerus fractures found that noncemented RSA resulted in worse American Shoulder and Elbow Surgeon score and satisfaction scores but no difference in pain, shoulder range of motion, tuberosity healing, or Disabilities of the Arm, Shoulder and Hand score scores.[30] Based on these findings, patients with good quality bone can be treated with noncemented stems. If, however, any doubts persist with stability following impaction, especially in patients with poor bone quality, surgeons should strongly consider reimplanting components using cement.

Tuberosity Fixation and Healing

Although good outcomes with RSA for proximal humerus fractures are much less dependent on tuberosity healing when compared with hemiarthroplasty, some studies have highlighted the importance of tuberosity repair and healing. Initially, some surgeons proposed tuberosity excision since the RSA biomechanics were designed to work in a cuff-deficient shoulder. Unfortunately, this can lead to increased rates of complications such as instability, infection, and implant loosening.[23,31,32] The authors of a 2018 study found that patients with excised tuberosities had significant worse functional outcomes and increased rate of instability compared with patients with anatomically healed or malunited/resorbed tuberosities (12% versus 1.2% versus 2.3%, respectively).[23] Tuberosity excision may also compromise the stabilizing effect of the soft tissues around the prosthesis, specifically with regard to the subscapularis.

Tuberosity healing rate ranges from 47% to 88%, and efforts to enhance tuberosity healing after RSA in complex

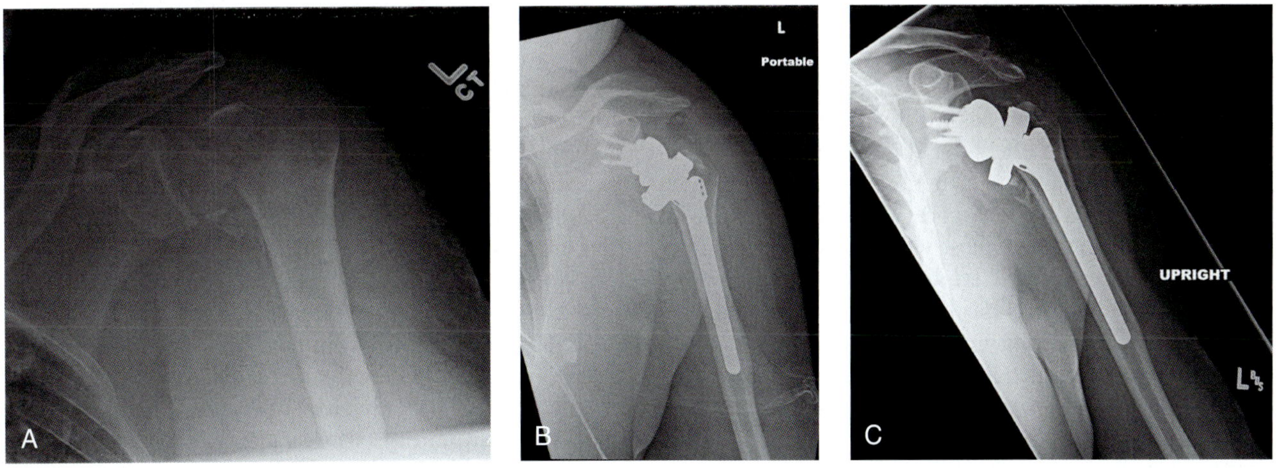

FIGURE 2 **A**, AP radiographs showing a proximal humerus fracture-dislocation in a 68-year-old man. **B**, AP radiograph showing treatment with a noncemented reverse shoulder arthroplasty with reduced tuberosities. **C**, AP radiographs 2 years postoperatively demonstrating healed tuberosities and well-fixed implants.

Section 6: Trauma and Fractures

fractures include suture constructs,[24,33-35] bone grafting techniques,[36] and partial cementation techniques.[19] Principles of tuberosity repair include multiple points of fixation from the rotator cuff at the bone tendon cuff region into the humeral shaft and/or the humeral component. Further stability is then achieved with horizontal sutures to reattach the tuberosities to each other (**Figure 2**). Pointed reduction clamps may be used to assist with anatomic reduction of the tuberosities. Regardless of what technique is used, stable fixation much be achieved to allow early range of motion with minimal motion at the level of the fracture.

Several studies have reported increased rates of the tuberosity healing and improved outcomes with using autograft from the fractured humeral head to augment the tuberosity fixation.[19,27,36,37] The authors of a 2017 study reported a healing rate of 78% for patients who had grafted tuberosity repair compared with 40% healing in those who were not grafted (P = 0.048).[37] Various grafting techniques have been described including a wedge horseshoe graft, cancellous block autograft, and the black and tan technique where a transition zone between the cement mantle and proximal end of stem is created with bone graft to prevent thermal necrosis of the tuberosity repair. Humeral implant design has also been found to help with tuberosity healing. The use of a low-profile fracture stem provides room for grafting of the tuberosities, allows for a more anatomic repair, and provides a large ingrowth surface for tuberosity healing.[38,39] The bulky design of the standard reverse shoulder prostheses may result in malpositioning of the tuberosities and increase shoulder stiffness.[18]

As a general rule, patients with anatomically healed tuberosities have improved shoulder motion, particularly with forward flexion and external rotation, when compared with patients with resorbed or malunited tuberosities[14,17,21-25,27] (**Table 2**). The loss of shoulder motion as a result of tuberosity malunion or resorption may lead to difficulties with performing simple daily tasks.[41] Most studies have been consistent in demonstrating that anatomic tuberosity healing has positive effect on shoulder motion; however, its effect on clinical outcomes is unknown. Some studies report better Subjective Shoulder Value and Constant-Murley scores[14,21,23,27] in patients with healed tuberosities than in those with tuberosity malunion/resorption, whereas other studies report no statistically significant difference in clinical outcomes[22,24,40,42] (**Table 3**). Despite these conflicting findings, routine repair of the tuberosities is recommended both for its potential impact on function and help with early postoperative stability.

Complications

Overall complication rates after RSA for all indications vary among studies and range from 5% to 68%.[34,43-48] The most common clinical complications include instability and infection. Other complications include intraoperative fracture, acromial stress fractures, nerve palsy from lengthening tension or iatrogenic injury, pain syndromes, and stiffness. Radiographic complications include scapular notching, humeral and glenoid component lucency, tuberosity malunion or nonunion, and heterotopic ossification. There are few studies reporting on complications of RSA for fracture, and most of the current data are reported separately in individual studies.

Scapular notching ranges from 19% to 96% and is the most commonly reported complication with RSA; however, its clinical relevance is unknown.[31,43] The clinical effects of notching remain controversial as some authors report that notching does not affect range of motion or functional scores whereas other reports indicate that scapular notching could be an independent variable predictive of an adverse outcome and baseplate failure.[31,49,50] Standard methods to reduce eventual notching include inferior baseplate placement, placing the baseplate in 10° of inferior tilt, lateralizing the glenosphere with either a lateralized implant or a bony increased offset RSA, increasing glenosphere diameter, using a platform stem, and using a more varus humeral component.[51-53]

Although postoperative instability after standard RSA ranges from zero to 38%,[43,45,46] instability rates after RSA for proximal humerus fractures vary from 0.6% to 11%.[10,14,23,31,32,40,54-56] Dislocation or subluxation typically occurs within the first 6 months and 50% of cases can be addressed with closed reduction alone with short-term sling immobilization.[57] Risk factors for dislocation include obesity (body mass index > 30), prior surgery, and inadequate subscapularis repair.[58]

Prosthetic joint infections are a devastating complication and rates range from 2.2% to 10%.[14,17,21,23,32,37,40,54] Risk factors for postoperative infections include patients with rheumatic disease, revision surgery, or large hematoma.[54] Patients with proximal humerus fracture typically have traumatized soft tissue and preexisting hematoma. It is important to pay even more attention when handling soft tissues to prevent the risk of wound dehiscence and infection.

Studies specifically evaluating complications after RSA for fractures have also identified patient factors that increase their risk for postoperative complications. In a case series of 103 patients who underwent RSA for fracture, the overall complication rate was 25% with 7.6% major complications (infection, dislocation, perioperative fracture). Patients with higher American Society of Anesthesiologists physical status classification and a history of rheumatoid arthritis were at increased risk for a major complication with the first 90 days of surgery.[54] Another retrospective study found that the most common complications after RSA for fracture were instability

Table 2

Comparison of Shoulder Range of Motion Between Healed and Nonhealed Tuberosity Groups After Reverse Shoulder Arthroplasty for Proximal Humerus Fracture

	Study (Year)	Healed Tuberosity Mean Degree (Range) ± SD	Tuberosity Nonunion/Malunion Mean Degree (Range) ± SD	*P*
Forward flexion	Gallinet et al[14] (2013)	127.2	96.5	0.002
	Garofalo et al[17] (2015)	145.3 ± 19.3	114.1 ± 15.8	<0.0001
	Grubhofer et al[21] (2016)	123 (45-165)	94 (40-130)	0.01
	Chun et al[22] (2017)	125 ± 18	127 ± 14	0.647
	Ohl et al[23] (2018)	126.7 ± 27.6	113.8 ± 29.9	<0.001
	Boileau et al[27] (2019)	141 (50-170) ± 25	115 (90-150) ± 26	0.029
	Jain et al[40] (2019)	134.1	112.5	<0.05
	Reuther et al[25] (2019)	127.6 ± 28.8	129.1 ± 35.6	0.716
	Simovitch et al[24] (2019)	131.9 ± 32.1	126.5 ± 32.6	0.7056
Abduction	Gallinet et al[14] (2013)	112.8	90.4	0.011
	Grubhofer et al[21] (2016)	115 (40-165)	92 (40-140)	0.11
	Jain et al[40] (2019)	114.8	95.1	<0.05
	Reuther et al[25] (2019)	118.9 ± 30	120.6 ± 37.6	0.808
	Simovitch et al[24] (2019)	108.3 ± 30	114.1 ± 30.4	0.5444
External rotation at side	Gallinet et al[14] (2013)	19.7	1.6	0.0004
	Garofalo et al[17] (2015)	34.3 ± 11.8	12.9 ± 11.6	<0.0001
	Grubhofer et al[21] (2016)	21 (−10 to 60)	2 (0-10)	0.01
	Chun et al[22] (2017)	29 ± 8	10 ± 9	<0.001
	Ohl et al[23] (2018)	22 ± 16.2	16.7 ± 20.2	<0.001
	Boileau et al[27] (2019)	27 (0-50) ± 12	11 (0-30) ± 12	0.01
	Jain et al[40] (2019)	27.8	7.6	<0.05
	Reuther et al[25] (2019)	19.6 ± 16.4	14.2 ± 13.1	0.281
	Simovitch et al[24] (2019)	35.6 ± 20.4	28.6 ± 21.5	0.0415
External rotation at 90° abduction	Gallinet et al[14] (2013)	49.4	10.3	0.00001
	Chun et al[22] (2017)	25 ± 10	7 ± 9	<0.001
	Ohl et al[23] (2018)	43.2 ± 26.9	33 ± 26.8	<0.001
Internal rotation	Gallinet et al[14] (2013)	L4	Coccyx	0.43
	Garofalo et al[17] (2015)	45.6 ± 18.9	25.7 ± 19.1	<0.0001
	Grubhofer et al[21] (2016)	6 (0-10)[a]	3 (0-8)[a]	0.06
	Chun et al[22] (2017)	15 ± 2	17 ± 1	0.125
	Ohl et al[23] (2018)	4.8 ± 2.7[a]	4 ± 2.4[a]	0.014
	Boileau et al[27] (2019)	5.2 (2-10) ± 2.7[a]	4.3 (2-6) ± 1.5[a]	0.42
	Jain et al[40] (2019)	30 ± 21	21 ± 6	NR
	Reuther et al[25] (2019)	71.5 ± 20.8	73.9 ± 14.8	0.722
	Simovitch et al[24] (2019)	3.4 ± 1.4[a]	3.8 ± 1.2[a]	0.6616
Internal rotation at 90° abduction	Gallinet et al[14] (2013)	55.6	36.8	0.004

[a]Indicates range of motion based on points system as part of the Constant-Murley score.

Table 3

Comparison of Patient-Reported Outcome Scores Between Healed and Nonhealed Tuberosity Groups After Reverse Shoulder Arthroplasty for Proximal Humerus Fracture

Outcome Score	Study (Year)	Healed Tuberosity Mean (Range) ± SD	Tuberosity Nonunion/Malunion Mean (Range) ± SD	*P*
CMS	Gallinet et al[14] (2013)	65.3	50.1	0.0005
	Grubhofer et al[21] (2016)	65 (33-83)	50 (21-65)	0.01
	Chun et al[22] (2017)	67.9 ± 11.6	63.9 ± 8.2	0.228
	Ohl et al[23] (2018)	61 ± 13.1	54.5 ± 15.2	<0.001
	Boileau et al[27] (2019)	64 (28-80) ± 15	51 (30-73) ± 12	0.018
	Reuther et al[25] (2019)	60.3 ± 12.3	61.5 ± 13.5	0.906
	Simovitch et al[24] (2019)	64.6 ± 12.5	63.2 ± 7.4	0.4552
ASES	Chun et al[22] (2017)	74.3 ± 10.7	70.7 ± 7.2	0.231
	Reuther et al[25] (2019)	73.7 ± 14.8	78.6 ± 16.4	0.283
	Simovitch et al[24](2019)	79.1 ± 17.2	77 ± 14.7	0.5058
DASH	Gallinet et al[14] (2013)	30.1	39.3	0.14
SSV	Grubhofer et al[21] (2016)	86 (30-100)	68 (45-100)	0.03
	Ohl et al[23] (2018)	75.5 ± 14.8	69.1 ± 18.2	<0.001
	Boileau et al[27] (2019)	83 (50-100) ± 15	65 (40-80) ± 15	0.029
SST	Simovitch et al[24] (2019)	9.2 ± 2.1	8.2 ± 2.8	0.2851

ASES = American Shoulder and Elbow Surgeon score, CMS = Constant-Murley score, DASH = Disabilities of the Arm, Shoulder and Hand score, SST = simple shoulder test, SSV = subjective shoulder value.

and intractable shoulder stiffness. Those with a higher Charlson Comorbidity Index, diabetes, and resection or resorbed greater tuberosities were associated with higher rates of these complications.[55]

Future Directions

Current data demonstrate promising results with the management of proximal humerus fractures using RSA, but the literature is limited to retrospective cohort studies, case series, or meta-analyses. There are no published randomized studies directly comparing nonsurgical management with RSA for severe proximal humerus fractures; however, there are at least two on-going studies. The ReShAPE (Reverse Shoulder Arthroplasty for the treatment of Proximal humeral fractures in the Elderly) trial is a multicentered combined randomized and observational study of patients aged 70 years and older with three-part and four-part proximal humerus fracture who are treated nonsurgically or with RSA.[59] The Nordic Innovative Trials to Evaluate osteoPorotic Fractures Collaboration is conducting a prospective, single blinded, randomized control trial comparing RSA with nonsurgical management of displaced proximal humerus fractures in patients aged 65 to 85 years.[60] The results of these and other studies will hopefully help guide treatment going forward.

SUMMARY

Severe proximal humerus fractures present several reconstructive challenges, and the ideal treatment for these injuries remains controversial. Although some may argue that these injuries should be managed nonsurgically, RSA is a good treatment option in elderly patients with complex proximal humerus fractures and numerous studies have consistently reported good, reproducible functional outcomes supporting the increased use of RSA for proximal humerus fractures. It has been found to be a more cost-effective treatment option when compared with open reduction and internal fixation or hemiarthroplasty. Tuberosity repair is critical to restoring functional shoulder motion, specifically rotation, and techniques to help with healing include bone grafting, partial cementation techniques, and use of a fracture stem. Further studies are needed to better delineate patient benefit and ideal indications of RSA for the management of irreparable proximal humerus fractures.

KEY STUDY POINTS

- RSA is a reliable surgical treatment option for high functioning elderly patients with complex proximal humerus fractures.
- Tuberosity repair and anatomic healing is important to help restore functional shoulder range of motion after RSA for proximal humerus fractures; however, a good, reliable clinical outcome is independent of tuberosity healing.
- Clinical and radiographic outcomes for cemented versus noncemented stems for proximal humerus fractures are inconclusive. Recent studies have reported good short-term results with noncemented stems with stable humeral fixation and low rates of radiographic lucency up to 3-year follow-up.
- Complications with RSA for fracture resemble those with standard RSA although rates can differ slightly. Infection and instability remain the most common complication, and standard precautions should be taken to prevent them, which may include repair of the tuberosities.

Annotated References

1. Schairer WW, Nwachukwu BU, Lyman S, Craig EV, Gulotta LV: Reverse shoulder arthroplasty versus hemiarthroplasty for treatment of proximal humerus fractures. *J Shoulder Elbow Surg* 2015;24(10):1560-1566. doi:10.1016/j.jse.2015.03.018.

This study using the Nationwide Inpatient Sample database for 2011 found that RSA is becoming widely used to manage proximal humerus fractures and was more likely to be used in small, rural, nonteaching hospitals and in areas that perform a high volume of RSA procedures for other diagnoses. Level of evidence: III.

2. Rajaee SS, Yalamanchili D, Noori N, et al: Increasing use of reverse total shoulder arthroplasty for proximal humerus fractures in elderly patients. *Orthopedics* 2017;40(6):e98 2-e989. doi:10.3928/01477447-20170925-01.

This database study using the Nationwide Inpatient Sample data from 2011 to 2013 found a 1.8-fold increase in the use of RSA for proximal humerus fracture with a concomitant reduction in the rate of open reduction and internal fixation and hemiarthroplasty. Those who were treated with RSA were also more likely to be discharged home when compared with patients treated with hemiarthroplasty.

3. Foruria AM, de Gracia MM, Larson DR, Munuera L, Sanchez-Sotelo J: The pattern of the fracture and displacement of the fragments predict the outcome in proximal humeral fractures. *J Bone Joint Surg Br* 2011;93(3):378-386. doi:10.1302/0301-620X.93B3.25083.

4. Rangan A, Handoll H, Brealey S, et al: Surgical vs nonsurgical treatment of adults with displaced fractures of the proximal humerus: The PROFHER randomized clinical trial. *J Am Med Assoc* 2015;313(10):1037-1047. doi:10.1001/jama.2015.1629.

This multicentered, randomized clinical trial evaluated the clinical effectiveness of surgical and nonsurgical treatment for adults with displaced proximal humerus fractures involving the surgical neck. There was no difference in patient-reported outcomes between the two groups over a 2-year period following fracture occurrence. Level of evidence: I.

5. Mao F, Zhang D-H, Peng X-C, Liao Y: Comparison of surgical versus non-surgical treatment of displaced 3- and 4-part fractures of the proximal humerus: A meta-analysis. *J Invest Surg* 2015;28(4):215-224.

This meta-analysis study compared the clinical outcomes of surgical versus nonsurgical management of displaced three-part or four-part proximal humerus fractures. There was no difference in functional outcome based on the Constant-Murley score between the two groups; however, patients who were treated surgically had improved health-related quality of life. Level of evidence: I.

6. Lange M, Brandt D, Mittlmeier T, Gradl G: Proximal humeral fractures: Non-operative treatment versus intramedullary nailing in 2-, 3- and 4-part fractures. *Injury* 2016;47(suppl 7):S14-S19. doi:10.1016/S0020-1383(16)30848-8.

This comparative study found no difference between nonsurgical management and intramedullary nailing of two-part, three-part, and four-part proximal humerus fractures. Level of evidence: III.

7. Fjalestad T, Hole MØ, Hovden IAH, Blücher J, Strømsøe K: Surgical treatment with an angular stable plate for complex displaced proximal humeral fractures in elderly patients: A randomized controlled trial. *J Orthop Trauma* 2012;26(2):98-106. doi:10.1097/BOT.0b013e31821c2e15.

8. Boons HW, Goosen JH, van Grinsven S, van Susante JL, van Loon CJ: Hemiarthroplasty for humeral four-part fractures for patients 65 years and older: A randomized controlled trial. *Clin Orthop Relat Res* 2012;470(12):3483-3491. doi:10.1007/s11999-012-2531-0.

9. Roberson TA, Granade CM, Hunt Q, et al: Nonoperative management versus reverse shoulder arthroplasty for treatment of 3- and 4-part proximal humeral fractures in older adults. *J Shoulder Elbow Surg* 2017;26(6):1017-1022. doi:10.1016/j.jse.2016.10.013.

In a retrospective study of 19 patients treated nonsurgically and 20 patients treated with RSA for three-part and four-part proximal humerus, the authors found no difference in shoulder motion or patient-reported outcomes. Level of evidence: III.

10. Chivot M, Lami D, Bizzozero P, Galland A, Argenson J-N: Three- and four-part displaced proximal humeral fractures in patients older than 70 years: Reverse shoulder arthroplasty or nonsurgical treatment? *J Shoulder Elbow Surg* 2019;28(2):252-259. doi:10.1016/j.jse.2018.07.019.

In patients aged 70 years or older with three-part or four-part proximal humerus fracture, those who were treated with RSA had higher Constant-Murley scores, better shoulder motion, and higher satisfaction than who were treated nonsurgically in this multicentered, retrospective comparative study. Level of evidence: III.

11. Wolfensperger F, Gruninger P, Dietrich M, et al: Reverse shoulder arthroplasty for complex fractures of the proximal humerus in elderly patients: Impact on the level of independency, early function, and pain medication. *J Shoulder Elbow Surg* 2017;26(8):1462-1468. doi:10.1016/j.jse.2017.01.021.

    A prospective case series of 33 patients found that primary RSA for complex proximal humerus fractures in elderly patients (≥70 years) provides good early function, reliable pain control, and restoration of independence. Level of evidence: IV.

12. Osterhoff G, O'Hara NN, D'Cruz J, et al: A cost-effectiveness analysis of reverse total shoulder arthroplasty versus hemiarthroplasty for the management of complex proximal humeral fractures in the elderly. *Value Health* 2017;20(3):404-411. doi:10.1016/j.jval.2016.10.017.

    This was a cost-utility analysis study comparing RSA and hemiarthroplasty for proximal humerus fractures in the elderly using data from current literature and decision tree and Markov modeling techniques. The authors found that RSA was a more cost-effective treatment option within 2 years of the initial procedure. In their model, they also found that the RSA group would need a complication rate of 38% before the hemiarthroplasty group would provide more quality-adjusted-life-year. Level of evidence: I.

13. Chalmers PN, Slikker W, Mall NA, et al: Reverse total shoulder arthroplasty for acute proximal humeral fracture: Comparison to open reduction–internal fixation and hemiarthroplasty. *J Shoulder Elbow Surg* 2014;23(2):197-204. doi:10.1016/j.jse.2013.07.044.

    Patients with three-part and four-part proximal humerus fractures treated with RSA had greater forward elevation and significant Medicare care cost reduction when compared with those treated with hemiarthroplasty and open reduction and internal fixation. Level of evidence: III.

14. Gallinet D, Adam A, Gasse N, Rochet S, Obert L: Improvement in shoulder rotation in complex shoulder fractures treated by reverse shoulder arthroplasty. *J Shoulder Elbow Surg* 2013;22(1):38-44. doi:10.1016/j.jse.2012.03.011.

    This retrospective study reported anatomic tuberosity healing in 66% of patients. When compared with patients without repair or nonunion/malunion of the tuberosities, those with healed tuberosities had significantly better shoulder motion and Constant-Murley scores. Level of evidence: III.

15. Sebastia-Forcada E, Cebrian-Gomez R, Lizaur-Utrilla A, Gil-Guillen V: Reverse shoulder arthroplasty versus hemiarthroplasty for acute proximal humeral fractures. A blinded, randomized, controlled, prospective study. *J Shoulder Elbow Surg* 2014;23(10):1419-1426. doi:10.1016/j.jse.2014.06.035.

    In this blinded, randomized controlled trial of 62 patients, those who underwent uncemented RSA for proximal humerus fractures had better pain relief, better function, and lower rate of revision surgery than those who underwent uncemented hemiarthroplasty. Level of evidence: I.

16. Cazeneuve J-F, Cristofari D-J: Grammont reversed prosthesis for acute complex fracture of the proximal humerus in an elderly population with 5 to 12 years follow-up. *Orthop Traumatol Surg Res* 2014;100(1):93-97. doi:10.1016/j.otsr.2013.12.005.

    This retrospective study of 23 patients demonstrated good long-term outcomes with treatment of complex proximal humerus fractures with cemented RSA but a 48% rate of scapular notching. Mean Constant score was 60 and active forward flexion was >120°. Those with tuberosity repair had improved external and internal rotation. Level of evidence: IV.

17. Garofalo R, Flanagin B, Castagna A, Lo EY, Krishnan SG: Reverse shoulder arthroplasty for proximal humerus fracture using a dedicated stem: Radiological outcomes at a minimum 2 years of follow-up—Case series. *J Orthop Surg Res* 2015;10(1):129. doi:10.1186/s13018-015-0261-1.

    This case series of 87 patients who underwent RSA for proximal humerus fracture with a fracture stem demonstrated a tuberosity healing rate of 75%. Those with healed tuberosities had significantly greater forward elevation, external rotation, and internal rotation. Tuberosity nonunions or resorption was seen in female patients; however, this was not statistically significant. Very comminuted tuberosity fractures were associated with resorption. Level of evidence: IV.

18. Ross M, Hope B, Stokes A, Peters SE, McLeod I, Duke PFR: Reverse shoulder arthroplasty for the treatment of three-part and four-part proximal humeral fractures in the elderly. *J Shoulder Elbow Surg* 2015;24(2):215-222. doi:10.1016/j.jse.2014.05.022.

    This retrospective study of 21 patients with three-part and four-part proximal humerus fracture managed with RSA demonstrated good clinical and radiographic outcomes with a mean ASES score of 89.3 and a mean Constant score of 88.03. Complication rates in this cohort were low and there are no dislocations. The authors also noted a higher rate of shoulder stiffness earlier in their study and modified their technique to excise the supraspinatus and anterior greater tuberosity to accommodate the bulky design of the reverse stem. Level of evidence: IV.

19. Formaini NT, Everding NG, Levy JC, Rosas S: Tuberosity healing after RSA for acute proximal humerus fractures: The "black and tan" technique. *J Shoulder Elbow Surg* 2015;24(11):e299-e306. doi:10.1016/j.jse.2015.04.014.

    This case series reported an 88% tuberosity healing rate in patients who underwent RSA for proximal humerus fractures using the black and tan technique, which creates a transition zone between the cement mantle and the proximal aspect of the humeral stem using cancellous autograft from the fractured humeral head. Level of evidence: IV.

20. Youn S-M, Deo S, Poon PC: Functional and radiologic outcomes of uncemented reverse shoulder arthroplasty in proximal humeral fractures: Cementing the humeral component is not necessary. *J Shoulder Elbow Surg* 2016;25(4):e83-e89. doi:10.1016/j.jse.2015.09.007.

    Uncemented RSA for the management of comminuted proximal humerus fractures in a cohort of elderly patients resulted in satisfactory functional and radiologic outcomes at a mean of 3-year follow-up. Only two patients (10%) in this case series had radiographic signs of being at risk for loosening (>3 lucent zones that were 2 mm or greater in width); however, none of these patients were asymptomatic and did not require revision surgery. Level of evidence: IV.

21. Grubhofer F, Wieser K, Meyer DC, et al: Reverse total shoulder arthroplasty for acute head-splitting, 3- and 4-part fractures of the proximal humerus in the elderly. *J Shoulder Elbow Surg* 2016;25(10):1690-1698. doi:10.1016/j.jse.2016.02.024.

    This retrospective multicentered study found good mid-term clinical results in 51 patients with acute, complex proximal humerus fractures who were treated with RSA. Patients with healed tuberosities had more anterior shoulder elevation, more external rotation, and better Subjective Shoulder Values and Constant-Murley scores. Level of evidence: IV.

22. Chun Y-M, Kim D-S, Lee D-H, Shin S-J: Reverse shoulder arthroplasty for four-part proximal humerus fracture in elderly patients: Can a healed tuberosity improve the functional outcomes? *J Shoulder Elbow Surg* 2017;26(7):1216-1221. doi:10.1016/j.jse.2016.11.034.

    This cohort study of 38 patients with four-part proximal humerus fracture treated with RSA reported anatomic healing of the tuberosities in 37% of patients. Patients with healed tuberosities had better external rotation but no difference in forward flexion, internal rotation, Constant-Murley scores, or American Shoulder and Elbow Surgeons score. Level of evidence: III.

23. Ohl X, Bonnevialle N, Gallinet D, et al: How the greater tuberosity affects clinical outcomes after reverse shoulder arthroplasty for proximal humeral fractures. *J Shoulder Elbow Surg* 2018;27(12):2139-2144. doi:10.1016/j.jse.2018.05.030.

    This was a retrospective, multicenter study of 420 elderly patients who underwent RSA for acute proximal humerus fractures. Patients with anatomic tuberosity healing had improved forward elevation, external rotation, Constant-Murley scores, and Simple Shoulder Value when compared with patients with tuberosity excision or malunion/nonunion. Patients with excised tuberosities had a significantly higher rate of instability (12.5%). Level of evidence: III.

24. Simovitch RW, Roche CP, Jones RB, et al: Effect of tuberosity healing on clinical outcomes in elderly patients treated with a reverse shoulder arthroplasty for 3- and 4-part proximal humerus fractures. *J Orthop Trauma* 2019;33(2):e39-e45. doi:10.1097/BOT.0000000000001348.

    Tuberosity healing was seen in 83% of patients in this retrospective cohort study of 55 patients with proximal humerus fractures were treated a low profile onlay fracture stem. Greater tuberosity union resulted in greater external rotation but no statistical difference in patient-reported outcomes as measured by ASES, Constant, simple shoulder test, or UCLA score. Level of evidence: IV.

25. Reuther F, Petermann M, Stangl R: Reverse shoulder arthroplasty in acute fractures of the proximal humerus: Does tuberosity healing improve clinical outcomes? *J Orthop Trauma* 2019;33(2):e46-e51. doi:10.1097/BOT.0000000000001338.

    This multicentered case series study of 81 patients compared the outcomes of healed, partially healed, and unhealed tuberosities after RSA for proximal humerus fractures and found no difference in shoulder motion, Constant-Murley scores, or ASES scores. Level of evidence: IV.

26. Wright JO, Ho A, Kalma J, et al: Uncemented reverse total shoulder arthroplasty as initial treatment for comminuted proximal humerus fractures. *J Orthop Trauma* 2019;33(7):e263-e269. doi:10.1097/BOT.0000000000001465.

    Management of comminuted proximal humerus fractures in elderly patients with uncemented RSA results in good clinical outcomes with most (97%) demonstrating stable humeral stem fixation on follow-up radiographs. Level of evidence: IV.

27. Boileau P, Alta TD, Decroocq L, et al: Reverse shoulder arthroplasty for acute fractures in the elderly: Is it worth reattaching the tuberosities? *J Shoulder Elbow Surg* 2019;28(3):437-444. doi:10.1016/j.jse.2018.08.025.

    Thirty-eight elderly patients with displaced or dislocated proximal humerus fractures were treated with reattachment of the tuberosities around a specific reverse fracture stem and cancellous bone autograft. Tuberosity healing rate was 84% and patients with healed tuberosities had improved forward flexion, external rotation, and better satisfaction. Level of evidence: III.

28. Molé D, Wein F, Dézaly C, Valenti P, Sirveaux F: Surgical technique: The anterosuperior approach for reverse shoulder arthroplasty. *Clin Orthop Relat Res* 2011;469(9):2461-2468. doi:10.1007/s11999-011-1861-7.

29. Krishnan SG, Bennion PW, Reineck JR, Burkhead WZ: Hemiarthroplasty for proximal humeral fracture: Restoration of the Gothic arch. *Orthop Clin North Am* 2008;39(4):441-450, vi. doi:10.1016/j.ocl.2008.05.004.

30. Schoch B, Aibinder W, Walters J, et al: Outcomes of uncemented versus cemented reverse shoulder arthroplasty for proximal humerus fractures. *Orthopedics* 2019;42(2):e236-e241. doi:10.3928/01477447-20190125-03.

Noncemented RSA for proximal humerus fractures was associated with worse ASES and satisfaction scores when compared with cemented RSA. However, there was no difference in pain scores, motion, tuberosity healing, or DASH scores between the two groups. Level of evidence: IV.

31. Cazeneuve JF, Cristofari D-J: The reverse shoulder prosthesis in the treatment of fractures of the proximal humerus in the elderly. *J Bone Joint Surg Br* 2010;92-B(4):535-539. doi:10.1302/0301-620X.92B4.22450.

32. Klein M, Juschka M, Hinkenjann B, Scherger B, Ostermann PAW: Treatment of comminuted fractures of the proximal humerus in elderly patients with the Delta III reverse shoulder prosthesis. *J Orthop Trauma* 2008;22(10):698-704. doi:10.1097/BOT.0b013e31818afe40.

33. Boileau P, Krishnan SG, Tinsi L, Walch G, Coste JS, Molé D: Tuberosity malposition and migration: Reasons for poor outcomes after hemiarthroplasty for displaced fractures of the proximal humerus. *J Shoulder Elbow Surg* 2002;11(5):401-412.

34. Acevedo DC, Vanbeek C, Lazarus MD, Williams GR, Abboud JA: Reverse shoulder arthroplasty for proximal humeral fractures: Update on indications, technique, and results. *J Shoulder Elbow Surg* 2014;23:279-289. doi:10.1016/j.jse.2013.10.003.

This review article provides a good overview of all the potential controversies and pitfalls regarding reverse shoulder arthroplasty for proximal humerus fractures. Level of evidence: V.

35. Frankle MA, Ondrovic LE, Markee BA, Harris ML, Lee WE: Stability of tuberosity reattachment in proximal humeral hemiarthroplasty. *J Shoulder Elbow Surg* 2002;11(5):413-420.

36. Levy JC, Badman B: Reverse shoulder prosthesis for acute four-part fracture: Tuberosity fixation using a horseshoe graft. *J Orthop Trauma* 2011;25(5):318-324. doi:10.1097/BOT.0b013e3181f22088.

37. Uzer G, Yildiz F, Batar S, et al: Does grafting of the tuberosities improve the functional outcomes of proximal humeral fractures treated with reverse shoulder arthroplasty? *J Shoulder Elbow Surg* 2017;26(1):36-41. doi:10.1016/j.jse.2016.05.005.

In this cohort study of 33 patients with three-part and four-part proximal humerus fracture treated with RSA, 18 patients underwent autologous bone block grafting of their tuberosity repair and had increased rates of healing compared with those who were not grafted (78% versus 40% [$P=0.048$], respectively). Patients with autograft augmentation also had better forward flexion motion, external rotation strength, ASES scores, and DASH scores. Level of evidence: III.

38. Krishnan SG, Reineck JR, Bennion PD, Feher L, Burkhead WZ: Shoulder arthroplasty for fracture: Does a fracture-specific stem make a difference? *Clin Orthop Relat Res* 2011;469(12):3317-3323. doi:10.1007/s11999-011-1919-6.

39. Li F, Zhu Y, Lu Y, Liu X, Wu G, Jiang C: Hemiarthroplasty for the treatment of complex proximal humeral fractures: Does a trabecular metal prosthesis make a difference? A prospective, comparative study with a minimum 3-year follow-up. *J Shoulder Elbow Surg* 2014;23(10):1437-1443. doi:10.1016/j.jse.2014.04.017.

This prospective study compared the outcomes of 35 patients who were treated with a trabecular metal shoulder prosthesis with those of 38 patients treated with a conventional prosthesis for proximal humerus fractures. They found that the trabecular metal group had lower rates of radiographic complication related to the greater tuberosity, better functional shoulder scores, and higher forward elevation and external rotation. Level of evidence: II.

40. Jain NP, Mannan SS, Dharmarajan R, Rangan A: Tuberosity healing after reverse shoulder arthroplasty for complex proximal humeral fractures in elderly patients—Does it improve outcomes? A systematic review and meta-analysis. *J Shoulder Elbow Surg* 2019;28(3):e78-e91. doi:10.1016/j.jse.2018.09.006.

In this meta-analysis of 381 patients with proximal humerus fractures treated with RSA, patients with healed greater tuberosities had better forward flexion, external rotation, and Constant-Murley scores than patients whose tuberosities did not heal. Level of evidence: IV.

41. Namdari S, Yagnik G, Ebaugh DD, et al: Defining functional shoulder range of motion for activities of daily living. *J Shoulder Elbow Surg* 2012;21(9):1177-1183. doi:10.1016/j.jse.2011.07.032.

42. Cuff DJ, Pupello DR: Comparison of hemiarthroplasty and reverse shoulder arthroplasty for the treatment of proximal humeral fractures in elderly patients. *J Bone Joint Surg* 2013;95(22):2050-2055. doi:10.2106/JBJS.L.01637.

This comparative study of 53 patients treated with either RSA or hemiarthroplasty for three-part and four-part proximal humerus fractures demonstrated better forward elevated, higher ASES and SST scores, and higher satisfaction in the RSA group. Level of evidence: II.

43. Cheung E, Willis M, Walker M, Clark R, Frankle MA: Complications in reverse total shoulder arthroplasty. *J Am Acad Orthop Surg* 2011;19(7):439-449.

44. Villacis D, Sivasundaram L, Pannell WC, Heckmann N, Omid R, Hatch GFR: Complication rate and implant survival for reverse shoulder arthroplasty versus total shoulder arthroplasty: Results during the initial 2 years. *J Shoulder Elbow Surg* 2016;25(6):927-935. doi:10.1016/j.jse.2015.10.012.

This database study reported higher rates of complications in patients with RSA than in those with total shoulder arthroplasty. The overall complication rate in the RSA group was 3%, 5.7%, 9.94%, and 21.8% at 30 days, 90 days, 1 year, and 2 years, respectively. Level of evidence: III.

45. Zumstein MA, Pinedo M, Old J, Boileau P: Problems, complications, reoperations, and revisions in reverse total shoulder arthroplasty: A systematic review. *J Shoulder Elbow Surg* 2011;20(1):146-157. doi:10.1016/j.jse.2010.08.001.

46. Boileau P: Complications and revision of reverse total shoulder arthroplasty. *Orthop Traumatol Surg Res* 2016;102(1 suppl):S33-S43. doi:10.1016/j.otsr.2015.06.031.

    This review article summarizes the complications seen with RSA and report that the most common causes of revision surgery after RSA include prosthetic instability (38%), infection (22%), humeral complications (21%), and glenoid complications (13%). Level of evidence: IV.

47. Jobin CM, Galdi B, Anakwenze OA, Ahmad CS, Levine WN: Reverse shoulder arthroplasty for the management of proximal humerus fractures. *J Am Acad Orthop Surg* 2015;23(3):190-201. doi:10.5435/JAAOS-D-13-00190.

    This review article discusses the role of RSA in the treatment of proximal humerus fractures and summarizes the outcomes and complications observed with RSA. It also includes the authors' preferred RSA technique and strategies for tuberosity repair. Level of evidence: V.

48. Jauregui JJ, Nadarajah V, Shield WP, Henn RF, Gilotra M, Hasan SA: Reverse shoulder arthroplasty: Perioperative considerations and complications. *JBJS Rev* 2018;6(8):e3. doi:10.2106/JBJS.RVW.17.00152.

    This review article summarizes the complications seen with RSA for all indications. Scapular notching, glenoid loosening, and instability were the most common postoperative complications. Level of evidence: V.

49. Simovitch RW, Zumstein MA, Lohri E, Helmy N, Gerber C: Predictors of scapular notching in patients managed with the Delta III reverse total shoulder replacement. *J Bone Joint Surg Am* 2007;89(3):588-600. doi:10.2106/JBJS.F.00226.\

50. Lévigne C, Boileau P, Favard L, et al: Scapular notching in reverse shoulder arthroplasty. *J Shoulder Elbow Surg* 2008;17(6):925-935. doi:10.1016/J.JSE.2008.02.010.

51. Berhouet J, Garaud P, Favard L: Evaluation of the role of glenosphere design and humeral component retroversion in avoiding scapular notching during reverse shoulder arthroplasty. *J Shoulder Elbow Surg* 2014;23(2):151-158. doi:10.1016/j.jse.2013.05.009.

    This cadaver study demonstrated that inferior scapular notching can be prevented by using a large-diameter glenosphere with lateralized center of rotation and by replicating the patient's native retroversion for the humeral component.

52. Erickson BJ, Frank RM, Harris JD, Mall N, Romeo AA: The influence of humeral head inclination in reverse total shoulder arthroplasty: A systematic review. *J Shoulder Elbow Surg* 2015;24(6):988-993. doi:10.1016/j.jse.2015.01.001.

    A systemic review of 38 studies and 2,222 shoulders found that the rate of scapular notching was higher with a 155° prosthesis than with a 135° prosthesis with a lateralized glenosphere. There was no difference in the rate of dislocation between the two types of prostheses. Level of evidence: IV.

53. Stephenson DR, Oh JH, McGarry MH, Rick Hatch GF, Lee TQ: Effect of humeral component version on impingement in reverse total shoulder arthroplasty. *J Shoulder Elbow Surg* 2011;20(4):652-658. doi:10.1016/j.jse.2010.08.020.

54. Noguera L, Trigo L, Melero V, Santana F, Torrens C: Reverse shoulder arthroplasty for acute proximal humeral fractures: Postoperative complications at 7 days, 90 days and 1 year. *Injury* 2019;50(2):371-375. doi:10.1016/j.injury.2019.01.002.

    The overall complication rate for elderly patients treated with RSA for proximal humerus fractures was 25% with 17.4% minor and 7.6% major complications. A major complication was defined as one that affects the final result or required additional surgery. Patients with an American Society of Anesthesiologists score of 3 or greater and those with rheumatic disease were at increased risk for a major complication within the first 90 days. Level of evidence: IV.

55. Klug A, Wincheringer D, Harth J, Schmidt-Horlohé K, Hoffmann R, Gramlich Y: Complications after surgical treatment of proximal humerus fractures in the elderly—An analysis of complication patterns and risk factors for reverse shoulder arthroplasty and angular-stable plating. *J Shoulder Elbow Surg* 2019;28(9):1674-1684. doi:10.1016/j.jse.2019.02.017.

    This retrospective study of patients who underwent RSA for proximal humerus fracture found a 22% complication rate with 5.1% of patients requiring revision surgery. The most common complications were instability and intractable shoulder stiffness. Higher Charlson comorbidity index, diabetes, and resection or resorbed greater tuberosities were associated with high rates of complications. Level of evidence: III.

56. Mata-Fink A, Meinke M, Jones C, Kim B, Bell J-E: Reverse shoulder arthroplasty for treatment of proximal humeral fractures in older adults: A systematic review. *J Shoulder Elbow Surg* 2013;22(12):1737-1748. doi:10.1016/j.jse.2013.08.021.

    This systematic review of 15 studies comparing RSA with hemiarthroplasty for proximal humerus fracture found improved forward flexion and functional outcomes scores in the RSA group with similar rates of complications. Level of evidence: IV.

57. Teusink MJ, Pappou IP, Schwartz DG, Cottrell BJ, Frankle MA: Results of closed management of acute dislocation after reverse shoulder arthroplasty. *J Shoulder Elbow Surg* 2015;24(4):621-627. doi:10.1016/j.jse.2014.07.015.

This retrospective study of 21 patients who underwent closed reduction for dislocation after RSA found that a majority of patients (62%) were stable and successfully treated without surgical intervention. Level of evidence: IV.

58. Chalmers PN, Rahman Z, Romeo AA, Nicholson GP: Early dislocation after reverse total shoulder arthroplasty. *J Shoulder Elbow Surg* 2014;23(5):737-744. doi:10.1016/j.jse.2013.08.015.

This retrospective study of 385 RSA demonstrated an early rate of instability (within 90 days) of 2.9% with a mean time to dislocation of 3.4 weeks. Patients who were male, had prior surgery, were overweight (mean body mass index 32.2 kg/m^2), or did not have satisfactory subscapularis repair were at increased risk of early dislocation. Level of evidence: IV.

59. Smith GCS, Bateman E, Cass B, et al: Reverse shoulder arthroplasty for the treatment of proximal humeral fractures in the elderly (ReShAPE trial): Study protocol for a multicentre combined randomised controlled and observational trial. *Trials* 2017;18(1):91. doi:10.1186/s13063-017-1826-6.

This is an ongoing multicentered, combined randomized and observational study of patients aged 70 years and older with three-part and four-part proximal humerus fracture who are treated nonsurgically or with RSA. Primary outcomes are the compare the pain and function of the two groups using the ASES score. Secondary outcomes include the DASH score, the ED-5Q (EuroQol Health Survey), the EQ-VAS, radiographic outcomes, and complications. Level of evidence: I.

60. Launonen AP, Fjalestad T, Laitinen MK, et al: Nordic Innovative Trials to Evaluate osteoPorotic Fractures (NITEP) Collaboration: The Nordic DeltaCon Trial protocol-non-operative treatment versus reversed total shoulder arthroplasty in patients 65 years of age and older with a displaced proximal humerus fracture: A prospective, randomised controlled trial. *BMJ Open* 2019;9(1):e024916. doi:10.1136/bmjopen-2018-024916.

This is an ongoing prospective, single-blinded, randomized control trial comparing RSA with nonsurgical management of displaced proximal humerus fractures in patients aged 65 to 85 years. The primary outcome is the quick-DASH score at 2 years. Secondary outcomes include VAS pain scale, grip strength, Oxford shoulder score, Constant score, revision surgeries, and complications. Level of evidence: I.

Chapter 31

Sequelae of Proximal Humeral Fractures

Robert Z. Tashjian, MD

ABSTRACT

Various complications are associated with the treatment of proximal humerus fractures including osteonecrosis, malunion, nonunion, arthritis, and stiffness. Osteonecrosis typically can be treated nonsurgically, with good results in stage I or II and a limited risk of progression, but stage III or IV disease typically requires surgical management. Arthroscopic débridement and core decompression are reasonable alternatives for persistently symptomatic stage I, II, or III disease, with the most promising results in stage I or II lesions. Proximal humeral malunion is uncommon. Persistently symptomatic surgical neck malunion with a neck-shaft angle of less than 110° can be treated with surgical neck osteotomy. Greater tuberosity malunion can be treated with osteotomy (usually for posterior displacement) or tuberoplasty with rotator cuff repair (for superior displacement). In a patient younger than 70 years, surgical neck nonunion with a viable humeral head and no arthritis can be treated with open reduction and internal fixation. Mild to moderate posttraumatic glenohumeral arthritis in a shoulder with concentric wear and some preserved joint space can be effectively treated with arthroscopic débridement and capsular release. Arthroscopic release is an excellent option for restoring motion and function in a patient who has posttraumatic adhesive capsulitis with minimal residual deformity.

Keywords: adhesive capsulitis; malunion; nonunion; osteonecrosis; posttraumatic arthritis; proximal humerus fracture

Introduction

Proximal humeral fractures account for approximately 5% of all fractures, and they are among the most commonly treated musculoskeletal injuries. Most of these injuries are minimally displaced and can be treated nonsurgically to achieve almost complete healing, a near-normal range of motion, and an excellent functional outcome.[1] Nonetheless, residual complications including osteonecrosis, nonunion, malunion, degenerative arthritis, and stiffness can ensue after nonsurgical or surgical care of a proximal humeral fracture.

Osteonecrosis

Osteonecrosis of the humeral head results from a loss of circulation that leads to bone cell death. Initially the bone of the avascular area attempts to repair itself with necrotic bone resorption and new bone deposition. Subchondral fracture may develop, leading to articular surface collapse and glenohumeral arthritis.[2] The etiology of proximal humeral osteonecrosis can be atraumatic, as in corticosteroid or alcohol use or sickle cell disease; or traumatic, as with proximal humeral fracture. Posttraumatic osteonecrosis can occur after nonsurgical or surgical care of proximal humeral fracture. The risk of osteonecrosis primarily is determined by the severity of the fracture.[3] Overall rates of osteonecrosis in large groups have been reported as 2% after nonsurgical management and 8% after surgical management.[1,4] Studies of three-part and four-part fractures reported osteonecrosis rates of 28% after nonsurgical management and 35% after surgical management.[3,5] These studies indicate a greater risk of osteonecrosis after a severe injury in comparison with the overall risk.

Posttraumatic osteonecrosis most often is associated with clinical disability, although the expected level of disability has improved over time from the dismal results once expected for patients with posttraumatic osteonecrosis. In a series of 166 operatively repaired proximal humerus fractures, 4.8% developed radiographic evidence of osteonecrosis and the average postoperative elevation and Disability of Arm, Shoulder and Hand scores were worse for those patients with osteonecrosis versus those without osteonecrosis.[6] In 25 patients with partial or complete collapse of the humeral head as a result of posttraumatic osteonecrosis, the clinical outcome depended on the extent of humeral head collapse and malunion of the fracture fragments.[7] Another study similarly found that the presence or absence of a

Dr. Tashjian or an immediate family member has received royalties from Shoulder Innovations, Wright Medical Technology, Inc., and Zimmer; serves as a paid consultant to or is an employee of Cayenne Medical and Mitek; and has stock or stock options held in Conextions, INTRAFUSE, and KATOR.

malunion was one of the major predictors of outcome in patients with posttraumatic osteonecrosis after a four-part fracture.[8] Although many patients with osteonecrosis without significant collapse or malunion have a reasonable clinical result, severe collapse and malunion often requires reconstruction with hemiarthroplasty or reverse total shoulder arthroplasty, depending on the residual malposition of the greater tuberosity.[9] In the absence of significant humeral head collapse or malunion, a more limited surgical procedure such as arthroscopic débridement or open or arthroscopic core decompression can be considered for a patient with persistent symptoms secondary to osteonecrosis.[10-13]

Evaluation and Classification

The initial symptom of osteonecrosis of the proximal humerus typically is a deep, poorly localized shoulder pain similar to that of early glenohumeral arthrosis. The pain often radiates to the elbow and is exacerbated by overuse. The typical location of the osteonecrotic lesion is superomedial, and abduction and forward flexion may elicit symptoms as the diseased portion of the humeral head contacts the glenoid surface. Some patients are relatively asymptomatic.

Standard shoulder radiographs and MRI are the main imaging diagnostic tools. The shoulder radiographs should include true AP views in internal and external rotation as well as an axillary lateral view. Radiographic changes typically occur during later stages of the disease, but early changes can be detected on MRI. Bone scanning is inadequate as a diagnostic tool for osteonecrosis of the shoulder.

The most commonly used classification is the Cruess system, which is a modification of the Ficat-Arlet classification of osteonecrosis of the hip.[14] Staging is extremely important because it dictates the treatment and predicts the outcome. The classification primarily is based on the severity of humeral head collapse (**Figure 1**). Stage I changes are not visible on plain radiographs and only can be seen as edema on MRI. Stage II changes are seen as a well-defined lesion on MRI and sclerosis on plain radiographs. A stage III lesion is a subchondral fracture with a loss of head sphericity. A stage IV or V lesion is characterized by humeral head collapse or glenoid involvement, respectively.

The Sakai classification system described in 2008 was based on lesion size as well as extent of collapse.[15] The size of an osteonecrotic lesion was evaluated by defining the so-called necrotic angle on midoblique-coronal and midoblique-sagittal MRI. A necrotic angle of more than 90° was found in 12 patients with Cruess stage I and II lesions and 92% of these humeral heads collapsed (4 to Cruess stage III and 7 to Cruess stage IV). None of the 34 patients with Cruess stage I and II lesions with a necrotic angle of less than 90° had progression to a Cruess stage III, IV, or V lesion.

Management Options

The management of posttraumatic osteonecrosis depends on three factors: the presence of symptoms, the stage of the lesion, and the extent of malunion. If the lesion is asymptomatic, observation is recommended, with the use of follow-up radiographs to monitor the lesion. If the lesion is symptomatic, it is reasonable to institute treatment. The management options include nonsurgical measures, such as physical therapy and anti-inflammatory drugs, as well as surgery. The nonarthroplasty surgical options include core decompression, arthroscopy with or without core decompression, and vascularized bone graft. In general, these options are reserved for symptomatic stage I, II, and III lesions with minimal evidence of malunion, after unsuccessful nonsurgical management. Arthroplasty is reserved for symptomatic stage IV and V lesions as well as stage III lesions with a significant malunion.

Natural History and Nonsurgical Management

The natural history of osteonecrotic lesions of the proximal humerus is poorly defined. The only available studies are of small, heterogeneous groups of patients with multiple etiologies and relatively poor radiographic categorization. The initial study reported that 78% of patients with steroid-induced osteonecrosis had a satisfactory long-term outcome. Only 22% required surgical treatment (in the form of shoulder arthroplasty); all of these patients initially had a Cruess stage IV or V lesion.[14] Higher lesion stage and larger lesion size were found to have a significant negative effect on lesion progression and the need for surgery in a study of 151 patients (200 shoulders).[16] Patients were treated nonsurgically and initially did not require future surgery; 77% had no or mild pain at an average 8.6-year follow-up. Three years after initial treatment, 78% of patients with traumatic osteonecrosis needed arthroplasty, compared with 47% of those with an atraumatic lesion. A study of 65 patients with osteonecrosis found worse long-term outcomes after nonsurgical treatment.[17] At a minimum 2-year follow-up, 20% of patients had undergone immediate surgery, 34% had surgery during the evaluation period, and 23% had a poor result after nonsurgical treatment, and only 23% had a satisfactory outcome after nonsurgical treatment. All of the patients who underwent surgery or had a poor outcome after continued nonsurgical treatment had a stage III, IV, or V lesion. Those with a stage I or II lesion did well long-term, with limited progression or need for surgery.[17] Another study reported no progression of stage I and II lesions with necrotic angles of less than 90° on midoblique-coronal and midoblique-sagittal MRI.[15]

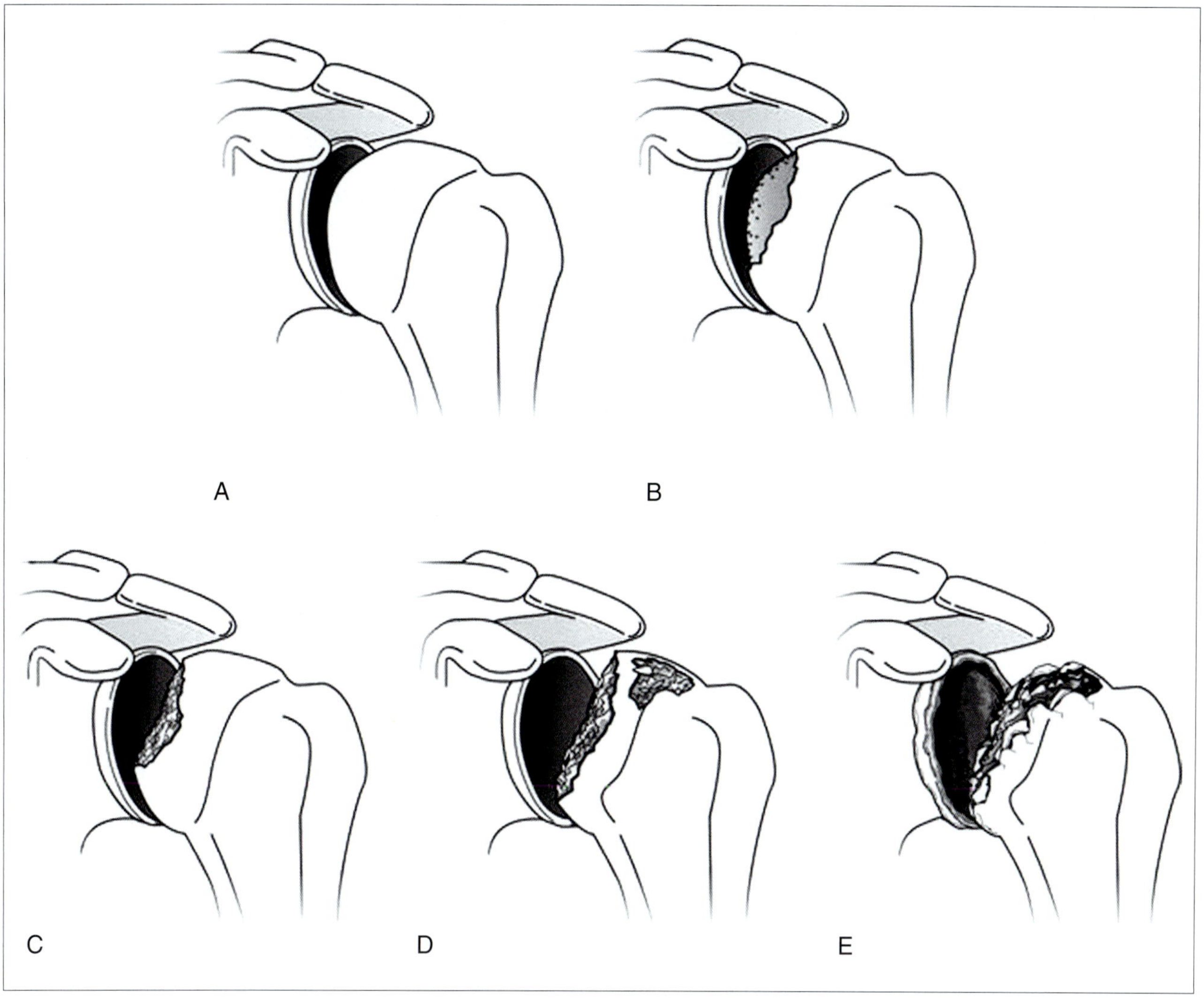

FIGURE 1 Schematic drawings showing the Cruess classification of proximal humeral osteonecrosis. **A**, Stage I: no radiographic evidence of shoulder osteonecrosis; the humeral head appears normal, with maintenance of curvature and no sclerosis. **B**, Stage II: signs of mottled sclerosis, but the curvature of the humeral head remains intact. **C**, Stage III: development of a crescent sign indicating subchondral fracture with loss of sphericity of the humeral head. **D**, Stage IV: progression to collapse of the subchondral bone and humeral head. **E**, Stage V: progression to early degenerative changes of the glenoid. (Reproduced with permission from Harreld KL, Marker DR, Wiesler ER, Shafiz B, Mont MA: Osteonecrosis of the humeral head. *J Am Acad Orthop Surg* 2009;17:345-355.)

The primary goals of nonsurgical management include pain relief and maintenance of motion. Physical therapy is recommended for prevention of adhesive capsulitis. Activity modification is necessary to limit heavy overhead lifting. In general, nonsurgical management can initially be considered for most patients. Initial nonsurgical management is most effective and therefore most appropriate for stage I or II disease, especially if the lesion is small, and offers a good chance for a satisfactory result. A relatively small stage III lesion also may respond to nonsurgical management, although most stage III, IV, or V lesions require some form of surgical intervention.

Nonarthroplasty Surgical Management

A limited number of nonarthroplasty surgical options exist for osteonecrotic lesions of the humeral head, including core decompression, arthroscopic débridement alone, and arthroscopic débridement with core decompression. The indications include a stage I or II lesion that is resistant to nonsurgical management and a stage III lesion with limited collapse. A severe stage III lesion or a stage IV or V lesion should be treated with partial or complete shoulder replacement.

Data are limited regarding the use of arthroscopic débridement for osteonecrotic lesions. The primary goals are to improve the lesion stage and to débride loose cartilage flaps or loose bodies. Short-term functional improvement and pain relief reasonably can be expected. In general, arthroscopic débridement is most useful for reducing pain from synovitis and relieving mechanical symptoms from chondral flaps or loose bodies, if it is performed in isolation without core decompression even in a stage III or IV lesion.

Core decompression for osteonecrosis has been extensively studied in patients with femoral head osteonecrosis. The treatment effect is a result of a reduction in bone marrow pressure that can reduce pain and possibly incite revascularization and deposition of new bone in the necrotic region. The rates of success have varied. Although the procedure is somewhat controversial, it appears to be effective in patients with a stage I or II lesion in the hip.[13] Several limited evaluations have been performed in patients with proximal humeral osteonecrosis.[13,18,19] The surgical techniques described for core decompression in the proximal humerus are both open and arthroscopic.[10,11,13]

In general, stage I and II lesions resistant to nonsurgical management had excellent long-term functional results and limited radiographic progression after core decompression, and none required arthroplasty.[13,19] It is unclear whether a reduction in radiographic progression results from the decompression or the normal natural history of a stage I or II lesion. Some success has been reported after core decompression of stage III lesions; 70% of patients had a good or excellent result at an average 5.6-year follow-up, with the remaining 30% requiring arthroplasty.[13]

Several techniques have been described for proximal humeral core decompression. In an open decompression technique, a small incision is made in the inferior deltopectoral interval just above the pectoralis major with blunt dissection carried just lateral to the bicipital groove.[13] A small, lateral deltoid-split approach can also be used, in which biplane radiographs are used to locate the lesion and a 5-mm coring device is used to perform the decompression; a large biopsy cannula (6 to 10 mm) also can be used, depending on the size of the lesion.[19] A percutaneous decompression technique reported in 2009 uses a 3.2-mm Steinmann pin with two or three passes in the lesion from a common entry site.[18] At a mean 32-month follow-up, 25 of 26 shoulders (96%) with stage I or II disease were successfully treated with the percutaneous technique, as measured on the UCLA scoring system. Only one patient had radiographic progression.[18] Reports of several arthroscopic techniques have emphasized the benefits of intra-articular visualization of the lesion to aid in staging, concomitant synovectomy, or débridement for pain relief; to improve localization for decompression; and to avoid joint penetration by the coring device (**Figure 2**). An anterior cruciate ligament guide was used through the anterior portal, followed by a guidewire from the lateral portal, which was overreamed with a 7-mm cannulated reamer.[10] A similar technique used an anterior cruciate ligament guide, with placement of several 3.2 mm Steinmann pins followed by overdrilling with a 4-mm coring device.[11] All four patients in the two combined studies had uneventful recovery and immediate pain relief. In general, both arthroscopic and open techniques are safe and effective for treating symptomatic stage I and II and possibly stage III lesions.

Proximal Humeral Malunions

Malunion of the proximal aspect of the humerus after fracture can be the result of inadequate reduction during surgical fixation, loss of reduction after surgical fixation, or nonsurgical management if the fracture is displaced or becomes displaced during treatment. A 2011 systematic review found a 7% incidence of varus malunion in 650 nonsurgically treated proximal humerus fractures.[1] Patients with a malunited fracture often have pain, limited range of motion, and impaired strength, depending on the fracture pattern and the presence of concomitant humeral head collapse or arthritis. The final deformity of the malunited fracture is dictated by muscle pull on the fracture fragments. A greater tuberosity malunion has superior and/or posterior displacement from the pull of the posterosuperior rotator cuff, which leads to subacromial impingement and weakness of the rotator cuff. The nonanatomic mechanics lead to pain and limited motion. Isolated surgical neck malunion typically results in varus and flexion deformity caused by the pull of the pectoralis major on the shaft fragment and the pull of the rotator cuff on the head fragment, leading to loss of flexion and abduction.

The clinical evaluation of a proximal humeral malunion should include the mechanism of injury and treatment history. Several conditions may predispose a patient to malunion, including osteoporotic bone, aggressive rehabilitation, or inadequate fixation. Radiographic evaluation should include plain radiographs (AP, AP in the plane of the scapula, axillary, and transscapular lateral views) as well as CT with three-dimensional reconstruction to allow accurate evaluation of the position and extent of any tuberosity displacement. MRI should be added if there is concern about early osteonecrosis or lack of rotator cuff integrity, which may necessitate altering the surgical management plan.

Several classification systems have characterized proximal humeral malunions, although none is universally accepted. A modification of fracture classification by the author of a 1970 study using parts categorization

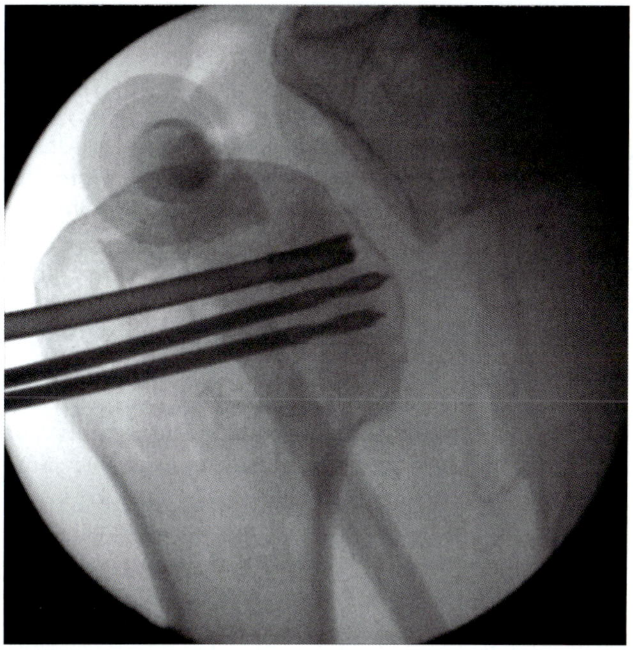

FIGURE 2 Intraoperative fluoroscopic image of a stage III osteonecrotic lesion undergoing arthroscopically assisted core decompression. (Courtesy of Pat Greis, MD, Salt Lake City, UT.)

probably is the most commonly used because of its simplicity.[20] The Beredjiklian system evaluates both bony and soft-tissue abnormalities.[21] A bony deformity is classified as a malposition of the lesser or greater tuberosity of more than 1 cm (type I), a step-off of the articular surface of more than 5 mm (type II), or a malalignment of the proximal humeral articular segment of more than 45° (type III). Soft-tissue abnormalities include stiffness, rotator cuff tearing, or impingement. The Boileau system specifies the indications for treatment and the outcomes of unconstrained arthroplasty.[22] Type I sequelae include impacted proximal humeral fractures progressing to head collapse or necrosis; type II, chronic dislocations or fracture-dislocations; type III, surgical neck nonunions; and type IV, severe tuberosity malunions requiring greater tuberosity osteotomy. Type I and II sequelae were found to have a satisfactory result after unconstrained arthroplasty because no greater tuberosity osteotomy was performed. Type III and IV sequelae had a poor result after unconstrained arthroplasty because a greater tuberosity osteotomy was required.

Although malunion can occur after any proximal humerus fracture, very few are amendable to isolated correction. Typically, an isolated greater tuberosity malunion or surgical neck malunion with an intact rotator cuff and no concomitant arthritic changes is optimal for surgical management. The nonarthroplasty surgical options for these injuries include (1) isolated arthroscopic débridement, (2) débridement with tuberoplasty, or (3) rotator cuff retensioning and osteotomy.[21,23-29] Malunion in a complex three-part or four-part fracture or malunion with associated arthritic changes, humeral head collapse, insufficient bone stock, or rotator cuff deficiency is better treated with anatomic shoulder arthroplasty or reverse total shoulder arthroplasty.

Greater Tuberosity Malunion

Isolated greater tuberosity malunion probably is the most common proximal humeral malunion. The surgical indications for fixation of greater tuberosity fractures include displacement of more than 1 cm; however, some surgeons suggest surgical fixation of fractures with more than 5 mm of displacement.[20,30] Symptomatic malunion can occur with a neglected fracture having more than 1 cm of displacement, failure of fixation of an internally fixed tuberosity, or unsuccessful nonsurgical management of a fracture having less than 1 cm of displacement. Posterior displacement often causes a rigid block to external rotation, and superior displacement can cause loss of abduction, impingement, and rotator cuff weakness. Indications for surgical management of the malunion include more than 5 mm of superior displacement or 1 cm of posterior displacement with pain, loss of motion, and impingement.

The surgical options for a malunited greater tuberosity fracture include open osteotomy, arthroscopic débridement, or arthroscopic tuberoplasty with rotator cuff repair. In a study of 11 patients with an isolated greater tuberosity malunion, two patients with superior displacement of 1 to 1.5 cm had a satisfactory result after management with arthroscopic acromioplasty alone.[21] The remaining nine patients had more than 1.5 cm of displacement and were treated with isolated osteotomy, rotator cuff repair, and capsular release to within 5 mm of anatomic restoration. The surgical repairs primarily used suture fixation. The authors of a 2014 study reported on a modified osteotomy of the greater tuberosity for symptomatic malunions with osteotomizing the fragment including the fracture bed and pushing the distal end of the osteomized fragment into the medullary cavity.[31] The authors reported on 10 patients who had an average final Constant score of 94 at an average of 42 months postoperative.

Several reports have described the arthroscopic management of isolated superiorly displaced greater tuberosity fractures using rotator cuff takedown, tuberoplasty, and repair. Four patients with isolated greater tuberosity malunion were treated with capsular release, lysis of subacromial adhesions, and subacromial decompression and rotator cuff takedown with tuberoplasty and rotator cuff repair.[25] The result was an average 52-point improvement in mean score on the American Shoulder and Elbow Surgeons Disability Index and a 4.5 point reduction in the visual analog scale pain score. Eight patients were treated in a similar fashion for a 5- to 10-mm posterosuperior displacement of the greater tuberosity; seven of the patients had a good or excellent result and returned to their previous occupation without restrictions.[26] Arthroscopic tuberoplasty and rotator cuff repair were recommended for symptomatic malunited greater tuberosity fractures with more than 5 mm of displacement.[32] A delay of at least 6 months after fracture was recommended to allow complete maturation of the malunion before tuberoplasty and rotator cuff repair.

Greater tuberosity malunion with significant (more than 1 cm) posterior displacement often requires open osteotomy, capsular and rotator cuff interval release, and fixation with suture or screws if the fragments are large enough. Preoperative CT with three-dimensional reconstruction is useful for planning the osteotomy. A deltopectoral approach is routinely used, but a second posterior approach may be required for mobilizing and detaching the fragment. A symptomatic malunion with 5 to 10 mm of superior displacement should be considered for arthroscopic acromioplasty, with or without tuberoplasty and rotator cuff reattachment.

Surgical Neck Malunion

Isolated surgical neck malunion is relatively uncommon, and limited data are available on the treatment indications and surgical options. Deformity typically results from acceptance of an imperfect open or closed reduction or from a loss of reduction during nonsurgical management. A neck-shaft angle of less than 120° is sufficient to reduce active shoulder range of motion and increase pain.[33] The author of 1970 study considered angulation of more than 45° to be an indication for surgical repair, which would result in a neck-shaft angle of approximately 90° to 100°.[20] All reported neck-shaft angles were less than 110°, and most were 90° to 105°; these reports can be used as a guide for the amount of proximal humeral varus necessary before corrective osteotomy is considered.[23,27,29]

Most surgeons recommend a simple lateral closing-wedge valgus osteotomy to restore a normal neck-shaft angle of 130° to 140°.[23,27,29] Although flexion and rotational deformity are common, restoration of valgus is of primary importance. The instrumentation options include a blade plate, T-plate, or a locking proximal humeral plate, but the locking plate appears to be the current instrument of choice (**Figure 3**). Preoperative templating using both radiography and CT is critical for exactly measuring the appropriate wedge size. Capsular release should be considered to restore passive motion before osteotomy. The osteotomized closing wedge can be used as bone graft. The osteotomy should be performed in the metaphyseal region at the location of greatest deformity.[23,27] Improvement of the neck-shaft angle by 20° has resulted after osteotomy, with a corresponding increase of 90° of forward flexion.[23] A more modest average improvement in elevation of 56° also has been reported.[29] Consequently, valgus closing-wedge osteotomy is a reasonable management option for improving pain, range of motion, and function in patients with an isolated surgical neck nonunion of the proximal humerus and a neck-shaft angle of less than approximately 110°.

Surgical Neck Nonunion

Surgical neck nonunions after a proximal humerus fracture are relatively uncommon but can cause significant disability and can be extremely challenging to treat. Surgical neck nonunion was found to occur in 1.1% of all proximal humeral fractures.[34] Successful surgical management dramatically improves function from that of a flail shoulder to that of a competent upper extremity.[35] The management options for surgical neck nonunions can be broadly categorized as open reduction and fixation (typically with associated bone grafting) or arthroplasty (anatomic and reverse).

Surgical neck nonunion can be classified as hypertrophic, in which the bone ends are viable with abundant callus formation, or atrophic, in which the bone ends have limited biologic viability. The predisposing factors include displacement, comminution, soft-tissue interposition of the biceps, systemic disease, osteopenia, or aggressive early rehabilitation.[34-36] Metaphyseal comminution or translation of more than one-third of the surgical neck increases the prevalence to 8% or 10%, respectively.[34] In the Boileau classification, proximal humeral nonunion is a type III sequela.[22] Based on this classification, unconstrained arthroplasty for surgical neck nonunion is likely to have a poor result because the greater tuberosity often needs to be osteotomized. Open reduction and internal fixation is recommended if the head remains viable, and reverse arthroplasty is recommended if the head is compromised in low demand patients older than 70 years. Surgical neck nonunion with a nonviable humeral head is difficult to manage in relatively young patients; unconstrained arthroplasty with a greater tuberosity osteotomy typically is the only available option, with an expectation of poor function.[22] Better results, specifically in forward elevation, have been shown when surgical neck nonunion was treated with unconstrained arthroplasty using calcar grafting and avoiding a greater tuberosity osteotomy.[37]

The management of a surgical neck nonunion depends on factors including patient age, bone quality, humeral head bone viability, glenohumeral arthritis, and status of the rotator cuff. In general, the three primary treatment

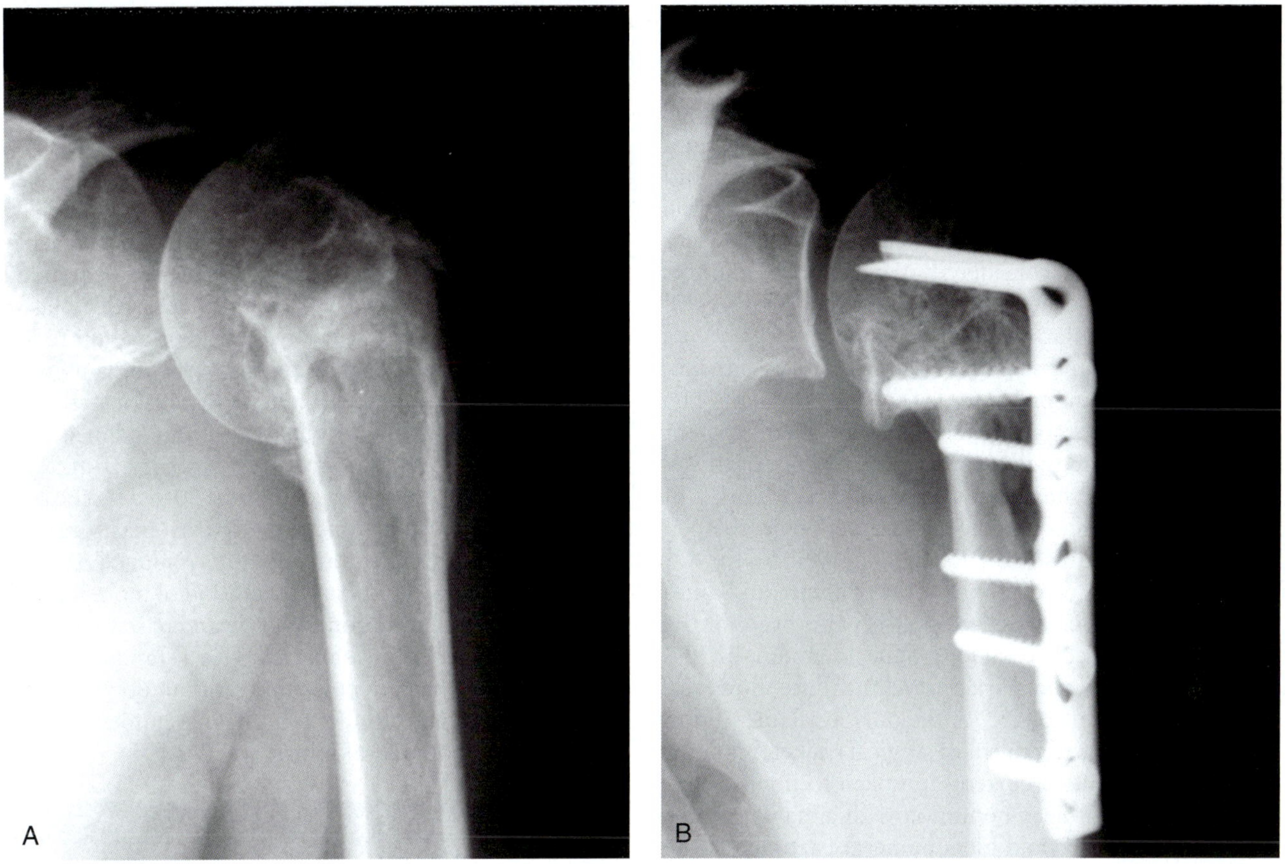

FIGURE 3 AP radiographs of the shoulder showing a surgical neck varus malunion before (**A**) and after (**B**) a valgus closing-wedge osteotomy using a proximal humeral blade plate for internal fixation. (Courtesy of Andrew Green, MD, Providence, RI.)

options for a surgical neck nonunion are open reduction and internal fixation with bone grafting, anatomic shoulder arthroplasty (total shoulder arthroplasty or humeral head replacement), or reverse total shoulder arthroplasty.

Open reduction and internal fixation with a plate is a reliable option in treating patients with a surgical neck nonunion who have sufficient humeral head bone stock and do not have arthritis. Of 13 patients, 12 healed after open reduction and internal fixation using a T-plate and rotator cuff tension banding with autogenous bone grafting.[36] Nine of the patients reported a good result, with no pain and a return to prefracture function, and four patients reported a fair result, with mild to moderate pain and without a return to prefracture work or function. In 25 patients who underwent blade plate fixation and autogenous bone grafting for a proximal humeral nonunion, the nonunion healed in 23 (92%), and 20 (80%) had a good or excellent outcome.[38] In 2009, 18 patients with a symptomatic proximal humeral nonunion were treated with open reduction and internal fixation using a proximal humeral locking plate augmented with an intramedullary cortical allograft.[39] Union was achieved in 17 patients (94%) at an average 5.4-month follow-up, and active forward elevation was an average 115°. Demineralized bone matrix and morcellized allograft cancellous bone were used as an adjunct in four patients. Suture fixation of the tuberosities with attachment to the plate was used to augment fixation. Finally, nine patients with a surgical neck nonunion were treated with open reduction and internal fixation without bone grafting and at final follow-up all fractures were confirmed healed based upon postoperative computer tomography scan.[40]

Several options exist to enhance bone healing in a repair of surgical neck nonunion, including bone grafting (autograft or structural allograft), extracorporeal shock wave therapy, pulsed electromagnetic field therapy, low-intensity pulsed ultrasonography, and bone morphogenetic proteins (BMPs). Autograft is the benchmark for grafting as it has osteoconductive, osteoinductive, and osteogenic properties. Autograft should be considered in the management of all surgical neck nonunions. Structural intramedullary cortical allograft is efficacious for augmenting the repair construct, and its use also should be considered.[39] Some evidence suggests a positive role for low-intensity pulsed ultrasonography, pulsed electromagnetic field therapy, and extracorporeal shock wave therapy in treating long bone nonunions; there are no data specifically on the use of these therapies after the management of proximal humeral nonunions. The data in favor of low-intensity pulsed ultrasonography and extracorporeal shock wave therapy are stronger than the data for pulsed electromagnetic field therapy.[41-43] These therapies should be considered as reasonable adjuncts to management because of their low risk profile and potential for stimulating healing.

BMP-7 was found safe and effective for the management of tibial nonunion in a type I collagen carrier.[44] The clinical and radiographic results of BMP-7 management were comparable to those of autograft, without graft site morbidity. BMP-2 has been shown to lower the risk of nonunion and infection in the management of fresh open tibial shaft fractures.[45] BMP-2 is approved by the US FDA only for use in acute open tibial fracture and anterior lumbar interbody fusion; BMP-7 is approved for the management of recalcitrant long-bone nonunion. BMP-7 has been taken off the market for clinical use, however, and off-label use of BMP-2 is the only available option for augmenting the treatment of surgical neck nonunions.

The recommended current approach to internal fixation of a surgical neck nonunion with a viable rotator cuff, humeral head, and glenohumeral cartilage is the use of a locking proximal humeral plate with autograft or allograft. A preoperative infection workup, including the erythrocyte sedimentation rate and C-reactive protein level, should be done if the nonunion resulted from earlier unsuccessful internal fixation. A deltopectoral approach is typical and can be extended distally into an anterolateral approach for greater exposure of the humeral shaft. A complete nonunion takedown with intramedullary reaming distally and proximally into the humeral head should be performed until bleeding bone is achieved. Tissue cultures and pathology specimens looking for signs of acute inflammation should be sent if the nonunion resulted from earlier unsuccessful internal fixation, and all hardware and other foreign material should be removed. Intramedullary cortical fibula allograft frequently is shaped to fit the intramedullary canal[39] (**Figure 4**). A proximal humeral locking plate often is used with an articulated tensioning device to aid in compression across the nonunion site. Suture augmentation through the rotator cuff and locking plate routinely is used. Autogenous bone graft is packed around the nonunion site, often with the addition of BMP-2 (used in an off-label manner). Low-intensity pulsed ultrasonography is used after surgery with a protective physical therapy regimen.

The initial choice of surgical management for a surgical neck nonunion should be based on the patient's age as well as shoulder-related factors. Open reduction and internal fixation with bone grafting should be considered if the patient is younger than 70 years and has an intact rotator cuff, a viable humeral head, and no arthritis. Reverse total shoulder arthroplasty should be considered if the patient is older than 70 years. If the patient is over 70 with a surgical neck nonunion and either a deficient rotator cuff or a nonviable humeral head then reverse total shoulder arthroplasty should be the surgical management of choice. Reverse total shoulder arthroplasty also can be considered if the patient is of age 60 to 70 years and has relatively low physical demands as well as a deficient rotator cuff or a nonviable or arthritic humeral head. Hemiarthroplasty, with avoidance of a greater tuberosity osteotomy and calcar grafting, can be considered for a patient aged 60 to 70 years who has higher demands. An unconstrained arthroplasty can be performed, with calcar grafting and avoidance of a tuberosity osteotomy, with an expectation of more limited goals including a limitation of active and passive motion and decreased function compared with a standard hemiarthroplasty, if the patient is younger than 60 years and has a deficient rotator cuff, a nonviable humeral head, or arthritic glenohumeral joint.

Glenohumeral Arthritis

Posttraumatic glenohumeral arthritis can be a difficult to treat, especially in relatively young patients for whom arthroplasty is not desirable. The nonarthroplasty surgical options include arthroscopic débridement with or without capsular release as well as arthroscopic biologic glenoid resurfacing. Several factors are used in making a decision, including patient age, work demands, the presence of limited motion or neurologic defects, the amount of joint space loss, the concentricity of wear, the presence of bipolar (humeral head and glenoid) disease, and the size and grade of osteochondral lesions. Each of these factors can affect the outcome of an arthroscopic procedure and should be considered in choosing a prosthetic or nonprosthetic surgical management of posttraumatic glenohumeral arthritis.

The history of a patient with posttraumatic arthritis should include earlier surgical management, patient age and activity level, hand dominance, severity of symptoms, mechanical symptoms, and future demands on the shoulder (such as physical labor or sports). The physical examination should specifically include an evaluation of range of motion loss, which is likely to influence the choice of surgical management and its outcome. A comprehensive neurologic examination should be performed, including the axillary nerve and the rotator cuff. The radiographic evaluation should include AP, true AP, scapular lateral,

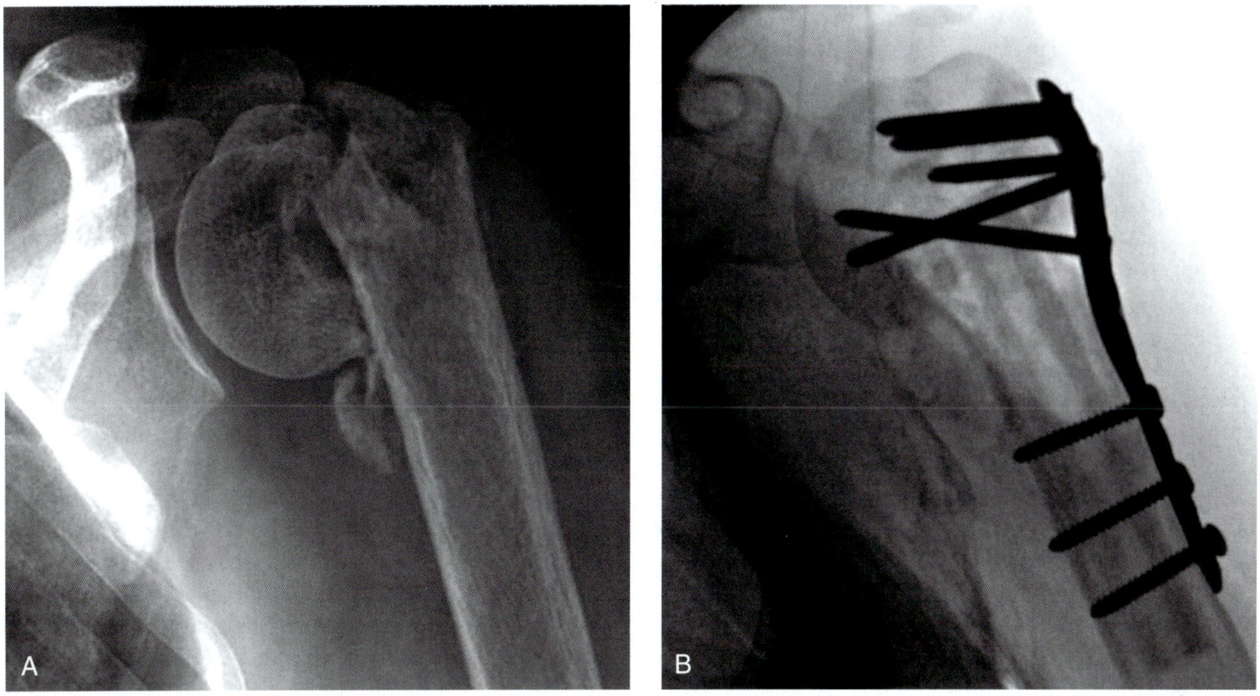

FIGURE 4 True AP radiographs of the shoulder showing a surgical neck nonunion with a viable humeral head and no arthritic changes before (**A**) and after (**B**) internal fixation using a locking proximal humeral plate augmented with intramedullary fibula and iliac crest allograft.

and axillary lateral plain radiographs. True AP radiographs should be used to evaluate joint space narrowing as well as the extent of any malunited fragments. The axillary radiograph should be used to evaluate the glenoid morphology and to detect an asymmetric wear pattern such as posterior subluxation or a posteriorly eroded glenoid. MRI can be useful for determining the status of the rotator cuff as long as no metallic fixation devices have been implanted. Otherwise, ultrasonography or CT angiography can be used. Both MRI and CT can be useful for further classifying glenoid morphology.

The early stages of posttraumatic osteoarthritis often can be treated nonsurgically with activity modification, NSAIDs, physical therapy, and corticosteroid injections. The American Academy of Orthopaedic Surgeons (AAOS) evaluated these treatment methods and concluded that current literature neither supports nor refutes their usefulness.[46] Consequently, it is reasonable to use these methods. Because evidence is lacking to support the efficacy of corticosteroid injections, it is recommended that injections into a single joint be limited to three unless there are special circumstances.[47] The AAOS also determined that viscosupplementation can be considered for patients with glenohumeral osteoarthritis.[46] Patients with glenohumeral osteoarthritis who were treated with hylan G-F 20 (Synvisc; Genzyme) reported improvements in pain relief, range of motion, and quality of life lasting up to 6 months after three weekly injections.[48] Patients with glenohumeral osteoarthritis who were treated with three to five nonguided intra-articular sodium hyaluronate injections had statistically significant more pain relief than with those treated with a placebo. Despite the statistical significance of the improvement (7.8-mm on a 100-mm visual analog scale), the clinical importance of the difference of such a small improvement is questionable.[49]

If nonsurgical management is unsuccessful, a patient with glenohumeral arthritis can be treated with arthroscopic débridement with or without capsular release, arthroscopic biologic glenoid resurfacing, or arthroplasty. The AAOS did not make a recommendation for or against arthroscopic treatment or biologic interposition in patients with glenohumeral osteoarthritis because of a lack of high-level evidence.[46]

Twenty-five patients with early glenohumeral arthritis underwent arthroscopic chondral and labral débridement with loose body removal, synovectomy, lavage, and subacromial bursectomy.[50] At 3-year follow-up, 80% had a good or excellent result. The researchers recommended arthroscopy only if some joint space was visible and the arthritis was concentric. Another study reported that 88% of patients reported pain relief at a minimum 2-year follow-up after arthroscopic débridement of grade IV osteochondral lesions.[51] If shoulder motion was within 15° of the opposite side, a capsular release was not performed. If decreased range of motion was found on examination (>15° loss of motion in elevation or external rotation as compared with the opposite side) then a capsular release was performed as well as the débridement. The average improvement in forward elevation and external rotation range of motion was 23° and 38°, respectively, in the patients who also received capsular release. The researchers recommended avoiding the procedure if the lesion was larger than 2 cm^2 because large size appeared to be associated with a return of pain and treatment failure. Another study reported similar increases in forward elevation and external rotation (of 21° and 17°, respectively) after capsular release.[52] The reduction in joint contact pressures after the release was believed to be the primary mechanism of pain relief. Reasonable results also were reported in a study of 36 patients, with significantly better results if the patient's Outerbridge changes were lower than grade 4.[53] Conversely, an evaluation of the extent of cartilage lesions found that monopolar Outerbridge grade 4 lesions did just as well as lower grade lesions.[54] Bipolar lesions had significantly worse outcomes than monopolar lesions. Similarly, the risk of failure after arthroscopic débridement was significant if the patient had bipolar grade 4 lesions; 87% of patient with bipolar grade 4 disease later required arthroplasty.[55] Other risk factors for failure included a joint space of less than 2 mm and large osteophytes (Samilson-Prieto grade 2; 3 to 7 mm on the humerus or glenoid). Skelley et al reported less impressive results after arthroscopic débridement reporting patients returning to preoperative pain levels at an average of 3.8 months following the procedure with 61% of patients stating they were unsatisfied with the surgery and 42% undergoing total shoulder arthroplasty at an average of 8.8 months after arthroscopy.[56] The reason for the poorer results compared with prior published reports is the more severe disease treated in this series with 24% of patients with bipolar grade III or IV lesions of the cartilage, 39% having grade 3 Samilson-Prieto scoring of their preoperative radiographs, 42% having posterior subluxation on preoperatively on radiographs with 27% having a noncentric glenoid erosion pattern. The authors of a 2015 study performed a systematic review including 32 studies of young patients with glenohumeral arthritis and concluded that arthroscopic débridement is efficacious and a safe alternative in the short term for young patients with arthritis with concerns about arthroplasty.[57] Arthroscopic débridement provided a lower risk of complication compared with arthroplasty with similar revision rates (18% to 20%) to arthroplasty over the same follow-up time frame.

A modification of the arthroscopic débridement procedure labelled the comprehensive arthroscopic management (CAM) procedure has been described by the authors of a 2013 study including arthroscopic chondroplasty, removal of loose bodies, humeral osteophyte resection, capsular release, axillary nerve neurolysis, subacromial decompression, and biceps tenodesis.[58] The authors originally reported on 30 shoulders after a mean of 2.6 years after the CAM procedure and reported 20% went on to arthroplasty at an average of 1.9 years after the procedure. Of the remaining patients, the final average American Shoulder and Elbow Surgeons (ASES) score was 83. Patients with <2 mm of joint space were more likely to progress to arthroplasty. Large humeral osteophytes preoperatively were associated with greater improvements in range of motion but worse satisfaction. The same group followed up on this report evaluating 49 shoulders at minimum of 5 years.[59] 26% of shoulders progressed to shoulder arthroplasty at a mean of 2.6 years with 76.9% survivorship at 5 years. Of the surviving shoulders, the average ASES score was 85 and the Single Assessment Numeric Evaluation was 82. The same group then evaluated a group of 107 shoulders at a minimum of 2 years after arthroscopic CAM procedure evaluating radiographic features associated with early failure with conversion to shoulder arthroplasty.[60] Patients with preoperative Kellgren-Lawrence grade 4, joint space narrowing under 2 mm, Walch type B2 or C glenoids, and older than 50 years were associated with failure and requirement for arthroplasty.

Based on the published studies, it is reasonable to consider arthroscopic débridement, without or without humeral osteophyte removal and axillary nerve neurolysis, for younger patients with concentric glenohumeral arthritis, at least 2 mm of preserved joint space, and relatively small unipolar lesions, up to and including grade 4 lesions with small humeral osteophytes. Capsular release may be added to reliably improve elevation and external rotation in a patient with stiffness and arthritis. Débridement is likely to have an inferior result, and later arthroplasty is more likely to be required, if the patient has nonconcentric wear (Walch B2 or C glenoids), higher grades of radiographic arthritis (Kellgren-Lawrence grade 4 or Samilson-Prieto grade 3 disease), less than 2 mm of preserved joint space, large (3- to 7-mm) osteophytes on the humerus or glenoid, and bipolar grade 4 lesions. Arthroscopic débridement alone should be avoided for such a patient.

Arthroscopic glenoid resurfacing was described as an option for patients who have severe disease and for whom arthroscopic débridement alone is unsuitable. During the procedure, arthroscopic débridement is followed by suturing of an interposition graft to the face of the

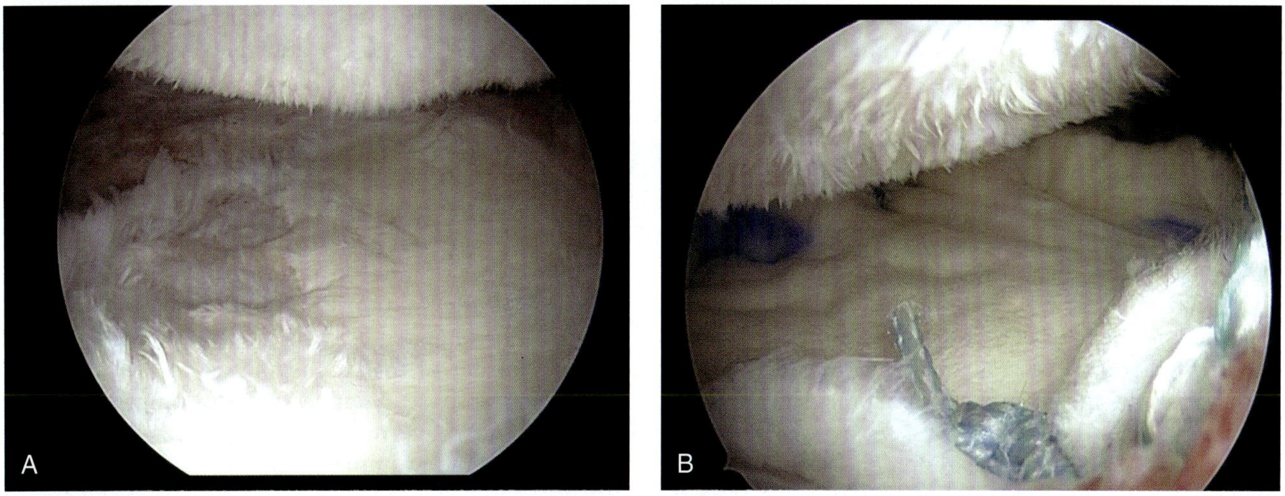

FIGURE 5 Arthroscopic images showing bipolar grade 3 humeral and grade 4 glenoid osteochondral lesions before (**A**) and after (**B**) humeral débridement with arthroscopic biologic glenoid resurfacing. (Courtesy of Robert T. Burks, MD, Salt Lake City, UT.)

glenoid (**Figure 5**). Thirty-two patients who underwent arthroscopic débridement and biologic glenoid resurfacing with an acellular dermal matrix had significant improvement in pain and functional outcomes, with a 72% success rate an average 3-year follow-up.[61] Ninety-four percent of these patients had a concentric wear pattern; 59% had moderate osteophytes and joint space narrowing; and 41% had large osteophytes, marked joint space narrowing, and severe sclerosis. Hand dominance in the affected extremity and systemic diseases such as diabetes, rheumatoid arthritis, or osteoarthritis were correlated with a poorer outcome, but radiographic grading was not. A study of 20 patients after arthroscopic glenoid resurfacing with a porcine small intestine submucosa patch found a 75% success rate at 3- to 6-year follow-up.[62] All patients had grade 4 bipolar lesions, and 25% had posterior subluxation on initial radiographs. Twenty-five percent required arthroplasty 1 to 5 years after the resurfacing. The data from these studies suggest that arthroscopic débridement with glenoid biologic resurfacing may be an alternative for a young patient who has bipolar grade 4 osteochondral changes with severe narrowing of a concentrically worn glenohumeral joint. It must be understood, however, that approximately 25% are likely to require arthroplasty within 3 to 5 years of the procedure. In 2017, 43 shoulders were evaluated at an average of 60 months follow-up after arthroscopic glenoid resurfacing using human acellular dermal matrix allograft.[63] Visual analog pain scores improved from 7 to 2 with improvements of median ASES scores from 47 to 76; 23% of patients required conversion to arthroplasty after a mean of 45 months. Increased age and lower preoperative ASES scores were risk factors for failure of arthroscopic glenoid resurfacing.

Posttraumatic Stiffness Without Arthritis

Loss of range of motion is common after treatment of a proximal humeral fracture and occurs in approximately 3% of surgically treated proximal humeral fractures.[64,65] The rangeof motion deficit typically is mild. At an average 3.5-year follow-up after minimally displaced proximal humeral fracture, forward elevation and external rotation averaged 89% and 87%, respectively, of that of the opposite shoulder.[66] This finding suggests mild permanent motion limitations. Such limitations are common after internal fixation of proximal humeral fractures. An average elevation of 156° and external rotation of 46° were reported after open reduction and internal fixation of proximal humerus fractures with a locking proximal humeral plate.[67]

Despite the acceptable results of both nonsurgical and surgical management, a small percentage of patients later have pathologic stiffness or adhesive capsulitis. Adhesive capsulitis can result from an extra-articular or intra-articular etiology. The intra-articular etiologies of stiffness include capsular contracture, arthritis, osteonecrosis, and articular malunion. The extra-articular etiologies include subacromial adhesions, hardware impingement, and tuberosity or surgical neck malunion. Appropriate management of posttraumatic adhesive capsulitis requires an understanding of the sources of stiffness.

A careful history for a patient with a nonsurgically treated fracture should include the duration of immobilization. Although the topic is controversial, some evidence suggests that immediate mobilization for a minimally displaced proximal humerus fracture treated nonsurgically leads to faster functional recovery, better short-term pain-relief and range of motion, and better long-term final function and range of motion compared with an initial 2- to 3-week period of sling immobilization.[66,68,69] A patient with stiffness should receive a thorough physical examination to evaluate earlier open surgical incisions and a neurologic examination to specifically evaluate the axillary and suprascapular nerves. The status of the rotator cuff and the passive and active range of motion should be documented. Patients typically report restricted motion and pain at the end range of motion. Concomitant impingement-related symptoms are not uncommon with postfracture stiffness, especially in patients treated with open reduction and internal fixation using a locking proximal humeral plate.

The shoulder radiographs should include AP, scapula plane AP, axillary, and scapular lateral views. The radiographs should be used to evaluate the presence and location of hardware from earlier surgical fixation, malunion of the tuberosities or surgical neck, or any articular cartilage injury resulting from arthritis or osteonecrosis. MRI can be obtained if there is concern about a concomitant rotator cuff injury or early osteonecrosis, especially if the patient has mechanical symptoms or pain with resisted rotator cuff testing. CT is helpful only if there is concern that malunion may be a source of pain or limited motion. CT arthrography may be beneficial for evaluating rotator cuff integrity if hardware is present from earlier internal fixation.

A management plan for a stiff postfracture shoulder should take into account all intra-articular or extra-articular etiologies. Nonsurgical management usually should be considered before surgical intervention. Physical therapy should focus on global passive and active-assisted stretching. NSAIDs can reduce intra-articular inflammation, thereby limiting pain and improving motion. Intra-articular steroid injections can be used to limit inflammation and provide early pain relief. Intra-articular sodium hyaluronate injection is not recommended for treating isolated adhesive capsulitis because it has no apparent benefit compared with placebo.[49]

Nonsurgical management should extend over a minimum of 2 to 3 months. At least 4 to 6 months should elapse after the fracture before surgical management is considered. Arthroplasty should be considered if significant osteonecrosis or arthritis is present. Corrective osteotomy should be considered, in conjunction with capsular release, if there is a tuberosity or surgical neck malunion without articular injury. Manipulation under anesthesia has been described as a possible treatment option for posttraumatic stiffness with no differences in outcomes between a control group with primary frozen shoulder although 17% required repeat surgery for persistent stiffness.[70] Surgical release of the capsular contracture can be considered if the fracture has healed with reasonable alignment and there is no significant articular cartilage injury.

Arthroscopic surgical release of a stiff posttraumatic shoulder has proved to be a reliable surgical solution leading to improvement in pain, function, and range of motion.[71-73] The first step in an arthroscopic release is diagnostic glenohumeral arthroscopy. The arthroscope initially is in a standard posterior portal; an anterior rotator cuff interval portal initially is developed as the working portal. The release is initiated by defining the anterior border of the supraspinatus and the superior margin of the subscapularis. An arthroscopic tissue ablator is used to remove all scarred rotator cuff interval tissue in the window until the underlying coracoacromial ligament can be identified to mark the superficial extent of the release. Care should be taken to avoid involving the bicipital sling and laterally destabilizing the biceps. Next, the interval between the subscapularis and middle glenohumeral ligament is bluntly developed using a blunt instrument. The middle and inferior glenohumeral ligaments and capsule are released just adjacent to the labrum. Caution should be used inferiorly as the dissection approaches the axillary nerve; proximity can be gauged by using electrocautery if the patient is not paralyzed. Visualization of the underlying subscapularis muscle indicates a complete release. The release should be continued inferior to the 6-o'clock position. The arthroscope should be placed anteriorly, and release of the posteroinferior capsule is continued with the cautery in the posterior portal (**Figure 6**). Subacromial débridement should be performed with removal of subacromial adhesions. Any screws used for internal fixation can be removed arthroscopically (**Figure 7**). If plate fixation was used at least 12 months earlier and the fracture has healed, a deltopectoral incision can be made to remove the plate after completion of the arthroscopic release and débridement. Manipulation under anesthesia may have a role in the management of idiopathic adhesive capsulitis, but it is not recommended for the management of posttraumatic adhesive capsulitis because most patients have both an intra-articular and extra-articular mechanisms of stiffness.

Physical therapy is initiated immediately after surgery, with a focus on passive and active-assisted stretching. Interscalene blocks using catheters typically provide pain relief for 24 to 48 hours and allow immediate physical therapy. In 200 consecutive patients, the use of an indwelling catheter placed under ultrasonography guidance had a reported 99% success rate and a 1% rate of transient neurologic deficit, with no permanent deficits.[74] Alternatively, NSAIDs, narcotics, and pregabalin can be prescribed for pain modulation. Continuous passive

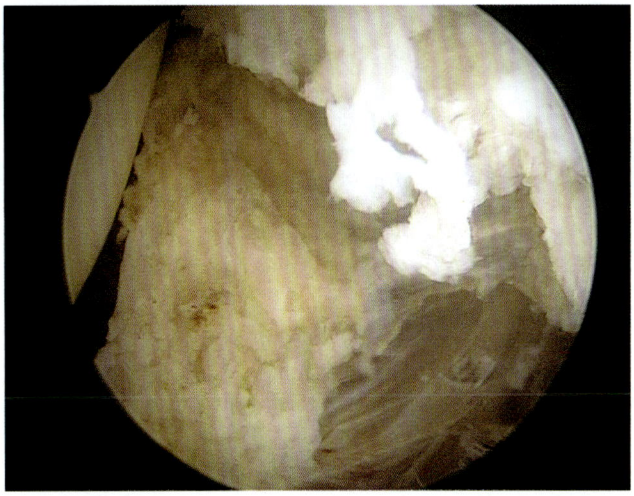

FIGURE 6 Arthroscopic image showing release of the posteroinferior glenohumeral ligament and capsule. The humeral head can be seen on the left. The glenoid is seen on the right (approximately the 6:30 position).

motion can be used as an adjunct to postoperative physical therapy, especially if the patient has limited social support for assistance with therapy.

Several studies have examined the results of arthroscopic capsular release for posttraumatic stiffness. A review of 21 patients with posttraumatic stiffness included 14 patients with stiffness after proximal humeral fracture.[72] The patients were treated with arthroscopic circumferential capsular and subacromial release of adhesions under interscalene block, with immediate physical therapy. At a mean 33-month follow-up (minimum follow-up, 12 months), 95% of patients were satisfied with the final result. The authors reported that at 6 months after surgery the patients had lost 48% of their gained motion although when evaluated at final follow-up the patients were able to recover 110% of their immediate postoperative motion. Fifty patients underwent arthroscopic capsular release for adhesive capsulitis classified as postsurgical (33 patients), postfracture (two patients with glenoid fracture, two with proximal humeral fracture, and two with proximal humeral fracture-dislocation), or idiopathic (11 patients).[71] At an average 20-month follow-up after surgery, all patients had a similar gain in range of motion; the patients with postfracture stiffness gained 39° of elevation and 38° of external rotation. Patients with postsurgical stiffness had worse pain, satisfaction, and functional activity scores than those with postfracture or idiopathic stiffness. Stiffness in 68 shoulders was categorized as idiopathic, posttraumatic, postsurgical, diabetic, or impingement. After arthroscopic release, the differences in pain, motion, and function were limited, except that patients with diabetes had significantly worse outcomes than patients in the other groups.[73] Fifty-eight patients were evaluated at an average of 23 months after arthroscopic glenohumeral arthrolysis and either open plate removal or arthroscopic nail removal for posttraumatic stiffness after fixation of a proximal humerus fracture.[75] Constant scores improved to an average of 68 with gains in forward flexion (37.6°), abduction (39.5°), and external rotation (24.3°) motion after release. In general, arthroscopic release of a posttraumatic frozen shoulder provides predictable pain relief and motion improvement (approximately 40° of elevation and 40° of external rotation) comparable to that for an idiopathic frozen shoulder. After surgery, the final improvements take more than 1 year to achieve.

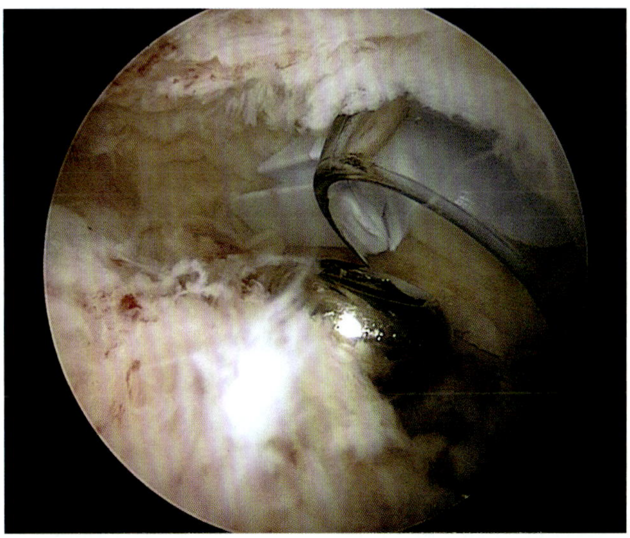

FIGURE 7 Arthroscopic image showing subacromial bursectomy and hardware removal after glenohumeral arthroscopic capsular release.

SUMMARY

A variety of complications can result from the surgical or nonsurgical management of proximal humerus fracture. Osteonecrosis typically can be treated nonsurgically, with good results in stage I or II and a limited risk of progression, but stage III or IV disease typically requires surgical management. Arthroscopic débridement and core decompression are reasonable alternatives for persistently symptomatic stage I, II, or III disease, with the most promising results in stage I or II lesions. Proximal humeral malunion is uncommon. Persistently symptomatic surgical neck malunion with a neck-shaft angle of less than 110° can be treated with surgical neck osteotomy. Greater tuberosity malunion can be treated with osteotomy (usually for posterior displacement) or tuberoplasty with rotator cuff repair (for superior displacement). In a patient younger than 70 years, surgical neck nonunion with a viable humeral head and no arthritis can be treated with open reduction and internal fixation with intramedullary strut graft and a locking proximal humeral plate. Mild to moderate posttraumatic glenohumeral arthritis in a shoulder with concentric wear, some preserved joint space, and minimal, primarily unipolar osteophytes can be effectively treated with arthroscopic débridement and capsular release. Arthroscopic release is an excellent option for restoring motion and function in a patient who has posttraumatic adhesive capsulitis with minimal residual bony deformity or arthritic changes. Restoration of function is similar to that of patients with idiopathic adhesive capsulitis.

KEY STUDY POINTS

- Osteonecrosis of the proximal humerus should be treated based upon symptom levels and stage. Arthroscopic débridement and core decompression is indicated for symptomatic stage I or II lesions resistant to nonsurgical management and a stage III lesion with limited collapse. A severe stage III lesion or a stage IV or V lesions should be treated with partial or complete shoulder replacement.
- Greater tuberosity malunion indicated for treatment includes a malunion of more than 5 mm of superior displacement or 1 cm of posterior displacement with pain, loss of motion, and impingement. For symptomatic malunions between 5 mm and 1 cm of displacement, arthroscopic tuberoplasty and rotator cuff repair is indicated while those with greater than 1 cm of displacement require greater tuberosity osteotomy.
- Arthroscopic débridement for glenohumeral osteoarthritis is most effective in patients with relatively preserved range of motion, the presence of 2 mm of joint space and a symmetrically aligned (nonsubluxated) glenohumeral joint relationship.
- Arthroscopic release of a posttraumatic stiff shoulder without arthritis is indicated for patients failing 6 months of therapy with relatively preserved glenohumeral architecture. Arthroscopic release provides predictable pain relief and motion improvement (approximately 40° of elevation and 40° of external rotation) comparable to that for an idiopathic frozen shoulder. After surgery, the final improvements take more than 1 year to achieve.

Annotated References

1. Iyengar JJ, Devcic Z, Sproul RC, Feeley BT: Nonoperative treatment of proximal humerus fractures: A systematic review. *J Orthop Trauma* 2011;25(10):612-617.
2. Harreld KL, Marker DR, Wiesler ER, Shafiq B, Mont MA: Osteonecrosis of the humeral head. *J Am Acad Orthop Surg* 2009;17(6):345-355.
3. Gerber C, Werner CM, Vienne P: Internal fixation of complex fractures of the proximal humerus. *J Bone Joint Surg Br* 2004;86(6):848-855.
4. Thanasas C, Kontakis G, Angoules A, Limb D, Giannoudis P: Treatment of proximal humerus fractures with locking plates: A systematic review. *J Shoulder Elbow Surg* 2009;18(6):837-844.
5. Yüksel HY, Yimaz S, Akşahin E, Celebi L, Muratli HH, Biçimoğlu A: The results of nonoperative treatment for three- and four-part fractures of the proximal humerus in low-demand patients. *J Orthop Trauma* 2011;25(10):588-595.
6. Belayneh R, Lott A, Haglin J, Knoda S, Zuckerman JD, Egol KA: Osteonecrosis after surgically repaired proximal humerus fractures is a predictor of poor outcomes. *J Orthop Trauma* 2018;32(10):e387-e393. doi:10.1097/BOT.0000000000001260.

   Prospective cohort study of 165 patients treated with open reduction internal fixation of a proximal humerus fracture. 4.8% of patients developed osteonecrosis. Patients who developed osteonecrosis had significantly worse forward elevation and Disabilities of Arm, Shoulder and Hand scores supporting that the development of osteonecrosis is a predictor of poorer outcome after open reduction internal fixation. Level of evidence: III.
7. Gerber C, Hersche O, Berberat C: The clinical relevance of posttraumatic avascular necrosis of the humeral head. *J Shoulder Elbow Surg* 1998;7(6):586-590.
8. Lee CK, Hansen HR: Post-traumatic avascular necrosis of the humeral head in displaced proximal humeral fractures. *J Trauma* 1981;21(9):788-791.
9. Boileau P, Chuinard C, Le Huec JC, Walch G, Trojani C: Proximal humerus fracture sequelae: Impact of a new radiographic classification on arthroplasty. *Clin Orthop Relat Res* 2006;442:121-130.
10. Chapman C, Mattern C, Levine WN: Arthroscopically assisted core decompression of the proximal humerus for avascular necrosis. *Arthroscopy* 2004;20(9):1003-1006.
11. Dines JS, Strauss EJ, Fealy S, Craig EV: Arthroscopic-assisted core decompression of the humeral head. *Arthroscopy* 2007;23(1):e1-e4.
12. Hardy P, Decrette E, Jeanrot C, Colom A, Lortat-Jacob A, Benoit J: Arthroscopic treatment of bilateral humeral head osteonecrosis. *Arthroscopy* 2000;16(3):332-335.
13. Mont MA, Maar DC, Urquhart MW, Lennox D, Hungerford DS: Avascular necrosis of the humeral head treated by core decompression: A retrospective review. *J Bone Joint Surg Br* 1993;75(5):785-788.

14. Cruess RL: Experience with steroid-induced avascular necrosis of the shoulder and etiologic considerations regarding osteonecrosis of the hip. *Clin Orthop Relat Res* 1978;130:86-93.

15. Sakai T, Sugano N, Nishii T, Hananouchi T, Yoshikawa H: Extent of osteonecrosis on MRI predicts humeral head collapse. *Clin Orthop Relat Res* 2008;466(5):1074-1080.

16. Hattrup SJ, Cofield RH: Osteonecrosis of the humeral head: Relationship of disease stage, extent, and cause to natural history. *J Shoulder Elbow Surg* 1999;8(6):559-564.

17. L'Insalata JC, Pagnani MJ, Warren RF, Dines DM: Humeral head osteonecrosis: Clinical course and radiographic predictors of outcome. *J Shoulder Elbow Surg* 1996;5(5):355-361.

18. Harreld KL, Marulanda GA, Ulrich SD, Marker DR, Seyler TM, Mont MA: Small-diameter percutaneous decompression for osteonecrosis of the shoulder. *Am J Orthop (Belle Mead NJ)* 2009;38(7):348-354.

19. LaPorte DM, Mont MA, Mohan V, Pierre-Jacques H, Jones LC, Hungerford DS: Osteonecrosis of the humeral head treated by core decompression. *Clin Orthop Relat Res* 1998;355:254-260.

20. Neer CS II: Displaced proximal humeral fractures: I. Classification and evaluation. *J Bone Joint Surg Am* 1970;52(6):1077-1089.

21. Beredjiklian PK, Iannotti JP, Norris TR, Williams GR: Operative treatment of malunion of a fracture of the proximal aspect of the humerus. *J Bone Joint Surg Am* 1998;80(10):1484-1497.

22. Boileau P, Trojani C, Walch G, Krishnan SG, Romeo A, Sinnerton R: Shoulder arthroplasty for the treatment of the sequelae of fractures of the proximal humerus. *J Shoulder Elbow Surg* 2001;10(4):299-308.

23. Benegas E, Zoppi Filho A, Ferreira Filho AA, et al: Surgical treatment of varus malunion of the proximal humerus with valgus osteotomy. *J Shoulder Elbow Surg* 2007;16(1):55-59.

24. Calvo E, Merino-Gutierrez I, Lagunes I: Arthroscopic tuberoplasty for subacromial impingement secondary to proximal humeral malunion. *Knee Surg Sports Traumatol Arthrosc* 2010;18(7):988-991.

25. Lädermann A, Denard PJ, Burkhart SS: Arthroscopic management of proximal humerus malunion with tuberoplasty and rotator cuff retensioning. *Arthroscopy* 2012;28(9):1220-1229.

26. Martinez AA, Calvo A, Domingo J, Cuenca J, Herrera A: Arthroscopic treatment for malunions of the proximal humeral greater tuberosity. *Int Orthop* 2010;34(8):1207-1211.

27. Gill TJ, Waters P: Valgus osteotomy of the humeral neck: A technique for the treatment of humerus varus. *J Shoulder Elbow Surg* 1997;6(3):306-310.

28. Porcellini G, Campi F, Paladini P: Articular impingement in malunited fracture of the humeral head. *Arthroscopy* 2002;18(8):E39.

29. Solonen KA, Vastamäki M: Osteotomy of the neck of the humerus for traumatic varus deformity. *Acta Orthop Scand* 1985;56(1):79-80.

30. Park TS, Choi IY, Kim YH, Park MR, Shon JH, Kim SI: A new suggestion for the treatment of minimally displaced fractures of the greater tuberosity of the proximal humerus. *Bull Hosp Jt Dis* 1997;56(3):171-176.

31. Ogawa K, Matsumura N, Yoshida A: Modified osteotomy for symptomatic malunion of the humeral greater tuberosity. *J Orthop Trauma* 2014;28(12):e290-e295. doi:10.1097/BOT.0000000000000093.

    A retrospective evaluation was performed of eight patients who underwent an osteotomy of the greater tuberosity for a malunion including various features into the surgical technique. At 2 years, the Constant scores ranged from 82% to 100% supporting the modified osteotomy in achieving boney union and improvement of clinical symptoms. Level of evidence: IV.

32. Kim KC, Rhee KJ, Shin HD: Arthroscopic treatment of symptomatic malunion of the greater tuberosity of the humerus using the suture-bridge technique. *Orthopedics* 2010;33(4):242-245.

33. Paavolainen P, Björkenheim JM, Slätis P, Paukku P: Operative treatment of severe proximal humeral fractures. *Acta Orthop Scand* 1983;54(3):374-379.

34. Court-Brown CM, McQueen MM: Nonunions of the proximal humerus: Their prevalence and functional outcome. *J Trauma* 2008;64(6):1517-1521.

35. Galatz LM, Iannotti JP: Management of surgical neck nonunions. *Orthop Clin North Am* 2000;31(1):51-61.

36. Healy WL, Jupiter JB, Kristiansen TK, White RR: Nonunion of the proximal humerus: A review of 25 cases. *J Orthop Trauma* 1990;4(4):424-431.

37. Lin JS, Klepps S, Miller S, Cleeman E, Flatow EL: Effectiveness of replacement arthroplasty with calcar grafting and avoidance of greater tuberosity osteotomy for the treatment of humeral surgical neck nonunions. *J Shoulder Elbow Surg* 2006;15(1):12-18.

38. Ring D, McKee MD, Perey BH, Jupiter JB: The use of a blade plate and autogenous cancellous bone graft in the treatment of ununited fractures of the proximal humerus. *J Shoulder Elbow Surg* 2001;10(6):501-507.

39. Badman BL, Mighell M, Kalandiak SP, Prasarn M: Proximal humeral nonunions treated with fixed-angle locked plating and an intramedullary strut allograft. *J Orthop Trauma* 2009;23(3):173-179.

40. Quadlbauer S, Hofmann GJ, Leixnering M, Rosenauer R, Hausner T, Reichetseder J: Open reduction and fixation with a locking plate without bone grafting is a reasonable and safe option for treating proximal humerus nonunion. *Int Orthop* 2018;42(9):2199-2209. doi:10.1007/s00264-018-3820-3.

Nine patients were treated using open reduction and locking plate stabilization without bone grafting and were retrospectively reviewed at an average of 31 months postoperative with outcome scores. CT scan of the shoulder was performed to analyze union of fracture. All patients showed fracture union on CT scan with significant improvements in range of motion in all planes except adduction. Three of nine patients required plate removal but otherwise there were no complications. Therefore, open reduction and locking plate fixation without bone grafting is a reasonable and safe option for treating proximal humerus nonunion. It leads to a high union rate, significant improvement in ROM, and in the majority of the cases to an "excellent" and "good" functional outcome without an increased risk of complications. Level of evidence: IV.

41. Goldstein C, Sprague S, Petrisor BA: Electrical stimulation for fracture healing: Current evidence. *J Orthop Trauma* 2010;24 suppl 1:S62-S75.

42. Watanabe Y, Matsushita T, Bhandari M, Zdero R, Schemitsch EH: Ultrasound for fracture healing: Current evidence. *J Orthop Trauma* 2010;24 suppl 1:S56-S61.

43. Zelle BA, Gollwitzer H, Zlowodzki M, Buhren V: Extracorporeal shock wave therapy: Current evidence. *J Orthop Trauma* 2010;24 suppl 1:S66-S70.

44. Friedlaender GE, Perry CR, Cole JD, et al: Osteogenic protein-1 (bone morphogenetic protein-7) in the treatment of tibial nonunions. *J Bone Joint Surg Am* 2001;83-A suppl 1(pt 2):S151-S158.

45. Govender S, Csimma C, Genant HK, et al, BMP-2 Evaluation in Surgery for Tibial Trauma (BESTT) Study Group: Recombinant human bone morphogenetic protein-2 for treatment of open tibial fractures: A prospective, controlled, randomized study of four hundred and fifty patients. *J Bone Joint Surg Am* 2002;84(12):2123-2134.

46. Izquierdo R, Voloshin I, Edwards S, et al: American Academy of Orthopedic Surgeons: Treatment of glenohumeral osteoarthritis. *J Am Acad Orthop Surg* 2010;18(6):375-382.

47. Denard PJ, Wirth MA, Orfaly RM: Management of glenohumeral arthritis in the young adult. *J Bone Joint Surg Am* 2011;93(9):885-892.

48. Silverstein E, Leger R, Shea KP: The use of intra-articular hylan G-F 20 in the treatment of symptomatic osteoarthritis of the shoulder: A preliminary study. *Am J Sports Med* 2007;35(6):979-985.

49. Blaine T, Moskowitz R, Udell J, et al: Treatment of persistent shoulder pain with sodium hyaluronate: A randomized, controlled trial. A multicenter study. *J Bone Joint Surg Am* 2008;90(5):970-979.

50. Weinstein DM, Bucchieri JS, Pollock RG, Flatow EL, Bigliani LU: Arthroscopic debridement of the shoulder for osteoarthritis. *Arthroscopy* 2000;16(5):471-476.

51. Cameron BD, Galatz LM, Ramsey ML, Williams GR, Iannotti JP: Non-prosthetic management of grade IV osteochondral lesions of the glenohumeral joint. *J Shoulder Elbow Surg* 2002;11(1):25-32.

52. Richards DP, Burkhart SS: Arthroscopic debridement and capsular release for glenohumeral osteoarthritis. *Arthroscopy* 2007;23(9):1019-1022.

53. Guyette TM, Bae H, Warren RF, Craig E, Wickiewicz TL: Results of arthroscopic subacromial decompression in patients with subacromial impingement and glenohumeral degenerative joint disease. *J Shoulder Elbow Surg* 2002;11(4):299-304.

54. Kerr BJ, McCarty EC: Outcome of arthroscopic débridement is worse for patients with glenohumeral arthritis of both sides of the joint. *Clin Orthop Relat Res* 2008;466(3):634-638.

55. Van Thiel GS, Sheehan S, Frank RM, et al: Retrospective analysis of arthroscopic management of glenohumeral degenerative disease. *Arthroscopy* 2010;26(11):1451-1455.

56. Skelley NW, Namdari S, Chamberlain AM, Keener JD, Galatz LM, Yamaguchi K: Arthroscopic debridement and capsular release for the treatment of shoulder osteoarthritis. *Arthroscopy* 2015;31(6):1156-1166.e8. doi:10.1016/j.arthro.2014.11.012.

A retrospective review of 33 patients who underwent arthroscopic debridement and capsular release for shoulder arthritis was performed at a minimum of 2 years postoperatively. Although there were initial improvements in pain, 60.6% of patients reported they were not satisfied with the procedure at final follow-up. Total shoulder arthroplasty was performed on 42.4% of patients at an average of 8.8 months after arthroscopy. The authors concluded that isolated debridement and capsular release in the setting of arthritis may not provide substantial benefit to most patients. Level of evidence: IV.

57. Sayegh ET, Mascarenhas R, Chalmers PN, Cole BJ, Romeo AA, Verma NN: Surgical treatment options for glenohumeral arthritis in young patients: A systematic review and meta-analysis. *Arthroscopy* 2015;31(6):1156-1166.e8. doi:10.1016/j.arthro.2014.11.012.

A systematic review was performed comparing the surgical treatment options for young patients with glenohumeral arthritis. Thirty-two studies were included in the analysis. Revision surgery was noted to be equally likely after hemiarthroplasty, total shoulder arthroplasty, and arthroscopic debridement. Complications were less common after arthroscopic debridement than after hemiarthroplasty and total shoulder arthroplasty. Arthroscopic debridement and total shoulder arthroplasty resulted in better elevation and external rotation than hemiarthroplasty. Arthroscopic debridement was determined to be a safe surgical alternative in the short term for arthritis in the young patient. Level of evidence: IV.

58. Millett PJ, Horan MP, Pennock AT, Rios D: Comprehensive arthroscopic management (CAM) procedure: Clinical results of a joint-preserving arthroscopic treatment for young, active patients with advanced shoulder osteoarthritis. *Arthroscopy* 2013;29(3):440-448. doi:10.1016/j.arthro.2012.10.028.

    Twenty-nine patients (30 shoulders) were retrospectively reviewed after CAM procedure for advanced glenohumeral arthritis. Six shoulders progressed to arthroplasty at a mean of 1.9 years with patients having less than 2 mm of glenohumeral joint space having an increased risk to undergo arthroplasty. Survivorship at 1 year was 92% and 85% at years. The CAM procedure provides reliable short-term pain relief and functional improvement in young patients with advanced arthritis. Level of evidence: IV.

59. Mitchell JJ, Horan MP, Greenspoon JA, Menge TJ, Tahal DS, Millett PJ: Survivorship and patient-reported outcomes after comprehensive arthroscopic management of glenohumeral osteoarthritis: Minimum 5-year follow-up. *Am J Sports Med* 2016;44(12):3206-3213.

    Forty-seven patients were evaluated after CAM procedure for glenohumeral humeral arthritis at a minimum of 5 years postoperative; 26% of patients progressed to shoulder arthroplasty at an average of 2.6 years. Survivorship was 96% at 1 year and 77% at 5 years. The CAM procedure provides reasonable midterm outcomes in the setting of end-stage glenohumeral arthritis. Level of evidence: IV.

60. Mitchell JJ, Warner BT, Horan MP, et al: Comprehensive arthroscopic management of glenohumeral osteoarthritis: Preoperative factors predictive of treatment failure. *Am J Sports Med* 2017;45(4):794-802. doi:10.1177/0363546516668823.

    One hundred seven shoulders were evaluated at a minimum of 2 years after CAM for glenohumeral arthritis; 16% of patients progressed to shoulder arthroplasty at an average of 2 years. Patients with a narrower joint space (1.3 versus 2.6 mm), higher Kellegren-Lawrence grades for osteoarthritis, Walch B2 or C glenoids (as opposed to A1, A2 and B1), and age older than 50 years had a higher risk of failure going on to arthroplasty. Level of evidence: III.

61. de Beer JF, Bhatia DN, van Rooyen KS, Du Toit DF: Arthroscopic debridement and biological resurfacing of the glenoid in glenohumeral arthritis. *Knee Surg Sports Traumatol Arthrosc* 2010;18(12):1767-1773.

62. Savoie FH III, Brislin KJ, Argo D: Arthroscopic glenoid resurfacing as a surgical treatment for glenohumeral arthritis in the young patient: Midterm results. *Arthroscopy* 2009;25(8):864-871.

63. Hartzler RU, Melapi S, de Beer JF, Burkhart SS: Arthroscopic joint preservation in severe glenohumeral arthritis using interpositional human dermal allograft. *Arthroscopy* 2017;33(11):1920-1925. doi:10.1016/j.arthro.2017.04.005.

    The authors performed a multicenter retrospective review of 43 shoulders that underwent arthroscopic glenoid resurfacing at an average of 60 months follow-up; 23% of patients went on to having a shoulder arthroplasty at a mean of 45 months after surgery. Final ASES scores, active forward elevation, and external rotation for patients that survived were 76, 140°, and 20°, respectively. Patients were older (60 years versus 53 years) that needed revision. Arthroscopic glenoid resurfacing with dermal allograft is a safe option in selected patients and provides pain relief and has an acceptable revision rate at midterm follow-up. Level of evidence: IV.

64. Faraj D, Kooistra BW, Stappen WAH, Were AH: Results of 131 consecutive operated patients with a displaced proximal humerus fracture: An analysis with more than two years follow-up. *Eur J Orthop Surg Traumatol* 2011;21:7-12.

65. Yang H, Li Z, Zhou F, Wang D, Zhong B: A prospective clinical study of proximal humerus fractures treated with a locking proximal humerus plate. *J Orthop Trauma* 2011;25(1):11-17.

66. Koval KJ, Gallagher MA, Marsicano JG, Cuomo F, McShinawy A, Zuckerman JD: Functional outcome after minimally displaced fractures of the proximal part of the humerus. *J Bone Joint Surg Am* 1997;79(2):203-207.

67. Duralde XA, Leddy LR: The results of ORIF of displaced unstable proximal humeral fractures using a locking plate. *J Shoulder Elbow Surg* 2010;19(4):480-488.

68. Hodgson SA, Mawson SJ, Saxton JM, Stanley D: Rehabilitation of two-part fractures of the neck of the humerus (two-year follow-up). *J Shoulder Elbow Surg* 2007;16(2):143-145.

69. Lefevre-Colau MM, Babinet A, Fayad F, et al: Immediate mobilization compared with conventional immobilization for the impacted nonoperatively treated proximal humeral fracture: A randomized controlled trial. *J Bone Joint Surg Am* 2007;89(12):2582-2590.

70. Lancaster ST, Grove TN, Woods DA: Management of post-traumatic stiffness of the shoulder following upper limb trauma with manipulation under anaesthetic. *Shoulder Elbow* 2017;9(4):258-265. doi:10.1177/1758573217693974.

Sixty-four patients were retrospectively reviewed after manipulation under anesthesia for posttraumatic stiffness after a proximal humerus fracture. The authors compared outcomes between patients manipulated for posttraumatic stiffness due to a humeral fracture alone and primary frozen shoulder and determined there was no significant differences in Oxford Shoulder Scores. The authors recommend manipulation under anesthesia for posttraumatic stiffness for humeral fracturs when conservative methods fail. Level of evidence: IV.

71. Holloway GB, Schenk T, Williams GR, Ramsey ML, Iannotti JP: Arthroscopic capsular release for the treatment of refractory postoperative or post-fracture shoulder stiffness. *J Bone Joint Surg Am* 2001;83(11):1682-1687.

72. Levy O, Webb M, Even T, Venkateswaran B, Funk L, Copeland SA: Arthroscopic capsular release for posttraumatic shoulder stiffness. *J Shoulder Elbow Surg* 2008;17(3):410-414.

73. Nicholson GP: Arthroscopic capsular release for stiff shoulders: Effect of etiology on outcomes. *Arthroscopy* 2003;19(1):40-49.

74. Davis JJ, Swenson JD, Greis PE, Burks RT, Tashjian RZ: Interscalene block for postoperative analgesia using only ultrasound guidance: The outcome in 200 patients. *J Clin Anesth* 2009;21(4):272-277.

75. Maroun C, Aliani D, Hass A, Werthel JD, Vidil A, Valenti P: Shoulder arthroscopy combined to hardware removal in proximal humeral fractures: A series of 58 cases with a mean follow-up of 2 years. *Eur J Orthop Surg Traumatol* 2017;27(3):317-321. doi:10.1007/s00590-017-1938-4.

Fifty-eight patients were retrospectively reviewed after arthroscopic capsular release and open hardware removal after open reduction internal fixation for a proximal humerus fracture. At an average of 23 months postoperatively, Constant scores averaged 68, average forward elevation increased by 37°, and external rotation increased by 24°. The authors determined the procedure provides significant pain relief and improvement in motion. Level of evidence: IV.

Chapter 32

Clavicle Fractures

Brian W. Hill, MD • Michael A. Stone, MD • Joseph A. Abboud, MD

ABSTRACT

Clavicle fractures occur in patients of all ages but are most common in young, active individuals. Middle third fractures are the most common, and the majority can be treated nonsurgically; however, there continues to be significant debate regarding surgical indication for surgical fixation. Recent evidence has caused a paradigm shift and demonstrated that displaced midshaft fractures have lower rates of nonunion with improved short-term outcomes after surgical management. New technology has allowed for improved plate/nail design with less surgical insult. Even so, success is dependent on proper patient selection, meticulous surgical technique, and thoughtful rehabilitation. Nonsurgical and surgical management of middle, lateral, and medial clavicle fractures is discussed.

Dr. Abboud or an immediate family member has received royalties from DJ Orthopaedics, Globus Medical, Integra Life Sciences, and Zimmer; is a member of a speakers' bureau or has made paid presentations on behalf of Tornier; serves as a paid consultant to or is an employee of DJ Orthopaedics, Flexion Therapuetics, Globus Medical, and Zimmer; has stock or stock options held in Aevumed, Dolevium, Marlin Medical Alliance, LLC, OBERD, Parvizi Surgical Innovation LLC, and Shoulder JAM LLC; has received research or institutional support from Arthrex, Inc., Department of Defense, DePuy, A Johnson & Johnson Company, Integra, OREF, Orthospace, Tornier, and Zimmer; has received nonincome support (such as equipment or services), commercially derived honoraria, or other non–research-related funding (such as paid travel) from Curical Technologies LTD, Dolevium, Mininvasive, and Trice Medical; and serves as a board member, owner, officer, or committee member of the American Shoulder and Elbow Surgeons and the Mid Atlantic Shoulder and Elbow Society. Neither of the following authors nor any immediate family member has received anything of value from or has stock or stock options held in a commercial company or institution related directly or indirectly to the subject of this chapter: Dr. Hill and Dr. Stone.

Keywords: clavicle fracture nonunion; displaced clavicle fractures; precountoured plating

Epidemiology

Clavicle fractures have a reported annual incidence of 29.14 per 100,000 population.[1] Fractures are most common in males aged 13 to 20 years. Middle third fractures account for 69%, lateral fractures account for 28%, and medial third fractures account for only 3%.

Anatomy

The development of the clavicle is unique. It is the first bone to ossify (week 5 of fetus) and the only long bone to ossify through intramembranous ossification without a cartilaginous stage. It is sigmoidal in shape, with a round medial shape which flattens and widens laterally. The clavicle is in close proximity to the apical pleura, the brachial plexus, and the subclavian vessels. These structures can be injured by a fracture fragment or screw placement. The subclavian vein is most at risk during internal fixation as this structure sits anteriorly (and closer to the clavicle) than the subclavian artery.[2,3] In the medial third of the clavicle, the subclavian vein may be in intimate contact with the posterior aspect of the bone, and this proximity makes anterior-to-posterior screw placement perilous.[2] In the middle third of the bone, the vessels assume a posteroinferior position.[3] Abduction of the arm to 90° can increase the margin of safety during screw placement. Instrumentation can be most safely used in the lateral third of the clavicle.

The cutaneous branches of the medial, lateral, and sometimes intermediate supraclavicular nerves fan out to cover the subcutaneous surface of the entire clavicle. These nerves are at risk from a transverse incision or intraoperative traction. Chest wall numbness inferior to the incision is common after surgery affecting between 29% and 52% postoperatively.[4,5]

This chapter is adapted from Dunwoody JM, McKee MD: Clavicle fractures, in Nicholson GP, ed: *Orthopaedic Knowledge Update: Shoulder and Elbow*, ed 4. Rosemont, IL, American Academy of Orthopaedic Surgeons, 2013, pp 447-454.

Classification

The most common comprehensive classification of clavicle fractures is the Edinburgh system. In this reliable and reproducible system, the fracture is classified based on its location, displacement, comminution, and intra-articular extension.[1] In the less commonly used AO/Orthopaedic Trauma Association system, fractures are divided into types based on location and further subdivided into groups and subgroups based on the specific fracture pattern[6] (**Figure 1**).

Clinical Examination

Clavicle fractures frequently occur after a fall onto an outstretched hand or direct blow to the shoulder. Open fractures and true skin tenting are rare but can occur in elderly patients with minimal soft-tissue envelope, or after high-energy trauma[7] (**Figure 2**). Clavicular shortening can be clinically assessed by measuring from the suprasternal notch to the acromioclavicular joint and comparing the measurement to that of the contralateral side. Scapular winging and dyskinesia may be present with a malunion with shortening.[8] Any gapping or distraction of the clavicle fracture should prompt the clinician to evaluate for possible scapulothoracic dissociation, especially in the setting of a high-energy injury and associated neurologic deficits.

A careful neurologic and vascular examination should always be performed. Injuries to the subclavian vessels and the brachial plexus can occur, and associated shoulder girdle, chest wall, and upper extremity injuries should be closely evaluated. When a medial clavicle fracture is diagnosed, the patient should be closely examined for chest wall injury, pulmonary injury, and head or neck injuries.

Imaging

AP and 45° cephalad upshot views of the shoulder should be routinely obtained. Upright radiographs should be obtained to fully evaluate the effects of gravity on the progressive displacement of diaphyseal clavicle fractures.[9] CT may be useful in medial fractures but is not routinely used for other fractures. Angiography may be obtained if vascular trauma is suspected. For lateral clavicle fractures, weighted radiographs may be utilized to assess for ligamentous injury.

Nonsurgical Management

Nonsurgical management leads to uneventful healing in most patients with a nondisplaced clavicle fracture.[10] The figure-of-8 bandage has been used in the past but has no advantage over simple treatment using a sling for comfort.[11] Most patients will be able to remove the sling and begin range of motion exercises at 2 to 3 weeks.

There is not a universal agreement on the best management for displaced diaphyseal clavicle fractures and certainly not all displaced fractures require surgical intervention. Children have greater healing potential than adults, and patients older than 65 years may achieve satisfactory function in the setting of a nonunion.[12] Higher rates of functional deficit and complications have been reported after nonsurgical management of a displaced midshaft clavicle fracture than after surgical management.[4,10,13,14]

Surgical Management

Several randomized trials have demonstrated the benefits of surgical management for displaced midshaft clavicle fractures in patients aged 16 to 60 years to include lower rates of nonunion, a shorter time to fracture union, faster return to work in an active population, improved short-term functional outcomes, and possibly improved outcome scores at 1 year, although at the risk of higher complications if secondary interventions for plate removal is included.[14,15]

If plating is chosen, the plate can be placed superiorly or anteroinferiorly (**Figure 3**). The advantages of the anterior-inferior position include the ability to use longer screws, a potentially safer screw trajectory, less hardware prominence, and possible biomechanical superiority.[16-18] Superior plate placement has been shown to have a significantly higher rate of secondary procedures compared with anterior inferior plating in a pooled analysis.[19] The 3.5-mm reconstruction plate should be avoided, especially in a relatively large and active patient, because it has less resistance to bending and torque than a precontoured or compression plate.[20]

Locking plates have become popular, but their use in clavicle fixation remains controversial.[18,21,22] The shallow threads used in locking plates may be more susceptible to failure when loads are applied in an axial direction.[22] No prospective randomized clinical studies have compared locking with conventional plates, and their use remains unclear.

Intramedullary devices have the theoretic advantage of causing less soft-tissue disruption, smaller scars, and less chest wall numbness compared with formal open reduction and plating techniques (**Figure 4**). Three classes of intramedullary implants are in current use. Titanium elastic intramedullary nails are typically inserted antegrade. Straight, larger diameter pins are inserted using a retrograde technique. A retrograde flexible locked nail has been introduced, although clinical data are lacking. Unlocked intramedullary devices are biomechanically inferior to plates, especially in rotation. In most clinical studies, the use of straight, larger diameter pins leads to a higher complication rate (5% to 40%) than

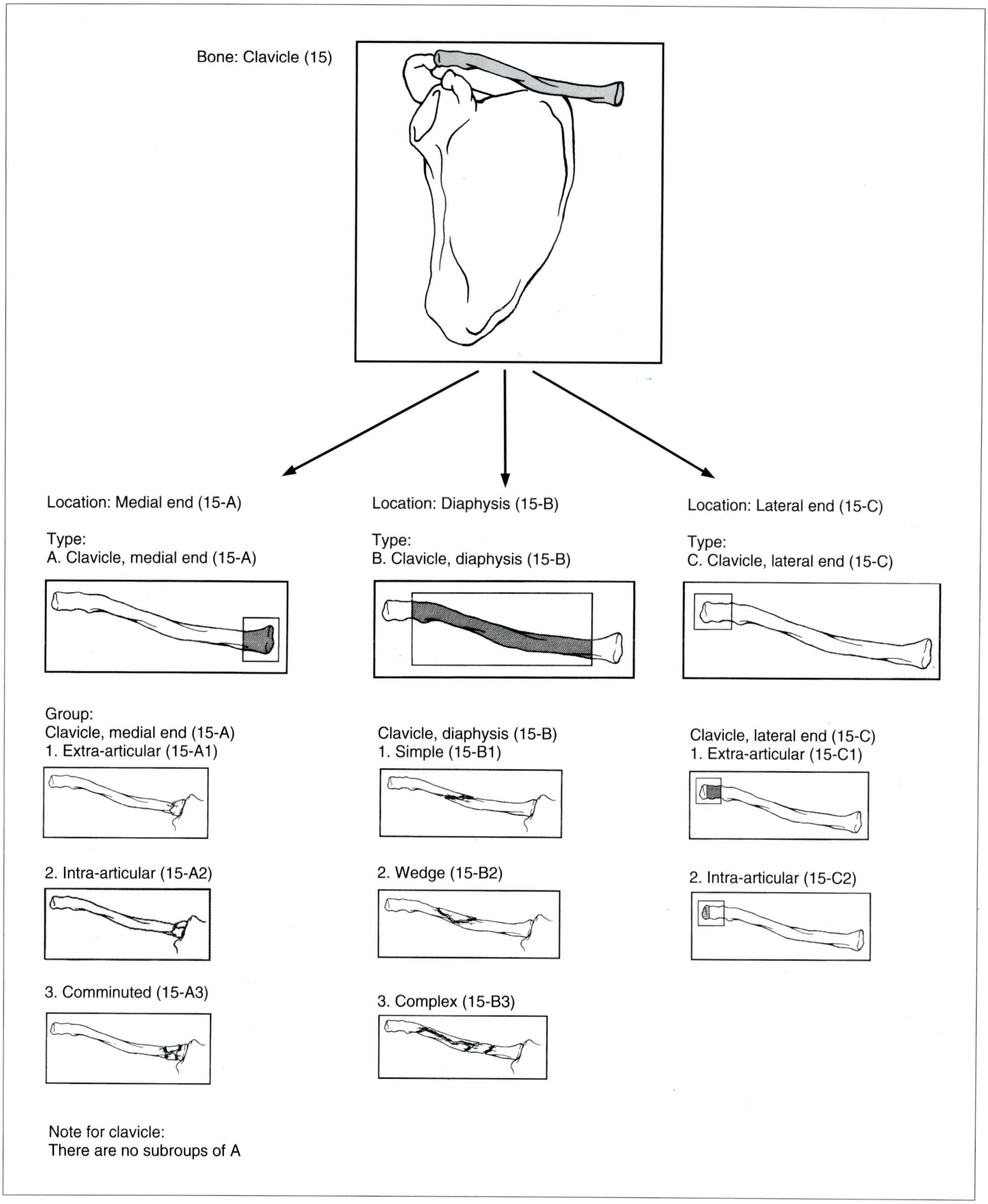

FIGURE 1 Illustration demonstrating the AO/Orthopaedic Trauma Association alphanumeric classification of clavicle fractures. The fractures are subdivided into type, group, and subgroup based on location and pattern. Subgroupings are not shown. (Reproduced with permission from Marsh JL, Slongo TF, Asel J, et al: Fracture and dislocation classification compendium – 2017: Orthopaedic Trauma Association classification, database and outcomes committee. *J Orthop Trauma* 2007;21(suppl 10):S1-S133.)

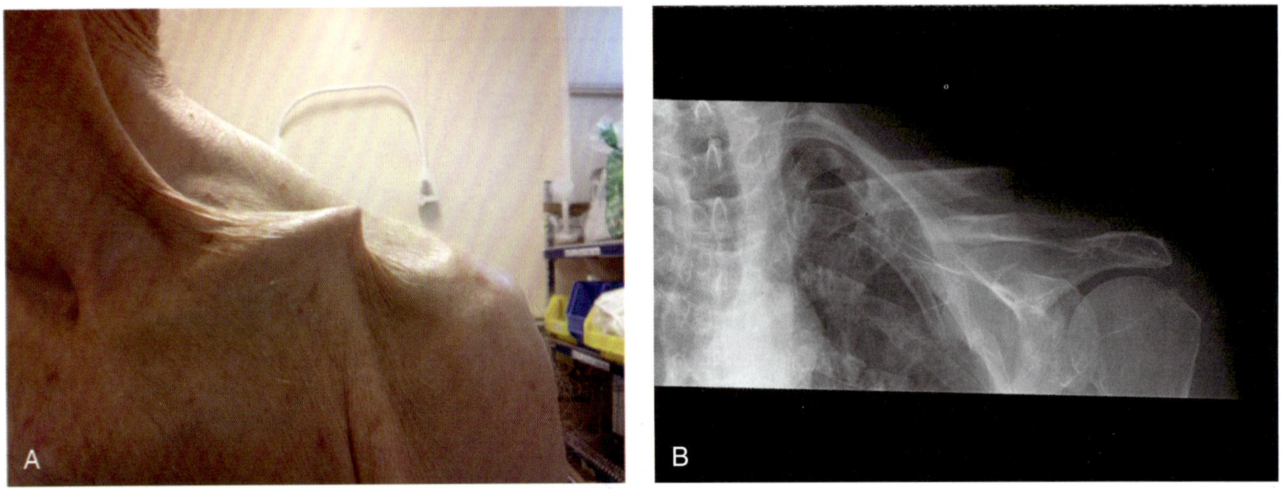

FIGURE 2 Photograph showing skin tenting (**A**) and AP 20° cephalad radiograph showing a displaced midshaft clavicle fracture (**B**) in a 79-year-old man 5 months after a fall down stairs. The patient also had fracture of ipsilateral ribs 2 through 10 and a hemothorax requiring tube thoracostomy drainage. Only the most superficial layer of skin was present over the medial spike of bone. True skin tenting with potential skin compromise, as seen in **A**, is rare.

plating.[20,23,24] Outcomes after elastic intramedullary fixation appear equivalent with plate fixation at one year; however, intramedullary fixation may be best reserved for patients with simple fracture patterns and minimal comminution.[25,26]

Anatomically precontoured plates in a superior configuration often are preferred. Some surgeons advocate vertical incisions to avoid the supraclavicular nerves; however, this approach has only been compared in smaller studies.[27] If utilizing a transverse incision, the branches of the supraclavicular nerves should be spared whenever possible. Attempts are made to achieve lag screw fixation followed by fracture stabilization, with a minimum of six cortices of fixation per fragment. A careful two-layer closure is performed, and the arm is kept in a sling for comfort. Contact sports are avoided for 3 months.[28] Plate removal is required in some patients but is deferred at least 1 to 2 years to avoid refracture.[29]

Malunion

Symptomatic malunion of a displaced midshaft clavicle fracture is uncommon.[8,30] The typical deformity includes shortening, inferior translation, and anterior rotation of the distal fragment. Shortening of at least 15 mm has shown to have the most functional significance, although this impact on functional outcomes has been questioned more recently.[31] The symptoms are proposed to be related to alterations in the musculotendinous relationships of the shoulder and narrowing of the costoclavicular space. Patients typically experience pain, scapular dyskinesis, easy fatigue of the shoulder musculature, and neurologic dysfunction. Unacceptable cosmesis may result from the ptotic, driven-in appearance of the clavicle.

During surgical planning, the clinical measurement of clavicular shortening is compared with the amount of radiographic overlap. If the clinical shortening is greater

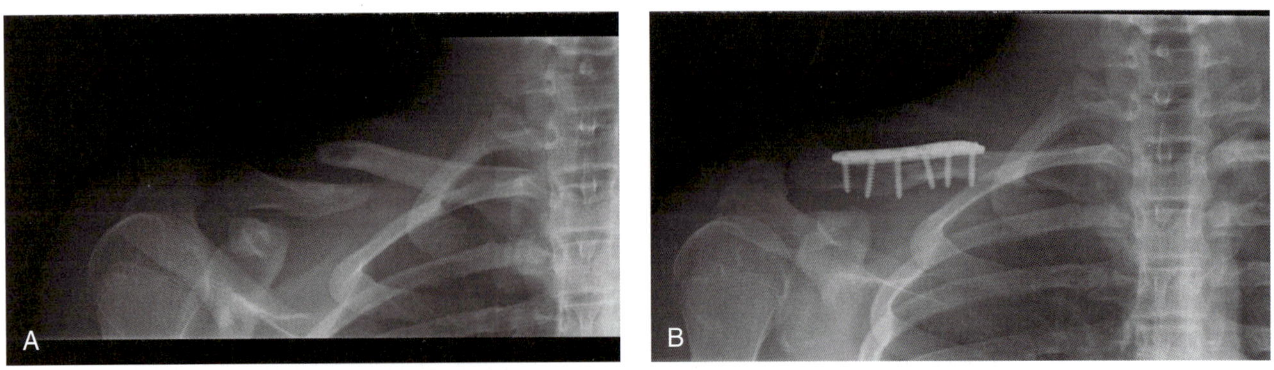

FIGURE 3 AP 20° cephalad radiographs showing a displaced midshaft clavicle fracture with significant shortening in a 16-year-old before (**A**) and after (**B**) open reduction and internal fixation using a superiorly positioned, precontoured plate.

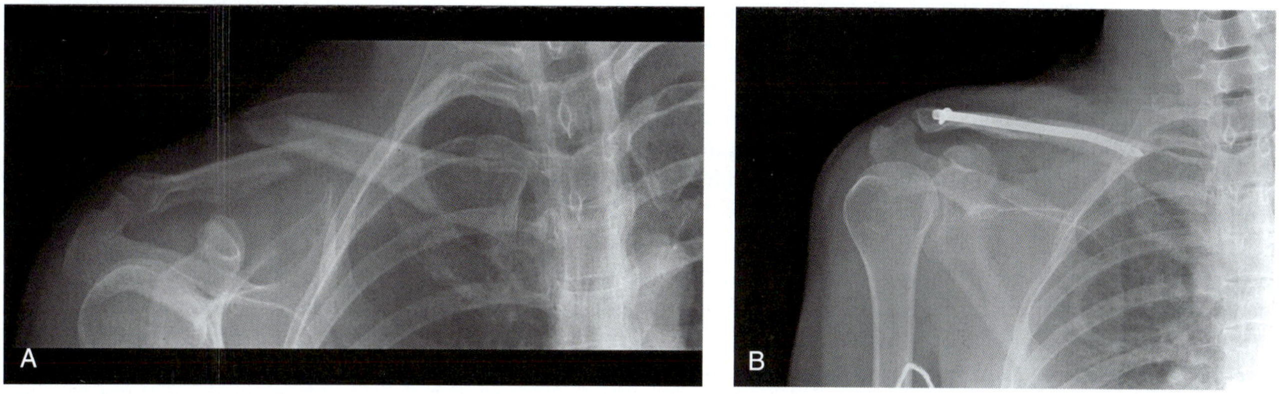

FIGURE 4 AP 20° cephalad radiographs showing a simple displaced midshaft clavicle fracture in a 28-year-old woman before (**A**) and after (**B**) treatment using a flexible, locked intramedullary nail. The advantages of this technique compared with formal open reduction and plate fixation include a smaller incision, less chest wall numbness, and minimal hardware prominence.

than the amount of radiographic overlap, an interpositional bone graft such as the iliac crest can be used to restore adequate length; however, this is not necessary in every case.[8] In most patients, surgery is successful for restoring function and relieving pain. The clavicle is osteotomized in the plane of the healed fracture, the fracture is re-created, and the deformity is corrected. Local bone graft can be used in almost all patients, and iliac crest bone graft is not necessary unless the clinical shortening exceeds that seen radiographically (eg, osteotomy and reorientation of the clavicle to its preinjury position will leave a significant bone defect at the osteotomy site). The preferred osteotomy stabilization is with a precontoured clavicle plate in a superior position and at least six cortices on each side of the osteotomy, if possible. Compression through the plate is applied whenever possible. Strengthening and resistance activities are allowed at 6 to 8 weeks. In one study, the average shortening was 2.9 cm before surgery and 0.4 cm after surgery.[8] Of the 15 patients, 14 patients healed at the osteotomy site and one patient had a nonunion. No iliac crest bone graft was needed. All patients with a healed osteotomy were satisfied with their surgery and functional outcome.

Nonunion

Nonunion has been defined as a condition in which bony union will not occur without surgical intervention. The exact timing of surgical intervention to correct a nonunion is a matter of debate and has been defined as both 24 weeks and 1 year.[4,32] Nonsurgically treated displaced midshaft clavicle fractures have a reported nonunion rate of approximately 15%; in comparison, the nonunion rate after fixation is 1% to 2%.[4,10] Factors associated with the development of midshaft nonunion include female sex, advanced age, fracture displacement, comminution, and smoking.[32,33]

In patients with a painful nonunion, surgery can be expected to have a high rate of success. Bone graft is required in a few patients.[34,35] Careful comparison of clinically assessed shortening with radiologic overlap may be helpful in predicting whether the patient requires an intercalary segment of iliac crest autograft. The bony ends are prepared by re-creating the medullary canals and feathering the edges. Local bone is saved and packed within the nonunion site. The use of superior anatomic plates with a minimum of six cortices per side is the treatment of choice. Interfragmentary compression with lag screws is performed if possible.

In the rare patient with failure of internal fixation, the possibility of infection must be considered. A two-stage approach may be necessary, in which eradication of the infection is followed by definitive reconstruction. These challenging procedures almost always require autogenous bone graft, occasionally augmented by osteoinductive osteobiologic material (bone morphogenetic protein).

Lateral Clavicle Fractures

Fractures of the lateral clavicle are less common than those of the midshaft clavicle, and they tend to occur in an older population compared with medial or middle third clavicle fractures.[1] The prevalence of nonunion in displaced lateral fractures is 28% to 44%, but the number of symptomatic nonunions is lower than that after a midshaft fracture.[1,12,36] A patient who is older than 65 years and has low physical demands may have satisfactory function after nonsurgical management.

The most commonly used classification for lateral clavicle fractures is the modified Neer system.[36] The management of Neer types IIA, IIB, and V is the most controversial. Other comprehensive classifications are the AO/Orthopaedic Trauma Association and Edinburgh systems.[1,6]

The management of a nondisplaced lateral clavicle fracture is nonsurgical, and good results can be expected. Management of displaced fractures relies on the integrity of the coracoclavicular and acromioclavicular ligaments. Specifically, if the conoid portion of the coracoclavicular ligament is still attached to the medial fracture fragment, significant displacement is often prevented. Displaced fractures may be amenable to surgical management. Although some authors prefer initial nonsurgical management for all fractures, there is evidence that more complications can be expected if fixation is delayed.[36] A myriad of fixation options has been described, with all having advantages and disadvantages.[36-40]

Plate fixation of the lateral clavicle is often difficult secondary to soft metaphyseal bone, a small lateral fragment, which limits screw fixation and significant forces on the distal clavicle fixation. Because of this, some surgeons have recommended hook plates for fractures in which there is inadequate purchase in the distal fragment (**Figure 5**). Care must be taken to appropriately size the hook to the morphology of the clavicle. In some instances, bending the hook down a few degrees may allow a better fit. The hook is placed under the acromion, posterior to the acromioclavicular joint. Even with these refinements, the use of a hook plate may be associated with shoulder pain, acromion osteolysis, and even fracture of the shaft of the clavicle medial to the plate. Symptoms are usually relieved by plate removal, and a high rate of union can be expected.[37,38,40,41]

Locking anatomic distal clavicle plates are the other common methods of fixation. If the distal fragment is small or bone quality is poor, fixation into the coracoid can be beneficial, although this is uncommon. This can be achieved with a screw through the plate or sutures around the coracoid.[37,39] It is preferable to fix most displaced lateral clavicle fractures in active, healthy patients. A rate of union higher than 90% and satisfactory functioned outcomes can be expected with this approach.

Subcoracoid fixation is an alternative method of fixation for lateral clavicular fractures with inadequate or tenuous fixation of the distal fragment. In acute setting, suture button fixation can be achieved in an arthroscopic-assisted manner. The subcoracoid region is débrided arthroscopically, and a suture button is passed (**Figure 6**). This is then retrieved from the superior clavicle and a button is placed while reducing the clavicle and then tensioned. In a chronic nonunion setting, tendon allograft may be used, looping the tendon under the coracoid and tying over the top of the clavicle. This is typically backed up with suture fixation into the coracoid as well. Alternatively, suture anchors can be embedded into the coracoid, with the suture passed around the clavicle. This technique, alone or in combination with standard methods, resulted in a high rate of union with excellent shoulder function and minimal hardware-related complications.[42]

Medial Clavicle Fractures

Medial-third clavicle fractures are rare, occurring in fewer than 3% of patients with clavicle fracture but may be associated with high-energy trauma.[1,43] A medial fracture frequently extends into the sternoclavicular joint. For this reason and because radiographs often are unclear, a CT is beneficial for defining the fracture pattern and extent of injury. The majority of medial clavicle fractures may be managed nonsurgically. Surgery may be considered for a posterior displaced fracture, particularly if the patient has impingement of nearby vital structures, such as the subclavian artery. In these circumstances, reduction should only be performed under general anesthesia with a thoracic surgeon available. Screws placed from anterior to posterior are at particular risk of causing injury to the subclavian vein.[2] These injuries must be approached on an individual basis.

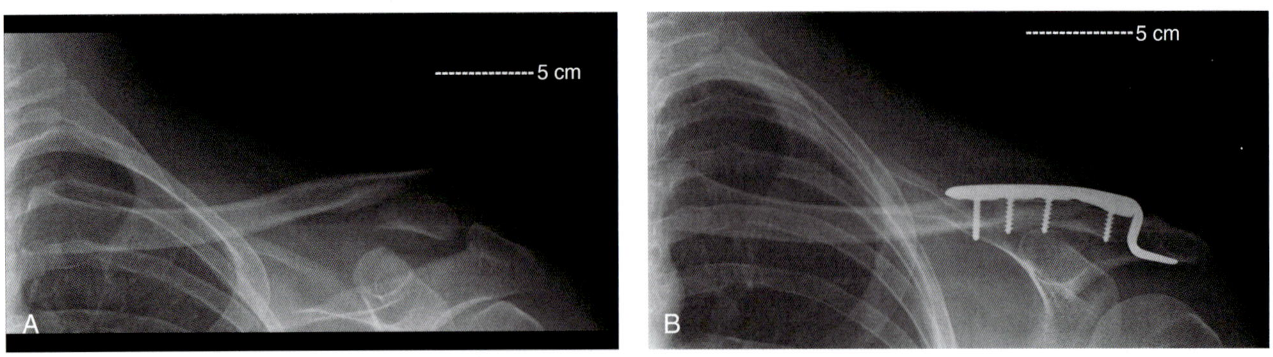

FIGURE 5 **A**, AP 20° cephalad radiograph showing a displaced type II lateral clavicle fracture in a 26-year-old man treated with open reduction and internal fixation (**B**) using a 3.5-mm locking compression plate (LCP) clavicle hook plate (Synthes). A hook plate was needed because of inadequate screw purchase in the distal fragment.

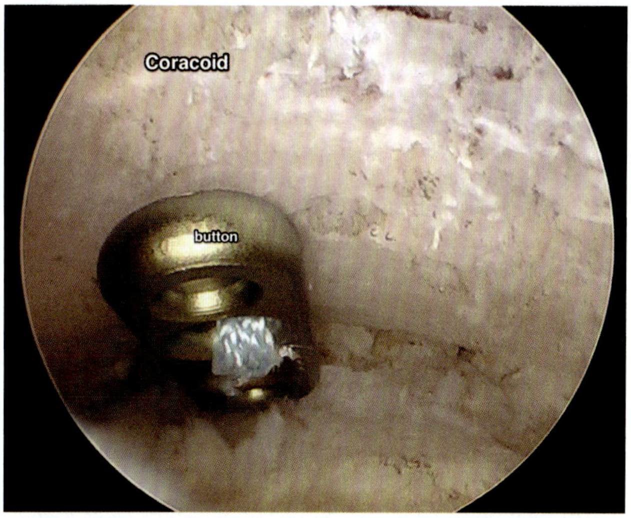

FIGURE 6 Arthroscopic image of subcoracoid suture button for a lateral clavicle fracture not amenable to plate fixation.

SUMMARY

Most fractures of the clavicle can be managed nonsurgically. However, several randomized clinical studies have found that primary surgical fixation of a displaced midshaft fracture of the clavicle in a healthy, active individual younger than 60 years was superior to nonsurgical management in functional outcomes and nonunion rates. As with other fractures, the decision to treat the injury surgically should include a shared decision-making model with the patient and surgeon. Careful patient selection and meticulous attention to surgical technique are mandatory for success. Open reduction and plate fixation with an anatomic plate is the most popular method of management, although intramedullary fixation has theoretic advantages and has had good results in some studies. Displaced lateral clavicle fractures have a high rate of nonunion, often with minimal symptoms in patients older than 65 years. A variety of surgical options, including precontoured distal plate fixation, hook plate fixation, and subcoracoid or coracoid repair, have had high rates of success in studies of relatively young, active patients.

KEY STUDY POINTS

- The majority of nondisplaced clavicle fractures can be managed nonsurgically.
- Displaced midshaft fractures should be considered for surgery to decrease the risk of nonunion and allow a shorter return to recovery and improved shoulder function.
- Careful patient selection with a shared decision-making model should be incorporated into the management of all clavicle fractures.

Annotated References

1. Robinson CM: Fractures of the clavicle in the adult. Epidemiology and classification. *J Bone Joint Surg Br* 1998;80(3):476-484.

2. Sinha A, Edwin J, Sreeharsha B, Bhalaik V, Brownson P: A radiological study to define safe zones for drilling during plating of clavicle fractures. *J Bone Joint Surg Br* 2011;93(9):1247-1252.

3. Werner SD, Reed J, Hanson T, Jaeblon T: Anatomic relationships after instrumentation of the midshaft clavicle with 3.5-mm reconstruction plating: An anatomic study. *J Orthop Trauma* 2011;25(11):657-660.

4. Canadian Orthopaedic Trauma Society: Nonoperative treatment compared with plate fixation of displaced midshaft clavicular fractures. A multicenter, randomized clinical trial. *J Bone Joint Surg Am* 2007;89(1):1-10.

5. Christensen TJ, Horwitz DS, Kubiak EN: Natural history of anterior chest wall numbness after plating of clavicle fractures: Educating patients. *J Orthop Trauma* 2014;28(11):642-647.

   This prospective observational study focused on the anterior chest wall numbness after plate fixation of 25 displaced middle clavicle fractures. Numbness at 2 weeks was common involving 83% of patients with the majority of patients (52%) still reporting numbness at 1-year follow-up. Level of evidence: IV.

6. Marsh JL, Slongo TF, Agel J, et al: Fracture and dislocation classification compendium – 2007: Orthopaedic Trauma Association classification, database and outcomes committee. *J Orthop Trauma* 2007;21(suppl 10):S1-S133.

7. Gottschalk HP, Dumont G, Khanani S, Browne RH, Starr AJ: Open clavicle fractures: Patterns of trauma and associated injuries. *J Orthop Trauma* 2012;26(2):107-109.

8. McKee MD, Wild LM, Schemitsch EH: Midshaft malunions of the clavicle. *J Bone Joint Surg Am* 2003;85(5):790-797.

9. Onizuka N, Anderson JP, Gilbertson JA, MacCormick LM, Cole PA: Displacement of diaphyseal clavicle fractures related to patient position and progressive displacement in the peri-injury period. *J Shoulder Elbow Surg* 2018;27(4):667-673.

   This is a prospective observational study of 50 patients with midshaft clavicle fractures. Patients initially had supine radiographs and then upright radiographs within 21 days demonstrating progressive displacement in 32% of the patients. Level of evidence: I.

10. McKee RC, Whelan DB, Schemitsch EH, McKee MD: Operative versus nonoperative care of displaced midshaft clavicular fractures: A meta-analysis of randomized clinical trials. *J Bone Joint Surg Am* 2012;94(8):675-684.

11. Andersen K, Jensen PO, Lauritzen J: Treatment of clavicular fractures. Figure-of-eight bandage versus a simple sling. *Acta Orthop Scand* 1987;58(1):71-74.

12. Robinson CM, Cairns DA: Primary nonoperative treatment of displaced lateral fractures of the clavicle. *J Bone Joint Surg Am* 2004;86(4):778-782.

13. McKee MD, Pedersen EM, Jones C, et al: Deficits following nonoperative treatment of displaced midshaft clavicular fractures. *J Bone Joint Surg Am* 2006;88(1):35-40.

14. Guerra E, Previtali D, Tamborini S, Filardo G, Zaffagnini S, Candrian C: Midshaft clavicle fractures: Surgery provides better results as compared with nonoperative treatment – A meta-analysis. *Am J Sports Med* 2019;47(14):3541-3551. doi:10.1177/363546519826961.

    This meta-analysis of 14 randomized trials compares nonsurgical and surgical management of displaced midshaft clavicle fractures. The pooled analysis found a lower risk of nonunion, quicker time to union, and improved Disabilities of the Arm, Shoulder and Hand scores at short-term and long-term follow-up after surgical management. Level of evidence: I.

15. Melean PA, Zuniga A, Marsalli M, et al: Surgical treatment of displaced middle-third clavicular fractures: A prospective, randomized trial in a working compensation population. *J Shoulder Elbow Surg* 2015;24(4):587-592.

    This prospective, randomized trial compares nonsurgical and surgical management of middle-third clavicle fractures and return to work. The patients treated with surgery had an earlier return to work and fewer cases of nonunions. Level of evidence: I.

16. Collinge C, Devinney S, Herscovici D, DiPasquale T, Sanders R: Anterior-inferior plate fixation of middle-third fractures and nonunions of the clavicle. *J Orthop Trauma* 2006;20(10):680-686.

17. Favre P, Kloen P, Helfet DL, Werner CM: Superior versus anteroinferior plating of the clavicle: A finite element study. *J Orthop Trauma* 2011;25(11):661-665.

18. Celestre P, Roberston C, Mahar A, Oka R, Meunier M, Schwartz A: Biomechanical evaluation of clavicle fracture plating techniques: Does a locking plate provide improved stability? *J Orthop Trauma* 2008;22(4):241-247.

19. Serrano R, Borade A, Mir H, et al: Anterior-inferior plating results in fewer secondary interventions compared to superior plating for acute displaced midshaft clavicle fractures. *J Orthop Trauma* 2017;31(9):468-471.

    This retrospective comparative study evaluates if plate position after midshaft clavicle fractures would affect the rate of secondary intervention. Superior plate placement resulted in a five times greater odds ratio of a secondary intervention. Level of evidence: III.

20. Drosdowech DS, Manwell SE, Ferreira LM, Goel DP, Faber KJ, Johnson JA: Biomechanical analysis of fixation of middle third fractures of the clavicle. *J Orthop Trauma* 2011;25(1):39-43.

21. Pai HT, Lee YS, Cheng CY: Surgical treatment of midclavicular fractures in the elderly: A comparison of locking and nonlocking plates. *Orthopedics* 2009;32(4).

22. Brouwer KM, Wright TC, Ring DC: Failure of superior locking clavicle plate by axial pull-out of the lateral screws: A report of four cases. *J Shoulder Elbow Surg* 2009;18(1):e22-e25.

23. Millett PJ, Hurst JM, Horan MP, Hawkins RJ: Complications of clavicle fractures treated with intramedullary fixation. *J Shoulder Elbow Surg* 2011;20(1):86-91.

24. Mudd CD, Quigley KJ, Gross LB: Excessive complications of open intramedullary nailing of midshaft clavicle fractures with the Rockwood Clavicle Pin. *Clin Orthop Relat Res* 2011;469(12):3364-3370.

25. Fuglesang HFS, Flugsrud GB, Randsborg PH, Oord P, Benth JS, Utvag SE: Plate fixation versus intramedullary nailing of completely displaced midshaft fractures of the clavicle: A prospective randomised controlled trial. *Bone Joint J* 2017;99-B(8):1095-1101.

    This prospective, randomized trial compares functional outcomes of plate fixation and elastic stable intramedullary nailing of displaced midshaft clavicle fractures. Plate fixation yielded a faster recovery at six months, but there were no differences after one year. The recovery after elastic stable intramedullary nailing was slower with comminution or if open reduction was required. Level of evidence: I.

26. Smekal V, Irenberger A, Attal RE, Oberladstaetter J, Krappinger D, Kralinger F: Elastic stable intramedullary nailing is best for mid-shaft clavicular fractures without comminution: Results in 60 patients. *Injury* 2011;42(4):324-329.

27. Chechik O, Batash R, Goldstein Y, et al: Surgical approach for open reduction and internal fixation of clavicle fractures: A comparison of vertical and horizontal incisions. *Int Orthop* 2018;43(8):1977-1982.

    This retrospective cohort study compares the results of clavicle fixation with standard horizontal incision versus vertical incision. There were no differences in functional outcomes, but the scar was shorter and a smaller region of hypoesthetic skin area was associated with a vertical incision. Level of evidence: IV.

28. Ranalletta M, Rossi LA, Piuzzi NS, Bertona A, Bongiovanni SL, Maignon G: Return to sports after plate fixation of displaced midshaft clavicular fractures in athletes. *Am J Sports Med* 2015;43(3):565-569.

    This retrospective case series follows athletes after clavicle fracture fixation and reports their ability to return to sport. The majority of patients returned to their similar level of play between 6 and 12 weeks. Level of evidence: IV.

29. Hsu SH, Ahmad CS, Henry PD, McKee MD, Levine WN: How to minimize complications in acromioclavicular joint and clavicle surgery. *Instr Course Lect* 2012;61:169-183.

30. Hill JM, McGuire MH, Crosby LA: Closed treatment of displaced middle-third fractures of the clavicle gives poor results. *J Bone Joint Surg Br* 1997;79(4):537-539.

31. Malik SS, Tahir M, Jordan RW, Malik SS, Saithna A: Is shortening of displaced midshaft clavicle fractures associated with inferior clinical outcomes following nonoperative management? A systematic review. *J Shoulder Elbow Surg* 2019;28(8):1626-1638.

    This systematic review of 16 studies analyzes the effect of clavicle fracture shortening on shoulder function or nonunion rates after nonsurgical management of midshaft clavicle fractures. The analysis failed to identify any association between shortening and nonunion or shoulder outcome scores. Level of evidence: III.

32. Robinson CM, Court-Brown CM, McQueen MM, Wakefield AE: Estimating the risk of nonunion following nonoperative treatment of a clavicular fracture. *J Bone Joint Surg Am* 2004;86(7):1359-1365.

33. Jarvis NE, Halliday L, Sinnott M, Mackenzie T, Funk L, Monga P: Surgery for the fractured clavicle: Factors predicting nonunion. *J Shoulder Elbow Surg* 2018;27(5):e155-e159.

    This is a retrospective review that demonstrated smoking was the only risk factor for failure after midshaft clavicle osteosynthesis. Level of evidence: IV.

34. Rosenberg N, Neumann L, Wallace AW: Functional outcome of surgical treatment of symptomatic nonunion and malunion of midshaft clavicle fractures. *J Shoulder Elbow Surg* 2007;16(5):510-513.

35. Endrizzi DP, White RR, Babikian GM, Old AB: Nonunion of the clavicle treated with plate fixation: A review of forty-seven consecutive cases. *J Shoulder Elbow Surg* 2008;17(6):951-953.

36. Banerjee R, Waterman B, Padalecki J, Robertson W: Management of distal clavicle fractures. *J Am Acad Orthop Surg* 2011;19(7):392-401.

37. Klein SM, Badman BL, Keating CJ, Devinney DS, Frankle MA, Mighell MA: Results of surgical treatment for unstable distal clavicular fractures. *J Shoulder Elbow Surg* 2010;19(7):1049-1055.

38. Good DW, Lui DF, Leonard M, Morris S, McElwain JP: Clavicle hook plate fixation for displaced lateral-third clavicle fractures (Neer type II): A functional outcome study. *J Shoulder Elbow Surg* 2012;21(8):1045-1048.

39. Andersen JR, Willis MP, Nelson R, Mighell MA: Precontoured superior locked plating of distal clavicle fractures: A new strategy. *Clin Orthop Relat Res* 2011;469(12):3344-3350.

40. Tiren D, van Bemmel AJ, Swank DJ, van der Linden FM: Hook plate fixation of acute displaced lateral clavicle fractures: Mid-term results and a brief literature overview. *J Orthop Surg Res* 2012;7:2.

41. ElMaraghy AW, Devereaux MW, Ravichandiran K, Agur AM: Subacromial morphometric assessment of the clavicle hook plate. *Injury* 2010;41(6):613-619.

42. Shin SJ, Roh KJ, Kim JO, Sohn HS: Treatment of unstable distal clavicle fractures using two suture anchors and suture tension bands. *Injury* 2009;40(12):1308-1312.

43. Throckmorton T, Kuhn JE: Fractures of the medial end of the clavicle. *J Shoulder Elbow Surg* 2007;16(1):49-54.

Chapter 33

Classification and Management of Acromioclavicular Separations

Steven Klepps, MD • Trenton Sprenkle, DO

ABSTRACT

Acromioclavicular joint separations are common in young athletes and trauma patients. Depending on the grade of injury as well as patient demographics, nonsurgical and surgical treatment can be provided. Current indications for which patients are best treated with surgery either early or late will be updated in this chapter. For those in need of surgical repair or reconstruction, many different techniques have been developed. These include arthroscopic and open techniques as well as various soft-tissue transfers and implants types. These various options will be discussed in detail throughout this chapter as well. Following stabilization, either surgically or nonsurgically a regimented recovery program is important to achieve full recovery.

Keywords: acromioclavicular joint; reconstruction; repair; separation

Mechanism of Injury and Classification

The acromioclavicular (AC) joint frequently is injured in physically active individuals, including athletes who participate in contact sports. The most common mechanism of injury is a direct blow onto the superior aspect of the shoulder. The most commonly used classification, the Rockwood system, is based on the anatomic structures injured. Rockwood type I and II injuries involve the AC joint capsule; types III, IV, and V injuries involve the coracoclavicular (CC) ligaments as well as the capsule.[1,2] A type III injury is displaced superiorly, and a type IV injury is displaced posteriorly. In addition to the CC ligament and capsular injuries, a type V injury involves deltotrapezial disruption leading to increased separation and often to incarceration of the clavicle into the deltotrapezial fascia. Type III and V separations that result in superior displacement of the clavicle are believed to be caused by drooping (ptosis) of the arm rather than by the clavicle rising superiorly. Therefore, a sling that bears part of the weight of the arm often reduces the separation. Recently type III separations have been further divided in IIIA (stable) and IIIB (unstable) subgroups with IIIBs having more pain, weakness in shoulder flexion, and scapula dyskinesia and may be more likely to need surgery.[2] A type VI injury is rare and involves clavicular displacement inferiorly in a subcoracoid position.

Clinical Evaluation

History and Physical Examination

The patient often describes a direct injury to the superior aspect of the shoulder, as in forceful contact with the ground or a fall from a height. There is pain and swelling in the superior aspect of the shoulder. The pain usually precludes the patient from raising the arm or continuing to be involved in sports. There may be associated neck pain or numbness and tingling.

The components of the examination depend on the level of separation. With a type I or II injury, the patient has pain with palpation of the AC joint. Cross-body adduction testing also is painful. The only deformity is slight swelling. With a type III or V injury, the patient has a painful deformity of the AC joint in which the clavicle sits superior to the acromion because of the downward force of the arm. A type III injury often can be reduced when the arm is simply pushed upward while the distal clavicle is held down or when the patient shrugs his or her shoulders. A type V injury usually cannot be reduced with this maneuver, because the clavicle is trapped within the trapezius.[1,2] This distinction is helpful in initial surgical decision making. A type V injury is best treated surgically; whereas a type III injury still is considered best treated nonsurgically.[3,4] However, the preferred treatment of type III injuries is controversial as will be discussed later in the chapter. A type IV injury is notable for the posterior protrusion of the clavicle. Often the protrusion is subtle and best seen radiographically, but in some patients, it can be seen on physical examination if the patient is closely evaluated for horizontal instability. Recently, attempts have been made to use ultrasonography to further assess instability, especially horizontal, which may be helpful in borderline cases.[5]

Neither of the following authors nor any immediate family member has received anything of value from or has stock or stock options held in a commercial company or institution related directly or indirectly to the subject of this chapter: Dr. Klepps and Dr. Sprenkle.

Imaging

Injury to the AC joint generally can be definitively diagnosed through radiographs. The AC joint view (also called the Zanca view) typically shows the separation well (**Figure 1, A**). This view is obtained with reduced radiation with the x-ray beam directed 15° cephalad to avoid overlap between the spine of the scapula and the AC joint. An axillary view is utilized to detect posterior displacement in a type IV injury (**Figure 1, B**). The treating physician cannot solely rely on the radiograph as recently the acromion has been noted to overhang the clavicle in up to 30% of axillary views and therefore should still correlate with physical examination.[6] In fact, dynamic radiographs as well as using "the AC width index" for comparison to the contralateral shoulder have been described to further assist with assessing horizontal instability.[7,8] Radiographs also are important in ruling out the main differential diagnosis, which is a distal clavicle fracture that can mimic an AC joint separation. In a young adolescent patient, a periosteal sleeve fracture can be identified if only a thin line of calcification from the periosteum is noted around a displaced distal clavicle. Imaging of the entire clavicle and scapula may be indicated to ensure the patient does not have an associated sternoclavicular injury (a bipolar clavicle) or a fracture within the clavicle or the scapula (a floating shoulder), especially if tenderness or swelling is noted within these areas.

In a type I injury, there is no evidence of separation on plain radiographs. In a type II injury, often there is slight widening or superior elevation that can be appreciated only by radiographically comparing the injured and contralateral AC joints. For a thin patient, one radiograph often is sufficient for obtaining an image of both joints. For a larger patient, bilateral views can be helpful if a type II separation is suspected. Although bilateral views showing type II separation do not significantly affect management, they can be useful for confirming the diagnosis for the patient. Weighted radiographs generally are not helpful and have fallen out of favor. The increase in CC distance (best seen on contralateral radiographs) is 25% to 100% in a type III injury and 100% to 300% in a type V injury.[1] Type IV injuries are best seen on axillary views with the clavicle sitting posterior to the anterior edge of the acromion.

Surgical Versus Nonsurgical Management

Type I and II separations are treated nonsurgically to achieve symptom relief and a gradual return to activity. Generally, these injuries heal well with a short course of rehabilitation. However, type II separations have been associated with persistent pain, and degenerative changes have been reported to develop 5 to 10 years after injury.[9] The patient should be made aware of these possible outcomes, but generally they do not affect the initial treatment. Distal clavicle resection and meniscus removal can be considered for a patient with a type II separation that remains symptomatic. If instability is noted at the time of surgery, AC joint stabilization should be performed; distal clavicle resection alone has been associated with persistent pain believed to result from the underlying instability.[9] For this reason, open resection should be considered for distal clavicle resection following type II separations, because it allows manual evaluation for subtle instability.

Although type III separations are controversial, in the United States, they are usually treated nonsurgically, with

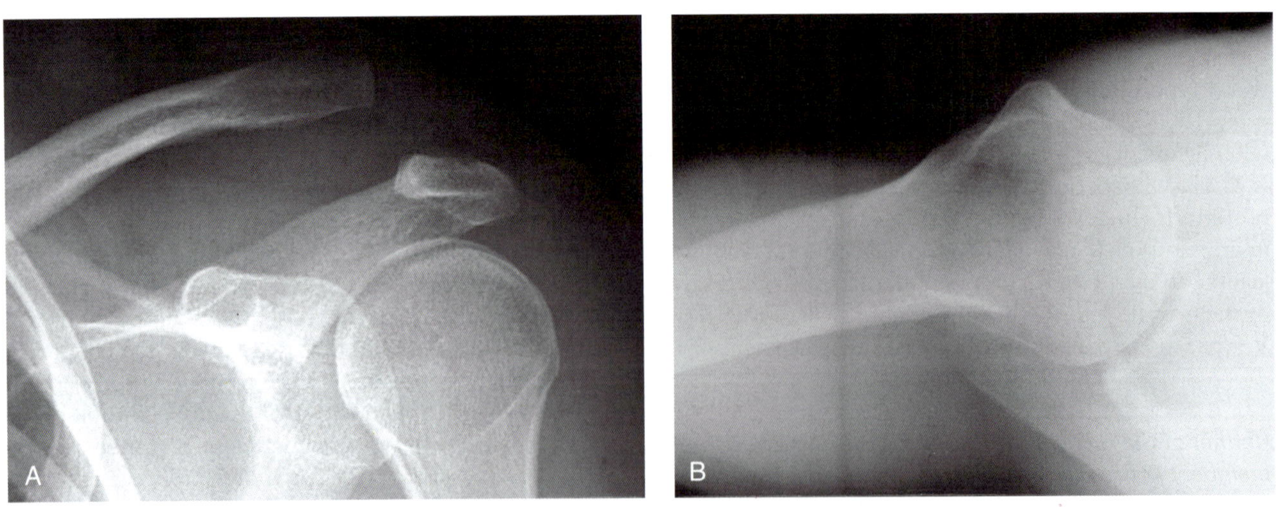

FIGURE 1 **A**, AP (Zanca) radiograph of the acromioclavicular (AC) joint showing a type III separation with 100% displacement of the clavicle superior to the acromion. **B**, Axillary radiograph of the shoulder showing the clavicle posteriorly displaced relative to the anterior edge of the acromion.

some exceptions.[4] For instance, patients who are overhead athletes or do heavy manual labor have been considered for early repair, but studies have reported good results with nonsurgical treatment even in these patients.[4,10,11] In fact, the authors of a 2011 study reported a 92% success rate with 21-year follow up in patients treated nonsurgically. However, in Europe, there is a much higher incidence of treating type III separations with initial surgical treatment with very good results as well.[10] There is still no definitive study to show better results after surgical or nonsurgical treatment, but a 2011 meta-analysis did find that surgical treatment led to better cosmesis but not to better results related to throwing, pain, or function.[12] Another meta-analysis study did not find sufficient randomized controlled studies to form an outcome-based conclusion.[13] One of the six studies examined within this study found that nonsurgical treatment led to an earlier return to sport or work and lower rates of complications such as infection or hardware failure, but surgical treatment led to higher Constant scores. Unfortunately, the studies in this meta-analysis involved treatment using Kirschner wires (K-Wires) (five studies) and hook plates (one study), neither of which is currently considered the best stabilization option. The question remains as to whether a more modern stabilization method would outperform nonsurgical treatment for type III injuries.

Nonsurgically treated patients with a type III injury generally require a longer time for complete recovery than those with a type I or II injury. Up to 3 months may be needed for return to full function and return to sport or work. For this reason, there is some question about the advisability of acute repair in athletes injured near the end of the season because a full course of nonsurgical treatment followed by surgery might not provide adequate time for recovery before the next season begins. Arthroscopic surgery and repair options, such as the use of cerclage sutures or hook plates, are less invasive than the typical reconstructions and have led to more early repairs being performed. These methods have for the most part replaced fixation with K-wires or Bosworth screws, although they work on the same principle. In general, type IV and V separations are initially treated surgically in healthy patient because these injuries tend to remain symptomatic if treated nonsurgically.

Surgical Management

Hundreds of surgical techniques have been described making it difficult to determine which surgical option is best. Surgeons should be aware of the various techniques so as to make an informed decision on the best option for an individual patient. Regardless of the surgical technique, the surgeon must decide whether the distal clavicle needs to be resected as part of the reconstruction. In general, the distal clavicle can be left in place during an acute repair because it has not developed significant hypertrophy or irregularity. Some authors describe removing the intra-articular disk if it is torn.[14] There is some risk of long-term pain or osteoarthritis at the AC joint if the distal clavicle is not resected, but in the short term, patients appear to do well regardless of whether distal clavicle resection is done with acute repair. Removing the distal clavicle may add to horizontal instability after repair.[6,14] For chronic separations, the distal clavicle typically is generally resected, especially if significant irregularity or hypertrophic changes are present.

Several important technical points apply to all AC joint reconstruction techniques; these were developed in part from biomechanical and clinical studies. To avoid slippage, it is important to place the sutures or the grafts that wrap around the coracoid at the base of the coracoid rather than at the tip. Placing suture anchors into the coracoid or a hole through the coracoid has been proposed as a means of avoiding slippage, but this technique is associated with an added cost for anchor placement and a risk of coracoid fracture because the hole weakens the coracoid.[15,16] When placing sutures or graft around the coracoid, it is important to pass them from medial to lateral to reduce the risk of neurologic injury.[17] Augmentation with tape (rather than suture fixation) has become common but can lead to coracoid or clavicle fracture because tape is stronger than suture and can cut through bone. The risk of suture failure has led to the use of multiple sutures; a 91% success rate was reported in suture-only acute repairs in which the suture was placed both in a cerclage fashion beneath the coracoid and either over or through the distal clavicle.[14] The clavicle holes for suture augmentation should not be placed too distally within the clavicle because doing so can lead to widening of the AC joint space as it pulls the clavicle medially. Essentially, the same clavicle drill hole location should be used for a Weaver-Dunn and an anatomic reconstruction. Over reduction of the clavicle is useful in compensating for stretching of the reconstruction. Wide stripping of the clavicle periosteum with débridement of any scar tissue below the clavicle is essential to allow mobilization and anatomic reduction before the repair. Oversewing the deltotrapezial fascia at the end of the procedure is important for stability, and, therefore, large, thick flaps of tissue should be mobilized during the exposure.

The Modified Weaver-Dunn Reconstruction

The modified Weaver-Dunn reconstruction has historically been the standard surgical option, although many variations of AC reconstruction have been proposed over the years. This method involves transferring the coracoacromial (CA) ligament from the acromion to the distal clavicle, with supplementation placed between the coracoid and the clavicle using heavy sutures or suture tapes (**Figure 2**). The modified Weaver-Dunn reconstruction has performed well, but its association with postoperative loosening has led to the development of multiple modifications, such as the Chuinard reconstruction (transfer of the acromion bone fragment with the CA ligament), suture reinforcement, and anatomic reconstruction (free graft transfer). In fact, a recent systematic review comparing multiple different reconstruction options reported that the Weaver-Dunn reconstruction had the highest reported revision surgery rate (5.4%).[18]

There are many potential advantages to performing reconstructions using local tissue. For instance, the use of local tissue with its vascular supply for the graft may maximize the healing potential. The sacrifice is minimal; the CA ligament often is taken down to treat impingement without significant effect. The use of local tissue also avoids the risk of reaction and the cost of using foreign material. However, with reported loosening and weaker biomechanics, this reconstructive option appears to be coming less commonly performed.

The Anatomic Reconstruction

The anatomic reconstruction has become popular during the past 15 years, primarily as a reaction to the risk of loosening after the Weaver-Dunn reconstruction. Anatomic reconstruction involves transferring a tendinous graft, such as the semitendinosus or gracilis, around or through the coracoid and through drill holes in the clavicle (**Figure 3, A**). The main advantages of graft placement below the coracoid is that it provides a stronger construct than a CA ligament transfer and is technically easier than the Weaver-Dunn reconstruction because mobilizing the CA ligament often leaves inadequate tissue for the reconstruction.[19-22] Autograft or allograft can be used. The graft can be fixed with either sutures or interference screws in the clavicle. Often, the graft is woven onto itself to avoid screw placement. Screws have been shown to provide the biomechanically strongest fixation, but the use of absorbable screws can lead to a reaction (osteolysis) and subsequent fracture. This factor has led some surgeons to use only sutures for fixation of the graft tissue[15,23] or to even avoid clavicle tunnels altogether referred to as a "nonanatomic" reconstruction. Other authors have begun using single tunnel reconstructions with good results as well to minimize the effects of multiple tunnels.[24]

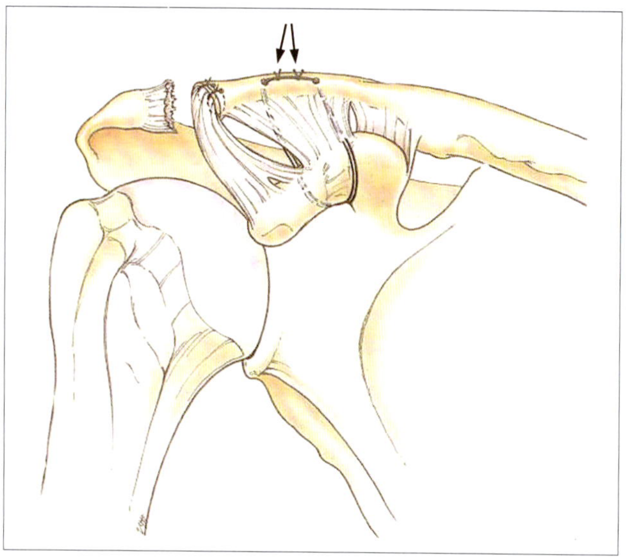

FIGURE 2 Schematic drawing of the Weaver-Dunn reconstruction, showing the coracoacromial (CA) ligament transferred to the distal end of the clavicle, with suture augmentation beneath the coracoid and through drill holes in the clavicle (arrows).

Another concept that has become much more commonly discussed and addressed surgically is horizontal instability. The reconstruction of coracoclavicular ligaments has been shown to provide good superior-inferior stability but leaves AP instability, which has been considered a limitation of standard reconstructions. Many different horizontal stabilizations have been described. The tendon autograft/allograft can be extended over the AC joint and attached to the acromion to provide horizontal stability[25,26] (**Figure 3, B**). Others have described placing an intramedullary graft.[23] Cerclage sutures can be placed around the AC joint. An additional button extending to the acromion from the coracoid can be added arthroscopically (triple button) to improve horizontal stability as well.[27-29] Several studies have evaluated these various supplemental horizontal techniques and have not shown one that is clearly superior biomechanically.[7,30,31] Also, despite this focus on improving horizontal instability, systematic review studies have still not shown clear clinical benefit with this addition to the construct with the authors of a 2018 study only reporting clinical improvement in 1/12 studies.[7,30,31] Despite the lack of proven clinical benefit, there definitely appears to be a movement toward more horizontal stabilization.

As with the Weaver-Dunn reconstruction, it is important to avoid too-distal placement of the clavicle screw holes, which can lead to a widened AC joint. Based on anatomic studies, the entire clavicle length is measured as a straight line to determine drill hole placement. The holes are placed at 20% and 30% of the clavicle length from the distal end of the clavicle.[19] Keeping the tunnels at least 15 mm apart also is believed to be useful for decreasing the risk of fracture.[15] Some authors promote a single-tunnel or no-tunnel reconstruction as a means of

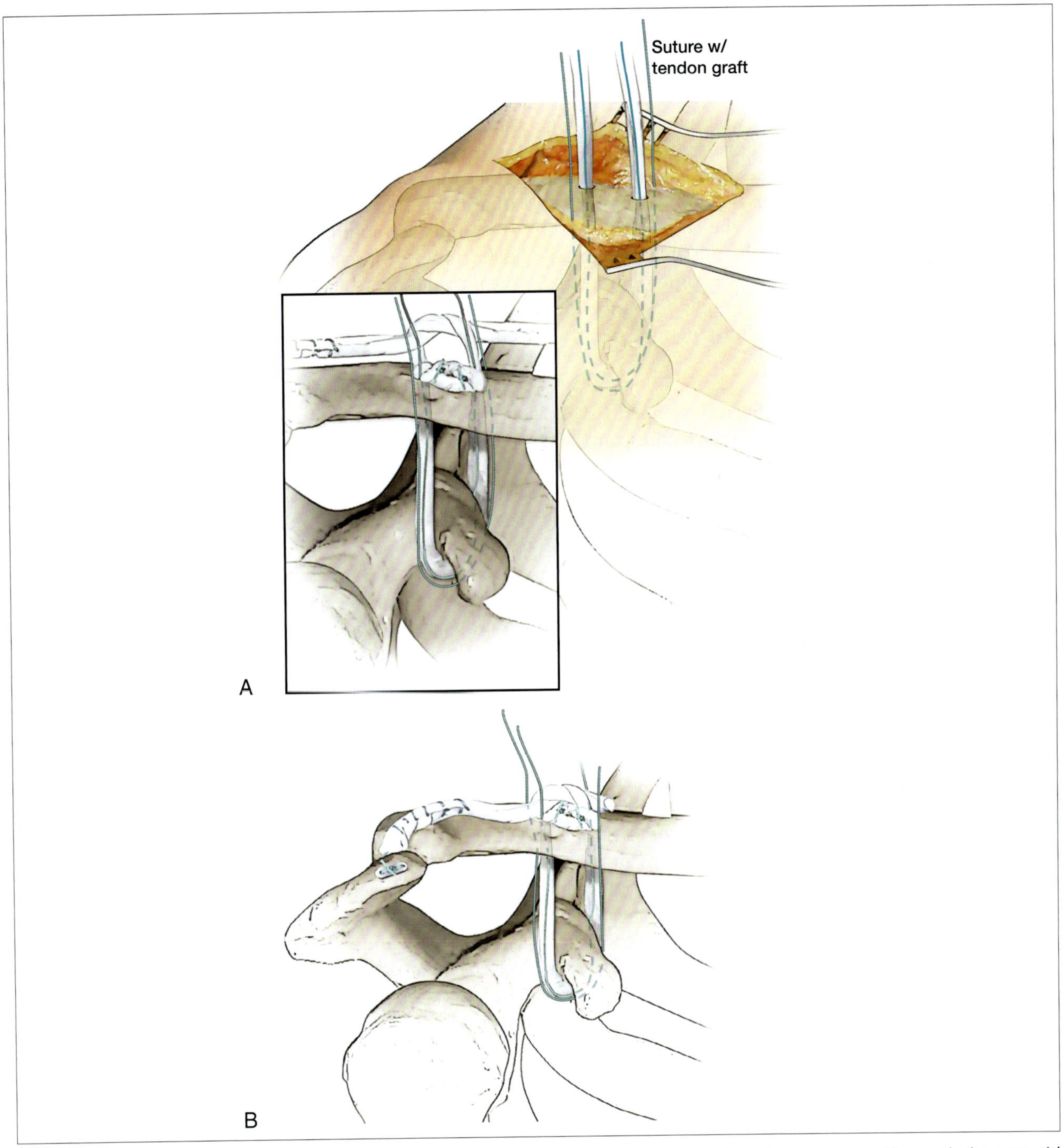

FIGURE 3 **A**, Schematic drawing of the anatomic reconstruction, showing the tendon graft and sutures passed beneath the coracoid and transferred through drill holes in the distal clavicle. Fixation is accomplished with tying the graft onto itself and suture fixation. **B**, Extension of graft to the acromion to stabilize the acromioclavicular (AC) joint thus providing horizontal stabilization.

further decreasing the risk of fracture, but this technique could lead to sawing through or loosening of the tendon.[20] Decreasing the size of the clavicle holes, with suture fixation only, has also been recommended.[15] Although several biomechanical cadaver studies have compared the anatomic reconstruction with the Weaver-Dunn reconstruction,[1,2,21,23] these have been time-zero studies using a variety of techniques, and they have not resolved the question of whether the anatomic reconstruction is clinically better than the Weaver-Dunn reconstruction.

One prospective clinical study directly compared the Weaver-Dunn and anatomic reconstructions in 24 patients.[22] The 12 anatomically treated patients had better American Shoulder and Elbow Surgeons Shoulder Indexes and Constant scores as well as a reduced CC interval. However, patients in both treatment groups had excellent results. Despite these positive results, the question remains as to whether the clinical benefit of anatomic reconstruction justifies the cost of graft and screws, donor site morbidity, and a possible foreign tissue reaction. Further studies are warranted before the anatomic reconstruction can be strongly recommended over the classic Weaver-Dunn reconstruction.

Arthroscopic Reconstruction

Arthroscopic techniques have been developed for AC joint repair and reconstruction, and studies on their results have increased significantly over the last 10 years suggesting increased performance of these techniques.[32] However, in this systematic review, there was no difference noted when comparing open and arthroscopic techniques in terms of level of reduction, complications, and rate of revision. Nonetheless, if comparable results can be obtained arthroscopically, then it certainly makes sense to transition to arthroscopic methods for reduced pain, cosmesis, etc. Acute repair fixation is performed using heavy sutures and locking metal clips, such as the TightRope device (Arthrex), placed between the clavicle and the coracoid. This fixation device allows motion through the sutures; unlike screw fixation, it is not rigid, and device removal therefore is not required. The principle is to place the clavicle in its native position in the hope that the CC ligaments will reconstitute themselves. This concept is similar to that of Bosworth screw or K-wire fixation, which are left in place for 6 weeks before removal, but with the advantage of not requiring a second surgery. The Bosworth screw and K-wire fixation methods also carried a risk of screw failure, pin migration, infection, or pullout. Unfortunately, disruption of TightRope-like devices has been reported.[17] As a result, these fixation devices have been modified by changing the shape or size of the button (eg, to a dog bone shape) or increasing the amount of fixation as with the double-tunnel/triple-tunnel technique. Unfortunately, the authors of a 2018 study showed worse results with the "dog bone" modifications with a higher failure rate and more symptomatic hardware.[33] Single tunnel as well as triple buttons have also been developed with good results reported.[24,28,29] Some manufacturers have added a tendon to the flip-button devices as well. Ultimately, there is no consensus as to the best construct using these various arthroscopic techniques, but it does appear the rate of their use will continue to increase.

Arthroscopic methods for reconstructing chronic separations have also been developed. These techniques include the GraftRope system, triple bundle, and tendon or CA ligament transfer (with or without a fleck of acromion).[29,34,35] A study of 57 patients treated with an arthroscopic Weaver-Dunn procedure for chronic instability reported an 88% success rate.[35] There is concern that arthroscopic surgery is inferior to open surgery in the ability to mobilize the distal clavicle or oversew the deltotrapezial fascia, which are believed to be key surgical components, especially for chronic instability. The technical challenges of the arthroscopic techniques for chronic instability have likely prevented them from being more widely used.

One advantage of the arthroscopic technique is that it allows the shoulder to be evaluated for intra-articular pathology at the time of the AC joint repair or reconstruction. Studies have found a 15% to 48% rate of pathology, such as rotator cuff and labral tearing, which can be corrected at the time of AC joint surgery.[35-37]

Hook Plates

Hook plates have been used for the treatment of AC separations especially in European studies most commonly performed by trauma surgeons as opposed to shoulder specialists. However, in the United States, they are more commonly used for distal clavicle fractures or complex injuries. As with Bosworth screw fixation, short-term placement allows the CC ligaments and other structures to stabilize.[18,37] The role of hook plate placement in primary AC joint separations has been further called into question by a report of hook plate-specific complications in a study of 313 patients. These complications included hook plate erosion into the acromion with possible acromial fracture (one patient), hook plate fracture (four patients), infection (six patients), and redislocation after hook plate removal (seven patients).[38] Complications of hook plates were again reported recently in a meta-analysis study, which showed hook plates and K-wires had the highest complication rates.[18] In addition, several studies have shown inferior results with hook plates than other reconstruction/repair options. Flip-button techniques have shown better results in terms of functional return and pain and do not require plate removal.[28,39] One advantage of hook plates was that they did allow earlier return to activity in one study.[39] Hook plates were found to perform best when used with a soft-tissue graft, but this method appears to defeat the purpose of minimally invasive plate placement. A comparison study found better results after Weaver-Dunn reconstruction than after hook plate treatment, including less pain at rest and better Constant scores.[40]

Although hook plates do not appear to have a major role in acute, isolated AC joint injuries, they may have a role in specific patients with complex injuries. For instance, hook plates may be useful for AC separations associated with coracoid or scapula fractures in which fixation cannot be placed between the coracoid and the clavicle (**Figure 4**). The hook plate is placed along the distal clavicle and under the spine of the acromion with

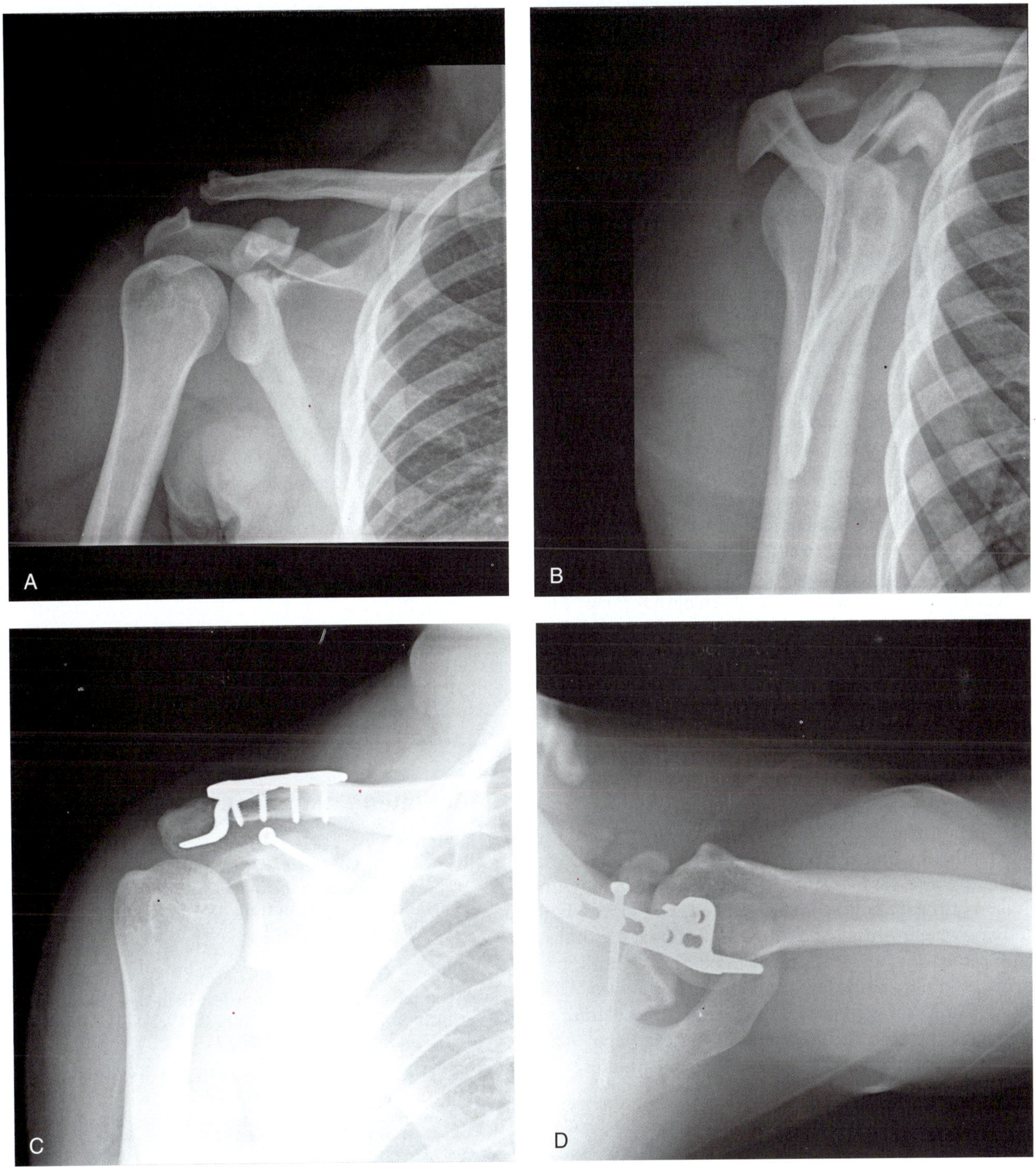

FIGURE 4 AP (**A**) and outlet (**B**) radiographs of a type III acromioclavicular (AC) separation with a displaced coracoid fracture. AP (**C**) and axillary (**D**) radiographs of the hook plate placed for stabilizing the AC joint and a single screw placed into the coracoid for fixation. Interval healing of the fracture can be seen.

the acromion rather than coracoid relied on for stability. Hook plates also have been used for revision AC reconstruction, especially if excess distal clavicle was resected and poor soft-tissue quality remains.

Rehabilitation

In patients who are nonsurgically treated, the higher grade type III, IV, and V injuries typically require more time for recovery than the lower grade type I and II injuries. A type I or II injury typically requires 2 to 3 weeks of nonsurgical treatment followed by a gradual return to sport, and a type III injury typically requires 4 to 6 weeks. Return to sport requires full range of motion and full strength as well as a nontender AC joint. Nonsurgical treatment is considered unsuccessful if the patient is unable to return to sport or work at 3 months; then surgery should be considered.[41]

A program of progressive rehabilitation developed in 2010 is organized into four phases.[42] In phase I, ice, NSAIDs, and minimal immobilization are used in an effort to reduce pain and swelling. Scapula stabilization treatment and lower extremity strengthening are begun. A sling is used for comfort only; patients having a type III injury typically require a longer period of sling use than those with a lower grade injury. Patients advance to phase II when they are at 75% of normal range of motion. Phase II treatment consists of restoring full range of motion, and early strengthening exercises are allowed. Patients proceed to phase III when 75% of strength returns. The goal of phase III is to regain full strength; power and endurance are emphasized. Patients advance to phase IV when the strength of the injured arm equals that of the contralateral arm. Phase IV involves sport-specific training. Patients who do not fully recover after 6 weeks of nonsurgical treatment are more likely to require surgery than patients who do recover fully.

Many different postoperative rehabilitation protocols have been proposed. Typically, the shoulder is immobilized for the first 6 weeks. During the next 6 weeks, full active and passive range of motion is pursued, with limited lifting. Strengthening is initiated at 3 months. Full activity, weight-lifting, and throwing begins at 4 months, with return to contact sports at 6 months. Overall, patients do have a fairly high return to sports with 92% to 100% returning to some sport and 62% returning to their previous sport in a recent systematic review.[43] The lowest rate of return was seen in overhead athletes.

SUMMARY

AC joint injuries are common among physically active individuals. Most patients recover well with nonsurgical management and regain full function. A stepwise approach to rehabilitation appears to best restore patient function. However, certain injury patterns, such as types IV, V, and VI, are best treated surgically. In addition, patients who do not recover after 3 months of nonsurgical treatment also are best treated surgically. Controversy still exists as to the best surgical option, but good outcomes can be expected as long as principles including adequate mobilization, augmented (suture/tape) fixation with appropriately placed screw holes, and appropriate rehabilitation are followed.

KEY STUDY POINTS

- Controversy still exists as to the best treatment approach for grade III AC joint separations, and therefore the treating physician should educate the patient based on the current literature to help the patient decide on the best individualized treatment.
- Anatomic reconstructions appear to have the best biomechanical and clinical results and appear to be becoming the standard reconstructive options as opposed to the Weaver-Dunn reconstruction.
- Arthroscopic techniques are becoming more popular especially in acute repairs.
- Horizontal stabilization techniques have become increasingly described, but questions remain as to the optimal technique and if clinical results are affected.
- Multiple surgical techniques continue to be described with a fair number of failures and complications, suggesting that surgeons will continue to search for the best surgical option for these injuries.

Annotated References

1. Johansen JA, Grutter PW, McFarland EG, Petersen SA: Acromioclavicular joint injuries: Indications for treatment and treatment options. *J Shoulder Elbow Surg* 2011;20(suppl 2):S70-S82.

2. Frank RM, Cotter EJ, Leroux TS, Romeo AA: Acromioclavicular joint injuries: Evidence-based treatment. *J Am Acad Orthop Surg* 2019;27(17):e775-e788. doi:10.5435/JAAOS-D-17-00105.

   This article is a modern review article that discusses anatomy and biomechanics of the AC joint with a review of current treatment options and outcomes. Level of evidence: III.

3. Nissen CW, Chatterjee A: Type III acromioclavicular separation: Results of a recent survey on its management. *Am J Orthop (Belle Mead NJ)* 2007;36(2):89-93.

4. Schlegel TF, Burks RT, Marcus RL, Dunn HK: A prospective evaluation of untreated acute grade III acromioclavicular separations. *Am J Sports Med* 2001;29(6):699-703.

5. Hobusch GM, Fellinger K, Schoster T, Lang S, Windhager R, Sabeti-Aschraf M: Ultrasound of horizontal instability of the acromioclavicular joint: A simple and reliable test based on a cadaveric study. *Wien Klin Wochenschr* 2019;131:81-86.

   This article discusses the role of ultrasonography in evaluation of both anterior/posterior and horizontal instability. However, the focus is on determining the amount of horizontal instability that occurs with transection of various ligaments of the AC joint. Level of evidence: IV.

6. Barth J, Boutsiadis A, Narbona P, et al: The anterior borders of the clavicle and the acromion are not always aligned in the intact acromioclavicular joint: A cadaveric study. *J Shoulder Elbow Surg* 2017;26:1121-1127.

   This article is a cadaver study that attempts to determine the anatomic position of the acromion compared with the clavicle and finds that 40% do not line up exemplifying anatomic variability. Level of evidence: III.

7. Aliberti GM, Kraeutler MJ, Trojan JD, Mulcahey MK: Horizontal instability of the acromioclavicular joint: A systematic review. *Am J Sports Med* 2020;48(2):504-510. doi:10.1177/0363546519831013.

   This systematic review identifies failed acromioclavicular repairs and assesses incidence of horizontal instability. Authors report variable reports and assessments with variable surgical techniques with no clear solutions but state authors should be aware. Level of evidence: IV.

8. Vaisman A, Villalón Montenegro IE, Tuca De Diego MJ, Valderrama Ronco J: A novel radiographic index for the diagnosis of posterior acromioclavicular joint dislocations. *Am J Sports Med* 2014;42:112-116.

   This radiographic study determined the AC joint width index for a series of patients and found an index greater than 60% was associated with posterior instability. Level of evidence: II.

9. Mouhsine E, Garofalo R, Crevoisier X, Farron A: Grade I and II acromioclavicular dislocations: Results of conservative treatment. *J Shoulder Elbow Surg* 2003;12(6):599-602.

10. Lizaur A, Sanz-Reig J, Gonzalez-Parreño S: Long-term results of the surgical treatment of type III acromioclavicular dislocations: An update of a previous report. *J Bone Joint Surg Br* 2011;93(8):1088-1092.

11. Bannister GC, Wallace WA, Stableforth PG, Hutson MA: The management of acute acromioclavicular dislocation: A randomised prospective controlled trial. *J Bone Joint Surg Br* 1989;71(5):848-850.

12. Smith TO, Chester R, Pearse EO, Hing CB: Operative versus non-operative management following Rockwood grade III acromioclavicular separation: A meta-analysis of the current evidence base. *J Orthop Traumatol* 2011;12(1):19-27.

13. Ceccarelli E, Bondì R, Alviti F, Garofalo R, Miulli F, Padua R: Treatment of acute grade III acromioclavicular dislocation: A lack of evidence. *J Orthop Traumatol* 2008;9(2):105-108.

14. Lädermann A, Grosclaude M, Lübbeke A, et al: Acromioclavicular and coracoclavicular cerclage reconstruction for acute acromioclavicular joint dislocations. *J Shoulder Elbow Surg* 2011;20(3):401-408.

15. Turman KA, Miller CD, Miller MD: Clavicular fractures following coracoclavicular ligament reconstruction with tendon graft: A report of three cases. *J Bone Joint Surg Am* 2010;92(6):1526-1532.

16. Gerhardt DC, VanDerWerf JD, Rylander LS, McCarty EC: Postoperative coracoid fracture after transcoracoid acromioclavicular joint reconstruction. *J Shoulder Elbow Surg* 2011;20(5):e6-e10.

17. Motta P, Maderni A, Bruno L, Mariotti U: Suture rupture in acromioclavicular joint dislocations treated with flip buttons. *Arthroscopy* 2011;27(2):294-298.

18. Moatshe G, Kruckeberg B, Chahla J. Provencher M, Laprade R: Acromioclavicular and coracoclavicular ligament reconstruction for acromioclavicular joint instability: A systematic review of clinical and radiographic outcomes. *Arthroscopy* 2018;34:1979-1995.e8.

    This systematic review compared various repair/reconstruction techniques with similar subjective outcomes after surgical treatment and low reoperation rates. However, treatment with hook plate/K-wires was associated with the highest complication rates, and modified Weaver-Dunn had the highest unplanned revision surgery rates. Level of evidence: IV.

19. Rios CG, Mazzocca AD: Acromioclavicular joint problems in athletes and new methods of management. *Clin Sports Med* 2008;27(4):763-788.

20. Grutter PW, Petersen SA: Anatomical acromioclavicular ligament reconstruction: A biomechanical comparison of reconstructive techniques of the acromioclavicular joint. *Am J Sports Med* 2005;33(11):1723-1728.

21. Thomas K, Litsky A, Jones G, Bishop JY: Biomechanical comparison of coracoclavicular reconstructive techniques. *Am J Sports Med* 2011;39(4):804-810.

22. Tauber M, Gordon K, Koller H, Fox M, Resch H: Semitendinosus tendon graft versus a modified Weaver-Dunn procedure for acromioclavicular joint reconstruction in chronic cases: A prospective comparative study. *Am J Sports Med* 2009;37(1):181-190.

23. Gonzalez-Lomas G, Javidan P, Lin T, Adamson GJ, Limpisvasti O, Lee TQ: Intramedullary acromioclavicular ligament reconstruction strengthens isolated coracoclavicular ligament reconstruction in acromioclavicular dislocations. *Am J Sports Med* 2010;38(10): 2113-2122.

24. Banffy MB, van Eck CF, ElAttrache NS: Clinical outcomes of a single-tunnel technique for coracoclavicular and acromioclavicular ligament reconstruction. *J Shoulder Elbow Surg* 2018;27:S70–S75.

    This clinical study reports the outcome of single-tunnel technique for repair of AC joint separations with good overall results and low complication rates. Level of evidence: IV.

25. Saccomanno MF, Fodale M, Capasso L, Cazzato G, Milano G: Reconstruction of the coracoclavicular and acromioclavicular ligaments with semitendinosus tendon graft: A pilot study. *Joints* 2014;2:6-14.

    This clinical series evaluates the use of a semitendinosus graft that reconstructs both the CC and AC capsule using the same graft with good results at 2 years follow-up. Level of evidence: IV.

26. Kibler WB, Sciascia AD, Morris BJ, Dome DC: Treatment of symptomatic acromioclavicular joint instability by a docking technique: Clinical indications, surgical technique, and outcomes. *Arthroscopy* 2017;33:696-708.e2.

    This clinical series evaluates an AC joint reconstruction technique that uses an allograft with docking into the clavicle with good overall results and small rate of failure. Level of evidence: IV.

27. Hann C, Kraus N, Minkus M, Maziak N, Scheibel M: Combined arthroscopically assisted coraco- and acromioclavicular stabilization of acute high-grade acromioclavicular joint separations. *Knee Surg Sports Traumatol Arthrosc* 2018;26:212-220.

    This cohort study assesses the results of arthroscopically assisted reconstructions for both primary and revision AC joint separations with good results in both subgroups of patients. Level of evidence: III.

28. Qi W, Xu Y, Yan Z, et al: The tight-rope technique versus clavicular hook plate for treatment of acute acromioclavicular joint dislocation: A systematic review and meta-analysis. *J Invest Surg* 2019;10:1-10. doi:10.1080/08941939.2019.1593558.

    This systematic review compared hook plate with tight rope repair of AC joint, showing better overall outcome and less pain with the tight rope technique. Level of evidence: III.

29. Tauber M, Valler D, Lichtenberg S, Magosch P, Moroder P, Habermeyer P: Arthroscopic stabilization of chronic acromioclavicular joint dislocations: Triple- versus single-bundle reconstruction. *Am J Sports Med* 2016;44: 482-489.

    This comparative cohort study compared triple-bundle and single-bundle reconstructive techniques. The triple-bundle technique showed superior clinical and radiologic results compared with isolated single-bundle reconstruction. The triple bundle showed better horizontal stability and outcome. Level of evidence: II.

30. Jordan RW, Malik S, Bentick K, Saithna A: Acromioclavicular joint augmentation at the time of coracoclavicular ligament reconstruction fails to improve functional outcomes despite significantly improved horizontal stability. *Knee Surg Sports Traumatol Arthrosc* 2019;27(12):3747-3763. doi:10.1007/s00167-018-5152-7.

    Authors of this systematic review compared coracoclavicular (CC) reconstruction with augmentation of the acromioclavicular (AC) joint to standard repairs. They concluded that CC reconstruction with augmentation of the AC joint has been shown to provide improved horizontal stability in both biomechanical and clinical studies compared with isolated CC reconstruction. However, comparative studies have shown no clinical advantage with respect to American Shoulder and Elbow Surgeon or Constant scores. Level of evidence: IV.

31. Dyrna F, Imhoff FB, Haller B, et al: Primary stability of an acromioclavicular joint repair is affected by the type of additional reconstruction of the acromioclavicular capsule. *Am J Sports Med* 2018;46:3471-3479.

    This cadaver study compared CC ligament reconstruction with addition of AC capsular repair and found better horizontal stabilization with the addition of the capsular repair. Level of evidence: III.

32. Gowd AK, Liu JN, Cabarcas BC, et al: Current concepts in the operative management of acromioclavicular dislocations: A systematic review and meta-analysis of operative techniques. *Am J Sports Med* 2019;47(11): 2745-2758.

    This systematic review compared various AC joint reconstruction techniques. Authors found equal results with open and arthroscopic techniques with no differences in loss of reduction, the complication rate, and the revision rate. There was a high rate of complications, and the surgeon should base treatment on patient profile. Level of evidence: III.

33. Vulliet P, Le Hanneur M, Cladiere V, Loriaut P, Boyer P: A comparison between two double-button endoscopically assisted surgical techniques for the treatment acute acromioclavicular dislocations. *Musculoskelet Surg* 2018;102:73-79.

    This comparison study assesses tight rope versus dog bone implants placed arthroscopically, which showed similar clinical results but better radiographic results in the tight rope subgroup. Level of evidence: IV.

34. DeBerardino TM, Pensak MJ, Ferreira J, Mazzocca AD: Arthroscopic stabilization of acromioclavicular joint dislocation using the AC graftrope system. *J Shoulder Elbow Surg* 2010;19(suppl 2):47-52.

35. Boileau P, Gastaud O, Wilson A, Trojani C, Bronsard N: All-arthroscopic reconstruction of severe chronic acromioclavicular joint dislocations. *Arthroscopy* 2019;35:1324-1335.

This case series study evaluates the incidence of intra-articular pathology in patients undergoing all-arthroscopic CC ligament reconstruction. 48% of patients were noted to have glenohumeral lesions. Higher-grade ACJ dislocations, previous ACJ surgery, and misplacement of bone tunnels were risk factors for recurrent instability. Level of evidence: IV.

36. Pauly S, Gerhardt C, Haas NP, Scheibel M: Prevalence of concomitant intraarticular lesions in patients treated operatively for high-grade acromioclavicular joint separations. *Knee Surg Sports Traumatol Arthrosc* 2009;17(5):513-517.

37. Arrigoni P, Brady PC, Zottarelli L, et al: Associated lesions requiring additional surgical treatment in grade 3 acromioclavicular joint dislocations. *Arthroscopy* 2014;30:6-10.

In this retrospective case series study, all patients undergoing AC joint reconstruction underwent arthroscopy for pathology. 42.8% were diagnosed with at least one additional pathologic lesion, and 29.5% required a dedicated additional treatment. SLAP and posterior rotator cuff tear management represented 24 of the 35 additional surgeries (68.5%). Patients aged 45 years or older had a greater risk of presenting with associated lesions that needed to be surgically managed. Level of evidence: IV.

38. Chiang CL, Yang SW, Tsai MY, Kuen-Huang Chen C: Acromion osteolysis and fracture after Hook plate fixation for acromioclavicular joint dislocation: A case report. *J Shoulder Elbow Surg* 2010;19(4):e13-e15.

39. Stein T, Müller D, Blank M, et al: Stabilization of acute high-grade acromioclavicular joint separation: A prospective assessment of the clavicular hook plate versus the double double-button suture procedure. *Am J Sports Med* 2018;46:2725-2734.

This prospective study compared hook plate to arthroscopic double-bundle repair. All patients showed significantly increased scores after surgery compared with preoperative status (all $P < 0.05$). Arthroscopic double-bundle repair had significantly better outcomes at 24 months. Clinically assessed horizontal instability was lower in the arthroscopic repair group as well. Loss of reduction is similar in both groups. It is stated that hook plate may be better for patients in need of less restriction postoperatively. Level of evidence: IV.

40. Boström Windhamre HA, von Heideken JP, Une-Larsson VE, Ekelund AL: Surgical treatment of chronic acromioclavicular dislocations: A comparative study of Weaver-Dunn augmented with PDS-braid or Hook plate. *J Shoulder Elbow Surg* 2010;19(7):1040-1048.

41. Trainer G, Arciero RA, Mazzocca AD: Practical management of grade III acromioclavicular separations. *Clin J Sport Med* 2008;18(2):162-166.

42. Cote MP, Wojcik KE, Gomlinski G, Mazzocca AD: Rehabilitation of acromioclavicular joint separations: Operative and nonoperative considerations. *Clin Sports Med* 2010;29(2):213-228, vii.

43. Kay J, Memon M, Alolabi B: Return to sport and clinical outcomes after surgical management of acromioclavicular joint dislocation: A systematic review. *Arthroscopy* 2018;34:2910-2924.e1.

This systematic review assessed rates of return to sport following AC joint treatment. Almost all patients returned to sport participation after surgical management of AC joint dislocations with most returning to their preinjury level of sport. The rates of return to sport were comparable across the different types of injuries and surgical procedures. Level of evidence: IV.

Section 7

Elbow Trauma, Fracture, and Reconstruction

SECTION EDITOR:
MARK S. COHEN, MD

Chapter 34

Tendon Injuries and Conditions of the Elbow: Biceps, Triceps, and Lateral and Medial Epicondylitis

Brandon Cincere, MD • Robert P. Nirschl, MD, MS

Section 7: Elbow Trauma, Fracture, and Reconstruction

ABSTRACT

Tendon injuries occur in three basic ways: repetitive overuse, high-intensity single-event trauma, and lower intensity single-event trauma superimposed on vulnerable tendons previously weakened by repetitive overuse. An additional factor is an apparent hereditary vulnerability noted in approximately 10% of patients with multiple tendon symptoms (shoulder, elbow, carpal tunnel, Achilles, plantar fascia) usually starting in the third decade of life.

The underlying histopathology of tendon overuse failure reveals no inflammatory cells. Disruptions of collagen in association with disrupted and dysfunctional vascular and tenocyte elements are the pathologic hallmarks (angiofibroblastic hyperplasia/tendinosis). The terms epicondylitis and/or tendinitis are therefore technically incorrect.

High-demand, single-event trauma can disrupt a normal tendon (more likely distal triceps and biceps) in collision-type sports. Overuse failure (such as angiofibroblastic hyperplasia/tendinosis) usually occurs with repetitive activity (such as racquet and throwing sports).

Management of major tendon ruptures consists of direct surgical repair. management of angiofibroblastic tendinosis can include nonsurgical or surgical intervention depending on the magnitude of the histopathology.

Keywords: angiofibroblastic hyperplasia/tendinosis; lateral and medial epicondylitis; nirschl elbow surgical techniques

Introduction

Elbow tendon injuries typically are categorized as resulting from single-event macrotrauma (acute injury), single-event trauma superimposed on tissue made vulnerable by overuse (acute-on-chronic injury), or multiple repetition overuse (chronic injury). Numerous pathologic conditions, ranging from acute to chronic injury, can occur around the circumference of the elbow. Ligament dysfunction, nerve dysfunction, and osteochondral injury may be associated with the condition. Elbow tendon overuse injury often is not an isolated event, and the entire extremity, from the cervical and thoracic spine to the shoulder and hand, should be evaluated.

Dr. Nirschl or an immediate family member has received royalties from Medical Sports and has stock or stock options held in TENEX. Neither Dr. Cincere nor any immediate family member has received anything of value from or has stock or stock options held in a commercial company or institution related directly or indirectly to the subject of this chapter.

Biceps Injuries

Evaluation

The distal biceps has two insertions on the radial tuberosity. The short head attaches distally on the tuberosity, allowing it to be a powerful elbow flexor. The long head attaches more proximally and ulnarly, farther from the axis of rotation of the forearm. This attachment enhances supination by increasing leverage. The biceps tendon spirals like a ribbon; its direction is clockwise in the left arm and counterclockwise in the right arm.[1]

Most distal bicep injuries occur as an acute avulsion from the radial tuberosity after sudden eccentric extension force while the elbow is in midflexion. The symptoms may include a tearing sensation and acute pain. Most such injuries occur in the dominant extremity in men aged 40 to 60 years. The risk of rupture is 7.5 times greater in people who use tobacco.[2] Pain and ecchymosis in the antecubital fossa are common findings, and tenderness and weakness with resisted supination and elbow flexion is also present. Palpation of a defect, a positive O'Driscoll hook test, or a positive squeeze test can reveal the injury unless there is a partial tear, an intact bicipital aponeurosis (a lacertus fibrosus), or bicipital tendinosis.[3,4] The O'Driscoll hook test was found to have 100% sensitivity and specificity.[3] A complete tear is diagnosed as acute if it occurred within the past 4 weeks or chronic if it occurred prior. Radiographic evaluation typically does not reveal an osseous injury but occasionally may show an irregularity, enlargement of the radial tuberosity, or avulsion.[5] Bicipital tendinosis without rupture can occur in isolation or in association with a cubital bursitis or a partial rupture. A partial tear is less common and can occur within the tendon or at its insertion (**Figure 1**). A clicking sensation near the tendon insertion

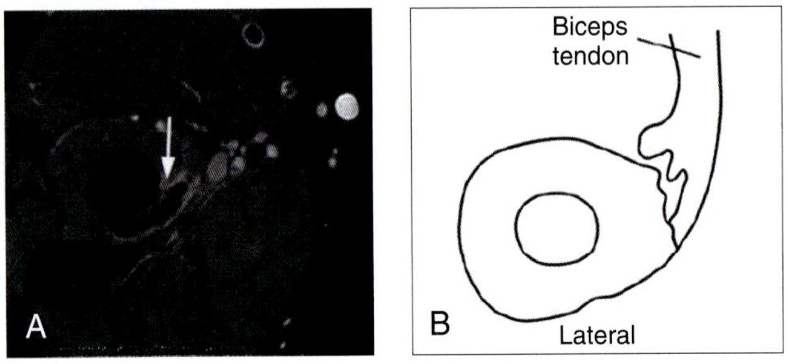

FIGURE 1 T2-weighted magnetic resonance image (**A**) and line drawing (**B**) showing a partial-thickness tear at the radial side attachment of the distal biceps tendon (arrow). (Reproduced from Sutton KM, Dodds SD, Ahmad CS, Sethi PM: Surgical treatment of distal biceps rupture. *J Am Acad Orthop Surg* 2010;18[3]:139-148.)

during forearm rotation may be caused by inflammation of the bursa between the tendon and the tuberosity. MRI can be helpful in identifying integrity and intrasubstance changes, but these are not always apparent.[5] MRI in the prone flexion, abduction, supinated position shows the full length of the biceps from the tuberosity to the musculocutaneous junction.[6] Diagnostic ultrasonography also can be considered.

Management

Most acute and complete distal biceps ruptures can be managed by reattachment. A variety of techniques have predictably good results superior to those of nonsurgical management.[5] The management of a chronic rupture can be challenging and is based on whether the bicipital aponeurosis is disrupted or intact. An intact tendon may be prevented from retracting more proximally. As time passes, retraction and scarring of the brachialis may limit the ability to achieve enough surgical length for a satisfactory primary repair. Semitendinosus graft reconstruction has been used to treat a chronic injury with inadequate length.[7] Repair and reconstruction to the radial tuberosity are less predictable in chronic injury and carry greater neurovascular risk. In such circumstances, a compromise method of soft-tissue attachment to the brachialis may be considered.

Partial tears can occur in association with tendinosis and bursitis. MRI can be useful in the diagnosis by showing partial tearing at the radial insertion of the radial tuberosity.[5] Endoscopy has been used to evaluate the potential for repairing a partial tear.[8] Injuries are considered for surgical intervention after unsuccessful nonsurgical management. Most partial ruptures can be successfully treated with release, débridement, and reattachment of the tendon, especially if the tear exceeds 50%. Débridement alone is less likely to have a successful outcome. Repair of a complete rupture is most likely to restore supination and flexion strength if it is done within 2 weeks of injury.[5]

Better functional and objective outcomes were found in patients treated surgically rather than nonsurgically.[2] Supination strength, but not flexion strength, was significantly improved in patients who underwent repair.[2] Patients treated nonsurgically had a higher incidence of activity pain and had decreased strength and endurance that was more severe in supination than in flexion. In general, nonsurgical treatment should be considered for a patient who has a chronic complex rupture, has a serious medical comorbidity, and is sedentary.[2]

Single-incision and two-incision techniques have been described. The Boyd-Anderson two-incision technique was developed to avoid the neurologic complications associated with a single incision. However, the use of this technique has led to various complications, including heterotopic ossification and radioulnar synostosis. Modification of the Boyd-Anderson technique into a muscle-splitting approach that does not violate the periosteum of the ulna has reduced the incidence of complications.[5] With this technique, virtually 100% improvement was reported in restoring flexion and supination strength, without loss of motion or rerupture.[9] Several other studies also reported that the technique led to successful results.[10-12] A systematic review documented an overall 16% complication rate with the two-incision technique and an 18% rate with the single-incision technique.[13] Patients who underwent a two-incision procedure were more likely to have a poor result compared with those who underwent a single-incision procedure (31% and 6%, respectively)[13] (**Table 1**).

The single-incision method has evolved with improvements in technique, devices, and repairs. Complications related to single-incision techniques include injuries to the posterior interosseous and lateral antebrachial cutaneous nerves.[2] The risk of nerve injury has been reduced by identifying the cutaneous nerve, maintaining the arm in supination, and using less invasive incisions. Multiple studies found a minimal risk of complications and good outcomes when cortical button fixation was used with single-incision techniques.[14-16] A meta-analysis found a 69% rate of satisfactory outcomes with the two-incision technique and a 94% rate with the single-incision technique.[13] The lower rate of satisfactory outcomes with the two-incision technique was attributable to loss of forearm rotation or rotational strength. The surgeon's level of training and experience should guide the decision as to the preferred technique.

A delay in diagnosis and treatment may complicate an anatomic repair. An intact bicipital aponeurosis can mask an acute rupture but also can limit proximal retraction and possibly allow a direct repair. Inadequate length should be anticipated in a chronic injury, and graft material should be available for reconstruction. The semitendinosus is anatomically similar to the distal biceps tendon.[7] A more extensive dissection is warranted,

Table 1

Complications After Two-Incision and Single-Incision Elbow Repairs

Complication	Technique: Two-Incision (N = 142)	Single-Incision (N = 165)	P
Heterotopic ossification[a]	8 (6%)	5 (3%)	0.45
Nerve palsy[b]	10 (7%)	20 (12%)	0.12
Loss of forearm rotation	13 (9%)	3 (2%)	0.01
Infection	0	3 (2%)	0.25
Flexion contracture	2 (1%)	1 (1%)	0.61
Total elbows with a complication	23 (16%)	29 (18%)	0.88

[a]Resulting in motion loss.
[b]Transient or permanent.
Adapted with permission from Chavan PR, Duquin TR, Bisson LJ: Repair of the ruptured distal biceps tendon: A systematic review. *Am J Sports Med* 2008;36:1618-1624. doi:10.1177/0363546508321482.

and nearby neurovascular structures should be identified and protected. Tenodesis to the brachialis also should be considered as a reasonable backup technique for treating a patient with a chronic injury and activity-related pain, with the expectation that supination strength may not improve.[5] This technique usually allows accelerated rehabilitation. At the time of repair or reconstruction, tension should be tested in elbow extension to assess the security of the repair as well as any limitations pertaining to the progression of the postoperative rehabilitation program.

Multiple studies have evaluated methods of radial tuberosity fixation. In a comparison of fixation strength in cyclic loading when transosseous tunnels and suture anchors were used, there was no specimen failure at 50 N over 3,600 cycles; the mean load to failure was significantly higher for osseous tunnels.[17] These results were confirmed in a second study.[18] A comparison of intact tendons and injured tendons repaired with interference screws found no significant difference, and interference screws had significantly higher mean failure strength and stiffness in comparison with interosseous tunnels.[19] An evaluation of several fixation techniques found that the use of cortical buttons achieved the highest load, stiffness, and cyclical load to failure, possibly allowing an earlier and more aggressive rehabilitation.[20,21] A systematic review of biomechanical studies found that the EndoButton (Smith and Nephew) was the best performing fixation device[13] (**Table 2**). When a cortical button and an interference screw were used for dual fixation to allow an aggressive rehabilitation protocol, most patients returned to normal daily activity within 4 weeks of surgery.[22]

After surgery, the elbow is typically immobilized for 7 to 10 days in 90° of flexion and supination. A hinged elbow brace may be used to protect the repair and block full extension for 6 to 8 weeks, based on the identified postrepair intraoperative tension. At this point, periods

Table 2

Biomechanical Studies of Distal Biceps Fixation

	Single Load-to-Failure Testing		Cyclic Testing	
Fixation Method	Ultimate Tensile Load (N)	Stiffness (N/mm)	Ultimate Tensile Load (N)	Displacement (mm)
Transosseous tunnel	125-210	15.9	195-310	3.55
Interference screw	131-192	30.4	232	2.15
EndoButton	159	—	249-440	2.58-3.42
Suture anchor	105-263	—	209-381	2.06-2.38

Adapted with permission from Chavan PR, Duquin TR, Bisson LJ: Repair of the ruptured distal biceps tendon: A systematic review. *Am J Sports Med* 2008;36:1618-1624. doi:10.1177/0363546508321482.

of unrestricted motion gradually are increased with the use of strengthening exercises. The patient usually is able to resume unrestricted activities 5 to 6 months after surgery, depending on the symptoms, strength, and endurance. Patients follow a similar course after repairs or reconstruction of a chronic injury. A patient who has undergone soft-tissue tenodesis to the brachialis is often able to resume unrestricted activities at 3 to 4 months.

Triceps Injuries

Evaluation

Approximately 0.8% of all tendon ruptures involve the distal triceps.[23] Most distal triceps ruptures occur in men and are associated with anabolic steroid use or weightlifting. The condition also is associated with metabolic bone disease, renal osteodystrophy, olecranon bursitis, Marfan syndrome, osteogenesis imperfecta, rheumatoid arthritis, and diabetes. The three heads of the triceps converge to insert over a wide footprint (average, 466 mm^2) on the olecranon, and most injuries occur at this osseous insertion.[23] The most common mechanism of injury is a sudden eccentric load to a contracted triceps. The patient has pain, swelling, and ecchymosis, with a palpable defect. Not all complete tears prevent active extension, but an absence of active extension signifies a complete tear. An intact lateral expansion or compensatory anconeus may allow active extension. A modified Thompson squeeze test may be positive if the patient is in the prone position with the arm hanging over the edge of the table. AP and lateral radiographs may reveal flecks of bone. MRI can be helpful in determining whether the rupture is complete or partial.[23] Eight of 10 partial ruptures were found to involve the medial insertion.[24] In 801 consecutive elbow MRI examinations, a triceps tear was found in 28 patients, including 5 women and 23 men. Partial tears were more common than complete tears.[25] The most common symptom was pain, typically after an athletic injury.

Management

The management of a triceps tear is dictated by patient-specific factors as well as the tear location and completeness and the patient's functional extension strength. A partial tear in a patient who is debilitated and has low physical demands can be managed nonsurgically. In general, tears smaller than 50% have been managed nonsurgically with satisfactory results.[24,26] A nonsurgically treated weightlifter with bilateral partial ruptures had normal function at 41 weeks and fatigue with lifting at 55 weeks.[27] Complete tears or tears of more than 50% are best treated surgically in an active patient. Chronic ruptures (of more than 6 weeks' duration) are more challenging, and multiple repair and reconstruction techniques have been described.[23]

Early primary repair (within 2 weeks of injury) is recommended for a complete tear with substantial loss of strength. Most commonly, transosseous holes are drilled, and whipstitch sutures are tied over a bone bridge. As an alternative, a bone anchor technique may be considered. An anatomic footprint repair technique has been described that resembles the suture-bridge technique for the rotator cuff[28] (**Figure 2**). When cylindrically loaded, this repair configuration had less repair site motion than a cruciate or a suture anchor repair, possibly allowing earlier rehabilitation.

The elbow is immobilized in 30° to 45° of flexion for 2 weeks after surgery. Passive extension and active guided flexion are begun at 2 weeks, with full active range of motion attained by 4 weeks. Aggressive weightlifting should be avoided for 4 to 6 months. Complications such as bursitis, flexion contractures, and rerupture can occur.

Posterior Elbow (Triceps) Tendinosis

Triceps tendinosis or posterior tennis elbow also is called boxer's elbow. This relatively uncommon overuse condition involves the insertion of the triceps into the posterior elbow with synovitis of the olecranon fossa. Repetitive rapid extensions of the elbow, such as

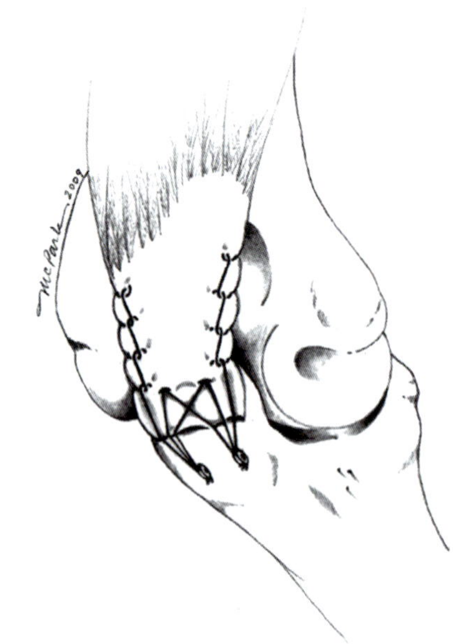

FIGURE 2 Schematic drawing showing a triceps repair with an anatomic technique. (Reproduced with permission from Yeh PC, Stephens KT, Solovyova O, et al: The distal triceps tendon footprint and a biomechanical analysis of 3 repair techniques. *Am J Sports Med* 2010;38[5]:1025-1033. doi:10.1177/0363546509358319.)

in throwing, punching, blocking (in football linemen), tennis serving, and weightlifting, are implicated in the pathology. Osteophyte and loose body formation with synovitis in the olecranon fossa frequently coexist as a result of the rapid and violent extension characteristic of boxing and overhead sports motions. Bursitis, posterior medial impingement, olecranon stress fracture, or olecranon apophysitis (in an adolescent) should be included in the differential diagnosis. The histopathology of triceps tendinosis is identical to that of medial and lateral tendinosis, with the potential for associated olecranon fossa synovitis and loose bodies. Extension blockade and flexion contractures may be encountered. The nonsurgical physical therapy methods are similar to those used for tennis elbow, but with extension blockade, the treatment plan should include posterior, medial, and lateral gliding of the ulna on the humerus.[29-31]

The recommended surgical approach for posterior tennis elbow is a small longitudinal posterior incision centered over the palpably sensitive area. An elliptical excision of the tissue with angiofibroblastic tendinosis changes is undertaken. A spur at the tip of the olecranon, if present, should be removed. In the throwing athlete, triceps tendinosis most commonly is associated with olecranon fossa synovitis, chondromalacia, osteophytes, and/or loose bodies, and it should be surgically treated.[32] The postoperative management is similar to that of lateral and medial elbow conditions.

Lateral Elbow Tendinosis

Lateral elbow tendinosis or tennis elbow most commonly is caused by tendon overuse and failure of tendon healing. This condition typically occurs during the fourth or fifth decade of life, affects the dominant extremity, and is equally common in men and women. The pathoanatomy is a noninflammatory, degenerative angiofibroblastic hyperplasia, possibly attributable to an inadequate healing response to microtearing. The tissue typically is dull, gray, and friable, and on gross examination, it often is edematous (**Figures 3** and **4**). The specific areas of the lateral elbow involve the extensor carpi radialis brevis (ECRB)–extensor digitorum communis (EDC) complex. The ECRB is involved in 100% of incidences, and the anterior edge of the EDC is involved in 65%. The primary goal of nonsurgical treatment is to revitalize the pain-producing unhealthy tissue so that it becomes healthy and does not produce pain. The patient risk factors for tendon overuse include age older than 35 years, a high activity level, a demanding activity technique, and an inadequate fitness level. Activities that can lead to lateral elbow tendinosis are listed in **Table 3**. The associated conditions include medial epicondylitis tendinosis, cubital tunnel syndrome, carpal tunnel syndrome, and rotator cuff tendinosis. A patient with all of these conditions is said to have mesenchymal syndrome. In approximately 5% of patients, anterolateral joint chondromalacia and synovitis are associated with lateral tennis elbow.[30,33-35]

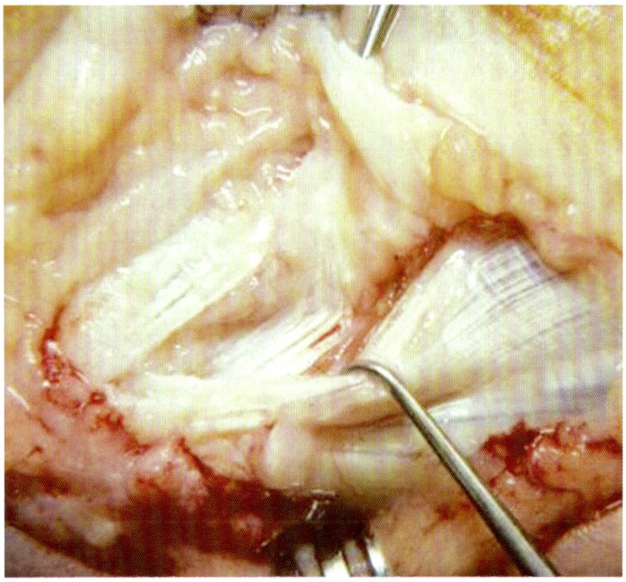

FIGURE 3 Intraoperative photograph showing gross pathologic angiofibroblastic hyperplastic tendinosis tissue. (Courtesy of Robert P. Nirschl, MD, MS, Photo file.)

Evaluation

An insidious onset of activity-related pain is followed by pain at rest and dysfunction as the pathologic change becomes extensive. The maximal tenderness on palpation is slightly (5 mm) distal and anterior to the lateral epicondyle. The patient has pain with provocative manual stress testing, such as resisted wrist and finger extension with the elbow in extended and flexed positions. Pain with the elbow flexed suggests substantial tendinosis damage. Functional strength loss can be measured using a dynamometer. Range of motion typically is within

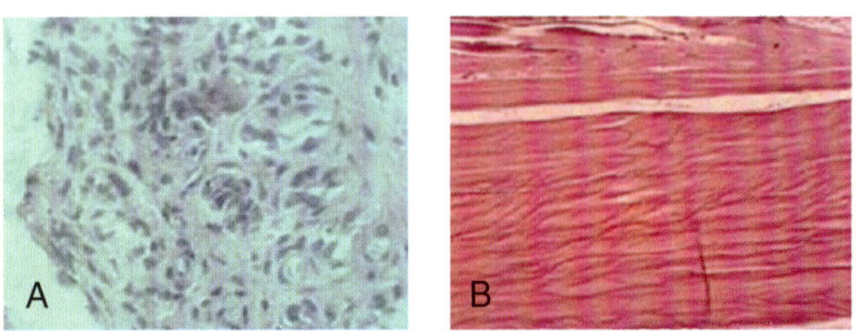

FIGURE 4 Histologic appearance of angiofibroblastic hyperplastic tendinosis (**A**) and normal tendon (**B**). (Reprinted from Clin Sports Med 2003;22[4]. Nirschl RP, Ashman ES: Tennis elbow tendinosis (epicondylitis), 813-836. Copyright © 2003 Elsevier, Inc. doi:10.1016/S0278-5919(03)00051-6.)

Table 3

Common Activities Leading to Epicondylitis

Activity	Lateral Epicondylitis	Medial Epicondylitis
Sports	Tennis (groundstrokes) Racquetball Squash Fencing	Golf Rowing Baseball (pitching) Javelin throwing Tennis (serving)
Occupational or other	Meat cutting Plumbing Painting Raking Weaving	Bricklaying Hammering Typing Textile production

Reproduced from Jobe FW, Ciccotti MG: Lateral and medial epicondylitis of the elbow. *J Am Acad Orthop Surg* 1994;2(1):1-8.

normal limits. The medial and posterior tendons should be assessed, with evaluation of the cubital tunnel, any posterior interosseous nerve (PIN) entrapment (3 to 4 cm distal), the cervical spine, and the carpel tunnel (a 10% association), each of which may represent an associated finding.[30] The strength of the rotator cuff should be assessed because weakness on the ipsilateral side is common and should be treated during rehabilitation. Elbow stability also should be evaluated and treated. The cervical and thoracic spine, the upper extremity, and sports mechanics should be assessed. Radiographic evaluation is recommended because 20% of patients have tendon calcification or lateral epicondyle reactive exostosis.[30] MRI is rarely needed for diagnosis, but it reveals edema and thickening at the extensor origin in 90% of patients with symptoms. Ultrasonography has moderate sensitivity and variable specificity, depending on the study and the examiner.[34]

The Posterior Interosseous Nerve

A 1972 report described surgical management of presumed tennis elbow by decompressing the PIN at the canal of Frohse, and lateral tennis elbow has been linked to PIN entrapment.[36] Nonetheless, there is no compelling evidence that PIN entrapment is a cause of lateral elbow tendinosis. Although the PIN is anatomically adjacent to the location of lateral elbow tendinosis, the possibility of an independent PIN condition should be considered. PIN entrapment is difficult to diagnose. The symptoms include a vague aching sensation over the extensor muscle mass and pain with resisted supination. Electromyography and a xylocaine block may aid in the diagnosis. Surgical nerve decompression often is unsuccessful, in part perhaps because of misdiagnosis.

Nonsurgical Management

The management of lateral elbow tendinosis should complement the natural biologic healing response in an ordered progression to enhance the sequence of neovascularization and collagen production. Treatment should begin by controlling inflammatory exudation and hemorrhage to relieve pain and then promoting specific tissue healing, general fitness, and control of force loads or violence. Some patients may require surgical removal of pathologic tissue, but the initial treatment should consist of protection, rest, ice, compression, elevation, medications (specifically, NSAIDs), and activity modification. Lateral elbow tendinosis histologically is not an inflammatory condition, but anti-inflammatory medications can control pain caused by chemical mediators and relieve associated synovitis or inflammation in the surrounding adipose and connective tissue.[30,32] When diclofenac was compared with placebo, patients receiving diclofenac reported lower levels of pain.[37] There was no significant difference when naproxen was compared with placebo.[38] Healing is promoted through concentric and eccentric rehabilitative exercise, high-voltage transcutaneous electrical nerve stimulation, aerobic and general conditioning exercise, absence from abuse, and possibly ultrasonography. General body conditioning can maintain or improve body fitness and stimulate healing of the injured tissue. Force load control is used to minimize potential injury-producing activities by counterforce bracing treatment, improvement in sports technique, control of the intensity and the duration of activity, and equipment evaluation.[30]

Steroid injections have been used for pain control but cannot be considered capable of tissue healing. Although steroid injections led to early good results, at 1-year follow-up, the results were no better or even worse than those of treatment with NSAIDs or physical therapy.[39] The excessive use of steroid injections (more than three focused injections) could cause harm to the underlying tissue, leading to further weakness and possibly tendon rupture. The injection technique is important; the needle should be placed under the ECRB, not at the epicondyle. The use of botulinum toxin A for pain control had conflicting results at 3 months, with no significant improvement in patients' grip strength.[40] It is possible that the use of botulinum toxin A could lead to muscle atrophy because of loss of use and worsening symptoms. A 2010 level I study found significant improvement in scores on the visual analog and Disabilities of the Arm, Shoulder and Hand scales when platelet-rich plasma (PRP) was used compared with steroid injection.[41] Patients treated with steroid injection had improved early results that were not sustained; patients treated with PRP had progressively improving results, with continued significant improvement at 1-year follow-up and no complications. A similar level I study reported similar results at 2-year follow-up.[42] PRP also was found to offer greater improvement than autologous whole blood.[43] A long-term biologic cure has yet to be found.

Extracorporeal shock wave therapy has been used for a variety of tendinopathies, but meta-analysis of nine placebo-controlled studies found conflicting results and no significant benefit over placebo.[44] Ultrasound-guided percutaneous radiofrequency lesioning led to a 78% reduction in symptoms.[45] Nitric oxide delivered with glyceryl trinitrate patches was found to offer no benefit over placebo in a 5-year prospective study.[46] General studies of nonsurgical treatment reported that 83% of patients had improvement at 1-year follow-up, but 40% continued to have minor discomfort at 5-year follow-up.[47,48] The negative prognostic indicators included manual work and a high level of baseline pain.

Surgical Management and Indications

Pain is the major indication for surgery. The answers to three questions should be considered: Is the pain of significant intensity to limit function? Does the pain interfere with the patient's daily activity or occupation? Is the pain and tenderness precisely located at the origin of the ECRB adjacent to the lateral epicondyle? Surgery may be considered after a period of high-quality nonsurgical management, usually of at least approximately 6 months' duration. Surgery may be contraindicated, and a careful reevaluation is necessary if the nonsurgical program was inadequate, the patient has been noncompliant, or the patient has a workers' compensation claim with a secondary gain component.[35]

The Nirschl mini-open techniques have gradually been refined since being originally described in 1979[35,49] (**Figure 5**). A 2.5-cm straight lateral incision is made, passing just anteromedial to the lateral epicondyle. A too-distal or too-medial incision is common by less experienced surgeons and should be avoided. The interface between the extensor carpi radialis longus (ECRL) and the aponeurosis of the EDC should be identified after dissection of bursal and adipose tissue; the ECRL typically is less firm than the extensor aponeurosis, and the fibers of the ECRL run more obliquely. The ECRL-EDC interval is vertically incised to a depth of 1 to 2 mm, just anteromedial to the epicondyle and in line with the EDC fibers. Sharp dissection proceeds in a more horizontal plane to allow medial retraction of the ECRL to expose the pathologic tissue in the ECRB. Dissection of the ECRL-EDC interval vertically beyond the 1- to 2-mm depth is a common error that distorts a clean exposure and identification of the ECRB. With anteromedial retraction of the ECRL, the diagonally oriented fibers of the ECRB come into view as they attach to the EDC and the anteromedial edge of the lateral epicondyle. The pathologic tissue can be identified in the ECRB as dull, gray, friable, and often edematous. This tissue is incised en block in an elliptical fashion, leaving the distal attachments of the ECRB. The ECRB has remaining distal attachments to the capsule, the orbicular ligament, the distal anterior extensor aponeurosis, and the underside of the ECRL and, as a result, does not retract more than 1 to 2 mm. An essentially normal mechanical ECRB working length thus is maintained. Suture repair of the remaining ECRB is therefore unnecessary and, if done, invites a flexion contracture. Any questionable tissue in the EDC can be evaluated and removed using the Nirschl scratch maneuver; normal tissue appears shiny and firm, with a yellowish white hue. Sixty-five percent of patients have tendinosis changes carry friable tissue at the anteromedial underside edge of the EDC, which constitutes approximately 15% of the EDC volume. Under no circumstances should the origin of the EDC be released from the epicondyle. Epicondyle bony exostosis is present in approximately 20% of patients and almost always is anteromedial; therefore, it is unnecessary to remove any of the epicondyle, but only the small anteromedial exostosis. When all pathologic tissue has been resected, one small hole can be drilled in the exposed cortical bone distal to the epicondyle but not in the epicondyle itself to enhance the vascular supply. If intra-articular pathology is suspected, the incision can be extended 0.5 cm distally, and a small longitudinal joint opening can be made in the capsule anterior to the radial collateral ligament.

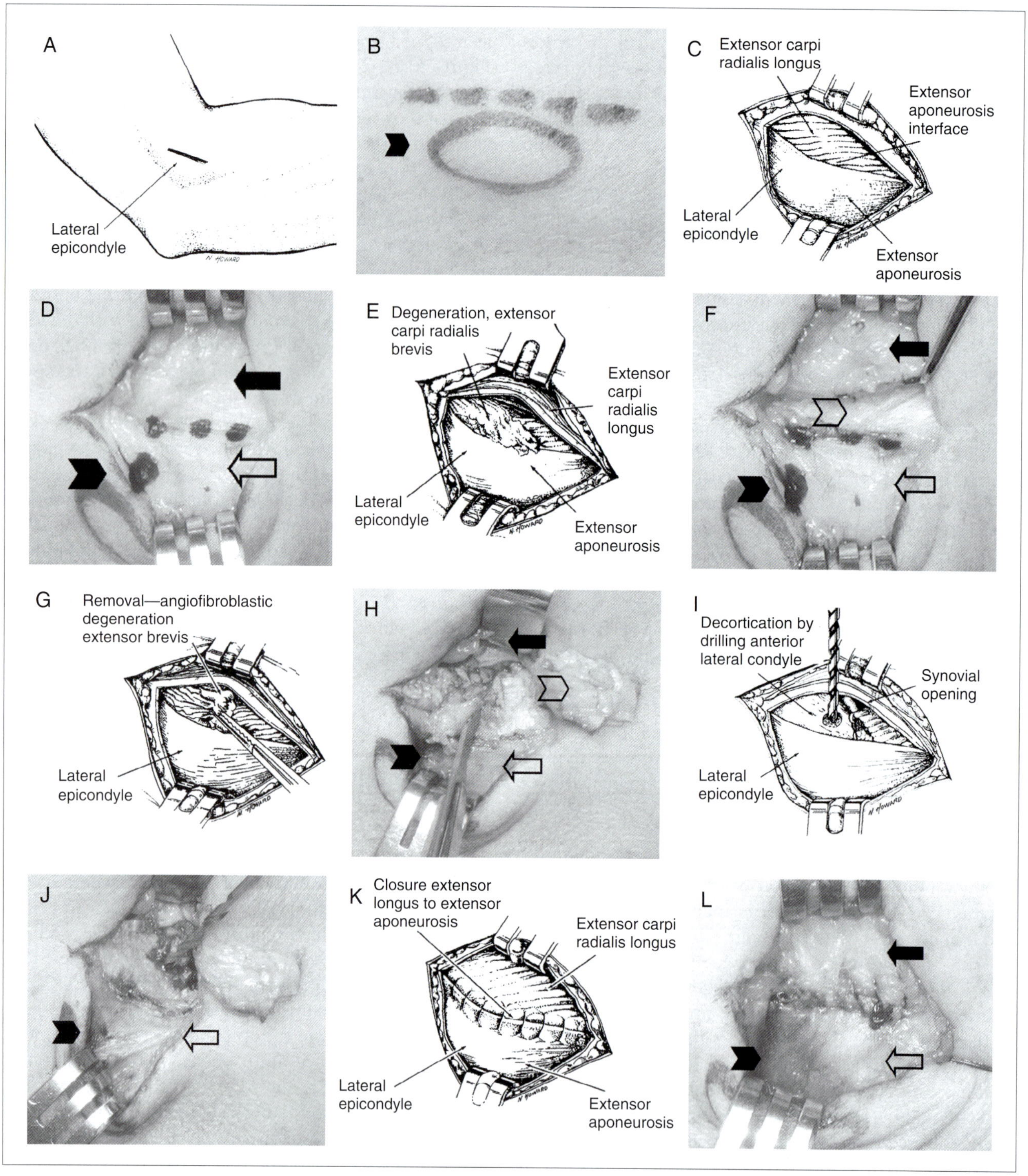

FIGURE 5 Matched schematic drawings and photographs showing the mini-open Nirschl technique for treating lateral tennis elbow. **A** and **B**, The 2.5-cm incision passes just anteromedial to the lateral epicondyle. **C** and **D**, The interface between the extensor carpi radialis longus (ECRL) and the extensor aponeurosis is identified. **E** and **F**, The incision is deepened to 2 to 3 mm, and the ECRL is retracted as the extensor carpi radialis brevis (ECRB) is seen. Grayish edematous pathologic tissue should be visible. **G** and **H**, Degenerated ECRB is removed. **I** and **J**, A hole is drilled through the cortical bone of the anterior lateral condyle to the cancellous bone level to enhance the vascular supply. **K** and **L**, The ECRL is firmly repaired to the anterior margin of the extensor digitorum communis (EDC). Because the ECRB is still attached to adjacent tissues, it is not necessary to suture the distal brevis. Black arrowheads = lateral epicondyle; black arrows = ECRL; clear arrowheads = tendinosis tissue; clear arrows = extensor aponeurosis. (Reprinted from Clin Sports Med 2003;22[4]. Nirschl RP, Ashman ES: Tennis elbow tendinosis (epicondylitis), 813-836. Copyright © 2003 Elsevier, Inc. doi:10.1016/S0278-5919(03)00051-6.)

Associated intra-articular pathology (most commonly synovitis or a plica) is found in only approximately 5% of patients with lateral tendinosis. Occasionally, a full-thickness tear of the ECRB extends into the joint. If this is present, any intra-articular pathology can be evaluated. The capsule should be repaired to prevent postoperative leakage of synovial fluid. The ECRB still has firm distal attachments as noted; therefore, repair is unnecessary. A side-to-side suture repair of the ECRL to the EDC is performed, burying the knots or using the Quill knotless closure device (Angiotech). In the uncommon situation in which the joint is opened, the capsule is closed with absorbable suture. A subcuticular closure is performed, and a sterile dressing is applied.[35] The postoperative management is similar to that of lateral, medial, or posterior tendinosis.

The Role of Arthroscopy

In comparison with an open or a mini-open procedure, arthroscopic débridement and release are reported to require less postoperative physical therapy, allow an earlier return to work, and provide the ability to treat associated intra-articular pathology.[50-54] The arthroscopic appearance of the lateral capsule was classified by the authors of a 2000 study.[55] The degenerative capsule and the undersurface of the ECRB are released from the lateral epicondyle by a mechanical shaver. The major concerns are iatrogenic cartilage injury, neurovascular injury, and inadequate débridement of the pathologic tissue. In a revealing study, open inspection after arthroscopic débridement revealed that 10 of 18 patients had residual gross pathologic tissue and an additional 4 patients had residual microscopic pathology.[56] In response, the technique was altered to use a curved radiofrequency probe rather than a shaver.[57] Other negative aspects of the arthroscopic technique compared with an open or a mini-open technique include increases in instrument costs, setup time, surgical time, and the learning curve. In comparison with the mini-open technique, the arthroscopic technique has no demonstrated advantages related to results or rehabilitation times. In addition, surgical failure is more likely as accurate resection of pain-producing pathologic tissue is often not accomplished.

Surgical Results

The ECRB open resection technique was found to lead to complete pain relief and return of full forearm strength in 85% of patients, and an additional 12% had significant pain relief.[49] The remaining 3% reported no pain relief or strength improvement; these patients included those with a workers' compensation claim. Complications were reported in 1% of patients. In a 10- to 14-year follow-up study using the Nirschl mini-open ECRB resection, the success rate was 97%.[58] A study of 19 patients who underwent open EDC release, excision, and reattachment found improvement in 18 patients, but 60% of those who played a high-demand sport and 15% of those with a high-demand job had changed their sport or job after the surgery.[59] A long-term prospective study of lateral EDC release found that 40% had persistent pain 6 weeks after surgery, 24% had persistent pain at 1 year, and 9% had persistent pain at 5 years.[60] A comparison of the old open Nirschl technique with a percutaneous EDC release technique found greater improvement in Disabilities of the Arm, Shoulder and Hand scores and patient satisfaction as well as a more rapid return to work in patients treated with the percutaneous technique.[61] Three studies of arthroscopic techniques found that 93% to 100% of patients had improvement at 2-year follow-up, but only 62% to 80% achieved complete pain relief.[51,52,54] At a minimum 2-year follow-up, a comparison of 44 patients treated with an arthroscopic procedure, 41 treated with a varying open procedure, and 24 treated with a percutaneous release identified no statistically significant differences; the 5.8% of patients who experienced a recurrence included three patients in the percutaneous group, one in the arthroscopic group, and two in the open group.[62] A comparison of open release and arthroscopic procedures found no statistically significant difference at 6-month follow-up; 70% of patients had a good or excellent result.[53]

The most common reason surgery is unsuccessful and the patient continues to have pain is the surgeon's failure to adequately remove the pathologic tendinosis tissue. This situation is common in an extensor release procedure, which is intended to weaken the force generator rather than resect pathologic tissue. It has been noted that the patients seeking second opinions following failed surgery invariably had variations of the aforementioned release techniques. Nirschl revision surgery, in which residual ECRB tendinosis tissue was resected, had an 83% success rate in 35 patients.[63] Other complications reflecting inadequate technique include excessive débridement with harm to the collateral ligament, which compromised stability; neuroma of a cutaneous radial branch as it crosses 1.5 cm anterior to the lateral epicondyle; reactive bone formation; and lateral epicondylar pain associated with epicondyle excision.[33]

Medial Elbow Tendinosis

Medial tendinosis (golfer's elbow) is caused by overuse-induced trauma to the wrist flexor-pronator muscle group. Pain and tenderness are centered about the common flexor origin at the medial epicondyle, which serves as the attachment point for the wrist flexor-pronator muscle groups and the ulnar collateral ligament. The primary tendons involved in the pathology are the flexor carpi radialis, the pronator teres, and, to a lesser extent, the flexor carpi ulnaris (in 5% of patients).[33,35] These three tendons have a confluent attachment site. The histologic changes are the same as in lateral tendinosis. The incidence of medial elbow tendinosis is approximately one-fifth that of lateral tendinosis. Young and middle-aged athletes are affected, and the condition has a peak incidence during the fourth and fifth decades of life.

Evaluation

Pain in medial elbow tendinosis can be reproduced with resisted wrist flexion and pronation, in which the elbow is extended while the wrist is extended and supinated. Palpable tenderness is present at and slightly distal to the epicondyle. Full range of motion is typical, but a slight loss of extension can occur. As with lateral elbow tendinosis, the medial elbow injury occurs as a result of failure of the tendon to adapt to overuse activity. Associated conditions include ulnar collateral ligament injury with valgus instability, which should be suspected in an overhead throwing athlete, and cubital tunnel syndrome. Ulnar nerve involvement, most notably in zone 3 of the medial epicondylar groove, is found in as many as 40% of patients and should be carefully evaluated.[33,35] The mechanics of overuse include repetitive wrist flexion and forearm pronation, as are common in racquet and throwing sports and in golf, in which the trailing arm is affected. Pronator syndrome and anterior interosseous nerve compression syndrome are uncommon but are included in the differential diagnosis. An adolescent athlete with medial elbow pain should be evaluated for Little Leaguer's elbow (medial apophysitis and lateral radial capitellar compression). The radiographs typically are normal but may reveal intra-articular issues, such as osteophytic spurs, in a high-demand athlete. MRI usually is unnecessary but may be helpful if an ulnar collateral ligament abnormality is suspected.[30,33,35]

Nonsurgical Management

The management of medial elbow tendinosis begins with nonsurgical treatment similar to that of lateral tendinosis, which has reported success rates of 88% to 96%.[64] In a level I comparison study, pain control was significantly improved at 6-week follow-up in patients treated with steroid injection rather than saline, but there was no difference at 3 months or 1 year.[65] Ultrasound-guided autologous blood injection led to improvement in scores on the visual analog and modified Nirschl scales at 4-week and 10-month follow-up.[66]

Surgical Management

A patient whose condition does not respond to high-quality nonsurgical management within 6 or more months can be considered for surgery. Surgical intervention through a mini-open approach is used to excise the degenerative tissue and reapproximate the normal healthy tissue (**Figure 6**). The skin incision is 4 cm long and parallels the medial epicondylar groove just posterior to the medial epicondyle, extending from 1 cm proximal to 3 cm distal. This **posteriorly** placed incision avoids branches of the medial antebrachial cutaneous nerve. The dissection is carried through the subcutaneous tissue to the deep fascia covering the ulnar head of the flexor carpi ulnaris, and then progresses anterolaterally, with retraction of subcutaneous tissue and skin over the medial epicondyle to expose the common flexor origin. Pathologic changes often are intratendinous, and most of the tendinosis may not be visible at this time. However, some tendinosis and softening almost always is detectable at the superficial layer. The most common pathologic areas are at the interface of the pronator teres and the flexor carpi radialis extending 2 to 3 cm distally from the tip of the epicondyle. It is important to understand the patient's primary area of palpable tenderness before anesthesia is administered because this information is useful for identifying the probable location of the tendinosis. A longitudinal split is made in the tendon at its origin and extending 2 to 3 cm distally, in line with the fibers. The tendon is separated, and the hidden pathologic tissue can be observed. This tissue is elliptically excised, and the Nirschl scratch test (eg, scraping briskly with the scalpel) is performed to evaluate the surrounding tissue. All normal tissue will resist the scratch maneuver and will remain intact. The common flexor origin is a key medial elbow stabilizer, and any release of a normal common flexor tendon is to be avoided. To enhance the potential for neovascularization, a drill bit no larger than 5/64 inch is used to drill one hole though the cortical bone distal to the epicondyle. Drilling into the epicondyle itself may lead to increased postoperative pain and is to be avoided.[30]

Forty percent of patients have concomitant cubital tunnel syndrome, and decompression of zone 3 of the medial epicondylar groove is undertaken. Zone 3 is distal to the epicondyle, and compression neurapraxia is most common in this zone (**Figure 7**). Nerve compression rarely occurs in zone 1 (proximal to the

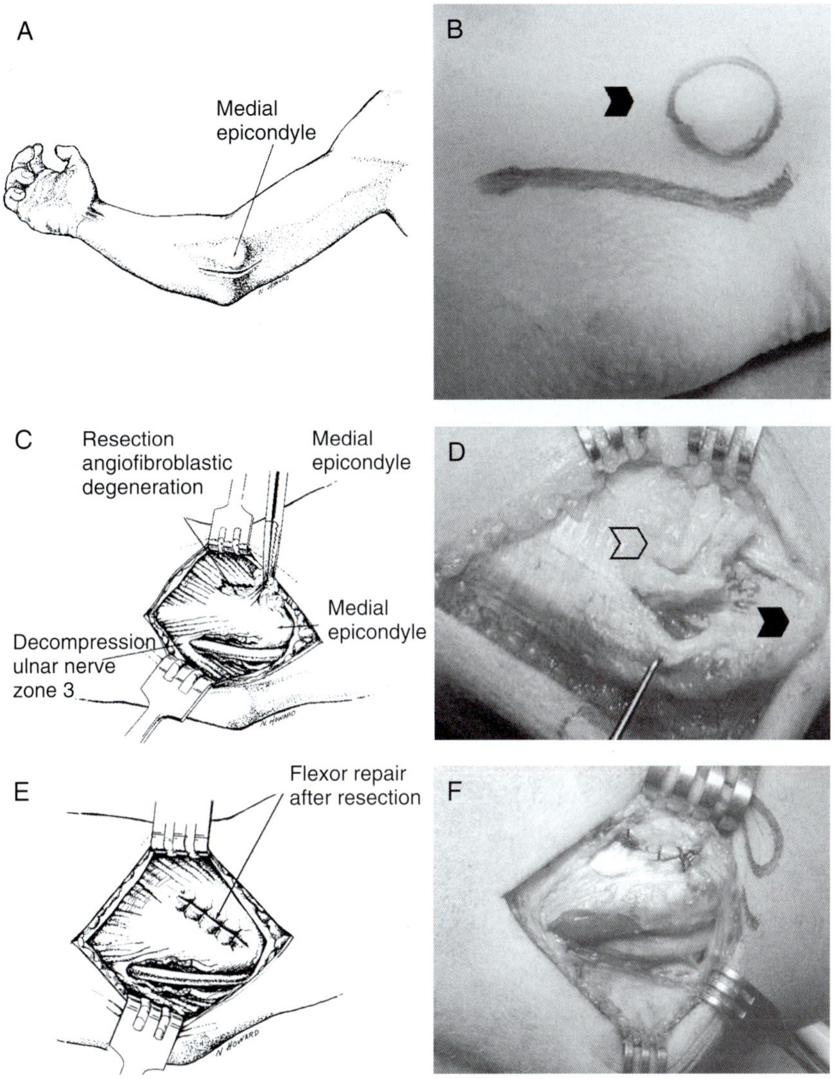

FIGURE 6 Matched schematic drawings and photographs showing the mini-open Nirschl technique for treating medial tennis elbow. **A** and **B**, The incision is made from the tip of the medial epicondyle distally for 3 to 4 cm, with care to avoid harming the sensory cutaneous nerve (medial antebrachial nerve) just anterior to the medial epicondyle. **C** and **D**, Resection of the angiofibroblastic tendinosis. The angiofibroblastic changes usually are located in the origin of the pronator teres and the flexor carpi radialis. The pathologic tissue is removed in a longitudinal and elliptical fashion, leaving normal tissue attachments intact. Ulnar nerve dysfunction is clinically detected in 60% of patients, and the ulnar nerve in zone 3 is decompressed. **E** and **F**, Repair of the common flexor origin. The medial epicondylar attachments of normal tissue are not disturbed. Black arrowheads = medial epicondyle; clear arrowheads = tendinosis tissue. (Reprinted from Clin Sports Med 2003;22[4]. Nirschl RP, Ashman ES: Tennis elbow tendinosis (epicondylitis), 813-836. Copyright © 2003 Elsevier, Inc. doi:10.1016/S0278-5919(03)00051-6.)

epicondyle) or zone 2 (at the epicondyle). Release of the cubital tunnel retinaculum and the flexor carpi ulnaris arcade is essential for adequately decompressing zone 3. After decompression, elbow flexion and extension are performed to ensure the nerve does not dislocate from the groove and is not under tension. If this uncommon instability is present or if nerve dysfunction is secondary to tension, full anterior ulnar nerve transfer can be considered.[33] The elliptical resection tendon defect is closed with a side-to-side suture repair while the knots are buried. This closure tends to enhance the decompression of the ulnar nerve at zone 3. A subcutaneous closure is performed, and a sterile dressing is applied.

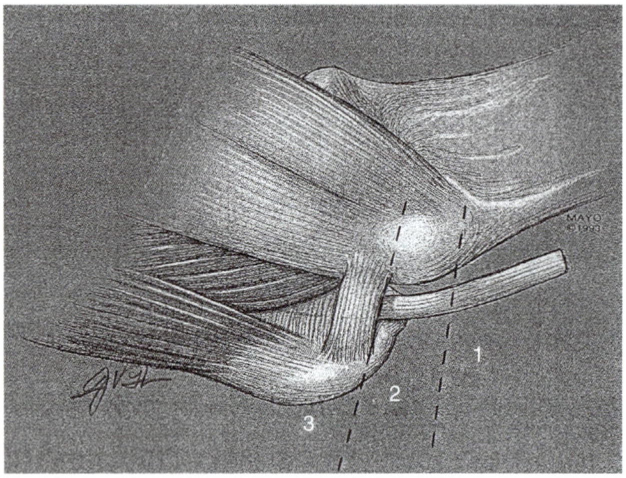

FIGURE 7 Schematic drawing showing the cubital tunnel zones of the ulnar nerve. Zone 1 is proximal to the epicondyle, zone 2 is at the medial epicondyle, and zone 3 is distal to the medial epicondyle (cubital tunnel retinaculum). Most ulnar nerve compression associated with medial elbow tendinosis occurs as compression of the cubital tunnel retinaculum in zone 3. (Reproduced with permission from Nirschl RP: Lateral and medial epicondylitis, in Morrey BF, ed: *Master Techniques in Orthopaedic Surgery: The Elbow*. New York, NY, Raven, 1994, pp 129-148.)

A medial epicondylectomy and a complete common flexor origin release are reported alternatives but are not recommended, as the authors have consulted on such patients with not only a failed result, but iatrogenic harm.

Reports on the outcomes of medial elbow tendinosis surgery are limited to only four studies. One study found involvement of the ulnar nerve in 23% of the patients and concomitant lateral epicondylitis in 20%. Objective function scores improved from 38% to 98% after surgery. In 86% of the patients, use of the elbow was not limited during daily activities or sports activities.[67] A 90% improvement also has been reported.[68] In a third study, at 7-year follow-up, 87% of the patients had a good or excellent result after débridement of the common flexor origin and decompression of the ulnar nerve (53% involvement); before surgery, 62% of these patients had a predisposition to overuse syndromes, as indicated by a concomitant musculotendinous dysfunction or a history of such dysfunction.[64] These findings emphasize the importance of evaluating and treating the entire patient and, specifically, the entire upper extremity. In the fourth study, the authors reported on 50 cases with an average follow-up of 37 months. Twelve patients (24%) all had concomitant ulnar nerve symptoms which were addressed at the time of surgery. Postoperatively, all patients reported partial or complete pain relief. Fourteen patients who had preoperative pain at rest had no rest pain postoperatively. Dynamometer grip strength testing increased from 92 to 107 lb on average. Ten patients decided not to return to their preinjury level of sports activity.[68]

Postoperative Management

Lateral, medial, and posterior elbow tendinosis require similar postoperative management. The arm is immobilized in 90° of flexion and neutral rotation for 48 hours, and active motion exercises are started after this time. The elbow immobilizer is used as needed during the next 3 to 5 days, with activities of daily living initiated at 3 to 4 days. Active range of motion without resistance is begun within 3 to 4 days, as are neck and shoulder exercises. At 3 weeks, resistance exercise is started with 1-lb weights. A counterforce brace is used during the next 2 months and later at the patient's discretion. A gradual return to high-demand activities begins 6 to 8 weeks after surgery. A full return to unrestricted activities usually is possible by 4 to 6 months. **Table 4** presents the three phases of rehabilitation after elbow tendinosis surgery.

Combined Medial and Lateral Elbow Tendinosis

The signs and symptoms of elbow tendinosis often occurring simultaneously include those of both medial and lateral tendinosis. This condition is most commonly diagnosed in recreational golfers and tennis players and is known as country club elbow. In the only reported study of country club elbow, 53 elbows were surgically treated after unsuccessful nonsurgical treatment and followed up for an average of 11.7 years (minimum, 5 years).[69] The average score on the Nirschl Tennis Elbow Scale, the Numeric Pain Intensity Scale, and the American Shoulder and Elbow Surgeons scale improved significantly, and 96% of the patients had returned to sports. No patients required revision surgery. One postoperative infection had resolved at 1 month.

The Role of Biologics and New Techniques

High-intensity ultrasonography ablation of tendinosis (Tenex) has been reported to offer a minimally invasive technique to remove tendinosis tissue in an office setting. The technique uses the established concepts of identification and removal of pathologic tissue in a less invasive manner and shows promise.[70]

In the past decade, the concept of regeneration of tendinosis tissue by biologics has received considerable attention and investigation. PRP studies have been widely circulated with very mixed results. Issues of PRP

Table 4

Physical Therapy Program for Medial and Lateral Elbow Tendinosis

Stage 1

Elbow position: Flexed to 90° and supported on the patient's lower extremities

Frequency: Once daily

Exercises: Isotonic wrist flexion, extension, and pronation-supination

Progression: Repetitions and resistance are increased as tolerated without an increase in symptoms until 30 repetitions with a 3-lb weight can be performed on for 2 consecutive days without an increase in symptoms.

Stage 2

Elbow position: More extended position with less support from the lower extremities

Frequency: Once daily

Exercises: Isotonic wrist flexion, extension, and pronation-supination. Resistance is decreased from 3 lb to 2 lb or 1 lb, depending on patient tolerance.

Progression: Repetitions and resistance are increased as tolerated without an increase in symptoms until 30 repetitions with a 3-lb weight can be performed for 2 consecutive days without an increase in symptoms.

Stage 3

Elbow position: Fully extended and unsupported

Frequency: Once daily

Exercises: Wrist flexion, extension, and pronation-supination. Resistance is decreased from 3 lb to 2 lb or 1 lb, depending on patient tolerance.

Progression: Repetitions and resistance are increased as tolerated without an increase in symptoms until 30 repetitions with a 3-lb weight can be performed for 2 consecutive days without an increase in symptoms. At this point, the frequency can be decreased to three or four times per week.

Additional Exercise

Finger abduction (splaying) against the resistance of a rubber band and squeezing of an egg, putty, or a stress ball frequently throughout the day to tolerance. Submaximal squeezes are recommended at first, with progressive intensity as the patient advances.

Modification

If the patient has pain during or after exercise persisting longer than 24 hr, the weight, the number of repetitions, or the range of motion is decreased.

Reproduced with permission from Johnson B, Nirschl RP: Overuse injuries of the elbow. *Orthop Phys Ther Clin North Am* 2001;10(4):617-634.

concentration, growth factors, leukocyte concentration, and more advanced methods of blood processing are in various stages of determination.[71] Stem cell therapy is another biologic receiving attention. Further study and clarity of outcomes, therefore, needs to occur in reference to the use of biologics.

SUMMARY

As the understanding of acute and chronic elbow tendon injuries becomes more complete, management is evolving to provide definitively satisfactory results with little morbidity. The development of mini-open surgical techniques is an example of this progress. The successful nonsurgical management of tendinosis begins with a correct diagnosis, an understanding of the injury, and a revitalization of the pathologic tissue through appropriate rehabilitation. Biologics have shown promise, but the current reported results are mixed and inconclusive. Successful surgical intervention focuses on identification of the pathologic tissue and appropriate resection. Further studies on PRP, stem cells, and others, as well as preclinical research, may lead to regenerative treatments at a cellular level.

KEY STUDY POINTS

- Partial or full rupture of distal triceps or biceps is best managed with surgical repair.
- The terms lateral and medial epicondylitis are inaccurate because the maladies are not in the epicondyle and there are no inflammatory cells in the histopathology of these failed tendons. The more accurate descriptive term for these maladies as described in the current literature is angiofibroblastic hyperplasia/tendinosis (eg, collagen disruption and immature dysfunctional vascular and tenocyte elements).
- Tendinosis tissue is pain producing.
- Low-volume tendinosis tissue can be repaired with nonsurgical rehabilitation and possibly biologic stimulation in selected cases.
- High-volume tendinosis tissue is best managed by accurate identification of location and surgical removal (Nirschl technique).

Annotated References

1. Kulshreshtha R, Singh R, Sinha J, Hall S: Anatomy of the distal biceps brachii tendon and its clinical relevance. *Clin Orthop Relat Res* 2007;456:117-120.

2. Miyamoto RG, Elser F, Millett PJ: Distal biceps tendon injuries. *J Bone Joint Surg Am* 2010;92(11):2128-2138.

3. O'Driscoll SW, Goncalves LB, Dietz P: The hook test for distal biceps tendon avulsion. *Am J Sports Med* 2007;35(11):1865-1869.

4. Ruland RT, Dunbar RP, Bowen JD: The biceps squeeze test for diagnosis of distal biceps tendon ruptures. *Clin Orthop Relat Res* 2005;437:128-131.

5. Ramsey ML: Distal biceps tendon injuries: Diagnosis and management. *J Am Acad Orthop Surg* 1999;7(3):199-207.

6. Giuffrè BM, Moss MJ: Optimal positioning for MRI of the distal biceps brachii tendon: Flexed abducted supinated view. *AJR Am J Roentgenol* 2004;182(4):944-946.

7. Hang DW, Bach BR Jr, Bojchuk J: Repair of chronic distal biceps brachii tendon rupture using free autogenous semitendinosus tendon. *Clin Orthop Relat Res* 1996;323:188-191.

8. Bain GI, Johnson LJ, Turner PC: Treatment of partial distal biceps tendon tears. *Sports Med Arthrosc* 2008;16(3):154-161.

9. Morrey BF, ed: *Master Techniques in Orthopaedic Surgery: The Elbow.* New York, NY, Raven, 1994, pp 115-128.

10. D'Alessandro DF, Shields CL Jr, Tibone JE, Chandler RW: Repair of distal biceps tendon ruptures in athletes. *Am J Sports Med* 1993;21(1):114-119.

11. Baker BE, Bierwagen D: Rupture of the distal tendon of the biceps brachii: Operative versus non-operative treatment. *J Bone Joint Surg Am* 1985;67(3):414-417.

12. Davison BL, Engber WD, Tigert LJ: Long term evaluation of repaired distal biceps brachii tendon ruptures. *Clin Orthop Relat Res* 1996;333:186-191.

13. Chavan PR, Duquin TR, Bisson LJ: Repair of the ruptured distal biceps tendon: A systematic review. *Am J Sports Med* 2008;36(8):1618-1624.

14. Bain GI, Prem H, Heptinstall RJ, Verhellen R, Paix D: Repair of distal biceps tendon rupture: A new technique using the EndoButton. *J Shoulder Elbow Surg* 2000;9(2):120-126.

15. Greenberg JA, Fernandez JJ, Wang T, Turner C: EndoButton-assisted repair of distal biceps tendon ruptures. *J Shoulder Elbow Surg* 2003;12(5):484-490.

16. Peeters T, Ching-Soon NG, Jansen N, Sneyers C, Declercq G, Verstreken F: Functional outcome after repair of distal biceps tendon ruptures using the EndoButton technique. *J Shoulder Elbow Surg* 2009;18(2):283-287.

17. Berlet GC, Johnson JA, Milne AD, Patterson SD, King GJ: Distal biceps brachii tendon repair: An in vitro biomechanical study of tendon reattachment. *Am J Sports Med* 1998;26(3):428-432.

18. Pereira DS, Kvitne RS, Liang M, Giacobetti FB, Ebramzadeh E: Surgical repair of distal biceps tendon ruptures: A biomechanical comparison of two techniques. *Am J Sports Med* 2002;30(3):432-436.

19. Idler CS, Montgomery WH III, Lindsey DP, Badua PA, Wynne GF, Yerby SA: Distal biceps tendon repair: A biomechanical comparison of intact tendon and 2 repair techniques. *Am J Sports Med* 2006;34(6):968-974.

20. Kettler M, Lunger J, Kuhn V, Mutschler W, Tingart MJ: Failure strengths in distal biceps tendon repair. *Am J Sports Med* 2007;35(9):1544-1548.

21. Mazzocca AD, Burton KJ, Romeo AA, Santangelo S, Adams DA, Arciero RA: Biomechanical evaluation of 4 techniques of distal biceps brachii tendon repair. *Am J Sports Med* 2007;35(2):252-258.

22. Heinzelmann AD, Savoie FH III, Ramsey JR, Field LD, Mazzocca AD: A combined technique for distal biceps repair using a soft tissue button and biotenodesis interference screw. *Am J Sports Med* 2009;37(5):989-994.

23. Yeh PC, Dodds SD, Smart LR, Mazzocca AD, Sethi PM: Distal triceps rupture. *J Am Acad Orthop Surg* 2010;18(1):31-40.

24. Mair SD, Isbell WM, Gill TJ, Schlegel TF, Hawkins RJ: Triceps tendon ruptures in professional football players. *Am J Sports Med* 2004;32(2):431-434.

25. Koplas MC, Schneider E, Sundaram M: Prevalence of triceps tendon tears on MRI of the elbow and clinical correlation. *Skeletal Radiol* 2011;40(5):587-594.

26. Vidal AF, Drakos MC, Allen AA: Biceps tendon and triceps tendon injuries. *Clin Sports Med* 2004;23(4):707-722, xi.

27. Harris PC, Atkinson D, Moorehead JD: Bilateral partial rupture of triceps tendon: Case report and quantitative assessment of recovery. *Am J Sports Med* 2004;32(3):787-792.

28. Yeh PC, Stephens KT, Solovyova O, et al: The distal triceps tendon footprint and a biomechanical analysis of 3 repair techniques. *Am J Sports Med* 2010;38(5):1025-1033.

29. Johnson B, Nirschl RP: Overuse injuries of the elbow. *Orthop Phys Ther Clin North Am* 2001;10(4):617-634.

30. Nirschl RP, Ashman ES: Tennis elbow tendinosis (epicondylitis). *Instr Course Lect* 2004;53:587-598.

31. Ellenbecker TS, Mattalino AJ: *The Elbow in Sport: Injury Treatment and Rehabilitation.* Champaign, IL, Human Kinetics, 1997.

32. Nirschl RP: Elbow tendinosis/tennis elbow. *Clin Sports Med* 1992;11(4):851-870.

33. Nirschl RP, Davis L: *Wrist and Elbow Reconstruction and Arthroscopy.* Rosemont, IL, American Society for Surgery of the Hand, 2006, pp 513-521.

34. Calfee RP, Patel A, DaSilva MF, Akelman E: Management of lateral epicondylitis: Current concepts. *J Am Acad Orthop Surg* 2008;16(1):19-29.

35. Nirschl RP: *Master Techniques in Orthopaedic Surgery: The Elbow.* New York, NY, Raven, 1994, pp 129-148.

36. Roles NC, Maudsley RH: Radial tunnel syndrome: Resistant tennis elbow as a nerve entrapment. *J Bone Joint Surg Br* 1972;54(3):499-508.

37. Labelle H, Guibert R, The University of Montreal Orthopaedic Research Group: Efficacy of diclofenac in lateral epicondylitis of the elbow also treated with immobilization. *Arch Fam Med* 1997;6(3):257-262.

38. Hay EM, Paterson SM, Lewis M, Hosie G, Croft P: Pragmatic randomised controlled trial of local corticosteroid injection and naproxen for treatment of lateral epicondylitis of elbow in primary care. *BMJ* 1999;319(7215):964-968.

39. Smidt N, van der Windt DA, Assendelft WJ, Devillé WL, Korthals-de Bos IB, Bouter LM: Corticosteroid injections, physiotherapy, or a wait-and-see policy for lateral epicondylitis: A randomised controlled trial. *Lancet* 2002;359(9307):657-662.

40. Wong SM, Hui AC, Tong PY, Poon DW, Yu E, Wong LK: Treatment of lateral epicondylitis with botulinum toxin: A randomized, double-blind, placebo-controlled trial. *Ann Intern Med* 2005;143(11):793-797.

41. Peerbooms JC, Sluimer J, Bruijn DJ, Gosens T: Positive effect of an autologous platelet concentrate in lateral epicondylitis in a double-blind randomized controlled trial: Platelet-rich plasma versus corticosteroid injection with a 1-year follow-up. *Am J Sports Med* 2010;38(2):255-262.

42. Gosens T, Peerbooms JC, van Laar W, den Oudsten BL: Ongoing positive effect of platelet-rich plasma versus corticosteroid injection in lateral epicondylitis: A double-blind randomized controlled trial with 2-year follow-up. *Am J Sports Med* 2011;39(6):1200-1208.

43. Thanasas C, Papadimitriou G, Charalambidis C, Paraskevopoulos I, Papanikolaou A: Platelet-rich plasma versus autologous whole blood for the treatment of chronic lateral elbow epicondylitis: A randomized controlled clinical trial. *Am J Sports Med* 2011;39(10):2130-2134.

44. Buchbinder R, Green SE, Youd JM, Assendelft WJ, Barnsley L, Smidt N: Shock wave therapy for lateral elbow pain. *Cochrane Database Syst Rev* 2005;4(4):CD003524.

45. Lin CL, Lee JS, Su WR, Kuo LC, Tai TW, Jou IM: Clinical and ultrasonographic results of ultrasonographically guided percutaneous radiofrequency lesioning in the treatment of recalcitrant lateral epicondylitis. *Am J Sports Med* 2011;39(11):2429-2435.

46. Bokhari AR, Murrell GA: The role of nitric oxide in tendon healing. *J Shoulder Elbow Surg* 2012;21(2):238-244.

47. Haahr JP, Andersen JH: Prognostic factors in lateral epicondylitis: A randomized trial with one-year follow-up in 266 new cases treated with minimal occupational intervention or the usual approach in general practice. *Rheumatology (Oxford)* 2003;42(10):1216-1225.

48. Binder AI, Hazleman BL: Lateral humeral epicondylitis—A study of natural history and the effect of conservative therapy. *Br J Rheumatol* 1983;22(2):73-76.

49. Nirschl RP, Pettrone FA: Tennis elbow: The surgical treatment of lateral epicondylitis. *J Bone Joint Surg Am* 1979;61(6A):832-839.

50. Kuklo TR, Taylor KF, Murphy KP, Islinger RB, Heekin RD, Baker CL Jr: Arthroscopic release for lateral epicondylitis: A cadaveric model. *Arthroscopy* 1999;15(3):259-264.

51. Owens BD, Murphy KP, Kuklo TR: Arthroscopic release for lateral epicondylitis. *Arthroscopy* 2001;17(6):582-587.

52. Mullett H, Sprague M, Brown G, Hausman M: Arthroscopic treatment of lateral epicondylitis: Clinical and cadaveric studies. *Clin Orthop Relat Res* 2005;439:123-128.

53. Peart RE, Strickler SS, Schweitzer KM Jr: Lateral epicondylitis: A comparative study of open and arthroscopic lateral release. *Am J Orthop (Belle Mead NJ)* 2004;33(11):565-567.

54. Baker CL Jr, Baker CL III: Long-term follow-up of arthroscopic treatment of lateral epicondylitis. *Am J Sports Med* 2008;36(2):254-260.

55. Baker CL Jr, Murphy KP, Gottlob CA, Curd DT: Arthroscopic classification and treatment of lateral epicondylitis: Two-year clinical results. *J Shoulder Elbow Surg* 2000;9(6):475-482.

56. Cummins CA: Lateral epicondylitis: In vivo assessment of arthroscopic debridement and correlation with patient outcomes. *Am J Sports Med* 2006;34(9):1486-1491.

57. Baker CL Jr, Baker CL III: Arthroscopy remains a viable, reliable method for treating lateral epicondylitis. *Orthopedics Today* February 2012. Available at: http://www.helio.com/orthopedics/arthroscopy/news/print/orthopedics-today. Accessed October 1, 2012.

58. Dunn JH, Kim JJ, Davis L, Nirschl RP: Ten- to 14-year follow-up of the Nirschl surgical technique for lateral epicondylitis. *Am J Sports Med* 2008;36(2):261-266.

59. Rosenberg N, Henderson I: Surgical treatment of resistant lateral epicondylitis: Follow-up study of 19 patients after excision, release and repair of proximal common extensor tendon origin. *Arch Orthop Trauma Surg* 2002;122(9-10):514-517.

60. Verhaar J, Walenkamp G, Kester A, van Mameren H, van der Linden T: Lateral extensor release for tennis elbow: A prospective long-term follow-up study. *J Bone Joint Surg Am* 1993;75(7):1034-1043.

61. Dunkow PD, Jatti M, Muddu BN: A comparison of open and percutaneous techniques in the surgical treatment of tennis elbow. *J Bone Joint Surg Br* 2004;86(5):701-704.

62. Szabo SJ, Savoie FH III, Field LD, Ramsey JR, Hosemann CD: Tendinosis of the extensor carpi radialis brevis: An evaluation of three methods of operative treatment. *J Shoulder Elbow Surg* 2006;15(6):721-727.

63. Organ SW, Nirschl RP, Kraushaar BS, Guidi EJ: Salvage surgery for lateral tennis elbow. *Am J Sports Med* 1997;25(6):746-750.

64. Gabel GT, Morrey BF: Operative treatment of medical epicondylitis: Influence of concomitant ulnar neuropathy at the elbow. *J Bone Joint Surg Am* 1995;77(7):1065-1069.

65. Stahl S, Kaufman T: The efficacy of an injection of steroids for medial epicondylitis: A prospective study of sixty elbows. *J Bone Joint Surg Am* 1997;79(11):1648-1652.

66. Suresh SP, Ali KE, Jones H, Connell DA: Medial epicondylitis: Is ultrasound guided autologous blood injection an effective treatment? *Br J Sports Med* 2006;40(11):935-939, discussion 939.

67. Vangsness CT Jr, Jobe FW: Surgical treatment of medial epicondylitis: Results in 35 elbows. *J Bone Joint Surg Br* 1991;73(3):409-411.

68. Olliviere C, Nirschl RP, Petrrone FA: Resection and repair for medial tennis elbow. A prospective analysis. *Am J Sports Med* 1995;23(2):214-221.

69. Schipper ON, Dunn JH, Ochiai DH, Donovan JS, Nirschl RP: Nirschl surgical technique for concomitant lateral and medial elbow tendinosis: A retrospective review of 53 elbows with a mean follow-up of 11.7 years. *Am J Sports Med* 2011;39(5):972-976.

70. Koh J, Mohan P, Morrey B, et al: Fasciotomy and surgical tenotomy for recalcitrant lateral elbow tendinopathy. *Am J Sports Med* 2013;4:636-644.

    At long-term follow-up, a combined surgical procedure for concurrent lateral and medial epicondylitis was found to improve surgical outcome scores, with 85% good to excellent results and 96% of the patients returning to their sport. Level of evidence: IV.

71. Muir S, Reisbig N, Baria M, Kaeding C, Bertone A: The concentration of plasma provides additional bioactive proteins in platelet and autologous protein solutions. *Am J Sports Med* 2019;47(9):1955-1963.

    In this descriptive laboratory study, the concentration of plasma as a potential additive biotherapy for the treatment of osteoarthritis was evaluated. Concentrated platelet-poor plasma was found to be a unique source of insulin-like growth factor 1 that may supplement orthopaedic biologic therapies. Level of evidence: IV.

Chapter 35

Elbow Injuries and the Throwing Athlete

Eric D. Haunschild, BS • James E. Hammond, DO, ATC • Brian J. Cole, MD, MBA

Section 7: Elbow Trauma, Fracture, and Reconstruction

ABSTRACT

The stress of repetitive overhead throwing on the elbow causes many injuries in throwers, requiring medical intervention ranging from conservative rest and physical therapy to surgery with lengthy postoperative recovery. Proper evaluation of throwing injuries with targeted history-taking, physical examination, and diagnostic imaging are essential in making correct diagnoses and guiding interventions. Most, if not all, of elbow injuries in throwers are amenable to conservative treatment options, which generally produce acceptable return-to-sport rates. If initial therapy fails, surgical techniques continue to advance with improved patient outcomes and more throwers returning to their prior level of play. Medical management of elbow injuries is continuously evolving, with improvements to existing interventions as well as novel new interventions on the horizon, which will continue to optimize elbow injury prevention and treatment in throwers.

The views expressed in this chapter are those of the authors and do not necessarily reflect the official policy or position of the Department of the Navy, Department of Defense, or the United States Government.

I (CDR James Hammond, DO, ATC, Medical Corps, Naval Medical Center Portsmouth, Portsmouth, VA) am a military service member. This work was prepared as part of my official duties. Title 17 U.S.C. 105 provides that "Copyright protection under this title is not available for any work of the United States Government." Title 17 U.S.C. 101 defines a United States Government work as a work prepared by a military service member or employee of the United States Government as part of that person's official duties.

Dr. Hammond or an immediate family member serves as a board member, owner, officer, or committee member of the Arthroscopy Association of North America. Dr. Cole or an immediate family member has received royalties from Arthrex, Inc. and Elsevier Publishing; serves as a paid consultant to or is an employee of Arthrex, Inc. and Regentis; has stock or stock options held in Ossio and Regentis; has received research or institutional support from Aesculap/B. Braun, Arthrex, Inc., National Institutes of Health (NIAMS & NICHD), and Regentis; has received nonincome support (such as equipment or services), commercially derived honoraria, or other non–research-related funding (such as paid travel) from Athletico, JRF Ortho, and Smith & Nephew; and serves as a board member, owner, officer, or committee member of the Arthroscopy Association of North America and the International Cartilage Repair Society. Neither Mr. Haunschild nor any immediate family member has received anything of value from or has stock or stock options held in a commercial company or institution related directly or indirectly to the subject of this chapter.

Keywords: epicondylitis; return-to-sport; ulnar collateral ligament; ulnar neuritis

Introduction

Overhead throwing imparts substantial stress to the elbow and can cause unique injuries. Biomechanical and clinical studies have elucidated the causative factors in these injuries and have allowed prevention and treatment strategies to evolve. The diagnosis of an elbow condition is facilitated by specific examination maneuvers, and radiography is useful for confirming the diagnosis. Prevention strategies, such as the monitoring of pitch counts, have been developed to decrease the risk of injury in young athletes. Evolving surgical strategies have contributed to changes in techniques for treating certain conditions in the throwing athlete.

Throwing-Related Elbow Anatomy and Biomechanics

The medial or ulnar collateral ligament (UCL) is the most clinically relevant anatomic structure in the elbow of the throwing athlete. The UCL is a complex composed of the anterior oblique, posterior oblique, and transverse ligaments. The anterior oblique ligament is the strongest ligament of the complex and the most important stabilizer to valgus stress in the throwing athlete. The anterior oblique ligament originates in the medial epicondyle. An evaluation of the ulnar insertion of the anterior oblique ligament in 2011 found that it extends distal to the sublime tubercle along a previously unnamed ridge and was present on all skeletal specimens.[1] Within the anterior oblique ligament, the anterior band and the posterior band alternately have primary responsibility for valgus stress throughout the ranges of flexion and extension; the anterior band is tight during extension, and the posterior band is tight during flexion.

The UCL receives dynamic support from the surrounding musculature. The flexor carpi ulnaris is the primary dynamic contributor to valgus stabilization of the elbow, and the flexor digitorum superficialis is a secondary stabilizer.[2] These two muscles help disseminate the substantial forces across the elbow during the throwing motion and thereby protect the UCL. Their relationship has implications for preventing and managing UCL injuries.

The throwing motion creates substantial energy and subsequent forces that are mediated by structures about the elbow. Moreover, different pitch types produce differing forces, with fastball, slider, and curveball pitches producing significantly greater elbow forces, torques, and injury risk when compared with the changeup.[3] Angular velocities as high as 3,000°/s have been observed at the elbow during the acceleration phase of the throwing motion. This velocity translates into 64 N/m of valgus torque. Because the tensile strength of the UCL is only 34 N/m, the other stabilizers of the elbow also are important for avoiding or minimizing injury.[4] The valgus load creates stress about the other aspects of the elbow: tensile forces occur on the medial aspect, shear and compressive stresses occur in the olecranon fossa as the elbow reaches extension, and compression forces occur laterally, primarily at the radiocapitellar joint. A 2011 cadaver study found that lateral contact pressures increased 67% after the UCL was transected.[5] Understanding these forces increases the ability to understand the relationships among the conditions that occur about the elbow.

Clinical Evaluation

History

A specific, detailed patient history is vital to understanding elbow pathology in a throwing athlete. Arm dominance and the duration, intensity, and location of symptoms should be noted as well as the type of activity that elicits symptoms (eg, does the pain occur at rest, with activities of daily living, or only with throwing?). Information should be elicited as to associated mechanical symptoms, paresthesia, or pain in other joints, especially the shoulder. It is important to determine the point in the throwing motion during which symptoms occur (windup, early cocking, late cocking, acceleration, deceleration, or follow through). The types of pitches, the number of pitches thrown per outing, and the throwing schedule should be determined. The curveball generates the greatest valgus stress at the elbow, the fastball and slider generate the greatest force, and the changeup generates less stress on the elbow and is considered a relatively safe pitch for athletes of all ages. However, skilled players are more likely to throw the fastball or the curveball, play on more teams, and pitch more frequently than other players.[6]

Physical Examination

General observations are easy to overlook during an evaluation of the elbow, but they can provide insight into stresses about the elbow. The patient's carrying angle should be observed to identify any side-to-side difference. The exact location and the medial, lateral, or posterior character of the pain should be determined. The range of motion should be evaluated; a lack of full extension is common in throwers.

Typically, the focus of the examination in a throwing athlete is on the medial elbow. An acute avulsion injury of the UCL usually occurs proximally at the medial epicondyle, and tenderness there or along the length of the anterior oblique ligament should be determined. Resisted strength testing of the flexor-pronator mass is done. Valgus stress at 0° and 30° of flexion also is typically assessed, but the instability is often more subtle in a throwing athlete. This test lacks the sensitivity needed to reliably identify a chronic injury. The milking maneuver and the moving valgus stress test also are used to assess valgus instability and UCL injury. The milking maneuver is performed by pulling on the patient's thumb with the forearm supinated and the elbow flexed beyond 90°. The moving valgus stress test begins in the same position, and the patient's thumb is pulled until the limit of external rotation is reached at the shoulder. The elbow is taken through a range of motion while the torque created by pulling on the thumb remains constant. Pain typically is most intense when the elbow is between 70° and 120°. The sensitivity of the moving valgus stress test is reported to be 100%, with 75% specificity.[7]

A patient with suspected UCL injury should be assessed for ulnar nerve pathology. Evidence of nerve subluxation, a positive Tinel sign, or symptoms with elbow hyperflexion testing should be noted. Pain associated with a flexor-pronator injury, as indicated by pain with resistance testing, should be differentiated from pain associated with medial epicondylitis, as indicated by tenderness over only the epicondyle with normal moving valgus stress.

Imaging

The initial imaging studies are plain radiographs in the AP, lateral, radiocapitellar, and axillary views. Valgus stress radiographs can be used to identify a medial joint line opening; an opening of more than 3 mm has been considered diagnostic.[8] The radiographs can be assessed for evidence of osteophytes, loss of joint space, loose bodies, or osteochondral defects. MRI can be used to confirm several diagnoses about the elbow, including osteochondritis dissecans (OCD), a UCL injury, avulsion of the flexor-pronator mass, and chronic thickening of the UCL. A 2011 study found that signal intensity on MRI can be used to predict rehabilitation outcomes; patients with a complete or high-grade UCL tear were most likely to require surgery[9] (**Figure 1**). A recent study for the first time classified UCL injury based on MRI imaging (**Table 1**). This classification system was applied to 240 patients and found to significantly predict the degree of valgus laxity and subsequently guide treatment.[10]

Ultrasonography and dynamic ultrasonographic examination have been described for defining UCL injury, but most available studies are small case studies or case reports. Several studies have found differences in UCL laxity among overhead throwing athletes as well as side-to-side differences between the athletes' throwing and nonthrowing arms.[11,12]

Arthroscopy has been used as a diagnostic tool primarily for closely evaluating a joint line opening with stress; 1 to 2 mm of joint line opening indicates a partial-thickness tear, and 4 to 10 mm of opening indicates a full-thickness tear. The ulnohumeral joint is viewed from the anterolateral portal, and the joint is stressed at 65° to 70° of elbow flexion with the forearm pronated.[13]

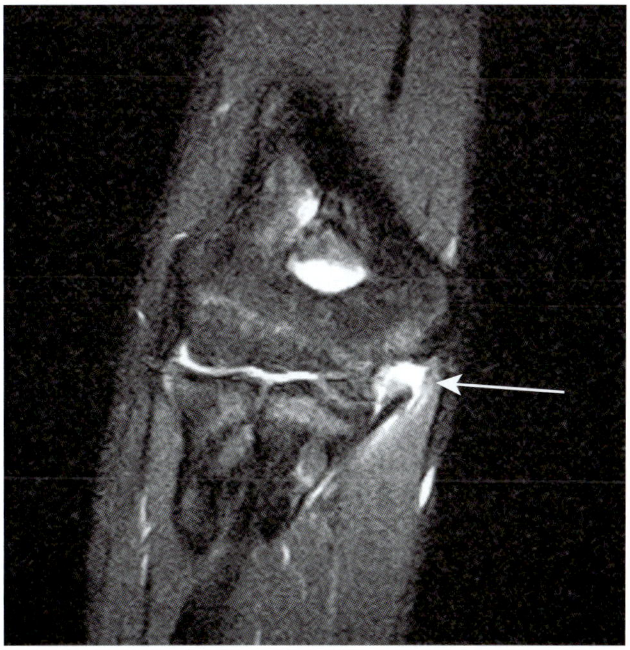

FIGURE 1 MRI showing a complete avulsion of the ulnar collateral ligament from the humeral epicondyle (arrow).

Table 1

Classification of Ulnar Collateral Ligament (UCL) Injury on MRI, as Proposed by Joyner et al[10]

Classification	Description of Injury
Type I	Edema limited to UCL only, low-grade partial UCL tear
Type II	High-grade partial-thickness tear of UCL with no extravasation of fluid on arthrogram
Type III	Full-thickness UCL tear with extravasation of fluid on arthrogram
Type IV	Tear or pathology in more than one location of the UCL

Conditions Causing Medial Elbow Pain

Medial Epicondylitis

Medial epicondylitis is less common than lateral epicondylitis and usually occurs as a result of repetitive wrist flexion and forceful pronation during golf, a racquet sport, or overhead throwing. Pain typically is elicited over the medial elbow and exacerbated by resisted forearm flexion and pronation. The diagnosis is primarily clinical, but ultrasonography and MRI are reported to be useful.[14] On MRI, increased signal is seen in the flexor muscular origin about the medial epicondyle.[15] Nonsurgical treatments have high success rates. The components of a typical nonsurgical treatment program include NSAIDs, flexibility exercises, ice, and guided physical therapy. Steroid injections have also been used. The use of iontophoresis was found to improve pain relief in a comparative study.[16] Ultrasound-guided autologous blood injection led to improved scores on the visual analog and modified Nirschl Pain Phase scales.[17] The use of platelet-rich plasma (PRP) has also shown promise as a nonsurgical intervention, with a recent randomized study showing significant improvements in both visual analog scale and Mayo Elbow Performance Score at 6 months compared with corticosteroid injection.[18] Another investigation demonstrated that PRP injections produce comparable outcomes to Tenex ultrasound-guided tenotomy in treating epicondylitis.[19] These investigations have included injections for both medial and lateral epicondylitis in the analysis, with future study required to further assess the use and efficacy of PRP. Surgical intervention typically involves resection of a portion of the diseased tendon by open, mini-open, or arthroscopic means. If the surgical goal has been accomplished, pain relief can be expected, but a strength deficit may remain.

UCL Injury

Incidence of both UCL injury and surgical procedures to address it are increasing in throwers of all ages, which is causing considerable concern. To categorize and mitigate this alarming trend, recent investigations have identified several risk factors predictive of UCL reconstruction in throwers. In Major League Baseball pitchers who had undergone UCL reconstruction, the following risk factors were identified: greater pitch speed, greater pitch count per game, fewer days between consecutive games, smaller repertoire of pitches, smaller stature, and a less pronounced horizontal pitch release location.[20] Another investigation on radiographic risk factors for failure of nonsurgical management of UCL injury found that distal UCL tears were 12 times more likely than proximal tears to eventually require surgical intervention.[21]

Regardless of the location of injury, the initial management of a UCL injury in an overhead throwing athlete should be nonsurgical. The regimen includes a 6-week period of rest from throwing as well as strengthening of the flexor-pronator musculature.[2] The athlete should be asymptomatic and have a normal examination before throwing activities are resumed. At that time, the athlete should optimize throwing mechanics and offset stress from the medial elbow. Late trunk rotation, reduced shoulder external rotation, and increased elbow flexion have been shown to increase valgus stress at the elbow.[22] Early investigations on the efficacy of physical therapy were not favorable, with a 42% return-to-sport rate for overhead throwing athletes at a mean 24.5-week follow-up.[23] However, recent reports have shown more promise, with a 90% return-to-sport rate reported for professional quarterbacks after 4 weeks, and 71% and 94% return-to-sport rates in professional baseball pitchers and position players, respectively.[24]

A developing area of interest in nonsurgical management of UCL injury is the use of PRP injections. Further investigation and standardization of PRP composition and administration are necessary, but early investigations have shown promise in the efficacy of PRP. One investigation in throwing athletes in whom 2 months of conservative management had previously failed had an 88% return-to-sport rate by 12 weeks following PRP injection and guided physical therapy. A similar investigation in professional baseball players in whom conservative management had previously failed showed a 67% return to preinjury level of competition. Notably, those in the investigation with distal tears all had poor outcomes.[24]

In the original Jobe technique for reconstructing the UCL, a figure-of-8 tendon graft was woven through bone tunnels and sutured back onto itself (**Figure 2**). This technique required takedown of the flexor-pronator mass and exposure of the posterior humeral cortex for one of the tunnels. An ulnar nerve transposition always was performed. The substantial morbidity of the exposure led to modification of this technique and development of new techniques. The modified Jobe technique consists of a muscle-splitting approach to decrease morbidity to the flexor-pronator musculature, a change in humeral tunnel direction, and ulnar nerve transposition only if the patient has preoperative symptoms. The humeral tunnel is directed somewhat anteriorly to avoid ulnar nerve injury with graft passage and decrease the dissection necessary for exposure. The outcomes and the biomechanical strength resulting from using the modified Jobe technique have become the standard for comparison with any other technique. A 93% return-to-sport rate was reported for overhead throwing athletes.[8] Another study reported an 83% return rate to the previous level of throwing at a minimum 2-year follow-up after a modified Jobe technique was used.[25]

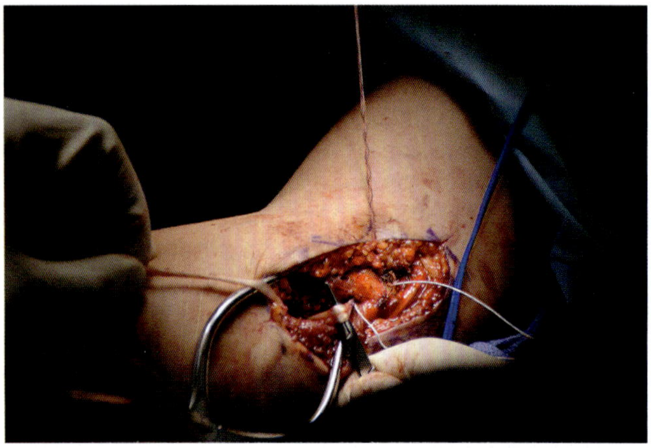

FIGURE 2 Intraoperative photograph showing anatomic reconstruction of the ulnar collateral ligament. One end of the graft is docked at the anterior-inferior aspect of the humerus and then looped through a tunnel at the sublime tubercle of the proximal ulna, and the second end of the graft is docked in the same tunnel at the distal humerus.

The commonly described docking technique also uses a muscle-splitting approach and two converging tunnels in the ulna. Only one primary tunnel is drilled in the humerus, and two smaller holes are drilled in the humerus to facilitate suture passage. One limb of the tendon graft is passed into the tunnel in the humerus. The second limb of the tendon graft is assessed for length and tension, sectioned to the appropriate length, and docked in the humeral socket. The sutures from each limb of the tendon graft are tied over a bone bridge after final tensioning. The use of the docking technique led to a good or excellent outcome in 19 of 21 athletes (90%).[26] An excellent result was defined as a return to previous level of play for at least 1 year, and a good result was defined as a return to throwing at a lower level for at least 1 year or the ability to throw at daily batting practice. A 92% rate of return to the preinjury level of throwing was reported at an 11.5-month follow-up after a quadrupled palmaris graft was used with the docking technique.[27]

Several techniques can be categorized as hybrid. A relatively new technique uses a single drill hole at the sublime tubercle and a single drill hole in the medial epicondyle. An interference screw is used at the sublime tubercle, with a docking technique on the humeral attachment. At 3-year follow-up after this technique was used, 19 of 22 patients (86%) had an excellent result.[28] Another technique uses the same single drill holes on the sublime tubercle and the medial epicondyle, with interference screws on each end of the construct. In a biomechanical study, this technique led to stability similar to that of intact UCL specimens.[4] These findings were corroborated by a 2014 investigation of 20 patients receiving the interference screw technique, which had a 90% return-to-sport rate.[29]

Although UCL reconstruction is the preferred surgical technique for UCL tear, recent developments in UCL repair have shown comparable outcomes in limited studies compared with reconstruction. A recent systematic review of UCL repair investigations found an 87% return-to-sport rate by 6 months after surgery. These results were far superior to early studies on UCL repair, which showed return-to-sport rates at only 71.4%.[30] The favorable postoperative timelines and recent outcome studies on repair are promising, but future investigations on outcome will be necessary before repair can be considered as an alternative to reconstruction.

Ulnar Neuritis

Approximately 40% of patients with UCL insufficiency have ulnar neuritis. A substantial valgus stress can create traction, friction, and compression on the nerve and induce neuritis. The presence of adhesions and/or osteophytes, nerve subluxation, a thickened medial triceps, or UCL injury also can increase stress on the nerve. Night pain and paresthesia into the ulnar nerve distribution can occur. Ulnar nerve symptoms can occur with throwing. On physical examination, a positive Tinel sign at the cubital tunnel, a positive elbow hyperflexion test, and/or evidence of ulnar nerve subluxation can be observed. Nonsurgical measures, including the use of night splinting, ice, NSAIDs, and activity modification, can be successful. Surgical management typically involves transposing the ulnar nerve into a subcutaneous position. This procedure has had great success with appropriate rehabilitation and a graduated return to throwing activities. The time to return to play with isolated ulnar nerve transposition is approximately 12 weeks.[31] If the patient has ulnar nerve symptoms associated with a UCL injury requiring reconstruction, ulnar nerve transposition should be done at the time of reconstruction. However, UCL reconstruction itself can have complications of ulnar neuropathy, with rates of 12% found at mean 3.3 years after surgery in a recent meta-analysis. Of those cases, 0.8% required surgical management to address ulnar neuritis. When looking at surgical techniques, the modified Jobe approach had complications of ulnar neuropathy in 16.9% of cases, whereas the docking technique had neuropathy in only 3.3% of cases.[32]

Recent investigations on the treatment of isolated ulnar neuritis in throwers have demonstrated mixed results. In one study, professional baseball players undergoing isolated ulnar nerve decompression/transposition had a 62% return-to-sport rate. Notably, those that did return performed statistically the same as matched control subjects.[33] However, another investigation on surgical outcomes in adolescent baseball players found that all of the players undergoing surgery returned to prior level of play at an average of 2 months postoperatively. This investigation also found a 60% return to prior play level following nonsurgical treatment, with UCL injury, ulnar nerve subluxation, and hand numbness on the ulnar side associated with poor nonsurgical outcomes.[34]

Conditions Causing Posterior Elbow Pain

Posteromedial Impingement or Valgus Extension Overload

Valgus extension overload is a relatively common condition in overhead throwing athletes in which posterior and, commonly, medial osteophytes impinge within the olecranon fossa as the elbow reaches extension. A review of 72 professional baseball players who underwent elbow surgery found that 65% had posterior olecranon osteophytes.[35] Athletes typically report posterior pain at the elbow during ball release and as the elbow reaches extension; this is the point at which osteophytes from the olecranon impinge within the fossa. The patient also commonly has some loss of terminal extension on examination. When valgus stress on the elbow is applied at 20° to 30° of flexion and the elbow is quickly taken to extension, a positive test re-creates the pain in the posteromedial elbow. Care must be taken to determine whether there is a concomitant UCL injury because there is a significant relationship between these diagnoses. Plain radiographs can reveal the posterior osteophyte.

Nonsurgical management begins with rest and 10 to 14 days of throwing restrictions followed by an interval throwing program to allow a gradual return to throwing. Pitching mechanics must be corrected during the interval throwing program to minimize stress at the elbow. A longer period of rest is recommended if symptoms persist or the patient cannot return to throwing at the earlier level. Intra-articular injection is not particularly helpful in patients with posteromedial impingement and should not be repeated.

Surgical management should be carefully considered. The medial elbow endures substantial valgus forces in the throwing athlete, and engagement of the olecranon in its fossa provides secondary stabilization to the elbow, particularly during extension. Any subtle laxity in the UCL may transfer stress to the posteromedial olecranon and cause it to impinge on the fossa as the elbow reaches extension. This stress induces osteophyte formation, which then increases impingement by shear mass effect. Overresection of the posteromedial olecranon can unmask or exacerbate symptoms of UCL injury. Twenty-five percent of professional baseball players who underwent osteophyte excision later had valgus instability requiring UCL reconstruction.[25] Studies conflict as to the amount of olecranon that can be excised before increased strain is seen at the UCL, and there is debate as to whether any excision of normal olecranon should be done. The procedure can be done in an arthroscopic or open fashion. In an open procedure, an osteotome is used to resect a portion of the olecranon tip, and a portion of the medial olecranon is removed. The arthroscopic procedure can be accomplished using a posterolateral portal for viewing and a central posterior portal for working. Care must be taken to remove osteophytes and minimize resection of normal olecranon. In addition, care must be taken to avoid ulnar nerve injury when resecting the medial aspect of the osteophyte as the ulnar nerve enters the cubital tunnel. A 2011 study reported an excellent outcome in seven of nine patients who underwent arthroscopic treatment of valgus extension overload.[36]

Olecranon Stress Fracture

Stress fractures of the olecranon have been described in javelin throwers and other throwing athletes.[37,38] These fractures are primarily described as transverse or oblique, with a mechanism of injury similar to that of a valgus extension overload injury. The olecranon is subject to increased stress as the elbow undergoes a valgus load and approaches extension. The substantial triceps forces at extension also have been implicated in this condition.

On physical examination, the athlete may have tenderness over the physis (if it is open), the posterior olecranon, or the posteromedial olecranon. Symptoms may be elicited by forceful extension of the elbow or resisted triceps muscle testing. Typically, the patient has less extension than in the contralateral elbow. Plain radiographs may show a sclerotic line of remodeling fracture if the condition is chronic. If the physis is open, it may be beneficial to obtain radiographs of the contralateral side to detect any physeal widening. A bone scan will reveal increased uptake in the area. MRI will show edema within the bone and allow characterization of the fracture line. MRI also is beneficial if an associated UCL injury is suspected.

The management of an olecranon stress fracture is somewhat controversial. Nonsurgical measures require rest from throwing and possibly temporary splinting. The return to an interval throwing program is delayed until symptoms have subsided and there is radiographic evidence of fracture healing. As a result, throwing can be restricted for as long as 6 months. Stress fractures may respond to bone stimulators, but this treatment has not been well defined. Recent surgical outcomes of olecranon stress fractures in the throwing athletes have been promising. In a recent systematic review where 98.1% of the cohort had an olecranon stress fracture, 76.9% of athletes underwent surgery and there was a 96.2% return-to-sport rate at or above preinjury levels.[39]

Some experts recommend early surgical treatment to reduce the time to resumption of throwing.[40] Surgical treatment also is recommended if nonsurgical management is unsuccessful. Tension-band wiring, tension-band wiring with a compression screw, and a compression screw alone have been used. A 6.5- or 7.3-mm cannulated compression screw typically is used. A 2012 case report described a persistent fracture after fixation in a college pitcher, in which bone grafting ultimately was required for healing.[41]

Persistent Olecranon Physis

The persistent olecranon physis is similar to an olecranon stress fracture and may be responsible for an athlete's posterior elbow pain. The olecranon physis has two ossification centers: the posterior center is oriented transverse to the longitudinal axis of the ulna and contributes to longitudinal growth; a second center is more anterior at the olecranon tip, contributing to the joint surface but not to longitudinal growth. These two centers fuse and create a single physis that persists until approximately age 14 years in girls and age 16 years in boys. This physis can become sclerotic during the process of closing and can be as wide as 5 mm.

Posterior elbow pain typically develops during the years from adolescence through the late teens. The pain occurs at terminal extension in the follow-through phase of throwing, and it can be relieved with rest. The physical examination may be benign; motion is normal, the elbow is stable, and there is no tenderness to palpation. Plain radiographs reveal a persistent physis in the olecranon that may be wider on the involved side than on the contralateral side. There may be evidence of sclerosis about the physis that is unexpected for the patient's age. T2-weighted MRI may show edema about the physis, but this finding is not diagnostic.

Treatment starts with nonsurgical measures, including a period of relative rest and cessation of throwing activities. NSAIDs and ice may be used as needed. Nonsurgical measures appear to be successful in most patients but may require as long as 4 months. The options for surgical treatment include open reduction and internal fixation, bone grafting, and open reduction and internal fixation with bone grafting. The fixation techniques include tension-band wiring, compression screws, and a combination of screws and tension-band wiring. The available studies are largely limited to case reports and small case studies.[42,43] It appears that the highest rates of successful union were in patients who underwent bone grafting with or without fixation. Those undergoing fixation alone had an approximately 66% failure rate. A 2010 study found that those with a persistent olecranon physis and evidence of sclerosis had a 100% failure rate with nonsurgical measures.[44]

Conditions Causing Lateral Elbow Pain

Capitellar Osteochondritis Dissecans

OCD is a local disorder of the subchondral bone that results in separation and fragmentation of articular cartilage and its underlying bone. It is important to differentiate this condition from Panner disease, which occurs in younger patients, is idiopathic, usually is self-limiting, and improves without surgical intervention. OCD typically occurs at the elbow in adolescents who are high-demand, repetitive overhead throwing athletes. The pathogenesis is not completely understood. Genetic factors, blood supply, repetitive trauma, and a vulnerable epiphysis have been implicated. The underlying bone undergoes degradation and can destabilize the overlying cartilage. Probably a combination of factors contributes to the process by which the lesion is created.

Typically, the athlete has elbow pain during activity. The pain is insidious in onset, is relieved by rest, and progresses if the activity is continued. The pain is difficult to localize and often is accompanied by loss of motion. Occasionally, the symptoms are mechanical, with catching or locking of the elbow joint. The most common finding on examination is tenderness over the radiocapitellar joint. Crepitus can be elicited in the lateral joint with pronation and supination, and there is loss of motion of 15° to 30°. In the active radiocapitellar compression test, the elbow is fully extended while the patient actively pronates and supinates the forearm and contracts the muscles about the elbow. A positive test reproduces the athlete's symptoms.

The initial imaging is with plain radiographs. The standard AP view in full extension and lateral views in 90° of flexion show typical capitellar radiolucency and flattening of the joint surface (**Figure 3**). The lesion commonly occurs in the anterolateral aspect of the capitellum. In the Minami classification system, a grade I lesion is a translucent cystic shadow in the middle or lateral capitellum, a grade II lesion has a split line or clear zone between the lesion and its subchondral bone, and loose bodies are present in a grade III lesion.[45]

MRI has become the modality of choice for evaluating these lesions. Early changes not found on plain radiographs can be detected on MRI, and the size, location, and stability of the lesion can be assessed. The key to making a treatment decision is to determine whether the articular surface is intact and the lesion is stable as seen on MRI. A peripheral ring of fluid or fluid under the articular surface suggests an unstable lesion; these findings are similar to those of an OCD lesion in another area of the body. The

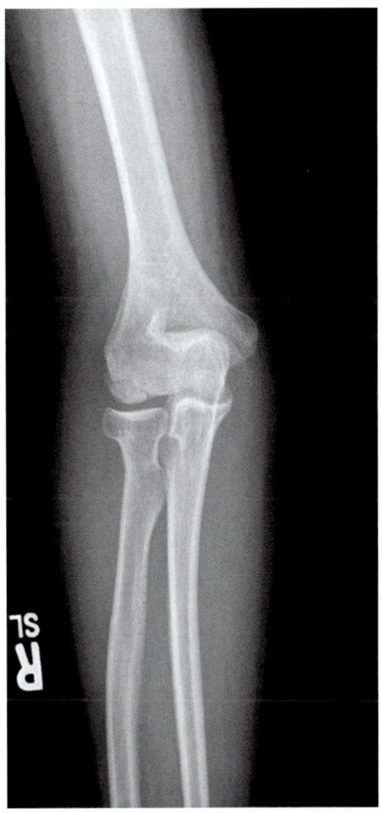

FIGURE 3 AP radiograph showing osteochondritis dissecans of the capitellum in which there is a complete fragment with subtle displacement. Such a lesion often has a relatively normal arthroscopic appearance because the articular cartilage is intact.

diagnosis sometimes is facilitated by the addition of an arthrogram or intravenously administered gadolinium.

OCD lesions are amenable to healing, and nonsurgical regimens are an option. The treatment begins with 6 months of elbow rest without throwing activity. Anti-inflammatory medications are used, and physical therapy is implemented to optimize motion and strength. Radiographs are assessed at 6-week intervals to ensure that the lesion is healing or is not progressing. MRI is repeated as needed at an approximately 3-month interval and compared with the initial studies. An interval throwing program is initiated at 6 months if the athlete has good motion, is asymptomatic, and has evidence of healing. Pitch counts initially should be monitored.[46] Patients with capitellar lucency or flattening have healing rates of 88% to 91%.[47,48] Those with open capitellar physes have a higher rate of healing. Advanced lesions have less capacity for nonsurgical healing. A stable lesion is characterized by an open capitellar epiphyseal plate, localized flattening or radiolucency of the subchondral bone, and good elbow motion. In an unstable lesion, the physis is closed, with radiographic fragmentation and loss of elbow motion of more than 20°.[49]

Surgical management is indicated if the patient has an unstable lesion or loose bodies or if nonsurgical treatment has been unsuccessful. Several surgical procedures have been described. Simple débridement can be effective for a contained lesion involving less than 50% of the capitellar surface. Microfracture or trephination of the subchondral base with a Kirschner wire also can be used after fragment excision and bed preparation (**Figure 4**). Fixation of a relatively large, unfragmented lesion can be achieved through different methods. Pullout wires, bone grafting, and Herbert screws have been successfully used. Several options exist for cartilage replacement, mirroring the options used in the knee and other joints. Mosaicplasty, osteochondral allograft, and autograft transplantation have been used to treat a relatively large OCD lesion or an uncontained lesion (in which there is loss of lateral column support).

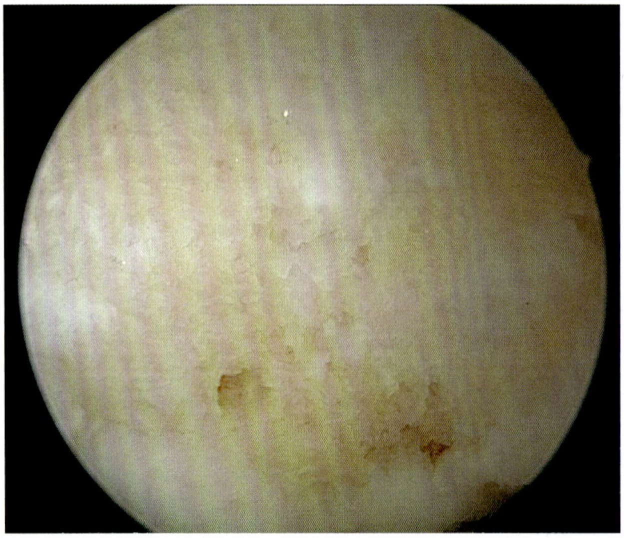

FIGURE 4 Arthroscopic image showing an osteochondritis dissecans lesion after microfracture.

Radiocapitellar Plica

Radiocapitellar plica, first described as a cause of a snapping elbow, essentially is a hypertrophic synovial plica that snaps over the edge of the radial head as the elbow moves from flexion to extension. The differential diagnosis includes intra-articular loose bodies, instability, lateral epicondylitis, and subluxation of the medial triceps over the medial epicondyle. Some of these conditions can be ruled out on the basis of location. The elbow examination typically is otherwise benign, with stability, full motion, and normal strength. The patient may have tenderness posterior to the lateral epicondyle and centered over the joint. Plain radiographs usually are not informative, and the plica frequently is missed on MRI.

Nonsurgical measures should be initially considered, including relative rest, NSAIDs, and gentle motion. Intra-articular steroid injections have been used in an attempt to relieve inflammation and decrease pain. Surgical management with an arthroscopic procedure has yielded good results. The snapping of the plica typically can be replicated on arthroscopic examination and allows the surgeon to locate the area to be released. The goal is to adequately release the synovial plica so that it no longer snaps over the radial head. The examination is repeated to ensure the release is complete. Postoperative management allows early range of motion and advancement of strength. An interval throwing program typically is started at 8 weeks and can advance as long as the patient remains asymptomatic.

SUMMARY

The elbow of a throwing athlete endures substantial stress during the phases of the throwing motion. The key to the correct diagnosis is to analyze the condition by elbow region, obtain a detailed history, apply specific examination maneuvers, and obtain appropriate imaging studies. Nonsurgical measures can be successful during specific phases of the disease process, and advances in surgical techniques have improved patient outcomes. Arthroscopic procedures have an increasing role in treating many conditions, with acceptable outcomes and return-to-play rates. Postoperative management is stepwise and specific to restore optimal mechanics, flexibility, and strength to the affected muscle groups.

KEY STUDY POINTS

- Overhead throwing motion places significant valgus torque on the UCL and supporting muscle stabilizers, increasing susceptibility to elbow injury in throwers.
- Always assess a new throwing injury by evaluating the region of elbow pain and conducting a targeted history, obtaining specific information about pitch counts/days throwing/types of pitches, physical examination, and imaging to narrow down the differential diagnosis of elbow pain in that region.
- In most throwers, consider initial nonsurgical treatment, as advances in conservative therapies have produced increasingly comparable return-to-sport rates to surgical management. Platelet-rich plasma has demonstrated promise in multiple pathologies about the elbow.
- In those that fail initial therapy, surgical management of most elbow injuries produce excellent return-to-sport rates in throwers. Ulnar collateral ligament repair is demonstrating promise compared with reconstruction, but more studies are needed to better understand reproducibility and longevity.

Annotated References

1. Farrow LD, Mahoney AJ, Stefancin JJ, Taljanovic MS, Sheppard JE, Schickendantz MS: Quantitative analysis of the medial ulnar collateral ligament ulnar footprint and its relationship to the ulnar sublime tubercle. *Am J Sports Med* 2011;39(9):1936-1941.

2. Park MC, Ahmad CS: Dynamic contributions of the flexor-pronator mass to elbow valgus stability. *J Bone Joint Surg Am* 2004;86(10):2268-2274.

3. Escamilla RF, Fleisig GS, Groeschner D, Akizuki K: Biomechanical comparisons among fastball, slider, curveball, and changeup pitch types and between balls and strikes in professional baseball pitchers. *Am J Sports Med* 2017;45(14):3358-3367.

   18 professional baseball pitchers were examined in a biomechanical laboratory to assess pitching biomechanics among different pitch types. It was found that changeups produce the least force and torque to the joint compared with fastballs, sliders, and curveballs.

4. Ahmad CS, Lee TQ, ElAttrache NS: Biomechanical evaluation of a new ulnar collateral ligament reconstruction technique with interference screw fixation. *Am J Sports Med* 2003;31(3):332-337.

5. Duggan JP Jr, Osadebe UC, Alexander JW, Noble PC, Lintner DM: The impact of ulnar collateral ligament tear and reconstruction on contact pressures in the lateral compartment of the elbow. *J Shoulder Elbow Surg* 2011;20(2):226-233.

6. Fleisig GS, Kingsley DS, Loftice JW, et al: Kinetic comparison among the fastball, curveball, change-up, and slider in collegiate baseball pitchers. *Am J Sports Med* 2006;34(3):423-430.

7. O'Driscoll SW, Lawton RL, Smith AM: The "moving valgus stress test" for medial collateral ligament tears of the elbow. *Am J Sports Med* 2005;33(2):231-239.

8. Thompson WH, Jobe FW, Yocum LA, Pink MM: Ulnar collateral ligament reconstruction in athletes: Muscle-splitting approach without transposition of the ulnar nerve. *J Shoulder Elbow Surg* 2001;10(2):152-157.

9. Kim NR, Moon SG, Ko SM, Moon WJ, Choi JW, Park JY: MR imaging of ulnar collateral ligament injury in baseball players: Value for predicting rehabilitation outcome. *Eur J Radiol* 2011;80(3):e422-e426.

10. Joyner PW, Bruce J, Hess R, Mates A, Mills FB IV, Andrews JR: Magnetic resonance imaging-based classification for ulnar collateral ligament injuries of the elbow. *J Shoulder Elbow Surg* 2016;25(10):1710-1716.

    An MRI assessment of 240 patients who underwent UCL reconstruction was carried out to create the first MRI classification system for UCL injury. This system described in this study identified radiographic criteria predictive of valgus laxity as well as improved postoperative outcome.

11. Nazarian LN, McShane JM, Ciccotti MG, O'Kane PL, Harwood MI: Dynamic US of the anterior band of the ulnar collateral ligament of the elbow in asymptomatic Major League Baseball pitchers. *Radiology* 2003;227(1):149-154.

12. Sasaki J, Takahara M, Ogino T, Kashiwa H, Ishigaki D, Kanauchi Y: Ultrasonographic assessment of the ulnar collateral ligament and medial elbow laxity in college baseball players. *J Bone Joint Surg Am* 2002;84(4):525-531.

13. Field LD, Altchek DW: Evaluation of the arthroscopic valgus instability test of the elbow. *Am J Sports Med* 1996;24(2):177-181.

14. Park GY, Lee SM, Lee MY: Diagnostic value of ultrasonography for clinical medial epicondylitis. *Arch Phys Med Rehabil* 2008;89(4):738-742.

15. Kijowski R, De Smet AA: Magnetic resonance imaging findings in patients with medial epicondylitis. *Skeletal Radiol* 2005;34(4):196-202.

16. Nirschl RP, Rodin DM, Ochiai DH, Maartmann-Moe C, DEX-AHE-01-99 Study Group: Iontophoretic administration of dexamethasone sodium phosphate for acute epicondylitis: A randomized, double-blinded, placebo-controlled study. *Am J Sports Med* 2003;31(2):189-195.

17. Suresh SP, Ali KE, Jones H, Connell DA: Medial epicondylitis: Is ultrasound guided autologous blood injection an effective treatment? *Br J Sports Med* 2006;40(11):935-939, discussion 939.

18. Varshney A, Maheshwari R, Juyal A, Agrawal A, Hayer P: Autologous platelet-rich plasma versus corticosteroid in the management of elbow epicondylitis: A randomized study. *Int J Appl Basic Med Res* 2017;7(2):125-128.

A prospective trial compared 50 patients with epicondylitis managed with steroid injections with 33 patients receiving PRP injections. At 6 months after injection, the PRP-treated cohort demonstrated significantly improved outcomes compared with the steroid cohort. Level of evidence: I.

19. Boden AL, Scott MT, Dalwadi PP, Mautner K, Mason RA, Gottschalk MB: Platelet-rich plasma versus Tenex in the treatment of medial and lateral epicondylitis. *J Shoulder Elbow Surg* 2019;28(1):112-119.

A retrospective review of 62 patients compared efficacy of PRP injections and percutaneous tenotomy for treatment of epicondylitis. Both groups showed significant improvements, but there was no difference in improvement between both groups. Level of evidence: III.

20. Whiteside D, Martini DN, Lepley AS, Zernicke RF, Goulet GC: Predictors of ulnar collateral ligament reconstruction in Major League Baseball pitchers. *Am J Sports Med* 2016;44(9):2202-2209.

104 Major League Baseball pitchers who underwent UCL reconstruction were compared with a matched cohort of position players to assess for predictors of UCL reconstruction. Six key factors were identified: fewer days between consecutive games, smaller repertoire of pitches, less pronounced horizontal release location, smaller stature, greater mean pitch speed, and greater mean pitch counts per game. Level of evidence: III.

21. Frangiamore SJ, Lynch TS, Vaughn MD, et al: Magnetic resonance imaging predictors of failure in the nonoperative management of ulnar collateral ligament injuries in professional baseball pitchers. *Am J Sports Med* 2017;45(8):1783-1789.

32 pitchers were followed up while undergoing a trial of nonsurgical treatment following UCL injury. In 34% of them, the treatment failed and they required reconstructive surgery, but the remainder returned to prior level of play for a minimum of 1 year after conservative therapy. Distal tears demonstrated significantly higher failure rates. Level of evidence: III.

22. Aguinaldo AL, Chambers H: Correlation of throwing mechanics with elbow valgus load in adult baseball pitchers. *Am J Sports Med* 2009;37(10):2043-2048.

23. Rettig AC, Sherrill C, Snead DS, Mendler JC, Mieling P: Nonoperative treatment of ulnar collateral ligament injuries in throwing athletes. *Am J Sports Med* 2001;29(1):15-17.

24. Clark NJ, Desai VS, Dines JD, Morrey ME, Camp CL: Nonreconstruction options for treating medial ulnar collateral ligament injuries of the elbow in overhead athletes. *Curr Rev Musculoskelet Med* 2018;11(1):48-54.

This article is a review on conservative management of UCL injury. Reconstruction remains the benchmark for UCL tears, but primary UCL repair and biologic augmentation of partial tears have demonstrated promise in cases of avulsion or partial tears. Level of evidence: V.

25. Cain EL Jr, Andrews JR, Dugas JR, et al: Outcome of ulnar collateral ligament reconstruction of the elbow in 1281 athletes: Results in 743 athletes with minimum 2-year follow-up. *Am J Sports Med* 2010;38(12):2426-2434.

26. Bowers AL, Dines JS, Dines DM, Altchek DW: Elbow medial ulnar collateral ligament reconstruction: Clinical relevance and the docking technique. *J Shoulder Elbow Surg* 2010;19(suppl 2):110-117.

27. Paletta GA Jr, Wright RW: The modified docking procedure for elbow ulnar collateral ligament reconstruction: 2-Year follow-up in elite throwers. *Am J Sports Med* 2006;34(10):1594-1598.

28. Dines JS, ElAttrache NS, Conway JE, Smith W, Ahmad CS: Clinical outcomes of the DANE TJ technique to treat ulnar collateral ligament insufficiency of the elbow. *Am J Sports Med* 2007;35(12):2039-2044.

29. Watson JN, McQueen P, Hutchinson MR: A systematic review of ulnar collateral ligament reconstruction techniques. *Am J Sports Med* 2014;42(10):2510-2516.

A systematic review of 21 studies investigated different techniques for UCL reconstruction. The docking technique was found to have higher return-to-sport rates with fewer complications than the Jobe or modified Jobe technique. Level of evidence: IV.

30. Erickson BJ, Bach BR Jr, Verma NN, Bush-Joseph CA, Romeo AA: Treatment of ulnar collateral ligament tears of the elbow: Is repair a viable option? *Orthop J Sports Med* 2017;5(1). doi:10.1177/2325967116682211.

A systematic review of four studies investigated UCL primary repair. The patients included had comparable return-to-sport rates and performance with reference to the published literature of UCL reconstruction and were able to return to sport within 6 months following surgery. Level of evidence: IV.

31. Rettig AC, Ebben JR: Anterior subcutaneous transfer of the ulnar nerve in the athlete. *Am J Sports Med* 1993;21(6):836-839, discussion 839-840.

32. Clain JB, Vitale MA, Ahmad CS, Ruchelsman DE: Ulnar nerve complications after ulnar collateral ligament reconstruction of the elbow: A systematic review. *Am J Sports Med* 2019;47(5):1263-1269.

A systematic review of 17 retrospective cohort studies investigated complications following UCL reconstruction. 12% of all cases developed ulnar neuropathy, which was most common with detachment of the flexor-pronator mass, modified Jobe technique, and concomitant ulnar nerve transposition. Level of evidence: IV.

33. Erickson BJ, Chalmers PN, D'Angelo J, Ma K, Romeo AA: Performance and return to sport after ulnar nerve decompression/transposition among professional baseball players. *Am J Sports Med* 2019;47(5):1124-1129.

52 Major League Baseball players were identified as undergoing isolated ulnar nerve decompression/transposition between 2010 and 2016. This study identified a lower than expected return-to-sport rate of 62%, but those who were able to return to the same level of play as matched control subjects. Level of evidence: III.

34. Maruyama M, Satake H, Takahara M, et al: Treatment for ulnar neuritis around the elbow in adolescent baseball players: Factors associated with poor outcome. *Am J Sports Med* 2017;45(4):803-809.

40 adolescent baseball players with ulnar neuritis were assessed at mean 23.6 months after presentation. 60% were able to return to sport with isolated conservative therapy after mean 2.4 months. The remainder underwent surgery, with excellent outcomes and return to sport within 2 months. Ulnar distribution hand numbness, ulnar nerve subluxation, and UCL injury were associated with poor outcomes of nonsurgical therapy. Level of evidence: IV.

35. Andrews JR, Timmerman LA: Outcome of elbow surgery in professional baseball players. *Am J Sports Med* 1995;23(4):407-413.

36. Cohen SB, Valko C, Zoga A, Dodson CC, Ciccotti MG: Posteromedial elbow impingement: Magnetic resonance imaging findings in overhead throwing athletes and results of arthroscopic treatment. *Arthroscopy* 2011;27(10):1364-1370.

37. Hulkko A, Orava S, Nikula P: Stress fractures of the olecranon in javelin throwers. *Int J Sports Med* 1986;7(4):210-213.

38. Nuber GW, Diment MT: Olecranon stress fractures in throwers: A report of two cases and a review of the literature. *Clin Orthop Relat Res* 1992;278:58-61.

39. Smith SR, Patel NK, White AE, Hadley CJ, Dodson CC: Stress fractures of the elbow in the throwing athlete: A systematic review. *Orthop J Sports Med* 2018;6(10):2325967118799262. doi:10.1177/2325967118799262.

This systematic review reported on return to sport rates following stress fractures of the elbow in throwing athletes. All but one patient analyzed was diagnosed with an olecranon stress fracture. 40 (76.9%) of the 52 athlete cohort underwent operative management and 50 (96.2%) returned to prior sporting levels. Level of evidence: IV.

40. Suzuki K, Minami A, Suenaga N, Kondoh M: Oblique stress fracture of the olecranon in baseball pitchers. *J Shoulder Elbow Surg* 1997;6(5):491-494.

41. Stephenson DR, Love S, Garcia GG, Mair SD: Recurrence of an olecranon stress fracture in an elite pitcher after percutaneous internal fixation: A case report. *Am J Sports Med* 2012;40(1):218-221.

42. Charlton WP, Chandler RW: Persistence of the olecranon physis in baseball players: Results following operative management. *J Shoulder Elbow Surg* 2003;12(1):59-62.

43. Skak SV: Fracture of the olecranon through a persistent physis in an adult: A case report. *J Bone Joint Surg Am* 1993;75(2):272-275.

44. Matsuura T, Kashiwaguchi S, Iwase T, Enishi T, Yasui N: The value of using radiographic criteria for the treatment of persistent symptomatic olecranon physis in adolescent throwing athletes. *Am J Sports Med* 2010;38(1):141-145.

45. Minami M, Nakashita K, Ishii S, et al: Twenty-five cases of osteochondritis dissecans of the elbow. *Rinsho Seikei Geka* 1979;14(8):805-810.

46. Baker CL III, Romeo AA, Baker CL Jr: Osteochondritis dissecans of the capitellum. *Am J Sports Med* 2010;38(9):1917-1928.

47. Mihara K, Tsutsui H, Nishinaka N, Yamaguchi K: Nonoperative treatment for osteochondritis dissecans of the capitellum. *Am J Sports Med* 2009;37(2):298-304.

48. Matsuura T, Kashiwaguchi S, Iwase T, Takeda Y, Yasui N: Conservative treatment for osteochondrosis of the humeral capitellum. *Am J Sports Med* 2008;36(5):868-872.

49. Takahara M, Mura N, Sasaki J, Harada M, Ogino T: Classification, treatment, and outcome of osteochondritis dissecans of the humeral capitellum. *J Bone Joint Surg Am* 2007;89(6):1205-1214.

Chapter 36

Medial and Lateral Recurrent Elbow Instability

Terry Bradly Clay, MD • Jeffrey R. Dugas, MD

ABSTRACT

Recurrent medial and lateral elbow instability affects certain patient populations. Lateral elbow instability is most often the result of a prior traumatic event and is treated with ligamentous reconstruction. Symptomatic medial elbow instability is essentially exclusive to overhead throwing athletes. Historically, ulnar collateral ligament (UCL) reconstruction has been the treatment of choice. However, the recent re-emergence of UCL repair seems promising. It is important to discuss the background, pertinent historical and physical examination findings, imaging characteristics, and treatment options for recurrent medial and lateral elbow instability.

Keywords: lateral elbow instability; medial elbow instability; posterolateral rotatory instability (PLRI); UCL reconstruction; UCL repair

Introduction

Varus elbow instability is more common in the general population, most often the result of a prior traumatic event or postsurgical in nature. This is poorly tolerated, as most activities of daily living require shoulder abduction, leading to varus loading of the elbow. This instability, therefore, often requires surgical management. In contrast, valgus loading is less common during routine activities, and thus ulnar collateral ligament (UCL) insufficiency is better tolerated. The exception is overhead throwing athletes, who require a competent UCL and often need UCL repair or reconstruction to throw effectively. The patient history, physical examination, imaging, and a high index of suspicion are essential in diagnosing and managing these conditions.

Dr. Dugas or an immediate family member has received royalties from Arthrex, Inc.; is a member of a speakers' bureau or has made paid presentations on behalf of Arthrex, Inc.; serves as a paid consultant to or is an employee of Arthrex, Inc. and Theralase; has stock or stock options held in Theralase and Topical Gear; has received research or institutional support from Arthrex, Inc., Biomet, DJ Orthopaedics, Mitek, and Smith & Nephew; and serves as a board member, owner, officer, or committee member of the ACGME Task Force, the American Orthopaedic Society for Sports Medicine, and the Fellowship Committee. Neither Dr. Clay nor any immediate family member has received anything of value from or has stock or stock options held in a commercial company or institution related directly or indirectly to the subject of this chapter.

Medial Elbow Instability

Ulnar Collateral Ligament Injuries

Background

UCL injuries most commonly occur as the result of repetitive stress during overhead throwing. During the late cocking and early acceleration phases of throwing, the valgus load applied to the elbow exceeds the tensile strength of the anterior bundle of the UCL[1,2] (**Figure 1**). Biomechanical studies have established the anterior bundle of the UCL as the primary restraint to valgus load of the elbow.[3-5] These studies also demonstrate that valgus loads during the throwing motion approach the ultimate tensile strength of the native UCL. Contact pressure of the radiocapitellar joint are restored to within 20% of intact elbows after UCL reconstruction,[6] further emphasizing the importance of the UCL in providing valgus stability.

Multiple factors have been associated with increased risk of injury to the UCL in throwing athletes, including maximal velocity[7] as well as increased height, weight, age, and position played.[8] Increased emphasis on sports specialization as well as year-round play has also increased the incidence of UCL injuries (**Figure 2**). Given this epidemic of UCL injuries, preventive measures are imperative, especially for the young overhead athlete. Multiple guidelines[9] have been recommended by the USA Baseball Medical and Safety Advisory Committee, including emphasis on monitoring pitch count, required rest periods, avoiding year-round play, proper pitching mechanics, not throwing while fatigued, and appropriate shoulder/core

This chapter is adapted from Armstrong AD: Medial and lateral recurrent elbow instability, in Nicholson GP, ed: *Orthopaedic Knowledge Update: Shoulder and Elbow*, ed 4. Rosemont, IL, American Academy of Orthopaedic Surgeons, 2013, pp 505-514.

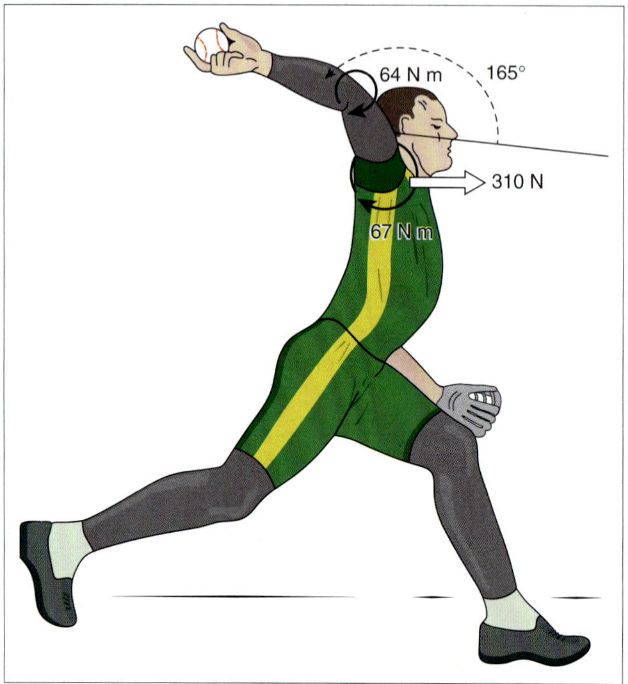

FIGURE 1 Illustration demonstrating the forces on the elbow during the acceleration phase of the throwing cycle. Shortly after maximum external rotation is achieved, the arm is externally rotated 165° and the elbow flexed 95°. The loads generated at this time are 67 N m of internal rotation torque, 310 N of anterior force at the shoulder, and 64 N m of varus torque at the elbow. (From Fleisig GS, Kingsley DS, Loftice JW, et al: Kinetic comparison among the fastball, curveball, change-up, and slider in collegiate baseball pitchers. *Am J Sports Med* 2006;34[3]:423-430, with permission. doi:10.1177/0363546505280431.)

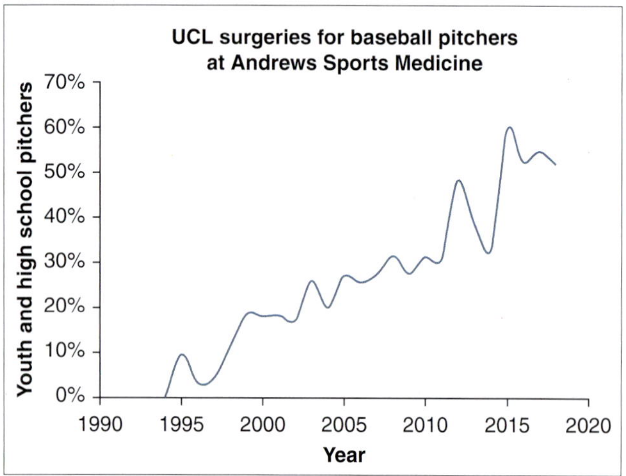

FIGURE 2 Graphic representation showing that since 1994, ulnar collateral ligament (UCL) surgeries among adolescent pitchers have increased tremendously, with a rapid rise in the last decade. (Adapted from American Sports Medicine Institute [ASMI]. UCL Surgeries on Adolescent Baseball Pitchers. Available at: http://asmi.org/research.php?page=research&section=UCL. Accessed February 1, 2019, with permission.)

strength and flexibility (Available at: https://www.mlb.com/pitch-smart/pitching-guidelines).

Although most UCL injuries occur in baseball, with pitchers and catchers most at risk, these occur in other overhead sports as well. Javelin throwers' distinct throwing motion, in conjunction with the weight of the javelin, places these athletes at risk for UCL injury. This uniquely weighted throwing motion also alters their postoperative rehabilitation, requiring a prolonged throwing program and rehabilitation period (15 months as opposed to approximately 1 year for UCL reconstruction).[10] Injuries have been reported in football quarterbacks. However, a 2010 review of the National Football League Injury Surveillance System revealed only 10 reported incidences from 1994 to 2008.[11] These athletes were successfully treated conservatively. Similarly, traumatic injuries such as dislocations in the nonthrowing athlete can typically be managed conservatively given the fact that most activities of daily living require little valgus load.

History and Physical Examination

Overhead athletes with medial elbow instability typically describe pain located over the medial elbow during the late cocking or early acceleration phase of throwing. They may describe an acute pop during throwing or may have an insidious onset of medial elbow pain often associated with decreased velocity and/or accuracy. The thrower should be asked about ulnar nerve symptoms and if present, whether they were transient or sustained. Ulnar nerve symptoms can be radicular or localized to the posteromedial elbow. Another cause of posteromedial elbow pain can be related to posteromedial osteophytes or valgus extension overload (**Figure 3**), and the athlete will complain of pain during deceleration or ball release.

The diagnosis of valgus elbow instability can be challenging, as the physical examination findings can be subtle. The patient often has point tenderness to palpation over the ligament, whether that be the medial epicondyle origin, ligament proper, or sublime tubercle insertion. A Tinel test should be performed to evaluate the ulnar nerve for ulnar radicular symptoms. Additionally, the ulnar nerve should be palpated during range of motion to evaluate for ulnar nerve subluxation, which should be addressed during surgical management. Preoperative range of motion is documented, as a number of throwing athletes have a flexion contracture. Palpation over the posteromedial olecranon will elicit pain in patients with valgus extension overload. Additionally, they often have a flexion contracture and pain with forced elbow extension while applying a valgus stress.

Medial elbow instability is assessed using multiple provocative tests including the valgus stress test, the

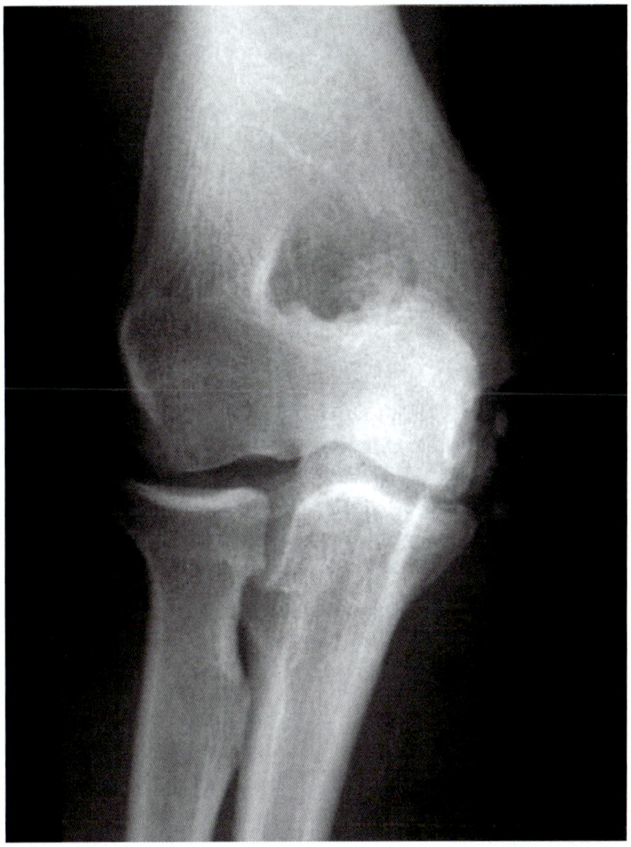

FIGURE 3 AP radiograph of the elbow of a former baseball pitcher showing posteromedial osteophytosis related to chronic valgus extension overload.

milking maneuver, and the moving valgus stress test.[12] The valgus stress test is performed with the elbow flexed to 30°, unlocking the olecranon from the fossa. With shoulder rotation controlled, gapping is compared with the contralateral limb while palpating the medial joint line during valgus stress. This often elicits pain as well. The milking maneuver statically loads the UCL. Again, with shoulder motion controlled, the patient's elbow is flexed to 90° and the forearm is supinated. The examiner then pulls the ipsilateral thumb to apply a valgus stress eliciting pain. The moving valgus stress test is a dynamic test that applies a constant valgus load to the elbow during an arc of motion. Athletes with UCL injury will describe pain at the medial elbow typically between 70° and 120° of flexion (**Figure 4**).

An elbow examination is not complete without evaluating the athlete as a whole. The ipsilateral shoulder must be examined and compared with the contralateral side. Overhead athletes with injury to their UCL often demonstrate glenohumeral rotation deficit and a tight posterior capsule.[13] As a result, shoulder therapy and posterior capsular stretching should be emphasized during postoperative rehabilitation to decrease stress on the UCL. The athlete's core musculature strength should also be assessed. The act of throwing is a complex motion with the transfer of energy from the thighs, buttocks, and trunk to the upper extremity, and weakness in the core can lead to increased stress on the shoulder and elbow.[14] Similarly, their mechanics must be evaluated to look for biomechanical flaws that predispose throwers to injuries.

Imaging

Although history and physical examination is the mainstay for detecting UCL injuries, proper imaging is imperative for establishing an appropriate preoperative plan. Plain radiographs are initially obtained including AP, lateral, internal oblique, external oblique, and axial views. These are often normal but may show additional areas of pathology including osteochondral defects, physeal injuries, stress fractures, evidence of valgus extension overload (**Figure 3**), degenerative changes, sequela of prior avulsion injuries, or ossification of the UCL. Stress radiographs can additionally be obtained but may not be well tolerated by the patient and therefore have been abandoned by some institutions. A 2014 study demonstrated that more than 0.4 mm of widening on stress radiographs correlated with injury and that increased gapping of more than 0.6 mm was associated with full-thickness tears.[15] MRI (with or without arthrography) has become the standard of care in identifying UCL injury and classifying the type of tear, which guide treatment options. Saline-enhanced magnetic resonance arthrography has been shown to have 86% sensitivity for detecting partial tears and 95% sensitivity for complete tears.[16] Dynamic ultrasonography has recently emerged as an additional diagnostic tool[17] and could help predict which players may be at increased risk for subsequent injury.[18,19]

Treatment Overview

There are numerous factors that should be considered when determining the best treatment algorithm including injury acuity, tissue quality, position played, level of competition, and timing to return to sport. High-demand athletes with complete tears or those with chronic injuries should consider reconstruction. Those with acute injury or avulsion injuries with good ligament quality can consider repair. In lower demand athletes or those with partial tears, conservative treatment can be attempted before discussing surgical options.

Nonsurgical Management

The mainstay of conservative management is rest and rehabilitation. Physical therapy is vital to fully restore normal function expeditiously but safely as well. Therefore, it must follow a progressive, sequential protocol each building on

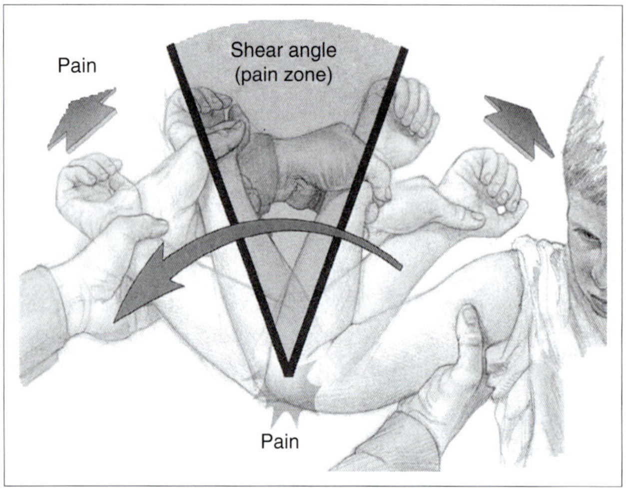

FIGURE 4 Schematic drawing showing the moving valgus stress test, in which a valgus load is applied to the elbow throughout an arc of motion. A patient with a ulnar collateral ligament tear will describe pain through the middle of the arc of motion, typically between 70° and 120° of flexion (the shear angle). (From Armstrong AD. Medial and lateral recurrent elbow instability, in Nicholson GP, ed: *AAOS Orthopaedic Knowledge Update Shoulder and Elbow*, 4th ed. Rosemont, IL, American Academy of Orthopaedic Surgeons, 2013; used with permission of Mayo Foundation for Medical Education and Research, all rights reserved.)

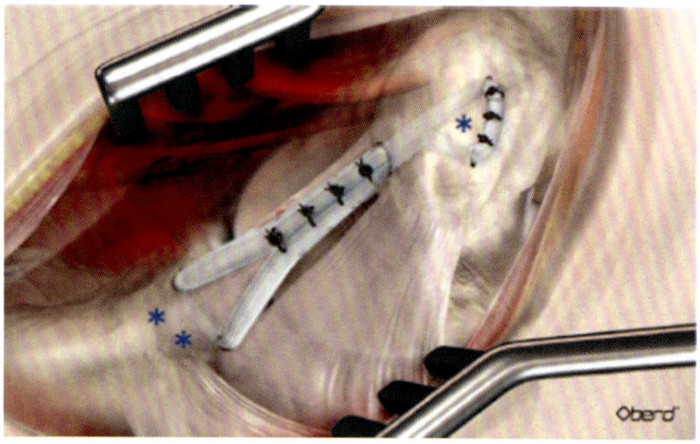

FIGURE 5 Illustration of ulnar collateral ligament (UCL) reconstruction using the figure-of-8 technique with a palmaris autograft through bone tunnels. Anatomic landmarks are labeled as the proximal UCL origin from the medial epicondyle (*) and the distal UCL insertion onto the sublime tubercle (**). (Reproduced with permission from Dugas JR, Walters BL, Beason DP, et al: Biomechanical comparision of ulnar collateral ligament repair with internal bracing versus modified Jobe reconstruction. *Am J Sports Med* 2016;44[3]:735-741.)

the previous phase to ensure proper healing. Immediate bracing treatment is applied to resist valgus force. This is coupled with progressive range-of-motion exercises increasing weekly until full painless motion is achieved, usually by week 4. Progressive strengthening is then begun early around week 6. This is followed by plyometric drills and an interval throwing program.[20] Glenohumeral and scapular strengthening, proprioceptive training, and lower body and core rehabilitation exercises are emphasized as well to improve the kinetic chain. This rehabilitation program is critical not only for the patient attempting conservative therapy but for postsurgical patients as well.

Historically, nonsurgical management of UCL injuries demonstrated poor return to sport with one study demonstrating 42%.[21] Thus additional modalities are being explored to improve outcomes. Similar to other areas of orthopaedics, biologics have gained recent interest to stimulate and enhance the tissue healing capability of the injured UCL. A 2016 study evaluated the efficacy of platelet-rich plasma injections in partial UCL tears in high-level athletes demonstrating 73% good to excellent outcomes.[22] Mesenchymal stem cells are another area of interest for repair because of their ability to differentiate into a variety of cell lineages. However, no clinical study has published results on the effectiveness in UCL injuries. More research is needed to clarify the role of biologics in UCL injury.

Ulnar Collateral Ligament Reconstruction

UCL reconstruction, as first described by Dr. Frank Jobe in 1974, has been considered the benchmark for management of UCL injuries in the overhead athlete.[23] Numerous techniques have been described with modern return-to-sport rates ranging from 83% to 95%, in part because of improvement in techniques as well as increased experience with the procedure.[23-36] The largest outcome study[36] of UCL reconstruction evaluated athletes with at least 2-year follow-up undergoing a modified Jobe (figure-of-8) technique using a muscle elevating approach with subcutaneous ulnar nerve transposition (**Figures 5** and **6**). The return-to-sport rate was 83% with an average return time of 11.6 months (range 3 to 72 months). In 2014, it has been shown that the time to return increases even more for Major League Baseball (MLB) players, averaging 16.8 months.[37]

Complication rates found using the modified Jobe technique in the aforementioned study[36] were 20%, with 16% minor complications and 4% major complications. Ulnar nerve symptoms were the most common complication with minor postoperative sensory neurapraxia in 16% of patients. Of these, 82% resolved within 6 weeks. In all of the remaining cases, except one patient, symptoms resolved by 1 year. These complications have been minimized with modifications of the technique including using an intermuscular split rather than elevating the entire flexor muscle fascia. With that said, the high reported ulnar nerve complication rate has led to the emergence

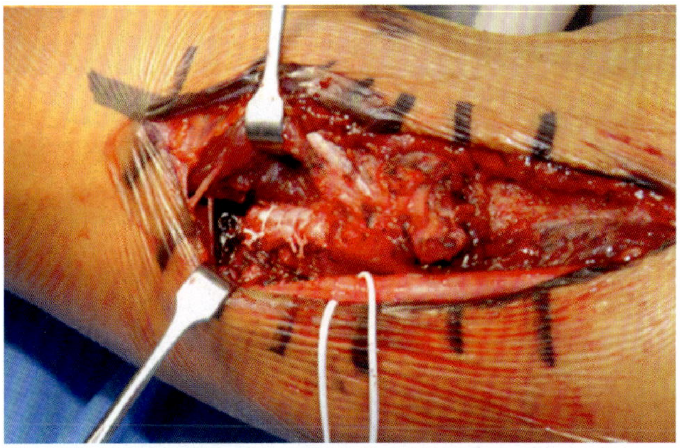

FIGURE 6 Intraoperative photograph of ulnar collateral ligament reconstruction using the figure-of-8 technique. The graft has been sewn together between the humeral and ulnar tunnels to increase tension within the graft and re-create the course of the native ligament. The ulnar nerve is ready for transposition using an intermuscular septum fascial sleeve. (Reproduced with permission from Andrews JR, Jost PW, Cain EL: The ulnar collateral ligament procedure revisited: The procedure we use. *Sports Health* 2012;4[5]:438-441.)

of alternative techniques[26-35] with similar return-to-sport rates and outcomes. This includes the docking technique, using a muscle-splitting approach without transposition of the ulnar nerve (**Figures 7** and **8**).

A recent systematic review evaluated the rate of ulnar nerve complications using all techniques.[38] The mean prevalence of postoperative ulnar neuropathy was 12%. The muscle-splitting approach had the lowest rate of neuropathy (3.9%) compared with muscle retraction (15.9%). The fixation technique associated with the highest rate of neuropathy was the modified Jobe (16.9%) compared with the modified docking technique (2.5%). Additionally, ulnar nerve transposition was associated with a high neuropathy rate (16.1%) compared with no handling of the ulnar nerve (3.9%). With that said, only 0.8% of all cases required revision surgery to address the ulnar nerve. Another study,[39] recently published, demonstrated that surgical outcomes in professional baseball players were not significantly different between UCL reconstruction technique and graft type with similar return to play and return to same level of play rates. The use of concomitant ulnar nerve transposition additionally did not affect outcomes. Therefore, although there may be a higher rate of ulnar nerve symptoms when using the modified Jobe technique with ulnar nerve transposition, this does not seem to affect outcomes or the need for revision surgery.

Ulnar Collateral Ligament Repair

Although UCL reconstruction has demonstrated excellent outcomes with consistent return to play over the past several decades, there are some limitations to the procedure. First, return to play is typically quoted at 12 to 18 months,[36,37] meaning the athlete will miss at least one season. In certain clinical situations, avoidance of UCL reconstruction and its associated year-long recovery may be beneficial. Additionally, there is a wide spectrum of injury to the ligament ranging from low-grade partial tears with good ligament quality to chronic complete tears with deficient ligament tissue. Therefore, there may be a subset of injuries that could be managed without undergoing a full reconstruction. These factors have led to the idea of possible alternative treatment options, including the reemergence of UCL repair.

Once conservative measures have failed, there are numerous indications for repair. These include overhead athletes who are young, acute avulsion injuries, partial tears with good ligament quality, and those with time restraints who would like an expedited return to play. The UCL tissue should appear healthy on MRI (**Figures 9** and **10**), but the final decision of performing a UCL repair is determined at surgery based on the intraoperative assessment of tissue quality. Patients with chronic attritional tears and those with bony ossicles that when removed would compromise the remaining tissue quality and quantity are poor repair candidates. Appropriate patient selection is critical for successful outcomes in UCL repair.

Historically, attempts at UCL repair yielded poor results, especially when compared with reconstruction. When looking at 13-year data in one study, the rate of return to same level of play in patients undergoing repair was 50%. This dropped to 29% in MLB players.[24] Likewise, in another study the return-to-play rate following repair was less satisfactory when compared with reconstruction (63% versus 81%).[25] Given the early poor results with repair, it was largely abandoned until recently. A renewed interest in UCL repair has emerged with advances in technologies and a better understanding of the spectrum of injuries. The author of a 2008 study demonstrated a 93% return to same level of sport with all but two patients returning at 6 months using mostly suture anchor repair.[40] These promising results led to a modification of the repair procedure with the addition of a collagen-coated FiberTape (Arthrex) to act as a backstop to valgus stress and provide a biologic augment for ligament healing (**Figures 11** through **14**).

Biomechanical testing of UCL repair with internal brace augmentation showed similar time-zero failure strength compared with the traditional Jobe reconstruction technique and greater resistance to gapping.[41] The first outcome study using this technique was recently published, with a 92% return to the same or higher level of play at a mean time of 6.7 months.[42] Kerlan-Jobe

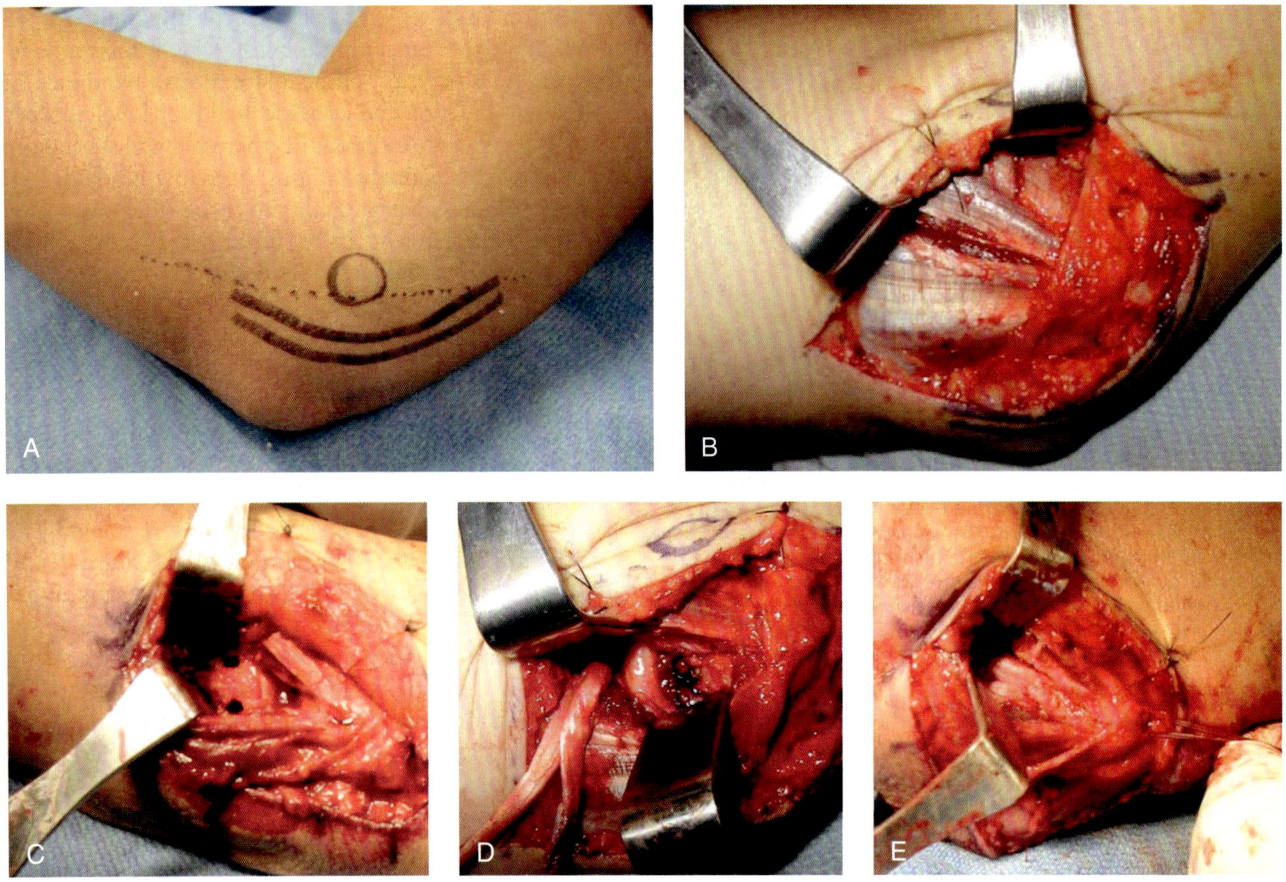

FIGURE 7 Photographs showing the docking technique for ulnar collateral ligament reconstruction. **A**, The medial-based incision (dotted line), the medial epicondyle (circle), and the ulnar nerve path (solid lines) are marked. **B**, The muscle-splitting approach requires care to protect the medial antebrachial cutaneous nerve. **C**, Two holes are drilled in the ulna, bridging the sublime tubercle. **D**, The medial epicondyle is exposed to drill one hole at the point of isometry, and the tendon graft is passed through ulna drill holes. **E**, In the completed reconstruction, both tendon ends are docked into the humerus with sutures passed through smaller drill holes placed more proximal than the isometric drill hole.

Orthopaedic Clinic scores averaged 88.2 at a minimum of 1 year and improved to 91.1 at 2 years, which approaches the asymptomatic mean value of a healthy pitcher (which should be in the low to mid 90s).[43] These reassuring results demonstrate that UCL repair with internal brace augmentation is a viable treatment option for overhead throwing athletes. However, further studies are indicated to establish the long-term effects of the procedure and determine the limits of the procedure's application.

Lateral Elbow Instability

Lateral Collateral Ligament Complex Injuries/ Posterolateral Rotatory Instability

Background

Unlike valgus elbow instability, which occurs in the overhead athletic cohort, posterolateral rotatory instability (PLRI) most commonly occurs in the general cohort after a traumatic event. This can be debilitating because activities of daily living place the lateral collateral ligament complex (LCLC) under constant stress. This usually develops after an elbow dislocation or a fall onto an outstretched hand, although there are additional much less common etiologies. These include iatrogenic injury from prior elbow surgery (aggressive lateral epicondylar release), multiple corticosteroid injection for recalcitrant lateral epicondylitis,[44] tardy PLRI due to cubital varus as a result from a prior malunion of a childhood supracondylar humerus fracture, or radial head resection.[45-47]

The classic mechanism for an elbow dislocation is axial compression, valgus force, and an external rotation moment (torque) to the elbow causing the radial head and proximal ulna to subluxate posterolaterally away from the humerus in a rotatory fashion.[48,49] If the LCLC then fails to adequately heal, this leads to PLRI. With

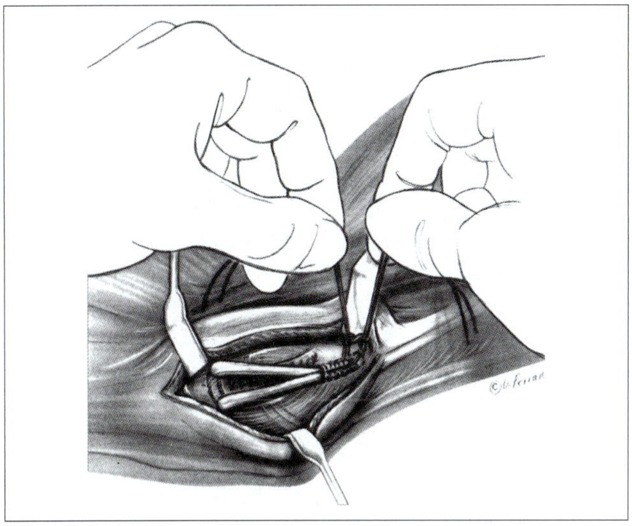

FIGURE 8 Drawing showing the docking technique for ulnar collateral ligament reconstruction, as it was first described. The tendon graft is passed through two drill holes in the ulna and one docking drill hole at the isometric point on the humerus. Sutures are passed through two smaller holes drilled more proximally. (© Hospital for Special Surgery. All rights reserved.)

posterolateral elbow dislocations, instability is rare, because it usually involves a stripping injury and the LCLC tends to return to its native position after reduction of the elbow. On the other hand, posteromedial dislocations tend to be distraction injuries resulting in more significant

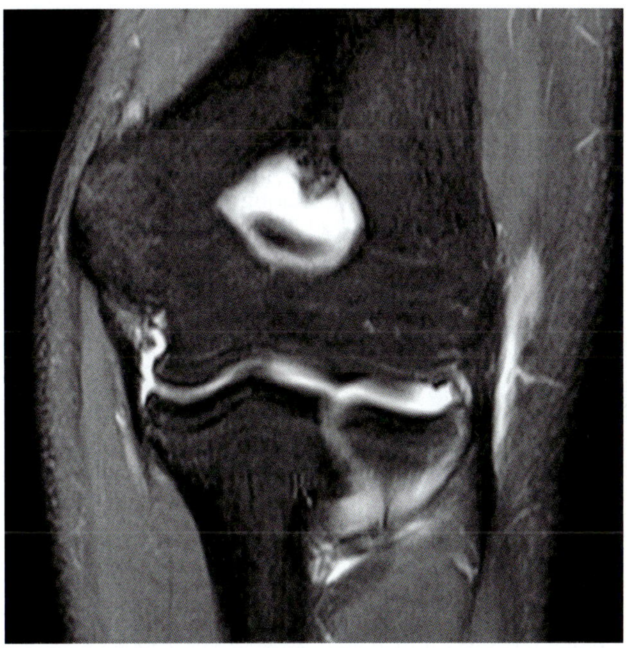

FIGURE 9 Preoperative magnetic resonance image with contrast of a pitcher with a partial distal ulnar collateral ligament (UCL) tear. Note the intra-articular dye undermining the distal UCL insertion forming the diagnostic T sign.

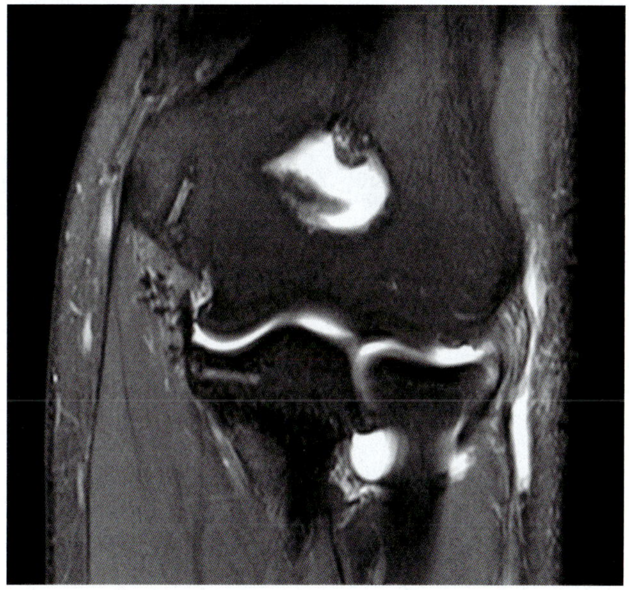

FIGURE 10 Postoperative magnetic resonance image with contrast of the same pitcher showing the healed distal end of the ulnar collateral ligament (UCL) to the sublime tubercle insertion without extravasation of the intra-articular dye and resolution of the previously seen "T" sign.

lateral soft-tissue damage. As a result, they may be associated with a higher risk for PLRI and recurrent instability.[50]

The LCLC is composed of the lateral ulnar collateral ligament (LUCL), the radial collateral ligament (RCL), the annular ligament, and the accessory collateral ligament. The LUCL is classically described as the primary restraint to PLRI although some biomechanical studies have suggested a significant role for the RCL as well.[45,51,52] One study[53] suggested the RCL, not the LUCL, is an isometric

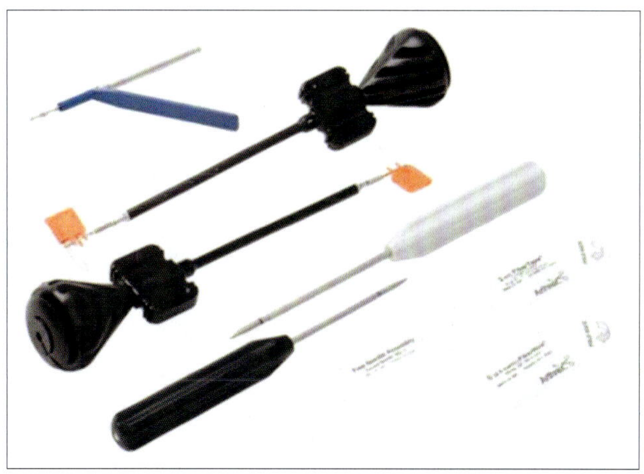

FIGURE 11 Photograph of ulnar collateral ligament internal brace kit (includes 3.5 mm PEEK [polyether ether ketone] SwiveLock, collagen-coated FiberTape, Fiberwire, free tapered needle, 2.7 mm drill, drill guide, 3.8 mm tap, and 3.45 mm punch/tap). (Courtesy of Arthrex®, Naples, Florida 2020.)

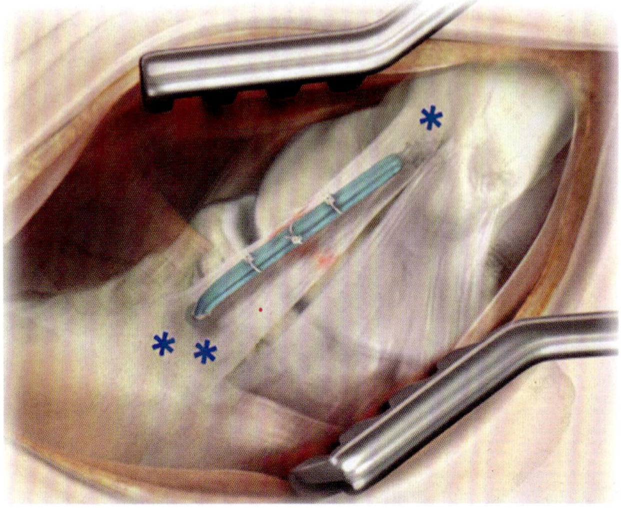

FIGURE 12 Illustration of ulnar collateral ligament (UCL) repair with internal brace (Arthrex). The augmentation integrated into the repair is visible. Anatomic landmarks are labeled as proximal UCL origin on the medial epicondyle (asterisk) and distal UCL insertion onto the sublime tubercle (double asterisk). (Reproduced from Dugas J, Walters B, Beason D, Fleisig G, Chronister J: Biomechanical comparison of ulnar collateral ligament repair with internal bracing versus modified Jobe reconstruction. *Am J Sports Med* 2016;44(3):735-741. doi:10.1177/0363546515620390.)

bundle. Another study[54] found no true isometric point for the LCLC and significant variability in the maximal isometric graft insertion point for LCLC reconstruction. There is likely a contribution of both the LUCL and the RCL for stability against PLRI. As a result, a dual reconstruction technique of the RCL and LUCL has been reported for the management of PLRI[55] with clinical outcomes similar to those of conventional LUCL reconstruction techniques.[56]

Diagnosis

The diagnosis of PLRI can be difficult. Most patients complain of mechanical symptoms of instability including snapping, clicking, or clunking in the elbow. They additionally may notice a prominence or dimple over the lateral elbow and may be able to reproduce their symptoms of instability with elbow extension and axial loading. Occasionally, they may present with lateral elbow pain only, usually a result of an iatrogenic etiology.

The classic examination test for PLRI is the lateral pivot-shift test[57] (**Figure 15**). This often is performed under anesthesia because patients cannot tolerate it in the clinic. With the patient supine, the arm is bent overhead. The elbow is then extended with an axial and valgus load with the forearm maximally supinated. The elbow will subluxate, and fluoroscopic imaging will show the radial head posterior to the capitellum and widening of the ulnohumeral joint. Flexion will reduce the joint with an appreciable clunk. This test is highly reproducible and independent of the examiner's level of training or experience.[58] The posterolateral drawer test, the chair push-up test, the floor push-up test, and the tabletop relocation test are additional examination maneuvers that are often better tolerated by the patient. Therefore, they are more commonly performed in the clinical setting and have become the examination of choice by some.[59,60] These tests simulate the lateral pivot shift test by producing an extended, supinated, axially, valgus-loaded elbow joint resulting in subluxation, reproducing the patient's symptoms.

Although the diagnosis of PLRI is clinical, imaging studies can be helpful. Static radiographs are often normal but may show indirect signs of injury including subluxation of the joint, fractures of the capitellum, coronoid, or radial head. MRI (with or without arthrography) can confirm the clinical suspicion and aid in surgical planning. This can show direct injury to the LCLC or more subtle signs of injury. A 2015 study showed that 2 mm of radiocapitellar incongruity (sagittal view) and 1 mm of ulnohumeral incongruity (axial view) are highly suspicious of elbow instability.[61] Similar to a Hill-Sachs lesion in the shoulder, a posterior capitellar

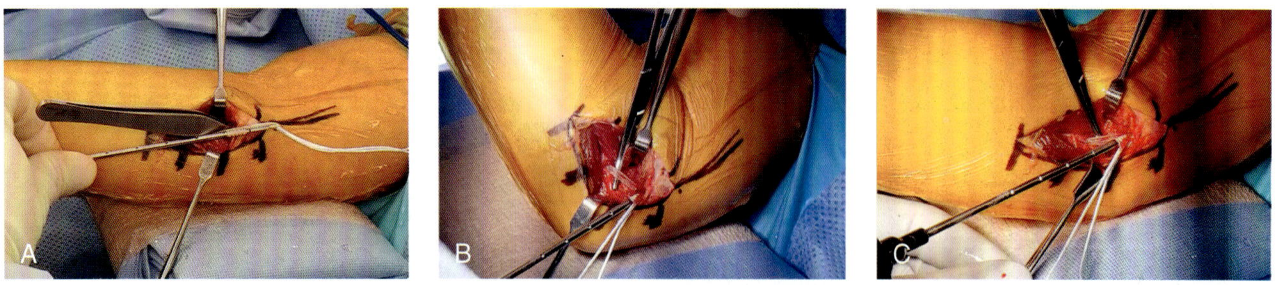

FIGURE 13 Intraoperative photographs showing the first anchor being inserted at the site of the tear and loaded with a 0 nonabsorbable suture and collagen-dipped FiberTape (Arthrex). The nonabsorbable suture is used to repair the ligament tear. **A**, The second anchor is tensioned by placing the threads of the anchor such that the third thread (or approximately half of the anchor) is at the level of the tunnel entrance. The anchor driver is inserted into the drilled hold, and tension is checked through full range of (**B**) flexion and (**C**) extension before advancing the screw over the driver. There should be no limitation of motion, and the anchor driver should not back out of the hole in flexion. (Reproduced from Dugas JR, Looze CA, Capogna B, et al: Ulnar collateral ligament repair with collagen-dipped FiberTape augmentation in overhead-throwing athletes. *Am J Sports Med* 2019;47(5):1096-1102. doi:10.1177/0363546519833684.)

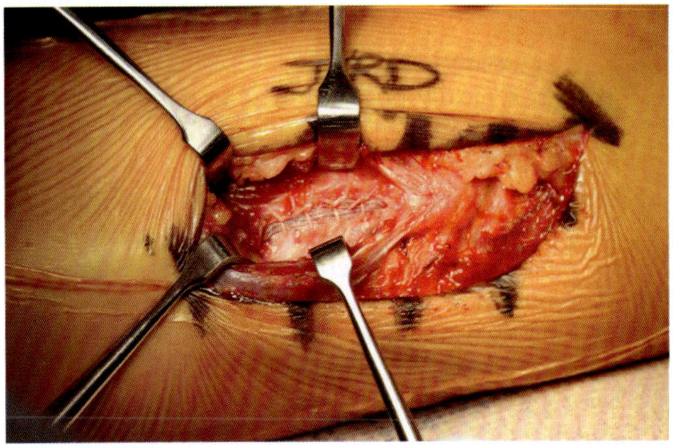

FIGURE 14 Intraoperative photograph of ulnar collateral ligament repair with internal brace and loosely tensioned FiberTape (Arthrex) sewn into the native ligament. (Reproduced from Dugas JR, Looze CA, Capogna B, et al: Ulnar collateral ligament repair with collagen-dipped FiberTape augmentation in overhead-throwing athletes. *Am J Sports Med* 2019;47(5): 1096-1102. doi:10.1177/0363546519833684.)

impression fracture may be visualized if associated with an elbow dislocation.[62] Additional abnormalities found on MRI can be a pseudodefect of the capitellum or a posterior capitellar impression fracture, also known as an Osborne-Cotterill lesion.[63,64] This represents an osteochondral fracture of the posterolateral capitellum, equivalent to a Bankart lesion of the glenoid. This defect is recognized as a cause of PLRI. Depending on the size of the osseous defect, a combined ligamentous and osseous reconstruction may be required.[65]

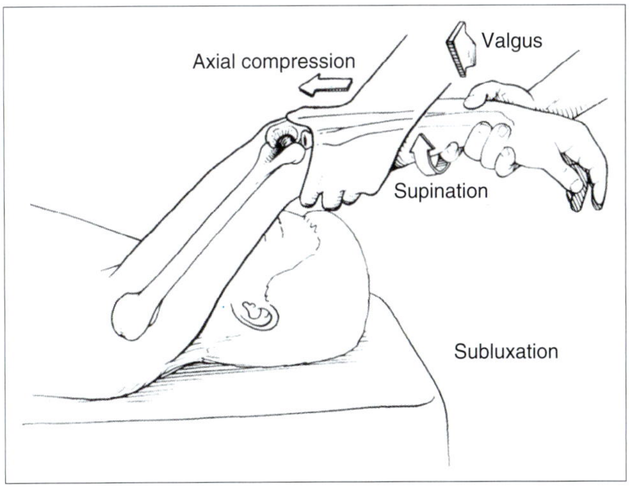

FIGURE 15 Drawing showing the lateral pivot shift test, which is the classic instability test for lateral collateral ligament complex insufficiency. An axial load is applied to the elbow at the same time as a forced supinated and valgus load. The elbow is subluxated when it is in extension, and often it is possible to visually and audibly observe elbow flexion to reduce the joint. (Reproduced with permission from O'Driscoll SW, Bell DF, Morrey BF: Posterolateral rotatory instability of the elbow. *J Bone Joint Surg Am* 1991;73[3]:440-446.)

Management

As most activities of daily living require valgus loading through the elbow, most patients with PLRI are symptomatic and require surgical treatment. It has been shown that the results of surgical repair are inferior to reconstruction, likely owing to attenuation of the ligaments and the resulting effect on the complex interworking of the LCLC.[66,67] At a mean 6-year follow-up on 44 patients, 86% of patients were satisfied with their outcomes, with posttraumatic etiology, subjective feelings of instability, and reconstructions demonstrating better results.[67] With the emergence of promising outcomes with ligament repair using suture tape augmentation techniques, including the medial elbow as described earlier, some have adapted the technique for application in lateral ligamentous injuries. Early data seem promising, with all 17 patients reporting a complete return to preinjury level of activities with the additional benefit of accelerated rehabilitation and early, brace-free initiation of full range of motion.[68] As this is only median 10-month follow-up data, further long-term studies are indicated to fully evaluate outcomes using this technique.

Classically, the LCLC is reconstructed using a figure-of-8 technique. This involves a bone tunnel in the ulna at the crista supinatoris and another bone tunnel at the isometric insertion of the LCLC on the humerus.[57] The tendon graft is passed in a figure-of-8 fashion and sutured to itself, similar to the technique described for UCL reconstruction. There are additional reconstruction options that have also been described including using the triceps tendon,[69,70] arthroscopic techniques,[71] interference screw techniques,[72] and the docking technique.[73] Biomechanical studies have shown no significant difference in stability among reconstruction techniques.[74]

Similar to the medial side of the elbow, the docking technique has increased in popularity[73,75] (**Figure 16**). A Kocher approach to the elbow is used. The ulnar tunnel is created by converging the base of two sockets. The first is immediately posterior to the supinator crest, whereas the second is located proximal and posterior to a bony bridge of at least 1.25 cm between the holes, near the base of the annular ligament. The bases of the sockets are connected and cleared of bone debris using an awl, and a looped suture is placed. Attention is then turned to the humeral socket, which should be isometric throughout the flexion-extension arc. This point is typically at the geometric center of a circle superimposed on the capitellar articular margin. The humeral socket is drilled toward, but not through, the posterior cortex to a depth of 15 mm. The center of the socket is placed approximately 1 mm proximal and posterior to the previously identified isometric point because once tensioned, the graft will drape along the anterior-inferior

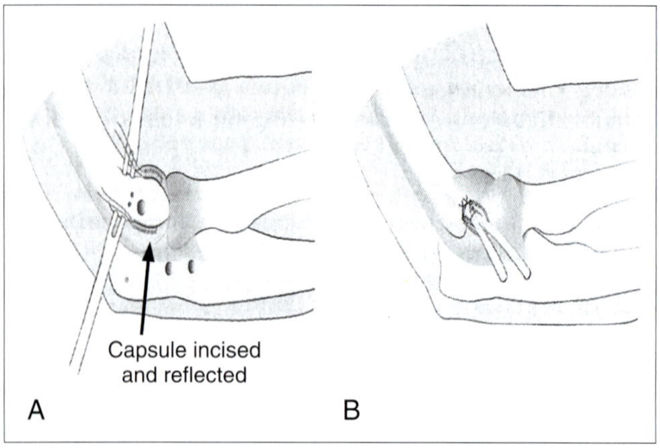

FIGURE 16 Schematic drawings showing the docking technique for reconstruction of the lateral collateral ligament complex. **A**, Two drill holes are created in the ulna, and one drill hole is created at the isometric point on the humerus, with two smaller exit drill holes proximal in the humerus for suture passage. **B**, In the completed reconstruction, the underlying capsuloligamentous complex is repaired, and tendon graft is passed through two ulnar drill holes and docked into a humeral drill hole. (Reprinted from *J Shoulder Elbow Surg* 21[3]. Jones KJ, Dodson CC, Osbahr DC, et al: The docking technique for lateral ulnar collateral ligament reconstruction: Surgical technique and clinical outcomes, 389-395. doi:10.1016/j.jse.2011.04.033. Copyright © 2012 Journal of Shoulder and Elbow Surgery Board of Trustees.)

rim of the socket, which brings it back to the isometric point. A second socket is drilled toward, but not through, the anterior cortex. Two smaller holes are drilled on either side of the supracondylar ridge, one anteriorly and one posteriorly with at least a 10 mm bony bridge. The graft is then passed through the ulnar tunnel from proximal to distal and then docked in the humeral tunnel. Before securing the graft, isometry is tested through a flexion-extension arc and the capsule is closed. The graft is then secured over the bony bridge. At a mean follow-up of 7 years using the docking technique, 75% of patients had no recurrent instability and 25% reported occasional instability during activities of daily living. All patients were satisfied with the outcome.

SUMMARY

Recurrent medial or lateral elbow instability is uncommon but can be disabling in certain patient populations. Nonsurgical management is often ineffective. The diagnosis relies on a focused patient history and physical examination, imaging, and a high index of suspicion. Ligament reconstruction is the benchmark for treatment with high rates of success although ligament repair has promising early results in certain subsets of patients.

KEY STUDY POINTS

- PLRI is typically posttraumatic in nature and often requires surgical reconstruction for definitive treatment.
- Symptomatic medial elbow instability is essentially exclusive to overhead throwing athletes, and surgical repair or reconstruction is the definitive treatment once nonsurgical management fails.
- UCL reconstruction, as first described by Dr. Frank Jobe in 1974, has been considered the benchmark for treatment of UCL injuries in the overhead athlete.
- There is a wide spectrum of UCL injuries ranging from acute, partial tears with good ligament quality to chronic, attritional tears with poor tissue substance.
- Early results of UCL repair seem promising with a 92% return to the same or higher level of play at a mean time of 6.7 months, compared with the typically quoted 12 to 18 months after UCL reconstruction.

Annotated References

1. Fleisig GS, Andrews JR, Dillman CJ, Escamilla RF: Kinetics of baseball pitching with implications about injury mechanisms. *Am J Sports Med* 1995;23(2):233-239.

2. Dillman CJ, Fleisig GS, Andrews JR: Biomechanics of pitching with emphasis upon shoulder kinematics. *J Orthop Sports Phys Ther* 1993;18(2):402-408.

3. Hotchkiss RN, Weiland AJ: Valgus stability of the elbow. *J Orthop Res* 1987;5(3):372-377.

4. Søjbjerg JO, Ovesen J, Nielsen S: Experimental elbow instability after transection of the medial collateral ligament. *Clin Orthop Relat Res* 1987;218:186-190.

5. Morrey BF, An KN: Articular and ligamentous contributions to the stability of the elbow joint. *Am J Sports Med* 1983;11(5):315-319.

6. Duggan JP Jr, Osadebe UC, Alexander JW, Noble PC, Lintner DM: The impact of ulnar collateral ligament tear and reconstruction on contact pressures in the lateral compartment of the elbow. *J Shoulder Elbow Surg* 2011;20(2):226-233.

7. Bushnell BD, Anz AW, Noonan TJ, Torry MR, Hawkins RJ: Association of maximum pitch velocity and elbow injury in professional baseball pitchers. *Am J Sports Med* 2010;38(4):728-732.

8. Han KJ, Kim YK, Lim SK, Park JY, Oh KS: The effect of physical characteristics and field position on the shoulder and elbow injuries of 490 baseball players: Confirmation of diagnosis by magnetic resonance imaging. *Clin J Sport Med* 2009;19(4):271-276.

9. Pitch Smart. USA Baseball. Pitching Guidelines. Available at: https://www.mlb.com/pitch-smart/pitching-guidelines. Accessed June 12, 2019.

10. Dines JS, Jones KJ, Kahlenberg C, Rosenbaum A, Osbahr DC, Altchek DW: Elbow ulnar collateral ligament reconstruction in javelin throwers at a minimum 2-year follow-up. *Am J Sports Med* 2012;40(1):148-151.

11. Dodson CC, Slenker N, Cohen SB, Ciccotti MG, DeLuca P: Ulnar collateral ligament injuries of the elbow in professional football quarterbacks. *J Shoulder Elbow Surg* 2010;19(8):1276-1280.

12. O'Driscoll SW, Lawton RL, Smith AM: The "moving valgus stress test" for medial collateral ligament tears of the elbow. *Am J Sports Med* 2005;33(2):231-239.

13. Dines JS, Frank JB, Akerman M, Yocum LA: Glenohumeral internal rotation deficits in baseball players with ulnar collateral ligament insufficiency. *Am J Sports Med* 2009;37(3):566-570.

14. Kibler WB, Sciascia A: Kinetic chain contributions to elbow function and dysfunction in sports. *Clin Sports Med* 2004;23(4):545-552, viii.

15. Bruce JR, Hess R, Joyner P, Andrews JR: How much valgus instability can be expected with ulnar collateral ligament (UCL) injuries? A review of 273 baseball players with UCL injuries. *J Shoulder Elbow Surg* 2014;23(10): 1521-1526.

    The authors hypothesized that valgus stress radiographs in patients with UCL injuries would show more valgus stress opening of the dominant elbow compared with the nondominant elbow.

16. Schwartz ML, al-Zahrani S, Morwessel RM, Andrews JR: Ulnar collateral ligament injury in the throwing athlete: Evaluation with salineenhanced MR arthrography. *Radiology* 1995;197(1):297-299.

17. Smith W, Hackel JG, Goitz HT, Bouffard JA, Nelson AM: Utilization of sonography and a stress device in the assessment of partial tears of the ulnar collateral ligament in throwers. *Int J Sports Phys Ther* 2011;6(1): 45 50.

18. Atanda AJ, Buckley PS, Hammoud S, Cohen SB, Nazarian LN, Ciccotti MG: Early anatomic changes of the ulnar collateral ligament identified by stress ultrasound of the elbow in young professional baseball pitchers. *Am J Sports Med* 2015;43(12):2943-2949.

    Stress ultrasonography was performed on the dominant arm in 127 asymptomatic professional pitchers, demonstrating a statistically significant increase in mean UCL thickness with increasing years of professional experience. Level of evidence: III.

19. Ciccotti MG, Atanda A Jr, Nazarian LN, Dodson CC, Holmes L, Cohen SB: Stress sonography of the ulnar collateral ligament of the elbow in professional baseball pitchers: A 10-year study. *Am J Sports Med* 2014;42(3):544-551.

    Stress ultrasonography was performed on 368 asymptomatic professional baseball pitchers over a 10-year period. Twelve players incurred a UCL injury and demonstrated increases in baseline ligament thickness, ulnohumeral joint space gapping with stress, and incidence of hypoechoic foci and calcifications. Level of evidence: III.

20. Wilk KE, Macrina LC, Cain EL, Dugas JR, Andrews JR: Rehabilitation of the overhead athlete's elbow. *Sports Health* 2012;4(5):404-414.

21. Rettig AC, Sherrill C, Snead DS, Mendler JC, Mieling P: Nonoperative treatment of ulnar collateral ligament injuries in throwing athletes. *Am J Sports Med* 2001;29(1): 15-17.

22. Dines JS, Williams PN, ElAttrache N, et al: Platelet-rich plasma can be used to successfully treat elbow ulnar collateral ligament insufficiency in high-level throwers. *Am J Orthop (Belle Mead NJ)* 2016;45(5):296-300.

    In this retrospective review, 44 baseball players (6 professional, 14 college, 24 high school) with partial UCL tears (22 proximal partial tears, 7 distal partial tears, 15 with diffuse signal) confirmed by MRI were treated with platelet-rich plasma injection. 73% had good to excellent outcomes. 67% of professional players (4 out of 6) returned to professional play. Mean time to competition was 12 weeks. There were no injection-related complications.

23. Jobe FW, Stark H, Lombardo SJ: Reconstruction of the ulnar collateral ligament in athletes. *J Bone Joint Surg Am* 1986;68(8):1158-1163.

24. Conway JE, Jobe FW, Glousman RE, Pink M: Medial instability of the elbow in throwing athletes: Treatment by repair or reconstruction of the ulnar collateral ligament. *J Bone Joint Surg Am* 1992;74(1):67-83.

25. Azar FM, Andrews JR, Wilk KE, Groh D: Operative treatment of ulnar collateral ligament injuries of the elbow in athletes. *Am J Sports Med* 2000;28(1):16-23.

26. Thompson WH, Jobe FW, Yocum LA, Pink MM: Ulnar collateral ligament reconstruction in athletes: Muscle-splitting approach without transposition of the ulnar nerve. *J Shoulder Elbow Surg* 2001;10(2):152-157.

27. Rohrbough JT, Altchek DW, Hyman J, Williams RJ III, Botts JD: Medial collateral ligament reconstruction of the elbow using the docking technique. *Am J Sports Med* 2002;30(4):541-548.

28. Bowers AL, Dines JS, Dines DM, Altchek DW: Elbow medial ulnar collateral ligament reconstruction: Clinical relevance and the docking technique. *J Shoulder Elbow Surg* 2010;19(suppl 2):110-117.

29. Hechtman KS, Zvijac JE, Wells ME, Botto-van Bemden A: Long-term results of ulnar collateral ligament reconstruction in throwing athletes based on a hybrid technique. *Am J Sports Med* 2011;39(2):342-347.

30. Vitale MA, Ahmad CS: The outcome of elbow ulnar collateral ligament reconstruction in overhead athletes: A systematic review. *Am J Sports Med* 2008;36(6):1193-1205.

31. Dines JS, ElAttrache NS, Conway JE, Smith W, Ahmad CS: Clinical outcomes of the DANE TJ technique to treat ulnar collateral ligament insufficiency of the elbow. *Am J Sports Med* 2007;35(12):2039-2044.

32. Dodson CC, Thomas A, Dines JS, Nho SJ, Williams RJ III, Altchek DW: Medial ulnar collateral ligament reconstruction of the elbow in throwing athletes. *Am J Sports Med* 2006;34(12):1926-1932.

33. Koh JL, Schafer MF, Keuter G, Hsu JE: Ulnar collateral ligament reconstruction in elite throwing athletes. *Arthroscopy* 2006;22(11):1187-1191.

34. Paletta GA Jr, Wright RW: The modified docking procedure for elbow ulnar collateral ligament reconstruction: 2-year follow-up in elite throwers. *Am J Sports Med* 2006;34(10):1594-1598.

35. Smith GR, Altchek DW, Pagnani MJ, Keeley JR: A muscle-splitting approach to the ulnar collateral ligament of the elbow: Neuroanatomy and operative technique. *Am J Sports Med* 1996;24(5):575-580.

36. Cain EL Jr, Andrews JR, Dugas JR, et al: Outcome of ulnar collateral ligament reconstruction of the elbow in 1281 athletes: Results in 743 athletes with minimum 2-year follow-up. *Am J Sports Med* 2010;38(12):2426-2434.

37. Makhni EC, Lee RW, Morrow ZS, Gualtieri AP, Gorroochurn P, Ahmad CS: Performance, return to competition, and reinjury after Tommy John surgery in Major League Baseball pitchers: A review of 147 cases. *Am J Sports Med* 2014;42(6):1323-1332.

    In assessing the likelihood of return to professional competition, reinjury rate, and change in performance after Tommy John surgery in Major League Baseball pitchers, the authors hypothesized that performance metrics and durability will decline after surgery. Level of evidence: III.

38. Clain JB, Vitale MA, Ahmad CS, Ruchelsman DE: Ulnar nerve complications after ulnar collateral ligament reconstruction of the elbow. A systematic review. *Am J Sports Med* 2019;47(5):1263-1269.

    This is a systematic review of 17 articles (n = 1,518 cases). The rate of postoperative ulnar neuropathy was 12.0% and 0.8% of cases required revision surgery. The surgical approach associated with the highest rate of neuropathy was detachment of flexor pronator mass (21.9%) versus muscle retraction (15.9%) and muscle splitting (3.9%). The fixation technique associated with the highest rate of neuropathy was the modified Jobe (16.9%) versus DANE TJ (9.1%), figure-of-8 (9.0%), interference screw (5.0%), docking technique (3.3%), hybrid suture anchor-bone tunnel (2.9%), and modified docking (2.5%). Concomitant ulnar nerve transposition was associated with a higher neuropathy rate (16.1%) compared with no handling of the ulnar nerve (3.9%). Submuscular transposition resulted in a higher rate of revision surgery for ulnar neuropathy (12.7%) compared with subcutaneous transposition (zero).

39. Griffith TB, Ahmad CS, Gorroochurn P, et al: Comparison of outcomes based on graft type and tunnel configuration for primary ulnar collateral ligament reconstruction in professional baseball pitchers. *Am J Sports Med* 2019;47(5):1103-1110.

    This is a cohort study of 566 Major League Baseball pitchers who underwent UCL reconstruction. Return to play (RTP) rate was 79.9% and return to same level of play (RSL) rate was 71.2%. There were no significant differences in RTP or RSL based on reconstruction technique or graft type. There was no significant difference of rate of subsequent elbow surgery or revision UCL reconstruction between surgical techniques. The use of concomitant ulnar nerve transposition did not affect outcomes. Level of evidence: III.

40. Savoie FH III, Trenhaile SW, Roberts J, Field LD, Ramsey JR: Primary repair of ulnar collateral ligament injuries of the elbow in young athletes: A case series of injuries to the proximal and distal ends of the ligament. *Am J Sports Med* 2008;36(6):1066-1072.

41. Dugas J, Walters B, Beason D, Fleisig G, Chronister J: Biomechanical comparison of ulnar collateral ligament repair with internal bracing versus modified Jobe reconstruction. *Am J Sports Med* 2016;44(3):735-741.

    In this controlled laboratory study, the authors performed a biomechanical comparison of a new technique of augmented UCL repair with a typical modified Jobe UCL reconstruction technique. The novel technique was found to have important biomechanical properties, including time-zero strength and ultimate failure load.

42. Dugas JR, Looze CA, Capogna B, et al: Ulnar collateral ligament repair with collagen-dipped FiberTape augmentation in overhead-throwing athletes. *Am J Sports Med* 2019;47(5):1096-1102.

A case series of 111 overhead athletes undergoing UCL repair with internal brace augmentation demonstrated this procedure is a viable option for select UCL injuries who wish to return to sport in a shorter time; 92% return to same or higher level of competition at a mean time of 6.7 months. Kerlan-Jobe Orthopaedic Clinic scores was 88.2. Level of evidence: IV.

43. Kraeutler M, Ciccotti M, Dodson C, Frederick R, Cammarota B, Cohen S: Kerlan-Jobe Orthopaedic Clinic overhead athlete scores in asymptomatic professional baseball pitchers. *J Shoulder Elbow Surg* 2013;22(3):329-332.

The authors hypothesized that healthy baseball pitchers would have high Kerlan-Jobe Orthopaedic Clinic (KJOC) scores. A total of 44 healthy asymptomatic pitchers were studied; of these, only 7 had KJOC scores lower than the mean.

44. Kalainov DM, Cohen MS: Posterolateral rotatory instability of the elbow in association with lateral epicondylitis: A report of three cases. *J Bone Joint Surg Am* 2005;87(5):1120-1125.

45. O'Driscoll SW, Spinner RJ, McKee MD, et al: Tardy posterolateral rotatory instability of the elbow due to cubitus varus. *J Bone Joint Surg Am* 2001;83-A(9):1358-1369.

46. Beuerlein MJ, Reid JT, Schemitsch EH, McKee MD: Effect of distal humeral varus deformity on strain in the lateral ulnar collateral ligament and ulnohumeral joint stability. *J Bone Joint Surg Am* 2004;86-A(10):2235-2242.

47. Hall JA, McKee MD: Posterolateral rotatory instability of the elbow following radial head resection. *J Bone Joint Surg Am* 2005;87(7):1571-1579.

48. O'Driscoll SW, Morrey BF, Korinek S, An KN: Elbow subluxation and dislocation: A spectrum of instability. *Clin Orthop Relat Res* 1992;(280):186-197.

49. Deutch SR, Jensen SL, Olsen BS, Sneppen O: Elbow joint stability in relation to forced external rotation: An experimental study of the osseous constraint. *J Shoulder Elbow Surg* 2003;12(3):287-292.

50. Rhyou IH, Kim YS: New mechanism of the posterior elbow dislocation. *Knee Surg Sports Traumatol Arthrosc* 2012;20(12):2535-2541.

51. Dunning CE, Zarzour ZD, Patterson SD, Johnson JA, King GJ: Ligamentous stabilizers against posterolateral rotatory instability of the elbow. *J Bone Joint Surg Am* 2001;83-A(12):1823-1828.

52. McAdams TR, Masters GW, Srivastava S: The effect of arthroscopic sectioning of the lateral ligament complex of the elbow on posterolateral rotatory stability. *J Shoulder Elbow Surg* 2005;14(3):298-301.

53. Moritomo H, Murase T, Arimitsu S, Oka K, Yoshikawa H, Sugamoto K: The in vivo isometric point of the lateral ligament of the elbow. *J Bone Joint Surg Am* 2007;89(9):2011-2017.

54. Goren D, Budoff JE, Hipp JA: Isometric placement of lateral ulnar collateral ligament reconstructions: A biomechanical study. *Am J Sports Med* 2010;38(1):153-159.

55. Rhyou IH, Park MJ: Dual reconstruction of the radial collateral ligament and lateral ulnar collateral ligament in posterolateral rotator instability of the elbow. *Knee Surg Sports Traumatol Arthrosc* 2011;19(6):1009-1012.

56. Jung HS, Lee JS, Rhyou IH, Lee HW, Park MJ: Dual reconstruction of lateral collateral ligament is safe and effective in treating posterolateral rotatory instability of the elbow. *Knee Surg Sports Traumatol Arthrosc* 2019;27(10):3284-3290.

This is a restrospective review of patients undergoing dual reconstruction over a 5-year period. All patients demonstrated resolved instability and achieved a fuctional arc of motion. Lateral pivot shift tests were negative in all patients. The median Mayo Elbow Performance Score significantly improved after surgery from 70 to 85. The median quick Disabilities of the Arm, Shoulder and Hand score improved from 38.6 to 11.4. Level of evidence: IV.

57. O'Driscoll SW, Bell DF, Morrey BF: Posterolateral rotatory instability of the elbow. *J Bone Joint Surg Am* 1991;73(3):440-446.

58. Lattanza LL, Chu T, Ty JM, et al: Interclinician and intraclinician variability in the mechanics of the pivot shift test for posterolateral rotatory instability (PLRI) of the elbow. *J Shoulder Elbow Surg* 2010;19(8):1150-1156.

59. Regan W, Lapner PC: Prospective evaluation of two diagnostic apprehension signs for posterolateral instability of the elbow. *J Shoulder Elbow Surg* 2006;15(3):344-346.

60. Arvind CH, Hargreaves DG: Tabletop relocation test: A new clinical test for posterolateral rotatory instability of the elbow. *J Shoulder Elbow Surg* 2006;15(6):707-708.

61. Hacki M, Wegmann K, Ries C, Leschinger T, Burkhart KJ, Muller LP: Reliability of magnetic resonance imaging signs of posterolatral rotatory instability of the elbow. *J Hand Surg Am* 2015;40(7):1428-1433.

The authors evaluated radiographic signs of PLRI using MRI, with the goal to determine objective radiographic criteria to aid in the diagnosis of PLRI. Level of evidence: IV.

62. Faber KJ, King GJ: Posterior capitellum impression fracture: A case report associated with posterolateral rotatory instability of the elbow. *J Shoulder Elbow Surg* 1998;7(2):157-159.

63. Rosenberg ZS, Blutreich SI, Schweitzer ME, Zember JS, Fillmore K: MRI features of a posterior capitellar impaction injuries. *AJR Am J Roentgenol* 2008;190(2):435-441.

64. Jeon IH, Micic ID, Yamamoto N, Morrey BF: Osborne-Cotterill lesion: An osseous defect of the capitellum associated with instability of the elbow. *AJR Am J Roentgenol* 2008;191(3):727-729.

65. Jeon IH, Min WK, Micic ID, Cho HS, Kim PT: Surgical treatment and clinical implication for posterolateral rotatory instability of the elbow: Osborne-Cotterill lesion of the elbow. *J Trauma* 2011;71(3):E45-E49.

66. Lee BP, Teo LH: Surgical reconstruction for posterolateral rotatory instability of the elbow. *J Shoulder Elbow Surg* 2003;12(5):476-479.

67. Sanchez-Sotelo J, Morrey BF, O'Driscoll SW: Ligamentous repair and reconstruction for posterolateral rotatory instability of the elbow. *J Bone Joint Surg Br* 2005;87(1):54-61.

68. Greiner S, Kock M, Kerschbaum M, Bhide PP: Repair and augmentation of the lateral collateral ligament complex using internal bracing in dislocations and fracture dislocations of the elbow restores stability and allows early rehabilitation. *Knee Surg Sports Traumatol Arthrosc* 2019;27(10):3269-3275.

    Seventeen patients with PLRI were treated with LUCL repair and suture tape augmentation. They were activitely mobilized immediately postoperatively and had a maximum bracing period of 3 days. At median 10-month follow-up, no patients showed signs of instability and all reported a complete return to preinjury level of activity. One patient required revision surgery for heterotopic ossification. Median range of motion 10° to 130° (0°-40° to 90°-150°), Oxford 41 (29 to 48), Mayo Elbow Performance Score 100 (70 to 100), Simple Elbow Value 83% (60° to 95°), and DASH score 18.5 (1.6 to 66), respectively. Level of evidence: IV.

69. Gong HS, Kim JK, Oh JH, Lee YH, Chung MS, Baek GH: A new technique for lateral ulnar collateral ligament reconstruction using the triceps tendon. *Tech Hand Up Extrem Surg* 2009;13(1):34-36.

70. Eygendaal D: Ligamentous reconstruction around the elbow using triceps tendon. *Acta Orthop Scand* 2004;75(5):516-523.

71. Savoie FH III, O'Brien MJ, Field LD, Gurley DJ: Arthroscopic and open radial ulnohumeral ligament reconstruction for posterolateral rotatory instability of the elbow. *Clin Sports Med* 2010;29(4):611-618.

72. Lehman RC: Lateral elbow reconstruction using a new fixation technique. *Arthroscopy* 2005;21(4):503-505.

73. Jones KJ, Dodson CC, Osbahr DC, et al: The docking technique for lateral ulnar collateral ligament reconstruction: Surgical technique and clinical outcomes. *J Shoulder Elbow Surg* 2012;21(3):389-395.

74. King GJ, Dunning CE, Zarzour ZD, Patterson SD, Johnson JA: Single-strand reconstruction of the lateral ulnar collateral ligament restores varus and posterolateral rotatory stability of the elbow. *J Shoulder Elbow Surg* 2002;11(1):60-64.

75. Camp CL, Sanchez-Sotelo J, Shields MN, O'Driscoll SW: Lateral ulnar collateral ligament reconstruction for posterolateral rotatory instability of the elbow. *Arthrosc Tech* 2017;6(4):e1101-e1105.

    The authors described some of the advantages of the docking technique in the treatment of recurrent symptomatic posterolateral rotatory instability.

Chapter 37

Elbow Stiffness: Pathogenesis, Evaluation, and Open Treatment

Rudy Kovachevich, MD • Hill Hastings II, MD

ABSTRACT

The elbow has a propensity to developing stiffness, especially after trauma. Increased expression of transforming growth factor-β has been implicated in the development of excessive scarring and the development of heterotopic bone formation following trauma. The incidence of heterotopic ossification increases with the magnitude of injury and occurs in 3% of simple elbow-dislocations, 20% of periarticular fracture-dislocations, and up to 75% to 89% of elbow injury associated with head trauma. Therapy can improve motion within 3 to 6 months of contracture development. When a persistent 30° extension deficit or inability to flex to 120° to 130° exists, surgical release may be considered. An arthritic or incongruous ulnohumeral joint is a contraindication to a simple release and is best managed by a salvage procedure such as interposition or replacement arthroplasty. With more common lateral pathology, a deep lateral approach surgical exposure is usually advised. A medial approach is indicated when pathology of the ulnar nerve and ulnar collateral ligament are involved. Postoperative therapy is essential for 3 to 6 months. Continuous passive motion has not been shown to be beneficial. Open release has been shown to provide a 52° increase in arc of motion with a complication rate of 10%. Inferior results are found in females, adolescents, those with high body mass index, and those with underlying brain injury.

Keywords: elbow contracture; heterotopic ossification; open treatment; results contracture release; surgical approaches

Dr. Hastings or an immediate family member has received royalties from Biomet, DJ Orthopaedics, and Zimmer; is a member of a speakers' bureau or has made paid presentations on behalf of Biomet and Synthes; and serves as an unpaid consultant to DJ Orthopaedics, Synthes, and Zimmer. Neither Dr. Kovachevich nor any immediate family member has received anything of value from or has stock or stock options held in a commercial company or institution related directly or indirectly to the subject of this chapter.

Introduction

The function of the upper extremity largely depends on the ability of the elbow to position the hand in space. Loss of elbow motion, therefore, can seriously interfere with daily activities and the ability to take care of oneself. Contracture and stiffness of the elbow can result from trauma, heterotopic ossification, burn injury, neurologic spasticity, prolonged immobilization, or postoperative scarring. The propensity of the elbow to become stiff has been attributed to numerous factors, including the highly congruous nature of the joint, the presence of three articulations within a single synovial cavity, and the proximity of the articular surface and capsule to the intracapsular ligaments and extracapsular muscles.[1] The etiology of elbow stiffness has been classified as extrinsic (extra-articular), intrinsic (intra-articular), or mixed[2] (**Table 1**).

Etiology

The anatomic structures and pathophysiologic mechanisms involved in a patient's elbow stiffness dictate the treatment and affect the prognosis. Soft-tissue contractures around the elbow, particularly the capsule and collateral ligaments, play a critical role in the development of arthrofibrosis, in which structural and biochemical alterations lead to thickening, loss of motion, and decreased tissue compliance.[3] Preclinical animal studies have found increased expression of transforming growth factor-β in rabbit elbow capsular tissue.[4] Transforming growth factor-β may have a role in the development of fibrotic scarring around the elbow secondary to cellular changes, such as elevated myofibroblast levels, increased extracellular matrix proliferation, and increased formation of collagen cross-links.[5-7]

Heterotopic ossification, defined as the inappropriate formation of mature lamellar bone in a nonosseous location, can contribute to the development of elbow stiffness, especially after traumatic injury. Heterotopic ossification must be distinguished from periarticular calcifications, which are amorphous calcium depositions in soft tissues that commonly occur after injury but do not necessarily affect motion.[8,9] The cause is not completely

Table 1

The Etiology of Elbow Stiffness

Classification	Types
Extrinsic (extra-articular)	Skin contracture Subcutaneous tissue contracture Capsule contracture Medial or lateral collateral ligament contracture Myostatic contracture Extra-articular malunion Heterotopic ossification
Intrinsic (intra-articular)	Articular malalignment Joint incongruity Arthritis Intra-articular adhesions Loose bodies Osteophyte impingement Coronoid Olecranon Fossa fibrosis Coronoid fossa Olecranon fossa
Mixed	Extrinsic contractures secondary to intrinsic pathology

understood, but it involves an osteoblastic differentiation of pluripotent mesenchymal stem cells thought to occur after injury or surgery or in an inflammatory state. The bone formed in heterotopic ossification is histologically identical to native bone although more metabolically active and without a true periosteal layer.

Evaluation

Elbow contractures are challenging to manage. Therefore, prevention is of paramount importance. The treatment of a patient with an elbow contracture is nonsurgical, followed by surgical treatment if necessary. A thorough history and physical examination complemented by plain radiographs are prerequisites to a full assessment of the causes of a loss of elbow motion. The character of end point resistance to motion should be noted; a hard, sudden end point suggests a bony block, and a softer end point suggests a soft-tissue constraint to motion.

It is helpful to supplement standard AP and lateral radiographs with coronoid and radiocapitellar views to better evaluate the coronoid and radiocapitellar joints. Evaluation of joint surfaces in the contracted elbow requires the AP view to be taken as two separate radiographs, one of which is perpendicular to the humerus and the other perpendicular to the radius and ulna. A lateral radiograph in full flexion can be useful for detecting bony impingement. Fluoroscopy can be used as an adjunct to distinguish between an osseous block to motion and a purely soft-tissue contracture. Advanced imaging studies, such as CT with two-dimensional or three-dimensional reconstruction, can identify the intra-articular blocks to range of motion for the purpose of surgical planning. This also helps define the integrity of the articular surfaces. MRI usually is not helpful.

Treatment Modalities

The goal of treatment for a patient with elbow stiffness and contracture is to provide and maintain a pain-free, functional, and stable joint. Nonsurgical measures can be helpful within the first 3 to 6 months after the contracture develops. These measures can include supervised physical therapy, static-progressive splinting, serial casting, and joint manipulation under anesthesia.

Surgical treatment is considered if the initial nonsurgical management is unsuccessful or if the patient has a significant osseous block to motion, as identified on examination and imaging studies. The typical indications for surgery include flexion contractures of more than 30° or the inability to flex the elbow to 120° to 130°. Patients who need greater motion for a vocational or sports activity may require surgical intervention for a smaller deficit.

The prerequisites for contracture release include a congruous joint with adequate ulnohumeral joint space, adequate soft-tissue coverage of the surgical site, resolution of soft-tissue posttraumatic inflammation, maturation of any heterotopic ossification, and the ability to comply with an aggressive postoperative rehabilitation regimen. The development of an incongruous or an arthritic ulnohumeral joint is a contraindication to simple surgical release because the release could worsen pain but only minimally improve motion. Severe posttraumatic arthritic changes are an indication for a salvage procedure, such as soft-tissue interposition arthroplasty, hemiarthroplasty, or total elbow arthroplasty.

Open Treatment

Surgical release of the elbow has proved to be an effective measure to restore range of motion and can be achieved with an open or an arthroscopic procedure. An open release typically is performed using an ultrasound-guided regional anesthetic block, with or without an indwelling catheter, and long-acting medications that provide postoperative pain control and muscular relaxation.

Open elbow contracture release should be tailored to the needs of the individual patient after determining whether the loss of elbow motion is in flexion, extension, or both. To improve elbow flexion, the posterior soft tissues that tether the joint, including the posterior joint capsule and triceps extensor mechanism, are released. Anterior bony restraints to flexion are removed, including loose bodies, osteophytes or overgrowth of the coronoid process, and scar or bone that may have filled the coronoid and radial fossae (**Figure 1**). There may be thickening and contracture of the posteromedial capsule (the posterior band of the ulnar collateral ligament), which requires release to restore full flexion. The steps for improving elbow extension are similar. Anteriorly, tethering soft tissues, such as joint capsule and brachialis adhesions, are released. Posterior impingement between the olecranon and olecranon fossa is corrected by partial olecranon excision and fossa débridement.

The ulnar nerve requires special consideration during contracture release. The normal tension and compression of the ulnar nerve during elbow flexion is more pronounced in a contracted elbow. If the patient has preoperative symptoms or ulnar nerve irritability, as shown by the Tinel sign, the elbow flexion test, or the ulnar nerve compression test, the nerve should be decompressed with or without transposition.

Numerous surgical approaches can be used for a contracture release. The skin incision to gain deep access to the joint can vary from a limited medial and/or lateral to a single extensile posterior approach that will provide access to both sides of the elbow. The approach typically is chosen based on the surgeon's preference, the presence of previous surgical incisions, the need for nerve decompression, and the location and extent of heterotopic ossification. A posterior incision is advisable if there is a possibility that elbow replacement eventually will be needed. Elevation of flaps to obtain medial and lateral deep exposure usually carries a greater chance of seroma formation than separate medial and lateral incisions. Regardless of the approach, it is important to protect and avoid injury to the medial brachiocutaneous, ulnar, median, radial, posterior interosseous, and median nerves during all dissections and releases.

The deep lateral approach, described initially as the lateral collateral ligament-preserving approach and subsequently as the column procedure, consists of open arthrolysis through a limited (6 cm) skin incision through the proximal aspect of a standard Kocher interval[10-12] (**Figure 2**). Dissection is carried down to the lateral column of the humerus. The triceps and the most proximal portion of the anconeus are reflected posteriorly to expose the olecranon, the olecranon fossa, and the lateral gutter (lateral ulnohumeral joint). The posterior capsule and scar are excised. The fossa is cleared of loose bodies, bone, and scar, and areas of bony overgrowth on the humerus and the olecranon are excised. The capsule can be excised from the soft area proximal and posterior to the radiocapitellar joint to inspect the radial head, excise proliferative synovitis, and remove any loose bodies that may be present. Any osteophytes on the posterior capitellum or the lateral olecranon that may be blocking extension are removed (**Figure 3**).

Anteriorly, exposure is obtained by reflecting the distalmost brachioradialis and extensor carpi radialis longus muscle origins from the supracondylar ridge of the humerus and distally splitting for 2 to 3 cm between the extensor carpi radialis longus and the extensor carpi radialis brevis distal to the lateral epicondyle. This distal extension facilitates exposure and can be used as needed to release the proximal supinator for decompression of the posterior interosseous nerve. At this point, the coronoid, olecranon, and radial fossae are débrided, osteophytes are resected, and loose bodies are removed. It is essential to restore a capacious coronoid fossa and capitellar recess with respect to depth and width. The elbow is manipulated first by extending and then flexing the elbow under direct visualization, using firm pressure on the proximal forearm. In long-standing contractures, the brachialis and triceps muscles typically have undergone myostatic contraction and can limit full terminal elbow extension and flexion, which can be stretched at the time of surgical release.

The advantages of the lateral approach include its simplicity, the use of a muscular plane that allows superficial sensory nerves to be avoided, and access to all three joint articulations. The lateral approach is limited, however, because it does not allow the posteromedial capsule and the ulnar nerve to be treated. A separate limited medial approach may be necessary for complete release in some patients and for simple decompression of the ulnar nerve. This approach usually involves a 3- to 5-cm posteromedial incision for in situ cubital tunnel release. If the ulnar nerve is not transposed, posteromedial olecranon residual osteophytes are exposed and débrided through a longitudinal incision in the medial triceps 1.5 cm posterior to the ulnar nerve.

A conceptually similar medial approach (Hotchkiss) is chosen if there is substantial ulnar nerve pathology that requires anterior transposition.[12] A medial or posterior incision is made to expose the flexor-pronator origin (**Figure 4**). The medial antebrachial cutaneous nerve is protected, and the ulnar nerve is released, mobilized, and transposed anteriorly. The triceps is elevated posteriorly from the intermuscular septum and the humerus to expose the posteromedial joint. The posterior capsule, including the posterior band of the medial collateral ligament, is released with care to preserve and protect the important and

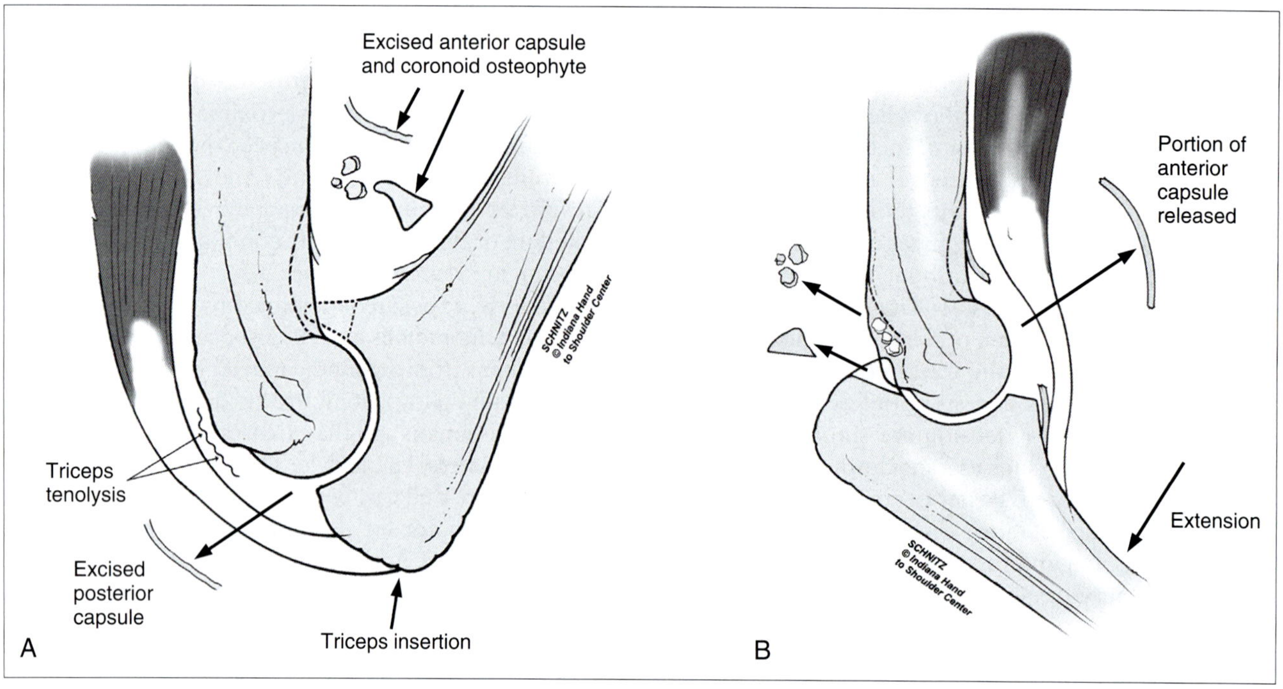

FIGURE 1 Schematic drawings showing anterior (**A**) and posterior (**B**) capsulectomy and débridement. (© G. Schnitz, Indiana Hand to Shoulder Center, Indianapolis, IN.)

more distal anterior band of the medial collateral ligament. The posterior joint and olecranon fossa then can be further débrided. The flexor pronator origin is longitudinally incised, and the anterior two-thirds are reflected from the medial epicondyle. The brachialis and the anterior portion of the flexor pronator mass are reflected from the medial humerus to expose the anterior capsule. The capsule is excised, and the coronoid and radial fossa are débrided. Enlarged or overgrown portions of the coronoid are excised. At this point, the elbow can be manipulated.

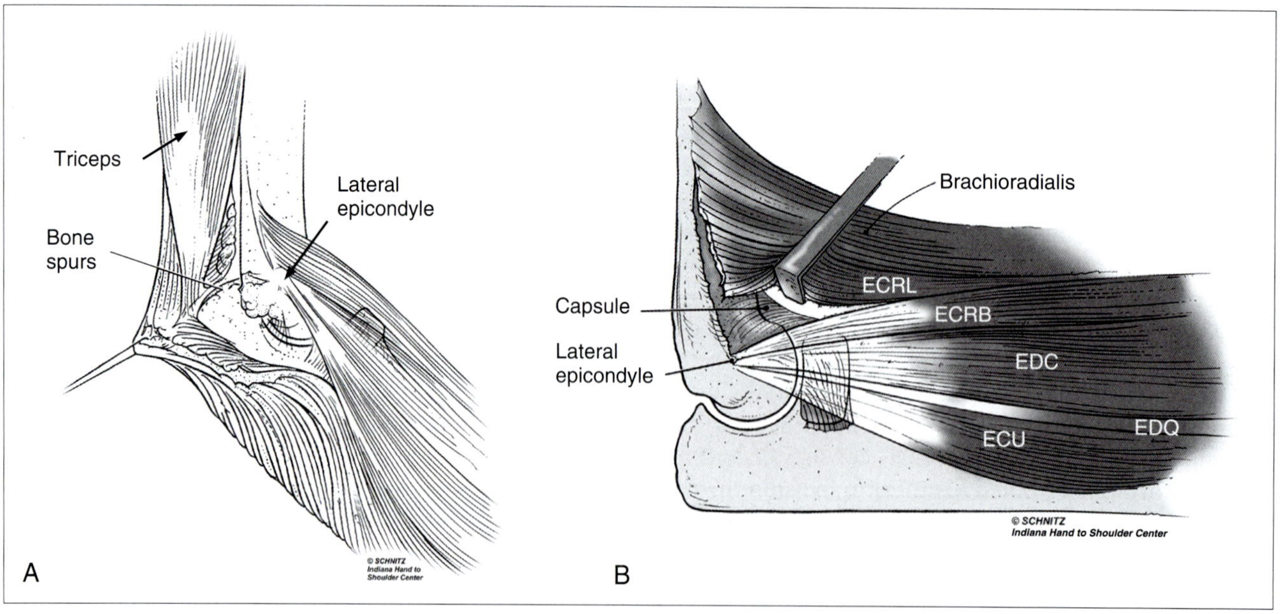

FIGURE 2 Schematic drawings showing the deep lateral (lateral collateral ligament–preserving) approach. **A**, Posterior exposure. **B**, Anterior exposure. ECRB = extensor carpi radialis brevis, ECRL = extensor carpi radialis longus, ECU = extensor carpi ulnaris, EDC = extensor digitorum communis, EDQ = extensor digiti quinti. (© G. Schnitz, Indiana Hand to Shoulder Center, Indianapolis, IN.)

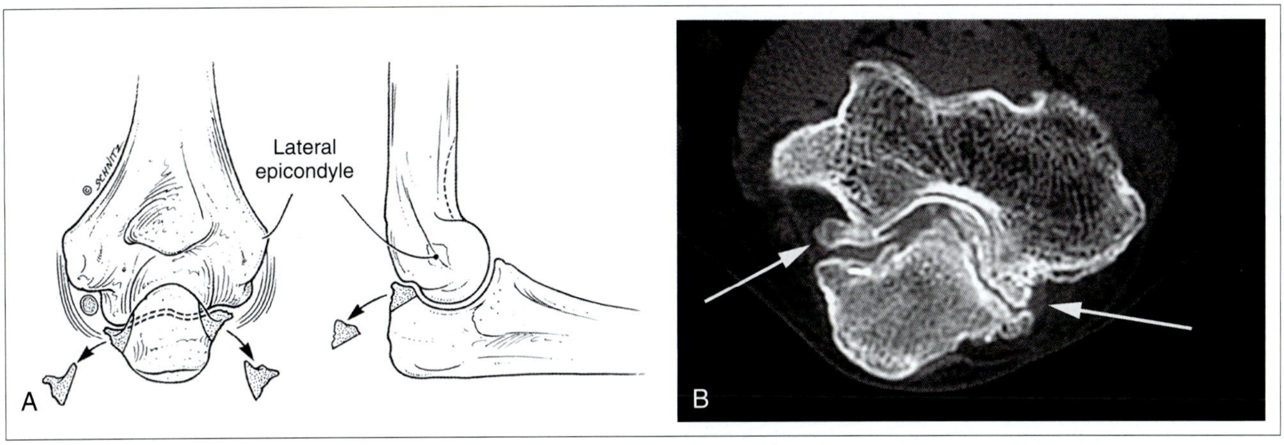

FIGURE 3 Débridement of gutter osteophytes. **A**, Schematic drawings showing typical osteophyte formations on the medial, lateral, and posterior aspects of the olecranon and proximal ulna. **B**, CT showing large medial and lateral gutter osteophytes (*arrows*). (© G. Schnitz, Indiana Hand to Shoulder Center, Indianapolis, IN.)

The advantages of the medial approach include the less visible postoperative scar, the ability to expose and decompress the ulnar nerve, and access for a direct release of the posterior band of the ulnar collateral ligament. The medial approach is limited because it does not facilitate exposure of common lateral pathology. The limitations of both the medial and lateral approaches, especially in patients with considerable heterotopic ossification, have led to the use of a combined medial and lateral approach. The outcomes of elbow contracture release are better if there is a discrete mechanical (osseous) block to motion rather than soft-tissue contracture alone.[13,14]

Heterotopic Ossification

Heterotopic ossification of the elbow most often occurs after direct joint trauma, surgery, burns, or traumatic brain injury. Its development appears to be partially related to the severity of the injury and the time between injury and surgery. It has been reported to occur in approximately 3% of simple elbow-dislocations and as many as 20% of periarticular fracture-dislocations.[15] After a closed head injury associated with elbow trauma, heterotopic ossification was documented to occur in 75% to 89% of patients.[11] Although heterotopic ossification around the elbow begins with the inciting insult, it is clinically manifested 2 to 12 weeks later. The initial findings include local soft-tissue swelling, tenderness, and warmth followed by progressive loss of elbow motion. Heterotopic ossification may be mistaken for infection during the perisurgical period. Its localized or diffuse pattern of formation may not follow anatomic tissue planes. The end points of elbow motion become rigid rather than compliant, as in soft-tissue contracture. Pain typically occurs with terminal flexion and/or extension rather than at the mid arc of motion, as is indicative of joint incongruity or arthrosis. The classification system of Hastings and Graham is useful for defining surgical planning and treatment[16] (**Table 2**).

The maturity of the bone and the time since bone production onset are important factors in evaluating heterotopic ossification and considering surgical intervention. In the past, laboratory studies (serum calcium, inorganic phosphate, and alkaline phosphatase) and technetium bone scans were used to follow the progression of heterotopic ossification. The prognostic value of these tests has not been proven, and they are no longer used for evaluation.[17,18] Plain radiography is the most effective means of evaluating for heterotopic ossification and following its progression. In patients with extensive ectopic bone formation, CT, particularly CT with three-dimensional reconstruction, can be useful for defining the geometry of ectopic bone formation, assessing ulnohumeral joint congruity, and planning the direction of surgical exposure. Within 4 to 6 weeks of the onset of heterotopic ossification, ill-defined fluffy periarticular densities can be identified radiographically. Over time, the margins become more distinct, and trabeculae appear. Smooth, well-demarcated cortical margins, the defining characteristic of radiographic maturity, typically do not appear for 3 to 6 months.[8] In most patients, surgical excision can be safely performed when the extent of heterotopic bone can be seen radiographically; it is not necessary to wait until full maturation. Early surgical intervention may be beneficial to limit capsular and ligamentous contracture, muscular atrophy, and cartilage degeneration, and it may be technically easier than later intervention.

Prevention of heterotopic ossification is key because there is no effective medical treatment. Diphosphonate

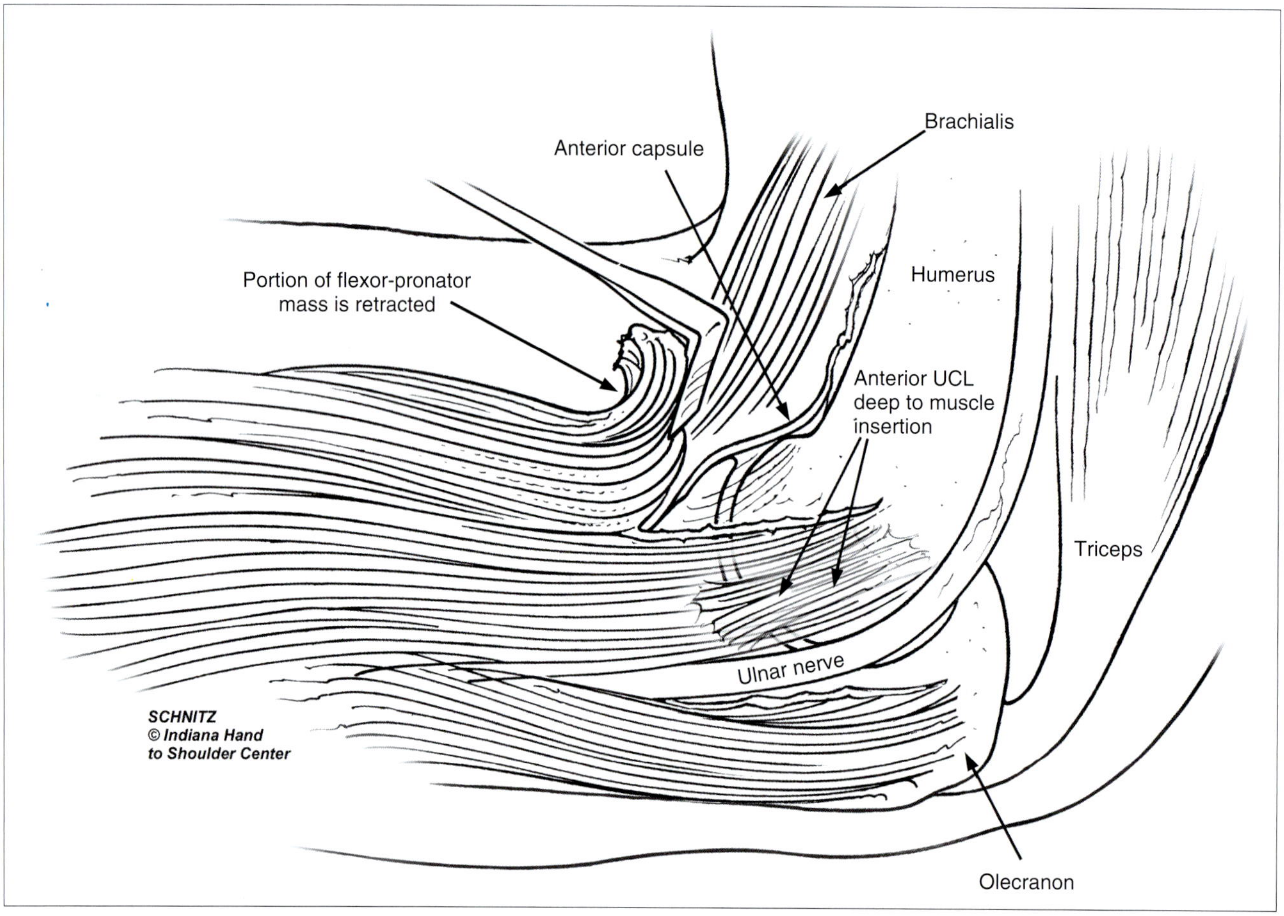

FIGURE 4 Schematic drawing showing the medial Hotchkiss approach. An anterior exposure through the flexor-pronator mass is used to gain access to the contracted anterior capsule. Care must be taken to preserve the anterior band of the ulnar collateral ligament (UCL). (© G. Schnitz, Indiana Hand to Shoulder Center, Indianapolis, IN.)

therapy was formerly used but was found to merely delay the mineralization of ectopic bone.[11] Prophylaxis consists of NSAIDs, such as indomethacin, ibuprofen, naproxen, or aspirin (Cox-1 NSAIDs have been shown to be ineffective against heterotopic ossification formation), and low-dosage external beam radiation. NSAIDs are effective if begun within 3 to 5 days of the inciting traumatic event. The treatment duration is controversial and ranges between 5 days and 6 weeks.[19] These agents work by inhibiting prostaglandin formation, and experimentally they have been found to inhibit stem cell differentiation and migration. Low-dosage external beam radiation therapy is administered using a limited-field technique, in a single dose of 600 to 700 cGy within 72 hours of surgery or trauma. The radiation therapy works by inhibiting the differentiation of stem cells.[16] Treatment with radiation, NSAIDs, or both has been proven safe and effective for preventing heterotopic ossification after surgical contracture release.[16] Results have been mixed after acute elbow trauma, however. Multiple studies found the treatment to be safe and efficacious,[20,21] but a later prospective randomized study was stopped because of increased rates of nonunion at fracture and olecranon osteotomy sites.[22]

Anteriorly located heterotopic ossification can be surgically resected using a medial, lateral, or combined approach. Anterior heterotopic ossification most commonly forms beneath the brachialis muscle and appears to be separated from the anterior articular surface by a radiolucent area. In contrast, posterior heterotopic ossification often forms in continuity with the articular surface beneath the triceps tendon. Care must be taken during resection to identify and protect the nearby radial, posterior interosseous, and median nerves. Burrs, curettes, osteotomes, and rongeurs typically are used to excise the bone. Because of the continuity of posterior bone with the joint surface, partial or complete elevation of the triceps from the olecranon is required. The ulnar nerve can be intimately involved and must be located and protected. Extensive restriction from heterotopic ossification is not necessarily a negative prognostic

Table 2

The Classification of Heterotopic Ossification

Class	Characteristics
I	Clinically insignificant No functional elbow motion limitation
II	Functional limitation to elbow motion
IIA	Ulnohumeral motion plane deficit smaller than 100° Flexion arc from 30° to 130°
IIB	Forearm rotation motion plane deficit smaller than 100° Arc from 50° pronation to 50° supination
IIC	Motion deficits in both ulnohumeral and forearm rotation planes
III	Elbow joint ankylosis
IIIA	Ulnohumeral motion plane
IIIB	Forearm rotation plane
IIIC	Both ulnohumeral and forearm rotation planes

factor; a 2010 study found comparable postoperative motion in completely ankylosed elbows and those with a partial motion restriction.[23]

Salvage Procedures

Elbow contracture release alone is contraindicated if the patient's elbow stiffness is associated with articular incongruity or arthrosis. In these patients, a salvage procedure typically is required for augmenting or replacing the damaged joint surface. Interposition arthroplasty is recommended to restore function and relieve pain in a patient who is physiologically young and has high physical demands. The goal of interposition arthroplasty is to improve and preserve functional stability and prevent re-ankylosis by placing a resurfacing material between the resected bone ends. Various interposition materials have been used to resurface the ulnohumeral joint, including fascia lata, cutis graft, Achilles tendon allograft, regenerative tissue matrix (AlloDerm [LifeCell]), bovine collagen, sterile absorbable gelatin sponge (Pfizer), and silicone. Patients with elbow instability have had poor results despite attempts at collateral ligament reconstruction.[24,25] A hinged external fixator can be used postoperatively to provide sufficient stability for soft-tissue healing without limiting early motion.[26] The use of external fixation to provide distraction on the interposed tissue had satisfactory results in 69% to 92% of patients by minimizing the load on the interposition material during early postoperative motion.[24,25,27] The complications can be significant and include bone resorption, nerve dysfunction, heterotopic ossification, triceps rupture, instability, and infection.

In patients who are older than approximately 60 years and have relatively low physical demands, hemiarthroplasty or total elbow arthroplasty should be considered for treating elbow contracture or arthrosis. Because such a patient may have poor bone stock, deformity, and capsuloligamentous instability, the use of a semiconstrained implant is recommended.[28] The surgical technique can be challenging because of anatomic distortion, and complications are likely, including mechanical failure, loosening, problematic wound healing, infection, triceps disruption, and fracture.[26] Despite these concerns, substantial functional improvement and pain relief can be expected.[27]

Postoperative Care

Numerous effective postoperative treatment programs have been described for patients who have undergone elbow contracture release surgery. The overall goals are to maintain a functional arc of motion, strengthen the muscles around the elbow, and reincorporate extremity use into functional activities.[1] Range-of-motion exercises are initiated postoperatively, with judicious use of regional anesthetic blockade, formal therapy, continuous passive motion, and/or static progressive splinting. Regional blockade is useful for immediate postoperative pain control and can facilitate the initiation of functional range-of-motion exercises. The use of continuous passive motion remains controversial; numerous authors have recommended this treatment despite the limited, low-level scientific evidence to support its use. A 2009 study examined the use of continuous passive motion in a matched split cohort of 32 patients after open elbow contracture release.[29] There was no demonstrable benefit to continuous passive motion in the postoperative management of contracture release at 6-month or final follow-up. The flexion-extension arc of motion improved a statistically nonsignificant average of 96° or 101° in the two groups. Although overall, open elbow contracture release is successful, numerous studies have shown inferior results in patients of female sex,[30] higher body mass index,[31] and in adolescent patients as well as those with underlying traumatic brain injuries.[32]

The postoperative rehabilitation regimen should be continued until a plateau in motion has been reached, typically at 3 to 6 months. If the patient's functional range of motion continues to be limited, formal manipulation under anesthesia has been described; however, few studies have documented an improved range of motion without complications. An examination under anesthesia described in 2010, consisting of an evaluation of passive motion arc; gentle manipulation in extension and flexion; evaluation of joint stability; and an assessment of smoothness of motion arc for crepitus, catching, or other surface irregularities, was performed in 51 patients at a mean 40 days after surgical release.[33] An average of 36° improved arc of motion was noted, with no permanent complications. The intent of this procedure is to overcome adhesions and contractures, thereby enhancing elbow motion, in patients undergoing external fixator removal or patients who have had limited progress in the first weeks after surgical release. In an article evaluating open elbow contracture release, an average increase in arc of motion of 52° was found with a complication rate of 10% and revision surgery rate of 11%.[34]

SUMMARY

The elbow joint is of critical importance to overall upper extremity function. Its high degree of constraint and associated soft tissues predisposes it for the development of stiffness and contracture. Recent preclinical and clinical research has shed light on the etiology and treatment options, although many questions remain unanswered. The prevention of elbow stiffness remains of paramount importance. Patient selection is essential when surgical intervention is being considered because the outcome partially depends on the patient's willingness and ability to participate in postoperative rehabilitation. In a properly selected patient, surgical release and débridement can restore a functional arc of elbow motion.

KEY STUDY POINTS

- Elbow function is compromised when there is a 30° loss of extension and limitation of flexion to less than 120° to 130°.
- The incidence of elbow heterotopic ossification following trauma increases with increased magnitude of injury and particularly with associated head trauma.
- Open contracture release in most cases is best performed through a lateral approach.
- Open medial approach is indicated when there is pathology of the ulnar nerve or ulnar collateral ligament at the elbow.
- Open surgical release of elbow contracture can improve arc of elbow flexion/extension motion by more than 50°.

Annotated References

1. Modabber MR, Jupiter JB: Reconstruction for posttraumatic conditions of the elbow joint. *J Bone Joint Surg Am* 1995;77(9):1431-1446.

2. Morrey BF: Post-traumatic contracture of the elbow: Operative treatment, including distraction arthroplasty. *J Bone Joint Surg Am* 1990;72(4):601-618.

3. Cohen MS, Schimmel DR, Masuda K, Hastings H II, Muehleman C: Structural and biochemical evaluation of the elbow capsule after trauma. *J Shoulder Elbow Surg* 2007;16(4):484-490.

4. Hildebrand KA, Zhang M, Hart DA: Myofibroblast upregulators are elevated in joint capsules in posttraumatic contractures. *Clin Orthop Relat Res* 2007;456:85-91.

5. Hildebrand KA, Zhang M, van Snellenberg W, King GJ, Hart DA: Myofibroblast numbers are elevated in human elbow capsules after trauma. *Clin Orthop Relat Res* 2004;419:189-197.

6. Unterhauser FN, Bosch U, Zeichen J, Weiler A: α-Smooth muscle actin containing contractile fibroblastic cells in human knee arthrofibrosis tissue. *Arch Orthop Trauma Surg* 2004;124(9):585-591.

7. Hildebrand KA, Zhang M, Hart DA: High rate of joint capsule matrix turnover in chronic human elbow contractures. *Clin Orthop Relat Res* 2005;439:228-234.

8. Viola RW, Hastings H II: Treatment of ectopic ossification about the elbow. *Clin Orthop Relat Res* 2000;370:65-86.

9. Summerfield SL, DiGiovanni C, Weiss AP: Heterotopic ossification of the elbow. *J Shoulder Elbow Surg* 1997;6(3):321-332.

10. Cohen MS, Hastings H II: Post-traumatic contracture of the elbow: Operative release using a lateral collateral ligament sparing approach. *J Bone Joint Surg Br* 1998;80(5):805-812.

11. Cohen MS, Hastings H II: Operative release for elbow contracture: The lateral collateral ligament sparing technique. *Orthop Clin North Am* 1999;30(1):133-139.

12. Mansat P, Morrey BF: The column procedure: A limited lateral approach for extrinsic contracture of the elbow. *J Bone Joint Surg Am* 1998;80(11):1603-1615.

13. Jupiter JB, O'Driscoll SW, Cohen MS: The assessment and management of the stiff elbow. *Instr Course Lect* 2003;52:93-111.

14. Kasparyan NG, Hotchkiss RN: Dynamic skeletal fixation in the upper extremity. *Hand Clin* 1997;13(4):643-663.

15. Thompson HC III, Garcia A: Myositis ossificans: Aftermath of elbow injuries. *Clin Orthop Relat Res* 1967;50:129-134.

16. Hastings H II, Graham TJ: The classification and treatment of heterotopic ossification about the elbow and forearm. *Hand Clin* 1994;10(3):417-437.

17. Lindenhovius AL, Linzel DS, Doornberg JN, Ring DC, Jupiter JB: Comparison of elbow contracture release in elbows with and without heterotopic ossification restricting motion. *J Shoulder Elbow Surg* 2007;16(5):621-625.

18. Park MJ, Kim HG, Lee JY: Surgical treatment of post-traumatic stiffness of the elbow. *J Bone Joint Surg Br* 2004;86(8):1158-1162.

19. McAuliffe JA, Wolfson AH: Early excision of heterotopic ossification about the elbow followed by radiation therapy. *J Bone Joint Surg Am* 1997;79(5):749-755.

20. Ellerin BE, Helfet D, Parikh S, et al: Current therapy in the management of heterotopic ossification of the elbow: A review with case studies. *Am J Phys Med Rehabil* 1999;78(3):259-271.

21. Strauss JB, Wysocki RW, Shah A, et al: Radiation therapy for heterotopic ossification prophylaxis afer high-risk elbow surgery. *Am J Orthop (Belle Mead NJ)* 2011;40(8):400-405.

22. Hamid N, Ashraf N, Bosse MJ, et al: Radiation therapy for heterotopic ossification prophylaxis acutely after elbow trauma: A prospective randomized study. *J Bone Joint Surg Am* 2010;92(11):2032-2038.

23. Brouwer KM, Lindenhovius AL, de Witte PB, Jupiter JB, Ring D: Resection of heterotopic ossification of the elbow: A comparison of ankylosis and partial restriction. *J Hand Surg Am* 2010;35(7):1115-1119.

24. Larson AN, Morrey BF: Interposition arthroplasty with an Achilles tendon allograft as a salvage procedure for the elbow. *J Bone Joint Surg Am* 2008;90(12):2714-2723.

25. Cheng SL, Morrey BF: Treatment of the mobile, painful arthritic elbow by distraction interposition arthroplasty. *J Bone Joint Surg Br* 2000;82(2):233-238.

26. Ring D, Jupiter JB: Operative release of complete ankylosis of the elbow due to heterotopic bone in patients without severe injury of the central nervous system. *J Bone Joint Surg Am* 2003;85(5):849-857.

27. Nolla J, Ring D, Lozano-Calderon S, Jupiter JB: Interposition arthroplasty of the elbow with hinged external fixation for post-traumatic arthritis. *J Shoulder Elbow Surg* 2008;17(3):459-464.

28. Mansat P, Morrey BF: Semiconstrained total elbow arthroplasty for ankylosed and stiff elbows. *J Bone Joint Surg Am* 2000;82(9):1260-1268.

29. Lindenhovius AL, van de Luijtgaarden K, Ring D, Jupiter J: Open elbow contracture release: Postoperative management with and without continuous passive motion. *J Hand Surg Am* 2009;34(5):858-865.

30. Cai J, Wang W, Yan H, Sun Y, Chen W, Fan C: Complications of open elbow arthrolysis in post-traumatic elbow stiffness: A systematic review. *PLoS One* 2015;10(9):e0138547.

This is a systematic review evaluating complications of open elbow arthrolysis in patients with posttraumatic elbow stiffness. Twenty-eight studies published between 1989 and 2013, involving 810 patients, were included. Total complication rate was found to be 24% with a revision surgery rate of 34%. Preoperative ROM and female sex were independent factors affecting outcomes. Level of evidence: II.

31. Zheng W, Chen S, Song J, Liu J, Fan C: The influence of body mass index on outcome of open arthrolysis for post-traumatic elbow stiffness. *J Shoulder Elbow Surg* 2017;26(5):809-814.

This retrospective study evaluated the effect of body mass index on functional outcomes and complications after open arthrolysis for posttraumatic elbow stiffness. One hundred twenty-two patients were evaluated, with all patients showing significant improvement after surgery. However, the normal weight group showed significantly better ROM and Mayo Elbow Performance Scores compared with their overweight counterparts. Complication rates were not different between groups. Level of evidence: III.

32. Streubel PN, Cohen MS: Open surgical release for contractures of the elbow. *J Am Acad Orthop Surg* 2015;23(6):328-338.

This JAAOS review article outlined the open surgery for contractures of the elbow. The authors noted a history of concomitant closed head injury and occurrence of burn injuries may increase the risk of heterotopic ossification. In addition, less predictable results are obtained in adolescent patients.

33. Araghi A, Celli A, Adams RA, Morrey BF: The outcome of examination (manipulation) under anesthesia on the stiff elbow after surgical contracture release. *J Shoulder Elbow Surg* 2010;19(2):202-208.

34. Haglin JM, Kugelman DN, Christiano A, Konda SR, Paksima N, Egol KA: Open surgical elbow contracture release after trauma: Results and recommendations. *J Shoulder Elbow Surg* 2018;27(3):418-426.

This retrospective record review article evaluated outcomes after surgical elbow contracture release for management of posttraumatic elbow contractures. The study included 103 patients and evaluated outcomes including arc ROM, complication rates, heterotopic ossification recurrence, and need for secondary surgeries. The study determined soft-tissue and bony elbow contracture release is effective and patients can expect to recover a functional elbow arc of motion. HO prophylaxis did not affect the rate of HO recurrence of ultimate elbow ROM. Level of evidence: IV.

Chapter 38

Elbow Arthritis

Julie E. Adams, MD • Scott P. Steinmann, MD

ABSTRACT

Elbow arthritis is a challenge to the orthopaedic surgeon. The complex anatomy about the joint, the propensity of the joint to stiffness following surgery or trauma, and the forces the joint must withstand for everyday activities make surgical treatment often difficult and associated with complications. This chapter explores concepts and critical points about evaluation and treatment of elbow arthritis.

Keywords: elbow arthritis; osteoarthritis; posttraumatic arthritis; rheumatoid arthritis; total elbow arthroplasty

Introduction

Elbow arthritis continues to be a challenging condition to treat. Rheumatoid arthritis and other inflammatory arthritides formerly were the most common forms of arthritis requiring surgical management. These conditions are becoming less problematic owing to the advent of disease-modifying antirheumatic drugs, which have been successful in limiting symptomatic joint changes in many patients. However, osteoarthritis and posttraumatic arthritis continue to be common conditions. Patients with hemophilia can also be affected by elbow arthritis. Although the lives of these patients have been prolonged and improved by the widespread use of blood factor replacement, persistent subclinical or clinical instances of bleeding in the elbow joint may set off changes that can develop into arthrosis.

The changing epidemiology of the elbow arthritis has led to a conundrum. Previously, most patients with symptomatic arthritis of the elbow who required surgical treatment were of advanced age and had low physical demands, often because of inflammatory disease. Currently, many patients with symptomatic arthritis are relatively young and healthy, and they expect to live long and active lives. These patients may not be amenable to complying with the typical restrictions required after total elbow arthroplasty (TEA). The implants used for the treatment of rheumatoid arthritis were designed for low activity levels and may not be optimal for patients with higher demands. Recent strategies have focused on alternative procedures or implants for such patients.

Nonsurgical Manangement

The nonsurgical treatment for all types of arthrosis of the elbow includes rest, bracing treatment, NSAIDs or oral analgesics, and injectable corticosteroids. As for hyaluronic acid, no benefit was seen 6 months after injection in the elbow joint.[1] A short-term benefit may be seen, as in other joints, but it may represent an anti-inflammatory effect.

Disease-modifying agents have altered the management of rheumatoid arthritis in the past few decades. Previously, a combination of NSAIDs and analgesics was used to reduce symptoms. The use of disease-modifying antirheumatic drugs has altered the course of disease treatment. These drugs are effective in reducing synovitis and systemic inflammation and in altering the course of joint destruction. Methotrexate, sulfasalazine, and leflunomide are often prescribed soon after diagnosis, and they may be used in combination. Corticosteroids often are used in the short term to alter joint inflammation or in the long term as an adjunctive treatment. The recent introduction of biologic agents to alter the inflammatory cascade in rheumatoid arthritis has revolutionized the treatment of this condition by targeting cytokines responsible for potentiating the disease process. The biologic drugs include tumor necrosis factor inhibitors such as adalimumab, etanercept, infliximab, certolizumab, and golimumab; interleukin-6 inhibitors

Dr. Adams or an immediate family member has received royalties from Arthrex, Inc., Biomet, and Zimmer; serves as a paid consultant to or is an employee of Arthrex, Inc.; and serves as a board member, owner, officer, or committee member of the American Association for Hand Surgery, the American Shoulder and Elbow Surgeons, and the American Society for Surgery of the Hand. Dr. Steinmann or an immediate family member has received royalties from Arthrex, Inc. and Biomet; serves as a paid consultant to or is an employee of Acumed, LLC, Arthrex, Inc., and Biomet; serves as a board member, owner, officer, or committee member of the American Shoulder and Elbow Surgeons, the American Society for Surgery of the Hand, and the Arthroscopy Association of North America.

such as tocilizumab; B-cell inhibitors such as rituximab; and T-cell costimulation inhibitors such as abatacept. These drugs can alter a patient's ability to mount an immune response to infection. Concern exists regarding the long-term effects of immunogenicity as well as the activation of latent viral infection and an increased risk of malignancy. To enhance surgical healing, most experts recommend discontinuing the use of these biologic agents for several half-lives before a planned procedure.[2]

The frequency and severity of intra-articular bleeding into the elbow in patients with hemophilic arthropathy may be decreased by the use of prophylactic and on-demand blood factor replacement. This treatment may limit synovitis and joint destruction in the long term and provide short-term symptomatic relief.[3]

Primary degenerative osteoarthritis of the elbow typically involves the dominant arm in men who have a history of manual labor. The use of crutches or a wheelchair for ambulation also increases the risk of primary degenerative osteoarthritis of the elbow. Most patients are older than 40 to 50 years and have mechanical symptoms, including catching and locking of the joint, symptomatic loose bodies, and lack of motion, particularly in terminal extension. Patients often describe pain at the ends of the arc of motion, although in advanced disease the pain exists throughout the arc of motion. This indicates more severe articular changes that may not be treatable with simple débridement.

Evaluation

A patient with arthrosis of the elbow often has concomitant ulnar nerve symptoms (cubital tunnel syndrome). It is important to specifically ask about symptoms and examine the patient with this condition in mind. Patient's symptoms are sometimes nerve related rather than the more obvious radiographic findings, and in some cases patients may more appropriately be treated by management of their nerve symptoms (such as with a cubital tunnel decompression) without any specific treatment of their concomitant arthritis. Plain radiographs in three views are helpful for the diagnosis of elbow arthritis. The osseous anatomy and subchondral cysts can be better delineated on CT scans. CT with three-dimensional surface renderings is the most helpful for understanding the three-dimensional anatomy, developing a surgical plan, and appropriately treating all areas of interest. MRI may be useful in the setting of evaluation of occult synovitis or cartilage defects.

Surgical Options

Surgical intervention may be considered for a patient who has functional limitations after unsuccessful nonsurgical management. The factors in determining the appropriate surgical treatment include the patient's activity level and age, the patient's preferences, the surgeon's experience and preference, and the extent of pathologic changes.

Open and arthroscopic débridement and synovectomy are effective treatment options for rheumatoid arthritis, osteoarthritis, posttraumatic arthritis, and hemophilic arthropathy. These procedures are most effective during earlier disease stages, before the joint space and the cartilage are totally obliterated. Synovectomy may delay disease progression and reduce the incidence of painful synovitis in inflammatory arthritis or symptomatic bleeding episodes in hemophilia. Arthroscopic débridement may be considered desirable because it is perceived to be minimally invasive and requires a shorter, less painful recovery period than open débridement. However, the outcomes of arthroscopic débridement have not been shown to be superior to those of open débridement, and the risks of arthroscopy may be greater than those of traditional open surgery. Open débridement is preferred if the surgeon lacks arthroscopic experience, the patient has very restricted motion, or a concomitant open procedure, such as ulnar nerve decompression or transposition, will be needed (although there is evidence that decompression of the ulnar nerve can be accomplished arthroscopically in selected patients).[4,5]

The approach for an open débridement can include a medial incision, a lateral incision, or both, depending on the pathology and the preference of the surgeon. A single posterior incision can be used, with the creation of full-thickness flaps to the medial and lateral sides. This approach necessitates a larger incision that can lead to seromas or wound complications.

TEA is a definitive means of improving pain and function in an arthritic elbow. However, TEA limits the use of the arm to light activity, and this restriction can be devastating for a young or an active patient. Therefore, TEA may be undesirable for such a patient.

When the entire ulnohumeral joint is compromised, other options are being sought to alleviate pain while preserving extensive use of the arm. Interposition arthroplasty has been suggested as such an option. A variety of materials have been used for interposition, including allograft and autograft dermis, Achilles tendon, and fascia lata. Outcomes of interposition arthroplasty were reported at a mean 6-year follow-up.[6] Of the 45 patients, 32 required revision surgery or had poor or fair results. Preoperative instability was associated with a relatively poor outcome. Several factors have been described as leading to a successful outcome after interposition arthroplasty, including preserved elbow stability, relatively well-preserved bony anatomy, intraoperative adequacy of joint release, stable resurfacing, and careful wound closure and management.[7] The patient should understand that improved motion and pain relief are the goals, but absolute improvement should not be expected.

Elbow Hemiarthroplasty and Arthroplasty

Humeral hemiarthroplasty of the elbow may be considered in selected patients (**Figure 1**). Most of the published reports are of small studies. Hemiarthroplasty may be indicated for a patient with rheumatoid arthritis who wishes to remain active and has preserved humeral and ulnar bone stock, a patient with an unreconstructable distal humeral fracture with preserved ulnar articulation, or a patient with nonunion or unsuccessful fixation of a distal humeral fracture. Early results were promising after hemiarthroplasty with a Kudo humeral component (Biomet) for unreconstructable distal humeral fracture in four patients (mean age, 80 years).[8] At a mean 4-year follow-up after hemiarthroplasty, eight women (mean age, 79 years) had a good to excellent Mayo Elbow Performance Score.[9] One patient had a periprosthetic fracture at 3 years, and another patient had an unsatisfactory range of motion. Radiographs revealed ulnar arthritic changes, but these were not correlated with functional outcomes. One report described outcomes of hemiarthroplasty of the elbow for a comminuted distal humeral fracture in 10 women (mean age, 75 years).[10] At 1-year follow-up, nine patients had a good to excellent Mayo Elbow Performance Score. There were five complications, most of which were minor, including transient ulnar nerve irritation, heterotopic ossification, and arthrosis at the ulna. In 2019, a series of 16 hemiarthroplasties for posttraumatic indications was published; minimum follow-up in the series was 2 years (range 25 to 124 months). This was a young cohort of patients, with a mean age of 45 years. There was a high rate of revision surgery in this cohort, at 31%, and a 13% conversion to TEA. Nevertheless, in the surviving implants, there was a 57% rate of good to excellent results and statistically significant improvements in arc of motion. It was concluded that "elbow hemiarthroplasty is an option for young or active patients with end-stage arthritis or unreconstructible distal humerus fractures in whom alternative procedures have failed or there are few other options for treatment."[11] The use of a humeral component without an ulnar component, as in hemiarthroplasty, has not been approved by the FDA and is considered an off-label use; such devices are limited in availability in the United States.

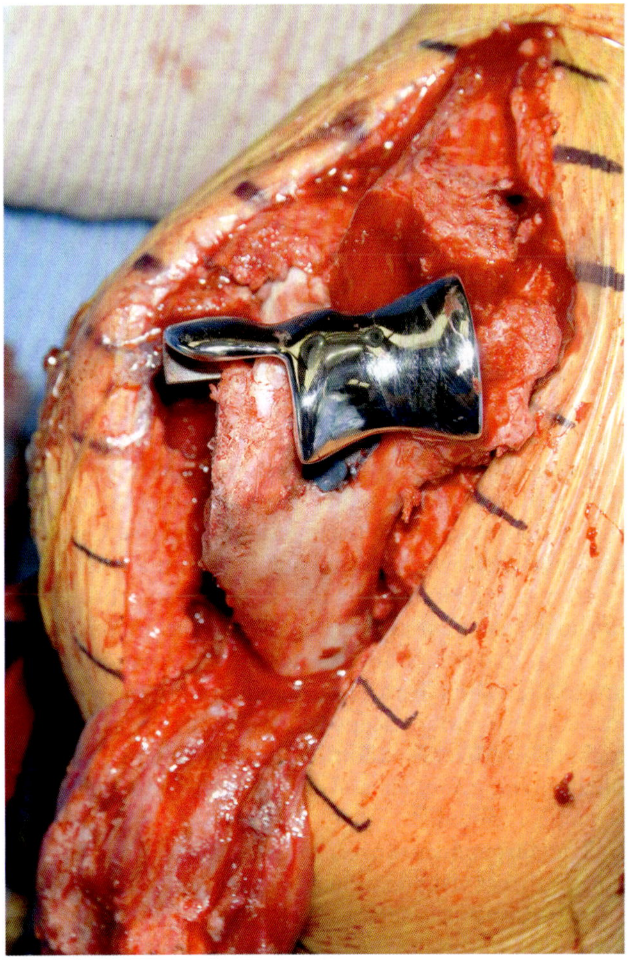

FIGURE 1 Photograph showing hemiarthroplasty of the elbow.

Hemiarthroplasty of the lateral compartment of the elbow (capitellar and radial head resurfacing or replacement) has been performed in selected patients (**Figure 2**). This procedure may be indicated for a patient with an Essex-Lopresti injury or a radial head fracture in association with articular impaction or a shear injury of the capitellum.[12] After an Essex-Lopresti injury, the native capitellar cartilage may not withstand surgical impaction of the radial neck, but a metallic articulation may be tolerated. Few reports have been published on

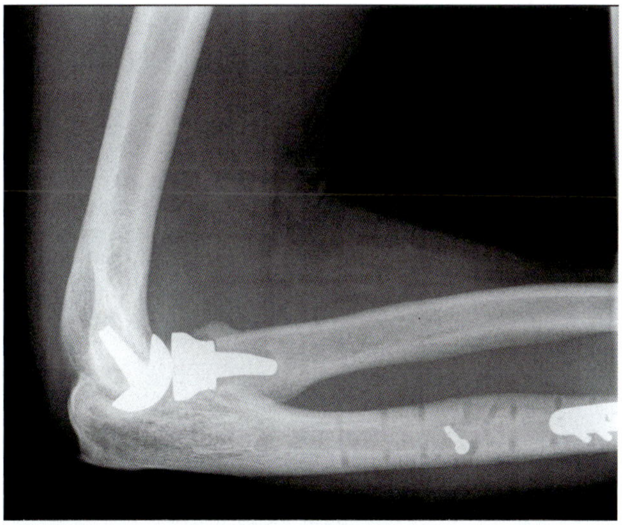

FIGURE 2 Lateral radiograph showing radiocapitellar arthroplasty in a patient with an Essex-Lopresti injury.

Section 7: Elbow Trauma, Fracture, and Reconstruction

the use of this procedure.[12-14] A 2019 report included` 15 patients with average age 52 years, and after an average of two previous surgical procedures. These patients underwent radiocapitellar replacement and were followed for a minimum of 2 years. Although there were significant improvements in Mayo Elbow Performance Score after surgery, the authors highlight the worrisome 31% revision rate, mostly due to the radial head component.[14]

Although there was a device available in the United States for this procedure, recently the radial head component of this implant underwent a voluntary recall, and there is no implant currently available for this procedure in the United States.

Convertible total elbow prostheses recently have become available. One implant allows conversion from distal humeral hemiarthroplasty to unlinked or linked TEA without removal of the humeral component. This implant is not commercially available in the United States at this time, but is available in other countries. Outcomes studies of these procedures are limited, but the outcomes of revision of unlinked TEA have been published.[13] Results were better after an unlinked prosthesis was revised to a linked prosthesis rather than to a second unlinked device, and overall survival was better when a primary procedure included a linked device rather than an unlinked device. However, the devices used in this study were older types, not the newer, currently available prostheses.[13,15]

Linked TEA is an acceptable option for a patient who is willing to comply with the severe restrictions placed on the activity of the arm (**Figure 3**). Patients who are relatively young must anticipate the need for revision of the prosthesis, and all patients must understand the high rate of complications associated with the procedure.[16,17]

Complications of TEA were studied in patients identified from a California discharge database.[18] High rates of short-term complications requiring inpatient treatment (10%) or revision surgery within 90 days of the initial prosthesis placement (8%) were reported. At a mean 4-year follow-up, 120 of the 170 patients had undergone revision, amputation, or fusion; 48 of these patients required revision within 12 months. These study results should temper enthusiasm for prosthesis placement. Nonetheless, the increased use of TEA was reported in a 2012 study of data from New York state.[19] Between 1997 and 2006, the use of TEA increased for patients with traumatic injury and greatly decreased for those with inflammatory arthritis. Within 90 days of the procedure, 6% of the patients required hospital readmission for a prosthesis-related complication. Revision rates were higher for patients who underwent a procedure for osteoarthritis (15%) rather than for trauma (5%) or inflammatory arthritis (8%). Revision may be required because of infection, bushing failure, fracture, or aseptic loosening. The failure of linked (semiconstrained) devices may be associated with the high demands the constraint places on the implant, which may be greatest in patients with posttraumatic arthritis or osteoarthritis.[20] A study of patients who underwent semiconstrained TEA for posttraumatic changes found a 70% survival rate at 15-year follow-up; 65% of the unsuccessful TEAs were in patients younger than 60 years. The use of unlinked implants may improve the durability of elbow arthroplasty, and further studies may provide additional information.[15,21]

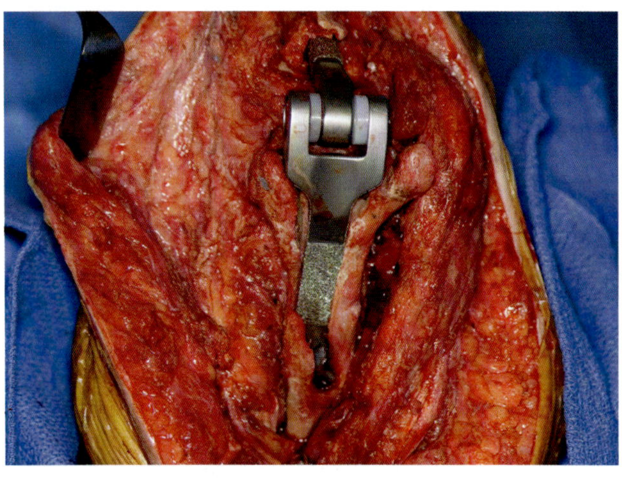

FIGURE 3 Photograph showing linked total elbow arthroplasty.

Recent advances in our understanding of the surgical approach used for elbow arthroplasty may limit complications of triceps insufficiency. The lateral para-olecranon approach involves keeping the majority of triceps in continuity and attached to the olecranon. The ulnohumeral joint is exposed through medial and lateral arthrotomies. Medially, the ulnar nerve is exposed and transposed, then the medial intermuscular septum is excised, and the surgeon exposes the interval between the medial head of the triceps and brachialis. Laterally, the interval between the anconeus and ulna is extended proximally and longitudinally; this separates the portion of the triceps tendon that blends into the anconeus fascia from that which inserts upon the olecranon.[22] This approach results in an easier rehabilitation protocol and less concern about triceps insufficiency than triceps detaching approaches; additionally, improved Disabilities of the Arm, Shoulder and Hand scores and functional strength is noted.[23]

The surgeon, however, must be aware that there is not the direct visualization and direct entry for the ulnar component that is seen in the setting of the triceps-off approach, and must beware malalignment or errors in placement of the ulnar component.[24]

Elbow Arthrodesis

Elbow arthrodesis is an option for the arthritic elbow if the patient is not a candidate for joint arthroplasty or if a salvage procedure is required after unsuccessful elbow arthroplasty. Most of the available studies regarding this procedure are small. Elbow arthrodesis causes profound functional limitations, and some believe there is no good position to fuse the elbow joint. Before planned, elective elbow arthrodesis, using casting to simulate the possible positions of fusion so that the patient can select the position allowing the best function is often worthwhile. Typically, the patient must choose between functional positioning of the arm for general activity or for bringing the hand to the mouth. One experienced surgeon's study of elbow fusion in patients with acute trauma or posttraumatic arthritis found that 10 of 12 patients required an additional procedure, 42% of the elbows had nonunion or delayed union, and infection developed in 33% of the elbows. The report states, "For the most part, this is a procedure of last resort and should be performed when no other options ... exist."[25]

SUMMARY

Elbow arthritis can be challenging to treat. The surgical options continue to evolve, but many procedures still sacrifice durability or function in favor of pain relief. Careful consideration of patient-specific and disease-specific factors is critical to successfully treating a patient with elbow arthritis.

KEY STUDY POINTS

- Use of elbow arthroplasty for patients with rheumatoid arthritis is diminishing, while there is an increased number of patients who present with end-stage elbow arthritis from posttraumatic or osteoarthritic etiologies.
- Because of this, many patients with end-stage arthritis may be younger and more active.
- Although joint replacement arthroplasty for many other large joints is a reliable and low-risk surgery associated with a low complication rate and a high survival as well as a high rate of subjective and objective excellent results at long-term TEA, particularly in younger or active patients, is associated with a high complication rate and high revision rate.
- Options for management of elbow arthritis include nonsurgical means, arthroscopic débridement, joint resurface seen such as interposition arthroplasty, or joint replacement arthroplasty.

Annotated References

1. van Brakel RW, Eygendaal D: Intra-articular injection of hyaluronic acid is not effective for the treatment of post-traumatic osteoarthritis of the elbow. *Arthroscopy* 2006;22(11):1199-1203.

2. Scott DL: Biologics-based therapy for the treatment of rheumatoid arthritis. *Clin Pharmacol Ther* 2012;91(1):30-43.

3. Adams JE, Reding MT: Hemophilic arthropathy of the elbow. *Hand Clin* 2011;27(2):151-163, v.

4. Kovachevich R, Steinmann SP: Arthroscopic ulnar nerve decompression in the setting of elbow osteoarthritis. *J Hand Surg Am* 2012;37(4):663-668.

5. Adams JE, Wolff LH III, Merten SM, Steinmann SP: Osteoarthritis of the elbow: Results of arthroscopic osteophyte resection and capsulectomy. *J Shoulder Elbow Surg* 2008;17(1):126-131.

6. Larson AN, Morrey BF: Interposition arthroplasty with an Achilles tendon allograft as a salvage procedure for the elbow. *J Bone Joint Surg Am* 2008;90(12):2714-2723.

7. Chen DD, Forsh DA, Hausman MR: Elbow interposition arthroplasty. *Hand Clin* 2011;27(2):187-197, vi.

8. Adolfsson L, Hammer R: Elbow hemiarthroplasty for acute reconstruction of intra-articular distal humerus fractures: A preliminary report involving 4 patients. *Acta Orthop* 2006;77(5):785-787.

9. Adolfsson L, Nestorson J: The Kudo humeral component as primary hemiarthroplasty in distal humeral fractures. *J Shoulder Elbow Surg* 2012;21(4):451-455.

10. Burkhart KJ, Nijs S, Mattyasovszky SG, et al: Distal humerus hemiarthroplasty of the elbow for comminuted distal humeral fractures in the elderly patient. *J Trauma* 2011;71(3):635-642.

11. Werthel JD, Schoch B, Adams JE, Steinmann SP: Outcomes after hemiarthroplasty of the elbow for the management of posttraumatic arthritis: Minimum 2-year follow-up. *J Am Acad Orthop Surg* 2019;27(19):727-735. doi:10.5435/JAAOS-D-18-00055.

    This series describes outcomes following hemiarthroplasty of the elbow for posttraumatic indications. Although there is a high revision surgical rate and high rate of conversion to TEA (>30% and >10%, respectively), this may be an option in those in whom alternative procedures have failed or there are few other options. Level of evidence: IV.

12. Heijink A, Morrey BF, Cooney WP III: Radiocapitellar hemiarthroplasty for radiocapitellar arthritis: A report of three cases. *J Shoulder Elbow Surg* 2008;17(2):e12-e15.

13. Steinmann SP: Hemiarthroplasty of the ulnohumeral and radiocapitellar joints. *Hand Clin* 2011;27(2):229-232, vi.

14. Spross C, Jak W, van Riet RP: Radiocapitellar arthroplasty: A consecutive case series with 2 to 6 years' follow-up. *J Shoulder Elbow Surg* 2019;28(1):131-136. doi: 10.1016/j.jse.2018.08.009.

    This series describes results following radiocapitellar replacement in 15 patients with minimum two-year follow-up. Although this procedure is a good option in certain clinical scenerios, the high revision rate (31%) prompts caution with existing implant designs. Level of evidence: IV.

15. Levy JC, Loeb M, Chuinard C, Adams RA, Morrey BF: Effectiveness of revision following linked versus unlinked total elbow arthroplasty. *J Shoulder Elbow Surg* 2009;18(3):457-462.

16. Celli A, Morrey BF: Total elbow arthroplasty in patients forty years of age or less. *J Bone Joint Surg Am* 2009;91(6):1414-1418.

17. Leclerc A, King GJ: Unlinked and convertible total elbow arthroplasty. *Hand Clin* 2011;27(2):215-227, vi.

18. Krenek L, Farng E, Zingmond D, SooHoo NF: Complication and revision rates following total elbow arthroplasty. *J Hand Surg Am* 2011;36(1):68-73.

19. Gay DM, Lyman S, Do H, Hotchkiss RN, Marx RG, Daluiski A: Indications and reoperation rates for total elbow arthroplasty: An analysis of trends in New York state. *J Bone Joint Surg Am* 2012;94(2):110-117.

20. Throckmorton T, Zarkadas P, Sanchez-Sotelo J, Morrey B: Failure patterns after linked semiconstrained total elbow arthroplasty for posttraumatic arthritis. *J Bone Joint Surg Am* 2010;92(6):1432-1441.

21. Ring D, Kocher M, Koris M, Thornhill TS: Revision of unstable capitellocondylar (unlinked) total elbow replacement. *J Bone Joint Surg Am* 2005;87(5):1075-1079.

22. Studer A, Athwal GS, MacDermid JC, Faber KJ, King GJ: The lateral para-olecranon approach for total elbow arthroplasty. *J Hand Surg Am* 2013;38(11):2219-2226.e3. doi:10.1016/j.jhsa.2013.07.029.

    The authors describe their technique for TEA using a triceps-on approach. Level of evidence: III.

23. Solarz MK, Patel MK, Struk AM, et al: A clinical comparison of triceps-sparing and triceps-detaching approaches for revision total elbow arthroplasty. *J Hand Surg Am* 2019;45(1):66.e1-66.e6. doi:10.1016/j.jhsa.2019.05.002.

    A comparison of triceps sparing and triceps detaching procedures indicated improved Disabilities of the Arm, Shoulder and Hand scores and triceps strength in those who underwent the triceps sparing approach. Level of evidence: V.

24. King A, Booker SJ, Thomas WJ, Smith CD: Triceps on, alignment off? A comparison of total elbow arthroplasty component positioning with a triceps-on and a triceps-off approach. *Ann R Coll Surg Engl* 2018;100:1-6. doi: 10.1308/rcsann.2018.0117.

    This series investigated malalignment of the ulnar component after triceps-off versus triceps-on approaches to TEA, finding there was a higher rate of malaligned components with triceps-on approaches, although it was not statistically significant between the two approaches. Level of evidence: III.

25. Reichel LM, Wiater BP, Friedrich J, Hanel DP: Arthrodesis of the elbow. *Hand Clin* 2011;27(2):179-186, vi.

Chapter 39

Radial Head and Neck Fractures

William R. Aibinder, MD • Graham J.W. King, MD, MSc, FRCSC, FAAOS

ABSTRACT

Radial head and neck fractures are the most common fracture around the elbow. These injuries can occur in isolation or with associated osseous and/or ligamentous injuries. A careful history and physical examination is required to determine if there is any additional pathology and to assess for a mechanical block to rotation. Advanced CT imaging may assist in understanding the fracture morphology and the pattern of concomitant injuries. Typically, isolated stable nondisplaced or partial articular fractures without a block to rotation can be treated with early self-directed mobilization. Surgical management options consist of open reduction and internal fixation, radial head arthroplasty, and radial head excision. Open reduction and internal fixation is preferred as long as stable fixation can be achieved. Radial head arthroplasty is preferred for unreconstructable comminuted fractures. Radial head excision is reserved as a salvage option.

Keywords: radial head arthroplasty; radial head excision; radial head fractures; radial neck fractures

Introduction

Radial head and neck fractures are the most common types of fracture around the elbow, with a combined incidence of 55.4 per 100,000 people per year. Radial head fractures are more common than radial neck fractures.[1] Although earlier studies found radial head fractures to be more common among men, more recent epidemiologic studies found either no sex-based difference in incidence or a 3:2 ratio of women to men.[1,2] The average age of patients with radial head fracture traditionally was reported as 30 to 40 years, but some studies narrow the age range to an average 43 to 48 years.[1,2] Nondisplaced fractures of the radial head and neck can be managed nonsurgically, but the treatment of displaced and comminuted fractures of the radial head and neck is controversial. Long-term outcome studies of the treatment options are emerging, and future randomized controlled studies may further guide patient management.

Dr. King or an immediate family member has received royalties from Wright Medical Technology, Inc.; serves as a paid consultant to or is an employee of Wright Medical Technology, Inc.; and serves as a board member, owner, officer, or committee member of the American Shoulder and Elbow Surgeons. Neither Dr. Aibinder nor any immediate family member has received anything of value from or has stock or stock options held in a commercial company or institution related directly or indirectly to the subject of this chapter.

Anatomy and Biomechanics

The radial head has a variably elliptical shape at its concave proximal surface, where it articulates with the convex capitellum to form the radiocapitellar joint, and at its margin, where a slightly flatter portion articulates with the lesser sigmoid notch to form the proximal radioulnar joint. The noncircular anatomy of the radial head and the variable offset of the head from the neck mean that a small amount of translation occurs at both joints during rotation.[3-5] These anatomic features need to be considered in radial head fracture repair or arthroplasty. A safe zone for hardware placement on the rounder, nonarticular margin of the radial head has been described as a 110° arc centered on a point 10° anterior to the lateral aspect of the radial head with the forearm in neutral rotation.[6]

The radial head contributes to the valgus, varus, and posterolateral rotatory stability of the elbow, especially in the presence of an associated elbow injury. The radial head also acts as an axial stabilizer of the forearm. Partial excision of radial head fracture fragments can reduce the stabilizing potential of the radial head, and total excision results in transfer of the normal radiocapitellar load transmission forces to the remaining ulnohumeral joint.[7]

The main extraosseous blood supply to the radial head is provided by a pericervical arterial ring formed around the radial neck by the radial recurrent artery (supplying

This chapter is adapted from Yoon A, King GJW: Radial head and neck fractures, in Nicholson GP, ed: *Orthopaedic Knowledge Update: Shoulder and Elbow*, ed 4. Rosemont, IL, American Academy of Orthopaedic Surgeons, 2013, pp 531-541.

the volar, lateral, and dorsal sides) and branches from the ulnar artery. Sequential plastination techniques have shown that this blood supply is more likely to be damaged by internal fixation with plates than by screws alone.[8]

As in other areas of the human skeleton, the microarchitecture of the radial head undergoes age-related and sex-related changes.[9] Osteoporotic changes may be responsible for the high proportion of patients who are female and older than 50 years as well as the differences in mechanism of injury and severity between men and women. Women with a radial head fracture had a mean age of 52 years, and a simple fall was the mechanism in 73% of fractures.[1,2] These demographic considerations mean that the fractures met the criteria for fragility fracture, and considerations related to osteoporosis investigation and management therefore were relevant. In contrast, 60% of men with a radial head injury had a high-energy mechanism of injury, and the injury occurred at a younger age (mean, 40 years).[1,2]

Assessment

The patient history should include the mechanism of injury, the level of energy involved, and the likelihood of associated injuries. The patient should be asked about concomitant pain in the shoulder or wrist as well as the presence of an elbow dislocation or a feeling of subluxation at the time of injury. The possibility of a neurovascular injury should be investigated through the history and physical examination. Stability testing of the elbow is difficult in the acute setting because of pain. Palpation of the bony prominences of the elbow and the collateral ligament landmarks may provide clues as to the presence of associated injuries. The assessment of forearm range of motion is important and guides the treatment of a nondisplaced or displaced radial head fracture. If the elbow does not have full rotational movement, it is important to determine whether the pain is from joint hemarthrosis or a mechanical block. Reevaluation in 1 week or aspiration of the intra-articular hemarthrosis under an injected local anesthetic can allow examination for clicking, crepitus, or a mechanical block.

Plain radiographs should be used to evaluate a radial head or neck fracture. The presence of an anterior or posterior fat pad sign should lead to a high level of suspicion for a nondisplaced fracture. Shoulder, forearm, and wrist radiographs may be required depending on the patient history and physical examination findings. CT defines fracture characteristics and associated osseous injuries more accurately than plain radiographs, and MRI is useful for detecting associated ligament injuries.[10,11] The additional information from MRI has not been proven to change treatment, however, and MRI does not need to be routinely used.[12]

Classification

There is poor interobserver agreement regarding the classification of radial head fractures, despite the introduction of CT and three-dimensional reconstruction.[10] Three types of radial head fractures were described in a 1954 study.[13] A type I fracture is a marginal sector or fissure fracture without displacement, a type II fracture is a marginal sector fracture with displacement, and a type III fracture is a comminuted fracture involving the entire radial head. A type IV fracture is any fracture of the radial head associated with an elbow dislocation; type IV does not classify the injury sustained by the radial head itself.[14] The original Mason classification was later modified to clarify the difference between types I and II by describing type II as displaced more than 2 mm and involving more than 30% of the articular surface.[15] Radial neck fractures also were included in this modification. In a further modification (the Mayo-Mason classification), a suffix is used to denote an associated bony, ligamentous, or dislocation injury.[16]

Associated Injuries

Associated injuries can be related to patient age, mechanism of injury, or fracture complexity.[1] A 2010 study found that 35 of 46 elbows with a radial head fracture (76%) had an associated injury on MRI.[11] All six Mason type III radial head fractures had associated injury (six lateral collateral ligament [LCL], one medial collateral ligament [MCL], and two capitellar); 17 of 23 Mason type II and 12 of 17 Mason type I fractures had associated injury, of which LCL and capitellar injuries were most common. Although these associated injuries are important, usually they can be observed during surgery (if surgical intervention is required), and MRI appears not to alter treatment decision making.[12] Although the likelihood of capitellar cartilage injury increases with the amount of displacement in a radial head fracture, often it is less severe than capitellar injury associated with a less displaced fracture.[17] Capitellar cartilaginous fragments have been found interposed between radial head fragments in Mason type I and type II fractures, and they can contribute to preoperative restriction in forearm rotation.[17,18] In Mason type II fractures, a complete loss of cortical contact of any fracture fragment strongly predicts the presence of an associated elbow fracture or ligamentous injury.[19] An associated bony injury was identified in 12.4% of radial head fractures.[2] Elbow dislocation occurs in as many as 10% of radial head fractures and is called a terrible triad injury when accompanied by a coronoid fracture. These injuries are associated with a relatively poor outcome.[20]

Management

Nonsurgical Management

A nondisplaced or minimally displaced radial head or neck fracture can be managed nonsurgically, with a good long-term result in most patients.[21] A long-term study evaluating the results of nonsurgical management of 100 Mason type I and II radial head and neck fractures at a mean of 10 years follow-up demonstrated reasonable outcomes with a mean DASH score of 5.8.[22] Ninety-two percent of patients were satisfied with their treatment and only two required additional surgery. Good long-term results also are reported for Mason type II radial head fractures that are moderately displaced (2 to 5 mm) without a block to rotation, although 12% of patients had a poor early outcome after nonsurgical management and subsequently were treated with radial head excision.[23] Recently, a study demonstrated no significant difference in outcomes for nonsurgical management of isolated radial head fractures with less than 2 mm of displacement compared with those with more than 2 mm of displacement.[24] Additionally, in a small series, patients with a displaced partial articular radial head fracture had comparable clinical outcomes when comparing open reduction and internal fixation (ORIF) with nonsurgical management.[25]

Elbow mobilization within 1 week of injury was found to lead to a significant decrease in pain, a better range of motion, and better elbow function, with none of the adverse effects related to longer immobilization.[26,27] There does not appear to be a difference in regard to functional outcomes of patients who were prescribed formal physical therapy compared with those who were instructed on a self-directed home exercise program.[28]

Aspiration of the hematoma that accompanies a Mason type I radial head fracture was reported to decrease the mean level of pain from 5.5 to 2.5 on the visual analog scale.[29] A randomized study compared patients with nondisplaced radial head fracture who were treated with aspiration alone and those who were treated with aspiration and bupivacaine injection. There was no functional benefit to local anesthetic use at any time from the first day through the first year after the procedure.[30]

Open Reduction and Internal Fixation

If surgical intervention is elected because of the presence of a mechanical block or an associated elbow injury, ORIF of the fractured radial head has good results as long as stable fixation is technically possible.[31,32] The results are better in a simple partial articular fracture than a complete articular fracture or a fracture with more than three displaced fragments, for which a primary radial head arthroplasty is recommended.[33,34] In a nonrandomized comparison, patients treated with radial head excision had poorer outcomes and a higher rate of osteoarthritis than those treated with ORIF.[31,35]

Low-profile fixation with countersunk screws, when feasible, is preferable to ORIF with plate and screw fixation, which is associated with more stiffness and high rates of hardware removal.[36,37] A posterior skin incision with elevation of a lateral full-thickness flap or a direct lateral skin incision can be used for any radial head surgery. If injury to the LCL is suspected on stress examination or visual examination of soft-tissue injury, using a Kocher approach simplifies the LCL repair as the surgery is completed. A common extensor origin-splitting approach is preferred in the setting of an intact LCL because it allows access to the commonly fractured anterolateral segment of the radial head. Keeping the forearm in pronation during the deep approach and avoiding the use of retractors on the anterior radial neck reduces the possibility of posterior interosseous nerve palsy. The fracture fragments are reduced while any soft-tissue attachments are maintained to preserve blood supply, and the fragments are provisionally held with Kirschner wires or pointed reduction forceps. Countersunk interfragmentary screws then can be used to maintain the reduction of a partial articular fracture (**Figure 1**). In a complete noncomminuted articular fracture or radial neck fracture, countersunk cannulated bouquet screws can be placed obliquely from the head to the neck in multiple planes to attain stability (**Figure 2**). The guidewire of the cannulated screw helps prevent the screw from glancing off the cortical bone of the radial neck during oblique placement.

If there is significant radial neck comminution and a plate is required for stability, a low-profile plate should be placed on the nonarticular portion of the head, with minimal soft-tissue stripping. The radial head and neck anatomy is complex and variable, and no anatomically precontoured plate can provide a reproducible perfect fit. However, such plates can be adjusted to fit by additional contouring during the surgery.[38] Plating can result in good functional outcome, with preserved motion in both the flexion-extension and pronation-supination planes; however, plate removal may be necessary to achieve this.[39]

Radial Head Arthroplasty

Radial head arthroplasty is preferred to ORIF if stable fixation cannot be achieved in a comminuted fracture. Radial head replacement has had good early and medium-term results with a variety of metal head designs.[40-45] A 2016 study demonstrated that the use of a smooth stem monopolar prosthesis maintains good clinical outcomes out to a mean of 8 years postoperatively.[45] Biomechanical testing revealed that monopolar radial head replacement stabilizes the radiocapitellar joint but that a bipolar prosthesis

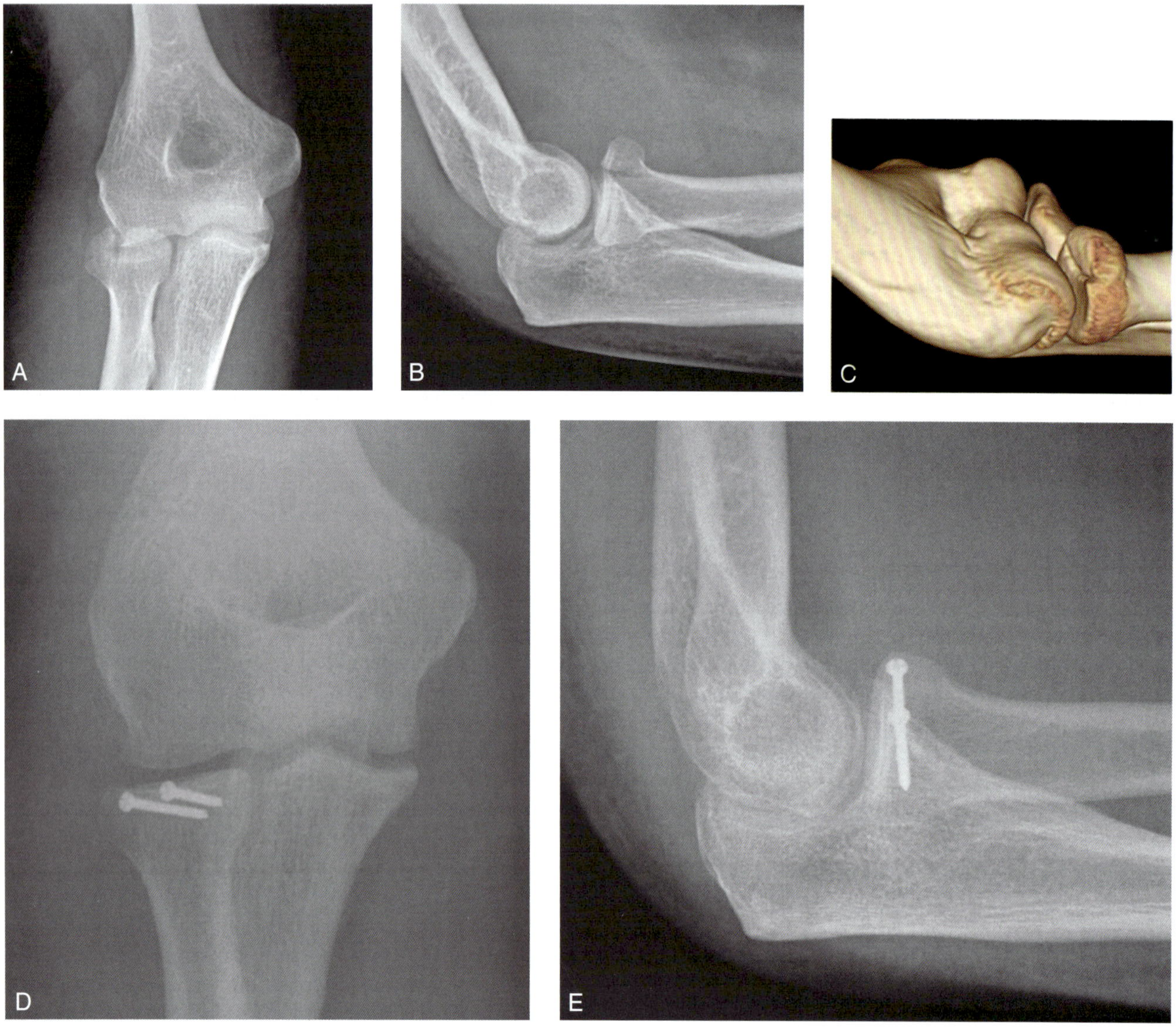

FIGURE 1 A partial articular radial head fracture in a 31-year-old man, as seen on an AP radiograph (**A**), a lateral radiograph (**B**), and three-dimensional CT (**C**). The patient was treated with open reduction and internal fixation of the displaced fragment. A significant chondral injury to the capitellum was observed during surgery, as well as an avulsion of the lateral collateral ligament, which was repaired. AP (**D**) and lateral (**E**) radiographs 3 months after surgery showing anatomic fixation. The patient had occasional discomfort but had returned to work as a truck driver. The elbow range of motion was 0° to 135°, with 70° of pronation and 70° of supination.

may facilitate subluxation.[46] Radiolucency is commonly seen around the stem of a noncemented smooth stem component but is not correlated with patient symptoms[45,47] (**Figure 3**). A recent systematic review and meta-analysis of 878 patients treated with a radial head arthroplasty compared unfixed (smooth stem noncemented) stems with fixed (cemented or press-fit) stems.[48] This study demonstrated no statistically significant difference in any functional outcome measured or final range of motion. An increased relative risk for revisions and complications was noted in implants with fixed stems.

Radiolucency around a rough ingrowth stem design is associated with pain and is a common reason for revision surgery.[49] Significant proximal radius osteolysis resulting from stress shielding was observed when a fully grit-blasted noncemented stem component was used.[50] Progressive osteolysis in cemented bipolar radial head replacement, presumably resulting from polyethylene wear, was reported to be common 8 years after surgery.[40] Noncemented smooth-stem bipolar radial head replacements had good results at 24- to 48-month follow-up, with no evidence of polyethylene wear and no reports of head-neck dissociation.[51] Additional reasons for the failure of metal radial head replacements include stiffness, instability, overlengthening, and infection.

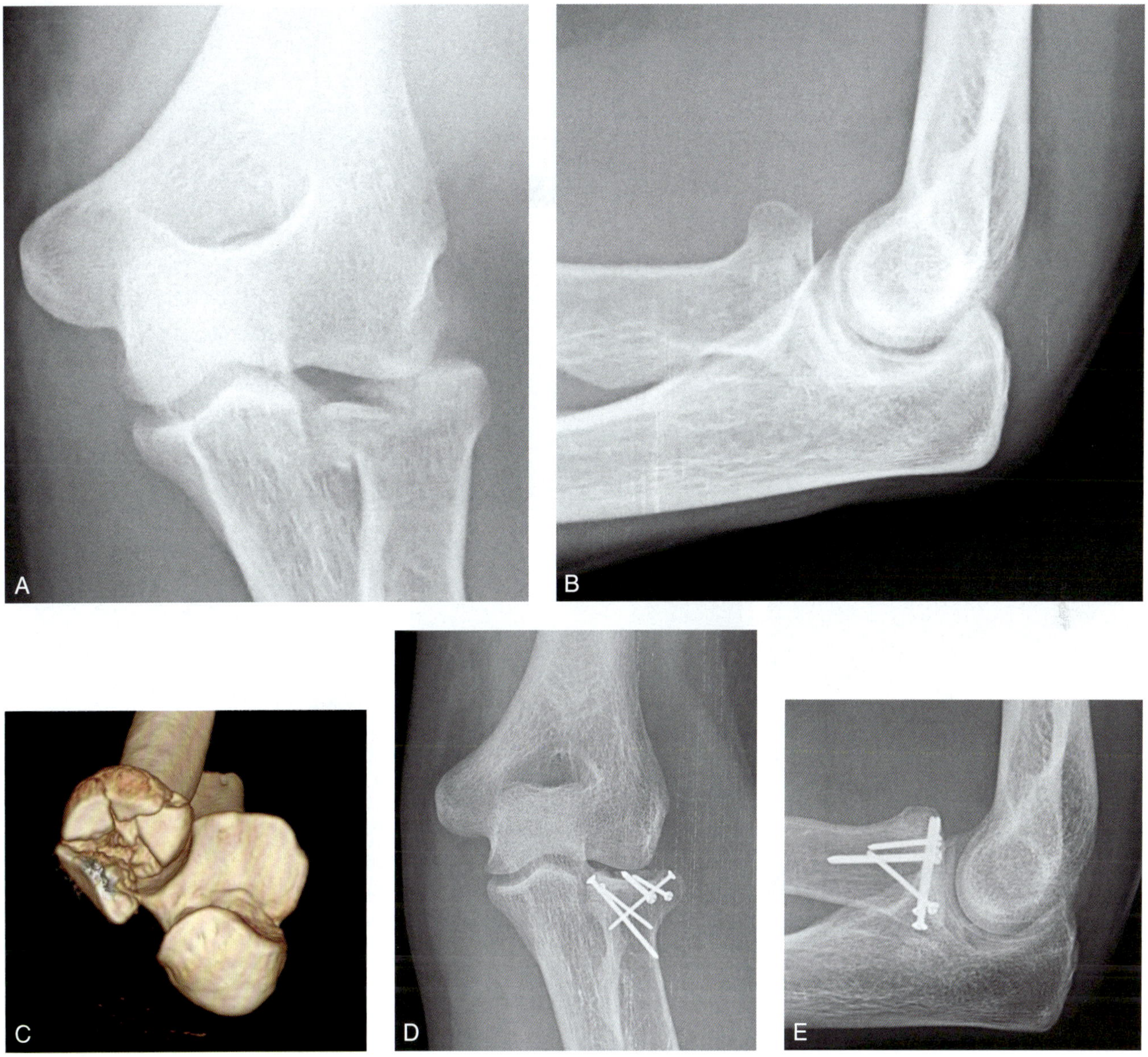

FIGURE 2 A full articular fracture of the radial head in a 31-year-old man who worked as heavy manual laborer, as seen on an AP radiograph (**A**), a lateral radiograph (**B**), and three-dimensional CT (**C**). The patient was treated with open reduction and internal fixation with bouquet fixation of the radial head fragments to each other and to the shaft, as seen on AP (**D**) and lateral (**E**) radiographs 5 months after surgery. The patient had an elbow range of motion from 17° to 144°, with 70° of pronation and 85° of supination.

Pyrocarbon, which has a similar modulus of elasticity to bone, is an emerging alternative to metal for the bearing surface in radial head replacement. Outcomes were good at a minimum 21-month follow-up, despite several early catastrophic failures at the head-neck junction.[52] A recent study of 18 cases with longer average follow-up of 6.5 years demonstrated capitellar changes in 89% of cases and a high rate of radial neck resorption.[53] Still, larger series are required for determining whether the theoretic advantages of pyrocarbon lead to satisfactory clinical outcomes.

Recent studies have improved the understanding of appropriate implant sizing in radial head arthroplasty.[54-57] The diameter and thickness of the implant should be based on the size of the native radial head. To avoid lateral trochlear wear, the implant diameter should be similar to the minor diameter of the native radial head, which typically is 2 mm less than the maximum diameter of the radial head. The prosthesis should articulate so that its proximal aspect is level with the proximal aspect of the radial notch of the ulna, which is approximately 2 mm distal to the tip of the coronoid[54] (**Figure 4**). The gap between

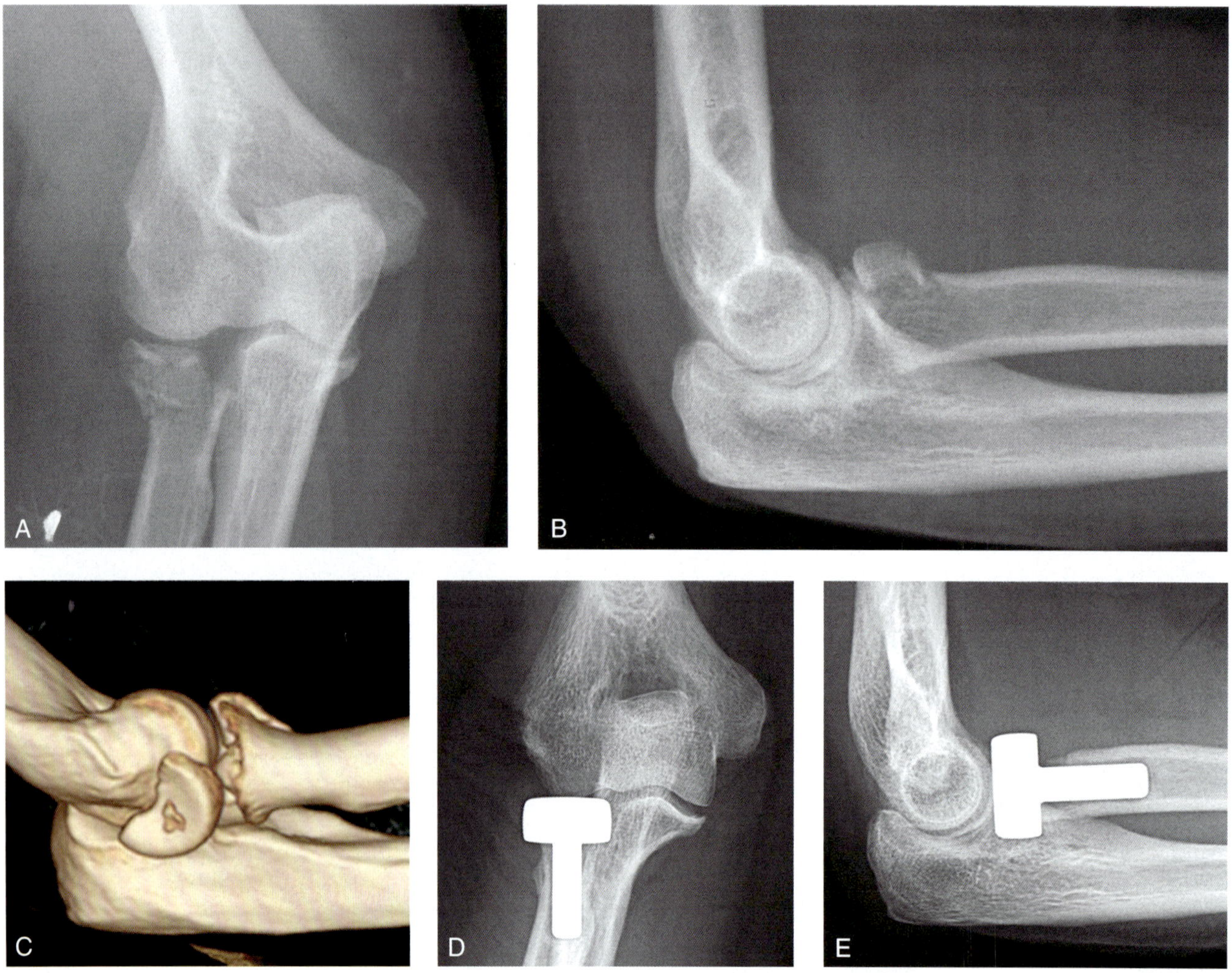

FIGURE 3 A highly comminuted and displaced full articular radial head fracture in the dominant arm of a 60-year-old woman, as seen on an AP radiograph (**A**), a lateral radiograph (**B**), and three-dimensional CT (**C**). At 3-month follow-up, AP (**D**) and lateral (**E**) radiographs show the radial head arthroplasty with a modular smooth-stemmed design. The implant length appears to be correct because the proximal aspect of the metal implant is articulating at the proximal aspect of the radial notch, the medial ulnohumeral joint is parallel, and there is no widening of the lateral ulnohumeral joint space. The typical mild radiolucency is seen around the implant stem. The patient had returned to all of her normal activities and had a full range of motion with no pain.

the capitellum and the radial head prosthesis should not be used to judge the optimal thickness of the radial head implant if the LCL was injured by the original fracture or the surgical approach. Intraoperative fluoroscopy and postoperative radiographs are useful for judging radial length. In uninjured elbows, the radiographically assessed lateral ulnohumeral joint space often is wider than the medial ulnohumeral joint space, and it may be nonparallel (becoming wider laterally). Therefore, the lateral ulnohumeral joint space is not a reliable measure of radial head arthroplasty overlengthening.[55] The medial ulnohumeral joint space usually is parallel in an uninjured elbow, but incongruity of the joint space may not be apparent on an AP radiograph until the radius is overlengthened at least 6 mm. In contrast, a dental mirror can be used during surgery to detect asymmetric widening of the lateral ulnohumeral joint space with as little as 2 mm of overlengthening of the radial head.[56] Contralateral radiographs are useful for quantifying radial head arthroplasty overlengthening because the measurements are consistent from side to side. A radiographic measurement technique described in 2011 had sensitivity of 98% for measuring radial head implant overlengthening as small as 1 mm.[57]

Radial Head Excision

Primary excision of unreconstructable radial head fractures is not commonly performed because of the high incidence of associated ligamentous injuries with more complex radial head fractures and the understanding of the key roles of the radial head in stabilization of a

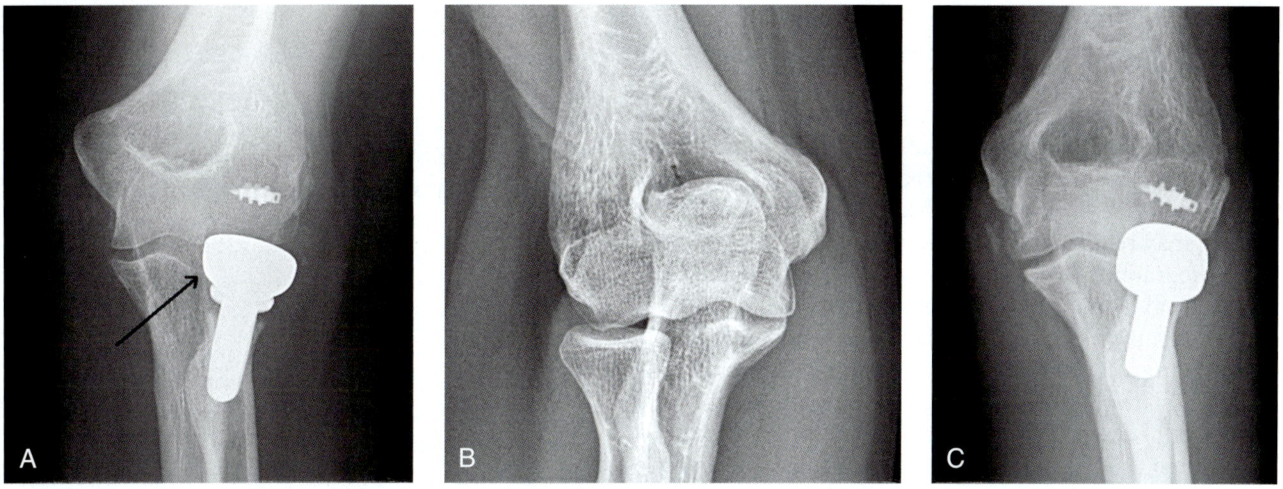

FIGURE 4 **A**, AP radiograph of a patient with significant pain and stiffness after radial head arthroplasty for fracture. Considerable overlengthening of the implant can be seen. The proximal aspect of the implant is proximal to both the proximal aspect of the radial notch (arrow) and the coronoid process. There is widening of the lateral ulnohumeral joint space but no widening of the medial ulnohumeral joint space. **B**, AP radiograph of the contralateral elbow shows the normal relationship of the radial head to the central ridge of the coronoid process in this patient. **C**, AP radiograph of the same patient 3 months after revision surgery with an appropriately sized implant. The ulnohumeral alignment and the relationship of the radial head implant to the radial notch and coronoid process have been restored.

ligament-deficient elbow and load transfer across the elbow. Despite the theoretic concerns, several long-term outcome studies found good functional outcomes after radial head excision for isolated fracture of the radial head or neck. Most of these elbows had degenerative changes on radiographs and a 7° to 11° increase in the carrying angle at the elbow.[58-60] Proximal radial migration is common after radial head excision and may result in symptomatic ulnar impaction symptoms at the wrist.[61] Because delayed radial head excision can be performed with good results, it is reasonable to consider excision as a late treatment option after unsuccessful initial management.[62]

Rehabilitation

Active range-of-motion exercises should be initiated within 1 week of injury in a patient who is being treated nonsurgically.[26,27] In a comparison of immediate mobilization, sling immobilization for 48 hours followed by range-of-motion exercises, and cast immobilization for 7 days before exercise initiation, the sling immobilization group demonstrated the least pain, and most motion, strength, and function.[27] Early active range-of-motion exercises also should be initiated after surgery to reduce the likelihood of stiffness. The range of motion may be restricted by the presence of associated bony or ligamentous elbow injury. If there is residual subluxation of the elbow with extension, rehabilitation is performed within the safe range, and a weekly increase of 10° to 15° of extension is allowed as muscle tone improves and ligaments heal.[63] Isometric muscle contractions are encouraged. If the LCL is deficient, supination is avoided and the elbow is splinted in pronation and 90° of flexion. The elbow should be extended only in pronation. Varus elbow stress, as is created by gravity in the common position of shoulder flexion and internal rotation with elbow flexion, should be avoided.[64] If the MCL is deficient, pronation is avoided and the elbow is splinted in supination and 90° of flexion. The elbow should be extended only in supination.[65] Valgus elbow stress should be avoided. If both the medial and lateral sides of the elbow are deficient, the elbow is splinted at 90° of flexion in neutral rotation, and extension is done in neutral elbow rotation. Rehabilitation with the patient supine and the arm overhead has been shown to improve elbow stability.[66] With any ligament deficiency, permitted rotation initially should be performed with the elbow in flexion.[66]

Serial radiographs are likely unnecessary and do not affect outcome or management for isolated stable Mason type I and II fractures.[67] In more displaced or unstable cases, radiographs should be used to monitor for fragment displacement and to determine when the bony union is sufficient to allow passive stretching and strengthening, typically at 6 weeks.[68] Patients who have residual instability or struggle with range of motion should receive formal physical therapy and splinting to reduce the risk of subluxation and stiffness.

Complications

Stiffness after radial head fracture is most common with surgical intervention and can be caused by prominent hardware in ORIF, improper sizing or technique in radial head arthroplasty, or the patient's noncompliance with postoperative rehabilitation. Stiffness can develop because of capsular contracture or heterotopic ossification even if the fracture is appropriately managed and the patient complies with rehabilitation. Soft-tissue stiffness often can be managed with physical therapy and static or dynamic splinting, but a firm mechanical block to range of motion may require surgical management.[68]

Radiographic malunion or nonunion is common after nonsurgical management and less common after ORIF, but frequently it is asymptomatic. For significant pain or mechanical symptoms, radial head excision and arthroplasty are well-recognized treatment options. Good results can be expected.[61,69] Intra-articular osteotomy is reported to be safe and effective for treating a symptomatic malunion of partial articular radial head fracture in the absence of significant degenerative change.[70]

Long-term outcome studies found that radiographic osteoarthritic changes are common after radial head fracture but are not correlated with a poor functional outcome.[23] Clinically significant osteoarthritis can be managed with radial head excision if the ulnohumeral joint is uninvolved. Instability is uncommon if associated elbow injuries are appropriately managed and the radial head is not excised. Significant proximal migration of the radius after radial head excision can cause symptoms at both the wrist and elbow. This complication is complex and has no simple or reliable treatment.

SUMMARY

Radial head and neck fractures are common and often are associated with other elbow injuries that may or may not require treatment. Nondisplaced fractures can be managed nonsurgically, with excellent results. Displaced fractures without significant comminution can be managed nonsurgically or with ORIF, with excellent expected results, but the optimal treatment remains unknown. Recent studies suggest that ORIF may not be superior to nonsurgical treatment in this subtype. Comminuted fractures can be managed with radial head arthroplasty, with good medium-term results, but long-term outcome studies are required. Radial head excision appears to be a good salvage option, although the patient should be warned that an increased carrying angle and degenerative radiographic changes are likely.

Recent longer term outcome studies have continued to increase our understanding of some treatment options. Nonetheless, there still remains a need for randomized controlled studies to guide the management of displaced and comminuted radial head and neck fractures.

KEY STUDY POINTS

- Isolated nondisplaced or minimally displaced radial head or neck fractures can be effectively treated with early self-directed active motion.
- Displaced radial head or neck fractures without a block to rotation have comparable results with ORIF and nonsurgical treatment; however, increasing displacement is associated with a poorer functional outcome.
- Radial head or neck fractures with a block to rotation or significant comminution often require surgical intervention, but the optimal treatment option remains unknown.
- Radial head arthroplasty is preferred in the setting of acute comminuted radial head fractures; excision should be reserved as a salvage option.
- Management of radial head or neck fractures requires thorough identification of any associated osseous or ligamentous injuries.

Annotated References

1. Duckworth AD, Clement ND, Jenkins PJ, Aitken SA, Court-Brown CM, McQueen MM: The epidemiology of radial head and neck fractures. *J Hand Surg Am* 2012;37(1):112-119.

2. Kaas L, van Riet RP, Vroemen JP, Eygendaal D: The epidemiology of radial head fractures. *J Shoulder Elbow Surg* 2010;19(4):520-523.

3. King GJ, Zarzour ZD, Patterson SD, Johnson JA: An anthropometric study of the radial head: Implications in the design of a prosthesis. *J Arthroplasty* 2001;16(1):112-116.

4. van Riet RP, Van Glabbeek F, Neale PG, Bortier H, An KN, O'Driscoll SW: The noncircular shape of the radial head. *J Hand Surg Am* 2003;28(6):972-978.

5. Galik K, Baratz ME, Butler AL, Dougherty J, Cohen MS, Miller MC: The effect of the annular ligament on kinematics of the radial head. *J Hand Surg Am* 2007;32(8):1218-1224.

6. Smith GR, Hotchkiss RN: Radial head and neck fractures: Anatomic guidelines for proper placement of internal fixation. *J Shoulder Elbow Surg* 1996;5(2 pt 1):113-117.

7. Beingessner DM, Dunning CE, Gordon KD, Johnson JA, King GJ: The effect of radial head excision and arthroplasty on elbow kinematics and stability. *J Bone Joint Surg Am* 2004;86(8):1730-1739.

8. Koslowsky TC, Schliwa S, Koebke J: Presentation of the microscopic vascular architecture of the radial head using a sequential plastination technique. *Clin Anat* 2011;24(6):721-732.

9. Gebauer M, Barvencik F, Mumme M, et al: Microarchitecture of the radial head and its changes in aging. *Calcif Tissue Int* 2010;86(1):14-22.

10. Guitton TG, Ring D, Science of Variation Group: Interobserver reliability of radial head fracture classification: Two-dimensional compared with three-dimensional CT. *J Bone Joint Surg Am* 2011;93(21):2015-2021.

11. Kaas L, Turkenburg JL, van Riet RP, Vroemen JP, Eygendaal D: Magnetic resonance imaging findings in 46 elbows with a radial head fracture. *Acta Orthop* 2010;81(3):373-376.

12. Kaas L, van Riet RP, Turkenburg JL, Vroemen JP, van Dijk CN, Eygendaal D: Magnetic resonance imaging in radial head fractures: Most associated injuries are not clinically relevant. *J Shoulder Elbow Surg* 2011;20(8):1282-1288.

13. Mason ML: Some observations on fractures of the head of the radius with a review of one hundred cases. *Br J Surg* 1954;42(172):123-132.

14. Johnston GW: A follow-up of one hundred cases of fracture of the head of the radius with a review of the literature. *Ulster Med J* 1962;31:51-56.

15. Broberg MA, Morrey BF: Results of treatment of fracture-dislocations of the elbow. *Clin Orthop Relat Res* 1987;(216):109-119.

16. van Riet RP, Morrey BF: Documentation of associated injuries occurring with radial head fracture. *Clin Orthop Relat Res* 2008;466(1):130-134.

17. Nalbantoglu U, Gereli A, Kocaoglu B, Aktas S, Turkmen M: Capitellar cartilage injuries concomitant with radial head fractures. *J Hand Surg Am* 2008;33(9):1602-1607.

18. Caputo AE, Burton KJ, Cohen MS, King GJ: Articular cartilage injuries of the capitellum interposed in radial head fractures: A report of ten cases. *J Shoulder Elbow Surg* 2006;15(6):716-720.

19. Rineer CA, Guitton TG, Ring D: Radial head fractures: Loss of cortical contact is associated with concomitant fracture or dislocation. *J Shoulder Elbow Surg* 2010;19(1):21-25.

20. Regan W, Morrey B: Fractures of the coronoid process of the ulna. *J Bone Joint Surg Am* 1989;71(9):1348-1354.

21. Herbertsson P, Josefsson PO, Hasserius R, Karlsson C, Besjakov J, Karlsson MK: Displaced Mason type I fractures of the radial head and neck in adults: A fifteen- to thirty-three-year follow-up study. *J Shoulder Elbow Surg* 2005;14(1):73-77.

22. Duckworth AD, Wickramasinghe NR, Clement ND, Court-Brown CM, McQueen MM: Long-term outcomes of isolated stable radial head fractures. *J Bone Joint Surg Am* 2014;96(20):1716-1723.

At a mean of 10-year follow-up, nonoperative management of 100 stable radial head fractures (57 Mason Type 1 and 43 Mason Type II) demonstrated good functional outcomes with a mean DASH score of 5.8 and mean Oxford Elbow score of 46. Older age, additional comorbidities, and fracture displacement were risk factors for worse DASH scores. Stiffness was reported in 14 elbows and persistent pain was noted in 24 elbows. Level of evidence: IV.

23. Akesson T, Herbertsson P, Josefsson PO, Hasserius R, Besjakov J, Karlsson MK: Primary nonoperative treatment of moderately displaced two-part fractures of the radial head. *J Bone Joint Surg Am* 2006;88(9):1909-1914.

24. Furey MJ, Sheps DM, White NJ, Hildebrand KA: A retrospective cohort study of displaced segmental radial head fractures: Is 2 mm of articular displacement an indication for surgery? *J Shoulder Elbow Surg* 2013;22(5):636-641.

At a mean 4.4-year follow-up, 36 radial head fractures managed conservatively were followed up and there was no difference in Patient-Rated Elbow Evaluation (PREE), DASH scores, or range of motion between those with 2 or 3 mm of displacement. Level of evidence: II.

25. Yoon A, King GJ, Grewal R: Is ORIF superior to nonoperative treatment in isolated displaced partial articular fractures of the radial head? *Clin Orthop Relat Res* 2014;472(7):2105-2112.

A retrospective study compared the clinical and functional outcomes of patients with isolated partial articular radial head fractures with 2 to 5 mm of displacement treated conservatively or with ORIF. There was no statistically significant difference between groups in regard to PREE scores, range of motion, or grip strength. Younger age was a risk factor for worse outcomes regardless of management. Level of evidence: III.

26. Liow RY, Cregan A, Nanda R, Montgomery RJ: Early mobilisation for minimally displaced radial head fractures is desirable. A prospective randomised study of two protocols. *Injury* 2002;33(9):801-806.

27. Paschos NK, Mitsionis GI, Vasiliadis HS, Georgoulis AD: Comparison of early mobilization protocols in radial head fractures. *J Orthop Trauma* 2013;27(3):134-139.

In this prospective randomized comparative study, 180 AO 21-B2.1 radial head fractures were assigned to three rehabilitation protocols: group 1, immediate mobilization; group 2, sling for 2 days and then active mobilization; and group 3, casting for 7 days and then active mobilization. Group 1 had a higher rate of pain the first 3 days; group 1 and 2 demonstrated improved functional outcomes compared with group 3 in regard to Broberg and Morrey score and ASES-Elbow score up to 2-year follow-up. Range of motion and grip strength showed no difference between 12-week follow-up. Level of evidence: I.

28. Egol KA, Haglin JM, Lott A, Fisher N, Konda SR: Minimally displaced, isolated radial head and neck fractures do not require formal physical therapy: Results of a prospective randomized trial. *J Bone Joint Surg Am* 2018;100(8):648-655.

In this prospective randomized study, 51 radial head fractures were assigned to either formal outpatient physical therapy or a self-directed home exercise program. Outcomes included DASH scores, pain, and range of motion at 6 weeks, 3 months, 6 months, and 1 year post-injury. There was no statistically significant difference in regard to any outcome measure aside from a lower DASH score in the formal physical therapy group at 6 weeks. Level of evidence: II.

29. Ditsios KT, Stavridis SI, Christodoulou AG: The effect of haematoma aspiration on intra-articular pressure and pain relief following Mason I radial head fractures. *Injury* 2011;42(4):362-365.

30. Chalidis BE, Papadopoulos PP, Sachinis NC, Dimitriou CG: Aspiration alone versus aspiration and bupivacaine injection in the treatment of undisplaced radial head fractures: A prospective randomized study. *J Shoulder Elbow Surg* 2009;18(5):676-679.

31. Lindenhovius AL, Felsch Q, Doornberg JN, Ring D, Kloen P: Open reduction and internal fixation compared with excision for unstable displaced fractures of the radial head. *J Hand Surg Am* 2007;32(5):630-636.

32. Lindenhovius AL, Felsch Q, Ring D, Kloen P: The long-term outcome of open reduction and internal fixation of stable displaced isolated partial articular fractures of the radial head. *J Trauma* 2009;67(1):143-146.

33. Ring D, Quintero J, Jupiter JB: Open reduction and internal fixation of fractures of the radial head. *J Bone Joint Surg Am* 2002;84(10):1811-1815.

34. Chen X, Wang SC, Cao LH, Yang GQ, Li M, Su JC: Comparison between radial head replacement and open reduction and internal fixation in clinical treatment of unstable, multi-fragmented radial head fractures. *Int Orthop* 2011;35(7):1071-1076.

35. Ikeda M, Sugiyama K, Kang C, Takagaki T, Oka Y: Comminuted fractures of the radial head. Comparison of resection and internal fixation. *J Bone Joint Surg Am* 2005;87(1):76-84.

36. Smith AM, Morrey BF, Steinmann SP: Low profile fixation of radial head and neck fractures: Surgical technique and clinical experience. *J Orthop Trauma* 2007;21(10):718-724.

37. Neumann M, Nyffeler R, Beck M: Comminuted fractures of the radial head and neck: Is fixation to the shaft necessary? *J Bone Joint Surg Br* 2011;93(2):223-228.

38. Burkhart KJ, Nowak TE, Kim YJ, Rommens PM, Muller LP: Anatomic fit of six different radial head plates: Comparison of precontoured low-profile radial head plates. *J Hand Surg Am* 2011;36(4):617-624.

39. Cronlein M, Zyskowski M, Beirer M, et al: Using an anatomically preshaped low-profile locking plate system leads to reliable results in comminuted radial head fractures. *Arch Orthop Trauma Surg* 2017;137(6):789-795.

In this retrospective study, 24 comminuted radial head fractures (Mason Type III and IV) treated with a precontoured locking plate at a mean follow-up of 30 months were reviewed. At final follow-up, 17 patients were highly satisfied and 3 were satisfied. The mean Mayo Elbow Performance score was 98 and mean QuickDASH score was 3. Only 10 elbows had an extension deficit of 10°. Level of evidence: IV.

40. Popovic N, Lemaire R, Georis P, Gillet P: Midterm results with a bipolar radial head prosthesis: Radiographic evidence of loosening at the bone-cement interface. *J Bone Joint Surg Am* 2007;89(11):2469-2476.

41. Grewal R, MacDermid JC, Faber KJ, Drosdowech DS, King GJ: Comminuted radial head fractures treated with a modular metallic radial head arthroplasty. Study of outcomes. *J Bone Joint Surg Am* 2006;88(10):2192-2200.

42. Dotzis A, Cochu G, Mabit C, Charissoux JL, Arnaud JP: Comminuted fractures of the radial head treated by the Judet floating radial head prosthesis. *J Bone Joint Surg Br* 2006;88(6):760-764.

43. Doornberg JN, Parisien R, van Duijn PJ, Ring D: Radial head arthroplasty with a modular metal spacer to treat acute traumatic elbow instability. *J Bone Joint Surg Am* 2007;89(5):1075-1080.

44. Chapman CB, Su BW, Sinicropi SM, Bruno R, Strauch RJ, Rosenwasser MP: Vitallium radial head prosthesis for acute and chronic elbow fractures and fracture-dislocations involving the radial head. *J Shoulder Elbow Surg* 2006;15(4):463-473.

45. Marsh JP, Grewal R, Faber KJ, Drosdowech DS, Athwal GS, King GJ: Radial head fractures treated with modular metallic radial head replacement: Outcomes at a mean follow-up of eight years. *J Bone Joint Surg Am* 2016;98(7):527-535.

In this retrospective study, 55 unreconstructible radial head fractures treated acutely with a modular smooth-stemmed metallic radial head implant at a mean follow-up of 8.2 years were reviewed. The mean Mayo Elbow Performance Index (MEPI) was 91. Elbow range of motion was significantly decreased compared with the contralateral extremity despite a mean flexion-extension arc of 11° to 137°. Ulnohumeral arthritis was noted in 38% of elbows. No implants were removed or revised. The MEPI score significantly improved from 2-year to 8-year follow-up with no change in motion or strength. Level of evidence: IV.

46. Moon JG, Berglund LJ, Zachary D, An KN, O'Driscoll SW: Radiocapitellar joint stability with bipolar versus monopolar radial head prostheses. *J Shoulder Elbow Surg* 2009;18(5):779-784.

47. Fehringer EV, Burns EM, Knierim A, Sun J, Apker KA, Berg RE: Radiolucencies surrounding a smooth-stemmed radial head component may not correlate with forearm pain or poor elbow function. *J Shoulder Elbow Surg* 2009;18(2):275-278.

48. Agyeman KD, Damodar D, Watkins I, Dodds SD: Does radial head implant fixation affect functional outcomes? A systematic review and meta-analysis. *J Shoulder Elbow Surg* 2019;28(1):126-130.

This systematic review and meta-analysis included 36 articles with 878 patients treated with a radial head arthroplasty for unreconstructible radial head fractures. Implants were unfixed in 356 or fixed (cemented or press-fit) in 572. The mean MEPS score was 88.2 and 85.9, respectively; the mean DASH score was 18.7 and 17.1, respectively; and the average flexion-extension arc was 116° and 119°, respectively. The revision rates were higher in the fixed group (7.9% versus 3.1%) and the complication rate was higher in the fixed group (25.5% versus 13.2%). Level of evidence: IV.

49. van Riet RP, Sanchez-Sotelo J, Morrey BF: Failure of metal radial head replacement. *J Bone Joint Surg Br* 2010;92(5):661 667.

50. Chanlalit C, Fitzsimmons JS, Moon JG, Berglund LJ, An KN, O'Driscoll SW: Radial head prosthesis micromotion characteristics: Partial versus fully grit-blasted stems. *J Shoulder Elbow Surg* 2011;20(1):27-32.

51. Zunkiewicz MR, Clemente JS, Miller MC, Baratz ME, Wysocki RW, Cohen MS: Radial head replacement with a bipolar system: A minimum 2-year follow-up. *J Shoulder Elbow Surg* 2012;21(1):98-104.

52. Sarris IK, Kyrkos MJ, Galanis NN, Papavasiliou KA, Sayegh FE, Kapetanos GA: Radial head replacement with the MoPyC pyrocarbon prosthesis. *J Shoulder Elbow Surg* 2012;21(9):1222-1228.

53. Ricon FJ, Lajara F, Fuentes A, Aguilar ML, Boix A, Lozano JA: Pyrocarbon arthroplasty in acute unreconstructable radial head fractures: Mid-term to long term results. *J Orthop Traumatol* 2018;19(1):13.

In this retrospective study, 18 unreconstructable radial head fractures treated acutely with a pyrocarbon radial head arthroplasty at a mean follow-up of 6.5 years were reviewed. The mean MEPS score was 89.5 with a median flexion-extension arc of 113°. Radiographic analysis demonstrated radiolucent lines in 38%, radial neck resorption in 83%, and arthritic changes in 78%. Radiographic bone adaptations did not affect clinical outcomes in this series. Level of evidence: IV.

54. Doornberg JN, Linzel DS, Zurakowski D, Ring D: Reference points for radial head prosthesis size. *J Hand Surg Am* 2006;31(1):53-57.

55. Rowland AS, Athwal GS, MacDermid JC, King GJ: Lateral ulnohumeral joint space widening is not diagnostic of radial head arthroplasty overstuffing. *J Hand Surg Am* 2007;32(5):637-641.

56. Frank SG, Grewal R, Johnson J, Faber KJ, King GJ, Athwal GS: Determination of correct implant size in radial head arthroplasty to avoid overlengthening. *J Bone Joint Surg Am* 2009;91(7):1738-1746.

57. Athwal GS, Rouleau DM, MacDermid JC, King GJ: Contralateral elbow radiographs can reliably diagnose radial head implant overlengthening. *J Bone Joint Surg Am* 2011;93(14):1339-1346.

58. Iftimie PP, Calmet Garcia J, de Loyola Garcia Forcada I, Gonzalez Pedrouzo JE, Gine Goma J: Resection arthroplasty for radial head fractures: Long-term follow-up. *J Shoulder Elbow Surg* 2011;20(1):45-50.

59. Antuna SA, Sanchez-Marquez JM, Barco R: Long-term results of radial head resection following isolated radial head fractures in patients younger than forty years old. *J Bone Joint Surg Am* 2010;92(3):558-566.

60. Karlsson MK, Herbertsson P, Nordqvist A, Hasserius R, Besjakov J, Josefsson PO: Long-term outcome of displaced radial neck fractures in adulthood: 16-21 year follow-up of 5 patients treated with radial head excision. *Acta Orthop* 2009;80(3):368-370.

61. Schiffern A, Bettwieser SP, Porucznik CA, Crim JR, Tashjian RZ: Proximal radial drift following radial head resection. *J Shoulder Elbow Surg* 2011;20(3):426-433.

62. Broberg MA, Morrey BF: Results of delayed excision of the radial head after fracture. *J Bone Joint Surg Am* 1986;68(5):669-674.

63. Coonrad RW, Roush TF, Major NM, Basamania CJ: The drop sign, a radiographic warning sign of elbow instability. *J Shoulder Elbow Surg* 2005;14(3):312-317.

64. Dunning CE, Zarzour ZD, Patterson SD, Johnson JA, King GJ: Muscle forces and pronation stabilize the lateral ligament deficient elbow. *Clin Orthop Relat Res* 2001;(388):118-124.

65. Armstrong AD, Dunning CE, Faber KJ, Duck TR, Johnson JA, King GJ: Rehabilitation of the medial collateral ligament-deficient elbow: An in vitro biomechanical study. *J Hand Surg Am* 2000;25(6):1051-1057.

66. Schreiber JJ, Paul S, Hotchkiss RN, Daluiski A: Conservative management of elbow dislocations with an overhead motion protocol. *J Hand Surg Am* 2015;40(3):515-519.

In this retrospective study, 27 patients with a simple elbow dislocation treated nonsurgically with an overhead motion protocol at a mean follow-up of 29 months were reviewed. At final follow-up the mean range of motion was from 6° to 137° with no recurrent instability. Level of evidence: IV.

67. Burton KR, Mellema JJ, Menendez ME, Ring D, Chen NC: The yield of subsequent radiographs during nonoperative treatment of radial head and neck fractures. *J Shoulder Elbow Surg* 2016;25(8):1216-1222.

In this study, 415 patients with Mason Type I and II radial head fractures treated nonsurgically were reviewed. Subsequent radiographs were performed on 262 fractures with only 1 of these patients (0.4%) being offered a change in management, which was declined. Displaced fractures were more likely to undergo subsequent radiographs; however, provider variation was more likely to influence whether a subsequent radiograph was to be obtained. Level of evidence: II.

68. Szekeres M, Chinchalkar SJ, King GJ: Optimizing elbow rehabilitation after instability. *Hand Clin* 2008;24(1):27-38.

69. Shore BJ, Mozzon JB, MacDermid JC, Faber KJ, King GJ: Chronic posttraumatic elbow disorders treated with metallic radial head arthroplasty. *J Bone Joint Surg Am* 2008;90(2):271-280.

70. Rosenblatt Y, Young C, MacDermid JC, King GJ: Osteotomy of the head of the radius for partial articular malunion. *J Bone Joint Surg Br* 2009;91(10):1341-1346.

Chapter 40

Fractures of the Distal Humerus

Carl Nunziato, MD • David Ring, MD, PhD

ABSTRACT

Arthroplasty and nonsurgical treatment are options for infirm and inactive patients with a fracture of the distal humerus. Surgical exposure does not have a clear relationship with adverse events after open reduction and internal fixation. Ulnar neuropathy is common after surgical management of a bicolumnar fracture and appears to be unrelated to where the nerve is left at the end of the surgery.

Keywords: fracture of the distal humerus; open reduction and internal fixation; prosthetic replacement

Introduction

Fractures of the distal humerus are relatively uncommon making them difficult to study and difficult to gain experience with. They are also difficult to repair and prone to adverse events and limited outcomes. Between 2013 and 2018, published data reported a decreasing incidence of fractures in the elderly, confirmed the trade-offs of olecranon osteotomy and triceps splitting or elevating approaches, and found comparable outcomes between parallel and orthogonal plating in type C fractures. Most patients experience limitation in motion after treatment of a distal humerus fracture.

Epidemiology

A recent study from Sweden found that fractures of the distal humerus represent 8% of all humerus fractures, with an incidence of 8.3 per 100,000 person-years. However, it is not clear if the authors included distal diaphyseal fractures in this review. Given the prevalence of proximal humerus fractures, it is suspected that the relative incidence of fractures of the distal humerus is much lower. The incidence was found to increase from the fifth decade of life onward, reflecting an association with osteoporosis.[1] A similar study in Finland found a decline in the incidence of distal humerus fractures in women older than 60 years from a peak of 35 per 100,000 person-years in 1998 to 23 in 2014.[2]

Classification and Characterization

Most research of distal humerus fractures continues to use the Arbeitsgemeinschaft für Osteosynthesefragen/Orthopaedic Trauma Association classification, which organizes these fractures into extra-articular metaphyseal (type A), partial articular, capitellum and trochlea, epicondyle, and single column (type B), or complete articular, bicolumnar (type C) (**Figure 1**).

Fractures of the distal humerus can be difficult to characterize on plain radiographs. One study of 614 observers (64 residents, 60 clinical fellows, trauma trained surgeons, 5 residents, 5 fellows) asked to classify 26 distal humerus fractures found the incidence of correct classification, defined by an independent panel of 16 observers, increased from 73% to 95% with the addition of a CT scan compared to radiographs alone.[3] Another study of nine observers (two upper extremity trained surgeons, one trauma surgeon, three upper extremity fellows, and three upper level residents) determined that CT scans improve interobserver and intraobserver reliability of classification and characterization when added to plain radiographs. Interobserver reliability for planned surgical treatment was not affected by the addition of CT scans. These findings were echoed in a third study where 3D reconstructions were added in addition to the 2D images.[4,5] A quantitative analysis of fracture fragment size and volume on 48 CT scans of distal humerus fractures found an average of nine fragments in bicolumnar fractures.[4,6]

Malalignment of intra-articular distal humerus fracture fragments may predispose patients to subluxation and arthritis. One study proposed evaluating extra-articular alignment via analysis of the trochlear

Dr. Ring or an immediate family member has received royalties from Skeletal Dynamics and Wright Medical Technology, Inc. and serves as a board member, owner, officer, or committee member of the American Academy of Orthopaedic Surgeons and the Orthopaedic Trauma Association. Neither Dr. Nunziato nor any immediate family member has received anything of value from or has stock or stock options held in a commercial company or institution related directly or indirectly to the subject of this chapter.

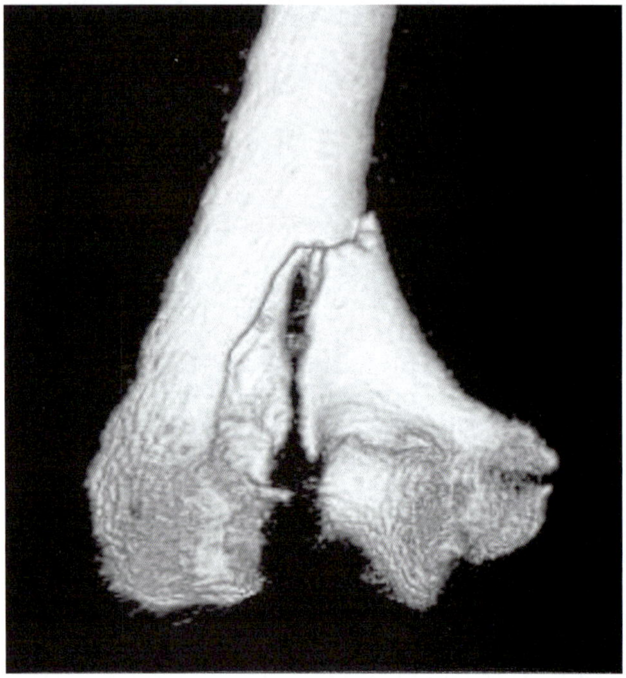

FIGURE 1 Three-dimensional CT showing a medial column fracture of the distal humerus. The medial trochlea is a separate impacted fragment.

capitellar index, a ratio of the humeral axis to the capitellum and trochlea, quantifying varus/valgus alignment. This radiographic marker demonstrated moderate ($\kappa = 0.56$) correlation with functional outcomes according to the Mayo Elbow Performance Scores (MEPS) 1 year after injury in 86 patients treated for distal humerus fractures.[7]

Management

Nonsurgical Management

The debate regarding the treatment of infirm and inactive patients is often between fixation and prosthetic replacement, but nonsurgical treatment is also a good option. One study of 19 low-demand patients evaluated an average 27 months after nonsurgical treatment with an average of 5 weeks of cast immobilization reported an average arc of elbow flexion and extension of 107° ± 16° and a mean score on the Mayo Elbow Performance Index of 90 (categorically excellent). Only two patients were described as having poor elbow function—one with a nonunion and one with concomitant radial head and coronoid fracture.[8]

A second study of nonsurgical treatment with splint immobilization followed by sling immobilization and passive range of motion starting 14 days after injury in 40 elderly and infirm patients reported functional (able to reach hand to mouth) motion an average of 46 months after injury in 95% of patients. They reported mean Disabilities of the Arm, Shoulder and Hand (DASH) score of 38 points (0 to 75) in the 20 surviving patients. Five patients underwent planned excision of potentially impinging fragments an average of 20 days after injury—a debatable intervention. Two patients had plate and screw fixation and two had total elbow arthroplasty (TEA) for painful nonunion. One patient with a united fracture chose TEA at 3 months because of stiffness and pain.[9]

Similar to the evolution in treatment of proximal humerus fractures, with additional experience and evidence, it might be found that initial nonsurgical treatment followed by the occasional salvage procedure is the optimal approach in infirm and inactive people with fractures of the distal humerus.

Surgical Exposure

Exposure of a fracture of the distal humerus varies by handling of the triceps muscle. Options include splitting the triceps with partial elevation of the triceps insertion off the olecranon (Campbell), elevation of the muscle off the lateral and medial borders of the humerus (paratricipital), elevation of the entire muscle insertion off the olecranon (Bryan/Morrey; used mostly for total elbow, but largely replaced by variations of the triceps splitting exposure), or olecranon osteotomy. There is debate regarding the added problems and adverse events associated with each exposure as well as the importance of visualization of the articular surface versus restoring the key elements of the medial ulnotrochlear and lateral capitellum–radial head articulations. Elevation of the extensor mechanism may risk extension weakness or triceps insufficiency, and olecranon osteotomy exposes the patient to increased risk of problems related to implants and nonunion of the osteotomy.

One prospective cohort study found no differences in motion or complications in 51 patients with type C fractures of the distal humerus treated through a paratricipital approach (27 patients) compared with olecranon osteotomy (24 patients) a year after surgery.[10] A similar retrospective comparison of surgical approaches for treatment of type C fractures resulting from low-energy falls in 36 elderly patients (average age: 69 years) found significantly longer surgical time (113 versus 89 minutes) and greater blood loss (222 versus 121 mL) in patients treated with olecranon osteotomy. In the 33 patients who underwent osteotomy, the authors reported 1 nonunion, 3 delayed union, 5 incidents of osteotomy implant loosening, and 6 cases of prominent implants causing symptoms.[11]

Olecranon osteotomy fared better when compared with outcomes achieved following a triceps elevating (Bryan/Morrey) approach in one retrospective study of 54 patients (average age 47 years) with intra-articular fractures. At an average 40 months after surgery, the 32 patients treated with triceps elevating approach had a significantly lower Mayo score (76.7 ± 13.4) than the 22 in the osteotomy group (85 ± 13.2), as well as a significantly less motion (triceps elevation, 22° to 88°; osteotomy, 13° to 99°). There was no significant difference in the complication rate.[12]

Type A: Extra-articular/Low Transcondylar Fractures

Extra-articular, bicolumnar fractures at the level of the base of the olecranon and coronoid fossae (low transcondylar) can be problematic. Even seemingly nondisplaced fractures can have healing issues. These most commonly occur in older individuals with poorer bone quality.

One case series, of 14 patients with low transcondylar fractures treated with plate and screw fixation, reported 2 patients with some screw migration and eventual union and 2 patients with nonunion. The two patients who developed nonunion received allograft for metaphyseal comminution at the time of surgery. One patient was treated with TEA, whereas the other declined further surgical intervention.[13] A second series of 10 elderly patients with low, extra-articular transcondylar fractures without significant comminution due to low-energy falls noted consistent healing after treatment with two crossed 4.5-mm screws.[14] A third case series of 46 elderly patients treated with varying internal fixation constructs demonstrated union in 41 of 43 surviving patients at 25 months with an average arc of motion greater than 100°. Another series of 15 patients with low-energy transcondylar fractures treated with bicolumnar orthogonal plating reported union in 14 patients and 1 patient was not evaluated to healing.[15,16]

Type B: Partial Articular/Single-Column and Capitellum/Trochlear Fractures

Single-column fractures of the distal humerus are uncommon. One study evaluating fracture patterns using CT scans of 133 patients with distal humerus fractures found only 9% of fractures corresponded with an AO type B1 or B2 fracture according to evaluation of CT scans. B1 and B2 fractures accounted for 5 of 50 (10%) high-energy fractures (motor vehicle collision, fall from greater than standing height) and 4 of 83 (5%) of lower energy fractures (eg, fall from standing).[17]

One study evaluated lateral column fractures in 20 patients treated with open reduction and internal fixation (ORIF). At follow-up, they reported an average flexion arc of 123° with a 15° flexion contracture at an average of 70 months after surgery.[18]

Capitellum/Trochlear Fractures

Capitellum fractures typically involve part of the lateral trochlea and often involve a greater part of the anterior

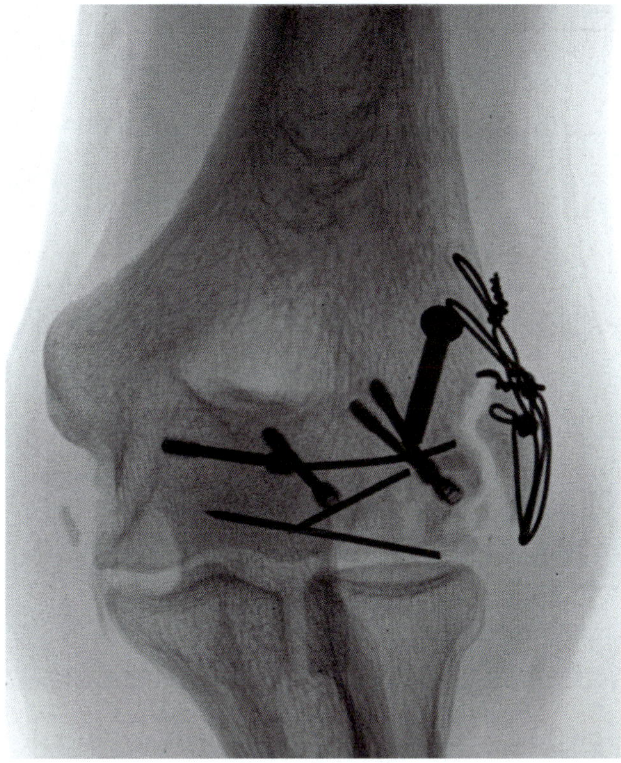

FIGURE 2 AP radiograph showing nonunion of the capitellum after open reduction and internal fixation of a complex Dubberley type 3B capitellum and trochlea fracture.

trochlea, the posterior part of the lateral column, and even the posterior and medial parts of the trochlea. It is useful to consider these as apparent capitellar fractures or capitellum-trochlea fractures to emphasize the potential complexity of the injury. Posterior comminution is associated with diminished function and higher rates of nonunion (**Figure 2**).

A study of 15 patients with Dubberley B injuries (trochlear/capitellar fractures with posterior comminution) treated with a dorsolateral anatomic plate with support of the distal humerus applied through an extended lateral approach to the elbow reported 100% union. The authors theorized the dorsal plate allowed for approximation of a stable posterior cortex and improved functional outcomes.[19] In another retrospective study of 18 patients with capitellar or trochlear fractures fixed with cannulated screws, 14 patients had returned to previous activity levels at final follow-up. The mean MEPS for this group was 87[20] (**Figure 3**).

Complete Articular, Bicolumnar/Type C Fractures

On the one hand, fixation in two orthogonal planes is a basic engineering concept long applied to the fixation of fractures of the distal humerus. On the other hand, placing of the plates parallel to each other on the direct medial and

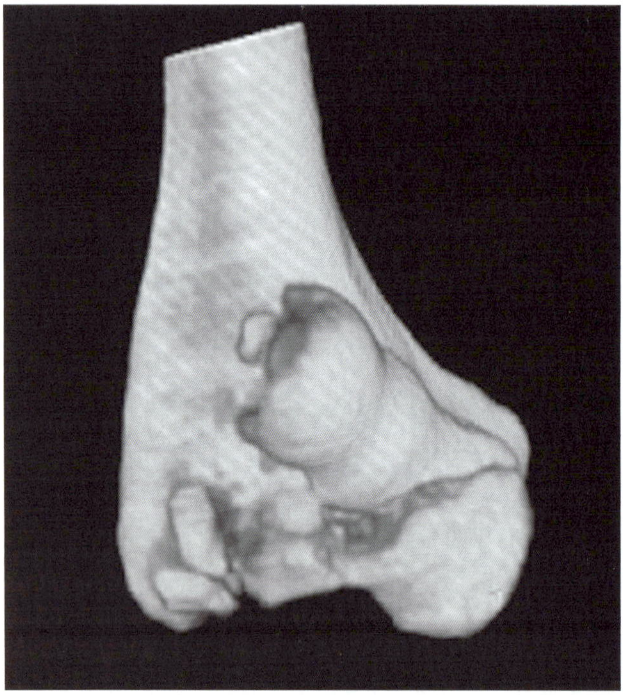

FIGURE 3 Three-dimensional CT showing a complex fracture of the capitellum and trochlea with fracture of the posterior part of the lateral column. The posterior trochlea also was fractured.

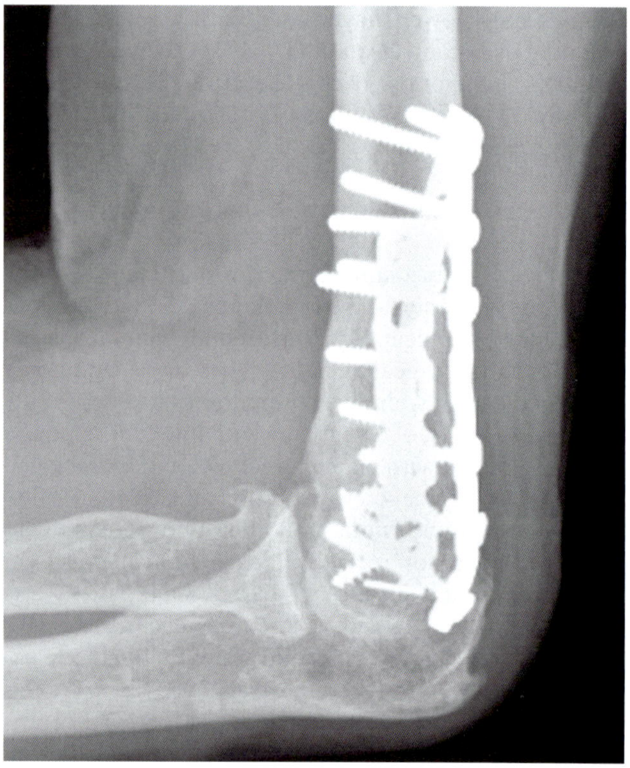

FIGURE 4 Lateral radiograph after open reduction and internal fixation of a distal humeral fracture, showing loss of the normal anterior translation of the distal humerus. The patient had only 90° of flexion.

lateral surfaces of the distal humerus allows for a larger number of screws and longer screws to engage the distal fracture fragments; each of these screws can go through a plate and contribute to stabilization across the columns; and most can contribute to securing articular fragments.

Since 2011, six biomechanical studies have examined parallel versus orthogonal plating: one concluded there was no difference in load to failure in any plane; one favored orthogonal plating undergoing axial torsion; and four favoring parallel plating, two of which noted high rates of screw loosening and failure in the posterior orthogonal constructs as a result of excessive axial stress or cyclical loading.[21-26] A systematic review of 17 studies concluded parallel plating was consistently stronger in response to axial stress.[27] Other biomechanical studies examining screw size and single versus dual plating confirmed the utility of larger 3.5 screws and dual plates.[28,29] Parallel plating results in more metal, so it is no surprise that it is stronger. But how much is enough and are there downsides to having more metal?

Case series studying the outcomes of patients treated with ORIF for bicolumnar/type C fractures are published with some regularity. They consistently report objective outcomes that inversely correlate with age and fracture complexity.[30] Two years after injury, elderly patients with type C3 fractures had less motion than patients with less articular involvement (24° to 113° versus 10° to 140°)[31] (**Figure 4**).

Five case series totaling 151 patients with an average age of 46 years and average follow-up of 37 months following intra-articular fractures of the distal humerus treated with ORIF reported an average arc of 104° (15° to 115°) with an average MEPS of 81. Three studies noted persistent pain and/or disability in more than 40% of patients. In another study, only 54% of patients (26/48) reported the ability to fully perform preoperative activities and work duties, whereas 31% patients (15/48) remained in their jobs but with persistent limitations, and 14% patients (7/48) reported having left their jobs because of limitations.[10,32-35]

Fourteen patients with type C open fractures had less motion on average (83° versus 109°), worse outcomes on the SF-36 survey (79 versus 57), and lower MEPS (84 versus 70) an average of 13 months after injury compared with 14 patients with closed type C fractures.[36]

A retrospective case study of 24 patients with type C3 fractures who underwent staged treatment with external fixation versus primary ORIF demonstrated worse range of motion in the staged group at 37 months. Only closed fractures and Gustilo I and Gustilo II open fractures were included to omit patients with significant soft-tissue damage; however, 4 of the 9 staged patients had experienced polytrauma, compared with none in the primary fixation group. This is consistent with earlier data regarding staged fixation in Gustilo III fractures, and likely is a manifestation of the fact that worse injuries are more likely to be treated with staged fixation.[37]

Open fractures are managed with early antibiotics and, when appropriate, tetanus prophylaxis. One study of 32 patients with an average age of 41 years and Gustilo I or II open distal humerus fractures compared outcomes in 15 patients treated with early (within 6 hours) surgery and 17 patients treated in a delayed setting (average time to surgery of 4.6 days). At final follow-up (average 40 months) the MEPS was not significantly different between the two groups (71 versus 64). Neither was there any significantly increased risk of postoperative infection (2 versus 3), or nonunion (1 versus 1).[38]

Hemiarthroplasty

Six case series of patients described 114 patients (average age 72 years) with distal humerus fractures evaluated an average 47 months after hemiarthroplasty. Most patients had capitellum and trochlea fractures with intact columns. A few patients had plate and screw fixation of column fractures along with hemiarthroplasty. The average arc of flexion and extension was 126°, average Mayo Elbow Performance Index 88 (good), and average DASH score of 24. Two of the three series that mentioned adaptive changes in the trochlear notch of the ulna observed them more than 50% of the time.[39-44]

Arthroplasty

One registry study evaluating 383 patients with an average age of 75 years treated with TEA following distal humerus fractures with an average follow-up of 67 months found an average overall 5-year implant survival rate of 99% and 10-year survival rate of 90%, although notably 23% and 40% of patients were deceased at the 5- and 10-year mark, respectively.[41] The authors reported a revision rate of 5% (18 patients) over the observation period, 7 for aseptic loosening, 3 because of periprosthetic fracture, 4 related to deep infection, and another 4 for mechanical failure not specified. Four additional case series of a total of 135 patients (average age: 79 years) at 39 months following TEA after distal humerus fracture reported an average MEPS of 85 (good) and arc of flexion of 97°.[45-48]

Two systematic reviews compared ORIF with TEA for the treatment of distal humerus fractures. One included 271 patients from 27 studies (ORIF = 10, TEA = 13, ORIF versus TEA = 4) and reported no significant difference in range of motion, MEPS, or complication and/or revision surgery rate at average follow-up of 44 months.[49] A second included 13 studies comparing ORIF versus TEA (5 studies), ORIF alone (5 studies), or TEA alone (3 studies) in 1,216 elderly patients with distal humerus fracture (766 ORIF, 450 TEA) found a significant difference in MEPS favoring TEA (88.8 versus 82.3) but a trend toward worse DASH scores (23.2 versus 29.8) and higher complication rate (25.0% versus 17.0%).[50]

Adverse Events

Fractures of the distal humerus seem particularly prone to adverse events. In the National Surgical Quality Improvement Database, the most common event within 30 days of injury was transfusion, and patients with an American Society of Anesthesiologists Physical Classification Score of 3 or greater are more likely to receive blood. The type of treatment (ORIF versus TEA) did not significantly affect rates of adverse events.[51]

A retrospective study based on insurance claims found obese patients had a 2.5 times increase in odds of wound separation or skin necrosis leading to additional surgical procedures and 6 times increase in systemic adverse events such as venous thromboembolism or exacerbation of medical comorbidities.[52]

A retrospective review of 89 patients who underwent ORIF for distal humerus fracture found an overall 15% incidence of wound complications such as separation or skin necrosis treated with at least one repeat irrigation and débridement, with 6.7% having soft-tissue coverage performed by a plastic surgeon. Gustilo grade III open fractures and use of an olecranon osteotomy for surgical exposure were associated with significantly higher rates of wound problems.[53] We find this rate of wound problems rather high, but we could not discern potential reasons for this.

Risks of nonunion and malunion remain significant complications for patients undergoing fixation of distal humerus fractures. One retrospective study of 129 patients and another of 636 patients documented 12% and 3% revision surgery rates for implant failure or nonunion.[54] Another retrospective study based on CPT codes associated with distal humerus fractures found 12% revision surgery, and a significant association between revision surgery rate and Charlson comorbidity index, smoking, obesity, diabetes mellitus, and radiographic osteoarthritis.[52]

Three studies describe potential pitfalls involved with use of anatomic, precontoured plates.[55-57] One case series described three patients with loss of fixation due to fixed screw angles limiting the length and trajectory of some of the distal screws.[55] An anatomic study found significant overlap between most medial and lateral distal humeral plates from common manufacturers with the medial and lateral collateral ligaments of the elbow.[56] Although the authors conclude they could not comment on the functional or clinical significance their findings, an older case series in 2011 describes four patients who developed aseptic osteonecrosis of the articular surface of the elbow after surgical fixation. The authors speculate the surgical dissection or implant placement may have disrupted the already tenuous blood supply to distal fracture fragments[57] (**Figure 5**).

Although a lot of emphasis is placed on technical factors, surgeon evaluation of postoperative radiographs have low sensitivity (63%) and specificity (53%) for prediction of implant loosening or breakage or nonunion after surgical treatment of a bicolumnar fracture of the distal humerus.[58]

The ulnar nerve is nearly always moved out of the way when repairing a fracture of the distal humerus. At the end of the surgery, some surgeons place it back in its anatomic position and others leave it in the anterior subcutaneous tissues. Most studies do not adequately report the degree to which the nerve was mobilized and handled. Recent studies—some not yet published—suggest that dysfunction of the ulnar nerve is extremely common (approaching 50%) after fixation of a fracture of the distal humerus, suggesting that the diagnosis is often overlooked and bringing all retrospective studies into question. Without careful and systematic prospective evaluation of the ulnar nerve, dysfunction is likely to be overlooked.

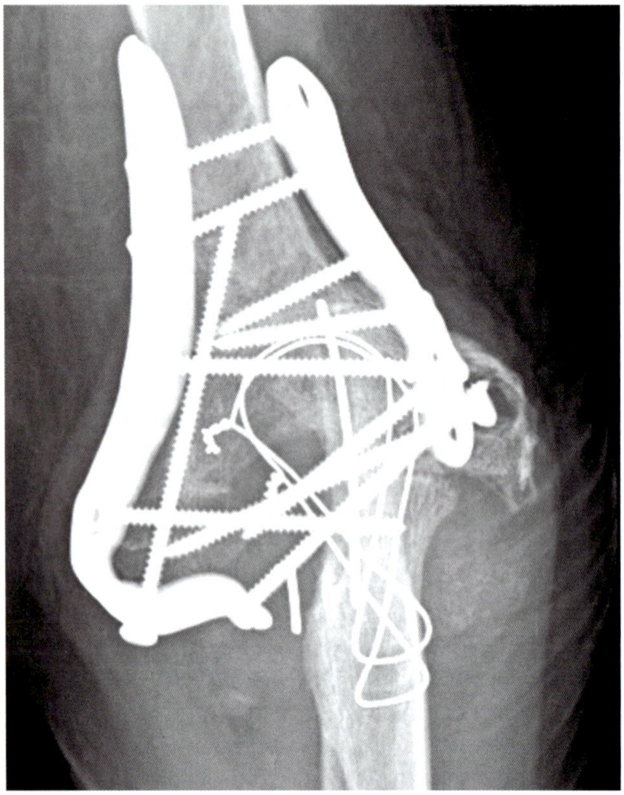

FIGURE 5 AP radiograph showing osteonecrosis of the trochlea after open reduction and internal fixation of the distal humerus.

Studies examining ulnar neuropathy following distal humerus fracture provided noncontributory evidence regarding the intraoperative management of the ulnar nerve to minimize ulnar neuropathy. Only one study, a meta-analysis of five retrospective studies with a total of 366 patients, found a higher incidence of ulnar neuritis in patients who underwent ulnar nerve transposition versus those in whom the nerve was managed in situ (23.5% to 15.3%).[59] Two other retrospective studies found no association between ulnar nerve symptoms and management of the nerve intraoperatively. One series of 24 patients noted an overall rate of 38% and an association with AO type C fractures. A larger retrospective review of 606 patients reported a 16% rate of ulnar neuropathy diagnosed and documented in the medical record after ORIF of distal humerus fracture. Fracture pattern—notably columnar involvement—was the only significant predictor of ulnar neuropathy.[60,61]

Perhaps the most compelling evidence regarding ulnar nerve management comes from a recent and not yet published multicenter prospective trial that randomized 58 patients with distal humerus fractures, treated with in situ management versus ulnar nerve transposition. These authors found no difference in ulnar nerve symptoms based on management technique (presented but not yet published). Additionally, although all patients did experience signs and symptoms consistent with ulnar nerve irritation, all did show significant improvement in elbow function and nerve symptoms at 2 years postoperatively (Emil H. Schemitsch, MD and Canadian Orthopaedic Trauma Society. Unpublished Data, October 2016).

Heterotopic ossification after surgical treatment of a fracture of the distal humerus is associated with male sex, ipsilateral forearm injury, and time between injury and surgery of greater than 7 days.[62] A retrospective study of 124 elbow fractures in 122 patients found a 35% rate of clinically relevant heterotopic ossification in patients with AO type A/B distal humerus fractures (6/19).[63]

SUMMARY

Areas for future study include (1) the role of nonsurgical treatment, in particular as an alternative to TEA; (2) the ability of TEA to successfully salvage nonunion after nonsurgical treatment in people who are infirm and inactive but would benefit from better arm function; (3) whether lesser degrees of surgical exposure and acceptance of less important articular incongruities placing attention instead on biology, fixation, and general alignment has advantages; (4) the prevalence of ulnar neuropathy after surgical treatment and whether there are any modifiable risk factors or if it is an integral part of operating on these injuries; and (5) the treatment of specific injuries, capitellum, and trochlea fractures in particular.

KEY STUDY POINTS

- Nonsurgical treatment is a viable option for infirm and inactive people. Any time arthroplasty is an option, nonsurgical treatment should also be considered.
- Surgical exposure might be balanced with the perceived importance of articular reduction and specific fragment fixation.
- Fixation methods can be tailored to surgeon preferences and fracture patterns pending evidence to the contrary.
- Ulnar neuropathy may be an unavoidable result of quality surgical treatment in a high percentage of patients. Where the nerve is placed at the end of the surgery might not be important.

Annotated References

1. Bergdahl C, Ekholm C, Wennergren D, Nilsson F, Möller M: Epidemiology and patho-anatomical pattern of 2,011 humeral fractures: Data from the Swedish Fracture Register. *BMC Musculoskelet Disord* 2016;17:159. doi:10.1186/s12891-016-1009-8.

   Distal humerus fractures represent 8% of all humerus fractures with increasing incidence in the elderly. Level of evidence: III.

2. Kannus P, Niemi S, Sievänen H, Parkkari J: Continuous decline in incidence of distal humeral fracture of older women in Finland. *Aging Clin Exp Res* 2017;29(3):467-471. doi:10.1007/s40520-016-0594-6.

   Distal humerus fractures represent 5% of all osteoporotic low-trauma fractures in patients older than 60 years. Level of evidence: III.

3. Jacquot A, Poussange N, Charrissoux J-L, et al: Usefulness and reliability of two- and three-dimensional computed tomography in patients older than 65 years with distal humerus fractures. *Orthop Traumatol Surg Res* 2014;100(3):275-280. doi:10.1016/j.otsr.2014.01.003.

   CT scan improves diagnostic accuracy of distal humerus fractures. Intraobserver reliability was improved with 3D modeling. Level of evidence: III.

4. Brouwer KM, Bolmers A, Ring D: Quantitative 3-dimensional computed tomography measurement of distal humerus fractures. *J Shoulder Elbow Surg* 2012;21(7):977-982. doi:10.1016/j.jse.2011.05.011.

5. Nolan BM, Sweet SJ, Ferkel E, Udofia AA, Itamura J: The role of computed tomography in evaluating intra-articular distal humerus fractures. *Am J Orthop (Belle Mead NJ)* 2015;44(9):E326-E330.

   When added to plain radiographic evaluation, CT evaluation changes classification and treatment plans.

6. Brouwer KM, Lindenhovius AL, Dyer GS, Zurakowski D, Mudgal CS, Ring D: Diagnostic accuracy of 2- and 3-dimensional imaging and modeling of distal humerus fractures. *J Shoulder Elbow Surg* 2012;21(6):772-776. doi:10.1016/j.jse.2012.01.009.

7. Rollo G, Rotini R, Eygendaal D, et al: Effect of trochleocapitellar index on adult patient-reported outcomes after noncomminuted intra-articular distal humeral fractures. *J Shoulder Elbow Surg* 2018;27(7):1326-1332. doi:10.1016/j.jse.2018.02.073.

   The postoperative Transcapitellar Index provides moderate ability to predict varus/valgus malunion and elbow function in adults. Level of evidence: III.

8. Desloges W, Faber KJ, King GJ, Athwal GS: Functional outcomes of distal humeral fractures managed nonoperatively in medically unwell and lower-demand elderly patients. *J Shoulder Elbow Surg* 2015;24(8):1187-1196. doi:10.1016/j.jse.2015.05.032.

   A case series of 19 low-demand patients treated with short term (<2 week) immobilization for distal humerus fracture demonstrated acceptable outcomes at 27 months. Level of evidence: IV.

9. Aitken S, Jenkins P, Rymaszewski L: Revisiting the "bag of bones": Functional outcome after the conservative management of a fracture of the distal humerus. *Bone Joint J* 2015;97-B(8):1132-1138. doi:10.1302/0301-620X.97B8.35410.

   Conservative management of distal humerus fractures in 40 elderly or low demand patients resulted in self-reported "functional" elbow motion in 95% of patients. Level of evidence: IV.

10. Singh R, Kanodia N, Singh H: Outcome following olecranon osteotomy versus paratricipital approach for complex intra-articular (AO 13-C) fracture of distal humerus: A prospective comparative study. *J Shoulder Elbow Surg* 2019;28(4):742-750. doi:10.1016/j.jse.2019.01.002.

    No significant differences were found in range of motion at 12 months in patients treated with olecranon osteotomy versus paratricipital approach for type C fractures. Level of evidence: II.

11. Zhang C, Zhong B, Luo CF: Comparing approaches to expose type C fractures of the distal humerus for ORIF in elderly patients: Six years clinical experience with both the triceps-sparing approach and olecranon osteotomy. *Arch Orthop Trauma Surg* 2014;134(6):803-811. doi:10.1007/s00402-014-1983-y.

    Olecranon osteotomy is associated with a higher rate of complications compared with triceps sparing approach. Level of evidence: III.

12. Elmadag M, Erdil M, Bilsel K, Acar MA, Tuncer N, Tuncay I: The olecranon osteotomy provides better outcome than the triceps-lifting approach for the treatment of distal humerus fractures. *Eur J Orthop Surg Traumatol* 2014;24(1):43-50. doi:10.1007/s00590-012-1149-y.

In intra-articular fractures, olecranon osteotomy provided better functional outcomes than triceps lifting approach. Level of evidence: IV.

13. Simone JP, Streubel PN, Sanchez-Sotelo J, Morrey BF: Low transcondylar fractures of the distal humerus: Results of open reduction and internal fixation. *J Shoulder Elbow Surg* 2014;23(4):573-578. doi:10.1016/j.jse.2013.12.013.

    Low transcondylar fractures treated with ORIF have a 79% union rate, which appears improved with modern parallel plating with locking constructs. Level of evidence: IV.

14. Park JS, Kim YT, Choi SJ: Crisscross-type screw fixation for transcondylar fractures of distal humerus in elderly patients. *Arch Orthop Trauma Surg* 2015;135(1):1-7. doi:10.1007/s00402-014-2116-3.

    In a case series of 10 elderly patients with low transcondylar fractures, crisscross screw fixation allowed for primary union in all patients by 3 months. Level of evidence: IV.

15. Ducrot G, Bonnomet F, Adam P, Ehlinger M: Treatment of distal humerus fractures with LCP DHP™ locking plates in patients older than 65 years. *Orthop Traumatol Surg Res* 2013;99(2):145-154. doi:10.1016/j.otsr.2012.12.011.

    Three of 46 elderly patients treated with ORIF of distal humerus fractures developed nonunion at 25 months. Level of evidence: IV.

16. Leigey DF, Farrell DJ, Siska PA, Tarkin IS: Bicolumnar 90-90 plating of low-energy distal humeral fractures in the elderly patient. *Geriatr Orthop Surg Rehabil* 2014;5(3):122-126. doi:10.1177/2151458514526882.

    Orthogonal bicolumnar fixation can result in good union and range of motion in elderly patients with transcondylar fractures and a low-energy mechanism. Level of evidence: IV.

17. Mitake T, Nishizuka T, Tatebe M, Hirata H: Adult distal humerus trauma with surgical intervention: CT analysis of fracture pattern, causes, and distribution. *Nagoya J Med Sci* 2018;80(2):199-205. doi:10.18999/nagjms.80.2.199.

    There were statistically significant association between fracture type and mechanism of injury in patients with distal humerus fractures. Level of evidence: III.

18. Keudell A, Kachooei AR, Moradi A, Jupiter JB: Outcome of surgical fixation of lateral column distal humerus fractures. *J Orthop Trauma* 2016;30(5):245-250. doi:10.1097/BOT.0000000000000496.

    Long-term follow-up of isolated lateral column distal humerus fractures treated surgically demonstrates good union rates with preservation of functional range of motion. Level of evidence: IV.

19. Wang P, Kandemir U, Zhang K, et al: Treatment of capitellar and trochlear fractures with posterior comminution: Minimum 2-year follow-up. *J Shoulder Elbow Surg* 2019;28(5):931-938. doi:10.1016/j.jse.2018.09.004.

    Capitellar and trochlear fractures with posterior comminution have good radiographic and functional outcomes if treated with dorsolateral plates supporting the distal humerus. Level of evidence: IV.

20. Bilsel K, Atalar AC, Erdil M, Elmadag M, Sen C, Demirhan M: Coronal plane fractures of the distal humerus involving the capitellum and trochlea treated with open reduction internal fixation. *Arch Orthop Trauma Surg* 2013;133(6):797-804. doi:10.1007/s00402-013-1718-5.

    Fourteen of 18 patients with coronal fractures of the elbow fixed with cannulated screws returned to previous level of activity at final follow-up. Level of evidence: IV.

21. Caravaggi P, Laratta JL, Yoon RS, et al: Internal fixation of the distal humerus: A comprehensive biomechanical study evaluating current fixation techniques. *J Orthop Trauma* 2014;28(4):222-226. doi:10.1097/BOT.0b013e3182a6693f.

    Parallel locking plates have a higher axial load to failure than nonlocking or orthogonal plates in cadavers.

22. Got C, Shuck J, Biercevicz A, et al: Biomechanical comparison of parallel versus 90-90 plating of bicolumn distal humerus fractures with intra-articular comminution. *J Hand Surg Am* 2012;37(12):2512-2518. doi:10.1016/j.jhsa.2012.08.042.

23. Koonce RC, Baldini TH, Morgan SJ: Are conventional reconstruction plates equivalent to precontoured locking plates for distal humerus fracture fixation? A biomechanics cadaver study. *Clin Biomech (Bristol, Avon)* 2012;27(7):697-701. doi:10.1016/j.clinbiomech.2012.03.008.

24. Taylor PA, Owen JR, Benfield CP, Wayne JS, Boardman N: Parallel plating of simulated distal humerus fractures demonstrates increased stiffness relative to orthogonal plating with a distal humerus locking plate system. *J Orthop Trauma* 2016;30(4):e118-e122. doi:10.1097/BOT.0000000000000477.

    Cadavers with parallel plates had higher load to failure compared with orthogonal plates when experiencing torsional and bending stresses.

25. Kudo T, Hara A, Iwase H, et al: Biomechanical properties of orthogonal plate configuration versus parallel plate configuration using the same locking plate system for intra-articular distal humeral fractures under radial or ulnar column axial load. *Injury* 2016;47(10):2071-2076. doi:10.1016/j.injury.2016.08.012.

    The posterolateral plate tends to fail anteriorly when subject to axial compression in cadaveric elbows.

26. Zalavras CG, Vercillo MT, Jun BJ, Otarodifard K, Itamura JM, Lee TQ: Biomechanical evaluation of parallel versus orthogonal plate fixation of intra-articular distal humerus fractures. *J Shoulder Elbow Surg* 2011;20(1):12-20. doi:10.1016/j.jse.2010.08.005.

27. Shih C-A, Su W-R, Lin W-C, Tai T-W: Parallel versus orthogonal plate osteosynthesis of adult distal humerus fractures: A meta-analysis of biomechanical studies. *Int Orthop* 2019;43(2):449-460. doi:10.1007/s00264-018-3937-4.

A meta-analysis of biomechanical studies concluded that parallel plating provides greater axial strength and stiffness compared with orthogonal plating. Level of evidence: IA.

28. Hungerer S, Wipf F, von Oldenburg G, Augat P, Penzkofer R: Complex distal humerus fractures-comparison of polyaxial locking and nonlocking screw configurations – A preliminary biomechanical study. *J Orthop Trauma* 2014;28(3):130-136. doi:10.1097/BOT.0b013e31829d19a4.

Construct stiffness significantly increased in osteotomized cadaver bones with use of 3.5 screws over 2.7 screws and placement of interfragmentary fixation.

29. Scolaro JA, Hsu JE, Svach DJ, Mehta S: Plate selection for fixation of extra-articular distal humerus fractures: A biomechanical comparison of three different implants. *Injury* 2014;45(12):2040-2044. doi:10.1016/j.injury.2014.08.036.

In sawbones, posterolateral plating was found to be mechanically superior to noncontoured locking compression plates in specimens with proximal osteotomy.

30. Nouraei M, Motififar M, Barazandeh M: Evaluation of outcomes of open reduction and internal fixation surgery in patients with type C distal humeral fractures. *Adv Biomed Res* 2018;7:3. doi:10.4103/abr.abr_283_15.

Case series of 46 patients demonstrated elbow stiffness in 29 patients (63%) at 12 months. Level of evidence: IV.

31. Biz C, Sperotto SP, Maschio N, Borella M, Iacobellis C, Ruggieri P: The challenging surgical treatment of closed distal humerus fractures in elderly and octogenarian patients: Radiographic and functional outcomes with a minimum follow-up of 24 months. *Arch Orthop Trauma Surg* 2017;137(10):1371-1383. doi:10.1007/s00402-017-2762-3.

Patients with type C3 fractures treated with ORIF demonstrated significantly decreased range of motion (24° to 114°) compared with those with less complex fracture patterns. Level of evidence: III.

32. Patel J, Motwani G, Shah H, Daveshwar R: Outcome after internal fixation of intraarticular distal humerus (AO type B & C) fractures: Preliminary results with anatomical distal humerus LCP system. *J Clin Orthop Trauma* 2017;8(1):63-67. doi:10.1016/j.jcot.2017.02.004.

Case series of 31 patients demonstrated 90% good or excellent outcomes on the MEPS scale at 10 months. Level of evidence: IV.

33. Chou Y-C, Hsu Y-H, Yu Y-H, Wu C-C: Triceps-reflecting anconeus pedicle approach with double precontoured locking plate fixation is efficient in the treatment of orthopaedic trauma association type C distal humerus fracture. *Injury* 2016;47(10):2240-2246. doi:10.1016/j.injury.2016.06.036.

Case series of 48 patients demonstrated mean arc of flexion/extension of 121° at 24 months. Level of evidence: IV.

34. Huang JI, Paczas M, Hoyen HA, Vallier HA: Functional outcome after open reduction internal fixation of intra-articular fractures of the distal humerus in the elderly. *J Orthop Trauma* 2011;25(5):259-265. doi:10.1097/BOT.0b013e3181dfd348.

35. Frattini M, Soncini G, Corradi M, Panno B, Tocco S, Pogliacomi F: Mid-term results of complex distal humeral fractures. *Musculoskelet Surg* 2011;95(3):205-213. doi:10.1007/s12306-011-0132-9.

36. Min W, Ding BC, Tejwani NC: Comparative functional outcome of AO/OTA type C distal humerus fractures: Open injuries do worse than closed fractures. *J Trauma Acute Care Surg* 2012;72(2):E27-E32.

37. Kösters C, Lenschow S, Schulte-Zurhausen E, Roßlenbroich S, Raschke MJ, Schliemann B: Management of comminuted fractures of the distal humerus: Clinical outcome after primary external fixation versus immediate fixation with locking plates. *Arch Orthop Trauma Surg* 2017;137(12):1693-1698. doi:10.1007/s00402-017-2792-x.

Patients who underwent staged fixation of closed and Gustilo I/II open fractures had worse outcomes at 37 months compared with those who had early ORIF. Level of evidence: III.

38. Radoičić D, Micić I, Dašić Z, Košutic M: Does timing of surgery affect the outcome of open articular distal humerus fractures. *Eur J Orthop Surg Traumatol* 2014;24(5):777-782. doi:10.1007/s00590-013-1358-z.

Patients with Gustilo I or Gustilo II open fractures treated at an average of 4.9 days postoperative do not have worse outcomes than those treated within 6 hours of injury. Level of evidence: III.

39. Schultzel M, Scheidt K, Klein CC, Narvy SJ, Lee BK, Itamura JM: Hemiarthroplasty for the treatment of distal humeral fractures: Midterm clinical results. *J Shoulder Elbow Surg* 2017;26(3):389-393. doi:10.1016/j.jse.2016.09.057.

Case series of 10 patients treated with hemiarthroplasty demonstrated mean MEPS of 89. Level of evidence: IV.

40. Phadnis J, Banerjee S, Watts AC, Little N, Hearnden A, Patel VR: Elbow hemiarthroplasty using a "triceps-on" approach for the management of acute distal humeral fractures. *J Shoulder Elbow Surg* 2015;24(8):1178-1186. doi:10.1016/j.jse.2015.04.010.

Case series of 16 patients treated with distal humeral hemiarthroplasty demonstrated MEPS of 89 at 35 months. Level of evidence: IV.

41. Nestorson J, Ekholm C, Etzner M, Adolfsson L: Hemiarthroplasty for irreparable distal humeral fractures: Medium-term follow-up of 42 patients. *Bone Joint J* 2015;97-B(10):1377-1384. doi:10.1302/0301-620X.97B10.35421.

    Elbow hemiarthroplasty demonstrated comparable medium-term functional outcomes to ORIF. Level of evidence: III.

42. Smith G, Hughes JS: Unreconstructable acute distal humeral fractures and their sequelae treated with distal humeral hemiarthroplasty: A two-year to eleven-year follow-up. *J Shoulder Elbow Surg* 2013;22(12):1710-1723. doi:10.1016/j.jse.2013.06.012.

    Case series of 26 patients with distal humeral hemiarthroplasty demonstrated MEPS of 90 at 80 months. Level of evidence: IV.

43. Adolfsson L, Nestorson J: The Kudo humeral component as primary hemiarthroplasty in distal humeral fractures. *J Shoulder Elbow Surg* 2012;21(4):451-455. doi:10.1016/j.jse.2011.07.011.

44. Argintar E, Berry M, Narvy SJ, Kramer J, Omid R, Itamura JM: Hemiarthroplasty for the treatment of distal humerus fractures: Short-term clinical results. *Orthopedics* 2012;35(12):1042-1045. doi:10.3928/01477447-20121120-06.

45. Ducrot G, Ehlinger M, Adam P, Marco DA, Clavert P, Bonnomet F: Complex fractures of the distal humerus in the elderly: Is primary total elbow arthroplasty a valid treatment alternative? A series of 20 cases. *Orthop Traumatol Surg Res* 2013;99(1):10-20. doi:10.1016/j.otsr.2012.10.010.

    Case series of 18 patients with type C distal humerus fractures treated with arthroplasty found good range of motion and excellent MEPS in 73%. Level of evidence: IV.

46. Linn MS, Gardner MJ, McAndrew CM, Gallagher B, Ricci WM: Is primary total elbow arthroplasty safe for the treatment of open intra-articular distal humerus fractures? *Injury* 2014;45(11):1747-1751. doi:10.1016/j.injury.2014.07.017.

    Case series of seven patients treated for open intra-articular distal humerus fractures with TEA because of poor bone quality had average arc of motion of 92° at 43 months. Level of evidence: IV.

47. Lami D, Chivot M, Caubere A, Galland A, Argenson J: First-line management of distal humerus fracture by total elbow arthroplasty in geriatric traumatology: Results in a 21-patient series at a minimum 2 years' follow-up. *Orthop Traumatol Surg Res* 2017;103(6):891-897. doi:10.1016/j.otsr.2017.06.009.

    Case series of 21 patients treated with TEA at 3.2-year follow-up reported average MEPS of 84. Level of evidence: IV.

48. Mansat P, Degorce NH, Bonnevialle N, Demezon H, Fabre T, SOFCOT: Total elbow arthroplasty for acute distal humeral fractures in patients over 65 years old – Results of a multicenter study in 87 patients. *Orthop Traumatol Surg Res* 2013;99(7):779-784. doi:10.1016/j.otsr.2013.08.003.

    Nine of 87 patients underwent revision surgery following total elbow arthroplasty. Level of evidence: IV.

49. Githens M, Yao J, Sox AH, Bishop J: Open reduction and internal fixation versus total elbow arthroplasty for the treatment of geriatric distal humerus fractures: A systematic review and meta-analysis. *J Orthop Trauma* 2014;28(8):481-488. doi:10.1097/BOT.0000000000000050.

    A meta-analysis of 271 patients in 27 studies found no significant difference in range of motion or complication rate between TEA and ORIF. Level of evidence: II.

50. Schindelar LE, Rondon AJ, Ilyas AM: Total elbow arthroplasty versus open reduction and internal fixation for the management of distal humerus fractures in the elderly. *Orthopedics* 2019;42(1):22-27. doi:10.3928/01477447-20181206-05.

    A meta-analysis of 13 studies found significantly greater flexion contracture in TEA versus ORIF. Level of evidence: II.

51. Medvedev G, Wang C, Amdur R, Neviaser R, Neviaser A: Operative distal humerus fractures in older patients: Predictors for early complications based on a national database. *HSS J* 2017;13(3):212-216. doi:10.1007/s11420-017-9547-7.

    Overall complications for ORIF or TEA after distal humerus fractures are low, and associated only with ASA score of >3. Level of evidence: IV.

52. Werner BC, Rawles RB, Jobe J, Chhabra A, Freilich AM: Obesity is associated with increased postoperative complications after operative management of distal humerus fractures. *J Shoulder Elbow Surg* 2015;24(10):1602-1606. doi:10.1016/j.jse.2015.04.019.

    Obesity is associated with a six times increase in systemic complications following distal humerus ORIF including infection, venous thromboembolism, and other medical complications. Level of evidence: III.

53. Lawrence TM, Ahmadi S, Morrey BF, Sánchez-Sotelo J: Wound complications after distal humerus fracture fixation: Incidence, risk factors, and outcome. *J Shoulder Elbow Surg* 2014;23(2):258-264. doi:10.1016/j.jse.2013.09.014.

    Surgery for distal humerus fracture is associated with 15% incidence of wound complication. Level of evidence: IV.

54. Claessen FM, Braun Y, Peters RM, Kolovich GP, Ring D: Plate and screw fixation of bicolumnar distal humerus fractures: Factors associated with loosening or breakage of implants or nonunion. *J Hand Surg Am* 2015;40(10):2045-2051.e2. doi:10.1016/j.jhsa.2015.07.009.

Higher revision surgery rates for implant failure and/or nonunion are associated with obesity, diabetes, radiographic arthritis, and smoking. Level of evidence: IV.

55. Jayakumar P, Ring D: A pitfall in fixation of distal humeral fractures with pre-contoured locking compression plate. *Arch Bone Jt Surg* 2015;3(2):130-133.

Precontoured fixed angle distal humerus plates may result in inadequate distal screw fixation and predispose patients to early implant failure. Level of evidence: IV.

56. Wegmann K, Burkhart K, Zimmermann J, et al: The interference of distal humeral plating with the medial and lateral collateral ligaments of the elbow. *Arch Orthop Trauma Surg* 2014;134(4):501-507. doi:10.1007/s00402-014-1952-5.

All anatomic distal humerus plates, except for posterolateral and posteromedial plates, interfere to some extent with the collateral ligaments of the elbow.

57. Wiggers JK, Ring D: Osteonecrosis after open reduction and internal fixation of a bicolumnar fracture of the distal humerus: A report of four cases. *J Hand Surg Am* 2011;36(1):89-93. doi:10.1016/j.jhsa.2010.09.001.

58. Claessen FM, Stoop N, Doornberg JN, et al: Interpretation of post-operative distal humerus radiographs after internal fixation: Prediction of later loss of fixation. *J Hand Surg Am* 2016;41(10):e337-e341. doi:10.1016/j.jhsa.2016.07.094.

Surgeons cannot reliably predict hardware failure based on postoperative radiographs of type C distal humerus fractures following open reduction and internal fixation. Level of evidence: III.

59. Shearin JW, Chapman TR, Miller A, Ilyas AM: Ulnar nerve management with distal humerus fracture fixation: A meta-analysis. *Hand Clin* 2018;34(1):97-103. doi:10.1016/j.hcl.2017.09.010.

Ulnar nerve transposition was associated with a higher incidence of postoperative ulnar neuritis than in situ management alone (23% to 15%). Level of evidence: II.

60. Wiggers JK, Brouwer KM, Helmerhorst GT, Ring D: Predictors of diagnosis of ulnar neuropathy after surgically treated distal humerus fractures. *J Hand Surg Am* 2012;37(6):1168-1172. doi:10.1016/j.jhsa.2012.02.045.

61. Worden A, Ilyas AM: Ulnar neuropathy following distal humerus fracture fixation. *Orthop Clin North Am* 2012;43(4):509-514. doi:10.1016/j.ocl.2012.07.019.

62. Douglas K, Cannada LK, Archer KR, Dean D, Lee S, Obremskey W: Incidence and risk factors of heterotopic ossification following major elbow trauma. *Orthopedics* 2012;35(6):e815-e822. doi:10.3928/01477447-20120525-18.

63. Hong C, Nashi N, Hey H, Chee Y, Murphy D: Clinically relevant heterotopic ossification after elbow fracture surgery: A risk factors study. *Orthop Traumatol Surg Res* 2015;101(2):209-213. doi:10.1016/j.otsr.2014.10.021.

Higher rates of heterotopic ossification following distal humerus ORIF were notable in males, combined floating elbow injuries, and longer time to surgery. Level of evidence: IV.

Chapter 41

Elbow Arthroscopy: Indications and Surgical Considerations

Aaron M. Chamberlain, MD, MSc, MBA • Ken Yamaguchi, MD, MBA • Brendan Patterson, MD, MPH

ABSTRACT

Elbow arthroscopy is a safe and reliable technique to effectively manage numerous pathologic conditions of the elbow. Clinical studies have demonstrated successful outcomes using arthroscopic techniques to manage loose bodies, inflammatory arthropathy, elbow stiffness (including in the setting of arthritis), osteochondritis dissecans lesions, lateral epicondylitis, and some fractures. Although there are well-known risks associated with elbow arthroscopy, these risks can be minimized with appropriate indications, understanding contraindications, appropriate setup and positioning, and safe arthroscopic technique.

Keywords: elbow arthroscopy; elbow stiffness; lateral epicondylitis; OCD lesion

Introduction

In 1931,[1] the elbow was described as unsuitable for arthroscopy based on a cadaver study. In 1985,[2] the successful use of elbow arthroscopy was described in 12 patients, concluding that safe, reproducible arthroscopy of the elbow was feasible as long as the surgeon paid close attention to detail. More recent advances in surgical technique, instrumentation, and equipment have contributed to an improvement in the usefulness of elbow arthroscopy, but careful consideration of surgical indications and the surgeon's experience are imperative to safe and effective arthroscopy of the elbow.

Dr. Chamberlain or an immediate family member serves as a paid consultant to or is an employee of Arthrex, Inc., DePuy, a Johnson & Johnson Company, Wright Medical Technology, Inc., and Zimmer; and has received research or institutional support from Zimmer. Dr. Yamaguchi or an immediate family member has received royalties from Biomet, Tornier, Wright Medical Technology, Inc., and Zimmer. Neither Dr. Patterson nor any immediate family member has received anything of value from or has stock or stock options held in a commercial company or institution related directly or indirectly to the subject of this chapter.

Indications

The indications for elbow arthroscopy have broadened substantially over time. In 1985, elbow arthroscopy was described as a diagnostic and therapeutic tool that could be used to remove loose bodies and perform radial head and capitellum chondroplasties.[2] The indications for elbow arthroscopy have since broadened to include the treatment of rheumatoid arthritis, elbow osteoarthritis and associated stiffness, osteochondritis dissecans (OCD), lateral epicondylitis, some fractures, symptomatic plica, and a variety of pathologic conditions encountered by throwing athletes.

A recent literature review found only fair-quality evidence to support the use of elbow arthroscopy for the treatment of rheumatoid arthritis or lateral epicondylitis and only poor-quality evidence to support arthroscopy for plica or annular ligament excision or for the treatment of osteoarthritis, OCD lesions, posterolateral rotatory instability, loose bodies, posttraumatic arthrofibrosis, or fractures.[3] High-quality evidence is lacking to support the use of arthroscopy in any elbow condition. However, elbow arthroscopy remains an evolving technique, and more high-quality research is needed to determine its usefulness.

Loose Body Removal

The removal of loose bodies is the most common indication for elbow arthroscopy.[4] The authors of a 1985 study[2] found that the removal of loose bodies was the most successful use of elbow arthroscopy compared with other indications, such as chondroplasty. In a study of 33 elbow arthroscopies for loose body removal, pain was improved in 85% of the patients, locking in 92%, and swelling in 71%.[5] Numerous published case studies have reported the clinical outcomes of loose body removal. A 2012 analysis of 12 case studies involving arthroscopic loose body removal found that 98 of 109 patients (90%) reported a good to excellent result or substantial improvement.[3] In nine studies of patients undergoing loose body removal during procedures such as débridement of osteophytes or chondroplasty, 110 of 150 patients (73%) had a good to excellent result or significant improvement. However, no published studies have compared arthroscopic and open loose body removal.

Synovectomy

Multiple researchers have found favorable results after arthroscopic synovectomy for rheumatoid arthritis.[6-8] In comparison with open synovectomy, arthroscopic synovectomy is less invasive, facilitates an earlier return to activity, and is associated with a lower risk of postoperative stiffness. However, two reports warned of the risk of incomplete synovectomy because of the limitations and technical challenges of the procedure.[6,9] Incomplete arthroscopic synovectomy may lead to a more rapid deterioration of results than open synovectomy. All 14 patients undergoing arthroscopic synovectomy for rheumatoid arthritis or juvenile idiopathic arthritis had mild or no pain at early postoperative follow-up, but only 8 (57%) had a good to excellent functional outcome at final follow-up (mean, 42 months).[6]

Advances in technique have improved the ability to achieve a more complete arthroscopic synovectomy. In 26 rheumatoid elbows undergoing arthroscopic synovectomy, the soft-spot portal and an accessory lateral portal were used to gain access to the posterior space of the radiocapitellar and proximal radioulnar joints. In addition, the standard proximal anteromedial and proximal anterolateral portals were used to gain access to the anterior joint space, and the posterolateral and posterior central portals were used for access to the posterior joint.[10] At a mean 34-month follow-up, the mean score on the visual analog pain scale had improved from 6.5 to 3.1, and the mean flexion arc had increased from 98° to 113°. For 19 elbows (73%), the patients reported good to excellent results. Clinically apparent synovitis recurred in only four elbows: two required repeat synovectomy, and one required total elbow arthroplasty. The fourth patient declined further surgery.

The overall results of arthroscopic synovectomy of the elbow are not as positive as those of arthroscopic synovectomy for other joints affected by rheumatoid arthritis. The limited case studies provide some weak evidence favoring arthroscopic synovectomy, with special attention to the need for a thorough and complete synovectomy.

Elbow Stiffness

Elbow stiffness is common and difficult to manage. Stiffness can result from a variety of traumatic and atraumatic conditions. Both intrinsic and extrinsic factors can contribute to stiffness. The intrinsic factors include pathology causing incongruity of the joint, such as arthritis, or incongruity resulting from fracture. Extrinsic causes in the context of a preserved joint include capsular tightness or contracture, heterotopic ossification, and skin or muscle contracture. Arthroscopic management of capsular contracture can be successful. Intrinsic pathology, such as arthritis with osteophyte formation, also can be treated arthroscopically with modern techniques and instrumentation.

Arthroscopic management of the stiff elbow is a challenging technical procedure. A study of the learning curve found no substantial decrease in operating time until the surgeon had completed 15 procedures.[11] Nonetheless, arthroscopic management of elbow stiffness is becoming more widely used.[11-20] A retrospective study of 14 consecutive patients with posttraumatic elbow stiffness who underwent arthroscopic capsulotomy found that only six of 14 patients had pain at a minimum 1-year follow-up.[12] The mean maximal pain score on the visual analog scale was 4.6. Elbow extension improved from 35.4° before surgery to 9.3° after surgery, and elbow flexion improved from 117.5° to 133°. The overall arc of motion improved from 82° to 123.6° (mean improvement, 41.6°). All patients stated they would choose to have the surgery again. A 2011 report described the results of arthroscopic capsular release and débridement of osteophytes in 27 elbows with posttraumatic elbow stiffness.[13] Preoperative extension and flexion were 24° and 123°, respectively. Postoperative extension improved to 7°, flexion improved to 133°, and total range of motion improved from 99° to 125°. No neurologic complications were noted.

Only one published study has directly compared arthroscopic and open débridement. A nonrandomized controlled study of the Outerbridge-Kashiwagi procedure (open débridement of osteophytes and fenestration of the olecranon fossa) compared with arthroscopic débridement and fenestration found that both procedures were effective and led to no major complications.[21] The patients treated with arthroscopic débridement and fenestration of the olecranon fossa had a trend toward better pain relief ($P < 0.10$), and those undergoing the open Outerbridge-Kashiwagi procedure had a greater range of flexion ($P < 0.05$). A retrospective review of 20 elbows at a mean 2-year follow-up after an arthroscopic Outerbridge-Kashiwagi procedure found that the total range of motion improved from 94° to 123° and visual analog scale pain scores improved from 5.8 to 1.8.[14] The overall results were good to excellent in 16 elbows, fair in 2, and poor in 2.

A retrospective study of 43 patients with primary osteoarthritis of the elbow demonstrated improvements in both pain and functional outcome after arthroscopic débridement.[22] At an average of 38 months follow-up, there were significant improvements in both pain as well as functional outcome as measured by the Mayo Elbow Performance Index. Additionally, the authors identified preoperative arc of motion to be an independent predictor of postoperative outcome. In another retrospective review of 21 elbows (in 20 patients) after arthroscopic débridement for elbow osteoarthritis, the authors describe a mean improvement of Disabilities of the Arm, Shoulder and Hand score at a mean 5.5 years follow-up. The Mayo score outcome for this cohort was excellent in 11 elbows and poor in only one. Of the 20 patients included in the study, 19 said they would have the surgery again.[23] A 2017 systematic review of nine studies including over 200 patients has demonstrated overall improvements in postoperative range of motion and functional outcome for patients with osteoarthritis of the elbow treated with arthroscopic débridement.[24]

Most studies describing arthroscopic management of the stiff elbow include patients with both intrinsic and extrinsic causes of joint stiffness, but exclude patients with articular incongruity or notable heterotopic ossification. No level I studies have analyzed the arthroscopic management of the stiff elbow. Despite their limitations, the existing published literature suggests that for experienced surgeons, arthroscopic release can be a safe and effective method of managing elbow stiffness that has been refractory to nonsurgical measures.

Osteochondritis Dissecans

OCD lesions in the elbow usually are localized lesions affecting the articular surface of the capitellum. These lesions are not uncommon in young athletes. The primary factors in considering surgical management include the integrity of the articular surface, the stability of the lesion, and whether the physis is open or closed. Surgical intervention may be indicated if the patient has unstable lesions, loose bodies, and/or had unsuccessful nonsurgical treatment.[25] The possible arthroscopic surgical interventions include transarticular drilling, loose body removal, drilling, microfracture, and mosaicplasty.[26] Numerous case studies have been published on the clinical results of arthroscopic management of OCD lesions.[25,27-35] A retrospective study including 71 patients with symptomatic OCD lesions undergoing arthroscopic débridement demonstrated improvements and pain and function after surgery.[36] The authors reported improved outcomes for patient with open epiphyseal plates, those undergoing loose body removal, and those with shorter duration of symptoms preoperatively. Despite the overall improvements seen in this cohort, the authors found that only 62% of patients returned to their primary sport. Two recent case series have reported promising results with arthroscopic fixation of symptomatic OCD lesions in adolescent baseball players.[37,38] At short-term and midterm follow-up, high rates of return to sport were demonstrated with arthroscopic fixation of OCD lesions in this highly active patient population. A systematic review of nine studies evaluated arthroscopic surgery in athletes with OCD lesions of the elbow.[39] The surgical interventions in the reviewed studies included débridement, fixation of the fragment, microfracture, and osteochondral autografting. Patients returned to sport 81% to 100% of the time, and 89% to 100% were pain free. Unfortunately, studies evaluating the arthroscopic management of OCD lesions of the elbow have used varied clinical outcome measures, so direct study comparisons are difficult. No study has compared nonsurgical and arthroscopic management.

Lateral Epicondylitis

Two retrospective cohort studies have compared open and arthroscopic release of the extensor carpi radialis brevis (ECRB) for the treatment of recalcitrant lateral epicondylitis.[40,41] Neither study found a significant difference between patients treated with an open or an arthroscopic procedure. The percentage of patients with a good to excellent result ranged from 60% to 75%. One study found an earlier return to work in patients treated arthroscopically versus those treated with an open procedure (1.7 or 2.5 weeks, respectively).[40] In a 2010 study of 36 patients treated with arthroscopic ECRB release for persistently symptomatic lateral epicondylitis, 31% reported mild pain with strenuous activities at a mean 3.5-year follow-up.[42] Two patients (6%) received no benefit from the procedure.

Overall, the existing data on arthroscopic ECRB release reveals results similar to those of open release. Most report consistently high levels of good to excellent outcomes, but no high-quality studies have examined arthroscopic ECRB release, and there are no comparisons of arthroscopic and nonsurgical management. Nonetheless, the existing results offer support for arthroscopic management of lateral epicondylitis.[40-43]

Fractures

Arthroscopic management of fractures about the elbow is a relatively recent and evolving indication for elbow arthroscopy. Most of the published material on arthroscopic fracture management is limited to small case studies and case reports. Arthroscopic management has been described for fractures of the capitellum (excision and fixation), coronoid (excision and fixation), and radial head.[44-49] However, no studies have been published comparing open and arthroscopic management of these fractures. At this time, there is no evidence to suggest poorer outcomes with arthroscopic management or to recommend arthroscopic over open management.

The Ulnar Nerve

In patients with elbow flexion limited to 90° to 100°, the ulnar nerve must be prophylactically treated to prevent nerve compression after release and improvement in flexion.[15] The ulnar nerve is located within the cubital tunnel, the floor of which is the posterior bundle of the ulnar collateral ligament. With flexion of the elbow beyond 90°, the dimensions of the cubital tunnel decrease, thus increasing pressure on the ulnar nerve.[50] Flexion cannot be restored in an elbow that has lost a substantial amount of flexion (retains less than 90° of flexion) if contracture of the posterior bundle is not treated. In addition, injury to the ulnar nerve may occur with manipulation of the elbow into a more flexed position as the posterior bundle becomes taut.

Prior ulnar nerve transposition, especially submuscular transposition, has been considered a relative contraindication to elbow arthroscopy.[51,52] The concern is that after ulnar nerve transposition, the ulnar nerve rests anteriorly relative to its normal anatomic position at the elbow and is in close proximity to the proximal anteromedial portal commonly used to visualize the anterior compartment of the elbow. However, with experience and a standardized approach, the proximal anteromedial portal can safely be used in an elbow with a prior ulnar nerve transposition. In 59 elbows with a subluxating or previously transposed ulnar nerve, arthroscopy was done using the standard anteromedial portal.[53] If the location of the transposed nerve was unequivocal, a 1-cm incision was made away from the nerve. If the location of the nerve was equivocal, a portal incision was made approximately 1 cm away from the apparent location of the nerve. Blunt dissection was performed down to the capsule, and a blunt switching stick was used to penetrate the joint capsule. If localization of the nerve was impossible, a 2- to 4-cm incision was made, the nerve was identified, and the portal was established. There were no surgical ulnar nerve injuries related to using the proximal anteromedial portal.[53]

Contraindications

Arthroscopic management is relatively contraindicated if the elbow has severe joint incongruity, anatomy distortion, heterotopic ossification, or muscle contracture. These elbows are best managed with an open surgical approach.[15] Because of the proximity of peripheral nerves, the most important contraindication perhaps is inadequate experience in the procedure, if it is expected to be difficult. Elbow arthroscopy is technically demanding, and increased surgeon experience is an important consideration when considering the safety of this procedure. A retrospective review of 417 patients undergoing elbow arthroscopy in the hands of highly experienced elbow arthroscopists reported a relatively low rate of nerve injury following surgery. The authors reported transient neurologic injuries in only 1.7% of cases with no nerve injury leading to a permanent nerve deficit or functional motor loss.[54] Severe elbow contractures often are associated with substantial soft-tissue adhesions and contractures of extra-articular soft tissues, which are difficult to manage arthroscopically. In an elbow with severe contracture, it can be difficult to insufflate the joint; this factor substantially increases the level of difficulty and the dangers associated with arthroscopy. Prior ulnar nerve transposition, especially submuscular transposition, is a relative contraindication and requires modification of the surgical technique to avoid nerve injury.

Surgical Considerations

Setup and Positioning

Elbow arthroscopy has the potential to cause serious injury to peripheral neurovascular structures and articular cartilage. Meticulous attention to detail is necessary in setup and positioning to minimize the risk of such complications.

Some surgeons perform elbow arthroscopy under regional anesthesia. General anesthesia is preferred, however, primarily because it allows immediate and repeated postoperative neurologic evaluation. In addition, regional anesthesia does not provide the complete relaxation of the patient that facilitates easy positioning into the lateral decubitus or prone position. Regional anesthesia may not be sufficient to prevent the patient from experiencing tourniquet pain during the procedure.

Antibiotic prophylaxis is a key consideration in elbow arthroscopy. The incidence of serious deep joint infection after elbow arthroscopy is reported to be 0.8%, and the incidence of prolonged drainage and superficial infection is reported to be 7%.[55] A first-generation cephalosporin can be used before tourniquet inflation. If an allergy must be considered, clindamycin or vancomycin can be substituted. At the conclusion of the procedure, the portal sites are closed with locked horizontal mattress stitches to prevent postoperative portal drainage and/or fistula formation. After surgery, some surgeons treat patients with oral antibiotic prophylaxis for 2 weeks until the wounds are fully closed and there is very little risk of drainage. The use of intra-articular steroids after surgery should be avoided as it has been demonstrated to increase the risk of postoperative infection.[54]

Elbow arthroscopy can be performed with the patient in the lateral decubitus, prone, or supine position.[2,56,57] The lateral decubitus position offers the advantages of readily accessible airway management during the procedure, greater intraoperative freedom of motion of the

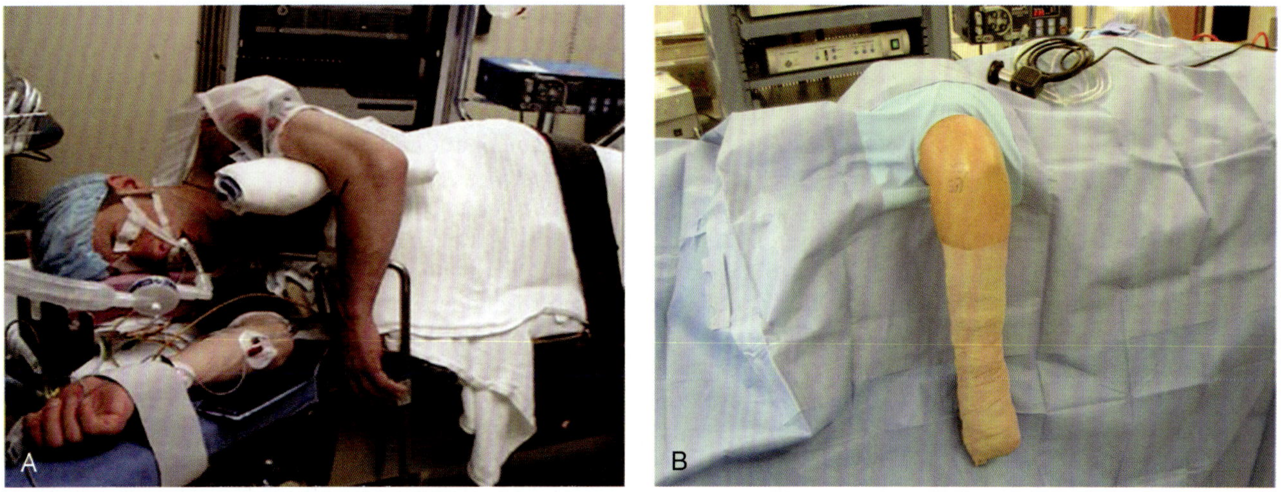

FIGURE 1 Intraoperative photographs showing patient positioning and setup for elbow arthroscopy before (**A**) and after (**B**) draping.

elbow, and better access to the posterior compartment. Ready access to the posterior compartment facilitates the use of osteotomes or large burrs to excise osteophytes from the olecranon tip when aggressive débridement of osteophytes is indicated.

After the patient is positioned in the lateral decubitus position, an axillary roll or gel pad is placed. A padded tourniquet is applied to the brachium proximally. The surgical extremity is positioned in a padded stationary arm holder with the elbow resting at approximately 90° of elbow flexion. To ensure there is enough space for instruments to fit between the elbow and the thorax, the arm should be abducted at least 90° from the body, and the elbow should be positioned slightly higher than the level of the shoulder. The patient's thorax should be positioned so that the anterior chest wall is at the edge of the bed. This positioning method allows full elbow flexion and extension during the procedure[58] (**Figure 1**).

Fluid Management

Proper fluid management is essential for the success and safety of elbow arthroscopy. Fluid distention is necessary to increase the working space in the joint. Just before a portal is created, the joint is distended with approximately 20 to 30 mL of normal saline injected with a needle through the soft spot located at the center of a triangle formed by the lateral epicondyle, the radial head, and the olecranon process (**Figure 2**). Distending the joint capsule improves safety by increasing the distance between the humerus and the joint capsule as well as nearby neurovascular structures. Capsular compliance in a very stiff elbow may be as low as 15% of that of a normal elbow; this means that joint space volume is substantially decreased, and the risk for injury is increased.[59] A lack of capsular distention (as indicated by an inability to inject more than 10 to 15 mL of normal saline) is an indication that the procedure is unusually dangerous and should be performed only by an appropriately experienced surgeon.

A pump-controlled or gravity flow fluid system can be used. A pump-controlled system is recommended, with the fluid pump pressure set to 35 mm Hg. However, it should be noted that actual pump pressures vary among products from different manufacturers. In general, the pump pressure is set approximately 30% lower for elbow arthroscopy than for shoulder arthroscopy. Low pump pressures should be used to minimize soft-tissue swelling, which can quickly occur in the elbow and can significantly impede elbow arthroscopy. Surgical time is important

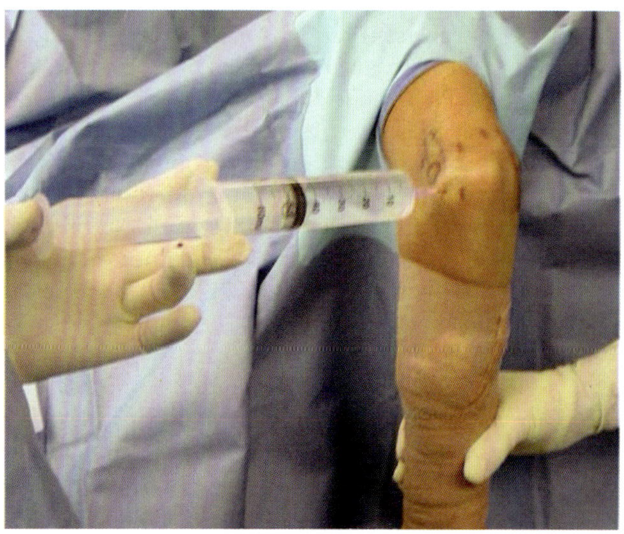

FIGURE 2 Intraoperative photograph showing insufflation of elbow with fluid before the arthroscopy is started.

in elbow arthroscopy because capsular tissues quickly become edematous and inhibit the intra-articular viewing and working space. Therefore, surgical efficiency is more important in elbow arthroscopy than in arthroscopy of other major joints.

Instrumentation and Equipment Advances

The use of modern instrumentation facilitates safe, effective, and efficient elbow arthroscopy. A standard 4.5-mm joint arthroscope is commonly used for elbow arthroscopy, although the smaller 2.7-mm arthroscope can be considered. A standard 30° lens is appropriate for most procedures. However, a 70° lens can provide more complete visualization of the coronoid fossa depth, some obscure loose bodies, and occult chondral lesions.[60] Cannulas may be used for fluid outflow as well as working, although the use of cannulas is not necessary and may contribute to insufflation and edema of the surrounding soft tissues. If cannulas are used, they should be low-flow cannulas without side fenestrations, to minimize soft-tissue insufflation. A variety of working cannulas are available, generally smaller than 5.5 mm.

Arthroscopy of the elbow is much more sensitive to deviations in portal placement than arthroscopy of other major joints, and imprecise portal placement will impede the surgeon's ability to effectively perform elbow arthroscopy. Guidewires and cannulated dilators are used to accurately and safely create portal sites. The use of these instruments to create the proximal anterolateral portal avoids repeated passage of cannulas and instruments through the surrounding soft tissues and thus reduces the chance of neurovascular injury. With the arthroscope placed in the proximal anteromedial portal for viewing the radiocapitellar joint, the guidewire is placed in the joint under direct visualization. A scalpel is used to incise skin around the wire, and cannulated dilators create the precise portal. Precise portal placement with guidewires and cannulated dilators is imperative because the radial nerve is, on average, 5 to 10 mm from the proximal anterolateral portal. After proximal anteromedial and proximal anterolateral portals have been established, a blunt trochar can be used to release intra-articular adhesions and lift the anterior capsule off the anterior humerus, thus increasing the working space.

A size 4.0 oscillating shaver is useful for débriding synovium and adhesions. Care should be taken to not direct the shaver toward the capsule. Judicious use of the suction in the shaver will prevent capsular tissue from being drawn into the shaver, possibly resulting in injury to adjacent neurovascular structures. Suction is rarely used in the anterior elbow.

Small-caliber burrs are useful for resecting large osteophytes or performing more aggressive osteocapsular arthroplasty. Specially designed osteotomes are useful for aggressive osteophyte resection in the posterior compartment and resecting osteophytes at the tip of the olecranon.

A 15° up-cutting basket resector can be safely used to develop a plane between the brachialis and the anterior capsule. With the plane developed, the basket resector is used to divide the anterior capsule, proceeding from lateral to medial. If necessary, the arthroscope can be switched to the proximal anterolateral portal, and the capsulotomy can be completed from the proximal anteromedial portal. When the deep surface of the brachialis is exposed, the anterior capsulotomy is complete. This step should be done after all other work in the anterior compartment is complete because soft-tissue edema will progress rapidly after the capsulotomy is performed, decreasing the intra-articular space for working and viewing.

Specially designed elbow arthroscopy retractors can be useful for safely retracting soft tissues, such as the anterior capsule, or protecting neurovascular structures, such as the ulnar nerve, while working posteriorly in the medial gutter.

SUMMARY

Elbow arthroscopy, once considered impossible, has evolved to become an increasingly valuable technique for treating a wide variety of elbow pathologies. Technical advances and modifications have allowed elbow arthroscopy to emerge as safe and reliable although technically demanding. A focus on surgeon education and technical advancement will be beneficial in the continuing evolution of elbow arthroscopy as a safe and beneficial technique.

KEY STUDY POINTS

- Arthroscopic débridement and release to manage stiffness in the setting of elbow osteoarthritis has been shown to provide lasting clinical benefit for range of motion and pain.
- Patient setup and positioning is critical to successful elbow arthroscopy.
- When performing a synovectomy for inflammatory arthropathy, special attention must be paid to débriding the synovium in the posterolateral gutter and posterolateral radiocapitellar joint space.

Annotated References

1. Burman MS: Arthroscopy or the direct visualization of joints: An experimental cadaver study. *J Bone Joint Surg* 1931;13:669-695.

2. Andrews JR, Carson WG: Arthroscopy of the elbow. *Arthroscopy* 1985;1(2):97-107.

3. Yeoh KM, King GJ, Faber KJ, Glazebrook MA, Athwal GS: Evidence-based indications for elbow arthroscopy. *Arthroscopy* 2012;28(2):272-282.

4. Baker CL, Brooks AA: Arthroscopy of the elbow. *Clin Sports Med* 1996;15(2):261-281.

5. Ogilvie-Harris DJ, Schemitsch E: Arthroscopy of the elbow for removal of loose bodies. *Arthroscopy* 1993;9(1):5-8.

6. Lee BP, Morrey BF: Arthroscopic synovectomy of the elbow for rheumatoid arthritis: A prospective study. *J Bone Joint Surg Br* 1997;79(5):770-772.

7. Nemoto K, Arino H, Yoshihara Y, Fujikawa K: Arthroscopic synovectomy for the rheumatoid elbow: A short-term outcome. *J Shoulder Elbow Surg* 2004;13(6):652-655.

8. Tanaka N, Sakahashi H, Hirose K, Ishima T, Ishii S: Arthroscopic and open synovectomy of the elbow in rheumatoid arthritis. *J Bone Joint Surg Am* 2006;88(3):521-525.

9. Horiuchi K, Momohara S, Tomatsu T, Inoue K, Toyama Y: Arthroscopic synovectomy of the elbow in rheumatoid arthritis. *J Bone Joint Surg Am* 2002;84-A(3):342-347.

10. Kang HJ, Park MJ, Ahn JH, Lee SH: Arthroscopic synovectomy for the rheumatoid elbow. *Arthroscopy* 2010;26(9):1195-1202.

11. Kim S-J, Moon H-K, Chun Y-M, Chang J-H: Arthroscopic treatment for limitation of motion of the elbow: The learning curve. *Knee Surg Sports Traumatol Arthrosc* 2011;19(6):1013-1018.

12. Ball CM, Meunier M, Galatz LM, Calfee R, Yamaguchi K: Arthroscopic treatment of posttraumatic elbow contracture. *J Shoulder Elbow Surg* 2002;11(6):624-629.

13. Cefo I, Eygendaal D: Arthroscopic arthrolysis for posttraumatic elbow stiffness. *J Shoulder Elbow Surg* 2011;20(3):434-439.

14. DeGreef I, Samorjai N, De Smet L: The Outerbridge-Kashiwaghi procedure in elbow arthroscopy. *Acta Orthop Belg* 2010;76(4):468-471.

15. Keener JD, Galatz LM: Arthroscopic management of the stiff elbow. *J Am Acad Orthop Surg* 2011;19(5):265-274.

16. Singh H, Nam KY, Moon YL: Arthroscopic management of stiff elbow. *Orthopedics* 2011;34(6):167.

17. Van Zeeland NL, Yamaguchi K: Arthroscopic capsular release of the elbow. *J Shoulder Elbow Surg* 2010;19(2 suppl):13-19.

18. Lapner PC, Leith JM, Regan WD: Arthroscopic debridement of the elbow for arthrofibrosis resulting from nondisplaced fracture of the radial head. *Arthroscopy* 2005;21(12):1492.

19. Nguyen D, Proper SI, MacDermid JC, King GJ, Faber KJ: Functional outcomes of arthroscopic capsular release of the elbow. *Arthroscopy* 2006;22(8):842-849.

20. Savoie FH III, Nunley PD, Field LD: Arthroscopic management of the arthritic elbow: Indications, technique, and results. *J Shoulder Elbow Surg* 1999;8(3):214-219.

21. Cohen AP, Redden JF, Stanley D: Treatment of osteoarthritis of the elbow: A comparison of open and arthroscopic debridement. *Arthroscopy* 2000;16(7):701-706.

22. Lim TK, Koh KH, Lee HI, Shim JW, Park MJ: Arthroscopic debridement for primary osteoarthritis of the elbow: Analysis of preoperative factors affecting outcome. *J Shoulder Elbow Surg* 2014;23:1381-1387.

    This is a retrospective study evaluating pain, flexion-extension motion, and Mayo Elbow Performance Index after elbow arthroscopic débridement in the setting of elbow osteoarthritis. Level of evidence: IV.

23. MacLean S, Oni T, Crawford L, Deshmukh SC: Medium-term results of arthroscopic debridement and capsulectomy for the treatment of elbow osteoarthritis. *J Shoulder Elbow Surg* 2013;22:653-657.

    This is a retrospective review of medium-term outcomes of 21 osteoarthritic elbows treated with arthroscopic débridement. Level of evidence: IV.

24. Sochacki KR, Jack RA, Hirase T, et al: Arthroscopic debridement for primary degenerative osteoarthritis of the elbow leads to significant improvement in range of motion and clinical outcomes: A systematic review. *Arthroscopy* 2017;33(12):2255-2262.

    This is a systematic review of articles describing clinical outcomes after elbow arthroscopic débridement for osteoarthritis. Level of evidence: IV.

25. Yadao MA, Field LD, Savoie FH III: Osteochondritis dissecans of the elbow. *Instr Course Lect* 2004;53:599-606.

26. Ahmad CS, Vitale MA, ElAttrache NS: Elbow arthroscopy: Capitellar osteochondritis dissecans and radiocapitellar plica. *Instr Course Lect* 2011;60:181-190.

27. Brownlow HC, O'Connor-Read LM, Perko M: Arthroscopic treatment of osteochondritis dissecans of the capitellum. *Knee Surg Sports Traumatol Arthrosc* 2006;14(2):198-202.

28. Jones KJ, Wiesel BB, Sankar WN, Ganley TJ: Arthroscopic management of osteochondritis dissecans of the capitellum: Mid-term results in adolescent athletes. *J Pediatr Orthop* 2010;30(1):8-13.

29. Micheli LJ, Luke AC, Mintzer CM, Waters PM: Elbow arthroscopy in the pediatric and adolescent population. *Arthroscopy* 2001;17(7):694-699.

30. Mihara K, Suzuki K, Makiuchi D, Nishinaka N, Yamaguchi K, Tsutsui H: Surgical treatment for osteochondritis dissecans of the humeral capitellum. *J Shoulder Elbow Surg* 2010;19(1):31-37.

31. Miyake J, Masatomi T: Arthroscopic debridement of the humeral capitellum for osteochondritis dissecans: Radiographic and clinical outcomes. *J Hand Surg Am* 2011;36(8):1333-1338.

32. Nobuta S, Ogawa K, Sato K, Nakagawa T, Hatori M, Itoi E: Clinical outcome of fragment fixation for osteochondritis dissecans of the elbow. *Ups J Med Sci* 2008;113(2):201-208.

33. Rahusen FT, Brinkman J-M, Eygendaal D: Results of arthroscopic debridement for osteochondritis dissecans of the elbow. *Br J Sports Med* 2006;40(12):966-969.

34. Takeda H, Watarai K, Matsushita T, Saito T, Terashima Y: A surgical treatment for unstable osteochondritis dissecans lesions of the humeral capitellum in adolescent baseball players. *Am J Sports Med* 2002;30(5):713-717.

35. Tis JE, Edmonds EW, Bastrom T, Chambers HG: Short-term results of arthroscopic treatment of osteochondritis dissecans in skeletally immature patients. *J Pediatr Orthop* 2012;32(3):226-231.

36. Bexkens R, van den Ende KIM, Ogink PT, van Bergen CJA, van den Bekerom MPJ, Eygendaal D: Clinical outcome after arthroscopic debridement and microfracture for osteochondritis dissecans of the capitellum. *Am J Sports Med* 2017;45(10):2312-2318.

    This is a case series describing clinical outcomes after arthroscopic débridement and microfractures for capitellar osteochondritis dissecans lesions. Level of evidence: IV.

37. Uchida S, Utsunomiya H, Taketa T, et al: Arthroscopic fragment fixation using hydroxyapatite/poly-L-lactate acid thread pins for treating elbow osteochondritis dissecans. *Am J Sports Med* 2015;43(5):1057-1065.

    This is a case series describing outcomes of 18 adolescent baseball players with OCD lesions managed with hydroxyapatite/poly-L-lactate acid thread pins to fix the OCD lesion. Level of evidence: IV.

38. Takeba J, Takahashi T, Watanabe S, et al: Short-term clinical results of arthroscopic osteochondral fixation for elbow osteochondritis dissecans in teenaged baseball players. *J Shoulder Elbow Surg* 2015;24:1749-1756.

    This is a case series of 13 adolescent baseball players who underwent arthroscopic osteochondral fixation in the setting of OCD. Level of evidence: IV.

39. de Graaff F, Krijnen MR, Poolman RW, Willems WJ: Arthroscopic surgery in athletes with osteochondritis dissecans of the elbow. *Arthroscopy* 2011;27(7):986-993.

40. Peart RE, Strickler SS, Schweitzer KM Jr: Lateral epicondylitis: A comparative study of open and arthroscopic lateral release. *Am J Orthop (Belle Mead NJ)* 2004;33(11):565-567.

41. Rubenthaler F, Wiese M, Senge A, Keller L, Wittenberg RH: Long-term follow-up of open and endoscopic Hohmann procedures for lateral epicondylitis. *Arthroscopy* 2005;21(6):684-690.

42. Lattermann C, Romeo AA, Anbari A, et al: Arthroscopic debridement of the extensor carpi radialis brevis for recalcitrant lateral epicondylitis. *J Shoulder Elbow Surg* 2010;19(5):651-656.

43. Savoie FH III, VanSice W, O'Brien MJ: Arthroscopic tennis elbow release. *J Shoulder Elbow Surg* 2010;19(2 suppl):31-36.

44. Feldman MD: Arthroscopic excision of type II capitellar fractures. *Arthroscopy* 1997;13(6):743-748.

45. Hardy P, Menguy F, Guillot S: Arthroscopic treatment of capitellum fracture of the humerus. *Arthroscopy* 2002;18(4):422-426.

46. Adams JE, Merten SM, Steinmann SP: Arthroscopic-assisted treatment of coronoid fractures. *Arthroscopy* 2007;23(10):1060-1065.

47. Hausman MR, Klug RA, Qureshi S, Goldstein R, Parsons BO: Arthroscopically assisted coronoid fracture fixation: A preliminary report. *Clin Orthop Relat Res* 2008;466(12):3147-3152.

48. Michels F, Pouliart N, Handelberg F: Arthroscopic management of Mason type 2 radial head fractures. *Knee Surg Sports Traumatol Arthrosc* 2007;15(10):1244-1250.

49. Rolla PR, Surace MF, Bini A, Pilato G: Arthroscopic treatment of fractures of the radial head. *Arthroscopy* 2006;22(2):e1-e6.

50. Gelberman RH, Yamaguchi K, Hollstien SB, et al: Changes in interstitial pressure and cross-sectional area of the cubital tunnel and of the ulnar nerve with flexion of the elbow: An experimental study in human cadavera. *J Bone Joint Surg Am* 1998;80(4):492-501.

51. Dodson CC, Nho SJ, Williams RJ III, Altchek DW: Elbow arthroscopy. *J Am Acad Orthop Surg* 2008;16(10):574-585.

52. Gramstad GD, Galatz LM: Management of elbow osteoarthritis. *J Bone Joint Surg Am* 2006;88(2):421-430.

53. Sahajpal DT, Blonna D, O'Driscoll SW: Anteromedial elbow arthroscopy portals in patients with prior ulnar nerve transposition or subluxation. *Arthroscopy* 2010;26(8):1045-1052.

54. Nelson GN, Wu T, Galatz LM, Yamaguchi K, Keener JD: Elbow arthroscopy: Early complications and associated risk factors. *J Shoulder Elbow Surg* 2014;23:273-278.

    Retrospective study of 417 elbow arthroscopy procedures with reporting of complications and associated risk factors. Level of evidence: IV.

55. Kelly EW, Morrey BF, O'Driscoll SW: Complications of elbow arthroscopy. *J Bone Joint Surg Am* 2001; 83-A(1):25-34.

56. O'Driscoll SW, Morrey BF: Arthroscopy of the elbow: Diagnostic and therapeutic benefits and hazards. *J Bone Joint Surg Am* 1992;74(1):84-94.

57. Poehling GG, Whipple TL, Sisco L, Goldman B: Elbow arthroscopy: A new technique. *Arthroscopy* 1989;5(3):222-224.

58. Yamaguchi K, Tashjian RZ: *Advanced Reconstruction: Elbow*. Rosemont, IL, American Academy of Orthopaedic Surgeons, 2007, pp 3-11.

59. Gallay SH, Richards RR, O'Driscoll SW: Intraarticular capacity and compliance of stiff and normal elbows. *Arthroscopy* 1993;9(1):9-13.

60. Bedi A, Dines J, Dines DM, et al: Use of the 70° arthroscope for improved visualization with common arthroscopic procedures. *Arthroscopy* 2010;26(12):1684-1696.

Chapter 42

Advanced Elbow Arthroscopy

James A. Hurt III, MD, FAAOS • Felix H. Savoie III, MD, FAAOS, FAOA

ABSTRACT

A detailed summary of elbow arthroscopy including the history, preoperative evaluation, workup, indications, conditions, new techniques, and complications has been provided. Advances in elbow techniques over the past 10 years have been reviewed. Specific procedures covered include the arthroscopic management of lateral epicondylitis, elbow arthrofibrosis, osteoarthritis, osteochondritis dissecans, fractures, and elbow instability.

Keywords: arthroscopy; contracture; elbow; nerve; portal; tennis

Introduction

Elbow arthroscopy was originally used to visualize the intra-articular anatomy and pathology of the elbow joint before open surgery or to aid in the removal of loose bodies within the joint. The accepted indications for elbow arthroscopy have multiplied over the years to include management of arthritis, elbow stiffness, arthrofibrosis, lateral epicondylitis, posterolateral rotatory instability (PLRI), posteromedial rotatory instability, osteochondritis dissecans (OCD), posterior impingement, intra-articular fractures, triceps tears, synovectomy for inflammatory arthritis, olecranon bursitis, distal biceps ruptures, and septic arthritis. Although the literature supports the use of elbow arthroscopy for these conditions, the quality of the evidence generally is poor.[1] Arthroscopy of the elbow is technically demanding and requires an intimate knowledge of the surrounding anatomy and especially the neurovascular structures.

Dr. Hurt or an immediate family member serves as a paid consultant to or is an employee of Smith & Nephew and serves as a board member, owner, officer, or committee member of the Arthroscopy Association of North America. Dr. Savoie or an immediate family member has received royalties from Exactech, Inc.; is a member of a speakers' bureau or has made paid presentations on behalf of Exactech, Inc. and Smith & Nephew; serves as an unpaid consultant to Biomet, CONMED Linvatec, Exactech, Inc., Mitek, Rotation Medical, and Smith & Nephew; has received research or institutional support from Mitek; and serves as a board member, owner, officer, or committee member of the American Shoulder and Elbow Surgeons and the Arthroscopy Association of North America.

Patient History and Examination

Every patient with elbow pain or dysfunction should have a complete history and physical examination. The patient's age, hand dominance, occupation, sports involvement, level of activity, and history of trauma should be obtained. The timing of the onset of the symptoms, precipitating activity, and the nature of the symptoms (eg, pain, instability, stiffness, and catching and locking) should be sought. The location of pain (ie, anterior, posterior, medial, or lateral) and the history often lead the examiner to the diagnosis even before the physical examination or imaging.

A thorough physical examination should include the cervical spine and the neck, the ipsilateral shoulder, the contralateral elbow, and the involved elbow. A neurovascular examination of the extremity should include pulses, reflexes, and motor and sensory testing. Range of motion (ie, flexion, extension, pronation, and supination) should be measured and documented. Stability testing of the elbow should be performed through the arc of flexion and extension and with varus and valgus load. Other provocative tests should be carried out as dictated by the patient's history and examination.

Plain radiographs including AP, lateral, and oblique views are helpful for determining overall alignment and identifying fractures, OCD lesions, and degenerative joint disease. CT helps to define fracture patterns and identify loose bodies. MRI allows a much better assessment of the soft tissues than CT, including cartilage and ligamentous structures.

Elbow arthroscopy requires skill, experience, and detailed knowledge of the elbow and its anatomy. One of the most common and most feared complications of elbow arthroscopy is injury to a peripheral nerve. Therefore, the surgeon must be familiar with elbow anatomy and confident of the correct placement of portals. The prone patient position is recommended for most arthroscopic surgery of the elbow. Although the lateral decubitus position is equally effective, it requires a special device to stabilize the arm.

Arthroscopically Managed Conditions

Lateral Humeral Epicondylitis

Lateral humeral epicondylitis originally was described in 1873. Its association with lawn tennis led to the commonly used name tennis elbow.[2] After 140 years, there is still a lack of consensus as to the best surgical and nonsurgical management of this condition. Most patients with lateral epicondylitis respond well to a variety of nonsurgical treatments, but 4% to 11% of patients require surgical intervention for continuing symptoms[3] (**Figure 1**).

The most commonly accepted theory of lateral epicondylitis is that repetitive use of the elbow causes microtears in the extensor carpi radialis brevis (ECRB) tendon. The absence of histologic signs of inflammation led to the use of the terms angiofibroblastic hyperplasia and angiofibroblastic tendinosis to describe the condition.[4,5] Another theory is that pain is generated from impingement of the synovial fold onto the radiocapitellar joint.[6] In a cadaver study, the synovial fold was found to be a distinct entity from the annular ligament, but it has an extremely close relationship with the common extensor enthesis.[7] It is also believed that lateral epicondylitis is caused by a combination of intra-articular and extra-articular lesions.

The exact origin of the ECRB tendon was characterized in both cadaver studies and surgical specimens as being just anterior to the distal-most tip of the lateral supracondylar ridge.[7,8] The tendon was found to be diamond shaped with a mean length of 13 mm (±2 mm) and a mean width of 3 mm (±1 mm) proximally, 7 mm (±2 mm) in the midportion, and 4 mm (±1 mm) distally.[7,8]

A wide assortment of percutaneous, endoscopic, and open procedures can be used to surgically manage lateral epicondylitis. Surgical intervention is indicated after unsuccessful nonsurgical management options including activity modification, physical therapy, NSAIDs, corticosteroid and platelet-rich plasma injections, and counterforce bracing treatment.

For arthroscopic management of lateral epicondylitis, it is helpful to create a specific tennis elbow portal 2 mm anterior to the tip of the lateral epicondyle. This portal will traverse the Nirschl lesion and allow resection from the top down rather than from the middle up, thus limiting resection to the pathologic tissue and decreasing the risk of radial nerve injury. When the portals are established, a portion of the lateral capsule is resected using a shaver to reveal the underlying common extensor origin. The ECRB origin is released completely using a shaver or an electrocautery. The lateral ligamentous structures are posterior to a line bisecting the radial head, and the release should not be carried past this line. A 70° arthroscope can be used to obtain the best view of the ECRB insertion and lateral ligamentous structures around the corner of the capitellum.[9] An extra-articular lateral release can be performed using a middle anterolateral portal that requires creating only a small hole in the joint capsule. The arthroscope is backed out of the capsule to directly visualize the diseased tissue and its débridement with a shaver entering from a proximal anterolateral portal.[10]

After the entire lesion is resected, the damaged tendon can be directly repaired to the bone or septum. This step can be done by placing a small anchor into the anterior

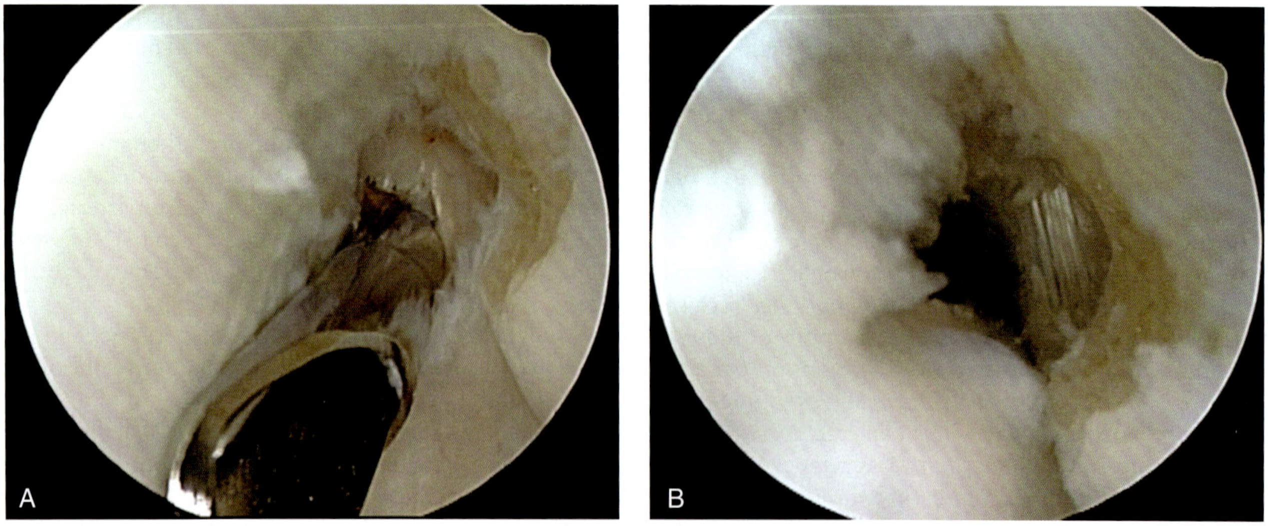

FIGURE 1 Arthroscopic images from the proximal anteromedial portal, showing the management of lateral humeral epicondylitis. **A**, The gray, amorphous angiofibrotic dysplasia of the extensor carpi radialis brevis tendon can be seen. **B**, The dysplasia has been excised, leaving the normal tendon intact.

lateral epicondyle and retrieving the sutures through the ECRB using a standard anterior lateral portal. The ECRB also can be plicated to the overlying extensor carpi radialis longus using a needle retriever technique.[11] It is unclear if this is necessary. Decortication of the underlying bone has been believed to increase healing potential. However, a previous study found that patients who underwent ECRB release and decortication had more pain postoperatively and required more time before return to work than patients who had a release alone.[3]

A case study of 36 patients who underwent arthroscopic treatment for recalcitrant lateral epicondylitis found improvement in pain, and the procedure appeared to be safe and effective.[3] A long-term follow-up study of 30 patients who underwent arthroscopic treatment for lateral epicondylitis found that no patients required further surgery, and 87% were satisfied with the outcome.[12] A review of 31 patients with 33 elbows showed that 93.5% were satisfied after arthroscopic débridement and resection of the radiocapitellar capsular complex.[6]

Although most studies have had good results, not all patients have a favorable outcome. The results of ECRB débridement at times can be unpredictable, and some patients continue to have lateral elbow symptoms including pain.[8] Patients with a workers' compensation claim and those with a high-demand, repetitive-stress job were found to have inferior results.

Arthrofibrosis

The elbow is extremely prone to stiffness, especially after trauma, and loss of motion is the most common complication after injury to the elbow joint. The elbow with its three articulations is an extremely congruous joint. Even a small alteration in this congruity often will be magnified and lead to stiffness. The elbow capsule can thicken and lose compliance after only a minor insult. The olecranon or coronoid fossae, if filled with loose bodies or scar tissue, limits terminal extension or flexion, respectively. Muscle contracture also can limit motion about the elbow. Pain often exacerbates posttraumatic elbow stiffness because the voluntary and involuntary guarding resulting from pain leads to worsening capsular and muscular contractures.[13] Loss of terminal extension is much more common than loss of flexion. The normal elbow range of motion is 0° to 145° of flexion and 90° of both pronation and supination. The functional range of motion is 30° to 130° of flexion and 50° of both pronation and supination.[14] A candidate for surgery should have a loss of terminal extension of 25° to 30° and/or less than 110° to 115° of flexion. Before surgical release, the patients should undergo several months of preoperative physical therapy and have a documented plateau in motion gains. Preoperative compliance is important to document, because compliance with postoperative therapy is paramount for retaining the motion gains achieved during surgery. However, overly aggressive physical therapy and manipulation can worsen the patient's symptoms and can even worsen the contracture.[13]

The arthroscopic release of a posttraumatic stiff elbow is complicated, and advanced arthroscopic skills are required to obtain motion while preserving the neurovascular structures. Heterotopic ossification is a relative contraindication to arthroscopic release. The advantages of arthroscopic treatment over open treatment include better visualization of intra-articular structures, less trauma to the surrounding tissues, and the potential for earlier postoperative motion and therapy. Knowledge of the location of the ulnar nerve is mandatory for arthroscopy about the elbow. If there is significant loss of flexion or any doubt as to the exact location of the ulnar nerve, a separate open procedure should be performed to locate and protect the ulnar nerve.[15]

The key principles of arthroscopic release of a posttraumatic stiff elbow are listed in **Table 1**. It is the surgeon's preference as to whether to begin the procedure in the anterior or posterior compartment. Most surgeons prefer to begin in the anterior compartment, where visualization and close proximity to neurovascular structures may limit the surgeon later, as swelling increases. In the anterior compartment, a synovectomy and débridement are performed, and all loose bodies are removed. The capsule is removed from the anterior humerus. Bony osteophytes should be removed from the coronoid, the coronoid fossa, radial fossa, and the radial head. A complete anterior capsulectomy is performed using a biter and/or shaver without suction. Care must be taken to avoid injury to the posterior interosseous nerve at the lateral border of the brachialis.[16] Posteriorly, a synovectomy is performed, and all loose bodies are removed. Proximally, the capsule can be elevated with a retractor and any

Table 1

The Key Principles of Arthroscopic Release of a Posttraumatic Stiff Elbow

Use a standard and reproducible technique.
Perform a prophylactic ulnar nerve decompression.
Control the inflow of fluid to avoid excessive swelling.
Remove bone to re-create conforming joint surfaces.
Perform a capsulectomy.
Always use retractors.
Stay under the learning curve.

adhesions between the triceps and the humerus can be released. Osteophytes are removed as needed from the tip of the olecranon and the olecranon fossa. The capsule of the medial and lateral gutters is carefully released. Release of the medial gutter and posterior band of the medial ulnar collateral ligament (MUCL) is important for improving flexion.

Arthroscopic release in elbows with high-grade contractures can be safely performed with careful technique and preoperative range of motion can be improved;[17] However, high-grade contractures have been a relative contraindication to arthroscopic release because of the small amount of working space available for instrumentation and the decreased compliance of the capsule. In contractures with less than 50° of motion, an extracapsular capsulectomy has been described in which a periosteal elevator is introduced through the proximal medial portal and a working space is created between the anterior humeral cortex and the anterior brachialis musculature.[13] The anterior capsule can then be dissected and excised under direct visualization.

Several level IV case studies report good functional results with arthroscopic management of elbow arthrofibrosis.[15,16,18] A high percentage of patients were able to return to sports or work and were able to maintain surgical gains over a 24-month period. Patients with a traumatic etiology and those with a shorter duration of symptoms before surgical intervention had better results. In a comparison of traumatic and degenerative elbow contractures, arthroscopic elbow arthrolysis showed a similar restoration of range of motion.[19]

The complication rates of open and arthroscopic procedures about the elbow are similar. In comparison with open procedures, however, arthroscopic procedures appear to be associated with a greater risk of permanent injury. Several incidences of neurovascular injury during arthroscopy have been documented.[20] This risk necessitates the use of a careful stepwise routine during all arthroscopic elbow procedures, especially if the working space has been altered or is decreased.[20] Prevention of nerve injury by a stepwise strategy has been described by a therapeutic level III study in 502 patients undergoing elbow contracture release. A standardized sequence was followed: (1) Enter the joint and establish a view; (2) Create a space in which to work; (3) Remove bone as necessary; and (4) Resect the capsule.[21]

Degenerative Joint Disease

Elbow osteoarthritis is an uncommon condition that typically presents as weakness, pain at the extremes of motion, and loss of motion. Like arthritis in other joints, elbow arthritis typically involves bony osteophytes and loose bodies that can decrease the range of motion of the joint, with or without mechanical symptoms such as locking and catching. Unlike arthritis in other joints, elbow arthritis typically does not involve joint space narrowing or loss of cartilage centrally.[22]

Degenerative joint disease of the elbow often is caused by rheumatoid arthritis or posttraumatic degenerative changes. Primary osteoarthritis of the elbow is almost exclusively seen in men who are athletes or do manual labor or heavy lifting. Patients with rheumatoid arthritis most often have pain throughout the range of motion, not limited to the extremes of motion. Plain radiographs are helpful in identifying arthritis in the elbow. Joint space narrowing, bony spurs, and loose bodies often can be identified. When surgical intervention is being considered, CT is helpful in planning débridement, removal of loose bodies, and ulnohumeral or osteocapsular arthroplasty. This better shows areas of bone overgrowth and impingement.

Nonsurgical treatment always should be attempted before surgical intervention. The use of NSAIDs, disease-modifying antirheumatic drugs (in patients with rheumatoid arthritis), corticosteroid injections, bracing treatment, physical therapy, and activity modification are alternatives to surgery. Surgical intervention should be considered if nonsurgical treatments do not provide pain relief or a functional range of motion about the elbow and if the patient is limited in the ability to work or perform activities of daily living. Arthroscopic débridement of osteophytes and loose body removal, along with selective capsular release, has had good short-term to midterm results.[13]

The path of the ulnar nerve should be traced before the portals are established. There are typically several loose bodies in the anterior compartment, which can be removed if they are small. A level IV study in 43 patients showed similar postoperative range of motion in patients regardless of whether the posterior band of the medial collateral ligament was released.[23] If the loose bodies are large, their removal can be deferred until a later time to preserve joint distention. A synovectomy is performed, and osteophytes are most easily removed from the coronoid with the shaver from the medial portal. The radial head can be excised, at the surgeon's discretion, if the patient has radiocapitellar symptoms. However, most patients with osteoarthritis have cartilage loss on the end bearing surface of the radial head. In these individuals, radial head resection is rarely necessary. A fenestration hole connecting the coronoid and olecranon fossa can then be drilled.[24]

Posteriorly, osteophytes are removed from the olecranon and the olecranon fossa. The medial and lateral gutters are débrided and cleared of loose bodies. The Outerbridge-Kashiwagi procedure is then completed (if favored by the surgeon) by enlarging the fenestration hole to 1 to 2 cm, and the tip of the olecranon is excised broadly to achieve full extension.[24] The ulnar nerve should be decompressed or transposed in patients with a large preoperative motion loss. Motion is started immediately after surgery. The patient can be treated to prevent heterotopic ossification with 700 cGY of radiation during the first 48 hours after surgery. This is typically not necessary in primary cases.

The original Outerbridge-Kashiwagi procedure was open, but the arthroscopic procedure has had good results when used for elbow arthritis.[25,26] In a retrospective review, 19 patients with mild to moderate elbow arthritis underwent an arthroscopic Outerbridge-Kashiwagi procedure. The patients had improved range of motion and pain scores at a mean 2-year follow-up. A retrospective chart review of 41 patients who underwent arthroscopic osteophyte resection and capsulectomy found decreased pain and increased range of motion at a mean 176-week follow-up.[27] A review found that 12 of 13 patients with concomitant elbow arthritis and ulnar nerve compression at the elbow had a good or excellent result at a mean 47-month follow-up after arthroscopic ulnar nerve release, osteophyte resection, and capsulectomy.[28]

Osteochondritis Dissecans

Repetitive trauma to the lateral compartment of the immature elbow often is observed in children who participate in baseball and gymnastics, and OCD often is seen in adolescents (age 11 to 15 years) who participate in overhead sports. The disease process most likely is multifactorial; it results from repetitive microtrauma and vascular susceptibility, but the exact etiology is unknown. The blood supply to the capitellum is provided by two end arteries with minimal collateral blood flow, and the structure is predisposed to an avascular state in an elbow repeatedly subjected to microtrauma. Patients often have vague lateral elbow pain and stiffness. A 15° to 20° flexion contracture is not uncommon. Both OCD lesions and tears of the MUCL can be caused by valgus overload. The integrity of the MUCL should be examined. Imaging of the elbow should include AP radiographs at full extension and at 45° of flexion, as well as oblique and standard lateral views. If an OCD lesion is suspected on plain radiographs, MRI should be obtained to further delineate the lesion. CT scans with three-dimensional reformatting is also very helpful in preoperative planning.

Management of OCD lesions depends on their size and location as well as the stability of the overlying cartilage. Lesions involving the lateral aspect of the capitellum (unconstrained or shoulder lesions) require more extensive surgery and have a worse prognosis than lesions involving only the central capitellum. A stage I OCD lesion is stable; the osteochondral lesion is intact and has not displaced. A stage I lesion often heals in 3 to 6 months and should be managed nonsurgically. Throwing and other activities that are stressful for the affected arm should be discontinued. Repeating the MRI at 2 to 3 months is helpful in monitoring healing. A stage II lesion is unstable but connected, with fractured cartilage. A stage II lesion should be managed surgically, with the size of the lesion dictating the surgical management. A relatively small lesion can be débrided, with good immediate pain relief.

There is debate over management of a stage II or larger lesion with débridement, repair, or osteochondral autograft. The location of the lesion on the capitellum can affect the outcome; a lesion with lateral column involvement has a relatively poor prognosis. Fragments can be fixed using headless screws, and the use of absorbable pins has been described.[29] A stage III lesion is unstable and fully displaced, and it must be managed surgically. Débridement with drilling or microfracture or osteochondral autograft replacement is chosen, as it is for a stage II lesion.[30] Microfracture is indicated for a small stage I lesion that did not respond to nonsurgical management or a stage II lesion without lateral column involvement. Osteochondral autograft should be used for a larger lesion, a lesion that involves more than 6 to 7 mm of the lateral column, or a lesion engaged by the radial head. Short-term outcomes after surgical management of OCD lesions tend to be good, but long-term outcomes for stage II and III lesions are much less favorable.[31]

The angle of approach from the portal is of utmost importance for thoroughly débriding, drilling, or placing osteochondral plugs. Dual direct lateral portals do not damage the lateral ligamentous complex and allow access to 78% of the capitellum with instrumentation.[32] A distal ulnar portal also allows good exposure to the capitellum and easy access for drilling, burring, or débridement during arthroscopy.[33] In a cadaver study, there was no significant difference between the percentage of capitellum seen among the dual lateral, distal ulna, and posterolateral approaches.[34] A novel approach to drilling OCD lesions uses a 1.8-mm Kirschner wire drilled into the radial head from 3 cm distal. By pronating, supinating, flexing, and extending the elbow, the lesion can be drilled without the creation of a large arthrotomy.[35] Usually the lesion is best visualized through a 70° arthroscope in the proximal posterior lateral portal, using mid and distal soft-spot portals for instrumentation and retractors.

A level III review of the literature concluded that surgery is indicated when nonsurgical treatment is unsuccessful, but the published studies have a low methodologic quality.[30] The short-term results of débridement, fixation, microfracture, and autografting are promising, but the long-term results are unclear. Although evidence is lacking, autografting appears to have better results than the other surgical treatments in the long term.

A retrospective review of results in 106 patients who underwent arthroscopic débridement of OCD lesions after closure of the capitellar physis found that patients with a large lesion and an open radial physis had both poor radiographic and clinical outcomes.[30,32,33,35,36] Other patients had excellent short-term outcomes. A retrospective review of 13 patients at a minimum 1-year follow-up after débridement of an OCD lesion found subjective symptom relief and a functional elbow, although many patients reported they had ended their earlier sports activity.[36] Twenty-five consecutive patients were treated with arthroscopic débridement and drilling of an OCD lesion; 12 patients also required a mini arthrotomy for bone grafting.[31] These patients had a statistically significant postoperative increase in flexion (10°) and extension (17°), and 18 of the 21 patients available for follow-up had returned to their sport at the preinjury level.

Case studies have described the use of a micronized allogeneic cartilage scaffold in conjunction with marrow stimulation techniques in an effort to promote hyaline cartilage formation and fixation of OCD fragments using hydroxyapatite/poly-L-lactate acid thread pins.[37,38]

Triceps Injury

The triceps functions to straighten the elbow. The triceps tendon inserts on the proximal and posterior aspects of the olecranon on the proximal ulna. The incidence of injury to the triceps tendon insertion has increased as aging individuals remain active, but it is more common in individuals who lift weights. The patient often experiences an acute onset of pain at the insertion during press-type activities such as pushing up from a seated position or performing a bench-press weight lift. Partial tears tend to have a more insidious onset of pain that is more noticeable at the beginning of extension from a fully flexed position.

The physical examination often reveals swelling and ecchymosis at the triceps insertion site. Elbow extension can be weakened in a partial tear. The triceps stress test reproduces pain over the site of injury when the patient attempts to extend the elbow from a fully flexed position. Surgical intervention is indicated if nonsurgical treatment is unsuccessful.

Arthroscopic fixation is a less invasive method than open repair of the triceps tendon. The patient is positioned prone or in the lateral decubitus position, and a diagnostic arthroscopy is performed. For the repair, an initial posterior central portal is placed (**Figure 2**), often through the triceps tendon tear. A posterior lateral portal is established, and the triceps tear is identified when the arthroscope is moved to this portal. The insertion at the olecranon is débrided. A dual suture anchor is inserted at the tip of the olecranon. Two mattress sutures are tied to repair the proximal aspect of the tear. A second suture anchor is placed more distally in the olecranon, and these sutures are retrieved through the tendon to complete the repair. Techniques have also been described that use passage of suture through the torn tendon with placement of the suture into a lateral row anchor distally on the olecranon.[39]

The ulnar nerve should be mapped out before portal placement in any arthroscopic elbow procedure (**Figure 3**). The bone in the olecranon can be extremely hard, and care must be taken to avoid breaking off the anchors during insertion. The arthroscopic repair should be converted to an open procedure if swelling becomes too great for completing the procedure arthroscopically. After surgery, the elbow should be held in extension. Motion should be limited, with an increase in flexion slowly over a period of 6 to 8 weeks.[40]

Fractures

One of the emerging uses of elbow arthroscopy is in fracture fixation and reduction. Innovative techniques continue to be developed to manage fractures with less invasive methods that preserve the soft-tissue envelope and minimize dissection. Arthroscopically assisted fracture fixation has been described for radial head fractures, coronoid fractures, pediatric lateral condyle fractures, capitellar fractures, and epicondylar and intercondylar fractures. The ability to obtain radiographs and physical examination often is limited because of the patient's pain. Aspiration of any hemarthrosis and injection of an intra-articular anesthetic can increase the ability to perform an accurate physical examination and position the extremity for radiographs, with greater patient comfort. CT and MRI should be ordered at the surgeon's discretion to define the fracture pattern and associated soft-tissue injuries for preoperative planning.

Unrecognized chondral injuries and other intra-articular pathology can be identified during arthroscopy. Fracture reduction can be directly visualized, thereby increasing its accuracy and decreasing the need for intraoperative fluoroscopy.

A patient with gross infection or contamination, neurovascular injury, or severely osteoporotic bone should be treated using an open procedure. The posterior interosseous nerve should be explored with an open technique in a patient with a radial head fracture that penetrates the capsule and brachialis anteriorly.[41]

Radial Head Fractures

Radial head fractures are the most common fractures about the elbow. Nondisplaced or minimally displaced Mason type I fractures often can be managed nonsurgically with early range-of-motion exercises. Mason type II and III fractures often are significantly displaced and

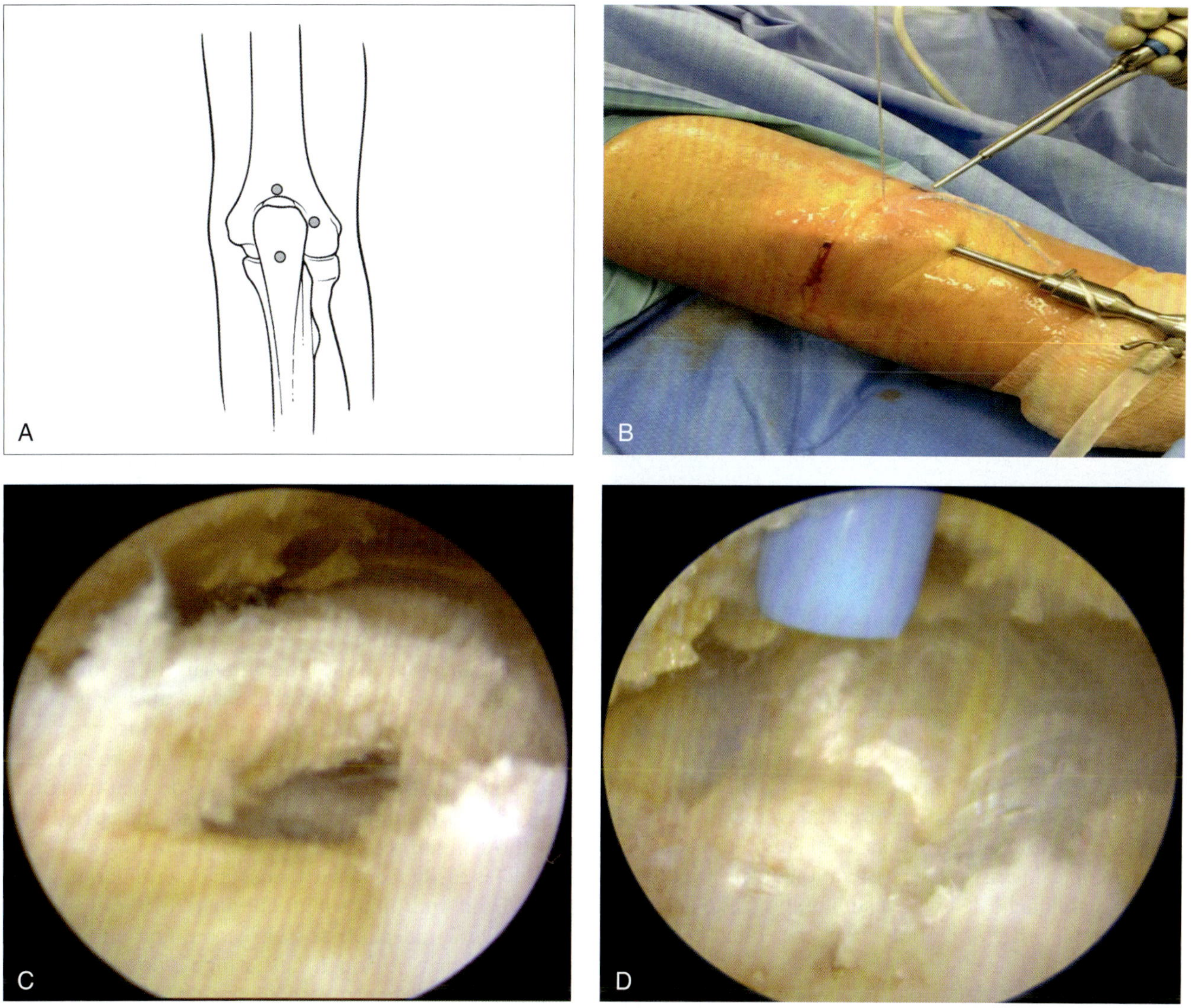

FIGURE 2 **A**, Schematic drawings of the elbow (PA view) showing the placement of arthroscopic portals for a triceps repair. **B**, Photograph showing the initial placement of the posterocentral portal may extend through the triceps tendon tear. **C**, The triceps tear is identified when the arthroscope is moved to the posterolateral portal. **D**, Arthroscopic triceps repair.

can block motion, and they are best managed surgically. Anteromedial and anterolateral portals allow an average of 220° visualized area of the radial head.[42] Addition of the midlateral portal allows for 360° visualization of the radial head.[43] During arthroscopy, a displaced two-part fracture is best viewed from the proximal anteromedial or posterolateral portal. After the fracture fragment is reduced, Kirschner wires can be placed through the anterolateral or soft-spot portal to stabilize the fracture, and the fracture then can be definitively fixed using percutaneously placed headless screws or absorbable pins. In a case study of Mason type II radial head fractures managed with arthroscopic reduction, percutaneous pinning, and placement of one or two headless screws, all 14 patients had a good to excellent result at 5.5-year follow-up.[44]

Coronoid Fractures

The coronoid plays an important role in maintaining the bony stability of the elbow joint. Fractures of the coronoid frequently are associated with axial loading and posterior dislocation of the elbow. Surgical intervention typically is recommended for a Regan-Morrey type III fracture or any fracture that interferes with joint motion or stability. Small fracture fragments or comminuted fractures not amenable to fixation with screws can be débrided or fixed using suture anchors at the fracture site. Larger coronoid fragments typically can be reduced with the aid of a tibial anterior cruciate ligament guide. The fracture can be stabilized by guidewires drilled through the guide, followed by definitive fixation with small cannulated screws. A retrospective review of arthroscopically aided coronoid

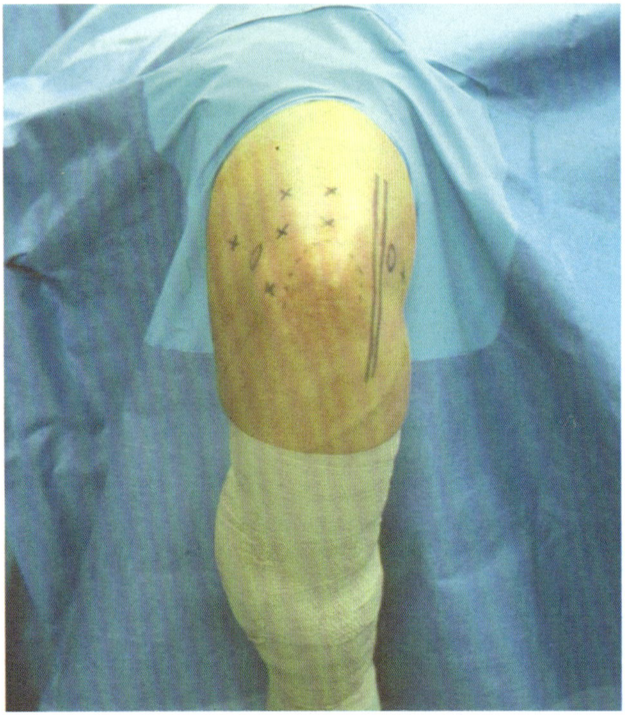

FIGURE 3 Photograph of the elbow showing the mapping of the ulnar nerve before portal placement.

fracture reduction found that all seven patients healed with a functional range of motion and were pain free.[45] A case study of four consecutive patients treated with either arthroscopically assisted screw fixation or suturing found that all patients healed with a stable elbow and achieved a functional range of motion about the elbow.[46]

Lateral Condyle Fractures

Lateral humeral condyle fractures often are seen in pediatric patients and typically are managed with a long arm cast (for a nondisplaced fracture), closed reduction and pinning, or open reduction using a Kocher approach. These fractures often are amenable to arthroscopic evaluation and assisted reduction followed by percutaneous pinning and long arm casting. Arthroscopy avoids a large soft-tissue dissection and decreases the risk of vascular insult to the fracture fragment, which can occur with an open procedure. Two small case studies found that this technique can be used with excellent short-term results.[47,48]

Posterolateral Rotatory Instability

PLRI, first described in 1991, involves insufficiency of the lateral ligamentous structures, specifically the radial ulnohumeral ligament (RUHL).[49] The RUHL is an important elbow stabilizer during supination and extension. Injury can cause difficulty even in simple activities of daily living. The RUHL has three separate components: the radial collateral ligament, the lateral ulnar collateral ligament, and the annular ligament. There appears to be a continuum between PLRI and frank elbow dislocation.[50] Pain with lateral elbow instability can often mimic lateral epicondylitis, and PLRI can be seen in association with lateral epicondylitis.[51] The close proximity of the ECRB tendon insertion and the RUHL may lead to iatrogenic PLRI during open ECRB débridement for tennis elbow.

Arthroscopic management of PLRI originally was described in 2001, and several variations had been described later.[50,52,53] The choice of treatment depends on whether the patient has an acute dislocation, recurrent dislocation, or chronic PLRI. In a simple dislocation, the RUHL complex is typically avulsed from its humeral attachment and heals with nonsurgical management. A diagnostic arthroscopy can be performed after an anteromedial portal is established. Hematoma should be removed, and a torn annular ligament can be sutured. A posterior central portal is created, and the posterior hematoma is evacuated. The site of avulsion from the lateral humeral epicondyle should be identified and débrided. An anchor is then placed into the humerus in the midline of the radiocapitellar joint, and a second anchor is placed more proximally at the two primary avulsion sites of the origin of the RUHL. The suture limbs are retrieved through the ligamentous complex. To prevent overtightening, the horizontal mattress sutures should be tied with the elbow in approximately 45° to 60° of flexion.

PLRI is easily seen on arthroscopic examination as the radial head and ulna subluxate posterolaterally during a pivot shift under anesthesia. A common finding with PLRI is the drive-through sign, which is not possible in a stable elbow. In the drive-through sign, the arthroscope can be moved from the posterolateral gutter across the ulnohumeral articulation from the posterior central portal.

Arthroscopic repair of chronic PLRI involves plication of the RUHL followed by repair to the humerus. Anchors are placed at the origin sites of the RCL and the RUHL for humeral fixation, and the ligament is plicated and repaired either by using these sutures or by placing additional plication sutures and repairing the plicated ligament complex to the humerus. The plication is performed by placing four to seven absorbable sutures from distal through the RUHL complex at its ulnar attachment and working proximally. The sutures are retrieved with a retrograde retriever that hooks under the radial collateral ligament from the posterolateral aspect of the lateral epicondyle. The sutures are individually retrieved percutaneously through the existing skin portals and tied sequentially. After tensioning, the drive-through sign should be eliminated.[53] The results of arthroscopic management of PLRI are equivalent to those of open repair.[52] Elbow arthroscopy allows for additional diagnostic techniques, with improved visualization of the joint and allows for coexisting intra-articular pathology to be addressed with minimal soft-tissue injury.[54]

Posteromedial Impingement

Overhead athletes generate high-level valgus and extension forces through their elbow during the throwing motion. The primary constraint to valgus stress at the elbow is the anterior band of the MUCL. An incompetent MUCL gives way to valgus instability of the elbow. Over time, posteromedial impingement (called thrower's elbow), ulnar nerve symptoms, ulnar stress fractures, OCD lesions, and even capsular contractures can develop in patients with valgus elbow instability. These symptoms constitute so-called valgus extension overload. The timing of pain during the different phases of throwing can alert the physician to the possible pathologic process. Surgical intervention should be considered if symptoms become disabling (preventing the athlete from performing the sports activity) and nonsurgical measures have been unsuccessful. Radiographs and MRI should be used for preoperative planning and 3D CT reconstructions are also helpful. In a case study of nine patients with posteromedial impingement, reproducible pathology was found when preoperative MRI findings were compared with intraoperative arthroscopic findings.[55]

Arthroscopic management of valgus extension overload consists of soft-tissue and bony débridement, loose body removal, and osteophyte resection.[56] The anterior compartment should be arthroscopically examined for bony spurs, cartilage lesions, and OCD lesions of the capitellum. The anterior capsule should be evaluated if the patient has a loss of terminal elbow extension. Athletes with a loss of terminal extension are able to return to their sport at the preinjury level after arthroscopic contracture release.[57] The medial collateral ligament should be evaluated using the arthroscopic valgus stress test. In the posterior compartment, the olecranon and the olecranon fossa are visualized and débrided of osteophytes. Spurs often are found on the posteromedial aspect of the olecranon. In 16 elbows of athletes with posterior impingement who underwent arthroscopic débridement of the posterior fossa, the extension deficit decreased from 8° to 2°.[58] If the MUCL has been torn, open reconstruction should follow arthroscopy.

Complications

Indications for elbow arthroscopy have continued to expand and elbow arthroscopy is now used to treat more and more complex cases. This demands an intricate knowledge of the traversing anatomic structures, especially the neurovascular structures. Multiple studies have reviewed the complication rate of elbow arthroscopy, which include both major (deep infection, permanent nerve injury) and minor (superficial infection, transient nerve palsies). Patients who receive an intra-articular steroid injection at the time of surgery are nearly three times more likely to develop a postoperative infection,[59] and major complication rates have been noted to be between 0.5% and 5%.[60-64] Obese patients have a significantly increased rate of complications in the Medicare population, including infection, nerve injury, stiffness, and medical complications.[65]

Multiple anatomic cadaver studies have been performed recently to help better define and improve the location and safety of portals.[66-69] Palpation of the ulnar nerve preoperatively was shown to only be accurate proximal to the medial epicondyle,[70] and ultrasonography has been used to assist in posteromedial portal placement.[71]

SUMMARY

Arthroscopy of the elbow requires advanced skills and intimate knowledge of the anatomy surrounding the elbow. The indications for elbow arthroscopy appear to be expanding constantly. Additional elbow conditions for which arthroscopy has been used include elbow chondromatosis, rheumatoid arthritis, distal biceps rupture, olecranon bursitis, septic arthritis, and medial epicondylitis.[72-75]

KEY STUDY POINTS

- Elbow arthroscopy requires a detailed knowledge of the elbow and its anatomy, especially the radial ulnar and median nerves and their location and course across the elbow joint.
- For arthroscopic management of lateral humeral epicondylitis, a tennis elbow portal 2 mm anterior to the tip of the lateral epicondyle allows complete intra-articular resection of the Nirschl lesion from the top down.
- If there is significant loss of flexion or any question as to the exact location of the ulnar nerve, a separate open procedure should be performed to locate and protect it.
- Patients receiving an intra-articular steroid injection at the time of surgery are three times more likely to develop a postoperative infection.

Annotated References

1. Yeoh KM, King GJ, Faber KJ, Glazebrook MA, Athwal GS: Evidence-based indications for elbow arthroscopy. *Arthroscopy* 2012;28(2):272-282.

2. Morris HP: Lawn-tennis elbow. *BMJ* 1883;2:557.

3. Kim JW, Chun CH, Shim DM, et al: Arthroscopic treatment of lateral epicondylitis: Comparison of the outcome of ECRB release with and without decortication. *Knee Surg Sports Traumatol Arthrosc* 2011;19(7):1178-1183.

4. Nirschl RP, Pettrone FA: Tennis elbow: The surgical treatment of lateral epicondylitis. *J Bone Joint Surg Am* 1979;61(6A):832-839.

5. Nirschl RP: Elbow tendinosis/tennis elbow. *Clin Sports Med* 1992;11(4):851-870.

6. Babaqi AA, Kotb MM, Said HG, AbdelHamid MM, ElKady HA, ElAssal MA: Short-term evaluation of arthroscopic management of tennis elbow; including resection of radio-capitellar capsular complex. *J Orthop* 2014;11(2):82-86. doi:10.1016/j.jor.2014.04.003. eCollection 2014 Jun.

   31 patients and 33 elbows underwent arthroscopic tennis elbow débridement of the ECRB with débridement of the capsular fringe complex. There was a 93.5% patient satisfaction at short-term follow-up. Level of evidence: IV.

7. Ando R, Arai T, Beppu M, Hirata K, Takagi M: Anatomical study of arthroscopic surgery for lateral epicondylitis. *Hand Surg* 2008;13(2):85-91.

8. Cohen MS, Romeo AA: Open and arthroscopic management of lateral epicondylitis in the athlete. *Hand Clin* 2009;25(3):331-338.

9. Arrigoni P, Zottarelli L, Spennacchio P, Denti M, Cabitza P, Randelli P: Advantages of 70° arthroscope in management of ECRB tendinopathy. *Musculoskelet Surg* 2011;95(suppl 1):S7-S11.

10. Brooks-Hill AL, Regan WD: Extra-articular arthroscopic lateral elbow release. *Arthroscopy* 2008;24(4):483-485.

11. Savoie FH III, VanSice W, O'Brien MJ: Arthroscopic tennis elbow release. *J Shoulder Elbow Surg* 2010;19(2 suppl):31-36.

12. Baker CL Jr, Baker CL III: Long-term follow-up of arthroscopic treatment of lateral epicondylitis. *Am J Sports Med* 2008;36(2):254-260.

13. Tucker SA, Savoie FH III, O'Brien MJ: Arthroscopic management of the post-traumatic stiff elbow. *J Shoulder Elbow Surg* 2011;20(2 suppl):S83-S89.

14. Morrey BF, Askew LJ, Chao EY: A biomechanical study of normal functional elbow motion. *J Bone Joint Surg Am* 1981;63(6):872-877.

15. Van Zeeland NL, Yamaguchi K: Arthroscopic capsular release of the elbow. *J Shoulder Elbow Surg* 2010;19(2 suppl):13-19.

16. Sahajpal D, Choi T, Wright TW: Arthroscopic release of the stiff elbow. *J Hand Surg Am* 2009;34(3):540-544.

17. Temporin K, Shimada K, Oura K, Owaki H: Arthroscopic release for the severely stiff elbow. *Musculoskelet Surg* 2019;104:81-86.

    Careful contracture release can be performed in the high-grade elbow contracture with improvements of both extension and flexion. Level of evidence: IV.

18. Degreef I, De Smet L: Elbow arthrolysis for traumatic arthrofibrosis: A shift towards minimally invasive surgery. *Acta Orthop Belg* 2011;77(6):758-764.

19. Lubiatowski P, Ślęzak M, Wałecka J, Bręborowicz M, Romanowski L: Prospective outcome assessment of arthroscopic arthrolysis for traumatic and degenerative elbow contracture. *J Shoulder Elbow Surg* 2018;27(9):e269-e278. doi:10.1016/j.jse.2018.02.068.

    Arthroscopic elbow arthrolysis shows similar range-of-motion restoration in traumatic and degenerative contractures. Range of motion achieved at surgery deteriorates early but recovers, yet may not recover to the level achieved at the time of surgery. Level of evidence: IV.

20. Park JY, Cho CH, Choi JH, Lee ST, Kang CH: Radial nerve palsy after arthroscopic anterior capsular release for degenerative elbow contracture. *Arthroscopy* 2007;23(12):1360.e1-1360.e3.

21. Blonna D, Wolf JM, Fitzsimmons JS, O'Driscoll SW: Prevention of nerve injury during arthroscopic capsulectomy of the elbow utilizing a safety-driven strategy. *J Bone Joint Surg Am* 2013;95(15):1373-1381. doi:10.2106/JBJS.K.00972.

    A series of 502 arthroscopic elbow contracture releases in 464 patients performed by one surgeon using a stepwise process retrospectively showed 24 patients (5%) with a transient nerve injury. All deficits resolved by 24 months. Level of evidence: III.

22. Cheung EV, Adams R, Morrey BF: Primary osteoarthritis of the elbow: Current treatment options. *J Am Acad Orthop Surg* 2008;16(2):77-87.

23. Kim SJ, Kim JW, Lee SH, Choi JW: Retrospective comparative analysis of elbow arthroscopy used to treat primary osteoarthritis with and without release of the posterior band of the medial collateral ligament. *Arthroscopy* 2017;33(8):1506-1511.

During arthroscopic management of elbow osteoarthritis, release of the posterior band of the medial collateral ligament showed improved range of motion at 6 months, but there was no significant difference at final follow-up. Level of evidence: IV.

24. Savoie FH III, O'Brien MJ, Field LD: Arthroscopy for arthritis of the elbow. *Hand Clin* 2011;27(2): 171-178, v-vi.

25. Kashiwagi D: Intra-articular changes and the special operative procedure, Outerbridge-Kashiwagi method, in Kashiwagi D, ed: *Elbow Joint*. Amsterdam, the Netherlands, Elsevier Science, 1985, pp 177-178.

26. Degreef I, De Smet L: The arthroscopic ulnohumeral arthroplasty: From mini-open to arthroscopic surgery. *Minim Invasive Surg* 2011;2011:798084.

27. Adams JE, Wolff LH III, Merten SM, Steinmann SP: Osteoarthritis of the elbow: Results of arthroscopic osteophyte resection and capsulectomy. *J Shoulder Elbow Surg* 2008;17(1):126-131.

28. Kovachevich R, Steinmann SP: Arthroscopic ulnar nerve decompression in the setting of elbow osteoarthritis. *J Hand Surg Am* 2012;37(4):663-668.

29. Takeba J, Takahashi T, Hino K, Watanabe S, Imai H, Yamamoto H: Arthroscopic technique for fragment fixation using absorbable pins for osteochondritis dissecans of the humeral capitellum: A report of 4 cases. *Knee Surg Sports Traumatol Arthrosc* 2010;18(6): 831-835.

30. Gonzalez-Lomas G, Ahmad C, Wanich T, ElAttrache N: Osteochondritis dissecans of the elbow, in Ryu RKN, ed: *AANA Advanced Arthroscopy: The Elbow and Wrist*. Philadelphia, PA, Saunders Elsevier, 2010, pp 40-54.

31. Jones KJ, Wiesel BB, Sankar WN, Ganley TJ: Arthroscopic management of osteochondritis dissecans of the capitellum: Mid-term results in adolescent athletes. *J Pediatr Orthop* 2010;30(1):8-13.

32. Davis JT, Idjadi JA, Siskosky MJ, ElAttrache NS: Dual direct lateral portals for treatment of osteochondritis dissecans of the capitellum: An anatomic study. *Arthroscopy* 2007;23(7):723-728.

33. van den Ende KI, McIntosh AL, Adams JE, Steinmann SP: Osteochondritis dissecans of the capitellum: A review of the literature and a distal ulnar portal. *Arthroscopy* 2011;27(1):122-128.

34. Trofa DP, Gancarczyk SM, Lombardi JM, Makhni EC, Popkin CA, Ahmad CS: Visualization of the capitellum during elbow arthroscopy: A comparison of 3 portal techniques. *Orthop J Sports Med* 2017;5(6):2325967117712228.

In the cadaveric comparison of three different portals for capitellar visualization, no difference was found for the dual lateral, distal ulna, and posterolateral approaches. Level of evidence: IV.

35. Arai Y, Hara K, Fujiwara H, Minami G, Nakagawa S, Kubo T: A new arthroscopic-assisted drilling method through the radius in a distal-to-proximal direction for osteochondritis dissecans of the elbow. *Arthroscopy* 2008;24(2):237.e1-237.e4.

36. Schoch B, Wolf BR: Osteochondritis dissecans of the capitellum: Minimum 1-year follow-up after arthroscopic debridement. *Arthroscopy* 2010;26(11):1469-1473.

37. Caldwell PE III, Auerbach B, Pearson SE: Arthroscopic treatment of capitellum osteochondritis dissecans with micronized allogeneic cartilage scaffold. *Arthrosc Tech* 2017;6(3):e815-e820.

Surgical technique of using micronized allogeneic cartilage scaffold in conjunction with marrow stimulation to help promote the formation of hyaline cartilage has been discussed. Level of evidence: V.

38. Uchida S, Utsunomiya H, Taketa T, et al: Arthroscopic fragment fixation using hydroxyapatite/poly-L-lactate acid thread pins for treating elbow osteochondritis dissecans. *Am J Sports Med* 2015;43(5):1057-1065.

Fixation of OCD fragments using hydroxyapatite/poly-L-lactate acid pins in adolescent baseball players with humeral capitellar OCD lesions has been discussed. Level of evidence: IV.

39. Ng T, Rush LN, Savoie FH III: Arthroscopic distal triceps repair. *Arthrosc Tech* 2016;5(4):e941-e945.

Arthroscopic triceps repair technique has been discussed. Level of evidence: V.

40. Savoie F III, Field L, O'Brien M: *AANA Advanced Arthroscopy: The Elbow and Wrist*. Philadelphia, PA, Saunders Elsevier, 2010, pp 132-135.

41. Peden JP, Savoie F III, Field L: Arthroscopic treatment of elbow fractures, in Ryu RKN, ed: *AANA Advanced Arthroscopy: The Elbow and Wrist*. Philadelphia, PA, Saunders Elsevier, 2010, pp 136-143.

42. Hodax JD, Blood TD, Kleinhenz DT, Gorman M, Biercevicz A, DaSilva M: An anatomic evaluation of arthroscopic access to the radial head. *Arthroscopy* 2017;33(5):953-958.

Use of the anterolateral and anteromedial portals allows for 220° of visualization of the radial head. Level of evidence: IV.

43. Cucchi D, Guerra E, Luceri F, et al: A combination of an anteromedial, anterolateral and midlateral portals is sufficient for 360° exposure of the radial head for arthroscopic fracture fixation. *Knee Surg Sports Traumatol Arthrosc* 2019;27(1):319-325.

Use of the anterolateral, anteromedial, and midlateral portals allows for 360° of visualization of the radial head. Level of evidence: V.

44. Michels F, Pouliart N, Handelberg F: Arthroscopic management of Mason type 2 radial head fractures. *Knee Surg Sports Traumatol Arthrosc* 2007;15(10):1244-1250.

45. Adams JE, Merten SM, Steinmann SP: Arthroscopic-assisted treatment of coronoid fractures. *Arthroscopy* 2007;23(10):1060-1065.

46. Hausman MR, Klug RA, Qureshi S, Goldstein R, Parsons BO: Arthroscopically assisted coronoid fracture fixation: A preliminary report. *Clin Orthop Relat Res* 2008;466(12):3147-3152.

47. Hausman MR, Qureshi S, Goldstein R, et al: Arthroscopically-assisted treatment of pediatric lateral humeral condyle fractures. *J Pediatr Orthop* 2007;27(7):739-742.

48. Perez Carro L, Golano P, Vega J: Arthroscopic-assisted reduction and percutaneous external fixation of lateral condyle fractures of the humerus. *Arthroscopy* 2007;23(10):1131.e1-1131.e4.

49. O'Driscoll SW, Bell DF, Morrey BF: Posterolateral rotatory instability of the elbow. *J Bone Joint Surg Am* 1991;73(3):440-446.

50. Smith JP III, Savoie FH III, Field LD: Posterolateral rotatory instability of the elbow. *Clin Sports Med* 2001;20(1):47-58.

51. Kalainov DM, Cohen MS: Posterolateral rotatory instability of the elbow in association with lateral epicondylitis: A report of three cases. *J Bone Joint Surg Am* 2005;87(5):1120-1125.

52. Savoie FH III, Field LD, Gurley DJ: Arthroscopic and open radial ulnohumeral ligament reconstruction for posterolateral rotatory instability of the elbow. *Hand Clin* 2009;25(3):323-329.

53. Savoie F III, Field L, Gurley DJ: Arthroscopic and open radial ulnohumeral ligament reconstruction for posterolateral rotatory instability of the elbow, in Ryu RKN, ed: *AANA Advanced Arthroscopy: The Elbow and Wrist*. Philadelphia, PA, Saunders Elsevier, 2010, pp 94-100.

54. Goodwin D, Dynin M, Macdonnell JR, Kessler MW: The role of arthroscopy in chronic elbow instability. *Arthroscopy* 2013;29(12):2029-2036.

Elbow arthroscopy is a useful adjunct in management of chronic elbow instability. It allows for diagnosis and management of intra-articular pathology. Level of evidence: IV.

55. Cohen SB, Valko C, Zoga A, Dodson CC, Ciccotti MG: Posteromedial elbow impingement: Magnetic resonance imaging findings in overhead throwing athletes and results of arthroscopic treatment. *Arthroscopy* 2011;27(10):1364-1370.

56. Noticewala MS, Vance DD, Trofa DP, Ahmad CS: Elbow arthroscopy for treatment of valgus extension overload. *Arthrosc Tech* 2018;7(7):e705-e710.

Arthroscopic management of valgus extension overload has been described stepwisely. Level of evidence: V.

57. Blonna D, Lee GC, O'Driscoll SW: Arthroscopic restoration of terminal elbow extension in high-level athletes. *Am J Sports Med* 2010;38(12):2509-2515.

58. Rahusen FT, Brinkman JM, Eygendaal D: Arthroscopic treatment of posterior impingement of the elbow in athletes: A medium-term follow-up in sixteen cases. *J Shoulder Elbow Surg* 2009;18(2):279-282.

59. Camp CL, Cancienne JM, Degen RM, Dines JS, Altchek DW, Werner BC: Factors that increase the risk of infection after elbow arthroscopy: Analysis of patient demographics, medical comorbidities, and steroid injections in 2,704 Medicare patients. *Arthroscopy* 2017;33(6):1175-1179.

Patients who receive an intra-articular steroid injection have a 2.79 times increased infection risk after surgery. Level of evidence: III.

60. Noticewala MS, Trofa DP, Vance DD, Jobin CM, Levine WN, Ahmad CS: Elbow arthroscopy: 30-Day postoperative complication profile and associated risk factors. *Arthroscopy* 2018;34(2):414-420.

Postoperative complication rates and need to return to the OR are very low after elbow arthroscopy. They are higher with preoperative steroid use and with diagnoses relating to trauma or inflammatory causes. Level of evidence: IV.

61. Jinnah AH, Luo TD, Wiesler ER, et al: Peripheral nerve injury after elbow arthroscopy: An analysis of risk factors. *Arthroscopy* 2018;34(5):1447-1452.

Minor nerve–related complication rate was 4.4%, with a 0.9% major peripheral nerve injury rate. Level of evidence: IV.

62. Desai MJ, Mithani SK, Lodha SJ, Richard MJ, Leversedge FJ, Ruch DS: Major peripheral nerve injuries after elbow arthroscopy. *Arthroscopy* 2016;32(6):999-1002.e8.

Major nerve injuries are rare occurrences, but likely underreported in the literature. Level of evidence: IV.

63. Elfeddali R, Schreuder MH, Eygendaal D: Arthroscopic elbow surgery, is it safe? *J Shoulder Elbow Surg* 2013;22(5):647-652.

Elbow arthroscopy has a 0.5% major complication rate, which is higher in patients with trauma or who have had previous elbow surgery. Level of evidence: IV.

64. Nelson GN, Wu T, Galatz LM, Yamaguchi K, Keener JD: Elbow arthroscopy: Early complications and associated risk factors. *J Shoulder Elbow Surg* 2014;23(2):273-278.

Complications were seen in 14% of cases with major complication in 5%. Intraoperative postsurgical steroid injections are associated with increased perioperative infections. Level of evidence: IV.

65. Werner BC, Fashandi AH, Chhabra AB, Deal DN: Effect of obesity on complication rate after elbow arthroscopy in a Medicare population. *Arthroscopy* 2016;32(3):453-457.

Obesity is associated with significantly increased rates of complications after elbow arthroscopy. Level of evidence: III.

66. Cushing T, Finley Z, O'Brien MJ, Savoie FH III, Myers L, Medvedev G: Safety of anteromedial portals in elbow arthroscopy: A systematic review of cadaveric studies. *Arthroscopy* 2019;35(7):2164-2172.

Proximal anteromedial portals put fewer structures at risk compared with the distal portal. Level of evidence: IV.

67. El Hajj F, Hoteit M, Ouaknine M: Elbow arthroscopy: An alternative to anteromedial portals. *Orthop Traumatol Surg Res* 2015;101(4):411-414.

Complication rates in elbow arthroscopy without an anteromedial portal are similar to reported complication rates in elbow arthroscopy. Level of evidence: IV.

68. Thon S, Gold P, Rush L, O'Brien MJ, Savoie FH III: Modified anterolateral portals in elbow arthroscopy: A cadaveric study on safety. *Arthroscopy* 2017;33(11):1981-1985.

The modified proximal and direct lateral portals provide adequate distance from the radial nerve and may be safe for clinical use. The distal anterolateral portal is in close proximity of the radial nerve. Level of evidence: IV.

69. Thaveepunsan S, Shields M, O'Driscoll SW: The needle-and-knife technique: A safe technique for anterolateral portal placement in elbow arthroscopy. *Orthop J Sports Med* 2019;7(1):2325967118817232.

Technique for safe anterolateral portal placement has been discussed. Level of evidence: IV.

70. Hilgersom NFJ, Cucchi D, Luceri F, et al: Locating the ulnar nerve during elbow arthroscopy using palpation is only accurate proximal to the medial epicondyle. *Knee Surg Sports Traumatol Arthrosc* 2019;27(10):3254-3260.

After an already initiated elbow arthroscopy, palpation of the ulnar nerve is only reliable proximal to the medial epicondyle. Level of evidence: IV.

71. Ohuchi H, Torres RJL, Shinga K, et al: Ultrasound-assisted posteromedial portal placement of the elbow joint to prevent ulnar nerve injury. *Arthrosc Tech* 2017;6(4):e1087-e1091.

Technique using ultrasound-guided identification of the ulnar nerve for posteromedial portal placement has been discussed. Level of evidence: V.

72. Flury MP, Goldhahn J, Drerup S, Simmen BR: Arthroscopic and open options for surgical treatment of chondromatosis of the elbow. *Arthroscopy* 2008;24(5):520-525.e1.

73. Kang HJ, Park MJ, Ahn JH, Lee SH: Arthroscopic synovectomy for the rheumatoid elbow. *Arthroscopy* 2010;26(9):1195-1202.

74. Bhatia DN: Endoscopic repair of acute and chronic retracted distal biceps ruptures. *J Hand Surg Am* 2016;41(12):e501-e507.

Technique for repair of distal biceps ruptures has been discussed. Level of evidence: V.

75. Meric G, Sargin S, Atik A, Budeyri A, Ulusal AE: Endoscopic versus open bursectomy for prepatellar and olecranon bursitis. *J Shoulder Elbow Surg* 2018;27(9):e269-e278.

Open versus endoscopic bursectomy shows that endoscopic bursectomy can be performed efficiently and quickly. Level of evidence: IV.

Section 8

Miscellaneous Shoulder and Elbow Topics

SECTION EDITOR:
EDWARD G. MCFARLAND, MD

Chapter 43

Suprascapular Neuropathy

Nicholas Jarmon, MD • Umasuthan Srikumaran, MD

ABSTRACT

Suprascapular neuropathy may result from traction, entrapment, or compression of the suprascapular nerve. Suprascapular neuropathy of the infraspinatus branch is the most common abnormality. Patients typically present with posterior shoulder pain and/or weakness in forward flexion or external rotation. Suprascapular neuropathy was first described in the English literature in 1959, and its true incidence and prevalence are unknown. The largest case series through 2019 included 87 patients, and a recent systematic review identified 21 studies with a total of 276 shoulders meeting the authors' inclusion criteria. Nonsurgical treatment remains the first line of treatment in the absence of space-occupying lesions. If this treatment fails, open and arthroscopic techniques for decompression have been described. Additional studies are needed to develop the ideal treatment algorithm.

Keywords: nerve decompression; paralabral cyst; spinoglenoid notch; suprascapular nerve

Introduction

Suprascapular neuropathy results from traction, entrapment, or compression of the suprascapular nerve (SSN). Most commonly, suprascapular neuropathy is an abnormality of the infraspinatus branch; however, the infraspinatus and supraspinatus branches can be affected independently or together. Patients typically present with posterior shoulder pain and/or weakness in forward flexion or external rotation. Suprascapular neuropathy was first described in the English literature in 1959,[1] and its true incidence and prevalence are unknown. The largest case series through 2019 included 87 patients,[2] and a recent and first systematic review identified 21 studies with a total of 276 shoulders meeting the authors' inclusion criteria.[3]

Anatomy

The SSN receives its primary contributions from C5 and C6, with occasional contribution from C4. Originating from the upper trunk of the brachial plexus, the nerve travels posterior to the clavicle, across the superior border of the scapula, and toward the suprascapular notch (**Figure 1**).

The SSN runs in the suprascapular notch—a bony depression medial to the base of the coracoid, below the transverse scapular ligament, which forms the roof of the suprascapular notch. The suprascapular artery typically runs above the ligament. Various morphologies of this notch have been described, ranging from a subtle bony depression to a bony tunnel with ossification of the transverse scapular ligament.[4] After exiting the tunnel, the nerve runs posterolaterally across the bony floor of the supraspinatus fossa, where it supplies motor branches to the supraspinatus muscle and sensory branches to the acromioclavicular and glenohumeral joints. The motor branches to the supraspinatus were found to originate, on average, 3 cm from the supraglenoid tubercle, whereas the motor branches to the infraspinatus originate, on average, 2 cm from the posterior rim of the glenoid.[5] At the posterolateral corner of the supraspinatus fossa, the nerve enters the spinoglenoid notch (SGN), passing under the spinoglenoid (inferior transverse scapular) ligament. Anatomic analysis[6] has shown wide variations in the presence of this ligament, but a 2005 study showed the ligament was present in 58 consecutive cadaver specimens[7] (**Figure 2**). A portion of this ligament inserts on the posterior capsule and becomes taut with adduction and internal rotation.[8] This position has been postulated to correspond with the follow-through phase of

Dr. Jarmon or an immediate family member is a member of a speakers' bureau or has made paid presentations on behalf of Zimmer. Dr. Srikumaran or an immediate family member is a member of a speakers' bureau or has made paid presentations on behalf of Conventus and FX Shoulder; serves as a paid consultant to or is an employee of Conventus and FX Shoulder; has stock or stock options held in Quantum OPS, ROM3, and Tigon Medical; and has received nonincome support (such as equipment or services), commercially derived honoraria, or other non–research-related funding (such as paid travel) from Arthrex, Inc., DePuy, a Johnson & Johnson Company, Smith & Nephew, Stryker, and Wright Medical Technology, Inc.

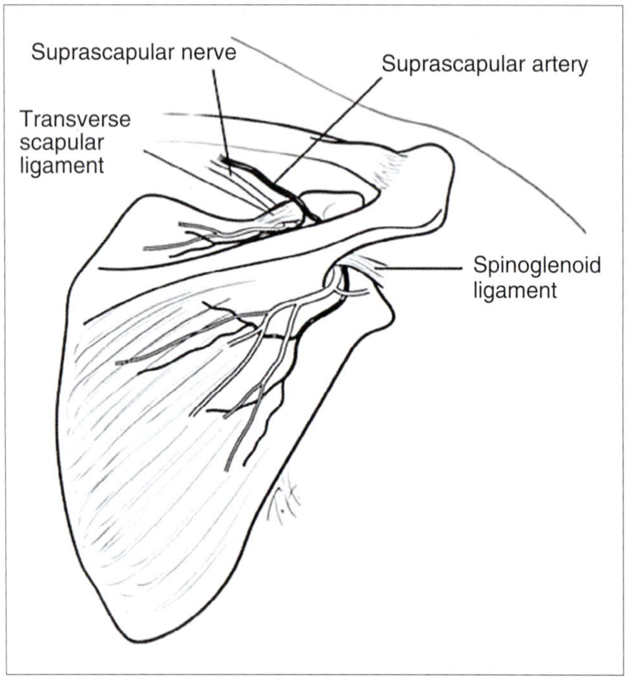

FIGURE 1 Illustration showing the anatomy of the suprascapular nerve. (Reproduced with permission from Safran MR: Nerve injury about the shoulder in athletes: Part 1. Suprascapular nerve and axillary nerve. *Am J Sports Med* 2004;32:803-819.)

throwing.[8] After exiting the notch, the nerve courses medially around the base of the scapular spine, sending motor branches to the infraspinatus muscle.

Mechanism of Injury

A variety of mechanisms have been identified as the causes of suprascapular neuropathy, including repetitive traction and microtrauma, compressive lesions, local anatomic variants, glenohumeral dislocation, scapula fracture, and surgical trauma.[9]

Multiple studies suggest that suprascapular neuropathy in overhead athletes is the result of repetitive traction and microtrauma,[10,11] possibly related to increased pressure on the nerve from tightening of the spinoglenoid ligament during the follow-through phase of the throwing motion.[8] Compression of the nerve can occur anywhere along its course. Suprascapular compression has been identified after fractures at the suprascapular notch and the distal clavicle.[12,13] Entrapment of the nerve at the SGN by paralabral cysts is common.[14] Although believed to be less common, paralabral cysts can extend more medially than the SGN and compress the nerve at the suprascapular notch.[15] Certain anatomic variations, such as narrow suprascapular or SGN,[16] an anterior coracoscapular ligament,[17] ossified transverse scapular ligaments,[16] or superiorly oriented fibers of the subscapularis,[18] may predispose patients to suprascapular neuropathy. Soft-tissue and bony tumors have also been implicated in suprascapular neuropathy.[19,20] A 29% incidence of SSN injury on electromyography (EMG) was found in patients with proximal humeral fractures or glenohumeral dislocation.[21]

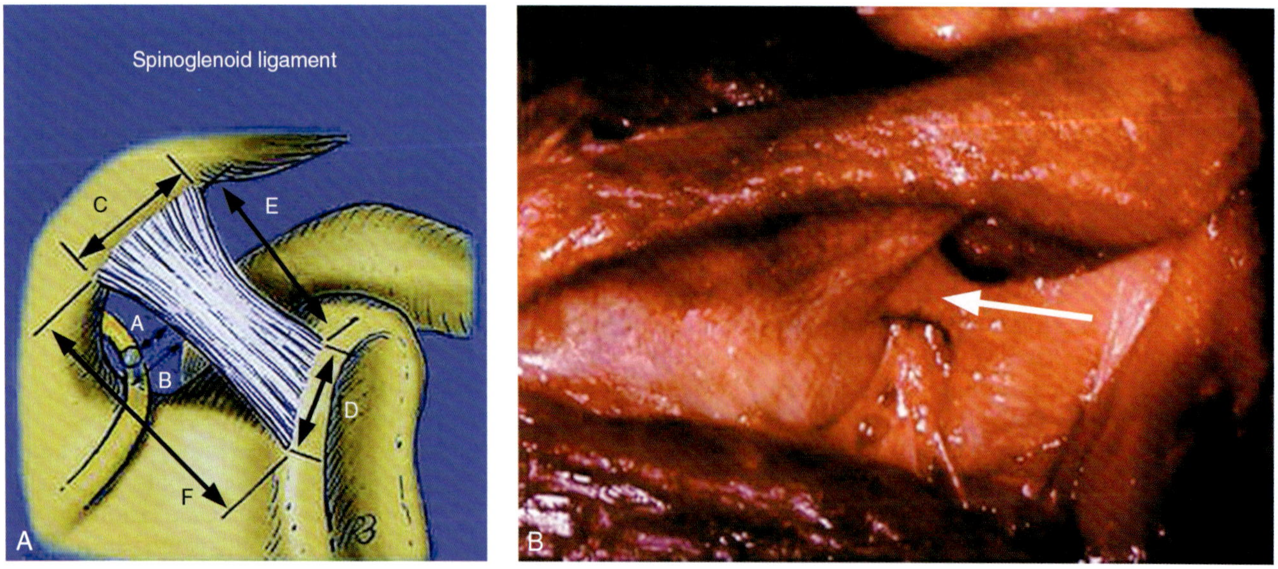

FIGURE 2 Anatomy of the spinoglenoid ligament from a posterior view. **A**, Artist's sketch. The lines shown are as follows: *A*, minimal distance from the ligament to the nerve; *B*, maximal distance from the ligament to bone; *C*, scapular spine insertion; *D*, glenoid insertion; *E*, superior border; and *F*, inferior border. **B**, Photograph of a cadaver specimen. Arrow: spinoglenoid ligament extending from the scapular spine to the posterior capsule. (The suprascapular nerve is seen running below the ligament.) (Reproduced with permission from Plancher KD, Peterson RK, Johnston JC, Luke TA: The spinoglenoid ligament: Anatomy, morphology, and histological findings. *J Bone Joint Surg Am* 2005;87[2]:361-365. doi:10.2106/JBJS.C.01533.)

The SSN can also become entrapped at the suprascapular notch or at the base of the scapular spine in the setting of a retracted rotator cuff tear.[22] Because the motor branches of the nerve are fixed within the muscle, retracted rotator cuff tears can increase medial tension on the nerve as it courses through the suprascapular notch and around the SGN.[22] A cadaver study demonstrated that over advancement of a tendon (>3 cm) can place tension on the motor branches.[5]

Suprascapular neuropathy has been described as a surgical complication secondary to direct injury. The authors of a recent study reported a patient who underwent repair of a type II superior labrum anterior to posterior (SLAP) lesion with two anchors.[23] Postoperatively, the patient had persistent pain. A repeat MRI study showed the posterior anchor protruding through cortical bone and abutting against the SSN, and an EMG study confirmed partial denervation of the SSN. At the second surgery, the anchor was shown to be directly compressing the nerve and was removed, after which the patient's symptoms resolved.[23] In a 2007 case report, suprascapular neuropathy caused by the penetration of screws from a Latarjet procedure into the SGN was described.[24] Penetration was confirmed with CT, and neuropathy was confirmed by EMG. The screws were removed, and at the time of final follow-up, the patient had complete resolution of symptoms, with a return to normal EMG findings. The SSN is also at risk with procedures requiring a posterior approach to the scapula.[25]

History and Physical Examination

Patients with SSN injuries may report a history of trauma or pain and/or weakness with overhead activities. The pain often is not localized. The patient will describe a dull or burning pain in the posterolateral, superior, or anterior aspect of the shoulder. As the pain is diffuse and nonlocalized, it is important to consider other potential causes of pain in these patients. Cervical spine involvement of the C5 or C6 nerve roots can also simulate pain in this area and may coexist with more peripheral compressive or traction injuries to the SSN or its branches. The SSN does not have sensory branches to the skin, so any paresthesias in the shoulder or in the upper extremity should not be ascribed to a SSN injury; other causes of the paresthesias should be explored.

When examining patients with shoulder pain, it is important and helpful to have both of the patient's shoulders exposed for comparative anterior and posterior visualization. Bilateral comparison, especially from behind, can allow the examiner to appreciate atrophy of the supraspinatus or the infraspinatus. Simple observation of the shoulders from behind will sometimes alert the examiner to involvement of the SSN at some level. Because the pain of suprascapular neuropathy is protean and may radiate down the arm or into the neck, neck pain may be present, and cervical spine involvement should be evaluated with the range of motion of the cervical spine. Similarly, in the presence of any suggestion of nerve injury, a neurologic evaluation of the entire upper extremity with sensory, motor, and reflex testing is appropriate. Comparison with the opposite extremity is also helpful when performing upper extremity neurologic testing because many conditions can simulate SSN neuropathy.

The best tests for SSN neuropathy are resisted manual stress testing of the involved muscles. The best test for involvement of the nerve at the level of the suprascapular notch would be resisted abduction of the shoulder. If the supraspinatus and the infraspinatus are involved, one study has shown up to 75% loss of abduction and external rotation strength.[26] Some patients may have a positive external rotation lag sign, but although this test is sensitive for supraspinatus and infraspinatus weakness, it is not specific for nerve injury, and other causes for profound weakness should be considered. Resisted external rotation with the arm at the side is the best test for strength of the infraspinatus.[27]

Other provocative tests of the shoulder may shed some light on the origin of pain, but most of these tests are neither specific nor sensitive for SSN involvement alone. In patients who have isolated infraspinatus nerve involvement, there may be signs of a coexisting SLAP lesion, but the examination for SLAP lesions remains inexact and controversial. A cadaver study has suggested that symptoms may be exacerbated with cross-arm adduction and internal rotation, but this suggestion has not been subjected to clinical verification.[8]

A detailed physical examination can help isolate the location of the lesion. Isolated atrophy of the infraspinatus is associated with injury at the SGN. Suprascapular neuropathy at the SGN will produce isolated weakness of external rotation at the side on physical examination. This weakness may be out of proportion to other physical examination, or even imaging, findings; that is, there will be no evidence of a ganglion cyst or a rotator cuff tear. Patients with atrophy of the supraspinatus and the infraspinatus are likely to have injury at the suprascapular notch (**Figure 3**). Global atrophy of the shoulder musculature suggests some other abnormality to account for a patient's symptoms. In the case of massive rotator cuff tears, the physical examination cannot determine whether the nerve is under tension based on weakness alone. In these cases, EMG and nerve conduction velocity studies are helpful.

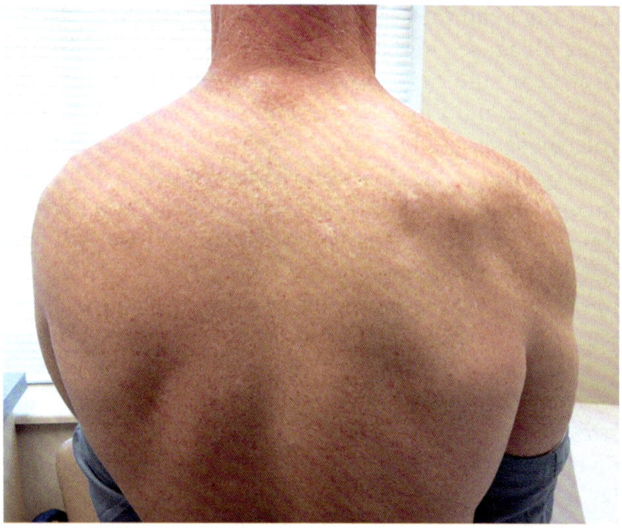

FIGURE 3 Clinical photograph of right-side supraspinatus and infraspinatus atrophy in a patient with electromyography (EMG)-documented suprascapular neuropathy.

Diagnostic Studies

Conventional radiographs are recommended in the initial evaluation of any patient with shoulder pain. Conventional radiographs are helpful for assessing the painful shoulder for fractures, previous surgically induced bone changes, tumors, dysplasia, or other bony variants that might account for nerve compression. CT defines osseous abnormalities, such as an ossified ligament or fracture callus, that may account for nerve entrapment better than does radiography.

MRI evaluation is considered the best next study for patients who have shoulder pain believed to be associated with SSN neuropathy. The MRI study will most accurately evaluate the rotator cuff for tendon tears but will also give important information about the presence and distribution of muscle atrophy. It will potentially give information about ganglion cysts or other space-occupying lesions that might be compressing the nerve. However, MRI will not identify the suprascapular notch unless specific images of that area are requested.[28]

Multiple studies have used ultrasonography to identify SSN abnormalities.[29,30] This modality has several advantages: (1) it can be used in conjunction with diagnostic and therapeutic injections; (2) it allows for the visualization of mass lesions, including ganglions, tumors, and bony abnormalities; and (3) in thin patients, the nerve itself can be seen along its course, whereas in heavier patients, vascular structures can be seen to approximate the location of the nerve. The disadvantages of this modality are that it is heavily operator dependent, and it may be less reliable in heavier patients.

The most important test standard for the diagnosis and confirmation of suprascapular neuropathy at any level is EMG/nerve conduction velocity studies of the upper extremity. The EMG/nerve conduction velocity study should include the entire upper extremity to rule out other potential causes of the patient's symptoms, such as cervical radiculopathy, brachial plexus lesions, myopathy, or other peripheral nerve involvements. When ordering this test to evaluate the SSN, it is often helpful to specify that the periscapular muscles, especially the infraspinatus, the supraspinatus, and the deltoid muscles, should be tested.[31] EMG may help to localize the site of compression. Increased latency and fibrillation potentials, as well as decreased amplitude, suggest nerve compression and denervation. The evaluation of sensory velocities is less reliable because sensory innervation is poorly defined. Normal values for the motor nerve conduction velocity study have been established for the SSN; what has not been clearly established is the sensitivity and the specificity of this study in detecting suprascapular neuropathy.[32] One potentially confounding variable is that many technicians may not be familiar with testing for the SSN and may not be testing for it properly.

Treatment Options

The treatment of suprascapular neuropathy depends on the severity of the symptoms and the physician's confidence that the neuropathy is the cause of the patient's symptoms. Many patients have coexisting lesions that might be contributing to the symptoms, such as symptomatic acromioclavicular arthritis or cervical spine disease. Treatment will also depend on the patient's degree of symptoms in terms of pain and disability for activities of daily living or sports participation.

In the absence of a space-occupying lesion, nonsurgical modalities, including activity modification, NSAIDs, and physical therapy, are widely accepted as the standard initial treatment of suprascapular neuropathy. The results of nonsurgical treatment were assessed in 15 patients whose suprascapular neuropathy was diagnosed clinically and confirmed with electrodiagnostic studies.[33] The outcome was excellent in five patients and good in seven, and only three required subsequent surgery for the persistence of symptoms. Of the three patients in the aforementioned study in whom nonsurgical treatment failed and who went on to have a decompression, there was one excellent, one good, and one poor result.

A 2013 study describing an open technique for SSN release at the SGN sought to emphasize that compression at the SGN can occur in isolation and that the spinoglenoid ligament can be the caustic agent in isolated infraspinatus weakness.[34] Of the 29 patients who underwent an open decompression of the SGN, six patients had ganglion cysts. Of the 29 patients, 23 (79%) showed improvement in external rotation strength within one week of surgery, and all patients improved their external rotation strength by at least one full strength grade.

However, in patients with proven compression of the nerve and a space-occupying lesion or cyst, nonsurgical treatment (although typically suggested as the initial treatment) may have less favorable results over time, and surgery will eventually be required. Of 19 patients treated nonsurgically for suprascapular neuropathy with known SGN cysts, only 10 were satisfied with their outcomes, whereas 26 of 27 patients treated with surgical excision of the cysts for the same abnormality were satisfied with their outcomes.[35]

In the absence of a space-occupying lesion, surgery may be considered if nonsurgical treatment fails or progressive weakness is noted. Ideally, an area of compression or abnormality should be localized to optimize outcomes. Data are limited with regard to determining how patients who undergo surgery fare after unsuccessful nonsurgical treatment in the absence of space-occupying lesions.

In the case of massive rotator cuff tears, it has been shown that there is a reversal of suprascapular neuropathy, tested by EMG/nerve conduction velocity study, with repair of the tendon tear.[22] It is unclear if there is any additional benefit to decompression of the nerve at the suprascapular notch in combination with rotator cuff repair.

A recent study looked at the utility of performing preoperative EMG in patients with retracted supraspinatus and infraspinatus tears. Of the 49 shoulders studied, only one patient demonstrated a suprascapular neuropathy. The authors suggest that the SSN need not routinely be released during rotator cuff repair.[36]

There are arthroscopic and open approaches to decompression of the SSN, depending on the location and the cause of the compression. The technique used will also depend on the experience of the surgeon.

For open suprascapular notch decompression,[37] a saber or a transverse incision along the scapular spine can be used (**Figure 4**). The trapezius is then split along its fibers, and the supraspinatus is retracted posteriorly. The transverse ligament is then localized and released (**Figure 5**), taking care to preserve the vascular structures running above and the nerve running below the ligament.[37] In addition to releasing the ligament, the notch may also be widened with the use of a burr, if indicated.

An arthroscopic approach for SSN release at the suprascapular notch has been described.[38-40] The procedure begins with the placement of standard portals for a routine diagnostic arthroscopy. After a subacromial bursectomy is performed, the anterior border of the supraspinatus is identified and traced medially when viewing from a lateral

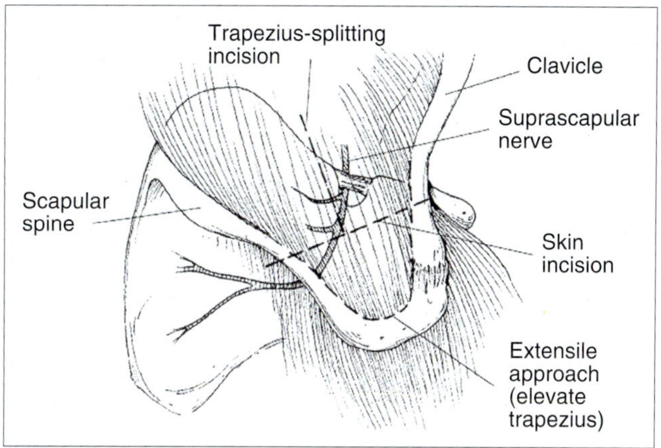

FIGURE 4 Illustration showing open approach to the suprascapular notch. (Reproduced from Romeo AA, Rotenberg DD, Bach BR Jr: Suprascapular neuropathy. *J Am Acad Orthop Surg* 1999;7[6]:358-367.)

or an anterolateral portal. The coracoclavicular ligaments are then identified and serve as an anterior landmark for further dissection medially and inferiorly along the coracoid base. A spinal needle is then used to localize a superior portal 1 to 2 cm medial to the acromioclavicular joint on the skin. The spinal needle should be directed toward the coracoid base and adjacent to the transverse suprascapular ligament. A blunt trocar is then placed through this portal to retract tissue medially along the transverse ligament, exposing the SSN and vessels (**Figure 6**). A second superior portal can be made just lateral to the first, allowing for additional instrumentation to release the transverse ligament. The blunt trocar may be placed inferior to the ligament to protect the nerve while it is released. If the suprascapular transverse ligament is partially or completely ossified, small osteotomes can be introduced to release the nerve. A Kerrison rongeur may also be used to remove bone above the nerve. This approach can be demanding for surgeons who are not familiar with the technique or the surrounding anatomy.

For open SGN decompression, a posterior incision is used, with a longitudinal incision 3 cm medial to the posterolateral corner of the acromion or with a vertical incision in the skin lines. The deltoid is then divided in line with its fibers, taking care not to split it too distally to avoid injury to the axillary nerve. The infraspinatus fascia is then identified and incised, and the infraspinatus muscle can then be retracted inferiorly. The dissection is then carried down the lateral aspect of the scapular spine, where the spinoglenoid ligament is identified and released.[41] An open decompression can also be accompanied by an arthroscopic examination of the joint to determine if there are any intra-articular abnormalities that might need to be addressed, such as an SLAP lesion or rotator cuff conditions.

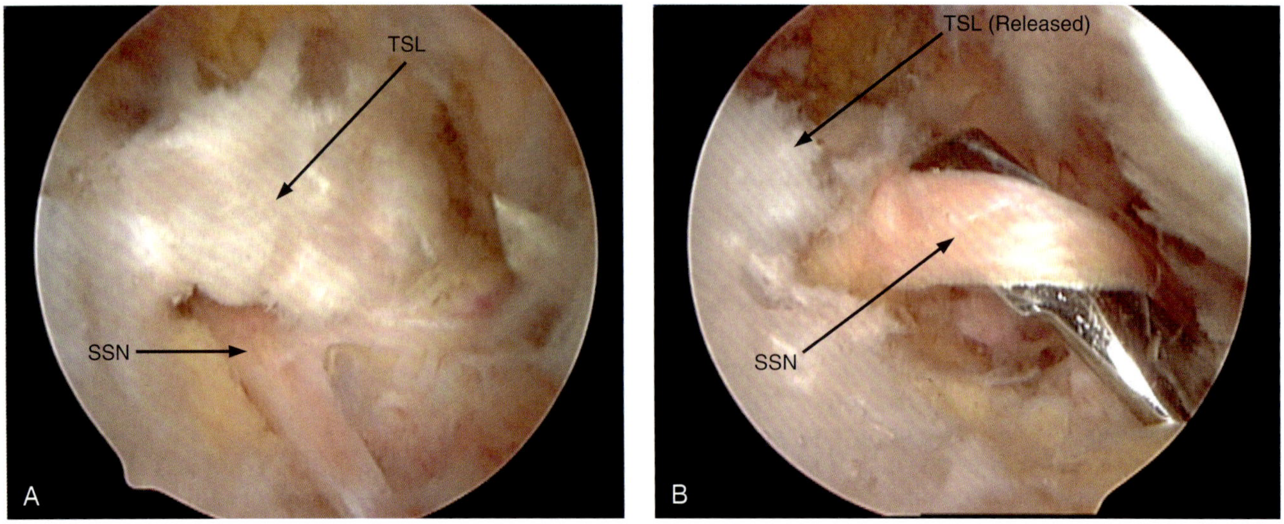

FIGURE 5 Intraoperative arthroscopic images of the transverse scapular ligament (TSL) and suprascapular nerve (SSN) before (**A**) and after (**B**) release of the ligament. (Reproduced with permission from Boykin RE, Friedman DJ, Higgins LD, Warner JJ: Suprascapular neuropathy. *J Bone Joint Surg Am* 2010;92[13]:2348-2364. doi:10.2106/JBJS.I.01743.)

An arthroscopic approach for SSN release at the SGN was first described in a 2007 study.[42] The procedure begins with the placement of standard portals for a routine diagnostic arthroscopy. After a subacromial bursectomy is performed, the SGN is visualized from the subacromial space. A second posterior portal is made, and a small Langenbeck retractor is used to gently retract the infraspinatus muscle belly inferiorly, allowing better visualization of the SSN and the paralabral cyst. The cyst can then be incised, and its contents can be aspirated with a shaver. A potential benefit of this technique is that it allows for evaluation of the intra-articular abnormality, which is often associated with cysts in this region. In some cases, it has been suggested that when a spinoglenoid cyst is found to be associated with a SLAP lesion or a posterior labral tear, it can be treated with labral repair alone.[43,44] In a 2006 study, of the 10 patients with SGN cysts associated with superior labral tears who underwent labral repair without cyst decompression, four had preoperative EMG studies confirming suprascapular neuropathy; all four had postoperative EMG studies showing return of normal function. Eight patients had postoperative MRI, all showing resolution of the cyst.[43]

When a single site of compression is not clearly identified on MRI, some authors have recommended empirical decompression of both notches.[45,46] Both arthroscopic[46] and open[5] techniques have been described for simultaneous decompression of the nerve at both locations.

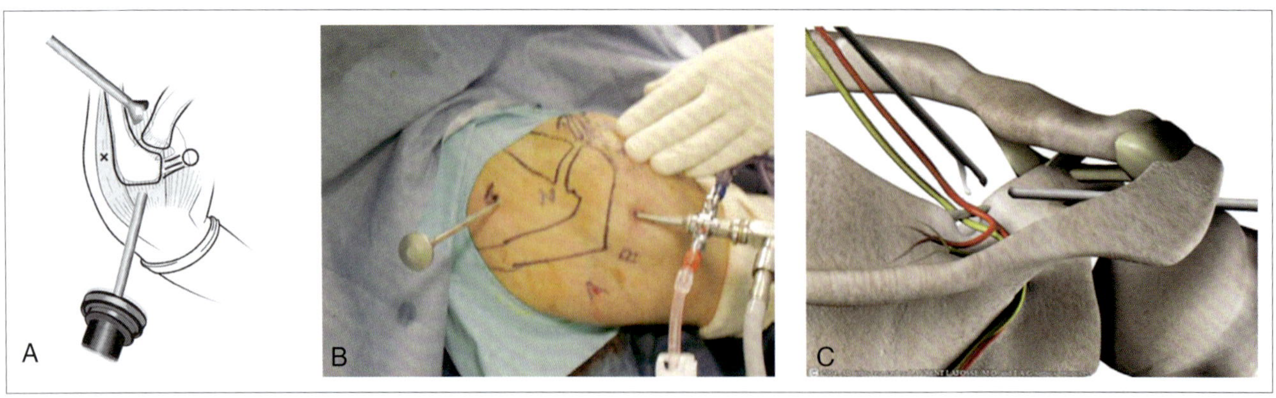

FIGURE 6 Portal placement for arthroscopic release of the suprascapular nerve as depicted on a right shoulder. **A**, Artist's sketch, superior view. **B**, Clinical photograph, superior view. **C**, Computer-generated image, posterior view. (Reproduced with permission from Boykin RE, Friedman DJ, Higgins LD, Warner JJ: Suprascapular neuropathy. *J Bone Joint Surg Am* 2010;92[13]:2348-2364. doi:10.2106/JBJS.I.01743.)

Table 1

Clinical Results

Study (Year)	Number of Patients	Mean Age (Years)	Mean Follow-up (Months; Range)	Treatment	Pre-EMG	Post-EMG	Outcome Measures	Clinical Outcomes
Martin et al[33] (1997)	15	35	47 (15-54)	Physical therapy: range of motion and periscapular strengthening	4 of 10 in nonsurgical group with abnormal findings	Normal after treatment	Activity, pain, strength	5 excellent, 7 good, 3 required surgery for persistent pain (1 good, 1 excellent, 1 poor).
Antoniou et al[52] (2001)	53	38	28 (12-91)	Surgical, 36; nonsurgical, 17	Yes	No	Modified ASES	Compressive lesions responded to surgical treatment; overuse injuries responded equally well to surgical and nonsurgical treatment.
Kim et al[48] (2005)	42	41	18 (12-48)	Open decompression	Yes	No	Pain and strength grade	Pain improved in 7 of 8 patients presenting with persistent pain. Preoperative supraspinatus strength 0 to 2 in all patients; postoperative supraspinatus 4 or better in 90% and 2 to 3 in 10%.

(continued)

Table 1

Clinical Results (continued)

Study (Year)	Number of Patients	Mean Age (Years)	Mean Follow-up (Months; Range)	Treatment	Pre-EMG	Post-EMG	Outcome Measures	Clinical Outcomes
Mallon et al[50] (2006)	8	68	24 (16-36)	Nonsurgical treatment, 4; partial repair of massive cuff tear with margin convergence, 4	All with denervation SS ± IS	2 follow-up EMGs obtained in surgical group: both showed partial nerve recovery	Clinical examination	Nonsurgical group, no change; surgical group, active elevation improved in 4 of 4 patients, and spinatus atrophy remained present clinically.
Westerheide et al[51] (2006)	14	41	51 (24-73)	Arthroscopic decompression	11 of 11 showed denervation of IS	No	SST, Constant, strength	SST improved (4.3-11.5), postoperative Constant score, 94; all improved strength.
Lafosse et al[40] (2007)	10	50	15 (6-27)	Arthroscopic decompression	10 of 10 with findings of chronic compression	7 of 8 had complete normalization, 1 of 8 partial recovery	Constant, strength, VAS, patient satisfaction	Improved Constant score and strength in external rotation and abduction, 9 of 10 excellent with complete pain relief, 1 of 10 satisfactory with moderate pain relief.
Shah et al[49] (2011)	27	49.3	22.5 (3-44)	Arthroscopic decompression	24 of 27 had positive findings	No	VAS, subjective shoulder value, ASES	17 of 24 pain relief, 17 of 24 improved, 18 of 24 improved ASES

ASES = American Shoulder and Elbow Surgeons score, EMG = electromyography, IS = infraspinatus, SS = supraspinatus, SST = simple shoulder test, VAS = visual analog scale.

Results

Making conclusive remarks about the best treatment of SSN neuropathy is difficult because these lesions are not common, the diagnostic criteria for making the diagnosis vary, the diagnosis is often not verified with EMG/nerve conduction velocity studies, and there are no randomized prospective studies analyzing the outcomes for the various treatment options. In a 2018 study, 47 patients underwent isolated labral repair for symptomatic posterior superior paralabral cysts. In the 20 patients presenting with clinical muscle atrophy and edema on MRI, the mean time to regression of muscle edema was 11 weeks.[44] Unfortunately, this study did not have any electrodiagnostic studies to confirm nerve compression. A meta-analysis from 2002 identified 88 cases of SSN entrapment from 1959 to 2001.[47] Unfortunately, fewer than 50% of the studies reported clinical outcomes. Although this meta-analysis suggested that earlier surgical intervention may help limit the amount of atrophy seen, additional conclusions could not be made because of the lack of reported outcomes. A recent systematic review of clinical outcomes of SSN decompression identified 21 studies (15 arthroscopic/6 open) including 275 patients and 276 shoulders meeting the authors' inclusion criteria. Eleven different outcome measures were used making it difficult to draw some comparisons between studies. However, all studies showed favorable outcomes with a low complication rate 2/276 (0.74%). The most commonly used outcome measure was visual analog scale, which was used in seven studies for a total of 123 patients. The mean visual analog scale score improved from 6.3 to 1.6. Nine of the 21 studies looked at return to support with 95.2% of athletes returning to sport, with 88% returning to preinjury level.[3]

Pain relief and strength improvement were reported in 28 of 31 patients treated with an open decompression at the suprascapular notch.[48] The authors of a 2011 study[49] reported on their results of 27 patients undergoing arthroscopic decompression at the suprascapular and/or SGN: of the 24 patients available for follow-up, 71% reported pain relief, 75% had a statistically significant improvement in the American Shoulder and Elbow Surgeons score, 71% had a statistically significant improvement in subjective shoulder value scores, and 71% would have the surgery again[33,40,49-52] (**Table 1**).

SUMMARY

Suprascapular neuropathy remains an uncommon diagnosis, although the true incidence is unknown. A thorough clinical evaluation is needed to properly identify this abnormality and appropriately rule out other possible conditions. After the disease process is identified and space-occupying lesions have been excluded, nonsurgical treatment remains the first line of treatment. If this treatment fails, open and arthroscopic techniques for decompression have been described. Randomized controlled trials to help guide treatment are lacking, and additional studies are needed to develop the ideal treatment algorithm.

KEY STUDY POINTS

- Various mechanisms of injury have been described including repetitive traction and microtrauma, compressive lesions, local anatomic variants, glenohumeral dislocation, scapula fracture, and surgical trauma.
- Resisted manual strength tests remain the most reliable physical examination findings for suprascapular neuropathy.
- The most important test standard for the diagnosis and confirmation of suprascapular neuropathy at any level is EMG/nerve conduction velocity studies of the upper extremity.
- Nonsurgical management is the first line of treatment provided a space-occupying lesion has been excluded.

Annotated References

1. Kopell HP, Thompson WA: Pain and the frozen shoulder. *Surg Gynecol Obstet* 1959;109(1):92-96.

2. Shi LL, Boykin RE, Lin A, Warner JJP: Association of suprascapular neuropathy with rotator cuff tendon tears and fatty degeneration. *J Shoulder Elbow Surg* 2014;23:339-346.

   This is a prospective cohort study of 87 patients. SSN was correlated with tendon tear size, but did not significantly influence fatty degeneration of supraspinatus or infraspinatus muscle bellies. Level of evidence: IV.

3. Momaya A, Kwapisz A, Choate WS, et al: Clinical outcomes of suprascapular nerve decompression: A systematic review. *J Shoulder Elbow Surg* 2018;27:172-180.

   This is a systematic review of suprascapular neuropathy. Surgical decompression leads to satisfactory patient-reported outcomes and return to sports rates with a low rate of complication. Level of evidence: IV.

4. Edelson JG: Bony bridges and other variations of the suprascapular notch. *J Bone Joint Surg Br* 1995;77(3):505-506.

5. Warner JP, Krushell RJ, Masquelet A, Gerber C: Anatomy and relationships of the suprascapular nerve: Anatomical constraints to mobilization of the supraspinatus and infraspinatus muscles in the management of massive rotator-cuff tears. *J Bone Joint Surg Am* 1992;74(1):36-45.

6. Rengachary SS, Burr D, Lucas S, Brackett CE: Suprascapular entrapment neuropathy: A clinical, anatomical, and comparative study. Part 3. Comparative study. *Neurosurgery* 1979;5(4):452-455.

7. Plancher KD, Peterson RK, Johnston JC, Luke TA: The spinoglenoid ligament: Anatomy, morphology, and histological findings. *J Bone Joint Surg Am* 2005;87(2): 361-365.

8. Plancher KD, Luke TA, Peterson RK, Yacoubian SV: Posterior shoulder pain: A dynamic study of the spinoglenoid ligament and treatment with arthroscopic release of the scapular tunnel. *Arthroscopy* 2007;23(9): 991-998.

9. Boykin RE, Friedman DJ, Higgins LD, Warner JJ: Suprascapular neuropathy. *J Bone Joint Surg Am* 2010;92(13):2348-2364.

10. Ferretti A, Cerullo G, Russo G: Suprascapular neuropathy in volleyball players. *J Bone Joint Surg Am* 1987;69(2):260-263.

11. Lajtai G, Pfirrmann CW, Aitzetmüller G, Pirkl C, Gerber C, Jost B: The shoulders of professional beach volleyball players: High prevalence of infraspinatus muscle atrophy. *Am J Sports Med* 2009;37(7):1375-1383.

12. Huang KC, Tu YK, Huang TJ, Hsu RW: Suprascapular neuropathy complicating a Neer type I distal clavicular fracture: A case report. *J Orthop Trauma* 2005;19(5):343-345.

13. Solheim LF, Roaas A: Compression of the suprascapular nerve after fracture of the scapular notch. *Acta Orthop Scand* 1978;49(4):338-340.

14. Tirman PF, Feller JF, Janzen DL, Peterfy CG, Bergman AG: Association of glenoid labral cysts with labral tears and glenohumeral instability: Radiologic findings and clinical significance. *Radiology* 1994;190(3): 653-658.

15. Moore TP, Fritts HM, Quick DC, Buss DD: Suprascapular nerve entrapment caused by supraglenoid cyst compression. *J Shoulder Elbow Surg* 1997;6(5):455-462.

16. Ticker JB, Djurasovic M, Strauch RJ, et al: The incidence of ganglion cysts and other variations in anatomy along the course of the suprascapular nerve. *J Shoulder Elbow Surg* 1998;7(5):472-478.

17. Avery BW, Pilon FM, Barclay JK: Anterior coracoscapular ligament and suprascapular nerve entrapment. *Clin Anat* 2002;15(6):383-386.

18. Bayramoglu A, Demiryürek D, Tüccar E, et al: Variations in anatomy at the suprascapular notch possibly causing suprascapular nerve entrapment: An anatomical study. *Knee Surg Sports Traumatol Arthrosc* 2003;11(6):393-398.

19. Hazrati Y, Miller S, Moore S, Hausman M, Flatow E: Suprascapular nerve entrapment secondary to a lipoma. *Clin Orthop Relat Res* 2003;411:124-128.

20. Yi JW, Cho NS, Rhee YG: Intraosseous ganglion of the glenoid causing suprascapular nerve entrapment syndrome: A case report. *J Shoulder Elbow Surg* 2009;18(3):e25-e27.

21. de Laat EA, Visser CP, Coene LN, Pahlplatz PV, Tavy DL: Nerve lesions in primary shoulder dislocations and humeral neck fractures: A prospective clinical and EMG study. *J Bone Joint Surg Br* 1994;76(3):381-383.

22. Costouros JG, Porramatikul M, Lie DT, Warner JJ: Reversal of suprascapular neuropathy following arthroscopic repair of massive supraspinatus and infraspinatus rotator cuff tears. *Arthroscopy* 2007;23(11):1152-1161.

23. Kim SH, Koh YG, Sung CH, Moon HK, Park YS: Iatrogenic suprascapular nerve injury after repair of type II SLAP lesion. *Arthroscopy* 2010;26(7):1005-1008.

24. Maquieira GJ, Gerber C, Schneeberger AG: Suprascapular nerve palsy after the Latarjet procedure. *J Shoulder Elbow Surg* 2007;16(2):e13-e15.

25. Wijdicks CA, Armitage BM, Anavian J, Schroder LK, Cole PA: Vulnerable neurovasculature with a posterior approach to the scapula. *Clin Orthop Relat Res* 2009;467(8):2011-2017.

26. Gerber C, Blumenthal S, Curt A, Werner CM: Effect of selective experimental suprascapular nerve block on abduction and external rotation strength of the shoulder. *J Shoulder Elbow Surg* 2007;16(6):815-820.

27. Kelly BT, Kadrmas WR, Speer KP: The manual muscle examination for rotator cuff strength: An electromyographic investigation. *Am J Sports Med* 1996;24(5):581-588.

28. Inokuchi W, Ogawa K, Horiuchi Y: Magnetic resonance imaging of suprascapular nerve palsy. *J Shoulder Elbow Surg* 1998;7(3):223-227.

29. Martinoli C, Bianchi S, Pugliese F, et al: Sonography of entrapment neuropathies in the upper limb (wrist excluded). *J Clin Ultrasound* 2004;32(9):438-450.

30. Yücesoy C, Akkaya T, Ozel O, et al: Ultrasonographic evaluation and morphometric measurements of the suprascapular notch. *Surg Radiol Anat* 2009;31(6):409-414.

31. Bredella MA, Tirman PF, Fritz RC, Wischer TK, Stork A, Genant HK: Denervation syndromes of the shoulder girdle: MR imaging with electrophysiologic correlation. *Skeletal Radiol* 1999;28(10):567-572.

32. Buschbacher RM, Weir SK, Bentley JG, Cottrell E: Normal motor nerve conduction studies using surface electrode recording from the supraspinatus, infraspinatus, deltoid, and biceps. *PM R* 2009;1(2):101-106.

33. Martin SD, Warren RF, Martin TL, Kennedy K, O'Brien SJ, Wickiewicz TL: Suprascapular neuropathy: Results of non-operative treatment. *J Bone Joint Surg Am* 1997;79(8):1159-1165.

34. Mall NA, Hammond JE, Lenart BA, Enriques DJ, Twigg SL, Nicholson GP: Suprascapular nerve entrapment isolated to the spinoglenoid notch: Surgical technique and results of open decompression. *J Shoulder Elbow Surg* 2013;22:e1-e8.

    A cohort of 29 consecutive patients underwent open SSN decompression at the SGN. The described open technique detaches no muscle and all cases resulted in improved ER strength. Level of evidence: IV.

35. Piatt BE, Hawkins RJ, Fritz RC, Ho CP, Wolf E, Schickendantz M: Clinical evaluation and treatment of spinoglenoid notch ganglion cysts. *J Shoulder Elbow Surg* 2002;11(6):600-604.

36. Collin P, Tresder T, Ladermann A, et al: Neuropathy of the suprascapular nerve and massive rotator cuff tears: A prospective electromyographic study. *J Shoulder Elbow Surg* 2014;23:28-34.

    This is a prospective study of two-center cohort of 49 patients using EMG to evaluate suprascapular neuropathy in the setting of RCT. Suprascapular lesions were not identified in the majority of patients with massive RCT. Level of evidence: III.

37. Post M: Diagnosis and treatment of suprascapular nerve entrapment. *Clin Orthop Relat Res* 1999;368:92-100.

38. Bhatia DN, de Beer JF, van Rooyen KS, du Toit DF: Arthroscopic suprascapular nerve decompression at the suprascapular notch. *Arthroscopy* 2006;22(9):1009-1013.

39. Lafosse L, Tomasi A: Technique for endoscopic release of suprascapular nerve entrapment at the suprascapular notch. *Tech Shoulder Elbow Surg* 2006;7:1-6.

40. Lafosse L, Tomasi A, Corbett S, Baier G, Willems K, Gobezie R: Arthroscopic release of suprascapular nerve entrapment at the suprascapular notch: Technique and preliminary results. *Arthroscopy* 2007;23(1):34-42.

41. Piasecki DP, Romeo AA, Bach BR Jr, Nicholson GP: Suprascapular neuropathy. *J Am Acad Orthop Surg* 2009;17(11):665-676.

42. Werner CM, Nagy L, Gerber C: Combined intra- and extra-articular arthroscopic treatment of entrapment neuropathy of the infraspinatus branches of the suprascapular nerve caused by a periglenoidal ganglion cyst. *Arthroscopy* 2007;23(3):328.e1-328.e3.

43. Youm T, Matthews PV, El Attrache NS: Treatment of patients with spinoglenoid cysts associated with superior labral tears without cyst aspiration, debridement, or excision. *Arthroscopy* 2006;22(5):548-552.

44. Schroder CP, Lundgreen K, Kvakestad R: Paralabral cysts of the shoulder treated with isolated labral repair: Effect on pain and radiological findings. *J Shoulder Elbow Surg* 2018;27:1283-1289.

    This is a prospective cohort of 47 patients with symptomatic paralabral cysts treated with isolated labral repair. Isolated repair led to pain relief with cyst resolution in most patients. Level of evidence: IV.

45. Sandow MJ, Ilic J: Suprascapular nerve rotator cuff compression syndrome in volleyball players. *J Shoulder Elbow Surg* 1998;7(5):516-521.

46. Soubeyrand M, Bauer T, Billot N, Lortat-Jacob A, Gicquelet R, Hardy P: Original portals for arthroscopic decompression of the suprascapular nerve: An anatomic study. *J Shoulder Elbow Surg* 2008;17(4):616-623.

47. Zehetgruber H, Noske H, Lang T, Wurnig C: Suprascapular nerve entrapment: A meta-analysis. *Int Orthop* 2002;26(6):339-343.

48. Kim DH, Murovic JA, Tiel RL, Kline DG: Management and outcomes of 42 surgical suprascapular nerve injuries and entrapments. *Neurosurgery* 2005;57(1):120-127.

49. Shah AA, Butler RB, Sung SY, Wells JH, Higgins LD, Warner JJ: Clinical outcomes of suprascapular nerve decompression. *J Shoulder Elbow Surg* 2011;20(6):975-982.

50. Mallon WJ, Wilson RJ, Basamania CJ: The association of suprascapular neuropathy with massive rotator cuff tears: A preliminary report. *J Shoulder Elbow Surg* 2006;15(4):395-398.

51. Westerheide KJ, Dopirak RM, Karzel RP, Snyder SJ: Suprascapular nerve palsy secondary to spinoglenoid cysts: Results of arthroscopic treatment. *Arthroscopy* 2006;22(7):721-727.

52. Antoniou J, Tae SK, Williams GR, Bird S, Ramsey ML, Iannotti JP: Suprascapular neuropathy: Variability in the diagnosis, treatment, and outcome. *Clin Orthop Relat Res* 2001;386:131-138.

Chapter 44

Scapular Kinematics, Dyskinesis, and Injuries

W. Ben Kibler, MD • Aaron Sciascia, PhD, ATC, PES, SMTC

ABSTRACT

Normal scapular kinematics are critical for optimal shoulder and arm function. Both coordinated muscular forces and the integrity of bony and joint anatomy are required for normal scapular motions. Alterations of the muscular forces or the bony anatomy create scapular dyskinesis, or abnormal motion of the scapula. Dyskinesis has been identified in almost every type of shoulder pathology, from impingement to bony injury, can be evaluated through a specific algorithm to identify the causative factors, and can be addressed through a coordinated rehabilitation protocol as part of the comprehensive management of the shoulder condition.

Keywords: dyskinesis; rehabilitation; scapula; shoulder injury

Introduction

Recent research and more experience with management have increased the scholarship regarding the role and function of the scapula in optimal shoulder function. Multiple studies have demonstrated the motions of the scapula during arm motion and function, showing the complex three-dimensional motions that occur to place the scapula in a position to act as a stabilizer for arm motion, as a base for glenohumeral motion and stability, and as a key element of scapulohumeral rhythm (SHR). Clinical studies have delineated reliable methods of examination of the scapula as part of the comprehensive evaluation of shoulder injury, have defined and classified the observable alteration of scapula motions as scapular dyskinesis, have clarified the multiple causative factors responsible for the dyskinesis, have identified the association of dyskinesis and multiple types of shoulder pathology, and have developed rehabilitation protocols to address the causative factors. The current concepts and practice relating the scapular function and scapular dyskinesis are summarized, an evaluation algorithm for causative factors is provided, the association of dyskinesis and shoulder injury is described, and rehabilitation protocols are demonstrated.

Dr. Kibler or an immediate family member serves as an unpaid consultant to Alignmed; has stock or stock options held in Alignmed; and serves as a board member, owner, officer, or committee member of the American Orthopaedic Society for Sports Medicine and the American Shoulder and Elbow Surgeons. Dr. Sciascia or an immediate family member serves as a board member, owner, officer, or committee member of the American Society of Shoulder and Elbow Therapists.

Scapular Kinematics

As an integral part of the anatomy of the glenoid and acromion, the scapula has key roles in normal shoulder and arm function. The scapula affects the movement of the glenohumeral joint and the acromioclavicular (AC) joint and is integrated with arm movement through the SHR that produces efficient kinematics. Scapular movement traditionally has been described using a single-plane, two-dimensional model in which scapular upward rotation and acromial elevation are the end points.[1,2] Upper trapezius activation to pull the acromion up and serratus anterior activation to move the inferior border laterally were described as the key muscle force couples.[1] The magnitude of the upward rotation has varied among studies but has averaged 60°, thus establishing the 1:2 scapula-humerus motion ratio for total SHR.

Research has found that scapular motion actually is multiplanar and three dimensional.[3] Motion-tracking systems and the use of indwelling bone pins have shown that total scapular movement is a composite of motions (rotations around axes) and translations (sliding motions along a surface); see **Figure 1**. The three observable rotary motions are upward-downward rotation around an axis perpendicular to the scapular body, internal-external rotation around a vertical axis along the medial border, and anterior-posterior tilt around a horizontal axis along the scapular spine.[3] Two translations can occur in the presence of an intact clavicular strut and AC joint: upward-downward sliding on the thorax (resulting from clavicular upward-downward motion at the sternoclavicular [SC] joint) and anterior-posterior sliding around the curvature of the thorax (resulting from clavicular anterior-posterior motion at the SC joint).

Bony and muscular structures adjacent to the scapula determine the scapular movement. The clavicle and the

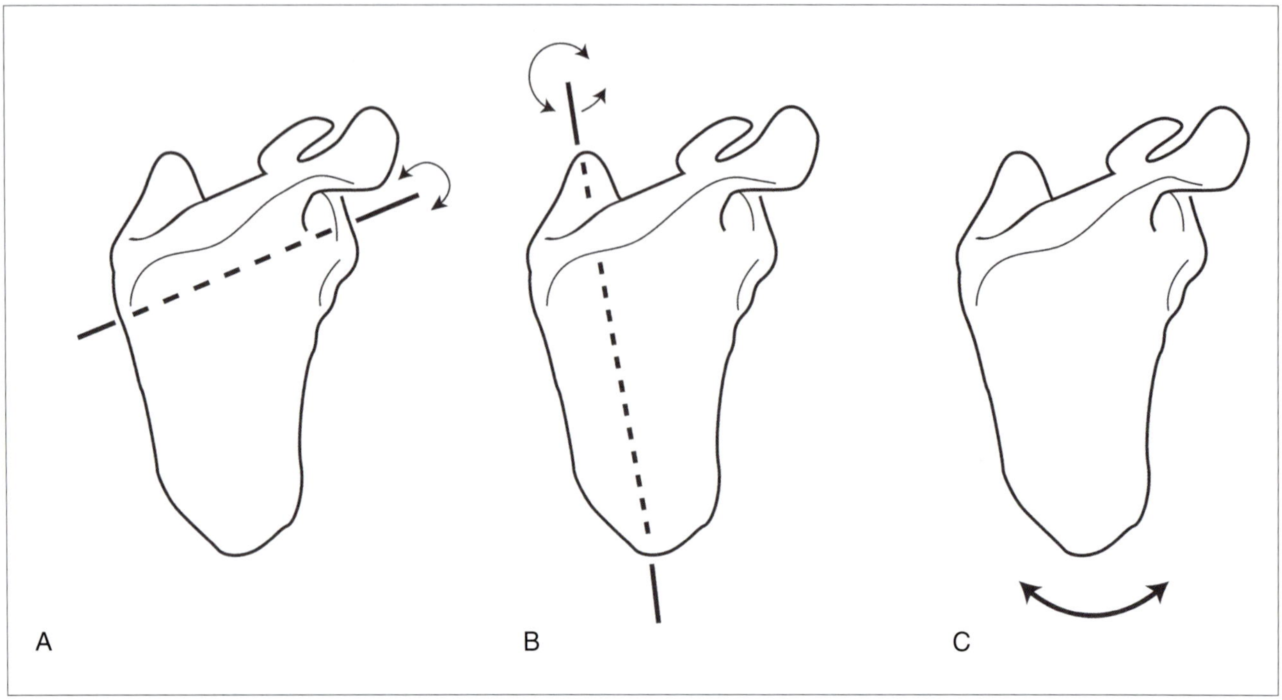

FIGURE 1 Schematic drawings showing the three-dimensional scapular motions. **A**, The horizontal axis allows anterior and posterior tilting to occur. **B**, The vertical axis allows internal and external rotation to occur. **C**, The sagittal axis allows upward and downward rotation to occur.

SC and AC joints are important in creating the scapular positions, motions, and translations.[4] The anatomy of the AC and SC joints and the clavicle must be almost normal to allow normal scapular motions. The clavicle is the only bony connection of the scapula to the axial skeleton. To maximize scapular movement and scapulohumeral motion during full arm elevation, the clavicle retracts 16°, elevates 6°, and posteriorly rotates 31° on its long axis.[4] All of these motions are based on the SC joint. AC joint motions resulting from acromial motion on the clavicle are 8° of internal rotation, 11° of upward rotation, and 19° of posterior tilting.[4] These constrained motions create a reproducible screw axis of motion between the clavicle and scapula through the AC joint and allow the three-dimensional motions.[5]

The primary muscular factors in scapular movement involve coupling of the upper and lower fibers of the trapezius muscle with the serratus anterior and rhomboid muscles. Elevation of the scapula with arm elevation is accomplished through activation and coupling of the serratus anterior and lower trapezius with the upper trapezius and rhomboids.[2,6] During this motion, the lower trapezius helps to maintain the instant center of rotation of the scapula through its attachment to the medial scapular spine.[2] The attachment of the lower trapezius to the scapular spine allows a straight line of pull as the arm elevates and the scapula upwardly rotates, and it creates a mechanical advantage to maintaining this position. The lower trapezius also has a role as a scapular stabilizer when the arm is lowered from an elevated position. The serratus anterior is multifaceted in that it contributes to all components of three-dimensional movement of the scapula; it helps to produce scapular upward rotation, posterior tilt, and external rotation while stabilizing the medial border and inferior angle.[6]

Because these stability and mobility muscles all attach to the axial skeleton, control of posture and stability in the core is as important for maximal activation of these muscles as control of the scapula is important for maximal rotator cuff activation. Maximal activation of the muscles and force couples occurs only through patterns of activation that begin from the core and proceed to the extremities. These patterns coordinate cocontractions and force couples and synergize activation to maximize developed strength. Lower trapezius and serratus anterior activation is maximized when the recruitment is in a diagonal direction, from the contralateral hip through the lumbodorsal fascia to the lower trapezius.[7] The most stable and efficient scapular position for function is retraction.[8-10] From this position, the subacromial space is at its widest, rotator cuff activation is maximal, internal impingement is minimized, and the association with injury is lowest.[8-13]

Most scapula-related shoulder dysfunction can be traced to loss of control of the normal resting scapular position and dynamic scapular motion, which results in alterations in position or motion that produce a position and motion of excessive protraction.[14] This protracted position causes the dysfunctional symptoms, or it contributes to and exacerbates dysfunctional symptoms (**Figure 2**).

The altered scapular position at rest has been described as the *s*capula malposition–*i*nferior medial border prominence–*c*oracoid pain–scapular dys*k*inesis (SICK) scapula.[15] The SICK scapula is characterized by apparent inferior drooping that actually represents anterior scapular tilting. This altered position suggests alterations in pectoralis minor flexibility and serratus anterior and lower trapezius strength, and it should alert the examiner to a possible scapula-related condition.

Scapular Dyskinesis

Altered dynamic motion is called scapular dyskinesis (the term combines *dys* [alteration of] and *kinesis* [motion]). Scapular dyskinesis is characterized by medial or inferomedial scapular border prominence, early scapular elevation or shrugging when the arm is elevated, and rapid downward rotation when the arm is lowered.[14-16] The salient clinical manifestation of the dyskinetic scapula is protraction, which appears as asymmetric prominence of the medial scapular border.

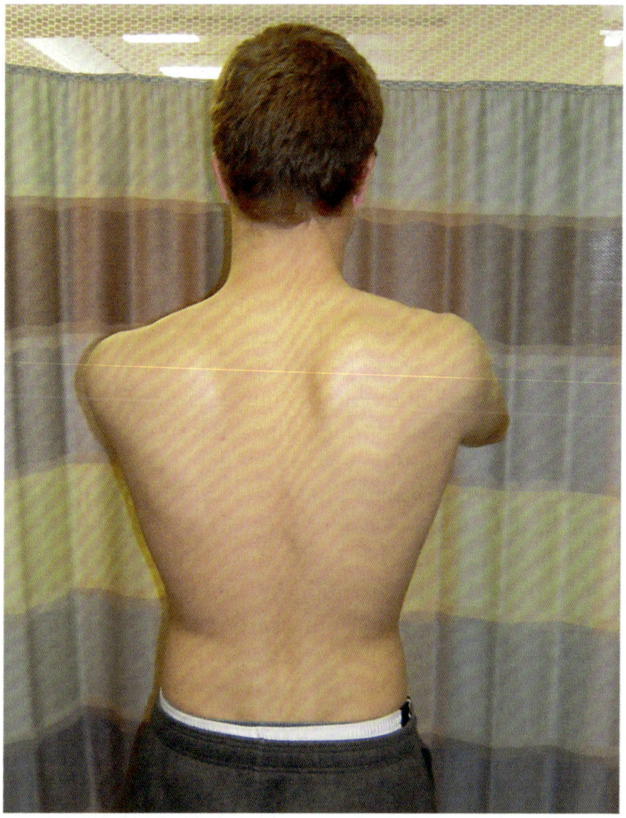

FIGURE 2 Photograph showing a patient with medial border prominence favoring the position of protraction.

Scapular dyskinesis is found in 67% to 100% of patients with shoulder injuries and has many causative factors including alterations in muscle activation, muscle or joint stiffness, scapular muscle detachment, clavicle fractures, and acromioclavicular and glenohumeral internal derangement.[12,13] Most often, scapular dyskinesis results from alteration in coupled muscle activation. The neurogenic causes include injury to the long thoracic or spinal accessory nerves, which appears to be relatively rare. More commonly, the muscle activation alterations are caused by inhibition of neural activation resulting from pain from a glenohumeral joint injury, a strength imbalance among the scapular stabilizers, fatigue of muscle activation, or a change in activation pattern. In almost every patient, the serratus anterior and lower trapezius are found to be weak, to have lower than normal activation intensity, or to be late in activation timing, and the upper trapezius has increased activation and abnormal activation timing.[17] This pattern results in less than normal posterior tilt, external rotation, and upward rotation motion, with greater than normal elevation and translation. These results have been found in patients with impingement, instability, and labral tears.[18-20]

Scapular dyskinesis also can result from muscle or glenohumeral joint stiffness. Dyskinesis is seen in almost all patients with significant degenerative arthritis of the shoulder or with adhesive capsulitis. In some patients, pectoralis minor inflexibility and tightness is believed to contribute to decreased scapular posterior tilt, upward rotation, and external rotation. Glenohumeral internal rotation deficit, which is related to posterior muscle stiffness and capsular tightness, creates dyskinesis by producing a windup of the scapula into protraction as the arm rotates into follow-through during throwing.[20]

Scapular muscle detachment is an uncommon but very painful and debilitating injury that may produce dyskinesis. It results from a tensile load on the scapular supporting muscles, mainly involving the lower trapezius and the rhomboids. It has characteristic history and physical findings that can lead to an accurate diagnosis and treatment. Early recognition of this injury can result in early treatment, to try to minimize the deleterious effects of the chronic pain on patient outcomes.[21,22]

Clavicle fracture can lead to dyskinesis if the anatomy is not almost completely restored. A malunion or nonunion with shortening decreases the length of the strut, especially if the shortening is more than 2 cm, and it can alter the scapular position toward internal rotation and anterior tilt.[23] Similarly, a significantly angulated clavicle fracture can result in functional shortening and loss of rotation. The distal fragment in a midshaft fracture often externally rotates, thereby affecting normal kinematics by decreasing the obligatory clavicular posterior rotation and scapular posterior tilt during arm elevation.

Type III to V AC joint injuries often lead to dyskinesis. These high-grade AC separations can disrupt the strut function and allow a so-called third translation, in which the scapula translates inferior to the clavicle and medial on the thorax.[24] Iatrogenic AC joint injury resulting from excessive distal clavicle resection and detachment of the AC ligaments shortens the bony strut and can allow excessive scapular internal rotation because of excessive anterior-posterior motion at the AC joint. Glenohumeral joint internal derangement, labral injury, biceps injury, or rotator cuff injury can cause dyskinesis through alteration in glenohumeral kinematics and inhibition of muscle activation.[25]

The final result of almost all of these causative factors is a protracted scapula at rest or an excessively protracting scapula with arm motion. This position, which usually results from increased internal rotation and anterior tilt, is unfavorable for every shoulder function except the so-called plus position in weight lifting. The malposition creates a decreased subacromial space and thereby may increase impingement symptoms.[11] In addition, the malposition decreases rotator cuff strength, and it increases strain on the anterior glenohumeral ligaments, strain on the scapula-stabilizing muscles, and the risk of internal impingement.[26] Most of the major goals of treatment of scapular dyskinesis relate to regaining functional retraction capability.

The relationship between dyskinesis and shoulder symptoms is not always clear. In a patient with nerve injury, fracture, AC separation, or muscle detachment, the injury creates the dyskinesis, which affects shoulder function. In some patients with a condition such as rotator cuff disease, labral injury, or multidirectional instability, the dyskinesis may be causative, creating pathomechanics that predispose the arm to injury. In other such patients, the dyskinesis may be a response to the injury, creating pathomechanics that increase the dysfunction. In either situation, the dyskinesis is present and must be treated with the patient's other pathologies.

The multiple causative mechanisms frequently are not isolated; several may be present in the same patient. Careful examination for the presence or absence of scapular dyskinesis and for each of the causative mechanisms should be part of the comprehensive evaluation of a patient with shoulder injury. The clinical evaluation of the scapula should include all possible local and distant contributors to dyskinesis, with a dynamic component because scapular motion is the key component of dyskinesis.

A clinically useful and reliable examination can identify dyskinesis and serve as a basis for treatment.[14,16,27] The goals of the physical examination of the scapula are to establish the presence or absence of a SICK scapula; to identify the presence of scapular dyskinesis; to evaluate joint, muscle, and bone causative factors; and to use dynamic corrective maneuvers to assess the effect of correcting the dyskinesis on the patient's symptoms.[16] An algorithm for the evaluation can serve as the outline (**Figure 3**). The first determination is for the presence or absence of dyskinesis. This can be accomplished through the yes/no observational evaluation of resting and dynamic scapular motion and position.[27] The next determination is whether the observed dyskinesis has relation to the clinical presentation and symptoms, through the scapular correctives maneuvers, the scapular assistance test (SAT) and the scapular retraction test (SRT).[28] A positive result for change of symptoms establishes the clinical importance of the dyskinesis in the dysfunction. The final determination is to evaluate the causative factors through a systematic evaluation (**Figure 4**). The results of the examination are useful in establishing the complete diagnosis of all elements of the dysfunction and in guiding treatment and rehabilitation.

Most of the scapular examination should be accomplished from the posterior aspect, with the scapula exposed for complete visualization. The patient's resting posture should be checked for side-to-side asymmetry and especially for evidence of a SICK position or inferomedial or medial border prominence. Marking the superior and inferomedial borders may be useful if it is difficult to determine the bony landmarks of the inferomedial or superomedial angles.

The SC and AC joints should be evaluated for instability, and the clavicle should be evaluated for angulation, shortening, or malrotation. Anterior and posterior AC joint laxity can be evaluated by stabilizing the clavicle with one hand, and then grasping and mobilizing the acromion in an anterior-posterior direction with the other hand (**Figure 5**).

Dynamic examination of scapular motion can reliably be done by clinical observation of the motion as the arm elevates and descends when viewed from behind the patient. This motion requires activation of the muscles to maintain the closed chain mechanism of SHR. Failure to maintain this rhythm can result in increased scapular internal rotation, with consequent medial border prominence. Clinical observation of medial border prominence in patients with symptoms was correlated with biomechanically determined dyskinesis, and this method has sufficient clinical reliability to be used as the basis for determining the presence or absence of dyskinesis.[27] The patient is asked to raise the arms in forward flexion to maximal elevation, and then to lower the arms three to five times, while holding a 3- to 5-lb weight in each hand.[29,30] Prominence of any aspect of the medial scapular border on the symptomatic side is recorded.

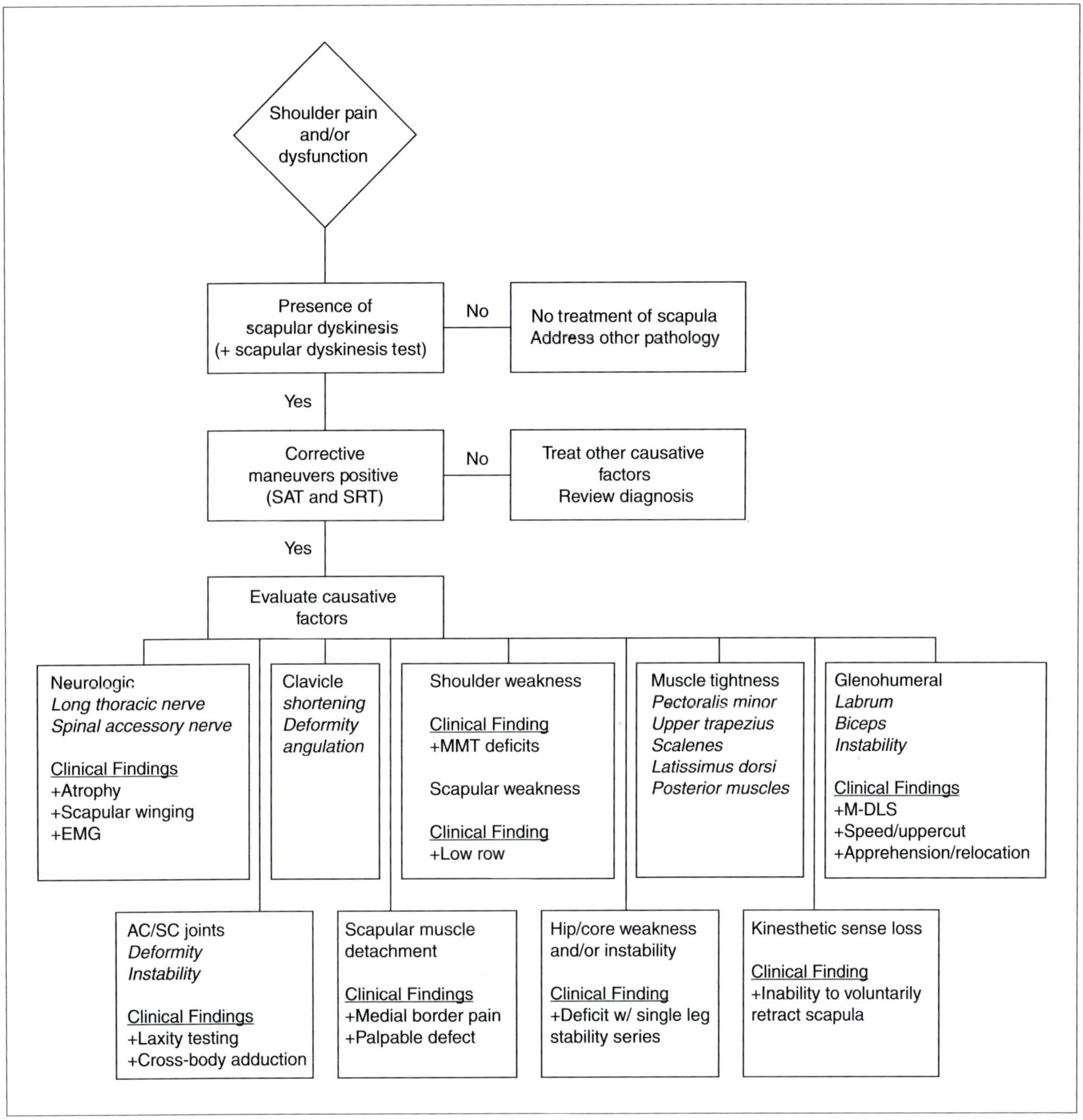

FIGURE 3 Scapular examination algorithm.

The SAT, SRT, and scapular reposition test are corrective maneuvers that can alter the injury symptoms and provide information about the role of scapular dyskinesis in dysfunction accompanying shoulder injury.[31] The SAT is useful in evaluating scapular contributions to impingement and rotator cuff strength, and the SRT is useful in evaluating contributions to rotator cuff strength and labral symptoms. In the SAT, the examiner applies gentle pressure to assist scapular upward rotation and posterior tilt as the patient elevates the arm (**Figure 6**). The most important biomechanical effect of the SAT is to increase scapular posterior tilt by 7° to 10° throughout the entire arc of arm elevation. This test has acceptable interrater reliability.[32] A positive result occurs when the painful arc of impingement symptoms is relieved and the arc of motion is increased. In the SRT, the examiner grades supraspinatus muscle strength using standard manual muscle testing procedures (**Figure 7**) or evaluates labral injury

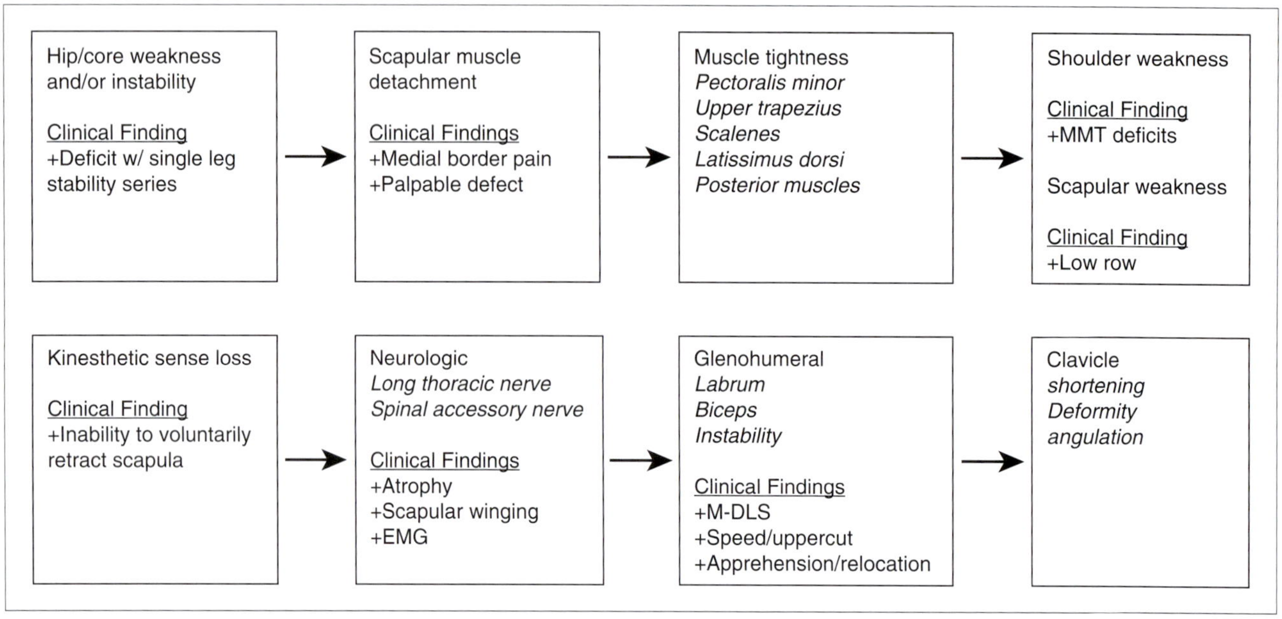

FIGURE 4 Scapular examination clinical decision making.

in association with the modified dynamic labral shear test.[9] The examiner then places and manually stabilizes the scapula in a retracted position. The biomechanical effects are a combination of increased external rotation and posterior tilt. A positive test occurs when demonstrated supraspinatus strength is increased or the symptoms of internal impingement related to the labral injury are relieved in the retracted position. Although a positive SAT or SRT is not diagnostic for a specific form of shoulder pathology, it proves that scapular dyskinesis is directly involved in producing the symptoms and indicates the need for early scapular rehabilitation exercises to improve scapular control.

A review of patients seen for shoulder problems in the authors' clinical practice who also had findings of scapular dyskinesis showed that two-thirds had findings that were not related to the need for surgical treatment. In the nonsurgical group, 63% had a grouping of findings, which included weakness of the lower trapezius and serratus anterior and inflexibility of the upper trapezius, pectoralis minor, and latissimus dorsi. This grouping has been termed lower trapezius insufficiency. Fifty-one percent of this group also demonstrated core weakness on one leg stability testing. This demonstrates that multiple deficits may be present and will need to be addressed.

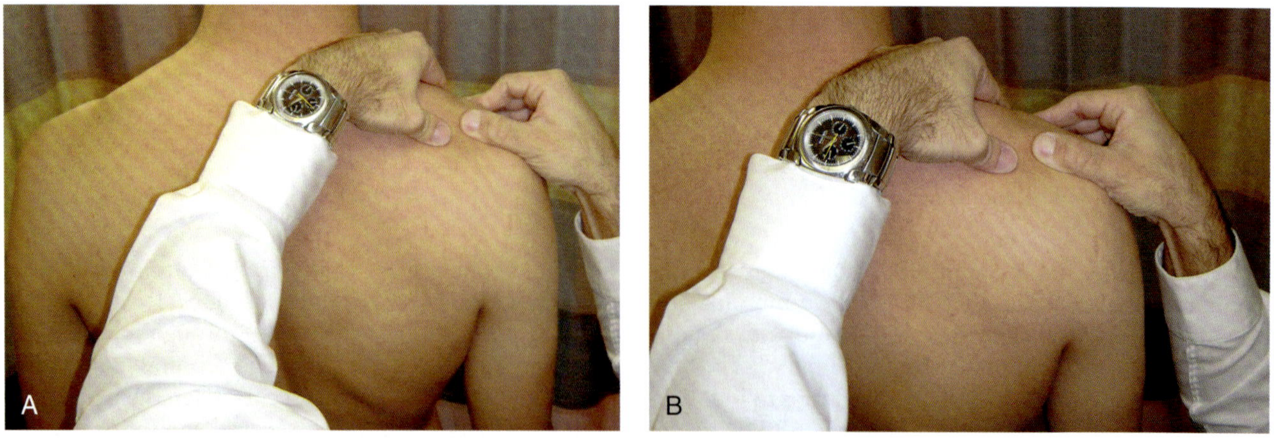

FIGURE 5 Photographs showing the clinical assessment of acromioclavicular (AC) joint laxity. The examiner stabilizes the clavicle while attempting to move the acromion to determine whether the AC joint is unstable. **A**, To assess AC joint laxity, the examiner begins by stabilizing the clavicle and grasping the acromion. **B**, The examiner then attempts to translate the acromion anteriorly and posteriorly to determine the amount of joint laxity (if any).

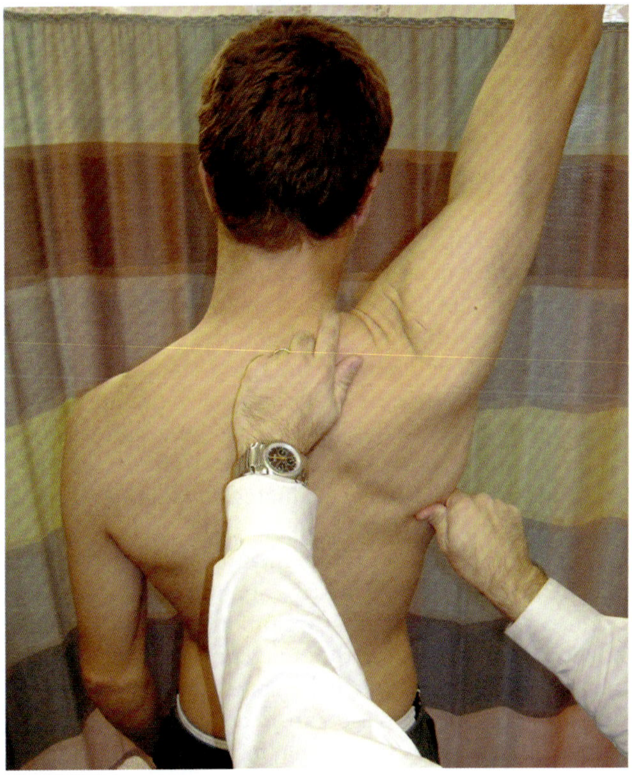

FIGURE 6 Photograph showing increased arm elevation during the scapular assistance test, which reveals the presence of a dysfunctional scapula.

Scapular Involvement in Shoulder Injuries

Winged Scapula

The winged scapula is a descriptive term usually used to identify the presence of an asymmetrically prominent medial scapular border at rest or with arm motion. The patient commonly has a deficit in shoulder function caused by the scapular instability. In the past, it was assumed that most incidences resulted from injury to a nerve supplying the scapula-stabilizing musculature or to an underlying neuromuscular problem such as muscular dystrophy.[33-35] Later research has shown that this biomechanical position or motion most frequently is associated with alterations in the supporting bony structure, the joints of the thoracoscapulohumeral complex, and/or in the strength, flexibility, activation sequencing, and attachment of the stabilizing musculature.[24] Therefore, the evaluation of a patient with a winged scapula must be sufficiently comprehensive to identify the factors causing the altered position and motion.

The exact frequency of neurologically based winging is poorly defined. The injury may be traumatic, iatrogenic, or idiopathic, and interpretation requires a careful patient history and examination. The long thoracic and spinal accessory nerves are most commonly involved. Long thoracic nerve injury and loss of serratus anterior muscle function lead to translation of the scapula superiorly and medially and disruption of normal scapulohumeral kinematics.

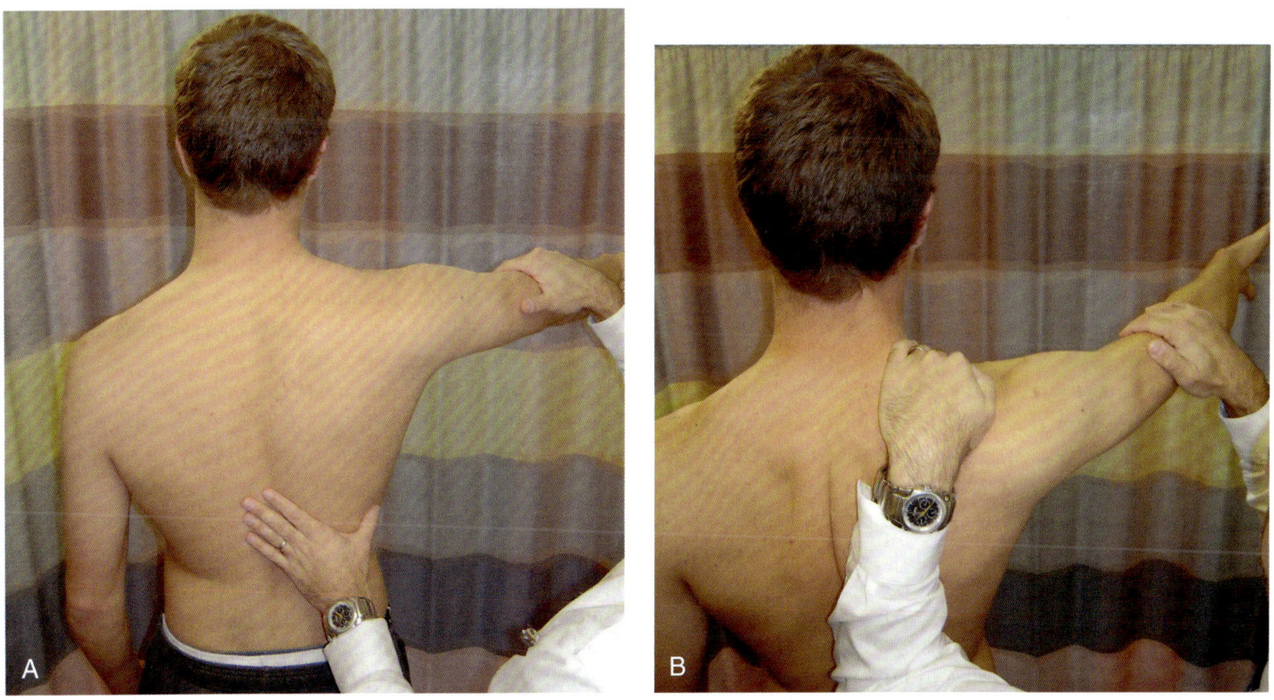

FIGURE 7 Photographs showing the scapular retraction test. **A**, The first component is manual muscle testing with the empty can maneuver. **B**, The second component is manual stabilization of the scapula, with the muscle test applied to the arm.

Clinically, this rotation causes the inferior angle to become notably prominent in both static and dynamic examination. The diagnosis can be confirmed on electromyography at approximately 6 weeks. The initial treatment includes observation with supportive care, rehabilitation, and possibly follow-up electromyography at 3-month intervals. Rehabilitation is focused on preserving glenohumeral motion and scapular stabilization by activating the rhomboids and lower trapezius. If there is no significant nerve recovery, maximal function is difficult to achieve because no other muscle can assume the roles of the serratus.

Surgery may be indicated for a patient with long thoracic nerve palsy after 1 year of symptoms and functional deficits, with no sign of recovery. Transfer of the sternocostal head of the pectoralis major has been the most successful procedure, with generally favorable results.[34] The selected portion of the tendon is reflected from its insertion on the humerus, tunneled ventral to the scapula, and attached to the inferior angle of the scapula by one of several techniques. The tendon length generally requires augmentation with fascia lata or other graft for length.

Scapular winging can result from injury to the spinal accessory nerve, which is susceptible to trauma from blunt force, traction, or penetrating injury. Iatrogenic injury can occur during lymph node biopsy or radical neck dissection. With loss of the trapezius activation, the scapula assumes a more inferior and lateral (drooping) posture. Winging often is less prominent than with serratus palsy, but atrophy in the upper trapezius, loss of muscle tone, and inability to shrug are easily discernible. Inability of the lower trapezius to achieve and maintain the retracted functional position of the scapula leads the patient to report pain and weakness with forward elevation and abduction. Compensatory muscle spasm in the rhomboids and levator scapulae are common. The diagnosis can be corroborated by electromyography, but the findings must be carefully interpreted. Occasionally, a false-negative report results from placement of the recording electrode in the normal underlying rhomboids instead of the thin, atrophic overlying trapezius. The treatment must be tailored to the particular cause; for neuritis or an idiopathic cause, supportive management and observation are recommended for as long as 1 year.

Surgery for spinal accessory nerve palsy surgery can be considered if nonsurgical management is unsuccessful. In the Eden-Lange transfer, which is intended to provide a dynamic medial and superior restraint, the levator scapula and rhomboids are transferred approximately 5 cm laterally and secured through drill holes to improve mechanical advantage and a substitute for trapezius function. Substantial improvement in average American Shoulder and Elbow Surgeons Disability Index and Constant Shoulder Scores have been reported.[36] A recent modification of the Eden Lange transfer, which involves a more superior transfer of the rhomboids and more closely replicates the direction of pull of the lower trapezius, has been shown to have superior outcomes.[37]

Snapping Scapula

Snapping scapula is a descriptive term for painful crepitus along the medial scapular border during arm motion. The symptoms traditionally were ascribed to osteochondromas or another bony pathology or to thickened bursitis in the thoracoscapular space, but more recent research found that alterations in normal SHR underlie most incidences of snapping scapula.[35,38] These alterations create increased compressive pressure along the medial border and contribute to the symptoms. The flexibility and strength of all surrounding musculature must be comprehensively evaluated to identify the causative factors.

The diagnosis and management of snapping scapula can be clinically challenging. Snapping scapula most frequently represents a disruption of the smooth gliding of the scapula over the thoracic cage and periscapular muscles. The normal coupled scapular motions of posterior tilt and external rotation are decreased as the arm elevates. Consequently, the normal movement of the instant center of rotation of the scapula from the superomedial border to the AC joint is disrupted, causing the scapula to rotate around the medial border, creating excessive pressure, and leading to symptoms.[24]

Patients generally report periscapular pain during overhead activities. The throwing motion, with its large scapular excursion, is particularly affected. Patients often notice an audible grinding or snapping, amplified by the thoracic cavity, which may be precipitated by the active range of motion or simply by shrugging. The superomedial border is most commonly cited as the location of pain. Because of the abnormal mechanics, the cause of crepitus is believed to be the chronically inflamed bursa. In a few patients, an anatomic abnormality such as osteochondromas or a malunited rib fracture disrupts the scapulothoracic articulation and creates a predisposition to snapping scapula.

The treatment of snapping scapula should begin with comprehensive nonsurgical management directed at the individual patient's etiologic factors. The cornerstone usually is physical therapy focused on proper postural and periscapular mechanics. The lower trapezius and serratus anterior are strengthened through isometric and dynamic endurance training. The contracted anterior muscles should be mobilized by massage and stretching. Activity modification and physical therapy modalities can be included. Scapular bracing treatment may be useful for some patients. Bursal inflammation can be treated using precise injections placed with appropriate technique and caution.

Surgery may be indicated for a patient who has undergone a thorough but unsuccessful program of nonsurgical management, is sufficiently disabled, and is willing to comply with postoperative care. Good success rates have been reported despite wide variance in techniques.[34,35] Both open and arthroscopic techniques have been successful, although there are concerns related to morbidity and cosmesis with open procedures. Arthroscopic techniques lead to more rapid recovery but are demanding and carry a greater neurovascular risk. With either technique, the surgeon can choose simple bursectomy or partial scapulectomy.

Impingement and Rotator Cuff Disease

Many studies have evaluated scapular kinematics in patients with rotator cuff weakness, rotator cuff tendinopathy or impingement, or rotator cuff tear. Most of these studies have found alterations in scapular kinematics.[39] It is not clear whether the observed dyskinesis is a cause, an effect, or a compensation for the pathology. If it is a cause, decreased upward rotation and posterior tilt may be altering the size of the subacromial space and changing rotator cuff clearance under the coracoacromial arch, producing mechanical abrasion and wear. Alternatively, increased anterior tilt and internal rotation may be creating glenoid antetilting during arm motion, predisposing the rotator cuff to internal impingement; or increased strain within the rotator cuff tendon because of decreased muscle activation may be increasing the observed apoptotic changes within the tendon cells. If the dyskinesis is an effect, probably there is an inhibitory effect of pain on individual muscle activation, a disruption of normal activation patterns, and an effect of pain avoidance on kinematic patterns.[39] One effect, the increased upward rotation in patients with rotator cuff tears, may represent a compensatory attempt to increase or maximize arm elevation or positioning in the face of weakened or absent rotator cuff activation. Whatever the relationship, scapular dyskinesis frequently is identified in rotator cuff disease and is associated with impaired function.

A positive SAT will show that the patient's excessive anterior scapular tilt is part of the pathophysiology producing external impingement symptoms. The treatment should include increasing the flexibility of the pectoralis minor and the short head of the biceps tendon as well as strengthening the serratus anterior as a scapular external rotator and the lower trapezius as a retractor. The scapular stability series of strengthening exercises is effective for achieving these goals (**Figure 6**). A positive SRT will show scapular involvement in the patient's muscle weakness; treatment is directed toward scapular stability in retraction, rather than the rotator cuff, as the first step in rehabilitation.

Labral Injury

Scapular dyskinesis was found to be associated with labral injury in one pathologic cascade model.[20] The altered position and motion of internal rotation and anterior tilt may change glenohumeral alignment, placing increased tensile strain on the anterior ligaments, increasing the peel-back of the biceps-labral complex on the glenoid, creating pathologic internal impingement, and weakening rotator cuff cocontraction strength. These effects are magnified in the presence of glenohumeral internal rotation deficit, which creates increased protraction because of the windup of the tight posterior structures during the follow-through phase of throwing. Evaluation of dyskinesis in a patient with suspected labral injury is key to rehabilitation. Elimination or reduction of the symptoms of pain found in the dynamic labral shear test can be frequently demonstrated by the SRT maneuver, which indicates that dyskinesis is part of the pathophysiology. Scapular rehabilitation is required to improve scapular retraction, including mobilization of tight anterior muscles and use of the scapular stability series of strengthening exercises. In addition, identification of scapular dyskinesis is an important part of preventing labral injury.

Acromioclavicular Joint Arthrosis and Injury

The bony components of the shoulder must be intact for optimal function. AC joint arthrosis with injury with resulting instability or high-grade AC separation alters the strut function of the clavicle on the scapula and changes the biomechanical screw axis of the SHR, allowing excessive scapular protraction and decreased dynamic acromial elevation when the arm is elevated.[5,24] This so-called third translation of the scapula allows the scapula to move in a inferomedial manner in relation to the clavicle, as is most often seen when a high-grade separation (type III to V) occurs. The protracted scapular position creates many of the dysfunctions associated with chronic AC separation, including impingement and decreased demonstrated rotator cuff strength. Scapular dyskinesis showing the third translation with arm elevation or forward flexion is a clinical examination finding that may help in determining the surgical treatment of a type III injury. Surgical treatment should be designed to reconstruct and reestablish the coupled AC joint function, which control scapular motion, and the restoration of the scapular position and motion should be one of the outcomes of the treatment.[40]

Clavicle Fracture

A fracture of the clavicle with a nonunion or shortened and rotated malunion alters the strut function and leads to a poor functional outcome. Muscle weakness and loss of range of motion are the functional deficiencies most often seen in association with a malunited or nonunited clavicle fracture.[23] The altered strut function of the clavicle allows excessive protraction of the scapula; this position limits rotator cuff function and the ability of the humerus to fully elevate. An assessment of scapular position in a patient with an acute or chronic fracture of the clavicle can help determine whether surgery is indicated for realigning the clavicular body and restoring the ability of the clavicle to serve as a strut.

Multidirectional Instability

One of the salient features of multidirectional instability is that symptoms and instability occur in the midranges of glenohumeral motion (where concavity-compression, bone alignment, and muscle activation play the most important roles), rather than at the end ranges of motion (where capsuloligamentous restraints are most important). Many patients with multidirectional instability simultaneously have increased protraction of the scapula and humeral head migration away from the center of the joint as the arm moves.[18,41] When the patient elevates the arm, the scapula deviates from the normal kinematic pattern of upward rotation, posterior tilting, and minimal internal rotation and instead follows a pattern of upward rotation, anterior tilting, and excessive internal rotation. This position allows the humeral head to translate inferiorly out of the glenoid socket, thus creating the instability. Inhibition of the subscapularis, lower trapezius, and serratus anterior, coupled with increased activation of pectoralis minor and latissimus dorsi, places the scapula in this protracted position.

In many patients with multidirectional instability, careful observation of the resting scapular position and the dynamic motion of the scapula with arm motion reveals protraction, especially in the positions associated with instability symptoms. By stabilizing the scapula in retraction, the SRT alters the glenoid position, decreases latissimus dorsi activation, and thereby decreases or eliminates the instability symptoms with arm motion. A positive SRT directs treatment toward strengthening the lower trapezius and serratus anterior and increasing the flexibility of the pectoralis minor and latissimus dorsi. The ability to achieve restoration of normal activation patterns accounts for the greater likelihood of successful rehabilitation in patients with multidirectional instability than in those with posttraumatic instability.

Rehabilitation of Scapular Dyskinesis

The three types of rehabilitation exercises for scapular control are proximal kinetic chain exercises to facilitate scapular muscle strength, flexibility exercises to minimize traction on scapular posture, and exercises specific for periscapular activation. Kinetic chain exercises for the trunk and hip start from and end at the ideal position of hip extension and trunk extension. Trunk and hip flexion-extension, rotation, and diagonal motions are included. The progressions include step up–step down and increasing weights. These exercises may be started before surgery when deficits have been identified and may be done while the shoulder is protected.

Flexibility exercises should focus on the anterior coracoid (pectoralis minor and biceps short head) and shoulder rotation. Tightness in these areas increases scapular protraction. The exercises include the open book and corner stretch for the coracoid muscles and the sleeper and cross-body stretches for shoulder rotation (**Figure 8**).

The goal of periscapular strengthening exercises should be to achieve a position of scapular retraction because this is the most effective position for maximizing scapular roles. Scapular retraction exercises may be done in a standing position to simulate normal activation sequences and allow kinetic chain sequencing. Scapular pinch and trunk extension–retraction exercises can be started early in rehabilitation while the shoulder is being protected because little tensile load or shear is imposed on the glenohumeral joint.

Several specific exercises are effective for activating the key scapular stabilizers (the lower trapezius and serratus anterior) and minimizing upper trapezius activation.[42] The low row, inferior glide, fencing, lawnmower, and robbery exercises, collectively called the scapular stability series, activate the target muscles to 18% to 30% of maximal activation[42] (**Figure 9**). This activation as well as arm angles limited to 90° abduction means that the scapular stability exercises are particularly effective during the early stages of rehabilitation after injury or surgery.

As healing progresses and loads can be applied to the shoulder, closed chain exercises also should be emphasized to restore the normal activations of the closed chain mechanism of the shoulder that stabilize the joint. In these exercises, the hand is supported on a stable or movable surface and the arm and scapula are loaded from distal to proximal. Rhythmic stabilization and wall washes are examples of closed chain exercises (**Figure 10**).

When scapular control is achieved, integrated scapula–rotator cuff exercises such as punches and shoulder dumps are added to stimulate rotator cuff activation from a stabilized scapula. These exercises can be done in various planes of abduction and flexion, with different amounts or types of resistance, and they can be modified to be sport specific.

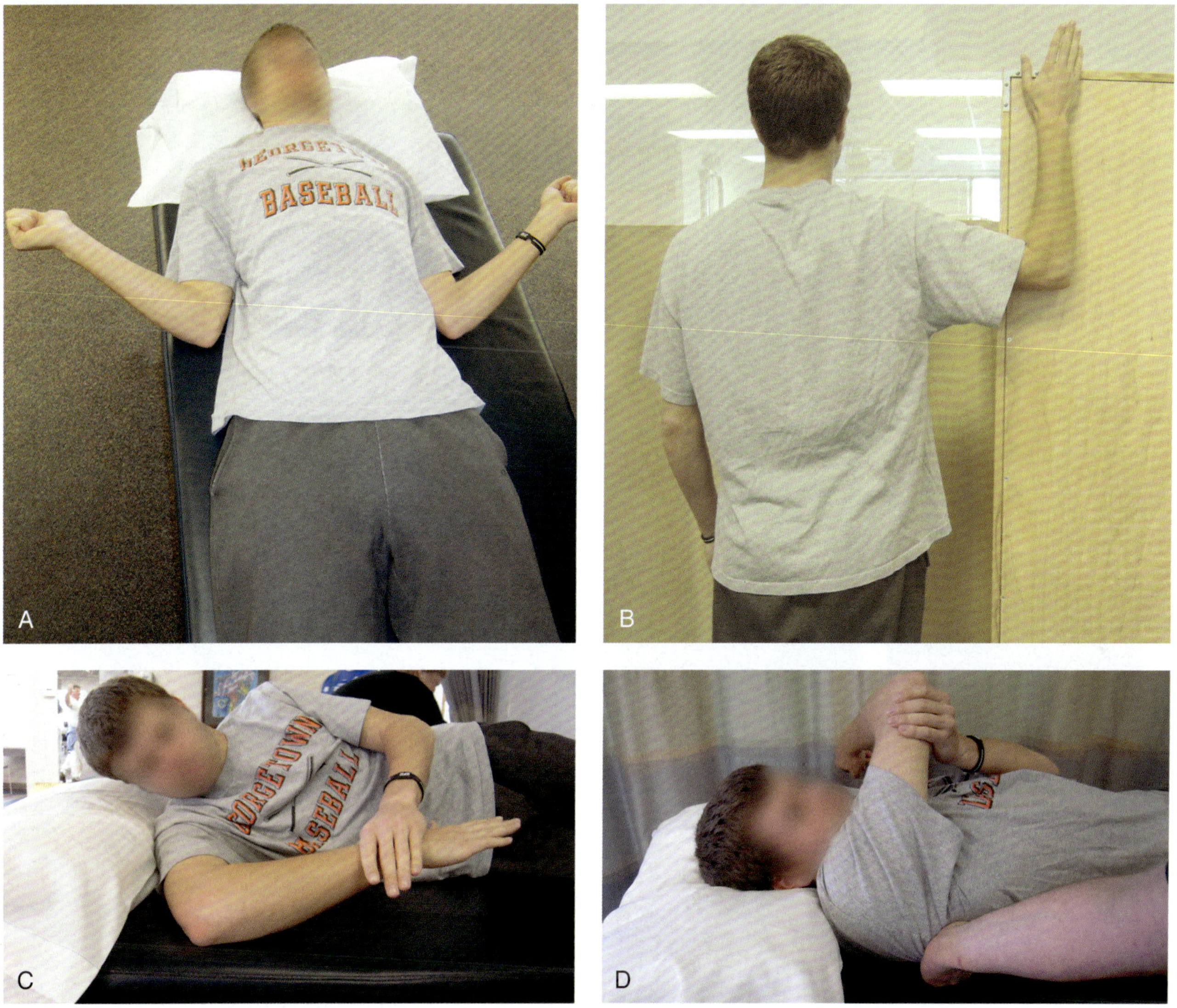

FIGURE 8 Photographs showing flexibility exercises. The open book stretch (**A**) and the corner stretch (**B**) for tight anterior soft-tissue structures. The sleeper stretch (**C**) and the cross-body stretch (**D**) for tight posterior rotator cuff muscles. The cross-body stretch is most effective when the scapula is stabilized.

Maximal integration of kinetic chain–scapula–shoulder coordination occurs when diagonal patterns of activation and loading are emphasized. Four-point, standing diagonal, and rotational exercises are used.

SUMMARY

The scapula is in a key position and plays a key role in all aspects of shoulder and arm function. Normal scapular kinematics places the glenohumeral joint in the most stable bony configuration, allows transfer of energy and force from the core to the hand, and maximizes muscle activation to move the arm and stabilize the joint.

Scapular dyskinesis, or alteration of the normal motion, is found in association with almost all shoulder pathology. It is not clear whether dyskinesis is a cause or an effect of the shoulder pathology, but dyskinesis frequently contributes to the clinical dysfunction, and therefore should be evaluated and treated as part of the comprehensive evaluation and treatment of the shoulder pathology.

Dyskinesis can be demonstrated by a clinically useful and reliable examination, and causative factors for dyskinesis can be identified. Treatment and rehabilitation protocols can then be developed to address the deficits demonstrated.

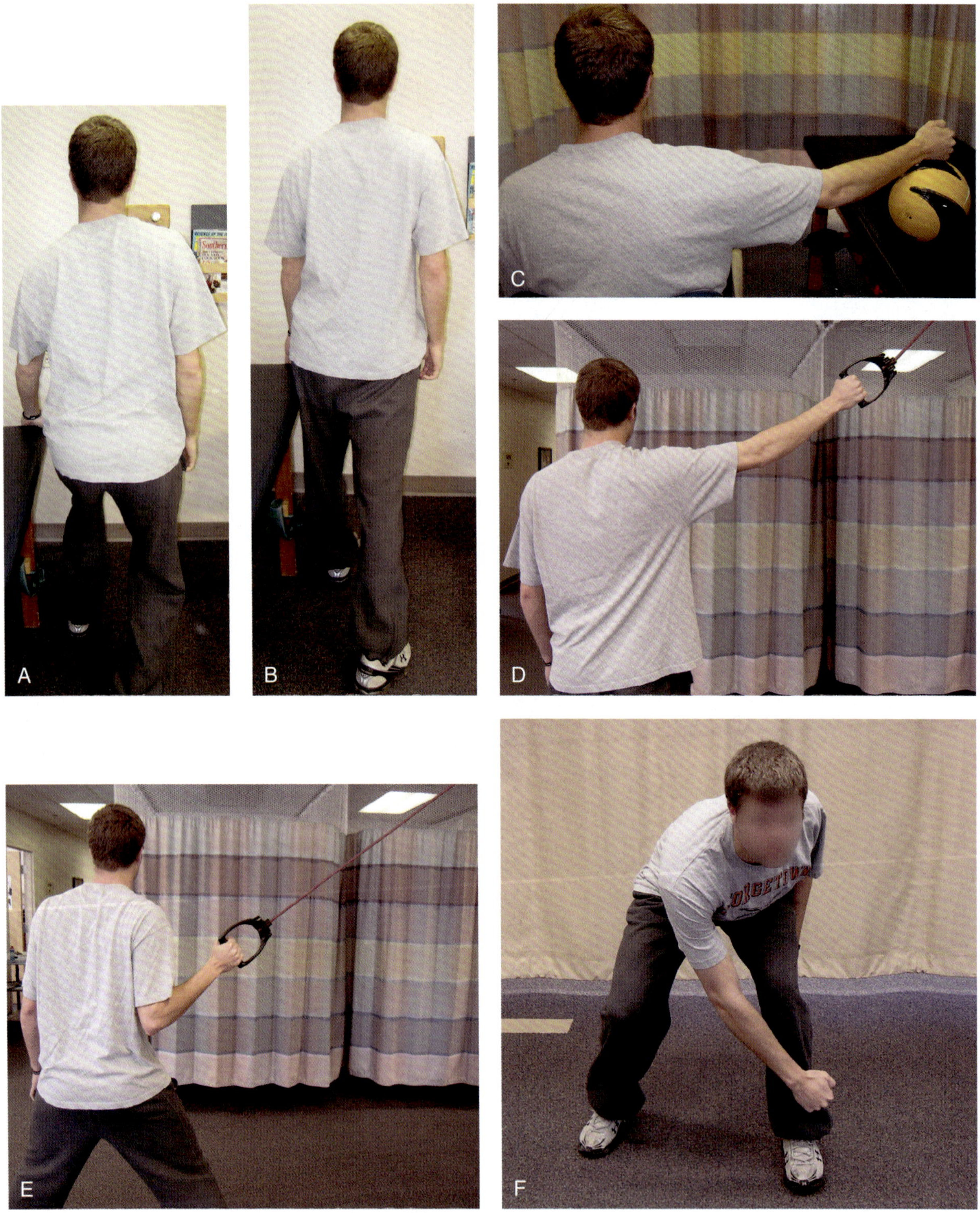

FIGURE 9 Photographs showing the scapular stability series of exercises. The low row in the starting position (**A**) and with extension of the hips and trunk to facilitate scapular retraction (**B**). The active inferior glide exercise, in which cocontraction of shoulder and scapular muscles helps depress the humerus and scapula (**C**). The fencing exercise in the starting position with the arm elevated above 90° in the frontal plane (**D**) and performed by side stepping and simultaneously retracting the scapula and adducting the arm (**E**). The lawnmower exercise begins with the patient standing (**F**) and continues the maneuver with extension of the hips and trunk followed by rotation of the trunk to facilitate scapular retraction (**G**); the lawnmower exercise is designed to integrate the lower extremity, trunk, and upper extremity. The robbery maneuver in the starting position, with the knees and trunk flexed and the arms held away from the body (**H**) and with extension of the hips and trunk and the patient instructed to attempt to place the elbows in the back pockets (**I**).

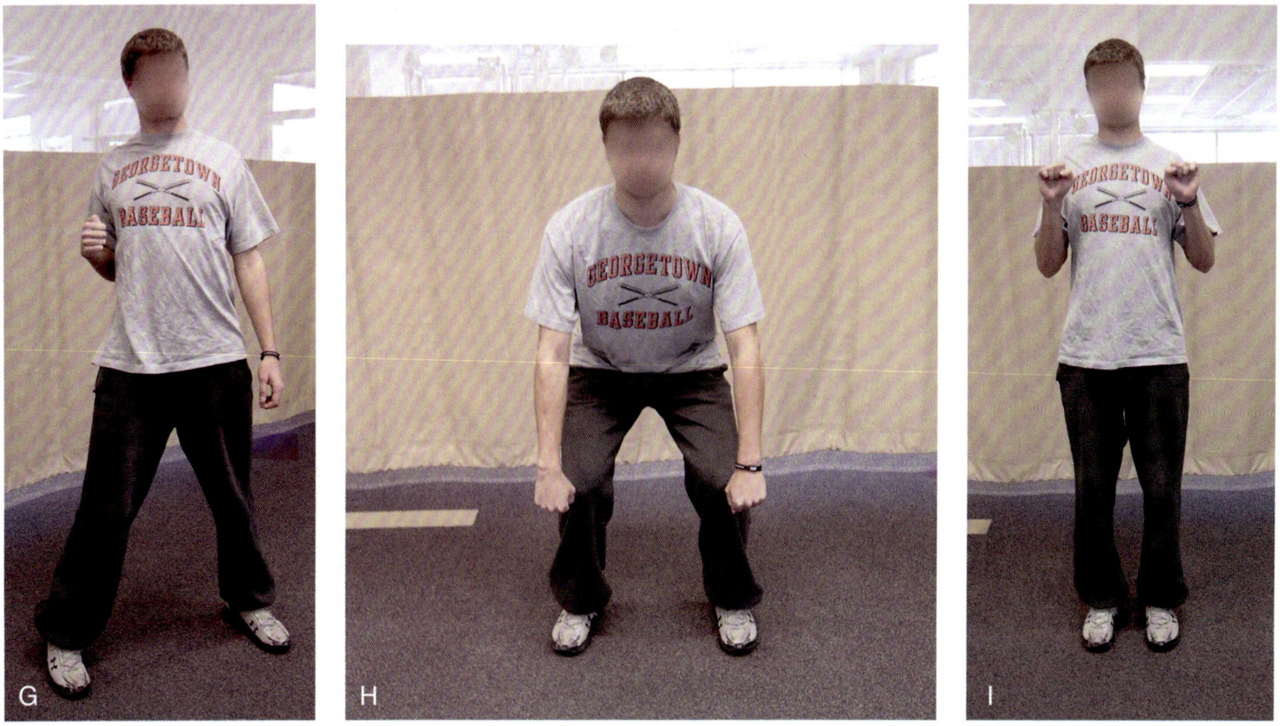

FIGURE 9 Cont'd

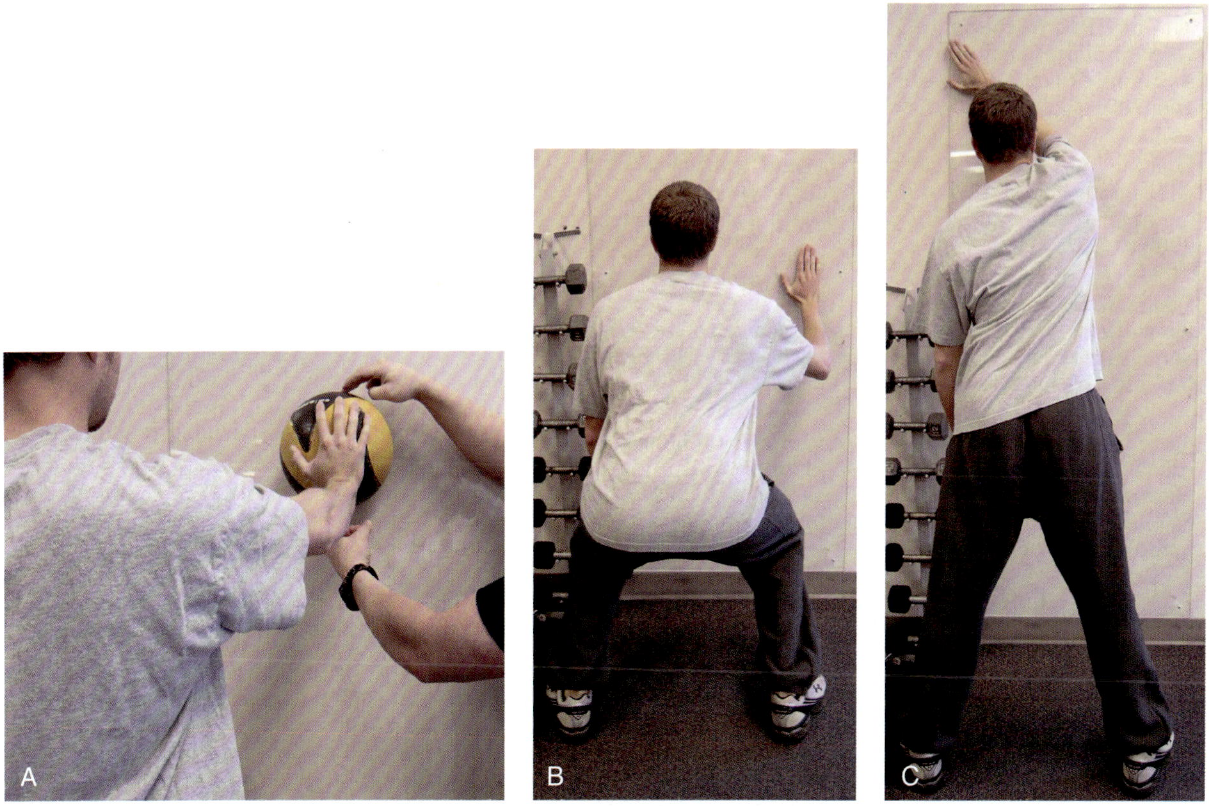

FIGURE 10 Photographs showing closed chain techniques, which aid in muscle reeducation and can be implemented in functional arm positions. **A,** Rhythmic stabilization is performed with the patient attempting to stabilize a ball while the clinician applies force from various directions. The wall wash exercise is closed chain by design where the patient begins in a half or full squat position with the hand of the involved arm on a wall. **B,** The patient stands using the legs and trunk to drive the arm through various ranges and planes of motion (**C**).

KEY STUDY POINTS

- Scapular dyskinesis occurs in a high percentage of shoulder injury.
- Dyskinesis can be a cause or an effect of the shoulder pathology, but should be managed as part of the comprehensive management.
- Clinical evaluation can be performed through an algorithm that can identify causative factors for the dyskinesis.
- Management should address the causative factors identified in the evaluation.

Annotated References

1. Bagg SD, Forrest WJ: Electromyographic study of the scapular rotators during arm abduction in the scapular plane. *Am J Phys Med Rehabil* 1986;65(3):111-124.

2. Bagg SD, Forrest WJ: A biomechanical analysis of scapular rotation during arm abduction in the scapular plane. *Am J Phys Med Rehabil* 1988;67:238-245.

3. McClure PW, Michener LA, Sennett BJ, Karduna AR: Direct 3-dimensional measurement of scapular kinematics during dynamic movements in vivo. *J Shoulder Elbow Surg* 2001;10:269-277.

4. Ludewig PM, Phadke V, Braman JP, Hassett DR, Cieminski CJ, LaPrade RF: Motion of the shoulder complex during multiplanar humeral elevation. *J Bone Joint Surg Am* 2009;91(2):378-389.

5. Sahara W, Sugamoto K, Murai M, Yoshikawa H: Three-dimensional clavicular and acromioclavicular rotations during arm abduction using vertically open MRI. *J Orthop Res* 2007;25:1243-1249.

6. Speer KP, Garrett WE: Muscular control of motion and stability about the pectoral girdle, in Matsen FA I II, Fu F, Hawkins RJ, eds: *The Shoulder: A Balance of Mobility and Stability*. Rosemont, IL, American Academy of Orthopaedic Surgeons, 1994, pp 159-173.

7. Cools AM, Dewitte V, Lanszweert F, et al: Rehabilitation of scapular muscle balance. *Am J Sports Med* 2007;35(10):1744-1751.

8. Smith J, Kotajarvi BR, Padgett DJ, Eischen JJ: Effect of scapular protraction and retraction on isometric shoulder elevation strength. *Arch Phys Med Rehabil* 2002;83:367-370.

9. Kibler WB, Sciascia AD, Dome DC: Evaluation of apparent and absolute supraspinatus strength in patients with shoulder injury using the scapular retraction test. *Am J Sports Med* 2006;34(10):1643-1647.

10. Tate AR, McClure P, Kareha S, Irwin D: Effect of the scapula reposition test on shoulder impingement symptoms and elevation strength in overhead athletes. *J Orthop Sports Phys Ther* 2008;38(1):4-11.

11. Solem Bertoft E, Thuomas KA, Westerberg CE: The influence of scapular retraction and protraction on the width of the subacromial space. An MRI study. *Clin Orthop Relat Res* 1993;(296):99-103.

12. Warner JJP, Micheli LJ, Arslanian LE, Kennedy J, Kennedy R: Patterns of flexibility, laxity, and strength in normal shoulders and shoulders with instability and impingement. *Am J Sports Med* 1990;18(4):366-375.

13. Warner JJP, Micheli LJ, Arslanian LE, Kennedy J, Kennedy R: Scapulothoracic motion in normal shoulders and shoulders with glenohumeral instability and impingement syndrome. *Clin Orthop Relat Res* 1992;(285):191-199.

14. Kibler WB, Sciascia AD: Current concepts: Scapular dyskinesis. *Br J Sports Med* 2010;44(5):300-305.

15. Burkhart SS, Morgan CD, Kibler WB: The disabled throwing shoulder: Spectrum of pathology. Part III: The SICK scapula, scapular dyskinesis, the kinetic chain, and rehabilitation. *Arthroscopy* 2003;19(6):641-661.

16. Kibler WB, Ludewig PM, McClure PW, Uhl TL, Sciascia AD: Scapula Summit 2009. *J Orthop Sports Phys Ther* 2009;39(11):A1-A13.

17. Cools AM, Witvrouw EE, DeClercq GA, Danneels LA, Cambier DC: Scapular muscle recruitment pattern: Trapezius muscle latency with and without impingement symptoms. *Am J Sports Med* 2003;31:542-549.

18. Ogston JB, Ludewig PM: Differences in 3-dimensional shoulder kinematics between persons with multidirectional instability and asymptomatic controls. *Am J Sports Med* 2007;35:1361-1370.

19. Michener LA, McClure PW, Karduna AR: Anatomical and biomechanical mechanisms of subacromial impingement syndrome. *Clin Biomech* 2003;18:369-379.

20. Burkhart SS, Morgan CD, Kibler WB: The disabled throwing shoulder: Spectrum of pathology. Part I: Pathoanatomy and biomechanics. *Arthroscopy* 2003;19(4):404-420.

21. Kibler WB, Sciascia A, Uhl T: Medial scapular muscle detachment: Clinical presentation and surgical treatment. *J Shoulder Elbow Surg* 2014;23(1):58-67.

    This article contains the surgical description and patient outcomes for patients undergoing surgical reattachment of detached lower trapezius and rhomboid muscles. Level of evidence: IV.

22. Kibler WB, Jacobs CA, Sciascia AD: Pain catastrophizing behaviors and their relation to poor patient-reported outcomes after scapular muscle reattachment. *J Shoulder Elbow Surg* 2018;27:1564-1571.

This article contains the long-term follow-up details of patients who underwent the scapular muscle reattachment procedure. A comparison was made between the patient outcomes and the presence of pain catastrophizing. Higher levels of catastrophizing led to significantly worse patient outcomes after surgery. Level of evidence: II.

23. McKee MD, Pedersen EM, Jones C, et al: Deficits following nonoperative treatment of displaced midshaft clavicular fractures. *J Bone Joint Surg Am* 2006;88:35-40.

24. Gumina S, Carbone S, Postacchini F: Scapular dyskinesis and SICK scapula syndrome in patients with chronic type III acromioclavicular dislocation. *Arthroscopy* 2009;25(1):40-45.

25. Kibler WB, Sciascia A, Wilkes T: Scapular dyskinesis and its relation to shoulder injury. *J Am Acad Orthop Surg* 2012;20(6):364-372.

26. Smith J, Dietrich CT, Kotajarvi BR, Kaufman KR: The effect of scapular protraction on isometric shoulder rotation strength in normal subjects. *J Shoulder Elbow Surg* 2006;15:339-343.

27. Uhl TL, Kibler WB, Gecewich B, Tripp BL: Evaluation of clinical assessment methods for scapular dyskinesis. *Arthroscopy* 2009;25(11):1240-1248.

28. Kibler WB, Ludewig PM, McClure PW, Michener LA, Bak K, Sciascia AD: Clinical implications of scapular dyskinesis in shoulder injury: The 2013 consensus statement from the "scapula summit". *Br J Sports Med* 2013;47:877-885.

    This consensus article on scapular function, dysfunction, evaluation, and treatment is the follow-up to the first published consensus report (see ref. 16). This current follow-up expanded on the research findings throughout the literature and discussed the role of the scapula within various types of shoulder pathologies. Level of evidence: V.

29. McClure PW, Tate AR, Kareha S, Irwin D, Zlupko E: A clinical method for identifying scapular dyskinesis. Part 1: Reliability. *J Athl Train* 2009;44(2):160-164.

30. Tate AR, McClure PW, Kareha S, Irwin D, Barbe MF: A clinical method for identifying scapular dyskinesis. Part 2: Validity. *J Athl Train* 2009;44(2):165-173.

31. Kibler WB: The role of the scapula in athletic function. *Am J Sports Med* 1998;26:325-337.

32. Rabin A, Irrgang JJ, Fitzgerald GK, Eubanks A: The intertester reliability of the scapular assistance test. *J Orthop Sports Phys Ther* 2006;36(9):653-660.

33. Kuhn J, Plancher K, Hawkins R: Scapular winging. *J Am Acad Orthop Surg* 1995;3:319-325.

34. Steinman S, Wood M: Pectoralis major transfer for serratus anterior paralysis. *J Shoulder Elbow Surg* 2003;12:555-560.

35. Kuhne M, Boniquit N, Ghodadra N, Romeo AA, Provencher MT: The snapping scapula: Diagnosis and treatment. *Arthroscopy* 2009;25(11):1298-1311.

36. Romero J, Gerber C: Levator scapulae and rhomboid transfer for paralysis of trapezius: The Eden-Lange procedure. *J Bone Joint Surg Br* 2003;85(8):1141-1145.

37. Elhassan BT, Wagner ER: Outcome of triple-tendon transfer, an Eden-Lange variant, to reconstruct trapezius paralysis. *J Shoulder Elbow Surg* 2015;24:1307-1313.

    This case series describes a modification to a traditional method of surgically transferring muscles to overcome neurologically derived scapular dysfunction. Level of evidence: IV.

38. Gaskill T, Millett PJ: Snapping scapula syndrome: Diagnosis and management. *J Am Acad Orthop Surg* 2013;21(4):214-224.

    This review article is a recent summation and iteration of snapping scapula, which encompasses the gamut of pathophysiology through management. Level of evidence: V.

39. Ludewig PM, Reynolds JF: The association of scapular kinematics and glenohumeral joint pathologies. *J Orthop Sports Phys Ther* 2009;39(2):90-104.

40. Kibler WB, Sciascia AD, Morris BJ, Dome DC: Treatment of symptomatic acromioclavicular joint instability by a docking technique: Clinical indications, surgical technique, and outcomes. *Arthroscopy* 2017;33:696-708.

    The benefits of anatomic reconstruction of high-grade AC injury is reviewed and buffetted by a modification of an accepted technique for reconstructing the coracoclavicular ligaments. This case series includes both reconstruction of the coracoclavicular ligaments and repair of the native AC ligaments as part of the same surgical procedures. The outcomes following surgery were positive. Level of evidence: IV.

41. Morris AD, Kemp GJ, Frostick SP: Shoulder electromyography in multidirectional instability. *J Shoulder Elbow Surg* 2004;13:24-29.

42. Kibler WB, Sciascia AD, Uhl TL, Tambay N, Cunningham T: Electromyographic analysis of specific exercises for scapular control in early phases of shoulder rehabilitation. *Am J Sports Med* 2008;36(9):1789-1798.

Chapter 45

Complex Regional Pain Syndrome of the Shoulder and Elbow

Mohammad A. Issa, MD • Paul J. Christo, MD, MBA

ABSTRACT

Complex regional pain syndrome (CRPS) is a debilitating neurologic condition with variable incidence and higher female prevalence reported in the literature, and rates of its occurrence in the upper extremity range from 2% to 5% after carpal tunnel surgery, 22% to 39% after distal radius fractures, and an even higher incidence in fractures treated with casting and closed reduction compared with percutaneous pinning. CRPS type I and type II differ only by the absence (type I) or presence (type II) of a specific nerve injury. Both are composed of a constellation of symptoms, including exaggerated pain accompanied by sensory, autonomic, motor, and trophic dysfunction.

The most common triggers are fractures, soft-tissue injuries (such as sprains, burns, cuts, or bruises), limb immobilization (such as the placement of a cast), and surgery. Multiple pathologic mechanisms likely play a role in the initiation and the propagation of CRPS including altered cutaneous innervation after injury, peripheral and central sensitization, inflammatory mediators, an altered sympathetic nervous system, and autoimmune etiologies.

CRPS is a complex disease that responds best to a multidisciplinary treatment approach involving physical/occupational therapy, pharmacologic, psychological, procedural interventions, and possibly surgery. The orthopaedic surgeon should be aware of CRPS implications preceding or following surgery of the shoulder and elbow to recognize and properly treat this debilitating illness. Through early recognition and intervention, orthopaedic surgeons can provide their patients with the best multimodal team-based approach and thereby the best chance for positive long-term outcomes.

Keywords: budapest diagnostic criteria; complex regional pain syndrome; multidisciplinary treatment; upper extremity surgery

Dr. Christo or an immediate family member serves as a paid consultant to or is an employee of Daiichi Sankyo and GlaxoSmithKline. Neither Dr. Issa nor any immediate family member has received anything of value from or has stock or stock options held in a commercial company or institution related directly or indirectly to the subject of this chapter.

Introduction

Complex regional pain syndrome (CRPS) is a rare, debilitating neurologic condition composed of a constellation of symptoms, including exaggerated pain accompanied by sensory, autonomic, motor, and trophic dysfunction.[1] It is commonly a limb-confined chronic pain condition that may be induced by minor injury, trauma, or surgery and clinically evolves following initial presentation. The condition may complicate a surgical procedure on an extremity by creating severe pain during the postoperative period. CRPS not only adversely affects quality of life but also is associated with large personal and societal healthcare costs.[2] It is imperative for the orthopaedic practitioner to both recognize and triage patients with CRPS for appropriate care; early treatment, including medication, physical and occupational therapy, and interventional pain management, is correlated with the best outcomes.

Definition and Epidemiology

CRPS is a term standardized by the International Society for the Study of Pain to bring together a disparate, idiosyncratic set of diagnostic schemes to describe the syndrome (previously referred to as shoulder-hand syndrome, reflex sympathetic dystrophy, causalgia, or algodystrophy).[1] The diagnostic criteria for CRPS include pain disproportional to any inciting event combined with signs and symptoms of sensory, vasomotor, sudomotor (sweat gland–stimulating), and motor/trophic changes[3,4] (**Tables 1** and **2**). CRPS types 1 and 2 are subdivisions of the syndrome based on the absence or the presence of identifiable nerve injury. It is important to ensure that there is no other diagnosis such

This chapter is adapted from Christo PJ, Wilhelmi BG: Complex regional pain syndrome of the shoulder and elbow, in Nicholson GP, ed: *Orthopaedic Knowledge Update: Shoulder and Elbow*, ed 4. Rosemont, IL, American Academy of Orthopaedic Surgeons, 2013, pp 599-611.

Table 1

International Society for the Study of Pain Orlando Criteria for Complex Regional Pain Syndrome

1. The presence of an initiating noxious event or a cause of immobilization
2. Continuing pain, allodynia, or hyperalgesia in which the pain is disproportionate to any known inciting event
3. Evidence at some time of edema, changes in skin blood flow, or abnormal sudomotor activity in the region of pain (can be a sign or a symptom)
4. Excludes the existence of other conditions that would otherwise account for the degree of pain and dysfunction

Data from Merskey H, Bogduk N: *Classification of Chronic Pain: Descriptions of Chronic Pain Syndrome and Definitions of Pain Terms*, ed 2. Seattle, WA, IASP Press, 1994.

as vascular compromise including deep vein thrombosis, infection, and nerve injury that can better explain the signs of symptoms before diagnosing a patient with CRPS.

There are few epidemiologic studies in which CRPS is defined by the agreed-on criteria, but a greater understanding of the epidemiologic effect of the disease appears likely in the future as a result of clarified diagnostic criteria. CRPS is a rare disease with an estimated annual incidence between 5.46 and 26.2 per 100,000 person-years and a prevalence of 20.7 to 26.2 per 100,000 persons.[5] One prospective study of 596 patients documented an incidence as high as 7% following a fracture when using the revised Budapest Criteria.[6] Multiple studies in literature have reported CRPS incidence ranging from 2% to 5% after carpal tunnel surgery, 22% to 39% after distal radius fractures, and an even higher incidence in fractures treated with casting and closed reduction compared with percutaneous pinning. Females are disproportionately affected, with a female-to-male ratio ranging from 2:3 to 5:1.[5] There is little agreement concerning the age demographic

Table 2

The Budapest Clinical Diagnostic Criteria for Complex Regional Pain Syndrome[a]

To make the clinical diagnosis, the following criteria must be met:

1. Continuing pain, which is disproportionate to any inciting event
2. Must report at least one symptom in three of the four following categories:
   - Sensory: Reports of hyperesthesia and/or allodynia
   - Vasomotor: Reports of temperature asymmetry and/or skin color changes and/or skin color asymmetry
   - Sudomotor/edema: Reports of edema and/or sweating changes and/or sweating asymmetry
   - Motor/trophic: Reports of decreased range of motion and/or motor dysfunction (weakness, tremor, dystonia) and/or trophic changes (hair, nail, skin)
3. Must display at least one sign at time of evaluation in two or more of the following categories:
   - Sensory: Evidence of hyperalgesia (to pinprick) and/or allodynia (to light touch and/or temperature sensation and/or deep somatic pressure and/or joint movement)
   - Vasomotor: Evidence of temperature asymmetry (>1°C) and/or skin color changes and/or asymmetry
   - Sudomotor/edema: Evidence of edema and/or sweating changes and/or sweating asymmetry
   - Motor/trophic: Evidence of decreased range of motion and/or motor dysfunction (weakness, tremor, dystonia) and/or trophic changes (hair, nail, skin)
4. No other diagnosis better explains the signs and symptoms

[a]CRPS is described as an array of painful conditions that are characterized by a continuing (spontaneous and/or evoked) regional pain that is seemingly disproportionate in time or degree to the usual course of any known trauma or other lesion. The pain is regional (not in a specific nerve territory or dermatome) and usually has a distal predominance of abnormal sensory, motor, sudomotor, vasomotor, and/or trophic findings. The syndrome shows variable progression over time.

Data from Harden RN, Bruehl S, Perez RS, et al: Validation of proposed diagnostic criteria (the "Budapest Criteria") for complex regional pain syndrome. *Pain* 2010;150(2):268-274.

with the greatest disease burden.[6] The disease appears to have a less severe clinical course when experienced at an older age of onset.[7] Although an individual health center's data or even multicenter epidemiologic data on CRPS are difficult to obtain, new instruments such as electronic web-based surveys or advocacy group websites may provide increased power to future studies.[7]

Pathophysiology

Although the exact mechanisms of CRPS have yet to be discovered, the scientific understanding of the pathophysiologic basis of the syndrome has increased greatly over the past decade.[8] Research has led to the theory that multiple pathologic mechanisms likely play a role in the initiation and the propagation of CRPS, and the variable expression of these mechanisms in various patients (and within the same patient over time) account for differences in clinical presentation.[1]

A neuronal injury trigger, however imperceptible, has been implicated with the development of CRPS (including CRPS type 1) and is part of the revised diagnostic criteria.[8] This trigger appears to alter the peripheral nervous system, given that patients with CRPS demonstrate fewer C-type and Aδ-type cutaneous afferent nerve fibers within the affected region as opposed to nonaffected regions of the body. Trauma to a limb also causes the peripheral nerves to increase the release of the neuropeptides substance P, bradykinin, and glutamate, which sensitize and increase the activity of local peripheral and secondary central nociceptive neurons and increase pain.

Repetitive stimulation and sensitization of nociceptors in the peripheral nervous system lead to changes in central nervous system (CNS) nociceptive processing. Patients with CRPS demonstrate windup, or increased excitability of wide-dynamic range central neurons. The windup of central sensitization is thought to be responsible for pain in response to nonnoxious stimuli (allodynia) and increased pain from noxious stimuli (hyperalgesia). Several mapping techniques of cortical brain activity, including functional MRI (fMRI), have demonstrated cortical reorganization in patients with CRPS.[9] These studies have shown a reduction in the distance between discrete activation areas of the thumb and the fifth finger in the brain cortex in response to tactile stimulation as well as decreased widespread cortical brain activation in response to pin-prick hyperalgesia and mechanical allodynia.[9] Follow-up of patients with cortical changes demonstrated a reversal of changes in patients who experienced a reduction of pain through therapy. These findings suggest that induced CNS changes may be responsible for reduced tactile discrimination and enhanced pain signaling seen in CRPS.

The clinical presentation of the acute phase of CRPS stimulates hypotheses about the role that inflammatory pathways play in the development of the syndrome.[10] The initial warm, erythematous, and edematous extremity is likely caused by plasma and protein extravasation accompanied by vasodilation. These tissue processes may be induced by proinflammatory cytokines such as interleukins-1β, -2, -6, and tumor necrosis factor α as well as the neuropeptides calcitonin gene-related peptide, bradykinin, and substance P. Studies of patients with CRPS have demonstrated increased proinflammatory cytokines in blister fluid, plasma, and cerebrospinal fluid. Proinflammatory neuropeptides may play a specific role in inflammatory pain because they not only directly increase nociceptive firing but also stimulate vasodilation, protein extravasation, and further release of other proinflammatory cytokines.

Sympathetic nervous system dysfunction has long been theorized to be a core component of CRPS pathophysiology.[8] During the acute or warm phase of clinical presentation, the affected limb is vasodilated and fails to vasoconstrict with cold stimuli, and sweating is often decreased. The limb concomitantly demonstrates decreased circulating plasma levels of norepinephrine. In time, transition to the chronic or cold phase of clinical presentation is that of vasoconstriction and sweating, even in the presence of decreased circulating plasma norepinephrine levels. This presentation suggests that adrenergic receptors are upregulated during the transition from acute to chronic disease, and the limb becomes hyperreactive to adrenergic stimulation in the chronic phase. Pain experienced by patients with CRPS also appears to be sympathetically mediated because stimuli such as cold or extreme emotion aggravate the pain experienced, and sympathetic blockade has been demonstrated to provide pain relief. Animal studies demonstrating adrenergic receptor expression on nociceptive fibers following nerve trauma have fueled speculation that such receptor expression in humans may be the mechanism of sympathetically mediated pain.

Research on predisposing factors that could predict which patients are susceptible to CRPS continues.[8] Recent genetic research on familial cases of CRPS has focused on the HLA molecules on the major histocompatibility complex gene and promoter regions of the tumor necrosis factor α inflammatory cytokines. Additional research has focused on the genetic inhibition of the successful transcription of angiotensin-converting enzyme, which aids in the degradation of bradykinin. No genetic factors have yet been proven to be a definitive link to CRPS.

Studies of the serum of patients with CRPS have demonstrated the presence of autoantibodies directed against surface antigens found on autonomic neurons.[10]

In a small pilot trial, the authors of a 2010 study demonstrated that intravenous immunoglobulin treatment can lead to a significant reduction in pain symptoms of patients with CRPS when compared with placebo.[11] These findings were not replicated in the subsequent randomized controlled trial (RCT), and low-dose intravenous immunoglobulin therapy for 6 weeks did not show effectiveness in relieving pain in patients with moderate to severe CRPS of 1 to 5 years duration.[12]

More recent in vivo and in vitro studies propose a role for functionally active noninflammatory autoantibodies[13,14] and indicate that immune therapies, which can either directly reduce autoantibody plasma levels or target lymphocytes,[15,16] may have a role in the treatment of CRPS. These findings, along with the potential of predisposing HLA genotypes, support the belief that CRPS has an autoimmune pathology.

Psychopathologic factors also have been examined for their role in the predisposition or propagation of CRPS because of the prevalence of anxiety and depression within this population.[8] No definitive causation has yet been demonstrated.

Clinical Features

CRPS is a clinical entity that has historically been described as an evolution of stages.[17] A study published in 2009, however, demonstrated more of a variable initial clinical presentation and variety in the subsequent clinical course among patients.[7] Despite this, the use of the classically described stages may someday provide phenotypic subgrouping for treatment tailored to the patient's current pathology and symptoms.[7]

Following neurologic injury, the most common initial presentation of CRPS is considered the acute or warm stage, in which the limb experiences exaggerated pain (both allodynia and hyperalgesia), warmth, erythema, decreased sweating, and extra-articular edema.[17] The second stage is the intermediate dystrophic stage, in which increased pain, sensory dysfunction, and continued evidence of vasomotor dysfunction are accompanied by significant motor and trophic changes (skin becomes glossy or thickened, nails become thickened or striated, and hair growth increases or decreases).[17] The third stage is the chronic, cold, or atrophic stage typified by decreased blood flow to the affected limb, thinning skin, muscle atrophy, decreased joint range of motion and contractures, and demineralization of bone[17] (**Figure 1**).

The onset of CRPS symptoms follows a neurologic insult that may result from mechanical, thermal, chemical, or ischemic events.[18] It is difficult for a surgeon to predict which upper extremity procedures are more likely to initiate CRPS, but any surgery or injury to the upper extremity could be considered a potential inciting event. Initial symptoms include temperature differences, edema, skin color or texture variations, sweat alterations, hair or nail texture changes, and motor weakness. Almost all individuals with CRPS experience constant pain with a burning, tearing, stinging, aching, or throbbing quality.[7] Exacerbations of constant pain occur with physical and emotional stress, cold weather, movement of the affected limb, and work. The pain is associated with the signs and the symptoms that define the disease, namely hypersensitivity (both allodynia and hyperalgesia), temperature differences, and swelling. Evolution of the clinical symptoms experienced by patients is common. The location

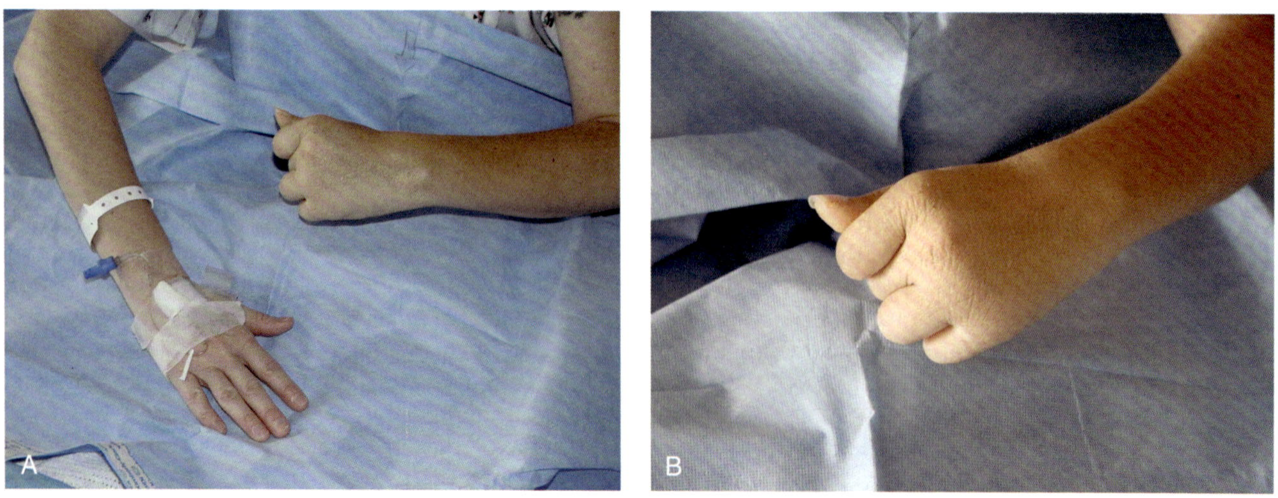

FIGURE 1 **A** and **B**, Photographs showing a hand with cold-type complex regional pain syndrome. Contractures, changes in skin color, muscle wasting, and trophic changes to skin and nails are seen.

and the extent of pain in an affected area tends to spread following the onset of symptoms. Clinical symptoms experienced also evolve as hypersensitivity, temperature differences, color variation, and swelling may decrease whereas motor weakness and disability of the affected limb may increase. There are patients in whom symptoms have been reported to resolve, but many of those experiencing resolution may experience subsequent relapse.

Approximately one-third of patients may suffer from sympathetically mediated pain, which is pain that is exacerbated by the increased release of catecholamines from the sympathetic nervous system.[19] The proposed mechanism is a pathologic coupling of the somatic afferent system and sympathetic nervous system, as discussed previously. These patients will experience pain triggered by cold, light mechanical stimulation, and emotional arousal. Sympathetically mediated pain has been a symptom of special interest in CRPS because of the possibility of either medical or surgical sympatholysis to provide relief.

The individual psychological, social, and financial toll of CRPS is substantial.[7] Pain negatively affects sleep, mobility, self-care, and activities of daily living. The disease is costly to diagnose and treat; an average patient will see more than four physicians before diagnosis and may undergo expensive diagnostic testing before establishing the diagnosis and the therapy plan. The costs of care are more difficult to bear because patients typically suffer loss of income due to impaired job performance and frequent unemployment. Psychiatric illness including anxiety and depression is common, and suicidal ideation may be reported in up to one-half of affected individuals at one point during the course of their disease.

Evaluation of the Patient Suspected of Having Upper Extremity CRPS

Orthopaedic practitioners are asked to evaluate upper extremity pain of various etiologies, and the ability to recognize the CRPS diagnostic pattern and initiate basic treatment is an important skill. CRPS is a rare diagnosis that may have subtle initial signs. A high index of suspicion is necessary in the setting of exaggerated pain following a recognized noxious event (such as trauma or surgery) or peripheral nerve injury. CRPS is a clinical diagnosis; therefore, a complete history and physical examination documenting the signs and the symptoms of CRPS provide the basis of diagnosis. Diagnostic testing provides additional evidence of the sequelae of CRPS, but it is more often useful in ruling out other pathology.

The physical examination of an upper extremity for signs of CRPS is an evaluation aimed at distinguishing expected inflammatory, neurologic, and orthopaedic changes from injury or surgery from those indicating a likely case of CRPS. The clinician should always have a high index of suspicion for CRPS when examining patients after an upper extremity injury or surgical procedure when the patient is describing disproportionate pain severity or a failure of pain to improve as predicted. Orthopaedic surgeons should conduct a full neurologic examination of the extremity, documenting sensory deficits, motor weakness, edema, spontaneous pain, or allodynia. Orthopaedic evaluation should document range of motion of joints proximal and distal to the injury and joint deformity. Limbs should be compared for asymmetric skin color or texture and hair or nail patterns, and changes in sweat patterns (an abnormally dry limb) should be questioned.

One of the simplest diagnostic tests for CRPS is the application of ice to the affected limb. The arm affected by CRPS is frequently sensitive to cold, and cooling the affected limb produces an increase in burning pain.[1] The use of the ice test is a simple, quick, in-office diagnostic test that should be performed during a first evaluation.

Electromyography and nerve conduction velocity studies quantify the amplitude and the transmission speed of neuronal signaling. Neurologic conditions such as diabetic peripheral neuropathy, ulnar nerve entrapment, myasthenia gravis, and Lambert-Eaton syndrome may be differentiated from CRPS on the basis of electromyography/nerve conduction velocity studies. Nerve injury after shoulder or elbow surgery, even if just neurapraxia, can initiate CRPS, and these individuals should be considered at risk after the nerve injury is appreciated by the clinician.

Radiographs are typically used to evaluate limb pain and may reveal osteopenia in chronic CRPS. CT or MRI of the cervical spine may reveal other causes of upper extremity neuropathic pain, including cervical stenosis or radiculopathy.[7] MRI of the painful limb may reveal brachial plexopathy, adhesive capsulitis, or other neurologic injury. MRI of the affected limb may demonstrate soft-tissue or marrow edema from acute CRPS, or the atrophy associated with chronic CRPS.

A variety of methods have been used to measure autonomic and sudomotor dysfunction in the patient with CRPS. Infrared thermography involves the use of infrared cameras to produce color mapping of the temperature of the skin of the affected limb for comparison with the unaffected limbs and normative control limbs.[20] A difference in temperature of 1°C between the affected and unaffected limbs is considered significant. A second quantitative test used in assessing sudomotor sweat production is the quantitative sudomotor axon reflex test. This test compares sweat produced following the topical application of a sweat-inducing agent, such as acetylcholine.

Sympathetically mediated pain is suggestive of but not necessary for a diagnosis of CRPS. Intravenous regional blockade with α-adrenergic receptor antagonists or local anesthetic blockade of the stellate ganglion, lumbar sympathetic chain, or thoracic sympathetic chain that relieves pain is considered a positive test for sympathetically mediated pain.

Triple phase bone scan is a series of radiographic images taken in a timed sequence following the injection of a radionuclide tracer.[20] The series demonstrates arterial blood, regional blood pooling, and bone uptake of the tracer in sequential fashion. Increased periarticular uptake of the tracer is associated with the acute phase of CRPS. This finding occurs as a result of increased blood flow and bone turnover during the acute phase of the disease. This scan can supplement rather than establish the diagnosis of CRPS.

Despite the potential benefits of diagnostic testing, diagnostic tests should be considered supplemental information to establishing a definitive diagnosis.[20] A 2007 prospective analysis of 158 patients for the first 16 weeks following a radial fracture found that thermography, plain radiographs, MRI, and triple phase bone scan lacked sufficient sensitivity and specificity to provide appropriate positive predictive value or negative predictive value for diagnosis[20] (**Table 3**).

Management

CRPS is a complex disease likely consisting of several pathologic mechanisms; therefore, multidisciplinary management involves physical, pharmaceutical, psychological, and possibly surgical/procedural intervention[2,3,23,26-49] (**Table 4**). All practitioners should strive to establish rapport with patients early because building a long-term strategy for intervention will be based on trust in the patient-physician relationship. Management is focused on the restoration of extremity function. Early initiation of CRPS therapy is a key component of an effective treatment strategy. Early range of motion of joints not affected directly by the surgery (eg, the elbow, the wrist, and fingers in the case of shoulder procedures) should be encouraged. Patients who delay treatment for longer than 6 months have a poorer long-term prognosis, and it is generally believed that early-stage CRPS symptoms may be reversible.[41]

Physical and Occupational Therapy

Physical medicine, including physical and occupational therapy, is a core component of rehabilitation designed to ensure positive functional outcomes. Pain can create a barrier of fear in the patient with CRPS who is attempting to use the affected limb (a condition known as kinesophobia). The goals of physical and occupational therapy

Table 3

Sensitivity, Specificity, Positive Predictive Value, and Negative Predictive Value of Selected Diagnostic Procedures Following Distal Radial Fracture

	Sensitivity (%)	Specificity (%)	Positive Predictive Value (%)	Negative Predictive Value (%)
2 wk after trauma				
Thermography	45	50	17	79
8 wk after trauma				
Thermography	50	67	26	85
Radiography—bilateral	36	94	58	86
MRI	43	78	31	85
Triple phase bone scan (TPBS)	19	96	58	86
16 wk after trauma				
Thermography	29	89	38	84
MRI	13	98	60	83
TPBS	14	100	100	83

Reproduced with permission from Schurmann M, Zaspel J, Löhr P, et al: Imaging in early posttraumatic complex regional pain syndrome: A comparison of diagnostic methods. *Clin J Pain* 2007;23(5):449-457. doi:10.1097/AJP.0b013e31805c9e66.

Table 4

Treatment Strategies for Complex Regional Pain Syndrome (CRPS) and Available Evidence

Treatment Class	Methods	Evidence
Pharmacologic (oral, intravenous, and transdermal)[21-35]	Varied	See **Table 5.**
Physical and occupational therapy[3,18]	Contrast baths Stress loading Isometric exercises Hot and cold water soaks Edema stockings	Physical therapy and occupational therapy provide improved quality of life and function to the affected limb.
Psychological therapy[36]	Relaxation Biofeedback	Insufficient evidence of efficacy for recommendation, but expert opinion encourages treatment of nonorganic contributions to chronic pain.
Sympathetic blockade and regional anesthesia[37-41]	Stellate ganglion block Interscalene block	Small retrospective studies demonstrate benefit when paired with physical therapy.
Intravenous regional blocks[42]	Guanethidine Lidocaine Clonidine Droperidol Reserpine	No evidence of benefit demonstrated when compared with placebo.
Neuromodulation[43-46]	Spinal cord stimulator Dorsal root ganglion stimulator Repetitive ttranscranial magnetic stimulation (rTMS) Transcutaneous electrical nerve stimulation (TENS)	Provides pain reduction and improved quality of life in carefully selected patients with refractory disease who have undergone successful trial stimulation. Noninvasive brain stimulation technique, which could have therapeutic utility (ongoing prospective studies). Insufficient evidence of efficacy for the use of TENS in CRPS.
Intrathecal medications[47-49]	Baclofen	Some evidence of efficacy for CRPS-related dystonia and improvement of function.
Surgical ablation[32,50]	Surgical sympathectomy Radiofrequency sympathectomy Chemical sympathectomy	Insufficient evidence of efficacy for pain relief in CRPS. Anecdotal reports of pain relief but with documented incidents of new neuropathic pain following sympathectomy.

are to overcome this fear of pain and return the patient to the best functional use of the limb. To accomplish this, physical therapists develop an incremental program designed to desensitize the affected limb and increase range of motion, flexibility, posture, and muscle strength.[3] Common modalities include contrast baths, alternating hot and cold water soaks, isometric exercises, and stress loading.[13] Occupational therapists encourage everyday use of the limb in activities of daily living. Specialized garments or wrappings may be enlisted to reduce edema and sensory overload of the affected limb. All physical medicine should allow for incremental increases in stress and patient breaks as needed to prevent catastrophic pain.

Graded motor imagery in the form of mirror box therapy has demonstrated promise in reducing neuropathic pain. This therapeutic technique utilizes a mirror to create a reflection of the unaffected limb (healthy limb) and serves as a healthy illusion for the affected limb by tricking the brain into believing that movement has occurred and without pain.

Psychological Therapy

The emotional burden of unrelieved chronic pain despite best therapeutic interventions creates a need for psychological therapy in the CRPS population.[33] At minimum, a patient with a new CRPS diagnosis should have a discussion with a psychological care provider to outline what is known about the pathophysiology and the course of the disease process and explain the need for active self-management and participation in a care plan. Psychological therapy is designed to reconstruct dysfunctional cognitive patterns and behaviors about CRPS pain into thought patterns that facilitate rehabilitation (cognitive-behavioral therapy). Further goals include skills in relaxation and biofeedback to be implemented when pain exacerbations occur. Assessment and treatment of concomitant axis I disorders, such as major depression, generalized anxiety disorder, or posttraumatic stress disorder, are important because these disorders complicate the goal of return to function.

Pharmacologic Therapy

Pharmacotherapy for CRPS is used in situations where the severity of pain is limiting participation in functional rehabilitation. The evidence for the use of pharmacologic agents is limited by a lack of prospective RCTs.[21] Clinicians are currently guided by available clinical trial data on CRPS and data from RCTs in neuropathic pain conditions to guide a sequential trial of medications.

Corticosteroids and NSAIDs have been used to treat the inflammation associated with CRPS. Randomized clinical trials have demonstrated that an oral regimen of corticosteroids has a clinically positive effect when taken during the acute phase following insult.[22] The only controlled trial of corticosteroids used in CRPS treatment trialed 30 mg oral prednisone daily (10 mg, three times daily) for up to 12 weeks.[22] In open trials, clinicians trialed initial doses of 40 to 60 mg oral prednisone with rapid taper over 4 weeks.[23] No studies have provided significant decrement of neuropathic pain from NSAIDs.[21]

Antioxidants have been used based on the perception that oxygen-free radicals created by inflammation may be a key component of CRPS propagation. A trial of vitamin C following a wrist fracture was found to lessen the incidence of postfracture CRPS development.[24] Yet, an RCT on the use of vitamin C after distal radial fractures showed no benefit to patients at 1 year.[25] Dimethyl sulfoxide and *N*-acetylcysteine have been demonstrated to provide significant pain relief in prospective trials when applied topically for 17 and 52 weeks.[26]

Anticonvulsant medications, such as gabapentin and pregabalin, have good evidence for effectiveness in neuropathic pain disorders, and this has prompted their use in CRPS. One prospective study of gabapentin in CRPS type 1 failed to provide significant benefit in pain reduction with this population, but sensory deficits improved.[27] A second study demonstrated a significant reduction of spontaneous and provoked pain in patients with CRPS with a mean disease duration of 2.7 months.[28]

Upregulation of inflammatory pathways sensitizes excitatory nociceptive pathways that use *N*-methyl-D-aspartic acid as a neurotransmitter.[29] Ketamine, an *N*-methyl-D-aspartic acid receptor blocker, is an attractive medication for the possible reversal of central sensitization and alteration of neural plasticity. Subanesthetic intravenous infusions, ketamine-induced comas, and topical ketamine ointments have proven effective at reducing numeric pain scores, although the duration of the effect remains uncertain.[29] Topical and subanesthetic ketamine currently have good if not stronger support and are much less intrusive.[23]

Adrenergic antagonists, such as phenoxybenzamine and phentolamine, have been used in the treatment of CRPS to block sympathetically mediated pain. Studies of oral use of adrenergic antagonists have shown promise in relieving pain based on retrospective review, but further prospective study is needed.[30] Intravenous regional phentolamine may be useful in the diagnosis of sympathetically mediated pain, though it is rarely used clinically anymore. Topically applied clonidine, an α-2 adrenergic agonist, has been demonstrated to relieve localized hyperalgesia in patients with sympathetically mediated pain.[31]

During CRPS progression, localized bone resorption occurs in the affected limb and is observable through triple phase bone scan (described previously). Diphosphonates and calcitonin have their clinical effect through the inhibition of the osteoclast bone resorption.[32] The use of diphosphonate therapy has proven to be superior to placebo for the relief of subjective pain as shown in a recently published systematic literature review and meta-analysis.[33] A study of 82 CRPS patients demonstrated significant and persistent reductions in pain after treatment with infusions of neridronic acid.[34] Calcitonin, however, has generated conflicting data with regard to its ability to reduce average pain scores.[32]

Opioid therapy for the treatment of CRPS may be needed if other treatments fail and is a topic of debate among physicians. Although potentially useful in the acute phases of tissue injury, the long-term use of opioids for either peripheral or central neuropathic pain may be less efficacious or at minimum would require large dosages.[35] At higher doses, adverse effects such as tolerance, addiction, immunosuppression, or endocrine dysfunction may become more prevalent[22-27,32,42,47-49,51-57] (**Table 5**).

Table 5

Pharmacologic Treatments of Complex Regional Pain Syndrome (CRPS)

Pharmaceutical	Mechanism of Action	Dosage Range Studied	Evidence for Effectiveness
Anti-inflammatory medications			
Corticosteroids[22,23]	Reduction in transcription of inflammatory cytokines	Oral prednisone 10 mg PO TID Methylprednisolone 32 mg PO QID × 14 d with 14-d taper	Improvement on CRPS rating scale Improvement on CRPS rating scale at 6 mo follow-up
Parecoxib[44]	Inhibition of cyclooxygenase 2 Reduction of prostaglandin formation	5 mg IV in combination with 1 mg/kg lidocaine/30 mg clonidine IV regional block once per week × 3 wk	Reduction in daily rescue medication and VAS pain score compared with control subjects
Free-radical scavengers			
Vitamin C[24]	Free-radical scavenging	500 mg PO daily × 50 d	Reduction in incidence of CRPS
DMSO[26]	Free-radical scavenging	50% DMSO cream topically to the affected area 5 times daily × 52 wk	Greater improvement than treatment with *N*-acetylcysteine in patients with warm CRPS Lower total treatment costs when compared with *N*-acetylcysteine Improvement in range of motion and vasomotor instability
N-Acetylcysteine[26]	Free-radical scavenging	600 mg PO TID × 52 wk	Greater improvement than treatment with DMSO in patients with cold CRPS
Pain medications			
Gabapentin[27]	Blocks calcium channels in neurons	600 mg PO daily × 2 d, then 600 mg BID × 2 d, then 600 mg TID × 17 d	No difference in treatment group versus placebo group after 3-wk course in pain scores but improvement versus placebo in global perceived pain
Opioids[35,53]	Activation of opioid receptors	90 mg PO daily sustained-release oral morphine Approximately 8.9 mg PO levorphanol	No significant data demonstrating a reduction of pain High-dose opioid therapy demonstrating a significant global reduction in neuropathic pain
Ketamine[54-56]	Antagonism of NMDA receptor	10% ketamine cream transdermally Intravenous ketamine-subanesthetic 30 mg/hr × 4.2 d Intravenous ketamine coma 7 mg/kg/hr + 0.15-0.4 mg/kg/hr IV midazolam × 5 d	Reduction in mechano allodynia and hyperalgesia Significant pain relief at up to 11 wk follow-up Complete remission of symptoms in 50% of patients at 10 yr posttreatment

(continued)

Table 5

Pharmacologic Treatments of Complex Regional Pain Syndrome (CRPS) (continued)

Pharmaceutical	Mechanism of Action	Dosage Range Studied	Evidence for Effectiveness
Antispasmotic agents			
Baclofen[47-49]	Inhibition of GABA-β receptors	Intrathecal baclofen up to 450 μg/d	Reduced dystonia and pain and increased quality of life
Osteoclast inhibitors			
Diphosphonates[32,34,57]	Inhibition of osteoclasts/bone remodeling	Ibandronate 6 mg IV daily × 3 d Alendronate 40 mg PO daily × 8 wk 7.5 mg IV daily × 3 d Pamidronate 60 mg IV once Clodronate 300 mg IV daily × 10 d Neridronate 100 mg IV daily × 4 d	Improvement in average and worst pain ratings Improvement in spontaneous pain, pressure tolerance, and joint mobility Significant reduction in spontaneous pain, tenderness, and swelling along with improvement in motion of involved extremity at 2 and 4 wk Improvement in pain score, global assessment of disease severity score, and physical function Improvement in pain score and clinical global assessment at 40 d Improvement in pain and physical function scores at 40 d
Calcitonin[32]	Release of β-endorphin Inhibition of osteoclasts/bone remodeling	200 IU intranasal daily 100 IU intramuscular 100 IU TID × 3 wk 100 IU BID × 4 wk 100 IU TID × 3 wk	No statistically significant benefits Significant reduction in pain scores and ROM Significant improvement in pain and ROM, significant improvement in upper extremity CRPS patients, no difference in level of edema No difference in improvement in pain scores, stiffness, swelling, and vascular instability Improvement in pain scores at 1 wk

BID = twice daily, DMSO = dimethyl sulfoxide, GABA = gamma-aminobutyric acid-β, IV = intravenous, NMDA = *N*-methyl-D-aspartic acid, PO = by mouth, QID = four times daily, ROM = range of motion, TID = three times daily, VAS = visual analog scale.

Sympathetic Blockade and Regional Anesthesia

The presence of sympathetically mediated pain has led to blockade of the primary sympathetic ganglion (the stellate ganglion), which provides sympathetic innervation for the upper extremity for both diagnosis and mitigation of sympathetically mediated pain. Current prospective studies support the use of stellate ganglion blocks with local anesthetic or botulinum toxin to reduce pain on a visual analog scale and increase participation in rehabilitation, especially when blocks are performed early (<16 weeks) following the onset of symptoms. Several questions remain concerning stellate ganglion blocks, including duration of pain relief and whether intermittent single-dose or continuous infusion administration are more effective.[37] Sympathetic blocks for diagnostic purposes have created large numbers of false-positive and false-negative results.[38] Although no positive predictors of sympathetic blockade are demonstrable, allodynia and hypoesthesia may be negative predictors for blockade success.[39]

Regional blockade of the brachial plexus has been demonstrated to provide pain relief and allow the medication-refractory patients with CRPS to participate in shoulder rehabilitation by blockade of somatic Aδ and C afferent nerve fibers.[40] The technique has been effective when used in continuous infusion settings lasting approximately 1 week. Although this technique has been used when sympathetic blockade fails, a pilot study comparing continuous stellate ganglion block with a continuous infraclavicular brachial plexus block demonstrated significant reduction in background neuropathic pain and pain exacerbations in both groups.[41]

Intravenous regional sympathetic blockade using the Bier block technique with various medications has been studied. Guanethidine, ketanserin, bretylium, atropine, droperidol, and reserpine have all been used as agents, but none have proven to have significant clinical benefit in decreasing pain over a significant length of time following meta-analysis.[42]

Surgical and Procedural Intervention

Neuromodulation through implantation of dorsal column spinal cord stimulators in the epidural space has been effective in decreasing the burning pain associated with chronic or cold CRPS (up to 70% success) and has been considered a positive treatment by patients undergoing this therapy at long-term follow-up appointments.[43] Undesirable outcomes may occur in up to 34% of patients with permanent stimulator implantations.[44] Most commonly, the revision is due to electrode repositioning rather than other complications, including equipment failure or infection.[44] Long-term follow-up has demonstrated diminishing relief at approximately 5 years.[43]

Another form of neuromodulation therapy that has shown significant CRPS pain reduction is dorsal root ganglion (DRG) stimulation. The DRG is a bundle of neurons located just outside the spinal cord and new evidence suggests that it is responsible for the hyperexcitability of the CNS that leads to many of the symptoms associated with CRPS such as allodynia. A recent randomized trial comparing dorsal column spinal cord stimulation and DRG stimulation showed that 74.2% of patients treated with DRG stimulation reported greater than 50% pain relief and approximately a third of those patients reported 80% or more reduction in pain.[45]

Locations other than the spinal cord along the pain pathway can also be a target for neurostimulation including injured peripheral nerves in patients with CRPS type 2, motor cortex stimulation with dural electrodes, and deep brain stimulation. Another treatment option that has shown promise involves the use of repetitive transcranial magnetic stimulation, using magnetic currents applied externally to the brain to induce neuroplastic cortical changes. There is a suggestion that this technique may offer therapeutic value, but more well-designed studies need to be conducted.[46]

Intrathecal medications have been suggested as a viable treatment to the CNS component of CRPS pain. Baclofen, a gamma-aminobutyric acid-β agonist, has been shown to reduce the dystonia and pain associated with chronic CRPS in prospective trials.[47-49]

Surgical sympathectomy involves the surgical severance of the sympathetic trunks or the stellate ganglion using chemical, radiofrequency, or open surgical techniques to reduce sympathetically mediated pain. These techniques are extensions of the temporary sympathetic block techniques described previously and may be used to prolong pain relief. A retrospective review of radiofrequency stellate ganglion sympathectomies identified 40% of patients with a greater than 50% reduction in pain at follow-up of approximately 1 year.[50] Despite positive findings, controversy over the long-term efficacy of surgical sympathectomy remains.[32]

Prevention

Primary prevention and prevention of secondary reactivation of CRPS in the postoperative/posttrauma patients are areas of ongoing study. One study documented administration of vitamin C for 50 days following wrist fracture and demonstrated a substantial decrement in the incidence of CRPS observed (7% vitamin C versus 22% control).[24] However, an RCT on the use of vitamin C after distal radial fractures showed no benefit to patients at 1 year.[25] Surgery on a limb previously affected by CRPS has been shown to cause exacerbation or relapse of symptoms. Perioperative calcitonin, stellate ganglion blockade, intravenous blockade, and multimodal anesthesia have all shown initial promise in reducing relapse.[21] Current recommendations support postponement of surgery until CRPS signs are minimal.[21]

SUMMARY

CRPS is a disease with a complex pathophysiologic basis. The orthopaedic surgeon should be aware of its implications preceding or following surgery of the shoulder and elbow to recognize and properly treat this debilitating illness. Through early recognition and intervention, orthopaedic surgeons can provide their patients with the best multimodal team-based approach and thereby the best chance for positive long-term outcomes.

KEY STUDY POINTS

- CRPS may affect up to 2% to 5% after carpal tunnel surgery and 22% to 39% after distal radius fractures.
- The diagnosis is clinical and based on the Budapest Criteria.
- Surgery or injury to the upper extremity can be an inciting event.
- Typical treatments consist of oral or topical agents, sympathetic blocks, neuromodulation, or IV ketamine aimed at restoring limb function and reducing pain.

Annotated References

1. Marinus J, Moseley GL, Birklein F, et al: Clinical features and pathophysiology of complex regional pain syndrome. *Lancet Neurol* 2011;10(7):637-648.

2. Goebel A: Complex regional pain syndrome in adults. *Rheumatology (Oxford)* 2011;50(10):1739-1750.

3. Merskey H, Bogduk N: *Classification of Chronic Pain. Descriptions of Chronic Pain Syndromes and Definitions of Pain Terms*, ed 2. Seattle, WA, IASP Press, 1994.

4. Harden RN, Bruehl S, Perez RS, et al: Validation of proposed diagnostic criteria (the "Budapest Criteria") for complex regional pain syndrome. *Pain* 2010;150(2): 268-274.

5. Sethna NF, Meier PM, Zurakowski D, Berde CB: Cutaneous sensory abnormalities in children and adolescents with complex regional pain syndromes. *Pain* 2007;131(1-2):153-161.

6. Beerthuizen A, Stronks DL, Van't Spijker A, et al: Demographic and medical parameters in the development of complex regional pain syndrome type 1 (CRPS1): Prospective study on 596 patients with a fracture. *Pain* 2012;153(6):1187-1192.

7. Sharma A, Agarwal S, Broatch J, Raja SN: A web-based cross-sectional epidemiological survey of complex regional pain syndrome. *Reg Anesth Pain Med* 2009;34(2):110-115.

8. Bruehl S: An update on the pathophysiology of complex regional pain syndrome. *Anesthesiology* 2010;113(3):713-725.

9. Cappello ZJ, Kasdan ML, Louis DS: Meta-analysis of imaging techniques for the diagnosis of complex regional pain syndrome type I. *J Hand Surg Am* 2012;37(2):288-296.

10. Kohr D, Tschernatsch M, Schmitz K, et al: Autoantibodies in complex regional pain syndrome bind to a differentiation-dependent neuronal surface autoantigen. *Pain* 2009;143(3):246-251.

11. Goebel A, Baranowski A, Maurer K, Ghiai A, McCabe C, Ambler G: Intravenous immunoglobulin treatment of the complex regional pain syndrome: A randomized trial. *Ann Intern Med* 2010;152(3):152-158.

12. Goebel A, Bisla J, Carganillo R, et al: Low-dose intravenous imuunoglobulin treatment for long-standing complex regional pain syndrome. *Ann Intern Med* 2017;167:476-483.

    A randomized, placebo-controlled, multicenter trial confirmed the efficacy of low-dose intravenous immunoglobulin compared with placebo in reducing pain during a 6-week period in adult patients who had CRPS from 1 to 5 years. Study showed that low-dose immunoglobulin treatment for 6 weeks was not effective in relieving pain in patients with moderate to severe CRPS of 1 to 5 years' duration. Level of evidence: I.

13. Tékus V, Hajna Z, Borbély É, et al: A CRPS-IgG-transfer-trauma model reproducing inflammatory and positive sensory signs associated with complex regional pain syndrome. *Pain* 2014;155:299-308.

    In this study, mice (5 to 7 per group) were treated with the IgG fractions obtained from six CRPS patients and six healthy volunteers. Flow-through-treated and saline-treated groups served as control groups. In this first IgG-transfer-trauma model for CRPS, serum IgG from patients with long-standing CRPS induced clinical and laboratory features of the human disease, indicating a relevant role for IgG autoantibodies. Level of evidence: III.

14. Dubuis E, Thompson V, Leite MI, et al: Longstanding complex regional pain syndrome is associated with activating autoantibodies against alpha-1a adrenoceptors. *Pain* 2014;155:2408-2417.

    A randomized crossover trial of low-dose intravenous immunoglobulin (IVIG) treatment, which point to a possible autoimmune mechanism, is presented. Purified serum immunoglobulin G (IgG) from patients with long-standing CRPS was tested for evidence of antibodies interacting with autonomic receptors on adult primary cardiomyocytes, compared with control IgG from healthy and diseased controls, and related the results to the clinical response to treatment with low-dose IVIG. The results suggest that patients with long-standing CRPS have serum antibodies to α-1a receptors, and that measurement of these antibodies may be useful in the diagnosis and treatment of the patients. Level of evidence: II.

15. Wigerblad G, Bas DB, Fernades-Cerqueira C, et al: Autoantibodies to citrullinated proteins induce joint pain independent of inflammation via a chemokine-dependent mechanism. *Ann Rheum Dis* 2016;75:730-738.

    In this study, antibodies purified from human patients with rheumatoid arthritis and from healthy donors and murinised monoclonal autoantibodies against citrullinated proteins, ACPA, were injected into mice. Painlike behavior was monitored for up to 28 days, and tissues were analyzed for signs of pathology. The results suggested that CXCL1/IL-8, released from osteoclasts in an autoantibody-dependent manner, produces pain by activating sensory neurons. Level of evidence: III.

16. Goebel A, Jones S, Oomman S, Callaghan T, Sprotte G: Letter: Treatment of long-standing complex regional pain syndrome with therapeutic plasma exchange: A preliminary case series of patients treated in 2008-2014. *Pain Med* 2014;15:2163-2164.

    This case series studied therapeutic plasma exchange (TPE) in the treatment of six patients with long-standing, refractory CRPS. TPE treatment appeared to induce remission in some patients, but for others repeat TPE treatment may not always be feasible, so the efficacy of immunosuppressant treatments should also be investigated in this group. These results add further credence to the concept that serum factors contribute to causing and/or maintaining some of the long-standing symptoms of CRPS. Level of evidence: IV.

17. Bonica JJ: *The Management of Pain, With Special Emphasis on the Use of Analgesic Block in Diagnosis, Prognosis and Therapy.* Philadelphia, PA, Lea & Febiger, 1953.

18. Patterson RW, Li Z, Smith BP, Smith TL, Koman LA: Complex regional pain syndrome of the upper extremity. *J Hand Surg Am* 2011;36(9):1553-1562.

19. Drummond PD: Sensory disturbances in complex regional pain syndrome: Clinical observations, autonomic interactions, and possible mechanisms. *Pain Med* 2010;11(8):1257-1266.

20. Schürmann M, Zaspel J, Löhr P, et al: Imaging in early posttraumatic complex regional pain syndrome: A comparison of diagnostic methods. *Clin J Pain* 2007;23(5):449-457.

21. Perez RS, Zollinger PE, Dijkstra PU, et al, CRPS I Task Force: Evidence based guidelines for complex regional pain syndrome type 1. *BMC Neurol* 2010;10:20.

22. Christensen K, Jensen EM, Noer I: The reflex dystrophy syndrome response to treatment with systemic corticosteroids. *Acta Chir Scand* 1982;148(8):653-655.

23. Kozin F, Ryan LM, Carerra GF, Soin JS, Wortmann RL: The reflex sympathetic dystrophy syndrome (RSDS): III. Scintigraphic studies, further evidence for the therapeutic efficacy of systemic corticosteroids, and proposed diagnostic criteria. *Am J Med* 1981;70(1):23-30.

24. Zollinger PE, Tuinebreijer WE, Kreis RW, Breederveld RS: Effect of vitamin C on frequency of reflex sympathetic dystrophy in wrist fractures: A randomised trial. *Lancet* 1999;354(9195):2025-2028.

25. Ekrol I, Duckworth AD, Ralston SH, Court-Brown CM, McQueen MM: The influence of vitamin C on the outcome of distal radial fractures: A double-blind, randomized controlled trial. *J Bone Joint Surg Am* 2014;96(17):1451-1459.

    This double-blind randomized controlled trial recruited adult patients with an acute fracture of the distal aspect of the radius over a 1-year period and randomized them to receive 500 mg of vitamin C or placebo daily for 50 days after the fracture. Results showed no significant difference at 1 year in the DASH (Disabilities of the Arm, Shoulder and Hand) score, other functional outcomes, the rate of CRPS, or osseous healing of nondisplaced or displaced distal radial fractures treated with vitamin C compared with placebo. Level of evidence: IV.

26. Perez RS, Zuurmond WW, Bezemer PD, et al: The treatment of complex regional pain syndrome type I with free radical scavengers: A randomized controlled study. *Pain* 2003;102(3):297-307.

27. van de Vusse AC, Stomp-van den Berg SG, Kessels AH, Weber WE: Randomised controlled trial of gabapentin in complex regional pain syndrome type 1 [ISRCTN84121379]. *BMC Neurol* 2004;4:13-22.

28. Tan AK, Duman I, Taşkaynatan MA, Hazneci B, Kalyon TA: The effect of gabapentin in earlier stage of reflex sympathetic dystrophy. *Clin Rheumatol* 2007;26(4):561-565.

29. Schwartzman RJ, Alexander GM, Grothusen JR: The use of ketamine in complex regional pain syndrome: Possible mechanisms. *Expert Rev Neurother* 2011;11(5):719-734.

30. Muizelaar JP, Kleyer M, Hertogs IA, DeLange DC: Complex regional pain syndrome (reflex sympathetic dystrophy and causalgia): Management with the calcium channel blocker nifedipine and/or the alpha-sympathetic blocker phenoxybenzamine in 59 patients. *Clin Neurol Neurosurg* 1997;99(1):26-30.

31. Davis KD, Treede RD, Raja SN, Meyer RA, Campbell JN: Topical application of clonidine relieves hyperalgesia in patients with sympathetically maintained pain. *Pain* 1991;47(3):309-317.

32. Sharma A, Williams K, Raja SN: Advances in treatment of complex regional pain syndrome: Recent insights on a perplexing disease. *Curr Opin Anaesthesiol* 2006;19(5):566-572.

33. Chevreau M, Romand X, Gaudin P, Juvin R, Baillet A: Bisphosphonates for treatment of complex regional pain syndrome type 1: A systematic literature review and meta-analysis of randomized controlled trials versus placebo. *Joint Bone Spine* 2017;84(4):393-399.

    This is a systematic literature review and meta-analysis of all randomized controlled trials to assess the benefit of diphosphonates on pain and function in patients with complex regional pain syndrome type 1. 258 articles were identified. Four trials of moderate to good quality comprising 181 patients (90 in the diphosphonate group and 91 in the placebo group) were included in this meta-analysis. The results suggested that diphosphonates reduce pain in patients with complex regional pain syndrome type 1. Level of evidence: I.

34. Varenna M, Adami S, Rossini M, et al: Treatment of complex regional pain syndrome type I with neridronate: A randomized, double-blind, placebo-controlled study. *Rheumatology (Oxford)* 2013;52(3):534-542.

In this randomized, double-blind, placebo controlled study, 82 patients with CRPS-I at either hand or foot were randomly assigned to IV infusion of 100 mg neridronate given four times over 10 days or placebo. After 50 days, the former placebo patients were given open label the same regimen of neridronate. Significant improvements versus placebo were observed in the indices of pain and quality of life. Level of evidence: I.

35. Rowbotham MC, Twilling L, Davies PS, Reisner L, Taylor K, Mohr D: Oral opioid therapy for chronic peripheral and central neuropathic pain. *N Engl J Med* 2003;348(13):1223-1232.

36. Bruehl S, Chung OY: Psychological and behavioral aspects of complex regional pain syndrome management. *Clin J Pain* 2006;22(5):430-437.

37. Yucel I, Demiraran Y, Ozturan K, Degirmenci E: Complex regional pain syndrome type I: Efficacy of stellate ganglion blockade. *J Orthop Traumatol* 2009;10(4): 179-183.

38. Krumova EK, Gussone C, Regeniter S, Westermann A, Zenz M, Maier C: Are sympathetic blocks useful for diagnostic purposes? *Reg Anesth Pain Med* 2011;36(6):560-567.

39. van Eijs F, Geurts J, van Kleef M, et al: Predictors of pain relieving response to sympathetic blockade in complex regional pain syndrome type 1. *Anesthesiology* 2012;116(1):113-121.

40. Detaille V, Busnel F, Ravary H, Jacquot A, Katz D, Allano G: Use of continuous interscalene brachial plexus block and rehabilitation to treat complex regional pain syndrome of the shoulder. *Ann Phys Rehabil Med* 2010;53(6-7):406-416.

41. Toshniwal G, Sunder R, Thomas R, Dureja GP: Management of complex regional pain syndrome type I in upper extremity-evaluation of continuous stellate ganglion block and continuous infraclavicular brachial plexus block: A pilot study. *Pain Med* 2012;13(1): 96-106.

42. Kingery WS: A critical review of controlled clinical trials for peripheral neuropathic pain and complex regional pain syndromes. *Pain* 1997;73(2):123-139.

43. Kemler MA, de Vet HC, Barendse GA, van den Wildenberg FA, van Kleef M: Effect of spinal cord stimulation for chronic complex regional pain syndrome type I: Five-year final follow-up of patients in a randomized controlled trial. *J Neurosurg* 2008;108(2):292-298.

44. Turner JA, Loeser JD, Deyo RA, Sanders SB: Spinal cord stimulation for patients with failed back surgery syndrome or complex regional pain syndrome: A systematic review of effectiveness and complications. *Pain* 2004;108(1-2):137-147.

45. Deer TR, Levy RM, Kramer J, et al: Dorsal root ganglion stimulation yielded higher treatment success rate for complex regional pain syndrome and causalgia at 3 and 12 months: A randomized comparative trial. *Pain* 2017;158(4):669-681.

This is a pivotal, prospective, multicenter, randomized comparative effectiveness trial, which was conducted in 152 subjects diagnosed with complex regional pain syndrome in the lower extremities. Subjects received neurostimulation of the DRG or dorsal column (spinal cord stimulation, SCS). The percentage of subjects receiving ≥50% pain relief and treatment success was greater in the DRG arm (81.2%) than in the SCS arm (55.7%, $P < 0.001$) at 3 months. Level of evidence: I.

46. Nardone R, Brigo F, Höller Y, et al: Transcranial magnetic stimulation studies in complex regional pain syndrome type I: A review. *Acta Neurol Scand* 2018;137(2): 158-164.

In this review, a systematic search of all studies using transcranial magnetic stimulation (TMS) was conducted to explore cortical excitability/plasticity and repetitive TMS (rTMS) for the treatment of CRPS. Changes in motor cortex excitability and brain mapping have been reported in CRPS-I patients. TMS examinations also revealed that the nature of motor dysfunction in CRPS-I patients differs from that observed in patients with functional movement disorders, limb immobilization, or idiopathic dystonia. This noninvasive brain stimulation technique could have therapeutic utility in CRPS. Level of evidence: III.

47. van Rijn MA, Munts AG, Marinus J, et al: Intrathecal baclofen for dystonia of complex regional pain syndrome. *Pain* 2009;143(1-2):41-47.

48. van der Plas AA, van Rijn MA, Marinus J, Putter H, van Hilten JJ: Efficacy of intrathecal baclofen on different pain qualities in complex regional pain syndrome. *Anesth Analg* 2013;116(1):211-215.

A prospective study examined the effects of intrathecal baclofen infusion pumps in six women. Three of six women had complete resolution of hand dystonia, four women had reduced painful muscle spasms, and two had marked reduction in myoclonic jerks. Level of evidence: IV.

49. van Hilten BJ, van de Beek WJ, Hoff JI, Voormolen JH, Delhaas EM: Intrathecal baclofen for the treatment of dystonia in patients with reflex sympathetic dystrophy. *N Engl J Med* 2000;343(9):625-630.

50. Forouzanfar T, van Kleef M, Weber WE: Radiofrequency lesions of the stellate ganglion in chronic pain syndromes: Retrospective analysis of clinical efficacy in 86 patients. *Clin J Pain* 2000;16(2):164-168.

51. Braus DF, Krauss JK, Strobel J: The shoulder-hand syndrome after stroke: A prospective clinical trial. *Ann Neurol* 1994;36(5):728-733.

52. Frade LC, Lauretti GR, Lima IC, Pereira NL: The antinociceptive effect of local or systemic parecoxib combined with lidocaine/clonidine intravenous regional analgesia for complex regional pain syndrome type I in the arm. *Anesth Analg* 2005;101(3):807-811.

53. Harke H, Gretenkort P, Ladleif HU, Rahman S, Harke O: The response of neuropathic pain and pain in complex regional pain syndrome I to carbamazepine and sustained-release morphine in patients pretreated with spinal cord stimulation: A double-blinded randomized study. *Anesth Analg* 2001;92(2):488-495.

54. Finch PM, Knudsen L, Drummond PD: Reduction of allodynia in patients with complex regional pain syndrome: A double-blind placebo-controlled trial of topical ketamine. *Pain* 2009;146(1-2):18-25.

55. Sigtermans M, Dahan A, Mooren R, et al: S(+)-ketamine effect on experimental pain and cardiac output: A population pharmacokinetic-pharmacodynamic modeling study in healthy volunteers. *Anesthesiology* 2009;111(4):892-903.

56. Kiefer RT, Rohr P, Ploppa A, et al: Efficacy of ketamine in anesthetic dosage for the treatment of refractory complex regional pain syndrome: An open-label phase II study. *Pain Med* 2008;9(8):1173-1201.

57. Breuer B, Pappagallo M, Ongseng F, Chen CI, Goldfarb R: An open-label pilot trial of ibandronate for complex regional pain syndrome. *Clin J Pain* 2008;24(8):685-689.

Chapter 46

Frozen Shoulder

Douglas Scott, MD • Andrew Green, MD

ABSTRACT

Frozen shoulder is a general term that refers to the presence of limited shoulder motion. Although a variety of conditions can lead to a frozen shoulder, many cases do not have an obvious cause or etiology and are considered to be idiopathic adhesive capsulitis. Although the natural history of this common condition is well established, the underlying etiology and pathophysiology are not fully understood. Most patients recover with nonsurgical treatment but should be advised of a protracted course. Various nonsurgical treatment modalities can help patients in the short term, but often little difference is seen in long-term follow-up, as typically this is a naturally self-limiting disease. Surgical intervention, including predominantly arthroscopic capsular release, provides reliable clinical improvement for refractory cases. Recent investigations into the pathophysiology have identified potential etiologic factors that may lead to advances in the understanding and improvements in management of this condition. For the purposes of this chapter, we are specifically referring to idiopathic adhesive capsulitis.

Dr. Green or an immediate family member has received royalties from Wright Medical Technology, Inc.; is a member of a speakers' bureau or has made paid presentations on behalf of DJ Orthopaedics; serves as a paid consultant to or is an employee of DJ Orthopaedics and Wright Medical Technology, Inc.; has stock or stock options held in IlluminOss Medical and Pfizer; has received research or institutional support from DJ Orthopaedics; has received nonincome support (such as equipment or services), commercially derived honoraria, or other non–research-related funding (such as paid travel) from Arthrex, Inc. and Smith & Nephew; and serves as a board member, owner, officer, or committee member of the American Academy of Orthopaedic Surgeons and the American Shoulder and Elbow Surgeons. Neither Dr. Scott nor any immediate family member has received anything of value from or has stock or stock options held in a commercial company or institution related directly or indirectly to the subject of this chapter.

Keywords: adhesive capsulitis; arthroscopic capsular release; diabetic shoulder; frozen shoulder; hydrodilatation; manipulation under anesthesia

Introduction

The term frozen shoulder is commonly used by medical professionals and the lay public to refer to conditions of shoulder pain and stiffness. The term periarthritis was first used in 1872 to refer to shoulders that had both limited active and passive shoulder motion.[1] Codman introduced the term frozen shoulder in 1934 to refer to a constellation of symptoms, and not necessarily a specific disease entity, understanding that many shoulder conditions can result in shoulder pain and limited motion.[2]

The term adhesive capsulitis was popularized by Neviaser and was based on surgical and autopsy findings of cases of frozen shoulder.[3] Differences between the various etiologies of secondary shoulder pain and stiffness have been discussed in previous chapters, but primary idiopathic adhesive capsulitis was defined by the authors of a 1993 study as "a condition of uncertain etiology characterized by substantial reduction of both active and passive shoulder motion that occurs in the absence of a known intrinsic shoulder disorder."[4]

Sustained inflammation of the synovial layer of the glenohumeral capsule leads to thickening and fibrosis, with contracture of the glenohumeral joint capsule. This typically begins with the patient experiencing the insidious onset of vague shoulder pain, followed by gradual loss of motion. The natural history evolves over months but is often self-limited, resolving over a period of 1 to 3 years.

Despite the prevalence of the condition and the extensive research on the subject, general practitioners and orthopaedic surgeons are often confused about the diagnosis and treatment of idiopathic adhesive capsulitis, and the inciting pathophysiology is still unclear. Other primary causes and underlying conditions of shoulder pain and stiffness must be considered and excluded before treating a patient. Nonsurgical management provides the mainstay of treatment, with surgical intervention showing improved outcomes in refractory cases.

Epidemiology

The incidence of idiopathic adhesive capsulitis is difficult to estimate because of ambiguity of application of diagnostic criteria and confusion with other shoulder disorders. Most studies report an incidence of 2% to 5% in the general population, although these figures may be inflated.[5] Approximately 60% to 80% of adhesive capsulitis patients are female and most are between 40 and 60 years of age.[6] The nondominant arm is affected in about 60% of cases, translating to left shoulder involvement in most cases.

Although recurrence in the same shoulder is rare, the same condition develops some time later in the contralateral shoulder in up to 30% of patients. A recent study reported the risk of subsequent contralateral development of adhesive capsulitis, with a higher incidence occurring in patients with diabetes and patients younger than 50 years old.[7]

A 2016 systematic review investigated a genetic predisposition to frozen shoulder.[8] An included study reported an 11.6% prevalence in twin pairs and demonstrated a heritability of 42% for frozen shoulder after adjusting for age. This study also reported that 20% to 30% of patients with frozen shoulder had a positive family history involving a first-degree relative. Furthermore, a meta-analysis also showed increased rates of HLA-B27 positivity in patients with frozen shoulder as compared with control subjects.

Etiology and Pathophysiology

Many primary disease processes affecting the shoulder ultimately result in painful loss of motion. Rotator cuff disease, primary glenohumeral arthritis, traumatic injuries (soft-tissue injuries and fractures), shoulder surgery, inflammatory joint and systemic diseases, and sequelae of neurologic conditions are among the many causes of acquired shoulder pain and stiffness. In contrast, idiopathic adhesive capsulitis occurs in the absence of major trauma, previous surgery, or other identifiable intrinsic or extrinsic pathology. The process that triggers idiopathic adhesive capsulitis has been difficult for researchers to define, leaving the true underlying etiology unknown.

Analyses of tissue obtained during arthroscopy for frozen shoulder show the presence of fibroblasts, proliferating fibroblasts, and myofibroblasts.[9] Some consider the process to be histologically similar to that seen in Dupuytren disease, and the two diseases are thought to share a common biochemical pathway that leads to contracture and fibrosis. The cell types identified have been shown to deposit a dense type III collagen matrix in the shoulder capsule. Capsular tissue from patients demonstrates fibroblastic proliferation, increased numbers of adipocytes, and increased subsynovial vascularity.[10]

Immunoreactivity of advanced glycation end products is found to be high in the capsule of adhesive capsulitis, meaning that overexpression of advanced glycation end products may help explain the fibroblastic proliferation and deposition of collagen matrix in idiopathic frozen shoulder.[11] Additionally, both human and animal studies suggest the involvement of matrix metalloproteinases associated with extracellular matrix remodeling, in the development of adhesive capsulitis.[12]

The findings of research investigating the pathophysiology of adhesive capsulitis are likely affected by the clinical stage of the patients from whom tissue is obtained. Tissue samples that are studied are commonly obtained from patients in the later stages of disease who have not responded to early nonsurgical treatment, and thus the findings may not directly relate to or identify the actual underlying etiology or trigger of the pathophysiologic process. Relating the findings of preclinical studies to the natural history of idiopathic adhesive capsulitis suggests the following clinical summary: a triggering event or process leads to an initial freezing phase, which involves a painful, inflammatory response that gradually progresses to a chronic, contracted, frozen phase.

A dynamic MRI study of frozen shoulder patients displayed an abnormal increase in blood flow from the acromial arterial network and the branches of circumflex humeral arteries into the axillary pouch and the rotator interval, highlighting the pathophysiologic activity and anatomic locations involved with the disease.[13] Abnormal neovessels and accompanying nerves are thought to be sources of pain, and an increase in immunostaining for vascular endothelial growth factor has been shown in adhesive capsulitis. Furthermore, a novel study showed that transcatheter arterial embolization of these neovessels can relieve pain associated with this condition.[14]

Cadaver studies have investigated the pathoanatomy implicated in frozen shoulder. A simulation of localized capsular contractures was done by performing selective capsular plication resulting in restrictions in passive range of glenohumeral motion.[15] The authors found that closure of the rotator interval, including the coracohumeral and superior glenohumeral ligaments, can restrict external rotation, particularly with the shoulder in an adducted position. The authors also found that tightening of the anterior-inferior aspect of the capsule, including the anterior-inferior glenohumeral ligament complex specifically, restricts rotation with increasing abduction of the arm. These findings correlate with the physical examination in practice, as well as intraoperative findings of patients with adhesive capsulitis, and provide a rationale for the selective release of specific anatomic structures during arthroscopic surgical treatment.

Associated Conditions

The importance of performing a thorough patient evaluation is highlighted by knowledge of the medical conditions that are associated with idiopathic adhesive capsulitis. Diabetes mellitus is the most notable and extensively studied medical condition associated with adhesive capsulitis. The incidence of adhesive capsulitis is reported to be as high as 10% to 36% among patients with diabetes.[16,17] Furthermore, the prevalence of frozen shoulder in individuals with type I diabetes has been found to be nearly twice that of patients with type II diabetes, and the duration of diabetes is correlated with the development of frozen shoulder. A 2018 retrospective cohort study added evidence of this association with diabetes, but also separately showed a link to obesity.[18]

Early research failed to show a direct correlation between glycemic control, evaluated with hemoglobin A1C (HbA_{1c}) level, and the actual prevalence of frozen shoulder.[19] However, a recent report considered cumulative HbA_{1c} that factors HbA_{1c} values over time to estimate the total burden of diabetes on a patient supporting the thought that patients with worse serum glucose control over a longer period are at an increased risk of the development of adhesive capsulitis.[20]

It is also commonly believed that patients with diabetes are at greater risk for failure of nonsurgical treatment and recurrence after manipulation under anesthesia (MUA) or surgical treatment. A 2019 study noted that intra-articular corticosteroid injections were less effective in patients with diabetes than those without diabetes.[21] Another study compared outcomes of arthroscopic capsular release of patients with diabetes with those of patients without diabetes.[22] Although both groups of patients had significant improvements in range of motion, pain scores, and shoulder scores 1 year postoperatively, patients with diabetes had less range of motion and poorer postoperative Constant scores. Appropriate counseling and expectations should be tailored to treat patients with diabetes and idiopathic adhesive capsulitis.

Hypothyroidism is also associated with adhesive capsulitis. A 2017 case-control study found that the prevalence of hypothyroidism was significantly higher in patients with adhesive capsulitis than in control subjects.[23] Furthermore, higher serum thyroid-stimulating hormone levels can be associated with bilateral and more severe cases.

Hypercholesterolemia and lipoproteinemias, particularly hyper-low-density lipoprotein (hyper-LDL) cholesterolemia and hyper-non-high-density lipoprotein (hyper-non-HDL) cholesterolemia, also have a significant association with idiopathic adhesive capsulitis.[24] This is consistent with the concept that underlying pro-inflammatory factors play a role in the development of the disease.[25,26]

Other medical conditions associated with frozen shoulder include hypertension, stroke, peripheral neuropathy, gout, and cardiopulmonary disease. Breast cancer with mastectomy and reconstruction also carries a high risk. In addition, frozen shoulder can develop in patients with other neurologic conditions such as cervical radiculopathy and brachial plexitis, and ipsilateral upper extremity trauma not involving the shoulder.

Clinical Evaluation

Adhesive capsulitis is primarily a clinical diagnosis that is based on the history and physical examination findings. Typically, either there is no noted event or the patient recalls a trivial traumatic event such as reaching quickly. Insidious onset of shoulder pain is a primary symptom, followed by a slow, but progressive, loss of shoulder motion. Pain at night is a common report and is often a troubling symptom for many otherwise relatively healthy and active patients. Patients are usually more comfortable in an upright stationary position, at rest, and with limited motion. Pain is usually localized to the shoulder and upper arm and occurs at the extremes of active and passive shoulder motion. Patients occasionally report neurologic symptoms of paresthesia and numbness.

Most patients eventually exhibit a marked loss of active and passive shoulder motion, especially with the shoulder in 90° of abduction. Often, a loss of external rotation of 50% or greater is present, and in the most severe cases, there is complete loss of glenohumeral motion. Manual stretching of the shoulder capsule at the extremes of motion reveals a firm end point and reproduces pain. Similarly, the capsular contracture results in a global limitation of translation of the shoulder. These findings should not be confused with painful weakness resulting from other conditions such as rotator cuff disease. Full strength is generally maintained in true idiopathic adhesive capsulitis. Nonspecific provocative testing such as impingement maneuvers may also elicit pain, confusing the underlying diagnosis. These at-times subtle distinctions during patient examination can prove valuable, but may be challenging to discern for even the experienced clinician.

A thorough clinical evaluation includes standard plain radiographs (true AP [Grashey view], outlet/Y-view, and axillary lateral views) to exclude other primary causes of shoulder pain and stiffness such as glenohumeral arthritis, acromioclavicular arthritis, and calcific tendinitis. Advanced imaging studies are not typically necessary or warranted in the primary evaluation of a patient with idiopathic frozen shoulder. Nevertheless, there are MRI and magnetic resonance arthrographic findings consistent with frozen shoulder.[27,28] This includes thickening of the coracohumeral ligament, thickening and increased signal in the capsule in the axillary recess, decreased overall capsular volume, and subcoracoid fat obliteration in the rotator cuff interval. Specifically, the thickness of the coracohumeral ligament has also been shown to correlate with the clinical loss of internal and external rotation. Overuse of advanced imaging should be avoided because the diagnosis can usually be reliably determined based on the history, physical examination, and plain radiography. Unnecessary advanced imaging has potentially deleterious clinical ramifications. A notable study reported a high false-positive rate of rotator cuff tears, especially partial-thickness tears, being interpreted from preoperative MRIs obtained in patients undergoing arthroscopic capsular release for frozen shoulder.[29] This illustrates the important principle of focusing on clinical judgment rather than on advanced imaging, particularly for a frozen shoulder.

The natural history of idiopathic adhesive capsulitis has three recognized phases: freezing, frozen, and thawing. However, the insidious nature of onset, variable course and severity, and frequent delay in presentation make such distinctions inexact. Generally, these phases progress from an initially intensely inflammatory, painful shoulder, to a shoulder with substantial limits of range of motion but oftentimes with less pain, and finally to recovery of motion and resolution of the condition. Although it is often difficult to pinpoint a patient's exact position on this clinical spectrum, the phases are a helpful, general guide to relay expectations of the anticipated clinical course.

Nonsurgical Management

Nonsurgical management is the mainstay of treatment of frozen shoulder, and much evidence has been reported to support this understanding. Nonsurgical options should be the primary approach to treatment with up to 95% of cases resolving without requiring surgery. Nevertheless, patients should be counseled that even with appropriate and eventually successful treatment, a prolonged course, often many months in length, should be expected.

Corticosteroids

Multiple studies support the role of corticosteroids in the management of frozen shoulder. In most reports, corticosteroid injection results in early reduction in pain without obvious longer term benefit.

A randomized clinical trial reported that intra-articular corticosteroid injection, combined with physiotherapy consisting of modalities and exercises, resulted in significantly greater improvement of Shoulder Pain and Disability Index scores and range of motion at 6-week follow-up compared with injection alone, saline injection with physiotherapy, and saline injection alone.[30] After 3 months, patients in the corticosteroid group had greater improvement in the Shoulder Pain and Disability Index score. Interestingly, however, at 12-month follow-up, there was no difference in outcomes between the groups. Furthermore, a meta-analysis published in 2017 including four randomized clinical trials demonstrated that, compared with placebo, intra-articular corticosteroid injections were more effective in reducing the pain score at 0 to 8 weeks, but there was no difference in pain between the injection group and the control group at 9 to 24 weeks.[31] Notably, improvement of shoulder range of motion in the injection group was greater than that of the control group both at 0 to 8, and 9 to 24 weeks from treatment.

Another prospective study compared a course of oral glucocorticoids with a series of three fluoroscopically guided intra-articular corticosteroid injections.[32] Patients in both groups also had a physical therapy program. Patients in the intra-articular injection cohort had superior Constant-Murley scores at all times up to the 1-year follow-up. Patients in the injection group also had consistently better range of motion at up to 8 weeks and variable differences beyond that. Visual analog scale scores for pain and function were no different, and the scores for patient satisfaction were better for those in the injection group.

A randomized controlled trial demonstrated that corticosteroid injections accelerated early pain relief and recovery of function compared with oral NSAIDs in patients with adhesive capsulitis.[33] Both groups also underwent a physical therapy program. However, at final follow-up of 12 weeks, there was no significant difference in pain. Correspondingly, shoulder function scores and most motion parameters improved faster in the injection group up to week 8, and there were no significant differences at final follow-up.

A 2019 systematic review and network meta-analysis showed that intra-articular corticosteroid, administered either alone or after distention of the shoulder capsule, provided clinically meaningful improvements in short-term follow-up.[34] Similarly, rotator interval corticosteroid injections yielded promising results in terms of pain relief. However, the benefits of corticosteroids were shown to dissipate over time in longer follow-up.

There is evidence to support the use of image-guided glenohumeral joint injection to improve the accuracy. One study reported that the accuracy of intra-articular glenohumeral injection from an anterior approach without radiographic guidance was only 26%.[35] Another study reported the accuracy of glenohumeral injection as 65% from an anterior approach, 46% from a posterior approach, and 46% from a superior approach.[36]

The effect of the location of injection has also been investigated. A comparison of the efficacy of ultrasound-guided glenohumeral and subacromial corticosteroid injections found that although the former had greater improvement in pain at 3-week follow-up, there was no difference at 6- and 12-week follow-ups.[37] In addition, there was no significant difference between the effect of subacromial and glenohumeral injections with respect to the Constant-Murley score or range of motion at any time point. A 2018 randomized controlled trial compared the effect of corticosteroid injection into the rotator interval with that of intra-articular or subacromial injection, for early frozen shoulder.[38] Improvements in pain visual analog scale, passive range of motion, Constant score, and DASH score were faster and significantly better in the rotator interval injection group at 4 weeks after injection.

A 2013 study that compared 40 mg glenohumeral joint injection with 20 mg of triamcinolone acetonide reported no difference in outcome scores (Shoulder Pain and Disability Index, visual analog scale for shoulder pain) and passive range of motion level at 1, 3, 6, and 12 weeks after treatment.[39]

In summary, the available evidence suggests that corticosteroids, most specifically glenohumeral joint injection, can provide short-term symptomatic relief but the available evidence does not demonstrate long-term benefit over the natural history of idiopathic adhesive capsulitis. Nevertheless, injections can be effective and should be considered for the treatment of idiopathic adhesive capsulitis. Clinicians should be aware that administration of oral or local corticosteroids temporarily increases serum glucose levels, especially in patients with diabetes, and these patients should be counseled appropriately.

Physical Therapy

Physical therapy, focusing on shoulder stretching exercises, is well accepted as a treatment of adhesive capsulitis. Pendulum circumduction and passive shoulder stretching exercises, including forward elevation, external rotation, horizontal adduction, and internal rotation, were performed by patients in a prospective study in which 90% of the patients were satisfied with their result at long-term follow-up. Diabetes and male sex were factors associated with a poor outcome. Few studies exist that compare stretching exercises with benign neglect, but it is logical that there are only minimal risks and disadvantages to attempting these exercises in all cases. The importance of focusing on gentle and gradual stretching over time, rather than forceful, aggressive therapy, should be highlighted. The objective literature is conflicting on whether home-based therapy or formal, professional therapy sessions are most beneficial. Treatment should be individualized for each patient.

In addition to traditional physical therapy exercises, there is interest in alternative treatments and the use of modalities in the management of frozen shoulder. A Cochrane review found moderate evidence supporting the use of mobilization techniques in short-term and long-term follow-up. The authors also found that when compared with placebo, laser treatment and both electroacupuncture and interferential acupuncture had a significantly positive short-term effect on pain, function, and range of motion. Other modalities, including extracorporeal shockwave therapy (ESWT),[40] ultrasonography, dynamic mobilization, temperature therapy, and massage, have been shown to accelerate patients' short-term functional outcomes. Future research in these areas can help define patient-specific treatment plans.

Hydrodilatation

Hydrodilatation, or arthrographic distention, which involves intra-articular glenohumeral fluid injection under pressure to disrupt the glenohumeral capsule, is considered to be safe and cost-effective, with a rapid and satisfactory outcome. One of several randomized clinical trials reported improved outcomes after hydrodilatation compared with either intra-articular or subacromial triamcinolone injection at 1- and 3-month follow-up.[41] Notable, however, was that outcome scores between these patient groups were equivalent at 6 months from treatment.

A 2016 prospective randomized controlled study showed that hydrodilatation combined with joint manipulation under an interscalene block provided earlier pain relief and restoration of shoulder range of motion and function compared with a single intra-articular corticosteroid injection in patients with primary frozen shoulder, at 3-month follow-up.[42] Nevertheless, there was no statistical difference in outcomes at 1 year after treatment, with most patients in both treatment arms satisfied.

Viscosupplementation

Hyaluron is a major component of hyaline articular cartilage and synovial fluid and is FDA approved for the treatment of knee osteoarthritis. Utilization for the treatment of shoulder disorders has been less extensive. Preclinical investigations suggest a possible basis for using viscosupplementation to manage adhesive capsulitis. The effect of hyaluron on fibroblasts harvested from the glenohumeral capsule of patients with idiopathic and secondary adhesive capsulitis was studied. Significant and dose-dependent inhibitory effects were found on cell proliferation, messenger RNA expression of adhesion-related procollagen, and cytokines.[43]

A 2012 prospective randomized clinical trial of 70 adhesive capsulitis patients that compared intra-articular hyaluronic acid injection with a physical therapy program versus physical therapy alone found equivalent improvement in pain, disability, and quality of life, and both active and passive range of motion after 3 months, indicating no significant additional benefit of hyaluronic acid injection.[44]

A systematic review of four level I and three level IV published studies investigating the use of hyaluronic acid injections for frozen shoulder found that at short-term follow-up (mean, 9 weeks), shoulder range of motion, Constant scores, and pain were significantly improved.[45] The authors also reported that isolated intra-articular hyaluronate injection had equivalent clinical outcomes and range of motion compared with intra-articular corticosteroid injection.

Suprascapular Nerve Block

In addition to motor innervation of the supraspinatus and infraspinatus muscles, the suprascapular nerve provides sensory innervation to the glenohumeral joint capsule. Suprascapular nerve blockade is thought to provide pain relief and allow for a more aggressive and tolerable stretching program.[46] Although limited current data show short-term pain relief, future research is needed to qualify long-term benefits in pain, disability, and patient satisfaction after this treatment.

Surgical Management

It should be emphasized that the vast majority of patients with idiopathic adhesive capsulitis achieve successful resolution with nonsurgical management. Most authors recommend at least 6 months of nonsurgical treatment before considering surgical intervention. However, in refractory cases, surgical intervention has been shown to provide reliable benefit to patients.

Manipulation Under Anesthesia

Although noninvasive, MUA is included in this section because it requires forceful manipulation of the shoulder and typically requires more than just a local anesthetic. Multiple studies have illustrated the short-term and midterm benefits of MUA for the treatment of frozen shoulder that is refractory to nonsurgical management.

When considering MUA, the clinician should understand the importance of delaying intervention until the frozen phase. Manipulation during the inflammatory, or freezing phase, can exacerbate the condition. Most manipulations are performed under a supplemental regional nerve block to ensure muscle paralysis and provide postprocedural analgesia. The scapula should be stabilized to isolate glenohumeral motion, and gradual stretching maneuvers are performed. Care must be taken to prevent iatrogenic injury, including glenohumeral dislocation, rotator cuff tear, and fracture, especially in older patients and patients with osteopenia. A guarded sequence of traction and flexion, cross-body adduction, internal rotation, external rotation, and abduction with external and internal rotation is safe and reliable. Rotational stretching that applies torsional forces to the proximal humerus is carried out after elevation, abduction, and adduction to minimize the risk of fracture. The importance of maintaining a diligent physical therapy stretching program after manipulation cannot be overemphasized. Plain radiographs are recommended after MUA to rule out bony injury.

A long-term (mean 15 years) retrospective study reported that improvements in pain relief, range of motion, and satisfaction were maintained after MUA for patients.[47] A retrospective case-control study compared the outcome of MUA for patients with diabetes with that of a nondiabetic control group.[48] The study included patients with primary and secondary frozen shoulder and found that 50% of the diabetic primary frozen shoulder required additional manipulation, compared with 14% of the patients without diabetes. Despite the high rate of secondary manipulation in the diabetic cohort, 85% of those patients were satisfied with the final outcome and, overall, the end point range of motion and outcome scores were not statistically different from their counterparts without diabetes.

In a prospective study, 30 patients who underwent MUA for primary frozen shoulder were examined afterward via arthroscopy.[49] The capsule was seen to be ruptured superiorly in 11 patients, anteriorly extending to the infraglenoid pole in 24 patients, and 16 patients also had posterior capsular tearing. In 18 patients, no additional joint damage was found after manipulation. Iatrogenic lesions reportedly included four patients with superior labrum anterior to posterior lesions, three fresh partial tears of the subscapularis tendon, four anterior labral detachments (one with a small osteochondral defect), and two tears of the middle glenohumeral ligament. The authors confirmed the general understanding that although MUA can effectively restore joint motion, there is a risk of iatrogenic injury, and a careful technique should be used. Particular caution should be used when manipulating a shoulder that does not easily release.

Arthroscopic Capsular Release

Arthroscopic capsular release provides consistent clinical improvement in the management of recalcitrant frozen shoulder.[50] The procedure is increasingly replacing isolated MUA because it provides a diagnostic inspection of the joint and a more precise capsulotomy/capsulectomy and minimizes the risk of iatrogenic injury. However, arthroscopy in the presence of a severe contracture can be technically challenging, and entering the glenohumeral joint can prove difficult because of the thickened and contracted capsule as well as the limited joint space, which along with abundant synovitis can make even basic arthroscopy difficult.

Following a standard diagnostic arthroscopy, a synovectomy of the rotator cuff interval is performed to facilitate visualization of the long head of the biceps, the subscapularis tendon, and the anterior capsule. Selective rotator cuff interval and capsular release can be performed with arthroscopic punches or guarded use of cautery devices. Care should be taken during the procedure to protect neurovascular structures, especially the axillary nerve inferiorly. Subsequently, confirmation of complete freedom of motion should be achieved via manipulation, during which the release of remaining contracted capsule can be palpated.[51] Associated procedures should be considered based on preoperative evaluation and diagnostic arthroscopy, such as concomitant surgical management of the biceps tendon complex or subacromial pathology. The vast majority of cases do not require additional surgical procedures.

Arthroscopy has essentially eliminated the need for open capsular releases in the management of idiopathic adhesive capsulitis. Nevertheless, open release still has a role in some cases of secondary shoulder stiffness related to an extrinsic cause, such as an overly tight repair for instability or a proximal humeral fracture with extra-articular scarring. An open approach is required if lengthening of the subscapularis tendon is needed to achieve external rotation. In addition, extensive subdeltoid scarring is often not amenable to arthroscopic capsular release. The disadvantages of an open approach include the need to protect the repaired or lengthened subscapularis tendon, which is counterproductive to the aggressive postoperative therapy required to maintain range of motion.

A 2016 study of arthroscopic capsular release for patients in whom nonsurgical management for idiopathic adhesive capsulitis had failed reported significant reductions in pain, improvements in range of motion, and improvements in overall shoulder function even in the first postoperative week.[52] These immediate improvements in pain and function continued to improve at 6, 12, and 24 weeks postoperatively. In addition, a prospective study of arthroscopic capsular release in 73 patients who were followed up for 1 year postoperatively reported that pain diminished at an average of 2.2 weeks, range of motion was within 10% of the contralateral shoulder at an average of 5.5 weeks, and patients were well enough to be discharged at an average of 8.9 weeks.[53] Nevertheless, 37% of the patients received a steroid injection for postoperative management, and 11% of the patients eventually developed recurrence of symptoms, the latter finding being consistent with multiple other studies. Furthermore, the results of a retrospective study of the long-term outcomes of arthroscopic capsular release indicated significant improvement in pain, function, and range of motion.[54] The range of motion was equivalent to that of the contralateral unaffected shoulder.

Although relative shoulder stiffness and loss of motion can be sequelae of traumatic shoulder injuries and shoulder surgery, surgical releases are not frequently required or performed in these cases. One study reported that only 3 of 345 patients who underwent rotator cuff repair were treated with arthroscopic capsular release.[55] Another study reported on 21 patients, 14 with proximal humeral fractures, who underwent arthroscopic capsular and subacromial release for posttraumatic frozen shoulder.[56] Substantial improvements were seen in shoulder motion and outcome. Patients with isolated soft-tissue injury without fracture had better results. In a 2010 study, the effect of etiology of frozen shoulders on the outcome of arthroscopic capsular release was evaluated, and no differences were found between idiopathic and posttraumatic stiffness.[5] In contrast, the cohort of patients undergoing arthroscopic capsular release after previous surgery had significantly worse outcomes.

In regard to the technical aspects of arthroscopic capsular release, recent studies have investigated the necessity of a pancapsular release, adding a posterior capsular release to the typical releases of the rotator interval and anterior-inferior capsular release. A randomized clinical trial reported no statistical benefit of pancapsular release in American Shoulder and Elbow Surgeons score, Simple Shoulder Test, and pain visual analog scale or range of motion[57] at 18-month follow-up. Another study reported that although the addition of a posterior capsular release improved immediate postoperative internal rotation scores, there were no significant differences in Constant score, pain visual analog scale score, and patient range of motion at subsequent follow-ups.[58]

SUMMARY

Idiopathic adhesive capsulitis is defined as painful limitation of glenohumeral motion without an identifiable cause. The natural history of this relatively common condition is well established, but the underlying etiology and pathophysiology are not fully understood. Most patients recover with nonsurgical treatment, but they should be advised that a protracted course is typical. Patients with diabetes should be advised of expected challenges to both nonsurgical and surgical outcomes. Surgical intervention, predominantly arthroscopic capsular release, provides reliable clinical improvement for refractory cases. Future study of the pathophysiology of idiopathic adhesive capsulitis will hopefully lead to improvements in patient treatment, especially affecting the long duration of the natural history of this condition.

KEY STUDY POINTS

- Idiopathic adhesive capsulitis is a relatively common cause of generalized shoulder pain and limited range of motion in the absence of other underlying diagnoses.
- Current research continues to investigate the histologic, genetic, and inflammatory factors that cause fibroblastic proliferation and neovascularization in this disorder.
- Nonsurgical management, including corticosteroids and physical therapy, provides the mainstay of care and leads to eventual resolution for the vast majority of patients.
- Corticosteroid injections provide short-term relief of symptoms.
- Hydrodilatation is a minimally invasive treatment for adhesive capsulitis.
- Arthroscopic capsular release provides reliable benefit for adhesive capsulitis refractory to nonsurgical management.

Annotated References

1. Duplay S: De la péri-arthrite scapula-humérale et des raideurs de l'épaule qui en sont al consequence. *Arch Gen Méd* 1872;20:513-542.

2. Codman EA: *The Shoulder: Rupture of the Supraspinatus Tendon and Other Lesions in or About the Subacromial Bursa.* Boston, MA, Thomas Todd and Co, 1934, pp 216-224.

3. Neviaser JS: Adhesive capsulitis of the shoulder: A study of pathological findings in periarthritis of the shoulder. *J Bone Joint Surg Am* 1945;27-A(2):211-222.

4. Zuckerman JD, Cuomo F: Frozen shoulder, in Matsen FA III, Fu FH, Hawkins RJ, eds: *The Shoulder: A Balance of Mobility and Stability.* Rosemont, IL, American Academy of Orthopaedic Surgeons, 1993, pp 253-267.

5. Elhassan B, Ozbaydar M, Massimini D, Higgins L, Warner JJ: Arthroscopic capsular release for refractory shoulder stiffness: A critical analysis of effectiveness in specific etiologies. *J Shoulder Elbow Surg* 2010;19(4):580-587.

6. Griggs SM, Ahn A, Green A: Idiopathic adhesive capsulitis: A prospective functional outcome study of nonoperative treatment. *J Bone Joint Surg Am* 2000;82(10):1398-1407.

7. Lamplot JD, Lillegraven O, Brophy RH: Outcomes from conservative treatment of shoulder idiopathic adhesive capsulitis and factors associated with developing contralateral disease. *Orthop J Sports Med* 2018;6(7):2325967118785169.

   This cohort study included 60 patients diagnosed with idiopathic adhesive capsulitis who were treated with a single intra-articular glenohumeral injection of local anesthetic and corticosteroid as well as 4 weeks of supervised physical therapy. After a minimum 2-year follow-up, this resulted in good clinical outcomes with a low incidence of surgical intervention. Young patients and patients with diabetes were shown to be more likely to develop contralateral disease later. Level of evidence: III.

8. Prodromidis AD, Charalambous CP: Is there a genetic predisposition to frozen shoulder?: A systematic review and meta-analysis. *J Bone Joint Surg Rev* 2016;4(2)e1-e9.

   This meta-analysis included research showing an 11.6% prevalence in twin pairs and demonstrated a heritability of 42% for frozen shoulder after adjusting for age. A second included study showed that 20% of patients with frozen shoulder had a positive family history involving a first-degree relative. The meta-analysis concluded that there is indeed limited evidence of a genetic link in frozen shoulder. Level of evidence: IV.

9. Hand GC, Athanasou NA, Matthews T, Carr AJ: The pathology of frozen shoulder. *J Bone Joint Surg Br* 2007;89(7):928-932.

10. Hettrich CM, DiCarlo EF, Faryniarz D, Vadasdi KB, Williams R, Hannafin JA: The effect of myofibroblasts and corticosteroid injections in adhesive capsulitis. *J Shoulder Elbow Surg* 2016;25(8):1274-1279.

    This preclinical study showed a higher prevalence of myofibroblast staining in patients with adhesive capsulitis, implicating activation of the myofibroblast in the pathophysiology of capsular contracture. Intra-articular steroid injection decreased the presence and amount of fibromatosis, vascular hyperplasia, fibrosis, and the presence of fibroblasts staining for α-smooth muscle actin.

11. Hwang KR, Murrell GA, Millar NL, Bonar F, Lam P, Walton JR: Advanced glycation end products in idiopathic frozen shoulders. *J Shoulder Elbow Surg* 2016;25(6):981-988.

    Shoulder capsule samples were collected from eight patients with idiopathic frozen shoulder and compared with those of 14 control group shoulders. The samples were hematoxylin and eosin stained and analyzed by immunohistochemistry using antibodies against advanced glycation end products. Hematoxylin and eosin–stained capsular tissue from frozen shoulder showed fibroblastic proliferation, increased numbers of adipocytes, and increased subsynovial vascularity, compared with control subjects.

12. Cho CH, Lho YM, Hwang I, Kim DH: Role of matrix metalloproteinases 2 and 9 in the development of frozen shoulder: Human data and experimental analysis in a rat contracture model. *J Shoulder Elbow Surg* 2019;28(7):1265-1272.

    The researchers obtained joint capsules from rats immobilized by molding plaster (a shoulder contracture model) at various time points. The expression of the inflammatory cytokine interleukin 6, metalloproteinase (MMP)-2, and MMP-9 was examined by immunohistochemistry and compared with controls. MMP-2 and MMP-9 were significantly overexpressed in the joint capsules of the frozen shoulders compared with those of controls.

13. Sasanuma H, Sugimoto H, Fujita A, et al: Characteristics of dynamic magnetic resonance imaging of idiopathic severe frozen shoulder. *J Shoulder Elbow Surg* 2017;26(2):e52-e57.

    This study evaluated dynamic three-dimensional MRI in the diagnosis of idiopathic severe frozen shoulder. Subjects consisted of 5 healthy control patients and 16 patients with idiopathic frozen shoulder. The frozen shoulder patients displayed an abnormal intake of blood flow from the acromial arterial network and the branches of circumflex humeral arteries into the axillary pouch and the rotator interval, dubbed the "burning sign," by the researchers. Level of evidence: IV.

14. Okuno Y, Oguro S, Iwamoto W, Miyamoto T, Ikegami H, Matsumura N: Short-term results of transcatheter arterial embolization for abnormal neovessels in patients with adhesive capsulitis: A pilot study. *J Shoulder Elbow Surg* 2014;23(9):e199-e206.

    Adhesive capsulitis was treated by transcatheter arterial embolization in seven patients and showed abnormal neovessels at the rotator interval in all subjects. The treatment decreased nighttime pain scores from 67 ± 14 to 27 ± 14 mm at 1 week after the procedure, with further improvement at 1 and 6 months. No major or minor adverse events were reported with the procedures. Level of evidence: IV.

15. Gerber C, Werner CM, Macy JC, Jacob HA, Nyffeler RW: Effect of selective capsulorrhaphy on the passive range of motion of the glenohumeral joint. *J Bone Joint Surg Am* 2003;85(1):48-55.

16. Bridgman JF: Periarthritis of the shoulder and diabetes mellitus. *Ann Rheum Dis* 1972;31(1):69-71.

17. Walker-Bone K, Palmer KT, Reading I, Coggon D, Cooper C: Prevalence and impact of musculoskeletal disorders of the upper limb in the general population. *Arthritis Rheum* 2004;51(4):642-651.

18. Kingston K, Curry EJ, Galvin JW, Li X: Shoulder adhesive capsulitis: Epidemiology and predictors of surgery. *J Shoulder Elbow Surg* 2018;27(8):1437-1443.

    In this retrospective cohort, 2,190 adhesive capsulitis patients were analyzed to evaluate variables associated with developing adhesive capsulitis. Obesity and diabetes were significantly associated with the condition. Level of evidence: III.

19. Yian EH, Contreras R, Sodl JF: Effects of glycemic control on prevalence of diabetic frozen shoulder. *J Bone Joint Surg Am* 2012;94(10):919-923.

20. Chan JH, Ho BS, Alvi HM, Saltzman MD, Marra G: The relationship between the incidence of adhesive capsulitis and hemoglobin A_{1c}. *J Shoulder Elbow Surg* 2017;26(10):1834-1837.

    In this retrospective analysis, researchers created a previously nonvalidated variable, cumulative HbA_{1c} that uses HbA_{1c} values over time to estimate the total disease burden a single individual experiences. The effect size of cumulative HbA_{1c} on adhesive capsulitis was significant; for each unit of time that the HbA_{1c} level was greater than 7, there was a 2.77% increase in the risk of adhesive capsulitis. Level of evidence: IV.

21. Barbosa F, Swamy G, Salem H, et al: Chronic adhesive capsulitis (Frozen shoulder): Comparative outcomes of treatment in patients with diabetes and obesity. *J Clin Orthop Trauma* 2019;10(2):265-268.

    This prospective cohort study of 210 idiopathic frozen shoulders over a 12-month period assessed functional outcomes before and after interventions, including steroid injections, arthroscopic release, and manipulation. Failure of initial injection therapy was higher in patients with diabetes (70%) than in those without diabetes (44%), but there was no statistical significance in outcomes of patients with body mass index of >30 and <30. Level of evidence: II.

22. Yanlei GL, Keong MW, Tijauw Tjoen DL: Do diabetic patients have different outcomes after arthroscopic capsular release for frozen shoulder? *J Orthop* 2019;16(3):211-215.

    This prospective study collected data of 56 consecutive patients with idiopathic frozen shoulder who underwent arthroscopic capsular release (360° arthroscopic capsulotomy). The procedure offered good outcomes in both patients with and without diabetes in terms of range of motion, pain relief, and shoulder function; however, patients with diabetes had poorer improvement in internal rotation and forward flexion postoperatively. Level of evidence: II.

23. Schiefer M, Teixeira PFS, Fontenelle C, et al: Prevalence of hypothyroidism in patients with frozen shoulder. *J Shoulder Elbow Surg* 2017;26(1):49-55.

    This case-control study measured serum thyroid-stimulating hormone and free tetraiodothyronine from 93 frozen shoulder patients and 151 control subjects. The prevalence of hypothyroidism diagnosis was significantly higher in the frozen shoulder group (27.2% versus 10.7%; $P = 0.001$). There was a trend toward independent association between high serum thyroid-stimulating hormone levels and bilateral frozen shoulder. Level of evidence: III.

24. Sung CM, Jung TS, Park HB: Are serum lipids involved in primary frozen shoulder? A case-control study. *J Bone Joint Surg Am* 2014;96(21):1828-1833.

    This case-control study comprised 300 patients diagnosed with frozen shoulder and compared the results with 900 control subjects. Univariate analysis showed total cholesterol, calculated LDL, measured LDL, HDL, and non-HDL cholesterol all to be significantly correlated with primary frozen shoulder.

25. Austin DC, Gans I, Park MJ, Carey JL, Kelly JD IV: The association of metabolic syndrome markers with adhesive capsulitis. *J Shoulder Elbow Surg* 2014;23(7):1043-1051.

This case-control, retrospective study investigated the relationship between metabolic syndrome components (insulin resistance, hypertension, dyslipidemia, and obesity) and the development of adhesive capsulitis. The prevalence of antihyperglycemia medications in the adhesive capsulitis cohort was 18.4%, twice the national rate of diagnosed diabetes. The overall prevalence of hypertensive medication use in the adhesive capsulitis group, 33.1%, was notably higher than the nationwide rate, 21.6%, but the prevalence of antilipid medication use and obesity was similar between the groups. Level of evidence: III.

26. Park HB, Gwark JY, Jung J: What serum lipid abnormalities are associated with adhesive capsulitis accompanied by diabetes. *Clin Orthop Relat Res* 2018;476(11):2231-2237.

    This case-control study evaluated 37 patients with newly diagnosed adhesive capsulitis accompanied by newly diagnosed diabetes, compared with control subjects. LDL and non-HDL were associated with adhesive capsulitis accompanied by diabetes, but it is yet unclear if these inflammatory lipoproteinemias are a cause, a related cofactor, or an aggravating factor in the development of adhesive capsulitis in patients with diabetes. Level of evidence: III.

27. Lee SY, Park J, Song SW: Correlation of MR arthrographic findings and range of shoulder motions in patients with frozen shoulder. *AJR Am J Roentgenol* 2012;198(1):173-179.

28. Song KD, Kwon JW, Yoon YC, Choi SH: Indirect MR arthrographic findings of adhesive capsulitis. *AJR Am J Roentgenol* 2011;197(6):W1105-W1109.

29. Loeffler BJ, Brown SL, D'Alessandro DF, Fleischli JE, Connor PM: Incidence of false positive rotator cuff pathology in MRIs of patients with adhesive capsulitis. *Orthopedics* 2011;34(5):362.

30. Carette S, Moffet H, Tardif J, et al: Intraarticular corticosteroids, supervised physiotherapy, or a combination of the two in the treatment of adhesive capsulitis of the shoulder: A placebo-controlled trial. *Arthritis Rheum* 2003;48(3):829-838.

31. Wang W, Shi M, Zhou C, et al: Effectiveness of corticosteroid injections in adhesive capsulitis of shoulder: A meta-analysis. *Medicine (Baltimore)* 2017;96(28):e7529.

    This meta-analysis included five studies with a sample size of 225 patients with adhesive capsulitis. The overall pooled data demonstrated that, compared with placebo as control treatment, intra-articular corticosteroid injections were more effective in reducing pain score at 0 to 8 weeks, but there was no difference between the injection group and the control group at 9 to 24 weeks. Improvement of patients' range of motion in the injection group was greater than that of the control group both at 0 to 8 and 9 to 24 weeks. Level of evidence: II.

32. Lorbach O, Anagnostakos K, Scherf C, Seil R, Kohn D, Pape D: Nonoperative management of adhesive capsulitis of the shoulder: Oral cortisone application versus intra-articular cortisone injections. *J Shoulder Elbow Surg* 2010;19(2):172-179.

33. Ranalletta M, Rossi LA, Bongiovanni SL, Tanoira I, Elizondo CM, Maignon GD: Corticosteroid injections accelerate pain relief and recovery of function compared with oral NSAIDs in patients with adhesive capsulitis: A randomized controlled trial. *Am J Sports Med* 2016;44(2):474-481.

    This randomized controlled trial included 74 patients with adhesive capsulitis, split into groups treated either with a single intra-articular corticosteroid injection before the beginning of a physical therapy program compared with a regimen of oral NSAIDs before the same physical therapy program. Patients treated with corticosteroid injections achieved faster pain relief compared with control patients during the first 8 weeks after treatment; however, no significant difference in pain was observed among the groups at final follow-up. Level of evidence: I.

34. Kitridis D, Tsikopoulos K, Bisbinas I, Papaioannidou P, Givissis P: Efficacy of pharmacological therapies for adhesive capsulitis of the shoulder: Systematic review and network meta-analysis. *Am J Sports Med* 2019;14:e1-e9.

    This 2019 network meta-analysis included 30 trials with a total of 2010 participants. Intra-articular corticosteroid injections, administered either alone or after distention of the shoulder capsule, provided clinically meaningful improvements in the short term. However, these short-term benefits of steroids dissipated over time. Study design: Network meta-analysis. Level of evidence: III.

35. Sethi PM, Kingston S, ElAttrache N: Accuracy of anterior intra-articular injection of the glenohumeral joint. *Arthroscopy* 2005;21(1):77-80.

36. Tobola A, Cook C, Cassas KJ, et al: Accuracy of glenohumeral joint injections: Comparing approach and experience of provider. *J Shoulder Elbow Surg* 2011;20(7):1147-1154.

37. Oh JH, Oh CH, Choi JA, Kim SH, Kim JH, Yoon JP: Comparison of glenohumeral and subacromial steroid injection in primary frozen shoulder: A prospective, randomized short-term comparison study. *J Shoulder Elbow Surg* 2011;20(7):1034-1040.

38. Sun Y, Liu S, Chen S, Chen J: The effect of corticosteroid injection into rotator interval for early frozen shoulder: A randomized controlled trial. *Am J Sports Med* 2018;46(3):663-670.

    In this randomized controlled trial, 97 adhesive capsulitis patients were randomized into three groups for corticosteroid injection in either rotator interval, intra-articular glenohumeral joint, or subacromial space. Rotator interval injections yielded better effects in terms of improvement in pain, passive ROM, and function. Level of evidence: I.

39. Yoon SH, Lee HY, Lee HJ, Kwack KS: Optimal dose of intra-articular corticosteroids for adhesive capsulitis: A randomized, triple-blind, placebo-controlled trial. *Am J Sports Med* 2013;41(5):1133-1139.

This randomized controlled clinical trial studied 53 patients with primary adhesive capsulitis in the freezing stage who were randomly assigned to receive ultrasound-guided intra-articular injections with 40 mg triamcinolone acetonide, 20 mg triamcinolone acetonide, or placebo. Repeated-measures analysis of variance and post hoc tests showed improvement in SPADI and VAS scores and in flexion, abduction, and internal rotation, especially for the low-dose and high-dose groups compared with the placebo. However, no significant difference was found between the two different corticosteroid dose groups. Level of evidence: I.

40. Chen CY, Hu CC, Weng PW, et al: Extracorporeal shockwave therapy improves short-term functional outcomes of shoulder adhesive capsulitis. *J Shoulder Elbow Surg* 2014;23(12):1843-1851.

In this prospective, randomized, controlled, single-blind clinical trial, 40 patients with primary adhesive capsulitis were treated with either extracorporeal shockwave therapy (ESWT) or oral steroid therapy. The total Clinical Severity Score (CSS) and range of motion parameter of the CSS in the ESWT group showed significant improvement from the fourth week that was better than that in the steroid group; the activities-of-daily-living parameter of the CSS achieved significance and was better than that in the steroid group at the sixth week. In addition, all of the adverse effects of ESWT were transient and tolerable. Level of evidence: I.

41. Yoon JP, Chung SW, Kim JE, et al: Intra-articular injection, subacromial injection, and hydrodilatation for primary frozen shoulder: A randomized clinical trial. *J Shoulder Elbow Surg* 2016;25(3):376-383.

In this randomized controlled trial, 90 patients with adhesive capsulitis were randomly allocated into the aforementioned three treatment arms. Although hydrodilatation yielded more rapid improvement at 1-month follow-up, the three injection methods for primary frozen shoulder resulted in similar clinical improvement in the final follow-up at 6 months. Level of evidence: I.

42. Mun SW, Baek CH: Clinical efficacy of hydrodistention with joint manipulation underinterscalene block compared with intra-articular corticosteroid injection for frozen shoulder: A prospective randomized controlled study. *J Shoulder Elbow Surg* 2016;25(12):1937-1943.

This prospective randomized controlled study included 121 patients presenting with primary frozen shoulder. Hydrodistention combined with joint manipulation under an interscalene block provided earlier pain relief and restoration of shoulder range of motion and function compared with single intra-articular corticosteroid injection. Level of evidence: II.

43. Nago M, Mitsui Y, Gotoh M, et al: Hyaluronan modulates cell proliferation and mRNA expression of adhesion-related procollagens and cytokines in glenohumeral synovial/capsular fibroblasts in adhesive capsulitis. *J Orthop Res* 2010;28(6):726-731.

44. Hsieh LF, Hsu WC, Lin YJ, Chang HL, Chen CC, Huang V: Addition of intra-articular hyaluronate injection to physical therapy program produces no extra benefits in patients with adhesive capsulitis of the shoulder: A randomized controlled trial. *Arch Phys Med Rehabil* 2012;93(6):957-964.

45. Harris JD, Griesser MJ, Copelan A, Jones GL: Treatment of adhesive capsulitis with intra-articular hyaluronate: A systematic review. *Int J Shoulder Surg* 2011;5(2): 31-37.

46. Dahan TH, Fortin L, Pelletier M, Petit M, Vadeboncoeur R, Suissa S: Double blind randomized clinical trial examining the efficacy of bupivacaine suprascapular nerve blocks in frozen shoulder. *J Rheumatol* 2000;27(6): 1464-1469.

47. Farrell CM, Sperling JW, Cofield RH: Manipulation for frozen shoulder: Long-term results. *J Shoulder Elbow Surg* 2005;14(5):480-484.

48. Jenkins EF, Thomas WJ, Corcoran JP, et al: The outcome of manipulation under general anesthesia for the management of frozen shoulder in patients with diabetes mellitus. *J Shoulder Elbow Surg* 2012;21(11):1492-1498.

49. Loew M, Heichel TO, Lehner B: Intraarticular lesions in primary frozen shoulder after manipulation under general anesthesia. *J Shoulder Elbow Surg* 2005;14(1):16-21.

50. Karas V, Riboh JC, Garrigues GE: Arthroscopic management of the stiff shoulder. *J Bone Joint Surg Rev* 2016;4(4):e21-e27.

This review article examines arthroscopic management of frozen shoulders. Current concepts are discussed, including the effect of stiff shoulder etiology on outcome, complications, and the senior author's preferred techniques.

51. Kim YS, Lee HJ: Essential surgical technique for arthroscopic capsular release in the treatment of shoulder stiffness. *JBJS Essent Surg Tech* 2015;5(3):e14.

This *JBJS Essential Surgical Technique* article provides a thorough and comprehensive stepwise guide for performing arthroscopic capsular release. Level of evidence: I.

52. Barnes CP, Lam PH, Murrell GA: Short-term outcomes after arthroscopic capsular release for adhesive capsulitis. *J Shoulder Elbow Surg* 2016;25(9):e256-e264.

This study included 133 patients with idiopathic adhesive capsulitis who underwent a complete arthroscopic release of the shoulder capsule. The procedure was found to result in immediate relative improvements in pain, functional outcomes, and range of motion, and no complications were reported. Level of evidence: IV.

53. Watson L, Dalziel R, Story I: Frozen shoulder: A 12-month clinical outcome trial. *J Shoulder Elbow Surg* 2000;9(1):16-22.

54. Le Lievre HM, Murrell GA: Long-term outcomes after arthroscopic capsular release for idiopathic adhesive capsulitis. *J Bone Joint Surg Am* 2012;94(13):1208-1216.

55. Namdari S, Green A: Range of motion limitation after rotator cuff repair. *J Shoulder Elbow Surg* 2010;19(2):290-296.

56. Levy O, Webb M, Even T, Venkateswaran B, Funk L, Copeland SA: Arthroscopic capsular release for posttraumatic shoulder stiffness. *J Shoulder Elbow Surg* 2008;17(3):410-414.

57. Moon N, Lee S, Shin W, Lee S, Suh K: Is pancapsular release more effective than selective capsular release for the treatment of adhesive capsulitis? *Clin Shoulder Elbow* 2015;18(1):28-35.

In this study, 35 patients with either primary or secondary adhesive capsulitis in whom nonsurgical management had failed were split into groups treated via either arthroscopic pancapsular release that comprised the release of the rotator interval, anteroinferior capsular, and the posterior capsular release, or a selective capsular release that comprised only the release of the rotator interval release and anteroinferior capsular release. The clinical outcomes, visual analog scale score, Constant score, and range of motion were assessed preoperatively and postoperatively. In both groups, the preoperative VAS score, Constant score, and ROM showed a significant improvement by the 6-month follow-up; however, pancapsular release did not show any advantage over selective capsular release in terms of overall clinical outcome. Level of evidence: I.

58. Kim YS, Lee HJ, Park IJ: Clinical outcomes do not support arthroscopic posterior capsular release in addition to anterior release for shoulder stiffness: A randomized controlled study. *Am J Sports Med* 2014;42(5): 1143-1149.

This randomized controlled trial included 75 patients who underwent arthroscopic capsular release for shoulder stiffness that were enrolled and randomized into two groups. In group I, capsular release was performed, including release of the rotator interval and anterior and inferior capsule. In group II, capsular release was extended to the posterior capsule. Both groups showed significantly increased ROM at the last follow-up compared with preoperative ROM, but at the last follow-up, no statistical differences were found between groups I and II in the American Shoulder and Elbow Surgeons score, Simple Shoulder Test, visual analog scale, and ROM. Level of evidence: I.

Chapter 47

Anesthesia and Analgesia for Shoulder and Elbow Surgery

E. David Bravos, MD

ABSTRACT

Anesthesia and analgesia for shoulder and elbow surgery are important components of patient care during the perioperative period. There are several anesthetic and analgesic considerations that should be taken into account that include preoperative comorbidities, patient positioning, intraoperative anesthetic choice, and analgesic techniques. Using multimodal and preventive analgesia is an effective approach.

Keywords: multimodal analgesia; peripheral nerve blockade; preventative analgesia

Introduction

Patients who require shoulder and elbow surgery can present several challenges for the perioperative team. Given the wide variety of patient ages, comorbidities, and the concern for neurologic evaluation, careful planning between the surgeon and the anesthesiologist is essential. One of the most significant concerns is managing postoperative pain. In addition to the traditional use of opioid and nonopioid analgesic agents, peripheral nerve blockade (PNB) of the brachial plexus is an excellent choice for postoperative analgesia because most surgeries can be covered with a single approach to the brachial plexus. The use of PNB has increased over the past decade secondary to the advancement of ultrasound guidance to perform it. When used as an analgesic agent, PNB can provide superior analgesia, decrease opioid-related adverse effects, and lead to greater patient satisfaction compared to intravenous opioids alone.[1,2] For certain surgeries of the elbow, PNB may serve as the intraoperative anesthetic, but for surgeries of the shoulder, it is commonly used as a postoperative analgesic and combined with a general anesthetic or heavy sedation. In cases where postoperative pain is expected to be moderate or severe, continuous PNB can be used. More recently, a liposomal formulation has been approved by the FDA which can potentially provide analgesia for 72 hours with a single injection.[3]

Dr. Bravos or an immediate family member has stock or stock options held in Pacira.

General Considerations for Preoperative Management

Given the wide range of patients who present for shoulder and elbow surgery, from the young healthy athlete to the elderly patient with significant comorbidities, careful preoperative evaluation must occur. In addition to the well-known contraindications to PNB, certain coexisting diseases may preclude their use. Patients known to have significant pulmonary disease may not be the best candidates for a brachial plexus block that can cause phrenic nerve paralysis. An interscalene block has been shown to cause blockade of the phrenic nerve 100% of the time and a supraclavicular block up to 80% of the time.[4-6] This can result in up to a 27% reduction in pulmonary mechanics, such as forced vital capacity and forced expiratory volume in the first second.[7] Additionally, patients with a contralateral diaphragmatic paresis would not be candidates for a brachial plexus block affecting the phrenic nerve. Other contraindications would include a recurrent laryngeal nerve palsy because of the potential blockade of the recurrent laryngeal nerve that can occur with interscalene or supraclavicular nerve blocks.

Patients with a preexisting nerve injury must be evaluated to determine if they are appropriate candidates for PNB. Careful communication between the anesthesiologist and the surgeon must take place if there is concern for potential nerve injury during the procedure or the need for immediate or ongoing postoperative neurologic evaluation.

Other preoperative considerations include whether patients will receive medications for preventive analgesia. Celecoxib, gabapentin, and acetaminophen have all been used.

General Considerations for Intraoperative Management

Intraoperative anesthetic management for shoulder and elbow surgery may be achieved with general anesthesia, regional anesthesia, or a combination of both. There are several factors that dictate whether a patient can have a regional technique alone as the intraoperative anesthetic or whether this must be combined with a general anesthetic requiring airway management with an endotracheal tube, a laryngeal mask airway, or heavy sedation. Understanding not only the anatomy and innervation of the upper extremity, but also the clinical distribution of the different blocks of the brachial plexus is essential.

Appropriate Selection of PNB

There are four major blocks of the brachial plexus, which are named according to the anatomic location of where these blocks are performed (**Figure 1**). Given that these blocks are located at different levels of the brachial plexus, they subsequently have different clinical distributions of anesthesia and analgesia of the upper extremity. Surgeries of the shoulder and the proximal humerus are best served by an interscalene block. This is because of blockade of the C3 and C4 nerve roots, which are not part of the brachial plexus, but rather help form the superficial cervical plexus. This, in turn, gives rise to the supraclavicular nerves, which provide sensation to the cape of the shoulder. These nerves are typically blocked by spread of a larger volume of local anesthetic when this block is performed at the level of C6. This will cover incisions that extend into the cape of the shoulder. A single-shot supraclavicular block has been used for surgery of the shoulder if enough volume of local anesthetic is given; however, it may not be the best block choice if continuous PNB is used because this type of block typically is run at a lower volume of local anesthetic postoperatively. Infraclavicular and axillary blocks are not appropriate for surgery of the shoulder or the proximal humerus. For surgeries of the distal humerus and the elbow, an infraclavicular block or a supraclavicular block would appropriately cover this area. An interscalene block may not be the best choice because of ulnar sparing caused by missing the C8 and T1 nerve roots. However, a low interscalene approach with a large enough local anesthetic volume may provide coverage. Axillary blocks are best suited for procedures below the elbow.

Other Local Anesthetic Techniques

In addition to PNB of the brachial plexus, other local anesthetic techniques may include subacromial (bursal) or intra-articular infiltration of local anesthetic, as well as suprascapular with or without axillary (circumflex) nerve blocks. In a systematic review, different local anesthetic techniques were studied to determine their efficacy and potential for opioid sparing.[8]

It is unclear if there is significant analgesic efficacy of subacromial/intra-articular infiltration. More importantly, concern for iatrogenic chondrolysis of continuous infusion of local anesthetic has caused this modality to fall out of favor. Suprascapular nerve blockade may provide clinically significant analgesia compared with placebo. The addition of an axillary nerve block may improve the analgesic efficacy of this technique. Although less efficacious compared with an interscalene nerve block, it may be used in patients with significant pulmonary disease in whom avoidance of phrenic nerve paralysis is preferred.[9] A continuous interscalene block with a basal rate infusion, along with patient-controlled boluses, is the most efficacious of all local anesthetic techniques for surgery of the shoulder.

Intraoperative Anesthetic Technique

For surgery of the shoulder, innervation of cutaneous and bony structures may not be covered by a brachial plexus block alone. Therefore, PNB is commonly performed for postoperative analgesia and combined with general anesthesia or heavy sedation. This is usually determined by the position in which the patient is placed (beach chair versus lateral) and the ability of the anesthesiologist to have access to the patient's airway.

For surgery of the elbow, a brachial plexus block may provide complete anesthesia of all the areas of surgical stimulation and may be used as the sole anesthetic technique, depending on the patient's position. This approach may allow the patient to be awake or minimally sedated if desired. For patients placed in a lateral or a prone position, more definitive airway management may be necessary.

Positioning

Position for surgery of the shoulder typically takes place in the beach chair or the lateral decubitus position. Regardless of technique, care in positioning and an understanding of the potential complications is paramount. Some advantages of the beach-chair position include ease of setup, decreased risk of nerve injury from traction, and ease of conversion to an open procedure.[10] Patients in the beach chair position are supine, with the head of the bed raised from 20° to 30° and up to 80° depending on the specific procedure. The table can also be positioned such that the hips are in a flexed position from 45° to 60° and the knees flexed to 30°. Alternatively, the legs may be kept in a more straight position at the knees to decrease venous pooling and increase venous return and cardiac output. Patients in the beach-chair position may experience sudden profound hypotension and bradycardia with reports of cardiovascular collapse.[11,12] This is thought to be a result of the Bezold-Jarisch reflex (**Figure 2**), whereby venous pooling in the lower extremities decreases venous return. Compensatory increases in heart rate and contractility can lead to the activation of receptors within the heart that paradoxically increase parasympathetic and decrease sympathetic output, leading

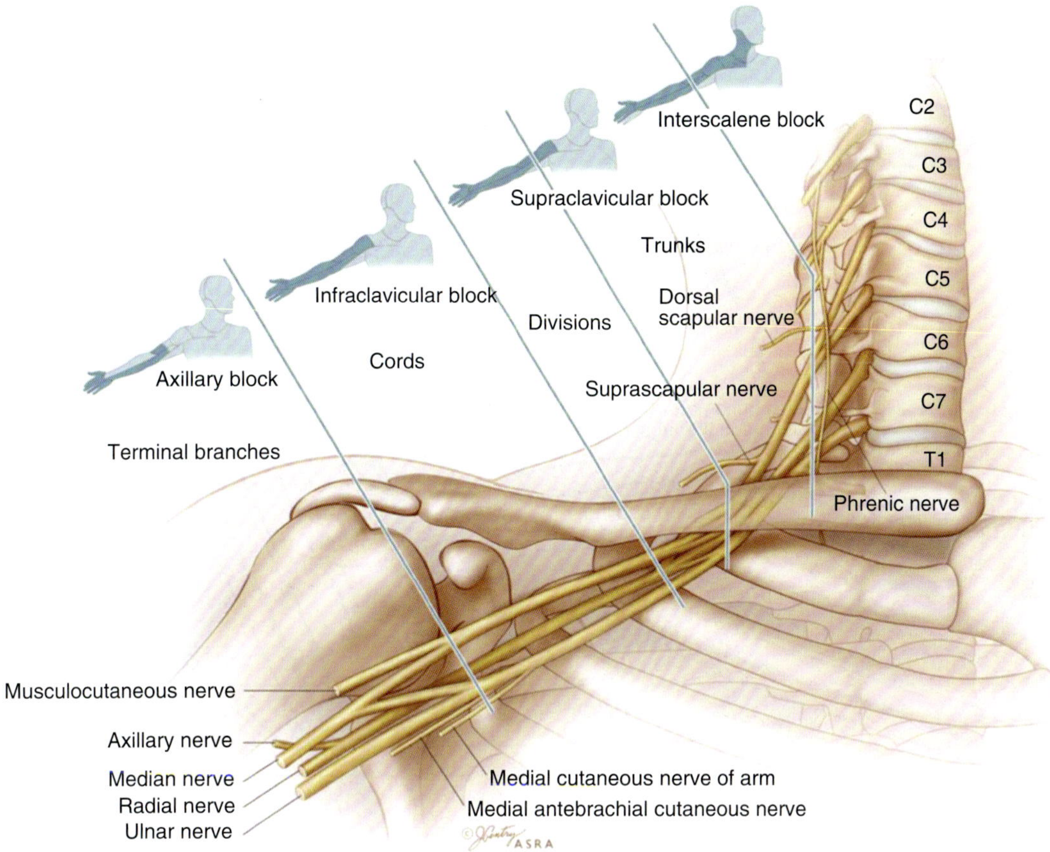

FIGURE 1 Illustration showing idealized brachial plexus. Various approaches define the individual brachial plexus blocks and their expected distribution of cutaneous anesthesia. (Reproduced with permission from *Reg Anesth Pain Med*. Neal JM, Gerancher JC, Hebl, JR, et al: Upper extremity regional anesthesia: Essentials of our understanding 2008, 34[2]:134-170. Copyright © 2009, with permission from the BMJ Publishing Group Ltd.)

to bradycardia, vasodilation, and resultant hypotension or cardiovascular collapse. This may be exacerbated by epinephrine containing local anesthetic solutions used for PNB.[13] Treatment may include adequate hydration, beta-blockers if the patient becomes reflexively tachycardic, and atropine or epinephrine for severe bradycardia.[14] Additionally, there is concern for central nervous system end-organ ischemia, including cerebral ischemia, ophthalmoplegia, and visual loss in the beach-chair position.[15,16] The exact mechanism is unknown, but has been purported to be from postural hypotension that can occur with the blood pressure being monitored from the patient's calf.[17] Cerebral perfusion pressure can be significantly different from what is measured intraoperatively because of the hydrostatic pressure difference from the head and the lower extremity. Exacerbation of this pressure can occur during arthroscopy, when the blood pressure may be further lowered to improve visualization in the surgical field. Another mechanism may include manipulation or positioning of the head, causing mechanical obstruction of the neck vessels.

The advantages of the lateral position include better visualization with arm traction, increased cerebral perfusion, and better access to the superior and posterior portals. The disadvantages of this position include the need for airway management and general anesthesia, risk of traction neuropathy, and difficulty with conversion to an open procedure.[10] Positioning for elbow surgery can be performed in the supine, lateral, or prone positions depending on the approach needed.

Neurologic Complications

Nerve injury can vary from a minor paresthesia to complete loss of motor function. Injury can be due to surgical-related, patient-related, or anesthesia-related factors. The overall incidence is low, but when it occurs,

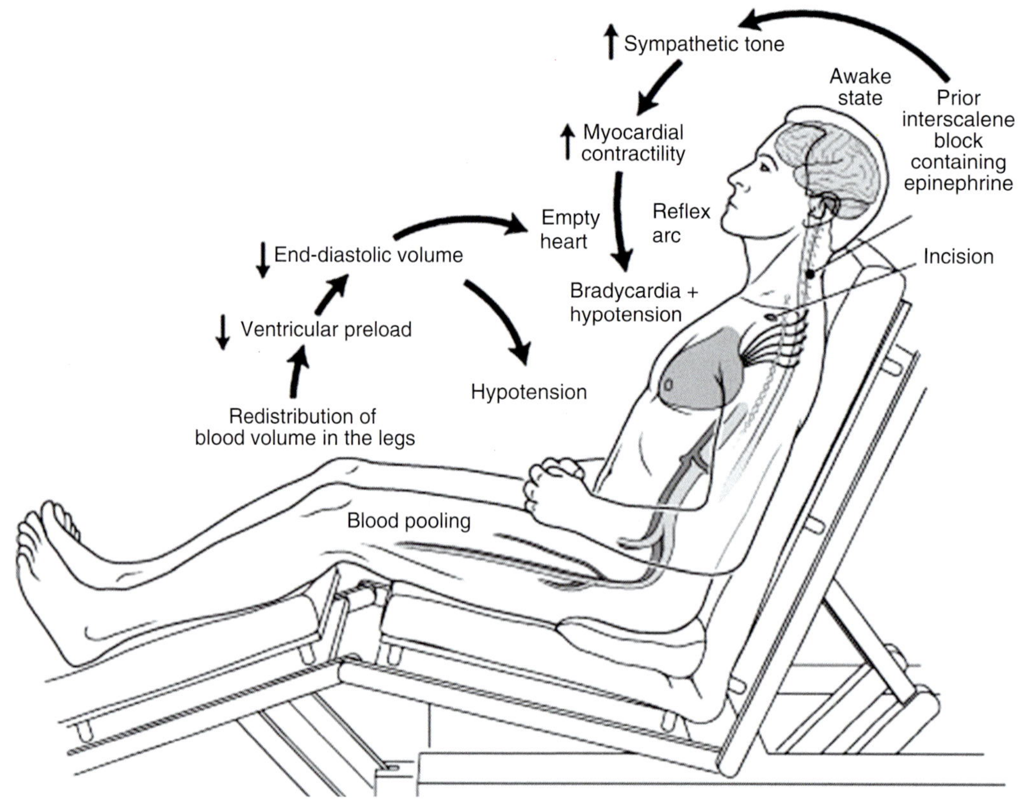

FIGURE 2 Illustration showing mechanisms of hypotension/bradycardia. Patients who receive interscalene brachial plexus block, are sedated, and are placed in the beach-chair position may develop hypotension and bradycardia during their anesthetic course. The proposed mechanism for this phenomenon is a relative preload deficit from the sitting position, combined with a hypercontractile ventricle, which occurs as a consequence of exogenous and endogenous epinephrine. The vigorously contracting empty heart causes reflex bradycardia and hypotension. (Reproduced with permission from *Reg Anesth Pain Med*. Neal JM, Gerancher JC, Hebl, JR, et al: Upper extremity regional anesthesia: Essentials of our understanding 2008, 34[2]:134-170. Copyright © 2009, with permission from the BMJ Publishing Group Ltd.)

nerve injury can cause significant distress to the patient and the perioperative team. The nerves most commonly injured from shoulder surgery include the axillary, musculocutaneous, suprascapular, and subscapular nerves. Injuries to these nerves most commonly occur during joint arthroplasty and surgery for anterior joint instability. The reported incidence is 1% to 2% in patients undergoing rotator cuff surgery, 1% to 8% in patients undergoing surgery for anterior instability, and 1% to 4% in patients undergoing arthroplasty.[18-21] Confounding any type of neurologic complication is the use of PNB. More specifically, an interscalene block is typically performed at the level of C6. The nerves most vulnerable during shoulder surgery come from the C5, C6, and C7 nerve roots. The incidence of nerve injury for PNB has been estimated to be less than 3%.[22] Therefore, open communication between the surgeon and the anesthesiologist is imperative if the patient is at increased risk of nerve injury. A thorough preoperative neurologic examination should be performed. If there is concern for neurologic injury or the need for postoperative neurologic monitoring, a single-shot nerve block can be performed postoperatively or a peripheral nerve catheter can be placed preoperatively, but not dosed until a normal postoperative neurologic examination has been documented.

Postoperative Analgesia

In addition to the unwanted psychological and physiologic effects of suboptimally treated pain, a lack of adequate postoperative analgesia can interfere with early physical therapy and rehabilitation, and possibly increase the risk of chronic postsurgical pain.[23-25] Perioperative opioids have been a mainstay for the treatment of pain despite many of the well-known adverse effects of nausea, vomiting, pruritis, sedation, constipation, and respiratory depression. In addition to these well-known adverse effects, surgeries with moderate to severe postoperative pain requiring larger amounts of opioids can delay discharge and create unanticipated hospital admissions in the outpatient setting. Although opioids may still have a role for treating postoperative pain, using several types of analgesic agents with different mechanisms and using multimodal and preventive analgesic strategies may minimize some of the unwanted side effects. In addition, limiting unnecessary exposure of opioids could decrease the risk of long-term use.[26]

Preventive and Multimodal Analgesia

Preventive analgesia refers to preventing or attenuating central sensitization that can occur after a traumatic insult and the inflammatory response that ensues.[27] Although it was initially thought that initiating analgesia before the insult was more efficacious than afterward, clinical trials have not consistently supported this finding.[28,29] More recently, it is thought that the most efficacious approach is to use a multimodal analgesic regimen during the entire perioperative period that can attenuate the firing of nociceptive input to the central nervous system before, during, and after a surgical procedure.[1] In turn, multimodal analgesia uses two or more analgesic agents with different mechanisms of action whose overall analgesic effects become additive or synergistic while decreasing the adverse effects of any one agent.[30] Greater emphasis has been placed on using nonopioid analgesic agents, including regional analgesic techniques, and using opioids for breakthrough pain.[31]

Opioids

Opioids are one of the most common analgesic agents used that have the benefit of being delivered by multiple routes (oral, intravenous, intramuscular, subcutaneous, intranasal, transmucosal, and neuraxial). They have no analgesic ceiling effect; however, their analgesic efficacy can be limited by the adverse effects of nausea, vomiting, sedation, pruritis, ileus, and respiratory depression. Patients undergoing shoulder and elbow surgery are typically treated with intravenous or oral regimens.

Parenteral Administration

Administration through the intravenous route produces a relatively rapid onset and reliable analgesia that can be quickly titrated compared with other routes. Patients with moderate to severe pain may require intravenous opioids, most commonly delivered in the form of intravenous patient-controlled analgesia (IV PCA). This method of delivery likely provides better pain relief and improved patient satisfaction compared with dosing as required by nursing staff.[32]

The variables that can be programmed into an IV PCA include the bolus or demand dose, lockout interval, and background infusion (**Table 1**). The optimal settings are not known, but following a few basic principles may increase analgesic efficacy and decrease the risk of potential overdosing. The optimal bolus or demand dose is based on the potency of the opioid and should be sufficient to decrease pain after a few patient-controlled doses. Too small of a dose can lead to inadequate analgesia, whereas too large of a dose can lead to increased adverse effects, including respiratory depression. The lockout interval should be based on the analgesic onset and the peak effect of the opioid and should allow the patient to determine the efficacy of the prior dose before another dose is self-administered. Too long of a lockout interval can lead to inadequate analgesia, and too short an interval can lead to stacking of doses. Continuous or background infusions are not typically recommended for opiate-naïve patients. It was thought that running a continuous infusion during periods of sleep while patients could not self-administer a dose may improve analgesia. However, this may lead to increased adverse events, such as respiratory depression, without a proven benefit of improved analgesia.[33,34] Continuous infusions may be of benefit in opioid-tolerant patients.

An important concept to realize when using an IV PCA is that one size does not fit all.[35] The process of treating a patient's pain is dynamic. Individuals may have different analgesic requirements, and these analgesic requirements may change during the perioperative period. This is especially true during the first 24 to 48

Table 1

Intravenous Opioid Patient-Controlled Analgesic Regimens

Opioid	Demand Dose	Lockout Interval (min)	Infusion Rate[a]
Morphine	0.5-2.5 mg	5-10	1-10 mg/hr
Fentanyl	10-20 μg	5-10	20-100 μg/hr
Hydromorphone	0.1-0.2 mg	5-10	0.1-0.2 mg/hr

[a]Continuous infusions are not recommended for opiate-naïve patients.

hours after surgery. A constant reassessment of a patient's pain control needs to be performed with adjustment of the analgesic regimen.

Enteral Administration

Oral opioids can be used to treat moderate to severe pain once a patient can tolerate oral administration, but they can be less reliable and titratable compared with intravenous opioids. They are available in both immediate-release and controlled-release formulations (**Table 2**). Although the immediate-release form has the ability to control moderate to severe pain, it needs to be given every 4 to 6 hours to maintain adequate plasma levels. Delays in administration when these medications are given as needed can result in an unnecessary increase in pain. Guidelines have been developed that recommend a fixed dosing schedule when using this formulation.[36] Controlled-release formulations are not generally recommended and do not confer any increased benefit to that of the immediate-release formulations unless a patient is on them preoperatively.[37,38]

Tramadol

Tramadol is a synthetic analgesic agent that is structurally related to codeine and morphine. It is thought to act directly on μ receptors as well as prevent the uptake of norepinephrine and serotonin, which are involved in spinal inhibition of pain.[39,40] Tramadol is less potent than morphine, but it has the benefit of a lower incidence of adverse effects such as respiratory depression, constipation, and dependence.[41,42] Its use has been shown to have a beneficial effect that is comparable with other opioids in managing patients with moderate postoperative pain. It may be used as part of a multimodal analgesic regimen or in patients who may not tolerate opioids.

Nonopioid Analgesic Agents

In congruency with a multimodal analgesic regimen, nonopioid analgesic agents play an important role in providing postoperative analgesia. A balanced regimen of nonopioid analgesic agents may lead to opioid sparing, decreased opioid-related adverse effects, and increased analgesic efficacy (**Table 3**).

Nonsteroidal Anti-Inflammatory Drugs

NSAIDs have effectively been used for treating nonsurgical pain because of their analgesic, anti-inflammatory, and antipyretic effects. Their role has increased in postoperative patients with the introduction of intravenous formulations such as ketorolac and diclofenac which have been shown to have similar analgesic efficacy to that of opioids.[43,44] These drugs act through inhibition of cyclooxygenase (COX) enzymes and ultimately the production of prostaglandins which are chemical mediators of the acute inflammatory and pain response. The main site of action is in the peripheral nervous system, but there may also be a central effect in nociception.[45] The COX-1 enzyme is constitutively expressed and is involved in gastric mucosal protection through prostaglandin E_2 and has a thromboxane-mediated effect on platelet aggregation. The COX-2 isoform is an inducible enzyme produced during inflammation and fever. Nonspecific COX inhibitors, such as ketorolac, block COX-1 and COX-2 isoenzymes, whereas selective COX inhibitors, such as celecoxib, inhibit only the COX-2 isoenzyme. COX-2 inhibitors have minimal effect on the coagulation system, allowing them to be safely used in the perioperative period with less concern for bleeding.

Although the use of NSAIDs as an analgesic agent has been shown to be beneficial, their use may be limited by some of their adverse effects. Of these, the most

Table 2

Oral Opioid Analgesic Agents

Opioid	Dose (mg)	Interval (hr)	Comments
Oxycodone (IR)	5-10	4-6	More than four doses should not be exceeded in a 24-hr period to avoid the stacking of doses with risk of adverse opioid side effects
Hydrocodone	5-10	4-6	Combined with acetaminophen
Hydromorphone	2-4	4-6	
Codeine	30-60	4	May be combined with acetaminophen or aspirin
Tramadol	50-100	6	

ER = extended release, IR = immediate release.

Table 3

Nonopioid Analgesic Agents

Analgesic	Dose (mg)	Interval (hr)	24-hr Maximum Dose (mg)	Comments
Aspirin	325-1,000	4-6	3,200	
Acetaminophen	500-1,000	4-6	4,000	
Ibuprofen	200-800	4-6	3,200	
Naproxen	500	12	1,000	
Celecoxib	200-400	12	800	
Ketorolac	15-30	6	60-120	15 mg if <50 kg or >65 yr; 30 mg if >50 kg or <65 yr; should not be given for more than 5 d
Gabapentin	300-1,200			Ideal analgesic dosing not known
Pregabalin	150-300			Ideal analgesic dosing not known

concerning for perioperative patients are platelet dysfunction, renal dysfunction, and gastrointestinal bleeding. Additionally, some concern for bone healing may exist when NSAIDs are used in orthopaedic procedures where an inflammatory response and prostaglandin production play a role in this process.[46] The adverse effects are due to the inhibition of COX enzymes. Inhibition of thromboxane synthesis can inhibit platelet aggregation and potentially increase surgical bleeding. Inhibition of prostaglandin production can lead to gastrointestinal bleeding through loss of mucosal protection and renal dysfunction from renal arteriolar vasoconstriction. The use of all COX inhibitors can lead to renal dysfunction; however, the use of selective COX-2 inhibitors can limit the risk of platelet dysfunction and gastrointestinal bleeding. The use of NSAIDs should be dictated by individual patients and the particular surgery they are having.

Acetaminophen

Acetaminophen is a nonopioid analgesic agent that is thought to act by inhibiting COX enzymes and decreasing central prostaglandin production.[47] Until recently, acetaminophen was available only in oral and rectal form in the United States, but it is now available in an intravenous formulation. Although it has weak anti-inflammatory properties, acetaminophen has significant analgesic and antipyretic properties with minimal gastrointestinal, renal, and platelet adverse effects. The use of acetaminophen has been studied in several surgery types, including orthopaedic surgery. When compared with placebo, acetaminophen decreased overall 24-hour morphine consumption, with improved pain scores and patient satisfaction.[48,49] Additionally, the combination of acetaminophen and NSAIDs has been shown to be more effective than either NSAIDs or acetaminophen alone[50] and more effective when given in scheduled doses rather than on an as-needed basis.[51] Despite its opioid-sparing and analgesic effect, acetaminophen has not been consistently shown to decrease opioid-related adverse effects.[52,53]

Gabapentin and Pregabalin

Gabapentin and pregabalin are gamma-aminobutyric analogues whose mechanism is thought to act on voltage-gated calcium channels, but whose true analgesic effect is unknown. Several studies suggest gabapentin, when given in a single preoperative dose, may have an opioid-sparing effect and may improve pain scores at rest and movement.[54-57] Additionally, one study has shown a decrease in opioid-related adverse effects, such as vomiting, but was not significantly reduced in others. Similarly, pregabalin has been shown to have a significant reduction in pain relief, pain intensity difference, and pain relief intensity difference compared with placebo and 400 mg of ibuprofen with dental pain from tooth extraction.[58,59]

Ketamine

Ketamine is an *N*-methyl-D-aspartic acid receptor antagonist and has been used as an anesthetic in the operating room. With the discovery of the *N*-methyl-D-aspartic acid receptor and its possible role in central sensitization and chronic postsurgical pain, it has also been used as analgesic adjunct.[60] Several studies have shown a possible analgesic and opioid-sparing effect when ketamine has been used in subanesthetic doses.[61,62] Patients undergoing total knee arthroplasty under general anesthesia who received low-dose ketamine intraoperatively and postoperatively for the first 48 hours had lower pain scores at rest and with movement, along with decreased time for flexion to 90° compared with placebo.[63] Its use has been limited out of concern for the psychomimetic and cardiovascular effects that may occur with anesthetic doses.

SUMMARY

Anesthesia and analgesia for shoulder and elbow surgery can be approached in several ways. Continuous communication between the anesthesiologist and the surgeon is essential to provide the best intraoperative and postoperative care. Using a multimodal analgesic approach with local anesthetic in the form of PNB and nonopioid analgesic agents while reserving opioids for rescue analgesia may be optimal. Patients may likely have superior analgesia, fewer opioid-related adverse effects, and overall greater satisfaction. This, in turn, can help the patient reach the ultimate goal of striving for the best functional and clinical outcome.

KEY STUDY POINTS

- Peripheral nerve blockade is an effective analgesic technique, but may have contraindications.
- Intraoperative anesthetic choice can depend on patient and surgical factors such as positioning.
- Using a multimodal and preventive analgesic approach may improve analgesic efficacy and decrease side effects from any particular analgesic agent.

Annotated References

1. Pogatzki-Zahn EM, Zahn PK: From preemptive to preventive analgesia. *Curr Opin Anaesthesiol* 2006;19(5):551-555.

2. Richman JM, Liu SS, Courpas G, et al: Does continuous peripheral nerve block provide superior pain control to opioids? A meta-analysis. *Anesth Analg* 2006;102(1):248-257.

3. U.S. Food & Drug Administration: FDA In Brief: FDA approves new use of Exparel for nerve block pain relief following shoulder surgeries. Available at: https://www.fda.gov/news-events/fda-brief/fda-brief-fda-approves-new-use-exparel-nerve-block-pain-relief-following-shoulder-surgeries.

4. Urmey WF, Talts KH, Sharrock NE: One hundred percent incidence of hemidiaphragmatic paresis associated with interscalene brachial plexus anesthesia as diagnosed by ultrasonography. *Anesth Analg* 1991;72(4):498-503.

5. Knoblanche GE: The incidence and aetiology of phrenic nerve blockade associated with supraclavicular brachial plexus block. *Anaesth Intensive Care* 1979;7(4):346-349.

6. Dhuner KG, Moberg E, Onne L: Paresis of the phrenic nerve during brachial plexus block analgesia and its importance. *Acta Chir Scand* 1955;109(1):53-57.

7. Urmey WF, McDonald M: Hemidiaphragmatic paresis during interscalene brachial plexus block: Effects on pulmonary function and chest wall mechanics. *Anesth Analg* 1992;74(3):352-357.

8. Fredrickson MJ, Krishnan S, Chen CY: Postoperative analgesia for shoulder surgery: A critical appraisal and review of current techniques. *Anaesthesia* 2010;65(6):608-624.

9. Dhir S, Sondekoppam RV, Sharma R, Ganapathy S, Athwal GS: A comparison of combined suprascapular and axillary nerve blocks to interscalene nerve block for analgesia in arthroscopic shoulder surgery: An equivalence study. *Reg Anesth Pain Med* 2016;41(5):564-571.

   Although an interscalene nerve block provides greater analgesia, combined suprascapular and axillary nerve blocks can be a clinically acceptable analgesic option with a different analgesic profile compared with an interscalene nerve block. Level of evidence: I.

10. Peruto CM, Ciccotti MG, Cohen SB: Shoulder arthroscopy positioning: Lateral decubitus versus beach chair. *Arthroscopy* 2009;25(8):891-896.

11. Aviado DM, Guevara Aviado D: The Bezold-Jarisch reflex. A historical perspective of cardiopulmonary reflexes. *Ann N Y Acad Sci* 2001;940:48-58.

12. Campagna JA, Carter C: Clinical relevance of the Bezold-Jarisch reflex. *Anesthesiology* 2003;98(5):1250-1260.

13. D'Alessio JG, Weller RS, Rosenblum M: Activation of the Bezold-Jarisch reflex in the sitting position for shoulder arthroscopy using interscalene block. *Anesth Analg* 1995;80(6):1158-1162.

14. Liguori GA, Kahn RL, Gordon J, Gordon MA, Urban MK: The use of metoprolol and glycopyrrolate to prevent hypotensive/bradycardic events during shoulder arthroscopy in the sitting position under interscalene block. *Anesth Analg* 1998;87(6):1320-1325.

15. Bhatti MT, Enneking FK: Visual loss and ophthalmoplegia after shoulder surgery. *Anesth Analg* 2003;96(3):899-902.

16. Pohl A, Cullen DJ: Cerebral ischemia during shoulder surgery in the upright position: A case series. *J Clin Anesth* 2005;17(6):463-469.

17. Rains DD, Rooke GA, Wahl CJ: Pathomechanisms and complications related to patient positioning and anesthesia during shoulder arthroscopy. *Arthroscopy* 2011;27(4):532-541.

18. Boardman ND III, Cofield RH: Neurologic complications of shoulder surgery. *Clin Orthop Relat Res* 1999;(368):44-53.

19. Wirth MA, Rockwood CA Jr: Complications of shoulder arthroplasty. *Clin Orthop Relat Res* 1994;(307):47-69.

20. Wirth MA, Rockwood CA Jr: Complications of total shoulder-replacement arthroplasty. *J Bone Joint Surg Am* 1996;78(4):603-616.

21. Zanotti RM, Carpenter JE, Blasier RB, Greenfield ML, Adler RS, Bromberg MB: The low incidence of suprascapular nerve injury after primary repair of massive rotator cuff tears. *J Shoulder Elbow Surg* 1997;6(3):258-264.

22. Brull R, McCartney CJ, Chan VW, El-Beheiry H: Neurological complications after regional anesthesia: Contemporary estimates of risk. *Anesth Analg* 2007;104(4):965-974.

23. Perkins FM, Kehlet H: Chronic pain as an outcome of surgery. A review of predictive factors. *Anesthesiology* 2000;93(4):1123-1133.

24. Wu CL, Fleisher LA: Outcomes research in regional anesthesia and analgesia. *Anesth Analg* 2000;91(5):1232-1242.

25. Wu CL, Rowlingson AJ, Partin AW, et al: Correlation of postoperative pain to quality of recovery in the immediate postoperative period. *Reg Anesth Pain Med* 2005;30(6):516-522.

26. Alam A, Gomes T, Zheng H, Mamdani MM, Juurlink DN, Bell CM: Long-term analgesic use after low-risk surgery: A retrospective cohort study. *Arch Intern Med* 2012;172(5):425-430.

27. Kissin I: Preemptive analgesia. *Anesthesiology* 2000;93(4):1138-1143.

28. Woolf CJ, Chong MS: Preemptive analgesia – Treating postoperative pain by preventing the establishment of central sensitization. *Anesth Analg* 1993;77(2):362-379.

29. Kissin I: Preemptive analgesia. Why its effect is not always obvious. *Anesthesiology* 1996;84(5):1015-1019.

30. Buvanendran A, Kroin JS: Multimodal analgesia for controlling acute postoperative pain. *Curr Opin Anaesthesiol* 2009;22(5):588-593.

31. Elvir-Lazo OL, White PF: The role of multimodal analgesia in pain management after ambulatory surgery. *Curr Opin Anaesthesiol* 2010;23(6):697-703.

32. Rathmell JP, Wu CL, Sinatra RS, et al: Acute post-surgical pain management: A critical appraisal of current practice. *Reg Anesth Pain Med* 2006;31(4 suppl 1):1-42.

33. Macintyre PE: Safety and efficacy of patient-controlled analgesia. *Br J Anaesth* 2001;87(1):36-46.

34. Smythe MA, Zak MB, O'Donnell MP, Schad RF, Dmuchowski CF: Patient-controlled analgesia versus patient-controlled analgesia plus continuous infusion after hip replacement surgery. *Ann Pharmacother* 1996;30(3):224-227.

35. Etches RC: Patient-controlled analgesia. *Surg Clin North Am* 1999;79(2):297-312.

36. US Department of Health and Human Services, US Public Health Service, US Acute Pain Management Guideline Panel: *Acute Pain Management: Operative or Medical Procedures and Trauma*. Rockville, MD, US Department of Health and Human Services, Public Health Service, Agency for Health Care Policy and Research, 1992.

37. Miller M, Barber CW, Leatherman S, et al: Prescription opioid duration of action and the risk of unintentional overdose among patients receiving opioid therapy. *JAMA Intern Med* 2015;175(4):608-615.

    Controlled-release formulations are not generally recommended for acute perioperative pain unless a patient is on them preoperatively. The authors provide evidence that unintentional overdose injury could be related to the prescribed opioid's duration of action. Level of evidence: III.

38. Dowell D, Haegerich TM, Chou R: CDC guideline for prescribing opioids for chronic pain – United States, 2016. *MMWR Recomm Rep* 2016;65(1):1-49.

    This guideline by the CDC primarily discusses opioid prescriptions for chronic pain, but also addresses high-risk prescribing practices leading to overdoses such as using extended-release/long-acting opioids for acute pain.

39. Halfpenny DM, Callado LF, Hopwood SE, Bamigbade TA, Langford RM, Stamford JA: Effects of tramadol stereoisomers on norepinephrine efflux and uptake in the rat locus coeruleus measured by real time voltammetry. *Br J Anaesth* 1999;83(6):909-915.

40. Bamigbade TA, Davidson C, Langford RM, Stamford JA: Actions of tramadol, its enantiomers and principal metabolite, O-desmethyltramadol, on serotonin (5-HT) efflux and uptake in the rat dorsal raphe nucleus. *Br J Anaesth* 1997;79(3):352-356.

41. Scott LJ, Perry CM: Tramadol: A review of its use in perioperative pain. *Drugs* 2000;60(1):139-176.

42. Edwards JE, McQuay HJ, Moore RA: Combination analgesic efficacy: Individual patient data meta-analysis of single-dose oral tramadol plus acetaminophen in acute postoperative pain. *J Pain Symptom Manage* 2002;23(2):121-130.

43. Ding Y, White PF: Comparative effects of ketorolac, dezocine, and fentanyl as adjuvants during outpatient anesthesia. *Anesth Analg* 1992;75(4):566-571.

44. McLoughlin C, McKinney MS, Fee JP, Boules Z: Diclofenac for day-care arthroscopy surgery: Comparison with a standard opioid therapy. *Br J Anaesth* 1990;65(5):620-623.

45. Moiniche S, Kehlet H, Dahl JB: A qualitative and quantitative systematic review of preemptive analgesia for postoperative pain relief: The role of timing of analgesia. *Anesthesiology* 2002;96(3):725-741.

46. Harder AT, An YH: The mechanisms of the inhibitory effects of nonsteroidal anti-inflammatory drugs on bone healing: A concise review. *J Clin Pharmacol* 2003;43(8):807-815.

47. Duggan ST, Scott LJ: Intravenous paracetamol (acetaminophen). *Drugs* 2009;69(1):101-113.

48. Sinatra RS, Jahr JS, Reynolds LW, Viscusi ER, Groudine SB, Payen-Champenois C: Efficacy and safety of single and repeated administration of 1 gram intravenous acetaminophen injection (paracetamol) for pain management after major orthopedic surgery. *Anesthesiology* 2005;102(4):822-831.

49. Sinatra RS, Jahr JS, Reynolds L, et al: Intravenous acetaminophen for pain after major orthopedic surgery: An expanded analysis. *Pain Pract* 2012;12(5):357-365.

50. Ong CK, Seymour RA, Lirk P, Merry AF: Combining paracetamol (acetaminophen) with nonsteroidal anti-inflammatory drugs: A qualitative systematic review of analgesic efficacy for acute postoperative pain. *Anesth Analg* 2010;110(4):1170-1179.

51. Sutters KA, Miaskowski C, Holdridge-Zeuner D, et al: A randomized clinical trial of the efficacy of scheduled dosing of acetaminophen and hydrocodone for the management of postoperative pain in children after tonsillectomy. *Clin J Pain* 2010;26(2):95-103.

52. Remy C, Marret E, Bonnet F: Effects of acetaminophen on morphine side-effects and consumption after major surgery: Meta-analysis of randomized controlled trials. *Br J Anaesth* 2005;94(4):505-513.

53. Maund E, McDaid C, Rice S, Wright K, Jenkins B, Woolacott N: Paracetamol and selective and non-selective non-steroidal anti-inflammatory drugs for the reduction in morphine-related side-effects after major surgery: A systematic review. *Br J Anaesth* 2011;106(3):292-297.

54. Dirks J, Fredensborg BB, Christensen D, Fomsgaard JS, Flyger H, Dahl JB: A randomized study of the effects of single-dose gabapentin versus placebo on postoperative pain and morphine consumption after mastectomy. *Anesthesiology* 2002;97(3):560-564.

55. Dierking G, Duedahl TH, Rasmussen ML, et al: Effects of gabapentin on postoperative morphine consumption and pain after abdominal hysterectomy: A randomized, double-blind trial. *Acta Anaesthesiol Scand* 2004;48(3):322-327.

56. Rorarius MG, Mennander S, Suominen P, et al: Gabapentin for the prevention of postoperative pain after vaginal hysterectomy. *Pain* 2004;110(1-2):175-181.

57. Dahl JB, Mathiesen O, Moiniche S: "Protective premedication": An option with gabapentin and related drugs? A review of gabapentin and pregabalin in in the treatment of post-operative pain. *Acta Anaesthesiol Scand* 2004;48(9):1130-1136.

58. Hill CM, Balkenohl M, Thomas DW, Walker R, Mathe H, Murray G: Pregabalin in patients with postoperative dental pain. *Eur J Pain* 2001;5(2):119-124.

59. Agarwal A, Gautam S, Gupta D, Agarwal S, Singh PK, Singh U: Evaluation of a single preoperative dose of pregabalin for attenuation of postoperative pain after laparoscopic cholecystectomy. *Br J Anaesth* 2008;101(5):700-704.

60. Schmid RL, Sandler AN, Katz J: Use and efficacy of low-dose ketamine in the management of acute postoperative pain: A review of current techniques and outcomes. *Pain* 1999;82(2):111-125.

61. Subramaniam K, Subramaniam B, Steinbrook RA: Ketamine as adjuvant analgesic to opioids: A quantitative and qualitative systematic review. *Anesth Analg* 2004;99(2):482-495.

62. Loftus RW, Yeager MP, Clark JA, et al: Intraoperative ketamine reduces perioperative opiate consumption in opiate-dependent patients with chronic back pain undergoing back surgery. *Anesthesiology* 2010;113(3):639-646.

63. Aveline C, Gautier JF, Vautier P, et al: Postoperative analgesia and early rehabilitation after total knee replacement: A comparison of continuous low-dose intravenous ketamine versus nefopam. *Eur J Pain* 2009;13(6):613-619.

Chapter 48

Advanced Imaging of the Shoulder and Elbow

Jan Fritz, MD, PD, DABR • John A. Carrino, MD, MPH • Ali Rashidi, MD

ABSTRACT

Accurate diagnosis of the various abnormalities of shoulder and elbow is important for optimal management, including selection of best treatment and prognosis. History, skilled clinical examination, and radiography can diagnose many shoulder and elbow abnormalities; however, when negative or indeterminate, advanced imaging techniques can aid in the diagnosis of a wide variety of abnormalities. In this chapter, the roles of MRI, MR arthrography, CT, CT arthrography, and ultrasonography in diagnosing abnormalities of the elbow and shoulder joints are reviewed.

Keywords: CT; elbow; MRI; shoulder; ultrasonography

Dr. Fritz or an immediate family member is a member of a speakers' bureau or has made paid presentations on behalf of Siemens AG; serves as an unpaid consultant to GE Healthcare and Siemens AG; has received research or institutional support from Siemens AG; has received nonincome support (such as equipment or services), commercially derived honoraria, or other non–research-related funding (such as paid travel) from BTG International Ltd, Microsoft, Synthetic MR Technologies AB, and Zimmer; and serves as a board member, owner, officer, or committee member of the American College of Radiology, the American Roentgen Ray Society, the International Society of Magnetic Resonance in Medicine, the Radiological Society of North America, the European Society of Musculoskeletal Radiology, the Society of Skeletal Radiology and the Association of University Radiologists. Dr. Carrino or an immediate family member serves as a paid consultant to or is an employee of Covera (Spreemo) Health, Pfizer, and Simplify Medical and serves as an unpaid consultant to Carestream, GE Healthcare, and Image Analysis Group. Neither Dr. Rashidi nor any immediate family member has received anything of value from or has stock or stock options held in a commercial company or institution related directly or indirectly to the subject of this chapter.

Introduction

Various abnormalities of the shoulder and elbow joint can cause pain and dysfunction. Continued advances in MRI, CT, and ultrasonography technology afford unprecedented image quality and anatomic detail that permit for the diagnosis of a wide spectrum of abnormalities. Consequently, the demand for imaging these complex joints has increased over the past few years. Radiography as the initial imaging technique carries a lower cost factor, is widely available, and can detect critical conditions such as fractures, calcific tendinitis, moderate to severe degenerative disease, and some neoplastic and tumorlike conditions. However, for more detailed diagnoses, for diagnosing subtle abnormalities, and especially for soft-tissue abnormalities, advanced imaging methods are superior. In this chapter, the roles of MRI, magnetic resonance arthrography (MRA), CT, CT arthrography (CTA), and ultrasonography for diagnosing abnormalities about the elbow and shoulder joints are reviewed.

MRI and MRA

Clinical MRI at 3.0 T has evolved to the preferred field strength for musculoskeletal MRI over the past decade. The most crucial advantage of 3 T MRI over MRI at 1.5 T is the approximately twofold higher signal yield, which allows MRI examinations with higher resolution within the same scan time, or up to four times faster with the same spatial resolution.[1] The amount of image contrast is also dependent on the magnetic field strength and is also higher at 3 T than at 1.5 T. As a result, on 3 T magnetic resonance images, the gray scale values between muscle and bone, bone and cartilage, and cartilage and fluid are wide apart, and structures can be better differentiated by the human eye. When applied appropriately, the sum of 3 T advantage often translates into higher image quality and better visibility of structures, which in some instances increases diagnostic accuracy. Especially MRI of small structures in the shoulder and

This chapter is adapted from Carrino JA, Thakkar RS: Advanced imaging of the shoulder and elbow, in Nicholson GP, ed: *Orthopaedic Knowledge Update: Shoulder and Elbow*, ed 4. Rosemont, IL, American Academy of Orthopaedic Surgeons, 2013, pp 633-642.

elbow, such as fibrocartilaginous and fine ligamentous anatomy and abnormalities, benefit from higher spatial resolution protocols. In general, 1.5 T MRI can achieve the same MRI signal and spatial resolution, but requires substantially longer acquisition times than 3 T. Advantages of 1.5 T over 3 T MRI include inherently less artifacts from metallic orthopaedic implants, breathing motion, and cerebrospinal fluid pulsation, and in select cases more homogenous fat suppression and lower cost of scanner and equipment.

Musculoskeletal MRI protocols used at most institutions consist of two-dimensional (2D) fast and turbo spin echo pulse sequences in multiple planes. The design and high signal yield of those sequences afford the combination of high tissue contrast of musculoskeletal structures and high in-plane spatial resolution. However, they require a slice thickness between 2.5 and 3 mm in the shoulder and 2 and 2.5 mm in the elbow, which leads to partial volume effects and potentially obscuration of small abnormalities. Modern three-dimensional (3D) turbo spin echo pulse sequences allow for substantially accelerated acquisition of MRI data and reduce partial volume averaging by acquiring thin, continuous, submillimeter slices through the joints.[2,3] 3D pulse sequence images can also be used to create multiplanar reformation images that allow joints to be evaluated in any orientation from a single parental 3D data set.[4]

Shoulder Joint

MRI is the imaging modality of choice for many indications because of its free choice of imaging planes and unparalleled soft-tissue contrast resolution. MRI provides detailed assessment and diagnosis of abnormalities of the rotator cuff, capsule-labral structures, tendons, muscles, bone, articular surfaces, as well as abnormalities associated with shoulder instability and impingement. Lesions of the subacromial bursa and extra-articular biceps tendon as well as morphologic abnormalities of the acromion, acromioclavicular joint, and coracoacromial ligament can be diagnosed.

On unenhanced MRI, the rotator cuff, labrum, joint capsule, and the cortical bone usually are dark appearing on all pulse sequences, and because of their close proximity and abutment, they may be difficult to distinguish from one another. The presence of either a joint effusion or joint distention through the intra-articular injection of a gadolinium contrast–containing sterile solution helps to separate coapted structures and further improve contrast by outlining anatomical structures with fluid that is of significantly higher signal.[5]

In 2009, a study examined in 150 patients the diagnostic accuracy of conventional 3 T MRI versus MRA for the detection of abnormalities of the shoulder in the same patient population.[6] On conventional MRI, sensitivities and specificities using arthroscopy as the reference standard were as follows: anterior labral tear, 83% sensitivity and 100% specificity; posterior labral tear, 84% and 100%; superior labrum anterior to posterior (SLAP) tear, 83% and 99%; supraspinatus tendon tear, 92% and 100%; partial-thickness articular surface tear, 68% and 100%; and partial-thickness bursal surface tear, 84% and 100%. On MRA, sensitivities and specificities using arthroscopy as the reference standard were as follows: anterior labral tear, 98% sensitivity and 100% specificity; posterior labral tear, 95% and 100%; SLAP tear, 98% and 99%; supraspinatus tendon tear, 100% and 100%; partial-thickness articular surface tear, 97% and 100%; and partial-thickness bursal surface tear, 84% and 100%. When compared with conventional MRI, MRA showed a statistical superior sensitivity for the detection of partial-thickness articular surface supraspinatus tendon tears, anterior labral tears, and SLAP tears.

Recent meta-analyses assessed the diagnostic accuracies of MRI and MRA for the diagnosis of shoulder abnormalities and found higher sensitivities of 3 T MRA compared with 3 T MRI for anterior labral (87% versus 83%), posterior labral (90% versus 83%),[7] and SLAP (80% to 85% versus 63% to 83%)[7,8] lesions, respectively, as well as superiority of 3 T MRI in diagnosis of SLAP lesions in comparison with 1.5 T MRI.[8]

In the shoulder joint, 2D fast and turbo spin echo pulse sequences are currently the sequence of choice for noncontrast MRI. However, 3D pulse sequences such as gradient echo steady-state free precession have been tried at many institutions. Recently, 3D MRI techniques have been used to decrease the time required to evaluate the shoulder joint during noncontrast MRI. Those new 3D techniques use fast pulse sequences (eg, turbo spin echo, which is a technique that allows acquiring magnetic resonance images substantially faster than conventional MRI techniques) with equal voxel dimensions in all three directions (isotropic, which permits reformation of multiple imaging planes), which permit high image quality and shorter acquisition times.

In 2018, a meta-analysis comparing the performance of isotropic 3D MRA and conventional 2D MRA for diagnosing labral lesions and rotator cuff tears found overall similar sensitivities and specificities.[9] For diagnosing rotator cuff tear, isotropic 3D MRA and conventional 2D MRA had sensitivities of 91% and 92%, respectively, and specificities of 90% and 90%, respectively. For diagnosing labral lesions, isotropic 3D MRA and conventional 2D MRA had sensitivities of 89% and 94%, respectively, and specificities of 89% and 94%, respectively. Accordingly, faster isotropic 3D MRA can replace conventional 2D MRA. Either technique can be used for accurate diagnoses, the choice of which will ultimately depend on local factors, such as MRI scanner and coil technology, as well as technologist and radiologist expertise. In addition, the newer 3D turbo spin echo sequences increased sensitivity when compared with older 3D gradient echo pulse sequences and were therefore recommended to achieve a more accurate diagnosis.

Rotator Cuff

Axial, sagittal oblique, and coronal oblique planes are typically used to image the rotator cuff. The sagittal oblique and coronal oblique planes are usually aligned with the supraspinatus tendon to achieve profile and true cross-sectional views, respectively. Routine MRI of the shoulder uses a combination of pulse sequences, including T1-weighted, proton density–weighted and intermediate-weighted, and T2-weighted images. T1-weighted pulse sequences are most accurate for the assessment of fatty tissues and are most useful for evaluating bone marrow, as well as fatty infiltration and atrophy of muscle bulk. Both, proton density–weighted or intermediate-weighted pulse sequences using long repetition times (in excess of 4 seconds) and intermediate echo times (30 to 40 ms), and T2-weighted pulse sequences are fluid sensitive and best suited to detect pathologic conditions of tendons, ligaments, articular and fibrocartilage, and bone, which are mostly accompanied by an abnormal increase in water signal. Full-thickness tears of the rotator cuff tendons can be accurately identified with T2-weighted pulse sequences by visualizing fluid signal intensity breaching and extending from the deep to the superficial surface of the tendon. In partial-thickness tears, the fluid signal only breaches one tendon surface (**Figure 1**). Additional morphologic abnormalities that might be associated with rotator cuff tears are tendon retraction, muscle atrophy, and fatty muscle infiltration, which are also important prognostic factors. Muscle atrophy and fatty infiltration is best seen on T1-weighted magnetic resonance images.

The degree of fatty degeneration of the rotator cuff muscle can be graded with the Goutallier classification (**Figure 2**), where grade 0 corresponds to a completely normal muscle without any fatty streak; grade 1 corresponds to muscle that contains few fatty streaks; grade 2 corresponds to muscle that contains more fatty streaks than in grade 1 but overall less than preserved muscle tissue; grade 3 corresponds to muscle with similar quantities of fatty streaks and muscle tissue; and grade 4 corresponds to muscle with more fatty streaks than muscle tissue.[10] MRI can provide this information about fatty atrophy as it is important in treatment decisions regarding conservative versus surgical repair, type of surgical repair, and providing a prognosis.

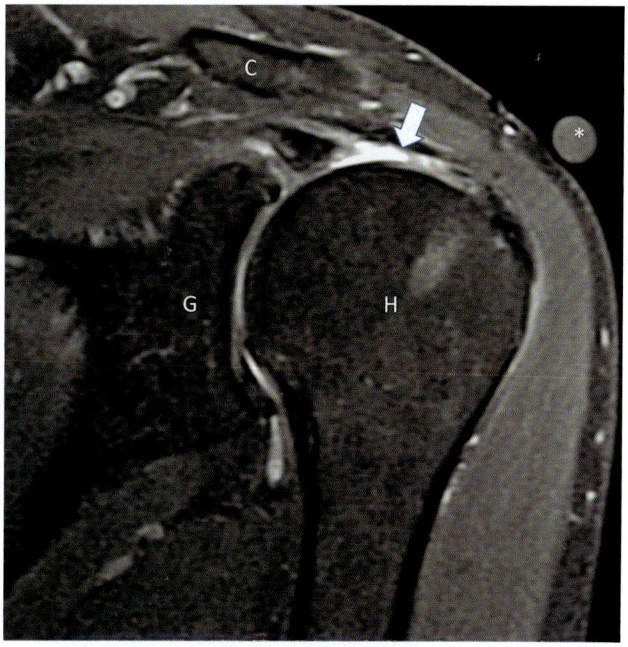

FIGURE 1 A 63-year-old man with a history of rotator cuff repair 8 years ago presenting with right shoulder pain following a falling injury. Coronal fat-suppressed T2-weighted turbo spin echo magnetic resonance image (repetition time/echo time [TR/TE], 4,000 ms/65 ms) shows a high-grade partial-thickness articular surface tear of the supraspinatus tendon (arrow). * = skin marker, C = clavicle, G = glenoid, H = humerus

MRA is recommended to differentiate full-thickness and articular surface partial-thickness tears,[11] whereas bursal surface partial-thickness tears may not be detected on T1-weighted magnetic resonance arthroscopic images because of the inability of intra-articularly injected contrast to outline the bursal surface of the rotator cuff. Detection of articular surface partial-thickness tears may be improved with the help of maneuvering certain technical aspects of imaging. The abduction and external rotation (ABER) view may increase the conspicuity of partial-thickness articular surface tears through lifting the tendon off the humeral head and reducing the compression of the articular surface fibers. However, considering that inclusion of the ABER view prolongs MRI examinations because of the need for repositioning of the shoulder and exchange or repositioning of the MRI coil with often no or only minimal increase in sensitivity, the ABER view may not be needed routinely. Partial volume averaging on coronal magnetic resonance images related to an oblique course of the rotator cuff tendons can be reduced with little time commitment by external rotation of the humerus, which brings the tendon course in the plane.

A 2009 meta-analysis compared the diagnostic accuracy of MRI, MRA, and ultrasonography for the diagnosis of rotator cuff tears.[12] Sixty-five articles met

Section 8: Miscellaneous Shoulder and Elbow Topics

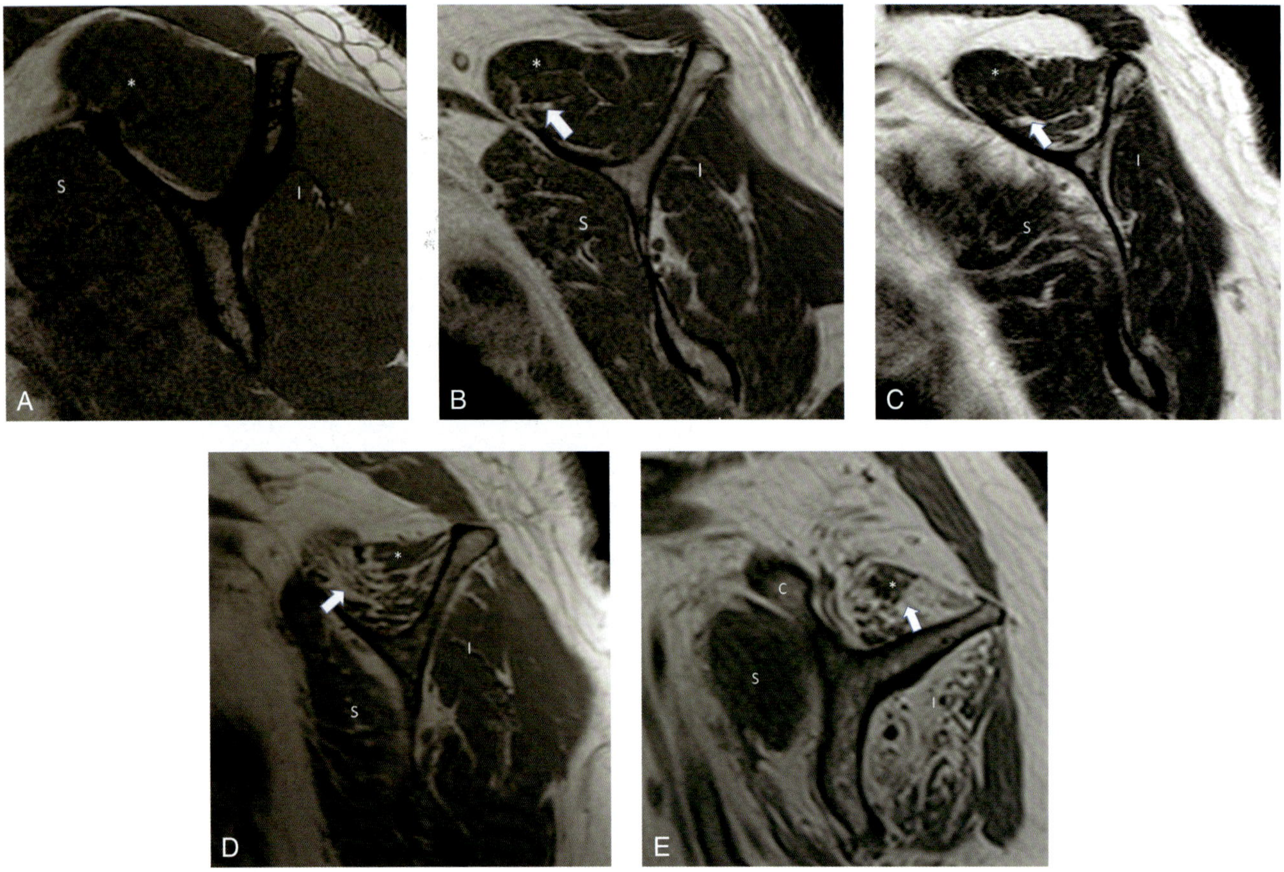

FIGURE 2 Sagittal T1-weighted magnetic resonance images show different degrees of fatty degeneration of supraspinatus muscle, which are graded with the Goutallier classification; grade 0 = normal muscle without any fatty streak (**A**), grade 1 = few fatty streaks in the muscle (arrow) (**B**), grade 2 = less fat than muscle (arrow) (**C**), grade 3 = muscle with similar quantities of fatty streaks and muscle tissue (arrow) (**D**), and grade 4 = muscle with more fatty streaks than muscle tissue (arrow) (**E**). * = supraspinatus muscle, C = coracoid process, I = infraspinatus muscle, S = subscapularis muscle

the inclusion criteria. In diagnosing a full-thickness and partial-thickness rotator cuff tear, MRA was found to be more sensitive and specific than either MRI or ultrasonography ($P < 0.05$). There were no significant differences in either sensitivity or specificity between MRI and ultrasonography in the diagnosis of partial-thickness and full-thickness rotator cuff tears ($P > 0.05$). Summary receiver operating characteristic (ROC) curves for MRA, MRI, and ultrasonography for all tears showed the area under the ROC curve was highest for MRA (0.935), followed by ultrasonography (0.889) and then MRI (0.878); however, pairwise comparisons of these curves showed no significant differences between MRI and ultrasonography ($P > 0.05$).

A 2015 meta-analysis investigating the diagnostic accuracy of MRA, MRI, and ultrasonography for the characterization of rotator cuff disorders[13] (**Table 1**) demonstrated similar performances of all three modalities in diagnosing full-thickness rotator cuff tears (sensitivity = 90% versus 90% versus 91%, respectively; and specificity = 95% versus 93% versus 93%, respectively). For the diagnosis of partial-thickness rotator cuff tears, all modalities had similar specificity (93% versus 94% versus 94%, respectively); however, MRA had higher sensitivity compared with MRI and ultrasonography (83% versus 67% versus 68%, respectively).

Capsulolabral Abnormalities

Direct MRA with the intra-articular injection of a dilute gadolinium solution distends the joint and helps to separate and better outline labral and capsular structures, which aid in the diagnosis, treatment planning, and follow-up (**Figure 3**).

3 T MRA is helpful if anterior labral tears, SLAP tears (**Figure 3**), and partial-thickness supraspinatus tendon tears are suspected clinically. MRA may also aid in the accurate identification and demonstration of the integrity of the glenohumeral ligaments, capsule, and labrum, and could aid in the grading of abnormalities.[14] It is also accurate for detecting a detached labral

Table 1

Diagnostic Accuracy of Ultrasonography, MRI, and MRA Imaging for the Diagnosis of Rotator Cuff Tears

	Overall		Full-Thickness Rotator Cuff Tear		Partial-Thickness Rotator Cuff Tear	
	Sensitivity (%)	Specificity (%)	Sensitivity (%)	Specificity (%)	Sensitivity (%)	Specificity (%)
Ultrasonography	91	86	91	93	68	94
MRI	90	90	90	93	67	94
MRA	90	90	90	95	83	93

MRA = magnetic resonance arthrography

fragment, labral degeneration, and lesions of the inferior part of labrum and of the inferior glenohumeral ligament.

SLAP injuries are best demonstrated in the oblique coronal plane on fluid-sensitive pulse images. Fluid or contrast insinuating into irregular defects between the labrum and superior glenoid is diagnostic (**Figure 4**). Ancillary findings to support a true SLAP tear include a lateral extension of abnormal signal intensity into the substance of the labrum, irregularity of the labral margin, and extension of the signal into the proximal biceps tendon. In distinguishing true labral abnormalities from variants, the sublabral recess tends to be more medial than SLAP tears, smoothly marginated, and located between the biceps tendon and the glenoid articular cartilage

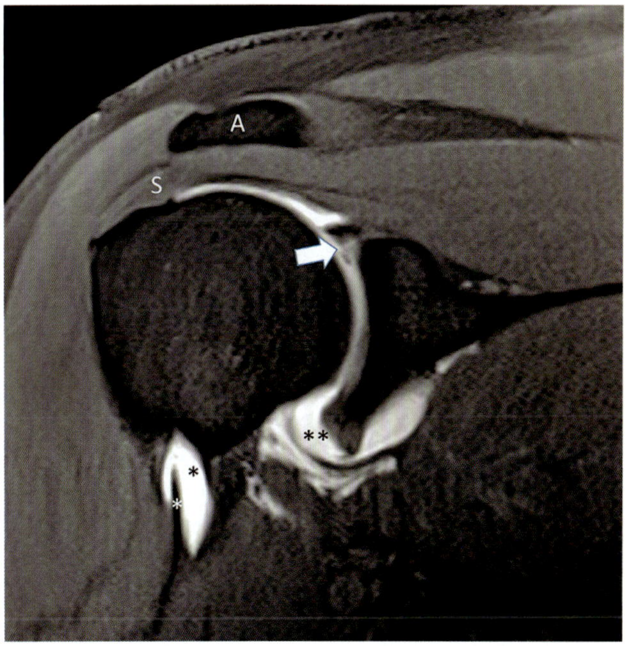

FIGURE 3 A 36-year-old man with shoulder pain after a work injury. Coronal fat-suppressed T1-weighted magnetic resonance arthrographic image (TR/TE, 780 ms/13 ms) shows a superior labral tear with a small displaced labral fragment (arrow), * (black asterisk) = injected contrast in the biceps tendon sheath, ** = injected contrast in the joint capsule, * (white asterisk) = long head biceps tendon, A = acromion, S = supraspinatus tendon

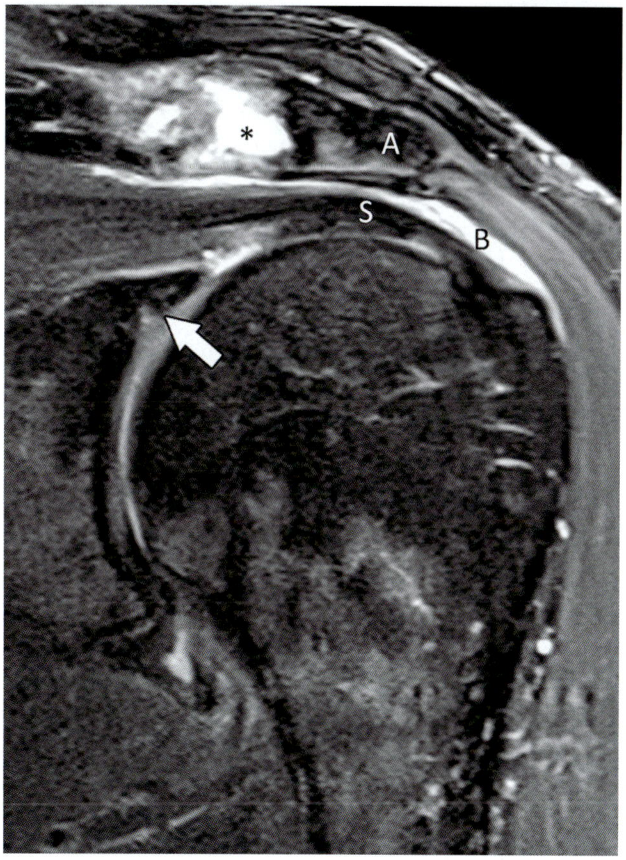

FIGURE 4 A 67-year-old man with shoulder pain. Coronal fat-suppressed T2-weighted turbo spin echo magnetic resonance image (TR/TE, 5,411 ms/83 ms) shows a degenerated superior labral tear (arrow). * = fluid in degenerated acromioclavicular joint, A = acromion, B = subacromial-subdeltoid bursal fluid, S = supraspinatus tendon

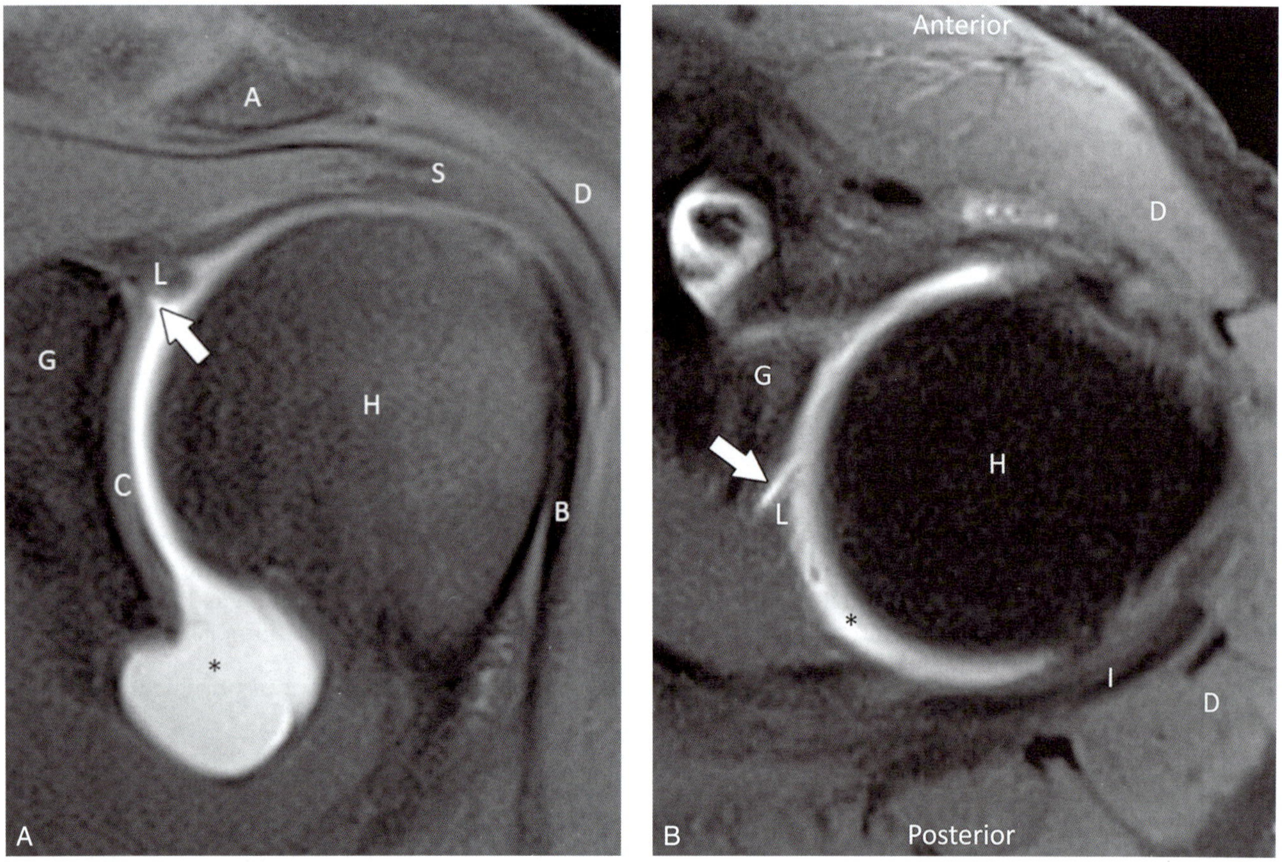

FIGURE 5 A 38-year-old man with left shoulder pain. Coronal (**A**) and axial (**B**) magnetic resonance arthrographic images show a labral sulcus (arrows). * = injected contrast in the glenohumeral joint space, A = acromion, B = long head of biceps tendon, C = glenoid cartilage, D = deltoid muscle, G = glenoid, H = humerus, I = infraspinatus tendon, L = glenoid labrum, S = supraspinatus tendon

(**Figure 5**). Conversely, SLAP tears will often extend posterior to the biceps tendon and more laterally than the sublabral recess. They are most likely to demonstrate laterally curved high signal intensity on oblique coronal images and anterior-posterior extension on axial images (**Figure 4**).

The anterior and posterior portions of the labrum are best evaluated on axial magnetic resonance images. MRI findings of a labral tear include abnormal signal within the labrum or interposed between the labrum and glenoid (**Figure 4**). Assessment of anterior capsule stripping without disruption is much more difficult because of the high variability of the normal capsular attachments along the anterior glenoid.

Articular Cartilage

Optimal evaluation of cartilage can be challenging, especially in the shoulder joint. Improving spatial resolution on 2D pulse sequences and obtaining different planes or arm positioning to better cover different areas of the curved humeral head offer improvements (**Figure 6**). The contrast of articular cartilage is best on intermediate-weighted proton density pulse sequences, which are most accurate.

Elbow Joint

Positioning a patient for MRI of the elbow can be accomplished either by the supine position with arm at the side, or prone position with arm extended overhead. The latter position is often preferred to have the elbow near the center of the bore of the MRI scanner, where the most homogenous signal and uniform fat suppression can be achieved. However, not all patients can tolerate this position for the duration for the MRI examination.

Similar to the shoulder joint, MRI protocols for the elbow usually include fluid-sensitive pulse sequences without and with fat suppression, which afford detection of abnormal conditions of tendons, ligaments, articular and fibrocartilage, and bone. Similar to T2-weighted magnetic resonance images with fat suppression, short tau inversion recovery pulse sequences are also fluid-sensitive,

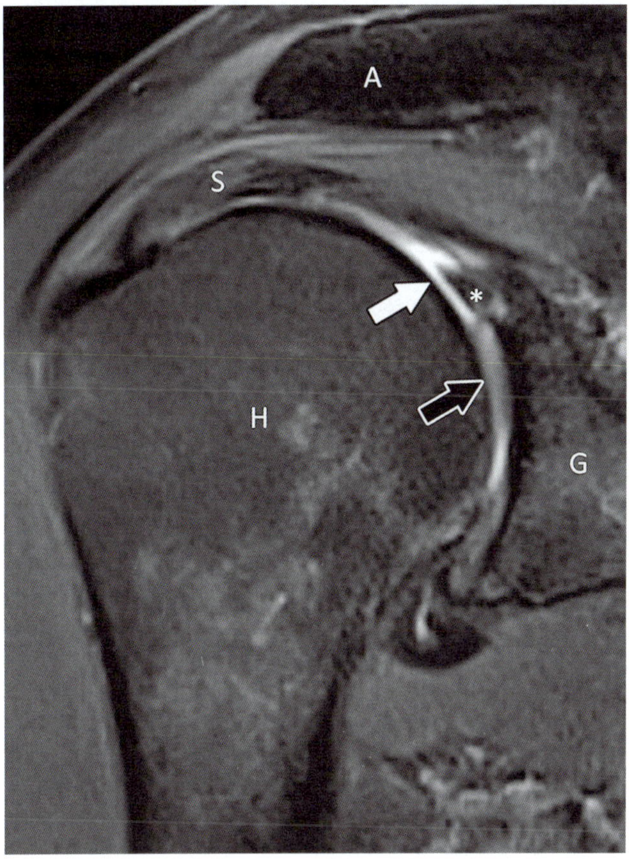

FIGURE 6 A 75-year-old man with right shoulder pain. Coronal fat-suppressed T2-weighted turbo spin echo magnetic resonance image (TR/TE, 3,650 ms/69 ms) shows full-thickness glenohumeral articular cartilage loss (white arrow) and adjacent preserved glenohumeral articular cartilage with surface wear (black arrow). * = superior glenoid labrum, A = acromion, G = glenoid, H = humerus, S = supraspinatus tendon

but offer more robust fat suppression, especially in the presence of metallic orthopaedic implants and prostheses. The inclusion of a T1-weighted pulse sequence is optional and can facilitate the assessment of fatty tissues, including bone marrow, muscle, and masses. To diagnose medial and lateral abnormalities of the elbow, axial and coronal plane images are best suited, whereas anterior and posterior abnormalities of the elbow are best evaluated in the axial and sagittal plane images.[15]

In the elbow joint, 3D pulse sequences are more challenging but can acquire much thinner slices than two-dimensional sequences, and 3D pulse sequences can improve the visibility of small anatomic detail. 3D pulse sequences can also be used to obtain multiplanar reformation images, which can be adjusted individually to any anatomic structure and hence improve visibility. This can be helpful when assessing the ulnar band of the lateral collateral ligament, which is often best visualized in its entirety by using 20° posterior oblique coronal plane. With 3D data sets, the orthopaedic surgeon and the radiologist can work together during postprocessing to ensure the best plane orientations are being used to visualize individual structures of interest. The combination of optimal tissue contrast and the ability to acquire thin contiguous slices is achieved through the isotropic resolution 3D turbo spin echo pulse sequences. Using this recently developed pulse sequences in the imaging of the elbow joint may improve the detection of collateral ligament tears. Intermediate-weighted and T2-weighted tissue contrast and multiplanar capabilities of these sequences are useful for evaluating tendons, muscles, and osseous structures of the elbow joint, especially when combined with fat suppression to improve fluid sensitivity.

Intra-articular contrast for MRA can be helpful in the evaluation of ligamentous injuries and when evaluating for the presence and suspicion of articular bodies that are not visible on conventional radiographs.[11] The sensitivity and specificity of MRA have been reported as 100% for the diagnosis of elbow ligaments when surgery is used as the standard of reference.[16] Despite the superior diagnostic accuracy of MRA when compared with conventional MRI, MRI is often preferred as the first in elbow injuries, because of the invasive nature of MRA.

Osteochondral Injury

The osteochondroses of the elbow represent a group of disorders that are well evaluated by MRI. Panner disease is of uncertain etiology but is thought to result from repetitive valgus stress resulting in compressive and shear forces, which lead to a vascular compromise in throwing athletes (usually adolescent boys). On radiographs, the epiphysis appears mottled and fragmented. On MRI it appears as patchy hypointensities on T1-weighted sequences. Articular bodies are not a frequent feature of Panner disease.

Osteochondritis dissecans of the capitellum generally affects adolescent athletes (12 to 16 years of age) and is seen more commonly in baseball players and gymnasts. They experience chronic lateral impaction forces because of repetitive microtrauma leading to lesions affecting both subchondral bone and overlying cartilage. Initial radiographs are normal, whereas MRI has the ability to detect this abnormality earlier. MRA with intra-articular contrast is especially useful for localizing the defect and demonstrating fragment stability. Fragments are considered unstable when any of the following findings exist: T2 hyperintensity surrounding the fragment, cysts are seen deep to the fragment, and T2 hyperintense edema is seen within the fragment. The bony defect can also be identified on CT.

Collateral Ligament Injury

Ulnar collateral ligament (UCL) injuries are a common source of medial elbow pain in the throwing athlete and are best evaluated with a combination of radiographs and MRI.[17] On fluid sensitive MRI, the abnormal findings of the UCL range from abnormally increased signal intensity within the ligament to frank discontinuity if completely torn. On magnetic resonance images, UCL tears can be classified into proximal (humeral attachment), midsubstance, and distal (ulnar attachment) partial-thickness and full-thickness tears.[18] Associated findings, such as bone contusion in the lateral compartment and injury to the common extensor tendons, may be seen. Bony avulsions often have an intraligamentous component. Thickening or attenuation of the ligament, with or without abnormal intrinsic signal intensity, and calcification or ossification is seen in chronic injury.

MRA is excellent in distinguishing partial and complete tears of the UCL. Diagnosis of a partial-thickness tear is made when the T sign of contrast, saline, or joint fluid is seen extending in a linear fashion along the medial margin of the coronoid process, through the disrupted deep UCL fibers, but confined by the intact joint capsule. Additionally, MRA can help to identify any cartilage abnormality present in the elbow joint.

The combination of MRA and ultrasonography was demonstrated to have higher accuracy than each modality alone in the evaluation of medial elbow pain.[19]

Laterally, the stabilizers include the radial collateral ligament, the annular ligament, the lateral UCL, and the accessory collateral ligament. The lateral stabilizing ligaments are less commonly injured than the UCL. If there is an interstitial injury or tear, MRI demonstrates high signal intensity within the substance of the ligament without (interstitial injury), whereas fiber disruption indicates partial-thickness and full-thickness tears. Additionally, periligamentous edema and hemorrhage may be present.

Muscles and Tendons Injury

Healthy tendons appear as uniformly low signal intensity on all pulse sequences. The tendon affected by degenerative tendinopathy usually demonstrates areas of thickening or thickening with mildly increased, intermediate T1 and T2 signal intensity. Partial or complete tears can occur as a result of acute traumatic events or as sequelae of advanced chronic tendinopathy. Fluid signal within the tendon substance but without extending beyond the tendon surface indicates intrasubstance or interstitial tearing. Partial tears require the loss of tendon fibers, which is indicated by tendon thinning and surface irregularity in the chronic stages, and fluid signal interposition between discontinuous fibers, edema, and hemorrhage in the acute and subacute phase. In complete tears, there is discontinuity of all fibers, which are separated by fluid signal in the acute setting or fatty tissues in the chronic phase. Scarring-in-continuity may occur with alternating episodes of tearing and healing and presents on MRI as seemingly continuous fibers with irregular surface and caliber.

Lateral epicondylitis is an overuse syndrome in which the involved tendons degenerate. The extensor carpi radialis brevis tendon is primarily involved (**Figure 7**). The anterior edge of the extensor digitorum communis tendon

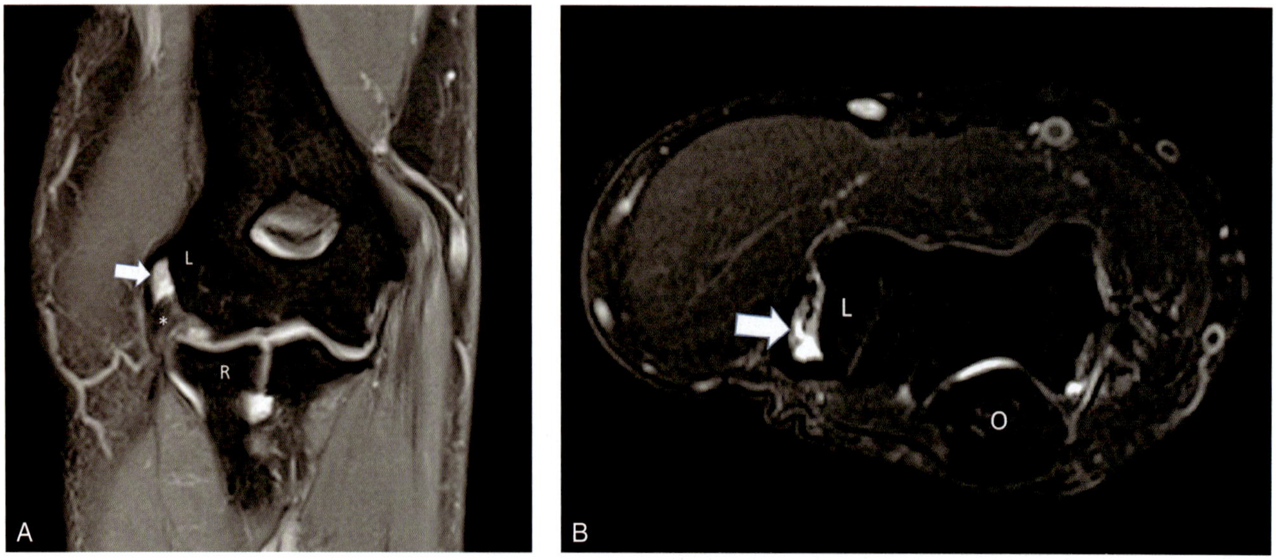

FIGURE 7 A 72-year-old man with right elbow pain. Coronal (**A**) fat-suppressed intermediate-weighted magnetic resonance images (TR/TE, 4,000 ms/33 ms) and axial (**B**) fat-suppressed T2-weighted magnetic resonance images (TR/TE, 4,100 ms/63 ms) show a deep high-grade partial-thickness tear (arrow) of the extensor carpi radialis brevis origin. * = radial collateral ligament, L = lateral epicondyle, O = olecranon, R = radial head

is involved 50% of the time, followed by extensor carpi radialis longus and extensor carpi ulnaris tendons. As the degree of injury increases, concomitant collateral ligament tears deep to the tendon attachment may be present.

The most common condition to affect the medial elbow is medial epicondylitis, also known as medial tennis elbow, golfer's elbow, and pitcher's elbow. The tendons involved are origins of pronator teres, flexor carpi radialis, and/or palmaris longus. There may be secondary involvement of flexor carpi ulnaris and flexor digitorum superficialis. As the degree of injury increases, the underlying anterior band of the medial collateral ligament should also be assessed.

In the skeletally immature athlete with medial elbow pain, MRI plays an important role in identifying underlying abnormalities. The medial epicondyle physis is weaker than the anterior band of the medial collateral ligament. This, in combination with the tensile forces generated by the common flexor tendon origin during valgus stress, can lead to a physeal injury known as little league elbow. MRI demonstrates physeal irregularity with widening and surrounding osseous edema to a frank displacement of the apophysis.

In the anterior compartment of the elbow, rupture of the distal biceps tendon is rare, accounting for less than 5% of biceps tendon injuries. Partial tears can be seen as an increase in fluid signal within an abnormally thickened or thinned tendon associated with the osseous finding of edema within the radial tuberosity and fluid within the radiobicipital bursa. In a complete tear with retraction beyond the joint line, the torn tendon and lacertus fibrosus attachment are separated by fluid signal in the acute setting (**Figure 8**). In cases where it is difficult to assess the insertion of the tendon on the radial tuberosity, a flexed elbow, abducted shoulder, and supinated forearms position may be helpful.[20] Sagittal images are then acquired of the humerus extending into the forearm, resulting in longitudinal images of the distal biceps tendon including its insertion. Isolated brachialis muscle tears are extremely rare. Brachialis musculotendinous tears have been described in rock climbers and are referred to as climber's elbow. Lastly, the most common condition to affect the posterior elbow is degeneration of the triceps tendon, which may lead to tears.

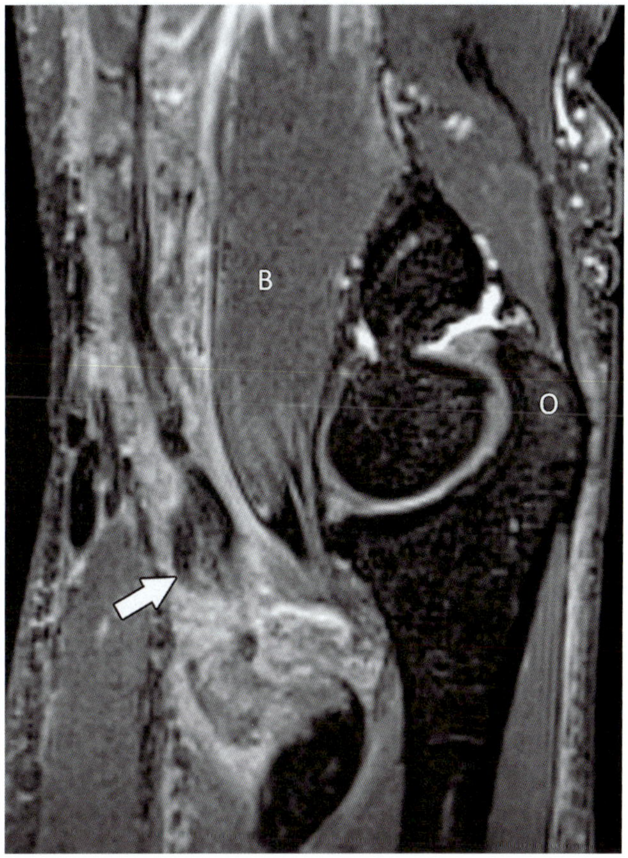

FIGURE 8 A 64-year-old man with elbow pain following a sudden fall and painful pop in his right elbow. Sagittal fat-suppressed T2-weighted turbo spin echo magnetic resonance image (TR/TE, 1,000 ms/29 ms) shows a full-thickness biceps tendon tear (arrow). B = brachialis muscle, O = olecranon

Nerve Entrapment

The three primary nerves at the elbow joint are the ulnar, radial, and median nerves. The most common nerve to get entrapped is the ulnar nerve at the cubital tunnel. Ulnar nerve compression is the most frequent peripheral neuropathy around the elbow and commonly occurs in throwing athletes. MRI can be helpful in assessing the integrity of nerves, as well as evaluating the muscle groups supplied by nerves for morphology and signal intensity. Axial magnetic resonance images depict the size and shape of the ulnar nerve, whereas fluid-sensitive magnetic resonance images may show an increase in signal intensity of the nerve in cases of entrapment (**Figure 9**). When an entrapment syndrome is present, the muscle group supplied in the acute phase may demonstrate abnormally increased T2-weighted signal intensity on fat-suppressed images. When the process is chronic, muscles will undergo atrophy and decrease in muscle bulk with fatty infiltration, which is best seen on T1-weighted magnetic resonance images.

CT and CTA

CT depicts osseous detail and combined with arthrography, also intra-articular, capsulolabral, tendinous, and ligamentous abnormalities in the shoulder and elbow joints. Modern multislice CT scanners provide excellent

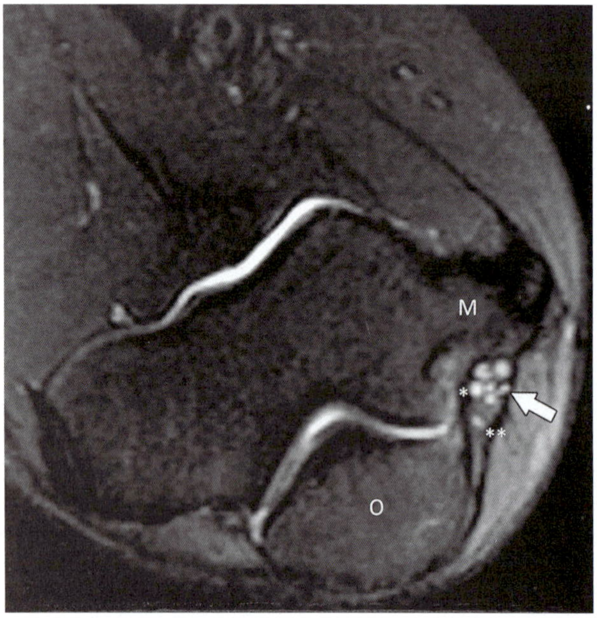

FIGURE 9 A 50-year-old woman with severe pain and weakness in an ulnar distribution of her right hand. Axial fat-suppressed T2-weighted turbo spin echo magnetic resonance image (TR/TE, 4,940 ms/86 ms) shows an ulnar neuropathy (arrow) with expanded nerve, abnormal T2 hyperintense signal, and enlarged central fasciclelike pattern. * = posterior band of ulnar collateral ligament, ** = Osborne ligament, M = medial epicondyle, O = olecranon

spatial resolution. When source data are obtained with isotropic spatial resolution, images can be reconstructed and reformatted in any arbitrary oblique plane that best shows complex joint anatomy and abnormalities. With postprocessing software, 3D models can also be created, which are helpful for surgical planning.[21]

Advantages of CT include the evaluation of soft-tissue calcification, myositis ossificans, and intra-articular bodies more readily than MRI. Osteoarthrosis can be diagnosed when there is joint space loss with bone-on-bone and apposition (**Figure 10**). Disadvantages of CT include the image acquisition–related radiation exposure, which requires careful consideration. CT has poor contrast resolution and thus limited soft-tissue characterization, which can obscure soft-tissue injuries. Metallic implants and prostheses within the bone or periarticular soft tissues can cause large image artifacts, which limit evaluation of the surrounding bone and soft tissues. However, now widely available clinically approved techniques based on dual-energy CT data and virtual monoenergetic extrapolation, as well as in-painting techniques to reconstruct missing data secondary to metal artifacts, can greatly reduce metal artifacts and improve image quality.[22,23] The detection of bone marrow edema pattern with CT is now possible with clinically approved algorithms for virtual noncalcium postprocessing of dual-energy data.

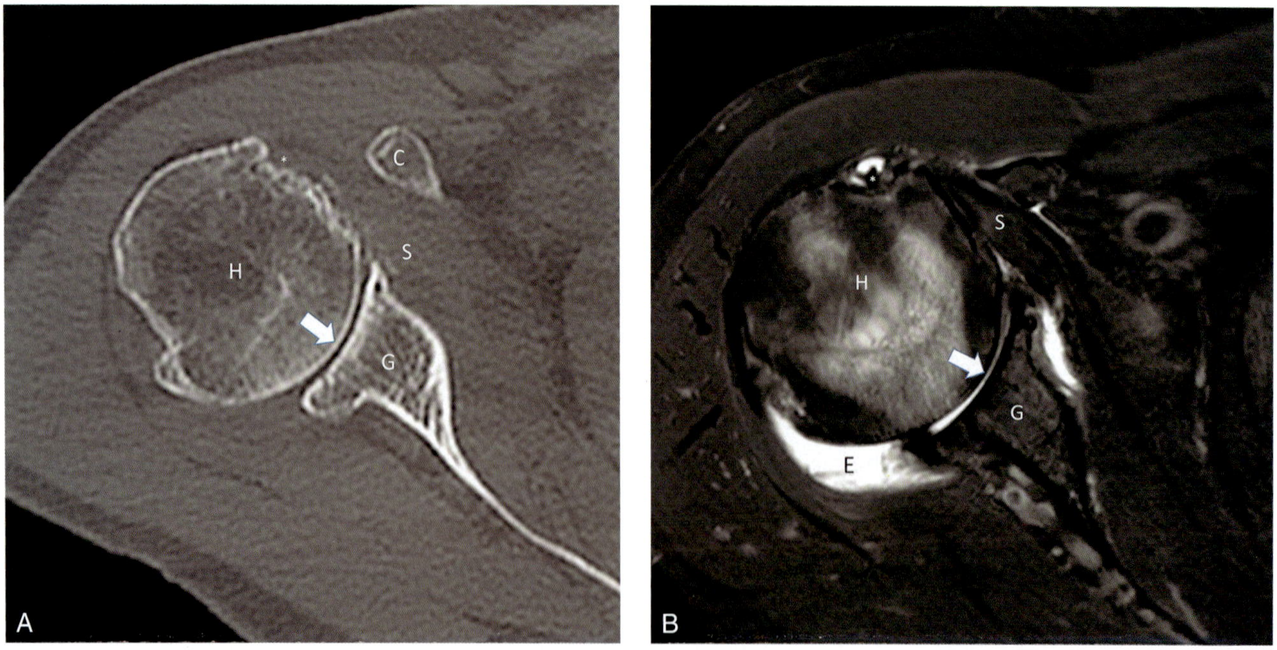

FIGURE 10 A 72-year-old man with shoulder pain. Axial CT image shows fine osseous detail. There is advanced glenohumeral osteoarthrosis with joint space loss (**A**, arrow), which is corroborated by the corresponding axial magnetic resonance image (**B**, arrow). * = long head of biceps tendon, C = coracoid process, E = joint effusion, G = glenoid, H = humeral head, S = subscapularis tendon

CTA indications includes the inability to perform MRI, such as contraindications to MRI, claustrophobia, and obesity, and failure of MRI in evaluating a suspected shoulder condition.[24] CTA requires two steps: the intra-articular injection of a sterile solution containing iodine-based contrast media and subsequent acquisition of CT images. The introduction of submillimeter isotropic multislice CT technology provided the basis for excellent spatial resolution in the 400 µm range and multiplanar reformation capabilities, which markedly improve the image quality and detail of CTA.

CTA has several advantages, including excellent spatial resolution and anatomic detail. With now widely available modern CT scanners, the scan time is substantially reduced, ranging within a few seconds. Fast scan modes substantially reduce motion artifacts, which renders it very useful for trauma and pediatric patients. Disadvantages of CTA are its invasive nature and exposure to ionizing radiation. CTA increases the detectability of lesions of cartilage, labrum, capsuloligamentous complex, and rotator cuff when compared with conventional CT.[25]

Shoulder Joint

Specific indications for CTA of the shoulder revolve around increasing the contrast resolution of images of the intra-articular soft tissues, which are not adequately visualized on unenhanced images. The indications include evaluation of the rotator cuff, the capsular-labral-ligamentous complex, and the articular cartilage, and especially in postoperative cases where the metal artifact interferes with MRI[26] (**Figure 11**).

A study assessed the diagnostic accuracy of CTA of the shoulder in patients with periarticular metal implants using surgical arthroscopy as the standard of reference.[27] A comparison between CTA and surgical arthroscopy in 42 patients showed sensitivities and specificities, ranging between 87% and 100%, respectively. In 28 patients, CTA had an accuracy of 94% when compared with open surgery. Interobserver agreement was high ($\kappa = 0.95$) in the evaluation of all types of lesions.

In a similar study that was performed for the detection of glenohumeral articular cartilage lesions, the diagnostic performances of 1.5 T MRA and CTA of the shoulder were compared with surgical arthroscopy in 56 patients.[28] Sensitivity and specificity of CTA and 1.5 T MRA for readers varied for cartilage lesions detection (46% to 82% versus 32% to 66%; and 89% to 96% versus 91% to 97%, respectively), whereas the accuracy of lesions detection by both modalities was moderate. Although MRA had statistically significant better performance for detection of the glenoid than humeral head articular cartilage areas ($P < 0.01$), the overall diagnostic performance of CTA was significantly better than that of 1.5 T MRA (all $P \leq 0.04$).

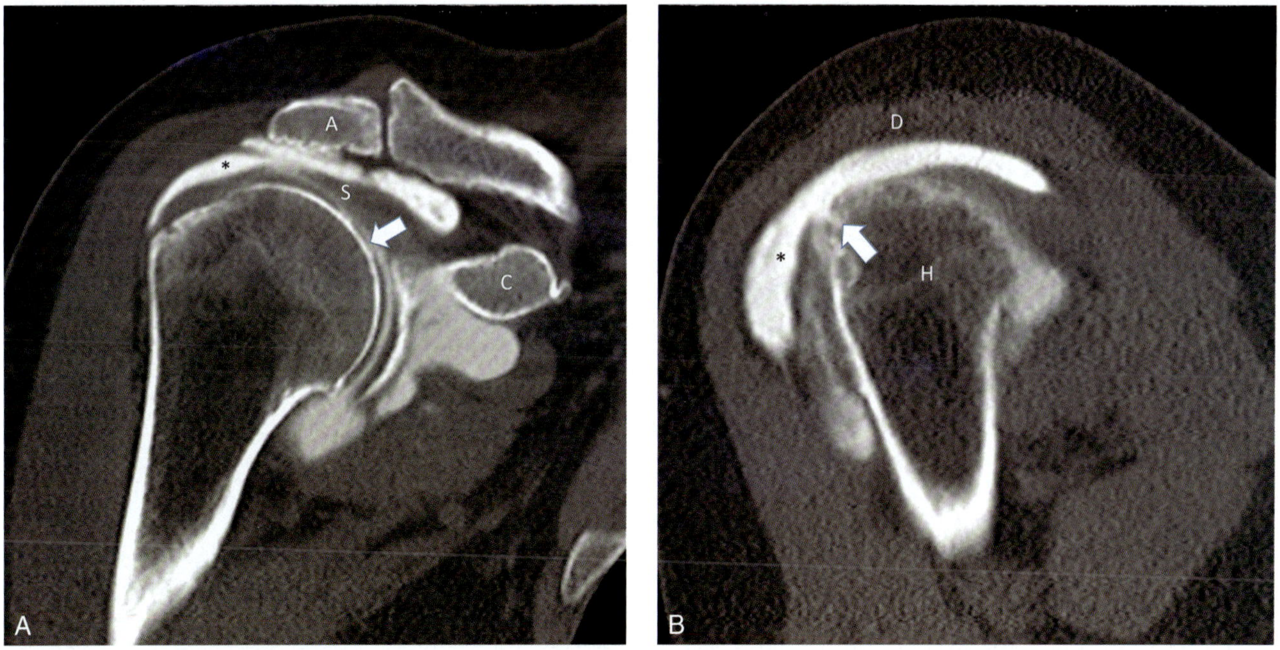

FIGURE 11 A 63-year-old woman with right shoulder pain. Coronal CTA image (**A**) shows high-grade partial-thickness articular cartilage loss of the superomedial humeral head (arrow). Sagittal CTA image (**B**) shows a small full-thickness anterior supraspinatus tendon tear (arrow) with iodine contrast material decompressing into the subacromial-subdeltoid bursa (**A** and **B**, asterisk). A = acromion, C = coracoid process, D = deltoid muscle, H = humeral head, S = supraspinatus muscle-tendon junction

Elbow Joint

CT is widely used for the elbow in the evaluation of fractures around the joints to detect and characterize intra-articular extension and small fracture fragments within the joint space. Intravenous iodine-based contrast agents can be administered to determine any vascular injury adjacent to the joint.[29] CTA with intra-articular injections of iodinated contrast is an excellent method of detecting disease in the overlying articular cartilage, although internal structural changes are not detected if the cartilage surface is intact.[24] CTA is an excellent alternative when there are contraindications in performing an MRI.

Ultrasonography

With the broader availability of high-frequency linear transducers in the range of 10 to 18 MHz, musculoskeletal ultrasonography is a rapidly growing field. Musculoskeletal ultrasonography has several advantages over MRI, such as being readily available, quick scan time, lower cost, and opportunity to perform dynamic imaging.[30] Ultrasonography is also noninvasive with no ionizing radiation exposure and allows quick and safe contralateral comparison. However, it is an operator-dependent modality, with a considerable learning curve. As ultrasonography is a focused imaging technique, rather than a large field-of-view technique as CT and MRI are, meticulous search patterns and operator experience are essential requirements. Ultrasonography limitations include a small field-of-view, which may interfere with a comprehensive image evaluation of the shoulder and elbow joint, and the inability to penetrate bone. Ultrasonography is best used to answer a specific question of a focused area of soft-tissue anatomy. It is less useful for the evaluation of deeper structures, osseous abnormalities, and osteochondral injuries. Although a recent study suggests that ultrasonography can be useful to detect bone tumors in children,[31] radiography, CT and MRI are required for complete characterization. Technological developments, including panoramic imaging (**Figure 12**), video storage, and (3D) image reformation, help to bridge the gap between static ultrasonographic and magnetic resonance images.

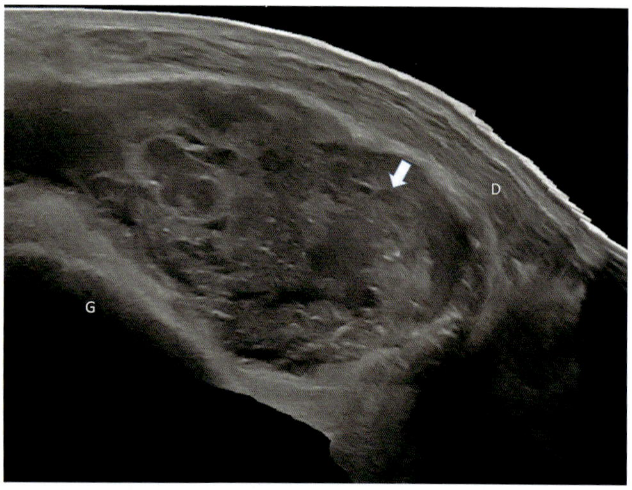

FIGURE 12 A 72-year-old woman with a long-standing history of rheumatoid arthritis. Panoramic ultrasonographic image of the posterior glenohumeral joint shows severe synovitis with marked capsular distention by synovial proliferation (arrow) and joint effusion. D = deltoid muscle, G = great tuberosity.

Shoulder Joint

Ultrasonography can be used to evaluate tendons of the rotator cuff and biceps (**Figure 13**) and diagnose bursitis, and it serves as a real-time tool for guiding procedures.

A 2011 study sought to determine the diagnostic accuracy of ultrasonography to detect partial-thickness and full-thickness rotator cuff tears based on all available clinical trials.[32] Sixty-two studies assessing 6,007 patients and 6,066 shoulders were included. Ultrasonography had good sensitivity and specificity for the assessment of partial-thickness (sensitivity, 84%; specificity, 89%), and full-thickness rotator cuff tears (sensitivity, 96%; specificity, 93%).

A 2018 meta-analysis studied the effectiveness and accuracy of shoulder 3D ultrasonography for detection of partial-thickness and full-thickness rotator cuff tears and found that 3D ultrasonography is more accurate for the detection of full-thickness rotator cuff tears than partial-thickness tears (sensitivity, 91% versus 82%; and specificity, 96% versus 88%, respectively).[33]

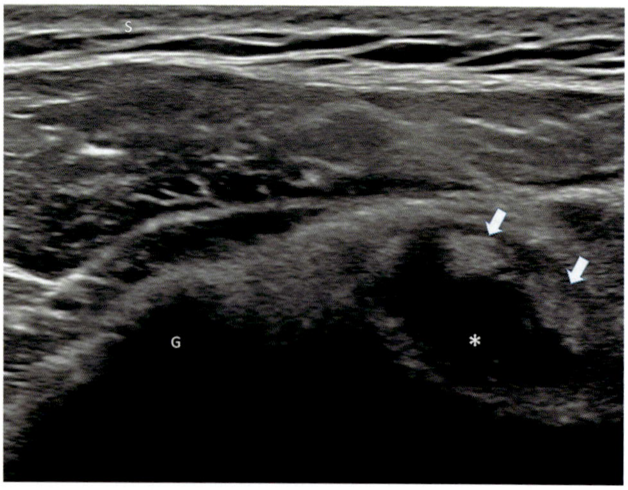

FIGURE 13 A 58-year-old man with right shoulder weakness and pain. Transverse ultrasonography image of the anterior shoulder shows a split long head biceps tendon (arrows) with fluid distention (*) of the tendon sheath. G = great tuberosity, S = subcutaneous fat

Ultrasonographic evaluation of the tendons should be performed in longitudinal and transverse planes. For each rotator cuff tendon, dedicated arm positions help to optimize the visibility and interpretation of the tendons. The healthy rotator cuff tendons appear as hyperechoic (bright) structures with a pattern of parallel fibrillary lines in the longitudinal plane and a hyperechoic ovoid structure in the transverse plane. Ultrasonography can distinguish between partial-thickness and full-thickness rotator cuff tears, by fluid intersecting into the tenderness defect, which appears as hypoechoic (dark) signal on ultrasonographic images. Signs of partial-thickness tears include focal anechoic or hypoechoic defects in the bursal or particular surface of the tendon.

Rotator cuff syndrome on ultrasonography can be diagnosed when dynamic scanning during abduction shows bursal distension, pooling of fluid in the bursa, or buckling of the bursa in patients with evidence of rotator cuff damage or bursal thickening.

Evaluation of the glenoid labral lesions is difficult because of the surrounding rotator cuff muscles and requires the expertise in shoulder ultrasonography. The diagnostic performance of ultrasonography in diagnosis of anterior[34] and posterior[35] labral lesions can be improved by performing ultrasonography after intra-articular injection (arthrosonography).

Elbow Joint

Ultrasonography is commonly used in the evaluation of soft-tissue disease around the elbow, enabling high-resolution imaging of superficial structures such as ligaments, tendons, and nerves.[36] Ultrasonography can be used to detect joint effusion, ligamentous and tendon tears, and ulnar nerve abnormalities, as well as serves as a guiding tool for performing various interventions around the elbow, including injections and soft-tissue biopsies. In addition, elbow ultrasonography can diagnose pediatric elbow fracture with a sensitivity and specificity of 96% and 89%, respectively.[37]

Dynamic sonography is helpful to assess for pathologic conditions that may only occur during joint motion, such as ulnar nerve subluxation or muscle herniation. Ultrasonography also has the ability to detect subtle calcifications and foreign bodies that may not be readily apparent on radiography or MRI.

Ultrasonography is a preferred guiding modality to perform procedures such as intra-articular, peritendinous, and perineural injections. Doppler imaging techniques visualize vascular structures, which is helpful to avoid inadvertent vessel injuries during ultrasonography-guided procedures.

SUMMARY

Both MRI and ultrasonography are accurate for the diagnosis of rotator cuff tears, whereas CTA can only accurately detect partial-thickness articular surface and full-thickness rotator cuff tendon tears. Both MRA and CTA are accurate methods for the detection of labrum tears and cartilage defects. **Table 2** depicts assessment ratings of abnormalities of the shoulder joint with various imaging modalities.

For the assessment of elbow joint abnormalities, MRI using pulse sequences with appropriate fluid-sensitivity is accurate for the diagnosis of radiographically occult osseous injuries, osteochondral and chondral defects, and soft-tissue abnormalities including tendons, ligaments, and nerves. MRA may improve the detectability of internal derangement and collateral ligament tears. CTA represents an

Table 2

Appropriate Assessment of Anatomic Regions of the Shoulder Joint on Various Imaging Modalities

	MRI	MRA	CT	CTA	US
Labral tears	++	+++	–	+++	–
Rotator cuff—partial-thickness tear (bursal surface)	++	++[a]	–	–	++
Rotator cuff—partial-thickness tear (articular surface)	++	+++	–	+++	++
Rotator cuff—full-thickness tear	+++	+++	–	+++	+++
Focal cartilage defects	++	+++	–	+++	–
Bone marrow edema	+++	+++[a]	++[b]	++[b]	–

CTA = computed tomography arthrography, MRA = magnetic resonance arthrography, US = ultrasonography

[a]Only when combining with fluid-sensitive pulse sequence. Interstitial and bursal surface rotator cuff tears, as well as bone marrow edema, may not be visible on T1-weighted arthrographic magnetic resonance images.

[b]Can now be diagnosed with virtual noncalcium postprocessing of dual-energy CT data.

alternative to MRA for the detection of articular cartilage defects and in case of contraindication to perform an MRI. Ultrasonography is accurate for the assessment of superficial structures, including ligaments, tendons, and nerves.

KEY STUDY POINTS

- MRI provides accurate and simultaneous diagnosis of many shoulder and elbow abnormalities, including early and advanced articular cartilage degeneration and defects, osteochondral lesions, capsulolabral lesions, abnormalities of the bursae and synovium, tendon avulsions and tears, muscle injuries and tears, ligamentous tears, osseous stress reactions with bone marrow edema pattern, radiographically occult and nondisplaced fractures, and abnormalities associated with instability.
- High spatial resolution 3 T MRI is more accurate than 1.5 T MRI for the diagnosis of SLAP tears of the shoulder.
- MRA can have higher accuracy than MRI for diagnosing of the rotator cuff tears and ligament injuries of the elbow.
- CTA is an alternative to MRI and MRA in patients with the inability to undergo MRI, affording high accuracy for the diagnosis of articular cartilage substance defects, glenohumeral labrum tears, partial-thickness articular surface and full-thickness rotator cuff tendon tears in the shoulder, and ulnar collateral ligament tears in the elbow.
- Ultrasonography is a noninvasive, widely available, and safe modality that is accurate for the diagnosis of the abnormalities of tendons, synovium, bursae, periarticular ligaments, and superficial soft tissues, but it is highly operator dependent and may not detect osseous lesions and glenoid labrum tears.

Annotated References

1. Bolog N, Nanz D, Weishaupt D: Muskuloskeletal MR imaging at 3.0 T: Current status and future perspectives. *Eur Radiol* 2006;16(6):1298-1307.

2. Fritz J, Fritz B, Thawait GG, Meyer H, Gilson WD, Raithel E: Three-dimensional CAIPIRINHA SPACE TSE for 5-minute high-resolution MRI of the knee. *Invest Radiol* 2016;51(10):609-617.

   This study reports the technique of rapid 3D turbo spin echo (TSE) MRI in 500 µm isotropic high spatial resolution for 3D knee MRI in an acquisition time of 5 minutes. Level of evidence: III.

3. Fritz J, Raithel E, Thawait GK, Gilson W, Papp DF: Six-fold acceleration of high-spatial-resolution 3D SPACE MRI of the knee through incoherent k-space undersampling and iterative reconstruction—First experience. *Invest Radiol* 2016;51(6):400-409.

   This study demonstrates the successful clinical implementation of sixfold accelerated, compressed sensing-based 500-µm high spatial resolution isotropic 3D MRI. The results of this study demonstrate similar image quality and diagnostic performance of a comprehensive 10-minute 3D TSE MRI prototype protocol and 20-minute 2D TSE MRI standard protocol. Level of evidence: II.

4. Fritz J, Ahlawat S, Fritz B, et al: 10-min 3D turbo spin echo MRI of the knee in children: Arthroscopy-validated accuracy for the diagnosis of internal derangement. *J Magn Reson Imaging* 2019;49(7):e139-e151.

   This study shows the high arthroscopy-validated diagnostic accuracy of 10-minute 3D CAIPIRINHA TSE MRI of the knee in diagnosis of internal knee derangements of children. Level of evidence: I.

5. Osinski T, Malfair D, Steinbach L: Magnetic resonance arthrography. *Orthop Clin North Am* 2006;37(3):299-319, vi.

6. Magee T: 3-T MRI of the shoulder: Is MR arthrography necessary? *AJR Am J Roentgenol* 2009;192(1):86-92.

7. Ajuied A, McGarvey CP, Harb Z, Smith CC, Houghton RP, Corbett SA: Diagnosis of glenoid labral tears using 3-Tesla MRI vs. 3-Tesla MRA: A systematic review and meta-analysis. *Arch Orthop Trauma Surg* 2018;138(5):699-709.

   This meta-analysis reports the diagnostic performance of 3 T MRI versus 3 T MRA with surgical inspection as the standard of reference. A total of 10 studies were included using 929 patients. Level of evidence: IV.

8. Symanski JS, Subhas N, Babb J, Nicholson J, Gyftopoulos S: Diagnosis of superior labrum anterior-to-posterior tears by using MR imaging and MR arthrography: A systematic review and meta-analysis. *Radiology* 2017;285(1):101-113.

   This meta-analysis of 32 studies compares the diagnostic accuracy of nonenhanced MRI and MRA for the diagnosis of superior glenoid labrum tears. Level of evidence: II.

9. Lee SH, Yun SJ, Jin W, Park SY, Park JS, Ryu KN: Comparison between 3D isotropic and 2D conventional MR arthrography for diagnosing rotator cuff tear and labral lesions: A meta-analysis. *J Magn Reson Imaging* 2018;48(4):1034-1045.

   This meta-analysis of 11 studies and 825 patients compares the diagnostic performance of 3D isotropic MRA and 2D conventional MRA for the diagnosis of rotator cuff tears and labral lesions. Level of evidence: II.

10. Goutallier D, Postel JM, Bernageau J, et al: Fatty muscle degeneration in cuff ruptures. Pre- and postoperative evaluation by CT scan. *Clin Orthop Relat Res* 1994;(304):78-83.

11. Shahabpour M, Kichouh M, Laridon E, Gielen JL, De Mey J: The effectiveness of diagnostic imaging methods for the assessment of soft tissue and articular disorders of the shoulder and elbow. *Eur J Radiol* 2008;65(2):194-200.

12. de Jesus JO, Parker L, Frangos AJ, Nazarian LN: Accuracy of MRI, MR arthrography, and ultrasound in the diagnosis of rotator cuff tears: A meta-analysis. *AJR Am J Roentgenol* 2009;192(6):1701-1707.

13. Roy JS, Braën C, Leblond J, et al: Diagnostic accuracy of ultrasonography, MRI, and MR arthrography in the characterisation of rotator cuff disorders: A systematic review and meta-analysis. *Br J Sports Med* 2015;49(20):1316-1328.

    This meta-analysis summarizes the diagnostic accuracy of ultrasonography, MRI, and MRA for the characterization of rotator cuff disorders by pooling data of 82 articles. Level of evidence: II.

14. Shah N, Tung GA: Imaging signs of posterior glenohumeral instability. *AJR Am J Roentgenol* 2009;192(3):730-735.

15. Brunton LM, Anderson MW, Pannunzio ME, Khanna AJ, Chhabra AB: Magnetic resonance imaging of the elbow: Update on current techniques and indications. *J Hand Surg Am* 2006;31(6):1001-1011.

16. Magee T: Accuracy of 3-T MR arthrography versus conventional 3-T MRI of elbow tendons and ligaments compared with surgery. *AJR Am J Roentgenol* 2015;204(1):W70-W75.

    This study reports the diagnostic accuracy of 3 T MRA versus 3 T MRI of elbow tendons and ligaments in 54 subjects, using surgical inspection as the standard of reference. Level of evidence: I.

17. Stevens KJ, McNally EG: Magnetic resonance imaging of the elbow in athletes. *Clin Sports Med* 2010;29(4):521-553.

18. Ramkumar PN, Frangiamore SJ, Navarro SM, et al: Interobserver and intraobserver reliability of an MRI-based classification system for injuries to the ulnar collateral ligament. *Am J Sports Med* 2018;46(11):2755-2760.

    This cohort study proposes an MRI-based classification for ulnar collateral ligament of elbow injuries based on the report of nine fellowship trained specialists. Level of evidence: II.

19. Roedl JB, Gonzalez FM, Zoga AC, et al: Potential utility of a combined approach with US and MR arthrography to image medial elbow pain in baseball players. *Radiology* 2016;279(3):827-837.

    This study reports improved diagnostic accuracy of combined ultrasonography and MRA for the evaluation of medial elbow pain in 144 baseball players. Level of evidence: I.

20. Chew ML, Giuffre BM: Disorders of the distal biceps brachii tendon. *Radiographics* 2005;25(5):1227-1237.

21. Rowe SP, Fritz J, Fishman EK: CT evaluation of musculoskeletal trauma: Initial experience with cinematic rendering. *Emerg Radiol* 2018;25(1):93-101.

    This article explains the role of cinematic rendering as a new 3D reconstruction technique of CT in the diagnosis of musculoskeletal trauma and provides clinical examples of the use of cinematic rendering in musculoskeletal imaging. Level of evidence: V.

22. Khodarahmi I, Isaac A, Fishman EK, Dalili D, Fritz J: Metal about the hip and artifact reduction techniques: From basic concepts to advanced imaging. *Semin Musculoskelet Radiol* 2019;23(3):e68-e81.

    This article reviews the general concepts of a spectrum of metal artifact reduction techniques for MRI and CT for advanced imaging of orthopaedic implants. Level of evidence: V.

23. Khodarahmi I, Fishman EK, Fritz J: Dedicated CT and MRI techniques for the evaluation of the postoperative knee. *Semin Musculoskelet Radiol* 2018;22(4):444-456.

    This article reviews conventional and advanced CT and MRI techniques for imaging of metallic orthopaedic implants. Level of evidence: V.

24. Fritz J, Fishman EK, Small KM, et al: MDCT arthrography of the shoulder with datasets of isotropic resolution: Indications, technique, and applications. *AJR Am J Roentgenol* 2012;198(3):635-646.

25. Fritz J, Fishman EK, Fayad LM: MDCT arthrography of the shoulder. *Semin Musculoskelet Radiol* 2014;18(4):343-351.

    This article reviews the role of CTA in the diagnosis of shoulder abnormalities. Level of evidence: V.

26. Oh JH, Kim JY, Choi JA, Kim WS: Effectiveness of multidetector computed tomography arthrography for the diagnosis of shoulder pathology: Comparison with magnetic resonance imaging with arthroscopic correlation. *J Shoulder Elbow Surg* 2010;19(1):14-20.

27. De Filippo M, Bertellini A, Sverzellati N, et al: Multidetector computed tomography arthrography of the shoulder: Diagnostic accuracy and indications. *Acta Radiol* 2008;49(5):540-549.

28. Omoumi P, Rubini A, Dubuc JE, Vande Berg BC, Lecouvet FE: Diagnostic performance of CT-arthrography and 1.5 T MR-arthrography for the assessment of glenohumeral joint cartilage: A comparative study with arthroscopic correlation. *Eur Radiol* 2015;25(4):961-969.

    This study shows the diagnostic performance of CTA and 1.5 T MRA in detecting glenohumeral hyaline cartilage lesions of the shoulder with arthroscopic correlation. Level of evidence: I.

29. Fritz J, Efron DT, Fishman EK: Multidetector CT and three-dimensional CT angiography of upper extremity arterial injury. *Emerg Radiol* 2015;22(3):269-282.

This article reviews the role of CTA in the diagnosis and management of upper extremity vascular injury in the setting of orthopaedic trauma. Level of evidence: V.

30. Jacobson JA: Musculoskeletal ultrasound: Focused impact on MRI. *AJR Am J Roentgenol* 2009;193(3):619-627.

31. Madej T, Flak-Nurzynska J, Dutkiewicz E, Ciechomska A, Kowalczyk J, Wieczorek AP: Ultrasound image of malignant bone tumors in children. An analysis of nine patients diagnosed in 2011–2016. *J Ultrason* 2018;18(73):103-111.

    This study evaluates the role of ultrasonography in the diagnosis of malignant bone tumors in children. Level of evidence: IV.

32. Smith TO, Back T, Toms AP, Hing CB: Diagnostic accuracy of ultrasound for rotator cuff tears in adults: A systematic review and meta-analysis. *Clin Radiol* 2011;66(11):1036-1048.

33. Teng A, Liu F, Zhou D, He T, Chevalier Y, Klar RM: Effectiveness of 3-dimensional shoulder ultrasound in the diagnosis of rotator cuff tears: A meta-analysis. *Medicine (Baltimore)* 2018;97(37):e12405.

    This meta-analysis describes the effectiveness of 3D ultrasonography in the detection of shoulder rotator cuff tears. Level of evidence: II.

34. Jeong WK, Ah Ryu J, Choi SH, et al: Shoulder sonography after intraarticular fluid injection for evaluation of anterior labral tears: Comparison with conventional sonography. *J Clin Ultrasound* 2013;41(2):94-100.

    In this study, the role of arthrosonography in the diagnosis of anterior labral tears is compared with the conventional ultrasonography. Level of evidence: II.

35. Park D: Evaluation of posterosuperior labral tear with shoulder sonography after intra-articular injection: A case series. *Am J Phys Med Rehabil* 2017;96(3):e48-e51.

    This study demonstrates the role of arthrosonography in the diagnosis of posterosuperior labral tears through a case series. Level of evidence: IV.

36. Lee KS, Rosas HG, Craig JG: Musculoskeletal ultrasound: Elbow imaging and procedures. *Semin Musculoskelet Radiol* 2010;14(4):449-460.

37. Lee SH, Yun SJ: Diagnostic performance of ultrasonography for detection of pediatric elbow fracture: A meta-analysis. *Ann Emerg Med* 2019;74(4):493-502.

    This meta-analysis included 10 articles and 519 patients to determine the diagnostic performance of sonography for detection of pediatric elbow fractures. Level of evidence: II.

Index

Note: Page numbers followed by "*f*" indicate figures and "*t*" indicate tables.

A

B

C

D

E

F

G

H

I

J

K

L

M

N

O

P

R

S

T

U

V

W

Y